GUIDE TO
CLINICAL TRIALS

GUIDE TO CLINICAL TRIALS

Bert Spilker, Ph.D., M.D.

President
Orphan Medical, Inc.
Minnetonka, Minnesota

Adjunct Professor of Medicine
Adjunct Professor of Pharmacology, and
Clinical Professor of Pharmacy
University of North Carolina Schools of Medicine and Pharmacy
Chapel Hill, North Carolina

Clinical Professor of Pharmacy Practice
University of Minnesota School of Pharmacy
Minneapolis, Minnesota

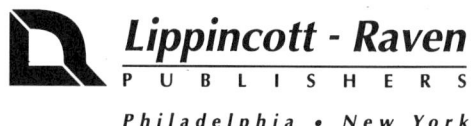
Lippincott - Raven
P U B L I S H E R S
Philadelphia • New York

Lippincott-Raven Publishers, 227 East Washington Square, Philadelphia, Pennsylvania 19106

Made in the United States of America

Library of Congress Cataloging-in-Publication Data

Spilker, Bert.
    Guide to clinical trials / Bert Spilker.
       p. cm.
    Includes bibliographical references and indexes.
    ISBN 0-88167-767-1
    1. Clinical trials. 2. Drugs—Testing. I. Title.
    [DNLM: 1. Clinical Trials. 2. Drug Evaluation. 3. Research
Design. QV 771 S756gb]
R853.C55S652 1991
615'.028'7—dc20
DNLM/DLC
for Library of Congress   91-7864
                            CIP

9 8 7 6 5 4

To my loving wife Arlene

Contents

Part II: Developing and Writing Clinical Protocols

Part III: Planning Special Types of Clinical Trials

Part IV: Planning and Conducting a Single Clinical Trial

Part V: A Nonmathematical Approach to Statistics and Data Processing

Part VI: Fundamental Principles, Considerations, and Techniques in the Interpretation of Clinical Data

Part VII: Interpretation of Safety and Efficacy Data

Part XI: Planning and Conducting Multiple Clinical Trials

Part XII: Management of Multiple Clinical Trials

Foreword

I cannot think of anyone who has been more prolific in his writings about clinical trial methodology than Dr. Spilker. His output is mind-boggling, and its high quality is attested to by the warm reception his work has received from thousands of grateful readers.

This latest comprehensive volume combines chapters from Dr. Spilker's first three books with more than 40 new chapters. It is instructive not only for its content, but for the message it sends about the science of clinical trials. In an era when cellular and molecular biology rules the roost as far as research funding is concerned, Spilker's excellent advice underscores the fact that molecular biology, although it will be increasingly important in our understanding of disease and the selection of drug candidates, has little to contribute to the delineation of drug efficacy and safety.

Equally clear is the fact that the formal training of basic scientists, physicians, dentists, veterinarians, pharmacists, nurses, statisticians, etc. does little to prepare these individuals for careers in pharmaceutical development and regulation. It is not necessary to deny categorically the utility of such formal training to conclude that the training is inevitably woefully inadequate for such careers. For the near future at least, "on-the-job training" will be the order of the day, with self-teaching an important component. This volume will be a major contribution to such training.

—*Louis Lasagna, M.D.*
Center for the Study of
Drug Development
Tufts University
Boston, Massachusetts

Preface

Objectives of this Book

This book has five major objectives: (1) to help the neophyte to the clinical trial environment gain knowledge about the complexities and procedures of planning, initiating, conducting, analyzing, interpreting, and publishing results of a successful clinical trial; (2) to assist the experienced individual who either seeks a series of checklists or desires to evaluate new variations on familiar themes (primarily those listed in the tables and illustrated in the figures); (3) to guide the university student in a pharmacy, pharmacology, or medical curriculum in his or her coursework on clinical trials, and to provide information that will prove helpful for making career decisions; (4) to orient marketing and sales personnel, journalists, and other nonscientists whose positions require the transfer of scientific and medical knowledge to other nonscientists; and (5) to serve as a reference source for any individual interested in clinical trials, whether based in government, pharmaceutical industry, academia, consulting companies, or elsewhere.

Contents

Over 40 new chapters have been added to the trilogy of books that were, essentially, combined to create this volume (*Guide to Clinical Studies and Developing Protocols, Guide to Clinical Interpretation of Data, Guide to Planning and Managing Multiple Clinical Studies*), and most of the original chapters have been rewritten or reorganized to reflect new information or modified views of the author. Some chapters focus primarily on current and future standards of conducting clinical trials, a topic that is worthy of its own book. Most chapters attempt to both tell a story and be autonomous so that chapters may be read in any order.

The twelve sections of this book lead the reader stepwise through the myriad of issues, factors, and considerations that relate to clinical trials. The twelve sections are listed below.

Part I. Developing Clinical Trial Designs. This section focuses on the steps involved in developing a clinical trial design by emphasizing the processes used in the trial's conceptualization.

Part II. Developing and Writing Clinical Protocols. This section describes the criteria and methodologies used to develop and write the clinical trial protocol.

Part III. Planning Special Types of Clinical Trials. Various types of specialized clinical trials are described, along with special considerations for their design.

Part IV. Planning and Conducting a Single Clinical Trial. This section traces the processes involved in a single clinical trial.

Part V. A Nonmathematical Approach to Statistics and Data Processing. Many issues and considerations are described from a clinical (i.e., nonstatistical) perspective.

Part VI. Fundamental Principles, Considerations, and Techniques of the Interpretation of Clinical Data. This section describes the processes used in the clinical interpretation of data.

Part VII. Interpretation of Safety and Efficacy Data. Both general and specific approaches are described.

Part VIII. Interpretation of Data from Special Trials, Modalities, and Populations. This section includes consideration of surgical trials, geriatric patients, radiation therapy, and many other groups for which consideration of specific factors is needed to interpret data adequately.

Part IX. Issues and Problems of Clinical Data Interpretation. Such issues include dealing with data that are difficult to interpret, reconciling differences in interpretation from multiple studies, and numerous other "real world" situations.

Part X. Publishing Clinical Data and Evaluating Published Literature. This section includes recommendations to enhance standards of clinical publication.

Part XI. Planning and Conducting Multiple Clinical Trials. Considerations underlying these activities are described and discussed.

Part XII. Management of Multiple Clinical Trials. This section provides considerations for academic or private physicians and management considerations for those in large business organizations.

Roles and Importance of Statistics

The volume intentionally avoids detailed discussions on the roles and applications of statistics in protocol development and data analysis. Virtually all protocols utilize statistical techniques for the development of clinical trial design and the analysis of data. The importance of statistics in clinical research is acknowledged, and the importance of working with a statistician throughout a protocol's planning, conduct, and analysis phases is stressed. There are, however, numerous books that focus on these areas (e.g., Hill, 1971; Lancaster, 1974; Feinstein, 1977; Friedman et al., 1981; Bailer and Mostellar, 1986; Ingelfinger et al., 1987), and one of these or other books should be consulted in conjunction with the current volume.

Over the last few decades there has also been a trend toward emphasizing the role of statistics in the interpretation of investigational data. This focus has been appropriate and has helped advance the standards of clinical study design, conduct, and interpretation. The *clinical* interpretation of data, however, has often not received its rightful recognition and emphasis for the role it plays in data interpretation in general. There are numerous well-written monographs and articles on statistics, formal logic, and causality, but none, prior to *Guide to Clinical Interpretation of Data* (Spilker, 1986), solely described the *clinical* interpretation of data. A number of texts emphasize the concepts of both statistics and logic, usually related to the field of epidemiology (Susser, 1973; Riegelman, 1981; Fletcher et al., 1988; Feinstein, 1985a; Sackett et al., 1985).

The importance of statistics in data analysis and as a basis for deriving an accurate clinical interpretation is affirmed and stressed. There is a natural progression from the statistical to the clinical evaluation of data. Involvement of both disciplines is usually necessary to attain an adequate interpretation of the data. Coordination and integration of the two approaches and disciplines are desirable.

Philosophical Orientation

The proper goal of individuals involved in clinical trials is the achievement of the highest appropriate standard to use in every case. Medicine itself may be viewed as a study of the balance between the fragility of life (almost invisible microorganisms or poisons can destroy healthy people in a matter of minutes) and the near indestructibility of life (as witnessed when the spark of life remains lit, despite the ravages of multiple severe diseases and afflictions).

Perspectives

Most of this book presents a clinical and nonmathematical perspective, making it applicable to professionals with any background or current affiliation. A few chapters, however, present a topic from the specific viewpoint of patients, contract organizations, academic clinicians, regulatory authorities, or pharmaceutical companies.

Overlap between Chapters

A certain amount of overlap and repetition occurs between sections and chapters in this book, primarily because some aspects of a clinical trial may be discussed in more than one of the categories described. An attempt had been made to minimize redundancy except when it provides useful emphasis to the discussion. One chapter (Chapter 71) presents a summary of information described in the subsequent chapters of Part VI.

Practical Approaches

A system of checklists, tables, and figures that detail practical information and issues render this book a guide for either medicine or nonmedicine trials. The points listed in tables are never placed in order of importance unless noted. The checklists enable the author of a protocol to ascertain whether he or she has forgotten any important detail in the planning, implementation, conduct, analysis, interpretation, or publication of a clinical trial. The checklists may also be used as a peripheral memory by individuals planning or conducting several trials at the same time, as opposed to either the use of a large variety of different papers/forms or reliance on memory. These checklists may be modified easily for trials with special requirements. Many succinct examples are provided. Long detailed examples to illustrate or prove a point are intentionally avoided.

The trial protocol is viewed as an expression of how the trial design will be implemented. The order of chapters in Part II reflects the general order in which an individual develops and writes a protocol rather than the order in which the separate parts of the protocol appear in the finished version. Therefore, the chapter dealing with a protocol's introduction appears near the end of Part II.

This book provides more practical details on most aspects of clinical trials than are found in previously published articles or books written prior to the first edition (Harris and Fitzgerald, 1970; Abrams, 1976; Chaput de Saintonge, 1977; Friedman et al., 1981; Cato, 1982) or subsequently (see appendix of Spilker, 1989a, for a complete bibliography).

Why This Book Is Not a Cookbook

This book is not a "how to" for carrying out clinical trials. Each company, academic group, or government agency differs in critical ways (e.g., standard operating procedures, approaches, standards used, objectives), and it is therefore not possible to present a single meaningful "how to" approach that may be directly used for conducting trials. Moreover, every medicine or project will also vary, and although the procedures followed at a single institution may be generally similar, the specific problems and issues that must be dealt with for each project are unique. This book presents many of the options that are available to those designing and conducting clinical trials. The best approach will be achieved by those who are most prepared to solve the novel challenges that arise in all clinical trials.

Acknowledgments

The author greatly appreciates the help of numerous people who assisted with the review and preparation of this combined and expanded book.

Dr. John Schoenfelder was the primary reviewer of most of the new chapters added to this volume. Ms. Laura Mansberg provided valuable copy editing of numerous chapters and also questioned many ambiguous portions of the text.

Others who generously reviewed one to three chapters in their area of specialty are: Dr. David Feeny, Dr. Michael Joseph, Dr. Allen Lai, Dr. Alan Lisook, Dr. Lloyd Millstein, Dr. George Szczech, and Dr. Hugh Tilson, Ms. Susan Tonascia is thanked for reviewing the Terminology section.

Technical assistance with the bibliography was provided by Mr. Allen Jones, assistance with literature searches by Mr. Rolly Simpson, and preparation of the manuscript by Msses. Anne Dwayne, Brenda Price, Jann Harding, Thomasine Cozart, Lynne Spencer, and Janice Wilson.

It is my pleasure to acknowledge the help of many people who assisted me with the three books on which this volume is based. The author owes a special debt of gratitude to Dr. John Schoenfelder, who gave his time unstintingly to help improve the quality of these books and removed many ambiguities that were present.

Other individuals also contributed to these books in terms of valuable discussions or review of selected segments or chapters. The author appreciates their important input: Mr. J. M. Arnold, Dr. David Barry, Ms. Nancy A. Bauer, Drs. Larry Bell, M. Robert Blum, Gilles Cloutier, Ms. Kathryn Crean, Drs. Walter B. Cummings, Joann Data, Ronald Deitch, Robert E. Desjardins, Howard C. Filston, Richard J. Fleck, Robert Fletcher, Donald T. Forman, Michael F. Frosolono, Eric H. Geiger, Ms. Pamela Griffin-Lyon, Dr. Steven H. Grossman, Messrs. Dan W. Heatherington, Robin K. Henning, Paul A. Holcomb, Jr., Drs. Heyward Hull, III, Kenneth B. Klein, Allen Lai, Jerome Levine, Walker Long, Mr. M. James Louis, Drs. Loren Miller, Lloyd G. Millstein, Donald H. Namm, Lawrence A. Nielson, Ms. Erika F. Nissman, Drs. Peter Palmer, J. Greg Perkins, Mr. David C. Pressel, Drs. Leonard R. Prosnitz, John Rogers, Warren C. Stern, Joel E. Sutton, George Szczech, Hugh Tilson, Richard L. Tuttle, Ms. Judy Van Wyck Fleet, Mr. Randy Vestal, Drs. Richard M. Welch, Tom Williams, Mrs. Cindy F. Wilson, and Dr. David Yeowell.

The author thanks Msses. Judy Appleton, Thomasine Cozart, Joyce B. Carpunky, Martha H. Fleming, Rosemary K. Freeman, and Sherron Paris for assistance in the preparation of these books; Messrs. David R. Price and Rolly Simpson for help with literature searches; and Mr. Allen Jones for help with the bibliographies.

The following table lists chapters in this volume that were originally published elsewhere. The author appreciates permission of the publishers to reprint the material (as modified) here. Each of the publishers is thanked. None of these references are listed in the bibliography at the end of this volume.

TABLE A. *Published materials used as the basis of selected chapters[a,b]*

Chapter number in this volume	Original title of article or book chapter	Original publisher and city	Reference
15	Methods of Assessing and Improving Patient Compliance in Clinical Trials	Raven Press, New York	In *Patient Compliance in Medical Practice and Clinical Trials*, J. Cramer and B. Spilker (eds.), 1991.
17	Data Review Committees	Prous Scientific, Barcelona	*Drug News and Perspectives*, 1990;3:417–420.
28	Remote Data Entry	Prous Scientific, Barcelona	*Drug News and Perspectives*, 1990;3:95–98.
31	Patient Refusers, Nonqualifiers, Dropouts, Dropins, and Discontinuers	Prous Scientific, Barcelona	*Drug News and Perspectives*, 1990;3:14–18.
38	On the Increasing Importance of Single-Patient Double-Blind Studies	Prous Scientific, Barcelona	*Drug News and Perspectives*, 1990;1:160–163.
40	National versus Multinational Clinical Trials	Prous Scientific, Barcelona	*Drug News and Perspectives*, 1990;3:469–474.
46	Development of Orphan Drugs: An Industry Perspective	Manchester University Press, Manchester, (UK)	In *Orphan Drugs and Orphan Diseases*, I. Scheinberg and J. Walshe (eds.), 1986:119–134.
54	Training Professionals in Clinical Trial Methods	Prous Scientific, Barcelona	*Drug News and Perspectives*, 1990;3:606–613.
58	Roles of Medical Contractors in Drug Development	Prous Scientific, Barcelona	*Drug News and Perspectives*, 1990;3:148–152.
63	Auditing a Clinical Trial	Prous Scientific, Barcelona	*Drug News and Perspectives*, 1990;3:280–286.
104	Meta-Analysis	Prous Scientific, Barcelona	*Drug News and Perspectives*, 1989;2:464–469.
107	Prospective Registration of Clinical Trials	Prous Scientific, Barcelona	*Drug News and Perspectives*, 1990;3:222–225.
108	Archiving Clinical Trial Data	Prous Scientific, Barcelona	*Drug News and Perspectives*, 1990;3:527–528.
109	Models of How Clinical Research is Conducted	Prous Scientific, Barcelona	*Drug News and Perspectives*, 1989;2:161–163.
110	Golden Rules of Clinical Drug Development	Prous Scientific, Barcelona	*Drug News and Perspectives*, 1988;1:222–225.
112	Missions, Objectives, Goals, Strategies, and Tactics Revisited	Prous Scientific, Barcelona	*Drug News and Perspectives*, 1989;2:281–286.
114, 115	Elements of a Clinical Strategy and Development Plan	Prous Scientific, Barcelona	*Drug News and Perspectives*, 1989;2:222–228.
119	Safety Profiles of New Drugs at the Time of Initial Marketing	Harvey Whitney Books, Cincinnati, OH	*Pharmacoepidemiology: An Introduction*, 2nd Ed. Hartzema, Porta, and Tilson (eds.), 1991.
120	Past, Present, and Future Standards of Post-Marketing Surveillance	Harvey Whitney Books, Cincinnati, OH	*Pharmacoepidemiology: An Introduction*, 2nd Ed. Hartzema, Porta, and Tilson (eds.), 1991.
133	Goals and Future Driections of Clinical Trials	Prous Scientific, Barcelona	*Drug News and Perspectives*, 1989;2:337–341.

[a] Each of these articles or chapters was written by Dr. Spilker.
[b] A portion of Part IV was originally published under the title, "Practical Considerations in Planning and Conducting Clinical Trials with Investigational or Marketed Drugs." *Clin Neuropharmacology*, 1983;6:325–347.

Terminology

Only a few terms of particular importance to this text are operationally defined in this section. Many additional terms are defined in the text.

   Definitions are unchanged from the original three volumes, with the following four exceptions. The usage of these four important terms is described.

1. **Clinical trials** is used throughout this book in lieu of clinical studies, because of common usage and because the term is more specific in that clinical trials emphasizes clinical investigations rather than all clinical evaluations. The term studies is retained for more general use or when discussing most clinical studies conducted during Phase IV.
2. **Clinical significance** is used instead of clinical importance, because the former term implies that the concept is being directly or indirectly compared with the term statistical significance. The term clinical importance is a reasonable term to use, except that it is not always interpreted or understood as being identical to clinical significance.
3. **Adverse reaction** is now used to imply some degree of causality with the treatment, rather than implying none. This is how the term has been used in most Phase IV clinical research, although even today it is not generally used that way in reports about Phases I to III clinical trials. The term adverse event is now used to include adverse reactions as well as all other nontreatment-related adverse experiences. The terms adverse medical event or adverse drug reaction are not used in this book.
4. **Medicine** is used instead of drug, because of the association of the latter term with abused, usually illegal, substances. There have been several editorials in the literature (Wright, 1987; Worthen, 1988) stating that the time has come to differentiate between therapeutic and abused substances. Social reasons dictate that the term drug be used for abused substances, and that the more positive word medicine be used for beneficial substances.

   The following definitions are preferred.

Abnormality. A sign, symptom, or laboratory result not characteristic of normal individuals.

Adverse event. Unwanted effects that occur and are detected in populations. The term is used whether there is or is not any attribution to a medicine or other cause. Adverse events may be known parts of a disease that are observed to occur within a period of observation, and they may be analyzed to test for their frequency in a given population or trial. This is done to determine if there is an unexpectedly increased frequency resulting from nondisease factors such as medicine treatment. The term adverse event or adverse experience is used to encompass adverse reactions plus any injury, toxicity, or hypersensitivity that may be medicine related as well as any medical events that are apparently unrelated to medicine that occur during the study (e.g., surgery, illness, and trauma). See definition of adverse reaction.

Adverse experience. See adverse event.

Adverse reaction. Unwanted effect(s) (i.e., physical and psychological symptoms and signs) resulting from treatment. A less rigid definition of adverse reaction includes the previous definition plus any undesirable effect or problem that is present during the period of treatment and may or may not be a well-known or obvious complication of the disease itself. Thus, many common personality, physical, psychological, and behavioral characteristics that are observed in medicine studies are sometimes characterized as adverse reactions even if they were present during baseline.

   Synonyms of adverse reactions generally include adverse medical effects, untoward effects, side effects, adverse drug experiences, and adverse drug reactions. Specific distinctions among some of these terms may be defined operationally. For example, the term adverse reaction is used to denote those signs and symptoms at least possibly related to a medicine, whereas the term adverse experiences is used to include nonmedicine-related medical problems in a trial such as those emanating from trauma or concurrent illness. Distinctions among side effects, adverse events, and adverse reactions are illustrated in the definitions of the two former terms.

Bias. (1) A point of view that prevents impartial judgment on issues relating to that point of view. Clinical trials attempt to control this through double blinding. (2) Any tendency for a value to deviate in one direction from the true value. Statisticians attempt to prevent this type of bias by various techniques, including randomization.

Clinical significance. The quality of a study's outcome that convinces physicians to modify or maintain their current practice of medicine. The greater the clinical significance, the greater is the influence on the practice of medicine. The assessment of clinical significance is usually based on the magnitude of the effect observed, the quality of the study that yielded the data, and the probability that the effect is a true one. Although this operational definition is presented from the physician's perspective, the term could operationally be defined from the patient's perspective. Patients are primarily concerned with results that will lead to an improved quality of life or a lengthening of their life. In addition, clinical significance may be applied to either positive data of efficacy or negative safety data such as for adverse reactions. Synonyms include clinical importance, clinical relevance, and clinical meaningfulness.

Clinical studies. The class of all scientific approaches to evaluate medical disease preventions, diagnostic techniques, and treatments. Investigational and marketed prescription medicine evaluations plus over-the-counter medicines are included.

Clinical trials. A subset of those clinical studies that evaluates investigational medicines in Phases I, II, and III. Phase IV evaluations of marketed medicines in formal clinical trials using the same or similar types of protocols to those used in Phases I and III are also referred to as clinical trials.

Compliance. 1. Adherence of patients to following medical advice and prescriptions. Primarily applied to taking medicine as directed, but also applies to following advice on diet, exercise, or other aspects of a patient's life. 2. Adherence of investigators to following a protocol and related administrative and regulatory responsibilities. 3. Adherence of sponsors to following regulatory, legal, and other responsibilities and requirements relating to a clinical trial.

Compound. A chemical synthesized or prepared from natural sources that is evaluated for its biological activities in preclinical tests.

Development of medicines. The term development as applied to medicines is used in several different contexts, even within the pharmaceutical industry. This often leads to confusion and misunderstanding. No single definition is preferred, but the particular meaning intended should be made clear by all people using the term. Three operational definitions are presented, from the broadest to the narrowest:

1. All stages and processes involved in discovering, evaluating, and formulating a new medicine, until it reaches the market (i.e., commercial sale).
2. All stages involving the evaluation and formulation of a new medicine (after the medicine has been discovered and has gone through preclinical testing), until it reaches the market.
3. Those stages after the preclinical discovery and evaluation that involve technical development. These processes include formulation work, stability testing, scaling-up the compound for larger-scale synthesis, and providing analytical support. Clinical trials are not included in this definition.

Disease. Disorders (e.g., anxiety disorders, seizure disorders), conditions (e.g., obesity, menopause), syndromes, specific illnesses, and other medical problems that are an acquired morbid change in a tissue, organ, or organism. Synonyms are illness and sickness.

Dosage regimen. (1) The number of doses per given time period (usually days), (2) the time that elapses between doses (e.g., dose to be given every 6 hours) or the time that the doses are to be given (e.g., dose to be given at 8 a.m., noon, and 4 p.m. each day), or (3) the quantity of a medicine (e.g., number of tablets, capsules, etc.) that are given at each specific time of dosing.

Drug. A licit or illicit substance that is abused. Medicines should be described as drugs when they are being purposely abused.

Efficacy. A relative concept referring to the ability of a medicine to elicit a beneficial clinical effect. This may be measured or evaluated using objective or subjective parameters, and in terms ranging from global impressions, to highly precise measurements. Efficacy is assessed at one or more levels of organization (e.g., subcellular, cellular, tissue, organ, whole body) and may be extrapolated to other levels.

Endpoint. An indicator measured in a patient or biological sample to assess safety, efficacy, or another trial objective. Some endpoints are derived from primary endpoints (e.g., cardiac output is derived from stroke volume and heart rate). Synonyms include outcome, variable, parameter, marker, and measure. See surrogate endpoint in the text. Also defined as the final trial objective by some authors.

Incidence rate. The rate of occurrence of new cases of a disease, adverse reaction, or other event in a given population at risk (e.g., the incidence of disease X is Y patients per year per 100,000 population).

Interpretation. The processes whereby one determines the clinical meaning or significance of data after the relevant statistical analyses have been performed. These processes often involve developing an explanation of the data that are being evaluated.

Medicine. When a compound or substance is tested for biological and clinical activity in humans, it is considered to be a medicine. Some individuals prefer to define a medicine as a compound that has demonstrated clinically useful properties in patients. This definition, however, would restrict the term to use sometime during or after Phase II. Others use the term loosely and apply it to compounds with biological properties during the preclinical period that suggest medical usefulness in humans. The author has adopted the first definition for use in this book.

Patient. The term patient is used almost exclusively throughout this book in preference to subject or volunteer. Patient is used to cover those cases in which the term volunteer would be appropriate.

Pharmacodynamics. The processes of the body's responses resulting from treatment with a medicine or compound. The processes include pharmacological, biochemical, physiological, and therapeutic effects. The pharmacodynamics of a response to treatment are presented with the scientific and/or clinical language of the disciplines involved in detecting, measuring, and describing the effects.

Pharmacokinetics. The processes of absorption, distribution, metabolism, and excretion of compounds and medicines.

Phases of clinical trials and medicine development. Four phases of clinical trials and medicine development exist and are defined below. Each of these definitions is a functional one and the terms are not defined on a strict chronological basis. An investigational medicine is often evaluated in two or more phases simultaneously in different clinical trials. Also, some clinical trials may overlap two different phases.

Phase I. Initial safety trials on a new medicine, usually conducted in normal male volunteers. An attempt is made to establish the dose range tolerated by volunteers for single and for multiple doses. Phase I trials are sometimes conducted in severely ill patients (e.g., in the field of cancer) or in less ill patients when pharmacokinetic issues are addressed (e.g., metabolism of a new antiepileptic medicine in stable epileptic patients whose microsomal liver enzymes have been induced by other antiepileptic medicines). Pharmacokinetic trials are usually considered Phase I trials regardless of when they are conducted during a medicine's development.

Phase IIa. Pilot clinical trials to evelute efficacy (and safety) in selected populations of patients with the disease or condition to be treated, diagnosed, or prevented. Objectives may focus on dose-response, type of patient, frequency of dosing, or numerous other characteristics of safety and efficacy.

Phase IIb. Well-controlled trials to evaluate efficacy (and safety) in patients with the disease or condition to be treated, diagnosed, or prevented. These clinical trials usually represent the most rigorous demonstration of a medicine's efficacy. Sometimes referred to as pivotal trials.

Phase IIIa. Trials conducted after efficacy of the medicine is demonstrated, but prior to regulatory submission of a New Drug Application (NDA) or other dossier. These clinical trials are conducted in patient populations for which the medicine is eventually intended. Phase IIIa clinical trials generate additional data on both safety and efficacy in relatively large numbers of patients in both controlled and uncontrolled trials. Clinical trials are also conducted in special groups of patients (e.g., renal failure patients), or under special conditions dictated by the nature of the medicine and disease. These trials often provide much of the information needed for the package insert and labeling of the medicine.

Phase IIIb. Clinical trials conducted after regulatory submission of an NDA or other dossier, but prior to the medicine's approval and launch. These trials may supplement earlier trials, complete earlier trials, or may be directed toward new types of trials (e.g., quality of life, marketing) or Phase IV evaluations. This is the period between submission and approval of a regulatory dossier for marketing authorization.

Phase IV. Studies or trials conducted after a medicine is marketed to provide additional details about the medicine's efficacy or safety profile. Different formulations, dosages, durations of treatment, medicine interactions, and other medicine comparisons may be evaluated. New age groups, races, and other types of patients can be studied. Detection and definition of previously unknown or inadequately quantified adverse reactions and related risk factors are an important aspect of many Phase IV studies. If a marketed medicine is to be evaluated for another (i.e., new) indication, then those clinical trials are considered Phase II clinical trials. The term postmarketing surveillance is frequently used to describe those clinical studies in Phase IV (i.e., the period following marketing) that are primarily observational or nonexperimental in nature, to distinguish them from well controlled Phase IV clinical trials or marketing studies.

Prevalence. The total number of people in a population that are affected with a particular disease at a given time. This term is expressed as the rate of all cases (e.g., the prevalence of disease X is Y patients per 100,000 population) at a given point or period of time.

Research (on medicines). Numerous definitions of research are used both in the literature and among scientists. In the broadest sense, research in the pharmaceutical industry includes all processes of medicine discovery, preclinical and clinical evaluation, and technical development. In a more restricted sense, research concentrates on the preclinical discovery phase, where the basic characteristics of a new medicine are determined. Once a decision is reached to study the medicine in humans to evaluate its therapeutic potential, the compound passes from the research to the development phase.

Research and development. When research and development are used together, it refers to the broadest definition for research (see above). Some people use the term research colloquially to include most or all of the scientific and medical areas (discovery, evaluation, and development) covered by the single term research and development. Medicine development has several definitions and, in its broadest definition, is exactly the same as the broad definition of research.

Risk. A measure of (1) the probability of occurrence of harm to human health or (2) the severity of harm that may occur. Such a measure includes judgment of the acceptability of risk. Assessment of safety involves judgment, and there are numerous perspectives (e.g., patients, physicians, company, regulatory authorities) used for judging it.

Safety. A relative concept referring to the freedom from harm or damage resulting from adverse reactions or physical, psychological, or behavioral abnormalities that occur as a result of medicine or nonmedicine use. Safety is usually measured with one or more of the following: physical examination (e.g., vital signs, neurological, ophthalmological, general physical), laboratory evaluations of biological samples (e.g., hematology, clinical chemistry, urinalysis), special tests and procedures (e.g., electrocardiogram, pulmonary function tests), psychiatric tests and evaluations, and determination of clinical signs and symptoms.

Satellite site. A secondary site at which patients in a clinical trial are seen, usually by the same investigator who sees patients at the primary site. A satellite site may be the same type of site (e.g., private office, hospital) or a different type from the primary site.

Serious adverse reaction. Multiple definitions are possible and no single one is correct in all situations. In general usage referring to patients in clinical trials, a serious adverse reaction may be (1) any bad adverse reaction that is observed, (2) any bad adverse reaction that one does not expect to observe, (3) any bad adverse reaction that one does not expect to observe and is not in the label, or (4) any bad adverse reaction that has not been reported with standard therapy. Definitions also may be based on the degree to which an adverse reaction compromises a patient's function or requires treatment (see Chapter 80, page 567).

Side effect. Any effect other than the primary intended effect(s) resulting from medicine or non-medicine treatment or intervention. Side effects may be negative (i.e., an adverse reaction), neutral, or positive (i.e., a beneficial effect) for the patient. This term, therefore, includes all adverse reactions plus other effects of treatment. See definition of adverse reaction.

Site. This refers to the place where a clinical trial is conducted. A physician who has offices and sees patients in three separate locations is viewed as having one site. A physician who is on the staff of four hospitals could be viewed as having one or four sites, depending on how similar or different the patient populations are and whether the data from these four locations will be pooled and considered a single site. For example, a single physician who enrolls groups of patients at a university hospital, private clinic, community hospital, and Veterans Administration Hospital should generally be viewed as having four sites, since the patient populations would be expected to differ at each site. See satellite site.

Statistical significance. This term relates to the probability that an event or difference occurred by chance alone. Thus, it is a measure of whether a difference is likely to be real, but it does not indicate whether the difference is small or large, important or trivial. The level of statistical significance depends on the number of patients studied or observations made, as well as the magnitude of difference observed.

Therapeutic window. This term is applied to the difference between the minimum and maximum doses that may be given patients to obtain an adequate clinical response and avoid intolerable toxic effects. The greater the value calculated for the therapeutic window, the greater a medicine's margin of safety. Synonyms are therapeutic ratio and therapeutic index.

Volunteer. A normal individual who participates in a clinical trial for reasons other than medical need and who does not receive any direct medical benefit from participating in the trial.

About the Author

Bert Spilker, Ph.D., M.D. is Director of Project Coordination at Burroughs Wellcome Co. and holds three faculty appointments as Professor at the University of North Carolina, Chapel Hill in the Schools of Medicine (Departments of Medicine and Pharmacology) and Pharmacy. Dr. Spilker has 18 years experience in the pharmaceutical industry, having worked for Pfizer Ltd. (United Kingdom), Phillips-Duphar B. V. (The Netherlands), Sterling Drug Inc. (Rensselaer, New York), and the Burroughs Wellcome Co. He worked for a private consulting company in the Washington, D.C. area and has additional experience in the private practice of general medicine. He is currently Chairman of the PMA's Commission on Drugs for Rare Diseases.

Bert Spilker received his Ph.D. in Pharmacology from the State University of New York, Downstate Medical Center in 1967, and did post-doctoral research at the University of California Medical School in San Francisco. He received his M.D. from the University of Miami Ph.D. to M.D. Program in 1977 and did a residency in internal medicine at Brown University Medical School. Bert Spilker is the author of over 80 publications plus ten books in a wide area of both pharmacology and clinical medicine.

Dr. Spilker is married and has two children.

CHAPTER 1

Introduction

An Overview of Approaches Used in This Book

The purpose of this introduction is to provide a perspective on the overall approach and types of concepts frequently used in the text. It is possible to divide the world into splitters and lumpers (i.e., those who analyze and break everything into components or who generalize and fold many aspects together). The author is a splitter, like most scientists and clinicians. Numerous aspects relating to clinical trials are described in terms of levels, spectra, flow diagrams, and matrixes. Some of the levels and types discussed are widely known and accepted, but the majority are proposed as a convenient means of conceptualizing specific topics. These models and descriptions are not intended to represent the truth about clinical trials, but rather to serve as a convenient categorization and frame of reference. They are a reflection of the author's view on specific topics. There is almost never a specific order of importance attached to the listing of points in tables or of examples described in the figures.

Levels or Hierarchies

The various aspects of clinical trials that are depicted in terms of a series of levels or hierarchies are listed in Table 1.1.

Spectra

Many aspects of medicine (and of life itself) are described in black and white terms that actually represent two poles (or extremes) on a continuum. The majority of opposites in clinical medicine represent such poles. Sometimes multiple discrete examples are described in this book that lie along a continuum or spectrum. Examples of spectra used are listed in Table 1.2.

Flow Diagrams

Almost any process or activity may be illustrated using a flow diagram. The flow diagrams in this book (Table 1.3) are therefore an arbitrary collection dependent on the author's personal preferences of selected pro-

TABLE 1.1 *Series of levels and hierarchies used in this book*

Chapter	Description
22	Types of data (e.g., nominal, ordinal, interval, ratio)
71	Evaluating clinical significance
71	Levels of organization
73	Cause and effect
73	Hierarchy of strength of evidence from different types of trial
74	Clinical significance
80	Adverse reactions
82	Interpretation of clinical data
82	Clinical levels of patient numbers
82	Clinical levels in the therapeutic process
88	Dose levels evaluated in toxicity
99	Benefits and risks
109	Levels of data interpretation
118	Clinical trial methodologies
123	Hierarchy of priorities

TABLE 1.2 *Spectra (i.e., continuums) used in this book*

Chapter	Description
38	Continuum along which results of single patient trials may be shown
41	Number of continuation protocols
41	Complexity of continuation protocols
41	Artificiality of a protocol
43	Types of validation
43	Degree of validity of a test
43	How well has a test's viability been evaluated
62	Style of monitoring
69	Time when an interim analysis is conducted
69	Amount and type of data evaluated in an interim analysis
69	Time when a decision is made to conduct an interim analysis
69	Formality of the interim analysis conducted
84	Pharmacokinetic training and orientation
116	Approaches to combining efficacy data
121	Organization of multinational companies from decentralized to centralized
122	Management styles
127	Regulatory standards: when during the Investigational New Drug Application (IND) to New Drug Application (NDA) program must certain information be submitted
127	Regulatory standards: how much detail must be provided on a point in a submission
127	Regulatory standards: amount of validation required

TABLE 1.3 *Flow diagrams used in this book*

Chapter	Description
28	Data processing and flow using remote data entry
30	Protocol development and approval
31	Patient entry into a clinical trial
63	The audit trail
68	Data processing

TABLE 1.4 *Examples of processes described as a series of steps*

Chapter	Item
20	Developing a protocol
42	Conducting a pharmacoeconomic evaluation
52	Designing quality of life trials
68	Data processing
71	Interpretation of clinical data
72	Decision analysis
99	Assessing risk
104	Conducting a meta-analysis
115	Designing a clinical development plan

TABLE 1.5 *Prototype agendas and tables of contents*

Chapter	Item
30	Table of contents for a protocol
60	Agendas for pretrial roundtable meetings (three examples)
125	Agendas for project meetings (three examples)
125	Table of contents of a final medical report (three examples)

TABLE 1.6 *Forms to track or report specific information*[a]

Chapter	Item
59	Investigator selection form
61	Clinical trial initiation: internal documents and procedures
61	Clinical trial initiation: information for investigator to send to the sponsor
61	Clinical trial initiation: information for the sponsor to send to the investigator
61	Conducting the clinical trial
62	Table formats to monitor multiple clinical trials
62	Graph format to track patient enrollment in a clinical trial
65	Disposition of medicine used in a clinical trial
66	Clinical trial data entry and analysis
66	Data collection form reconciliation
68	Monitoring activities during data processing, and analysis, and report writing
79	Logsheet of potential patients contacted about a clinical trial
79	Logsheet of potential patients disqualified at screen
79	Logsheet of potential patients entered in a clinical trial
103	Checklists to assess clinical trials (several examples)
123	Summarize work force allocation to specific trials (three examples)
125	Status of requests for medicine supplies to be sent to an investigator
125	Tracking clinical trials (six examples)
125	Individual patients in clinical trials
125	Grant payments on a clinical trial
125	Telephone conversation report
125	Periodic scheduled site visit report
125	Data collection form checklist
125	Evaluation of potential investigator
125	Shipment of clinical trial materials to site
126	Adverse reaction reporting forms (two examples)
130	Calculating costs of a clinical trial (13 examples)
130	Monitoring financial expenses for clinical trials

[a] Tables listing items or figures showing points to track in various situations are not listed.

TABLE 1.7 *Probabilities associated with various terms used in this book*

Term	Probability (%)
"Never"	0
"Rarely"	less than 1%
"Hardly ever"	1% to 5%
"Unusual"	5% to 10%
"Sometimes"	10% to 49%
"Frequently"	33% to 66%
"Generally"	50% to 75%
"Often"	50% to 75%
"Usually"	75% to 95%
"Invariably"	above 95%
"Virtually always"	above 98%
"Always"	100%

cesses to illustrate in this manner. Some individuals tend to describe most professional or personal activities in terms of flow diagrams. The author has attempted to avoid this extreme position.

Steps, Agendas, and Tables of Contents

Numerous processes may be described in terms of a few or many independent steps. While these may be illustrated with flow diagrams, many are simply listed and described (Table 1.4). Prototype agendas and tables of contents are listed in Table 1.5.

Forms to Track or Report on Specific Information

Numerous prototype forms and tables that can be readily used to track certain types of information are given in this book. A synopsis of these is given in Table 1.6. Many other tables or figures describe or list informa-

tion that may be (or should be) tracked, but these are not included in the list. These checklists are an important aspect of this book.

Probabilities as Represented by Various Terms

Chapter 72 contains a discussion about the great variation in the meaning that different people attach to the same word or term, such as *often*, *frequently*, *generally*, and *rarely*. Even absolute terms such as *always* and *never* are often used to cover a range of probabilities. Because all terms that have a probability associated with them are used many times in any book, the meaning of an author's usage should be helpful in understanding the meaning of various statements. Probabilities conceptualized by the author for various terms are given in Table 1.7. Some degree of overlap between the usage of these terms is unavoidable, particularly because exact probabilities are rarely known when one of the terms given in Table 1.7 is used.

PART I

Developing Clinical Trial Designs

All men naturally desire knowledge.

—*Aristotle*

The important thing is not to stop questioning. Curiosity has its own reason for existing. One cannot help but be in awe when he contemplates the mysteries of eternity, of life, of the marvelous structure of reality. It is enough if one tries merely to comprehend a little of this mystery every day. Never lose a holy curiosity.

—*Albert Einstein*

CHAPTER 2

Establishing the Overall Approach to a Clinical Trial

FACTORS INVOLVED

It is important to consider several factors in creating a trial design. A list of many of the factors that constitute a trial design is presented in Table 2.1. Some of these are more important in certain protocols than in others. For example, the major objective of a clinical trial might be to compare two routes of administration of a new medicine, whereas in other trials the choice of the route of administration may be a relatively minor factor or not subject to choice (e.g., if the medicine is only available in one form).

Establishing a rough hierarchy of the importance of the factors constituting the clinical trial design within a given trial is sometimes helpful in deciding which of these factors to consider initially. Once this decision is made, a design can be chosen by evaluating the possible variations for each of the relevant factors. One must ensure that the overall design created in this manner can be implemented within the resources available. If the design is complex and/or involves numerous options, it may be useful to construct algorithms or flow charts to help others to understand the trial design more easily. The criteria for the choices to be made at each decision point must be established in advance and clearly described in the protocol. Although algorithms may help to clarify complex trial designs, it is the author's opinion that they are rarely necessary.

There may be constraints on choosing a clinical trial design imposed by the objectives of the trial. One example is when investigational medicines are being evaluated in Phases I, II, or III. In such cases, the trial

design chosen must fit general regulatory authority guidelines for the specific phase of investigation. Also, if the data expected to be obtained from the clinical trial are to be combined with data from other trials, then the data collected should be able to be integrated with the other data. This may necessitate using a standard clinical trial design in multiple trials. This concern must also be reflected in the design of data collection forms in order to ensure that data collected are in the desired format. Careful attention must be paid to using compatible, if not completely identical, systems of disease classification and terminology to describe the classification, especially if the data sets obtained in the various clinical trials are to be merged.

TABLE 2.1 *Factors considered in constructing a clinical trial*

1. Preliminary considerations
2. Establishing the overall approach to a clinical trial
3. Establishing clinical trial objectives
4. Choosing the clinical trial's blind
5. Bias and confounding factors
6. Choice of an overall clinical trial design
7. Controls used in clinical trials
8. Sample size and number of parts of a clinical trial
9. Randomization procedures
10. Screening, baseline, treatment, and posttreatment periods
11. Patient populations, methodologies, and measurements
12. Patient recruitment
13. Dosing schedule
14. Compliance
15. Pharmacokinetics and medicine interactions
16. Data Review Committees
17. Dosage forms and formulations
18. Routes of administration

7

ROLE OF THE STATISTICIAN

Before discussing each of the elements of a basic clinical trial design, it is important to review the role of the statistician in the following areas:

1. Trial objectives. In most situations the statistician should review the objective(s).
2. Trial design. This is briefly discussed below.
3. Interim analyses. If these are to be performed, then their influence on the trial design must be determined. See Chapter 69.
4. Early termination of the trial. Criteria must be established in advance for trials using a sequential design and are sometimes established in advance for fixed-sample-size trials in which interim analyses are contemplated.
5. Analysis of the data. The statistician should prepare his or her approach(es) to the data in advance. Prototype tables and figures may be prepared.

TYPE I AND TYPE II ERRORS

Two statistical terms that should be familiar to investigators and clinical scientists are *type I error* (α) and *type II error* (β). The magnitudes of these errors are usually determined by the investigator before a clinical trial begins, often in collaboration with the statistician. These are important concepts, because they are used in the determination of sample size and also reflect how a trial will be viewed by the medical community.

Type I error (α) is the probability of declaring a statistical difference when in fact there is none. It may be viewed as the significance level necessary for the statistical test to detect a difference between treatments that is clinically meaningful (e.g., $\alpha = 0.05$). This also means that the probability of a false–positive result is not greater than 0.05. Type II error (β) is the probability of not detecting the difference that is looked for if it is present (i.e., the chance of missing a real effect). Power (defined as $1 - \beta$) is the probability of detecting this difference. It is desirable to have a high power or probability of detecting a difference between treatments, and the goal of any clinical trial is to have small type I (α) and small type II (β) errors. If the trial is limited by fixed resources, however, it will be difficult (or impossible) to achieve both goals. Since there is a tradeoff between the two types of errors, it will be necessary to decide which goal is more important.

CHOOSING THE MOST APPROPRIATE CLINICAL TRIAL DESIGN FOR A PARTICULAR TRIAL

Choosing the most appropriate design for a clinical trial is similar to choosing ready-made clothes. In this analogy, the clothes shopper is like the sponsor or group designing the trial. The shopper has to look the clothes over in the rack and pick out a few to try on for fit and appearance. Several will not fit; others may fit satisfactorily, but their appearance does not seem correct for the personality or purpose. The one chosen may need some alterations for the fit to be almost perfect.

Regarding a clinical trial design, the choice made is based on viewing the design from multiple perspectives. The first perspective usually considered is the medical one. The choice from the medical view focuses on the objective(s) of the clinical trial and addresses the question of which design is best suited to achieve the objectives. This perspective includes obtaining and evaluating all scientific and statistical opinions. Part of the medical perspective includes consideration of the statistical and clinical appropriateness of each possible trial design. Specific criteria exist and should be applied to determine when crossover trial designs may be used. Specific criteria also exist for sequential trial designs (see Chapter 6).

The second perspective one often considers is the marketing perspective. Even for pilot or pivotal Phase II and Phase III clinical trials, it is important to consider a marketing perspective. For instance, it is undesirable to enlist the world's foremost specialists at a tertiary care center to conduct a sophisticated clinical trial design when the data generated there will not be as useful for impressing general practitioners as would the data from a trial conducted by general practitioners in primary care practice, using a simple, but appropriate clinical trial design.

Third, one may evaluate the design from a regulatory perspective. Certain clinical trial designs, even in well controlled trials, have a poor history with the regulatory authorities regarding their appropriateness for pivotal clinical trials. Some guidelines issued by the FDA for specific therapeutic areas include suggestions about when to use certain clinical trial designs. Certain designs appear to facilitate medicine approval more than others.

Recently, political and social factors have had a greater influence than usual on the choice of clinical trial designs. The most obvious example of this influence involves the pressures exerted on pharmaceutical companies by AIDS activists to use compassionate plea protocols, open label designs, treatment-IND, and parallel-track procedures. Other pressures have been directed to modify interim analyses and early stopping rules.

PILOT TRIALS

There are situations in which a pilot trial is more appropriate to conduct than a full-scale or fully controlled trial. A pilot trial is used to obtain information, and work out the logistics and management, deemed necessary for further clinical trials. Although pilot trials are often unblind and use open-label medicines, they may also be single or double blind and may include tight control on all appropriate variables. The term "pilot" refers to the purpose of the trial. A number of common reasons that are advanced for conducting a pilot study are presented in Table 2.2.

Once a decision to conduct a pilot trial is reached, a further decision must be made as to whether it should be conducted as a separate trial or integrated into a controlled trial. If the finalization of details in the trial design of a controlled trial would depend on data generated in an open-label pilot trial, it is the author's view that the pilot and controlled trial should be separate. If, however, the pilot trial is intended to give the investigator experience with the medicine and the controlled trial has a finalized protocol and could be run independently, then combining these two parts may be beneficial from an administrative viewpoint.

The concept of using pilot patients as a vanguard may be relevant in some trials to confirm that the trial medicine is safe or that the procedures are suitable, safe, and operational before exposing a larger number of patients. This is especially relevant in Phase I trials, in which the safety of a new medicine may be almost completely unknown. The use of pilot patients is not advised in a well-controlled trial.

TABLE 2.2 *Common reasons for conducting pilot trials*

1. Dose ranging with a new medicine or with an old medicine being evaluated in a a new therapeutic area
2. Initial efficacy evaluation of a new medicine
3. Initial efficacy evaluation of an established medicine for a new indication
4. Determination or clarification of details requiring refinement prior to finalizing the protocol for a larger or similar clinical trial (e.g., to estimate the degree of variation in the measurements obtained); this information can help estimate the required sample size more accurately
5. Determination of details required to finalize plans for the conduct of the tiral (e.g., to conduct "dry runs" through complex protocols; to determine the duration required to conduct a medicine trial)
6. Evaluation of the methodology to be used in another trial
7. Evaluation of a variable related to the clinical pharmacology of a medicine (e.g., is total dose or blood level more important, b.i.d. versus t.i.d. dosing) in a rapid and noncontrolled manner
8. Development of clinical experience by research personnel with a medicine under open-label conditions prior to initiation of a double-blind clinical trial
9. Determination of the actual availability of patients for enrollment in a trial as opposed to the expected availability
10. Exploration of ethical questions relating to whether a specific placebo-controlled double-blind trial (or other trial design) is ethically acceptable to conduct with the trial medicine

Types of Pilot Trials

The major types of pilot trials depend on whether patients are treated or not. Those who are not treated stop after their baseline is assessed. Those who receive treatment may or may not continue into a full clinical trial after the completion of their trial, or their data may or may not be folded into the full clinical trial. This latter practice could only be considered if the protocol was unchanged.

Golden Rule of Pilot Trials

The term "pilot trial" sometimes has the connotation of being a "quick-and-dirty" evaluation. A sloppy approach, however, will not provide reliable information and may raise new questions (and problems) that have to be addressed. Therefore, a pilot trial must be planned with as much care as a full-scale controlled trial.

Can a Pilot Trial Become a Pivotal Trial?

Under some conditions the answer is clearly "yes." Those conditions are essentially that the pilot trial was well designed, controlled, conducted, and analyzed. The clinical trial originally must have been intended as a pilot or feasibility trial because it was uncertain whether the treatment would be effective, not because it was a quick-and-dirty trial.

Problems can arise if the clinical trial initially involved a small number of patients and, after their data were analyzed, a larger number of patients were then enrolled. The potential problems arising from such a scenario should be discussed with a statistician in advance of initiating the clinical trial.

When Are Pilot Trials Conducted?

Pilot trials may occur in all phases of a medicine's development, particularly when viewed as feasibility trials to test efficacy, safety, or a particular hypothesis. In Phase I, the vanguard group of a few volunteers or patients who receive higher doses than previously given are in a pilot trial. Phase II pilot trials are the ones that are most commonly discussed. In Phases III or IV, special populations may be exposed to a medicine as a pilot trial.

CHAPTER 3

Establishing Clinical Trial Objectives

INTRODUCTION

Before a total commitment is made to initiate and conduct a clinical trial, careful consideration should be given to the question of why the trial has been proposed. Is it based on someone's casual comment that such a clinical trial would be a "good idea" or an "important trial to undertake"? Whatever the reason(s) for the trial, they should be carefully evaluated from the point of view of whether that trial is truly necessary to answer the question(s) posed.

Establishing the Need for the Clinical Trial

The actual need for a clinical trial should always be addressed and demonstrated, since there are sometimes relatively simple alternatives to conducting a trial. The questions that prompted the proposal to conduct a clinical trial may sometimes be answered through a literature search and evaluation, or possibly one or more "experts" or consultants could be asked for their views. A third possibility is that the clinical trial may have already been performed. This could be

the case if a new question is raised on an established medicine. One should inquire with the company that developed or markets the medicine. If the potential author is in a pharmaceutical corporation, then older data in the files on the potential clinical trial medicine should be reviewed.

Balancing Breadth and Depth

A principle that many investigators consider fundamental is that one should seek the least complex approach to answering or addressing a clearly stated clinical problem, hypothesis, or question. In formulating an approach to the question to be addressed in the clinical trial and in establishing the trial design to answer that question, it may be helpful to think of the approach as a balance between breadth and depth. For example, if the objective of a trial were to examine the effect of a new medicine for its general analgesic properties, it would not be as valuable in the initial trial to evaluate a small group of patients intensively in great detail (in depth) as to study a larger group of patients more generally (in breadth). In-depth clinical trials are usually directed towards determining the answers to, or information on, specific questions, such as bioavailability or mechanism of action. Clinical trials that emphasize a broad approach (breadth) include many Phase III clinical trials, in which the objective is to gain information on how a large population of patients will react to the trial medicine under usual (and unusual) conditions. (The four phases of medicine trials in the United States are operationally defined in the terminology section of this book.)

Which Comes First: The Trial Objective or Design?

The clinical trial design is the framework by which the trial objectives will be met. The design is generally established after the trial objectives have been clearly elucidated. Otherwise, one may be in the position of attempting to fit the questions to be answered (i.e., trial objectives) to an imposed or fixed trial design. If it is not possible to implement a trial design acceptable for addressing the objectives posed, then it may be necessary to refine or modify the trial objectives.

There are several reasons why the specific clinical trial design required to address the trial objectives may be either unsuitable or impossible to adopt. The design might require (1) methods that are beyond the state of the art in the particular field of medicine involved, (2) equipment that is too expensive or too difficult to obtain or operate, (3) too many patients, (4) efforts that are too arduous for patients to meet comfortably, (5) too long a period to conduct, (6) too much manpower to conduct, or any other numerous possibilities. Thus, it may be necessary to revise the trial objectives to bring them within the limitations imposed on the trial design by resources, state-of-the-art considerations, or other factors.

TYPES OF CLINICAL TRIALS OF MEDICINES

Several classes of clinical trials of medicines address different types of purposes (goals). Although the exact number and description of these classes are arbitrary, a brief synopsis of each category will provide a basis for orienting one's major and minor trial objectives and for understanding the variety of different purposes for clinical trials of medicines.

Safety Evaluation

Although a safety evaluation constitutes an important part of almost all clinical trials of medicines, some trials are designed with a safety evaluation as their primary purpose. These trials include most of those conducted in Phase I. Safety is a broad topic that en-

compasses dose tolerance (i.e., how high a dose patients can receive without having clinically significant adverse reactions, physical signs, or laboratory abnormalities), dose frequency, and duration of exposure to a medicine.

Pharmacokinetic Evaluation

Establishing the relevant pharmacokinetic parameters in humans is an important part of the development of all medicines. This type of clinical trial concentrates on investigating one or more of the following basic pharmacological concepts: absorption, distribution, metabolism, and excretion.

Efficacy Evaluation

Clinical trials concentrating on efficacy are usually initiated in Phase II of clinical development, although important information can sometimes be gleaned from Phase I trials (e.g., when a medicine is expected to cause a specific change in a laboratory parameter in normals as well as in patients).

Mechanism of Action Evaluation

Clinical trials may be designed to elucidate the mechanism of action of an investigational or marketed medicine. This category would include evaluations of medicine interactions.

General Population Evaluation

The therapeutic use of a new medicine in a general patient population is primarily evaluated during Phase III and IV clinical trials.

Evaluation of Clinical Methodology

A medicine may be used as a research tool in developing and/or testing new techniques for the evaluation and/or validation of a specific methodology.

Evaluation of Clinical Pharmacology

Although this group of clinical trials overlaps to some degree with other types of trials, this category includes evaluation of new dosage formulations (e.g., tablets versus capsules), new routes of administration, new dosage regimens (e.g., b.i.d. versus t.i.d. dosing), and/or other characteristics of a medicine's pharmacological profile.

Postmarketing Evaluation

This category consists of the varied types of Phase IV studies that are designed to identify rare or infrequent adverse reactions as well as beneficial effects not previously known or evaluated with a new (or established) medicine. Specific types of epidemiological studies are described in Chapter 7.

The universe of clinical trials is divided differently by different scientists. Carter (1980) divided trials into three groups: exploratory (initial trials investigating a novel idea), confirmatory trials designed to replicate the results of the exploratory trials), and explanatory (trials designed to modify or better understand an established point). Other authors have used two groups: blazing and consolidating trials (Murphy, 1982), or pragmatic and explanatory (Weintraub, 1982).

CLINICAL TRIAL OBJECTIVES

What Are Objectives?

After one of these broad types of clinical trials has been identified as the major purpose or goal for the proposed trial, trial objectives must be established that are to be addressed within the framework of the above trial type.

Clinical trial objectives are concise statements of the major and minor questions that the trial is designed to answer. The author should reflect on the objectives and confirm that they represent valid and proper questions, or series of questions, to propose. If an underlying question is the basis of the proposed objective, then it may be desirable to modify the objective to reflect the underlying consideration. If other individuals will assist in developing the protocol, one should obtain their agreement that the established objectives are appropriate, correctly stated, and will meet the goals or purposes of the clinical trial. The overall trial goals (purposes) are differentiated from the objectives in that the former represent the type of trial to be conducted (see previous section), whereas the objectives are the concise statements that will enable the goals to be achieved.

Why Are Clinical Trial Objectives so Critical?

The objectives of a clinical trial are the questions a clinical trial asks and tries to answer. In all areas of research, asking the right question is perhaps the most important part of the research. How the research problem is stated determines the trial design used, the data collected, the analyses conducted, and the conclusions (i.e., interpretation) that can be drawn. It is therefore essential that the objective(s) be clearly, completely, and concisely expressed. If they are not, then the rest of the enterprise may be irrelevant and represent a significant waste of efforts.

How Are Trial Objectives Stated?

In all types of clinical trials, the objective should be stated as specifically and succinctly as possible in the protocol. It is not suitable to write that the objective is "to determine the mechanism of action of medicine X," since this objective is too general, vague, and merely restates the overall goal of the trial. It is preferable to write that the trial objective is to evaluate the effects of daily dose T of medicine W in population X on parameters Y and Z by continuous or daily recording of results obtained in tests A and B during time period C, as compared with medicine D at dose E, under the same experimental conditions. Table 3.1 lists information to include.

How Many Objectives May Be Posed?

Many methodological and statistical problems are created if too many questions are posed in one protocol. Posing many questions often creates an excessive number of subgroups of data, some of which may be insufficient in quantity to answer the questions posed. In addition, posing many questions often makes the clinical trial difficult to conduct and decreases the probability of having the trial completed successfully. Nonetheless, one must be sensitive to the large number of potential questions from which the most optimal ones are chosen and be aware of the many potentially informative analyses that may provide valuable insights for future trials.

TABLE 3.1 *Information to include (when relevant) in the statement of a clinical trial's objective[a]*

1. An expression describing the overall approach (e.g., *to assess, to compare, to evaluate, to determine*)[b]
2. Names of all medicines being evaluated
3. Specification of the dose(s) or dose range to be studied (e.g., 200 and 400 mg)
4. Identification of the dosage regimen (e.g., once a day for 3 weeks)
5. Disease(s) being evaluated
6. Type of patient(s) being evaluated (e.g., pediatric, renal failure)
7. General purpose (e.g., safety, efficacy, pharmacokinetics)
8. Specific purpose (e.g., dose-response, superiority to placebo)
9. Parameter(s) to be measured

[a] One or two *major* objectives are usually all that may be tested in a single clinical trial. One to three *secondary* objectives may also be tested. Each objective should be listed and is usually described in one or two sentences. The primary (major) objectives should be clearly delineated and separated from the secondary objectives so that *no* confusion develops.
[b] Do not use a term such as *to prove*, because it implies that results are known.

Primary and Secondary Objectives

A clinical trial often has both primary and secondary objectives, and these should be identified as such in the protocol. Ideally, no more than one or two of each should be included in a clinical trial. The more objectives posed the less the chance that a single clinical trial design will adequately address each objective. Also, a larger number of objectives will complicate the protocol and conduct of the clinical trial and make it less likely to be completed successfully. The analysis and interpretation of data will be compromised. The inclusion of numerous objectives should therefore be avoided whenever possible.

Feasibility of Objectives

After the objective is agreed on, it must be determined whether it is feasible to address the objective with known clinical methodology. If the clinical methodology exists, then one must determine whether it is possible, in terms of time, money, manpower, and other practical concerns, to mount the effort necessary to complete the clinical trial. It is understood that some practical considerations cannot be fully addressed until a general or detailed trial design has been chosen, evaluated, and reviewed with statisticians. It is thus possible that in subsequent stages of developing the trial design, the trial objectives may have to be modified. These modifications will allow a protocol to be written that will address its goals within the framework of available methodologies and resources.

Safety Objectives

If the objectives of the clinical trial relate to the evaluation of medicine safety, then the trial design chosen will depend on which aspects of safety are of particular interest for evaluation. Safety considerations may focus on the doses used, laboratory results, physical examinations, adverse reactions, or other areas. If the purpose of the trial is focused on determination of safe doses, then the trial objective may relate to evaluating the safety of doses for (1) dose ascension (e.g., a rapid and/or slow rate of dose ascension may be evaluated), (2) "loading" the patient, (3) determining the maximally tolerated maintenance dose, or (4) defining a safe rate of dose taper. Numerous other questions related to "safe doses" may also be posed, such as the safety of a sudden withdrawal of the medicine.

Other Objectives

There are numerous other purposes for conducting a clinical trial. Trial goals and objectives may be developed that relate to comparative claims with other medicines, labeling of the medicine, new dosage strengths or formulations, and establishment of various parameters related to pharmacokinetics. Although the trial's primary objective(s) may be focused on efficacy or pharmacokinetics, an evaluation of safety or medicine toxicity is virtually always performed at the same time, even if it is not a stated objective and is conducted in a nonrigorous manner.

May a Clinical Trial's Objective Be To Show Equivalence (i.e., no Difference) Between Treatments?

Many clinical trials conducted today, and an even greater proportion in the past, compare two or more different medicines in patients. One of those medicines was designated the standard therapy because it was assumed to be effective; it was thus chosen as the control for the clinical trial. If the outcome of the clinical trial demonstrated no difference between treatments, then the test medicine was assumed to be as effective as the standard therapy. The problems with this assumption are that there is no evidence that either treatment was effective, since both could have been ineffective, and there are no statistical methods that are generally accepted means of establishing the equivalence of two or more treatments. Moreover, the incentives to conduct the clinical trial at a high standard may be less for some investigators, since a poorly conducted trial that shows no differences between treatments because of its poor conduct will be interpreted as "positive." Finally, since there is an expectation that all patients will be doing well in a trial, a bias is introduced that may encourage less attention to careful observation and measurement.

Although there may be convincing reasons to conduct an equivalence type of clinical trial, it should only be used as a last resort measure if stronger clinical designs are either considered unethical or unfeasible. Modifications of traditional clinical trial designs should be sought to avoid using an equivalence objective. This type is discussed further in Chapter 6 on clinical trial designs.

Changing Objectives During a Clinical Trial

Modifying or changing objectives after a clinical trial has been initiated will usually cause major problems in the analysis and interpretation of the data obtained and in the acceptance of those data by the medical community. An example of this problem arose in the Anturane Reinfarction Trial (see Anturane Reinfarction Trial Research Group, 1980; Temple and Pledger, 1980, for a detailed description and discussion of the issues raised).

Anturane Reinfarction Trial

One of the most important lessons gained from the Anturane Reinfarction Trial is that a positive effect observed in a subgroup analysis that is not part of the trial's official objective(s) is not sufficient proof of activity in a well-controlled clinical trial. This means that the major objective must be clearly identified and defined in advance (i.e., in the protocol), and that any subgroup analyses conducted after the trial is completed that yield positive results may serve as a hypothesis to be tested in a subsequent clinical trial, but do not represent proof of activity for the original clinical trial.

Data from the trial demonstrated a reduction in cardiac mortality in patients given Anturane (sulfinpyrazone) after they had a myocardial infarction. A decrease in sudden deaths was observed in the treated group during the second through seventh month after infarction. The FDA conducted an audit of these data and rejected the official interpretation for several reasons. Briefly, Temple and Pledger of the FDA reported (1980) that the mortality data depended to a large degree on exclusion of certain deaths from analysis, that a full accounting of the patients was not presented in the publications, and that some important definitions (e.g., sudden death) were not made, which led to a poorly characterized patient group. In addition, some statistical weaknesses were described.

Conclusion and a Caution

Thus, it is essential at the outset of a clinical trial to consider the evaluations and trial objectives that may be important or useful after the data have been collected. It is also well known that as the number of statistical tests performed increases, the chances of finding at least one result that is statistically significant by chance alone also increases. If 100 independent statistical comparisons are made, then on the average, five will be significant (if the level of statistical significance is $\alpha = 0.05$ and there are no differences between the comparison groups). Thus, the number of measurements made and analyses performed will have at least some bearing on the significance of the data obtained.

PHASES OF CLINICAL TESTING

The purpose and objectives of a clinical trial are usually related in some degree to the phase of clinical testing in which the trial medicine is found. There are four phases of clinical testing, which are referred to frequently in this book. These phases may be defined in regulatory or operational terms. The operational definitions used throughout this book are presented in the terminology section.

It is usually possible to identify the phase of development in which an investigational or marketed medicine may be found. On the other hand, many medicines are in two or more phases at the same time. For example, a medicine could be evaluated for a new indication (Phase II), be on the market (Phase IV), and be undergoing a pharmacokinetic evaluation assessing a different patient population (Phase I) all at one time.

There are other examples in which specific phases of development have little meaning. A medicine that is to be used as an adjunct and is known to be safe may merely need to be tested in 1,000 patients to see if it works. Another example is a major breakthrough medicine that has a combined Phases I and II clinical program and does not require any Phase III clinical trials.

CHAPTER 4

Choosing and Validating the Clinical Trial's Blind

TYPES OF BLINDS: TRADITIONAL DEFINITIONS

The term "blind" refers to a lack of knowledge of the identity of the trial treatment. Patients, investigators, data review committees, ancillary personnel, statisticians, and monitors are the major groups of individuals who may be kept blind during a clinical trial of a medicine. Blinding is used to decrease the biases that occur in a clinical trial when patients are evaluated during treatment and to avoid a placebo effect that often occurs in open-label trials. The types of blind of patients and investigators in a clinical trial are described below and in Table 4.1.

1. Open label. No blind is used. Both investigator and patient know the identity of the medicine.
2. Single blind. The patient is unaware of which treatment is being received, but the investigator has this information. In unusual cases, the investigator and not the patient may be kept blind to the identity of the treatment.
3. Double blind. Neither the patient nor the investigator is aware of which treatment the patient is receiving. A double-blind design is generally considered to provide the most reliable data from a clinical trial. This type of clinical trial, however,

is usually more complicated to initiate and conduct than single-blind or open-label trials.
4. Combination of blinds. (a) In part 1 of a clinical trial, one type of blind may be used (e.g., single blind), and in part 2 of the same trial, another blind (e.g., double blind) may be used. A third part of the same trial may utilize the same blind as part 1 or use an entirely different type of blind. (b) Some patients may follow a protocol under one type of blind and others follow the same protocol under a different type of blind. (c) The blind used may be changed during the course of the clinical trial according to certain criteria (e.g., when inpatients are discharged, the double blind may be broken, and they may continue their treatment on open-label medication).

Amery and Dony (1975) proposed a design in which patients who respond to treatment with open-label medicine for a fixed period are switched to a double-blind part of the clinical trial, and the active medicine is then compared against placebo. This approach evaluates the possibility that beneficial effects observed during the open part of the trial represented a placebo response.

15

TABLE 4.1 *Situations and uses for various types of clinical trial blinds*

A. Open-label trial
1. Pilot trials conducted prior to a more definitive trial, when endpoints measured are objective and less subject to investigator and patient bias
2. Case studies in life-threatening situations
3. Unusual situations in which definitive data may be obtained (e.g., patients in a coma)
4. Exposure of medicine to a broad patient population to gain information of efficacy and safety for situations in which the medicine will be used (e.g., premarketing surveillance)[a]
5. Postmarketing surveillance studies to obtain data on medicine safety and general tolerance
6. Clinical trials in which ethical considerations do not permit blinding

B. Single-blind trial
1. Provides a degree of control when a double-blind trial is impossible or impractical to conduct
2. Provides a degree of assurance of the data's validity as compared with open-label trials

C. Double-blind trial
1. Best-controlled clinical trial design in most situations. Allows strong interpretation of data if:
   a. All other aspects of the trial were properly designed and conducted
   b. The blind remained intact
   c. The protocol was not seriously breached
   d. The power of the trial was adequate
   e. The patients were compliant
   f. All appropriate, relevant, and useful factors and data were considered

D. Triple-blind trial
1. Allows strongest interpretation of data if conditions described under C are met

[a] Definitive efficacy data are rarely obtained from open-label clinical trials.

TYPES OF BLINDS: NEW DEFINITIONS

Full Double Blind

Full double blind refers to efforts to maintain the double blind by keeping everyone blind who interacts directly with the patient (group A in Fig. 4.1), including staff and health care personnel.

Full Triple Blind

Full triple blind refers to efforts to maintain the double blind by keeping everyone blind who interacts directly with the patient or investigator (group B in Fig. 4.1). This definition is valuable in that it prevents the arbitrary choice of a single group (e.g., monitor, statistician) to include with the patient and investigator as constituting a triple blind. This definition also has the advantage of defining the relationships among all important participants in a clinical trial.

A facetious use of the term *triple blind* relates to a situation in which errors have occurred in packaging a medicine so that neither the investigator, patient, nor monitor (or sponsor) knows what medicine is in each package, and thus the container holds an unknown medicine or dose. When data from these patients reach a statistician in a randomized order, a "quadruple-blind" trial results.

Extremely few clinical trials are fully triple blinded

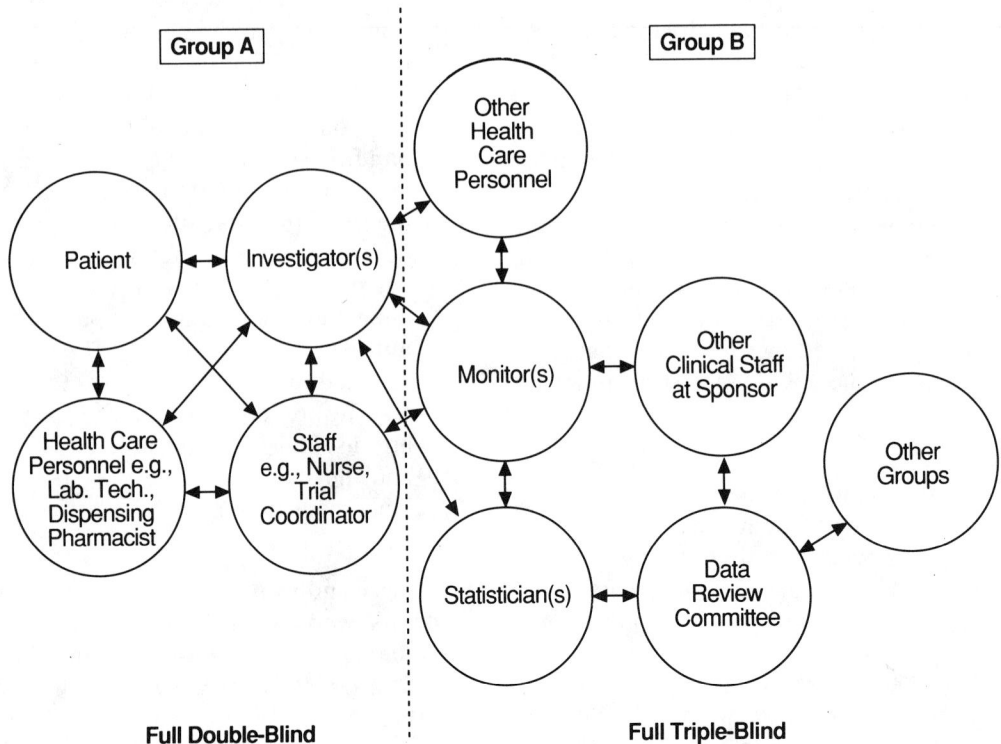

FIG. 4.1 Schematics of groups that remain blind to patient randomization during a full double-blind clinical trial (group A) or during a full triple-blind clinical trial (group B).

and it is not the author's contention that such blinding is either necessary or desirable in all cases. Nonetheless, it is certain that strong biases enter many trials because one or more of these groups were not blinded or were inadequately blinded. It is hoped that future clinical trials will pay greater attention to this issue and will more completely document the types of blinds used, as well as indicating how the effectiveness of the blind was ascertained.

Total Clinical Trial Blind

Total clinical trial blind refers to efforts to maintain the trial's blind by keeping everyone blind who interacts directly with the patient, the investigator, or the data. This definition has the advantages described under "Full Triple Blind," above, and includes pathologists who read slides, radiologists who interpret other tests, and statisticians who analyze the data, plus the group of blind participants. All groups and individuals associated with a clinical trial remain blind until the trial is completed and data are analyzed. The randomization code is prepared by someone unassociated with the clinical trial and statisticians analyze data for groups A and B without identifiers until after their analyses are completed, reviewed, and accepted, or possibly until after they have definitely chosen and confirmed that they will use specific statistical tests to analyze the data.

BLINDS IMPOSED ON INVESTIGATORS AND PATIENTS

The use of a blind in a clinical trial may adversely affect the physician—patient relationship, since in a double-blind trial neither one will know what treatment is being given, and one (usually the patient) will not know the treatment in a single-blind trial. This situation may create a strain on their relationship.

Two-Physician Method To Preserve Blind

Maintaining an effective double blind is extremely challenging or even impossible in some clinical trials. If certain data collected (e.g., blood levels of trial or concomitant medicines, specific adverse reactions) would effectively destroy the blind, then a system may be constructed to keep this information from the investigator in order to preserve the blind. One imaginative technique that has been used to maintain the double blind in some clinical trials may be referred to as the *two-physician method*. Physician 1 speaks with and examines patients at each visit. Physician 1 also evaluates the therapeutic response and possible medicine toxicity but does not receive any laboratory or other information that might unblind the trial. Physician 2, who is unblinded, receives the report from physician 1 as to possible medicine toxicity on each patient as well as all laboratory data. Physician 2 is then able to adjust the dose of medicine(s) the patient is receiving according to guidelines in the protocol.

Double-Placebo Method

In some clinical trials it may be necessary to use a separate placebo tablet (or other medicine form) for each trial or active medicine or for each size of two or more dose strengths of the trial medicine. In this *multiple-placebo* or *double-placebo* method, two (or more) separate containers are dispensed to each patient. Each bottle will contain either trial medicine or placebo and will provide the appropriate medication and dosage for patients when they take the required number of capsules or tablets from each bottle at each dosing time (i.e., group A receives medicine A and placebo B; group B receives placebo A and medicine B; and group C receives placebo A and placebo B). Two cases in which this technique is particularly useful are when two different routes of administration are being compared (e.g., a topical cream versus a tablet for treatment of a skin disorder) and when two different formulations are being compared (e.g., long- and short-acting medicines) that are taken at different intervals.

Approaches to Blinding a Clinical Trial in Difficult Situations

When a manufacturer will not supply the placebo of a marketed medicine plus the unmarked active medicine for a clinical trial, it is more difficult to create an effective blind. One approach is to use a generic version of the medicine, if one is available, and to make a placebo. Another approach is to use the two-physician method described above. Sponsors may also consider placing a marketed tablet in an opaque capsule, but this would change the dissolution characteristics. This approach would also require consideration of government regulations (e.g., is a new IND required?).

When a clinical trial involves a single dose of two or more medicines that cannot be easily blinded, it also creates a problem. Patients may be blindfolded and a study coordinator instructed to place the pills on the patients' tongues and to give them water to help swallow them.

BLINDS IMPOSED ON THE MONITORS

Monitors are individuals or groups who observe the conduct of a clinical trial to confirm that it is adhering to its protocol and to assist with problems that may arise in the conduct of the trial. These roles and other functions of the monitor are described in detail in Chapter 62.

The decision of whether to impose a blind on some or all monitors should be made prior to initiation of a study. If a monitor remains blind to patient treatment, it must also be determined whether or not the monitor will be privy to interim summarizations or analyses generated during the clinical trial. If monitors are made cognizant of such data, then a bias could be introduced into their relationship with investigators, even though the blind in a trial would literally remain intact. When an investigator notifies the sponsor of a patient's adverse reaction, the decision to unblind the patient's treatment to the investigator should not be made on the basis of the monitor's knowledge of the patient's true treatment. If the monitor has this information and somehow conveys it or an impression to physicians, then patients receiving placebo will tend to be kept in a clinical trial more than will patients who are receiving active treatment. Once a decision is made to remove a patient from a trial, then their treatment should be unblinded to assist in the treatment plan.

Some monitors may remain blind to individual patient treatment throughout a clinical trial but be privy to information on how well the overall trial is progressing in terms of efficacy through interim analyses. The wisdom of this partial unblinding must be questioned because of the possibility that the monitor may influence investigators either consciously or not.

BLINDS IMPOSED ON ANCILLARY PERSONNEL

In some double-blind trials, pharmacists or other personnel who package medicines must be unblinded. It is preferable that all individuals who normally interact with the investigator, patients, and others conducting the trial remain blind. Some results (e.g., ECGs, X-rays) may be interpreted by a person blind to the identity of the patients' treatment even in an open-label trial.

Professionals who interpret data within a clinical trial (e.g., pathologists who review tissue slides, radiologists who interpret X-rays) should generally remain blind to the treatment and/or diagnosis of the patient. Pharmacists who dispense medicines may remain blind by having the prescription filled by another pharmacist. Statisticians who analyze data may deal with treatments labeled as A, B, and so on, rather than with the name of the medicine or the term *placebo*. They could remain blind until they have chosen all of the statistical methods that will be used to analyze the data. Finally, clinicians who interpret data should in some instances be unaware of which result was from

the medicine group and which was from the placebo group.

IMPORTANCE OF FULLY DOUBLE-BLIND TRIALS: THREE EXAMPLES

The importance of utilizing double-blind trials whenever possible and practical is illustrated by two actual examples. In the first, an antidepressant was evaluated for anti-Parkinson's disease activity in two trials with identical study designs except that one was open-label and the other was double-blind (versus placebo). In the open-label trial, 8 of 12 (67%) patients significantly improved (by at least 30% in efficacy scores) on active medicine treatment, but in the double-blind phase (conducted at the same time in different patients), only 2 of 8 patients (25%) improved (C. G. Goetz, C. M. Tanner, and H. L. Klawans, personal communication). All patients received single-blind placebo for the first week of treatment in order to both identify and exclude early placebo responders from both the open-label and double-blind trials. These results are reminiscent of a report in the psychiatric literature stating that 83% of uncontrolled trials reported positive results, but only 25% of controlled trials were positive (Foulds, 1958). See Chapter 8 for additional examples.

The second example is that of a single-blind trial and a double-blind trial conducted by the same group of scientists, who evaluated the effect of zinc on hypogeusia (decreased taste acuity). In the single-blind trial, patients who failed to respond to placebo significantly improved their hypogeusia with zinc therapy (Shechter et al., 1972). This led the same authors to perform a randomized, double-blind, crossover trial in which no difference between zinc sulfate and placebo was observed (Henkin et al., 1976). Karlowski et al. (1975) reported that many patients broke the trial's blind by tasting the contents of the capsules. The authors described the significant impact that this event had on the data obtained.

CHECKING THE VALIDITY OF A DOUBLE-BLIND TRIAL

If a blind is to be incorporated into a clinical trial design, then it is important to check the validity of the blind prior to, during, and after the trial is completed.

Prior to the beginning of the clinical trial, the blind is "validated" by considering how it will be implemented and maintained plus a review of ways in which it may be challenged or broken during the trial. "What if" exercises may be useful in determining whether a sound system of blinding the trial has been created.

During the clinical trial, the monitor or other appropriate individual(s) may evaluate how well the blind is being maintained. Discontinued patients may be closely questioned on this point. If it is apparent that the blind in a trial is not effective, then measures may be taken to modify the protocol to strengthen the blind. Alternatively, nothing may be done, or the trial may be changed to an open-label one. Other possibilities certainly exist for dealing with the situation in which the integrity of the blind has been compromised.

After the clinical trial has been completed, all patients and the investigator may be asked to guess which treatment each patient received. This technique is described in the section on "End of Clinical Trial Questionnaire" in Chapter 65.

WHEN MAY OPEN-LABEL CLINICAL TRIALS BE CONDUCTED?

A basic tenet of this book is that controlled clinical trials should virtually never be conducted in an open-label manner. There are, however, a number of occasions when an open-label clinical trial design may be used. These are usually in uncontrolled clinical trials and include:

1. *Compassionate Plea Protocols.* These clinical trials are open-label by definition (see Chapter 41). The advantage of this design is the ability to provide patients a potentially valuable medicine earlier in its development.
2. *Treatment-IND Clinical Trials.* The same comments apply as those mentioned above.
3. *Uncontrolled Noncomparative Clinical Trials.* This category includes the above two types of clinical trials, plus other loosely controlled or uncontrolled trials. There is no pretext of control in these trials.
4. Phase I dose ranging trials in patients as opposed to volunteers (e.g., in severely or terminally ill cancer patients).
5. Phase I pharmacokinetic trials, particularly if no control group is used (that practice itself is generally unwise).
6. Phase II or III long-term continuation trials, particularly those initiated after a shorter term double-blind efficacy trial.
7. Clinical trials in which it would not be ethical to use a double-blind design.

Clinical trials that are open-label should use well-defined doses, dose-intervals, dose-adjustment criteria, and efficacy parameters, and should collect data using good clinical practices. Their design may be improved by having efficacy evaluated by an independent person who is either blinded to treatment assignment or to the hypothesis being tested.

Single-Blind Clinical Trials

The concept of a single-blind clinical trial has great appeal for selected situations. It usually keeps patients blind to their treatment, but data from many clinical trials demonstrate that results from single-blind trials are generally equivalent to open-label trials. Biases from investigators (or patients) who know the identity of their treatment clearly affect results (see Chapter 8, "Controls Used in Clinical Trials").

LeWitt et al. (1986) gave two dystonic patients tetrahydrobiopterin single-blind and a third patient received saline. Only the patients were kept blind to the treatment. Patients were examined by a physician who was unblinded and the physical examination was videotaped. This tape was rated by three blind clinicians. The relevant question is, were blind clinicians viewing an objectively conducted physical examination of three dystonic patients or was bias introduced? It is certain, in the author's view, that the physician conducting the examination could easily introduce bias, no matter how objective he was trying to be. This could occur by dwelling slightly on one or more "positive" findings in those patients who received the active medicine, or by being slightly more superficial in the patient who received saline. There is no reason why this type of clinical trial cannot be conducted double-blind.

The people who administer a medicine sometimes cannot be blinded to its identity (e.g., giving neonates a filmy white medicine versus giving a bolus of air intratracheally). It is possible to have a dose-administration team on call 24 hours a day to administer the medicine but not interact with investigators, patients, or staff.

Breaking the Blind

Many, if not most, patients and investigators enjoy playing a game during double-blind clinical trials called breaking the blind. In this game people look for clues to help them identify their treatment or the one each patient is receiving. Their prize is primarily an inner satisfaction. Although this seems innocent enough, it really is not. Biases that enter the clinical trial often affect its outcome. The antidote to this game of breaking the blind (by either patients or investigators) is to design a clinical trial whose blind is extremely hard to break. This is an important challenge for anyone who designs clinical trials.

How Blinds Are Broken

Many publications glibly state that their trial was conducted in a double-blind manner and do not provide information on (1) how well the blind was maintained, (2) whether it was verified, and (3) whether other individuals associated with the trial were kept blind. Insofar as a double-blind trial is defined as one in which neither the patient nor the investigator knows with absolute certainty what treatment the patient was randomized to receive, most trials remain truly double-blind. Nonetheless, many investigators and patients have a good to excellent idea of the specific treatment received by that patient.

A patient (or investigator) may unblind a clinical trial deliberately or inadvertently. Unblinding may occur based on clues provided by (1) adverse reactions, (2) efficacy, (3) lack of efficacy, or (4) laboratory analyte changes (e.g., specific changes observed in analytes or in plasma levels of concomitant medicines). If patients' urine turns blue with a medicine, it may be impossible to blind patients to treatment. Of course, a high- and low-dose group could be used to blind their knowledge of which group they are in. Other sources of unblinding include labeling errors, comments from unblinded monitors or investigators, or information presented in correspondence or reports. Some medicines cause specific adverse reactions that are difficult or impossible to mask (e.g., gingival hyperplasia), especially if the patient has been given information about them in the informed consent.

Consideration of the above factors and others discussed in this chapter should promote more tightly designed clinical trials that minimize the ability of patients or physicians to unblind them.

What Are the Clinical Consequences if the Double Blind in a Clinical Trial Is Broken?

There is no doubt that in many double-blind clinical trials the blind is partially or even totally broken (Karlowski et al., 1975; Lewis et al., 1975; Marini et al., 1976; Brownell and Stunkard, 1982). It is more important to ask whether this affects the data obtained. The consequences, if any, are usually noted because of biases introduced. These papers clearly show that there are important clinical consequences when patients break a trial's blind. It is not as easy to evaluate objectively the consequences for a trial when an investigator breaks the blind. Even when a totally blind trial can be designed, partial blinding may achieve many of the benefits of blinding (Deyo et al., 1990).

CHAPTER 5

Bias and Confounding Factors

BIAS VERSUS OBJECTIVITY IN INTERPRETATION OF DATA

It is common for authors or speakers to claim that their data have been interpreted with "objectivity." Most individuals believe that this is true about their own interpretations. In order to eliminate as much bias as possible from one's interpretation, it is essential to be able to recognize bias and to be able to decrease or at least to recognize the influence it has in the interpretation.

Necessary steps to achieve this goal are to (1) understand the types of biases that may influence the interpretation of data, (2) develop the ability to recognize these biases in one's own work as well as in reports or publications of others, and (3) be able to modify or qualify interpretations to account for and minimize biases.

Biases may occur at any stage of a clinical trial, but there are several that are particularly likely to occur at the point at which data are interpreted. Biases have been catalogued and classified in numerous ways. There is no a priori reason to use any one system except as it makes sense in a particular situation. In fact, it is not necessary to use any system. Biases occur as a consequence of the trial design used, the tests used, the people involved in the study, the patients, the analyses used, and/or the perspectives used in interpreting the data. Owen (1982) has proposed a list of 25 biases that may be introduced by readers when perusing the clinical literature.

OPERATIONAL DEFINITION OF BIAS

Bias indicates systematic error that enters a clinical trial and distorts the data obtained, as opposed to random error that enters a clinical trial. A bias may be a prejudice or leaning of one's opinion favoring one side of a question or issue too strongly before there are adequate data to support that conclusion or viewpoint. Biases may relate to errors introduced directly or indirectly into one or more aspects of a clinical trial. Biases may enter a trial either because of a factor or belief that is introduced or because a factor or belief is omitted and not introduced. When a bias enters a trial because it is introduced (or omitted), this event may occur either purposely on the part of an individual or group or as a result of ignorance on the individual or group's part. Anyone associated with a clinical trial who may exert influence on the results (e.g., sponsor, monitor, investigator, patient) may introduce biases. In statistical terms, bias has different meanings as it relates to a clinical trial. One definition is the tendency of a sample to be nonrepresentative of all patients or data in the trial.

CONSIDERATION OF TRIAL BIAS

The goal of a clinical trial is to minimize and attempt to eliminate most, if not all biases. There are some clinical trial designs (e.g., case control, retrospective) in which bias is inherent. Bias in decision making arises when using expert opinion, personal clinical experience, and published research. The question is to what degree it affects the interpretation of the results. If biases are undetected and not discussed insofar as they affect the interpretation, then the interpretation presented will probably be more susceptible to challenge.

One of the main purposes in choosing and developing a clinical strategy to develop a new medicine is to attempt to reduce known biases that may compromise the analysis and interpretation of the clinical data. When biases cannot be eliminated, it is important to define them so that they may be considered when conclusions are drawn from a trial. Relationships between bias and chance are illustrated in Fig. 5.1.

SOURCES OF BIASES IN A CLINICAL TRIAL

In the early planning stages of a clinical trial, one should be aware of biases that may either influence or become part of a trial. Biases may be introduced into a clinical trial at any stage in the planning, conduct, or analysis. Seven general stages or categories of bias were described by Sackett (1979). He indicated that the biases may occur in:

1. Examining the literature in the field
2. Specifying and selecting the clinical trial sample
3. Executing the experimental maneuver (or exposure)
4. Measuring exposures and outcome
5. Analyzing the data
6. Interpreting the analysis
7. Publishing the results

Sackett described 57 examples of biases in a "catalog" and gave a reference for many. This catalog (plus references) is presented in Table 5.1 later in this chapter.

Many biases may not be extirpated from a clinical trial if they are introduced as part of the trial design, and these often represent the primary reason why otherwise well-conducted and analyzed trials are not accorded credence by the medical community.

Potential biases range from the more obvious to the arcane. Among obvious sources of bias, three can briefly be mentioned as illustrative examples:

1. Extrapolation of data from one group of individuals to the entire population often leads to substantial errors. This may occur in clinical trials if the initial choice of the population sampled is not a true cross section of the desired (reference) population.

2. Patients with a known disease may be questioned many times about factors possibly relating to etiologies, but a control group may be questioned less intensely and less frequently. This may lead to a "recall bias," especially if the questions are difficult to answer or are sensitive. To avoid this bias an open-ended question may be used for all patients rather than a checklist followed by exploration of positive responses.

3. Patients with a worse prognosis may be overwhelmingly assigned to receive one treatment rather than another. This will make it much more difficult for that treatment group to demonstrate the response that would have been noted if the two treatment groups were equal.

These and additional biases are described in detail by Feinstein (1967) and Imperiale and Horwitz (1989).

Reducing Biases

In trying to reduce bias, the author of a protocol should be familiar with the most common sources of bias and

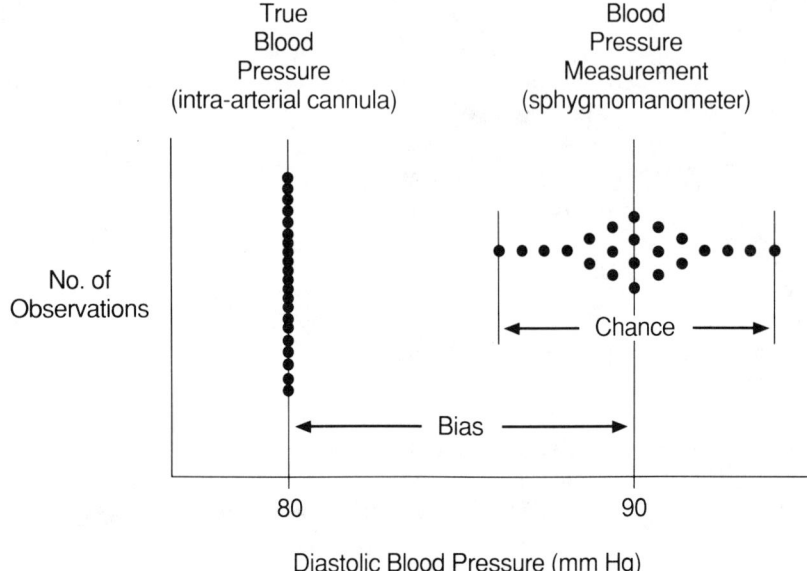

FIG. 5.1 Relationship between bias and chance: blood pressure measurements by intraarterial cannula and sphygmomanometer. (Reprinted from Fletcher et al., 1988, with permission of Williams and Wilkins.)

have a statistician evaluate the protocol, since many biases have a statistical basis. Randomized controlled trials have the greatest probability of reducing bias, and observational, cohort, case-controlled, or uncontrolled trials have the greatest propensity to include bias.

PROSPECTIVE VERSUS RETROSPECTIVE APPROACHES

It is widely accepted that well-designed prospective trials yield less biased, more scientifically acceptable data than do comparable retrospective trials. The retrospective (e.g., case-control survey) study is quite useful, however, under certain conditions. It is useful when the objective is to generate rather than to test hypotheses, and it is generally less expensive than a prospective trial. The retrospective survey is subject to a great deal of bias, and thus results are often seriously questioned. For example, the criteria for patient inclusion and adequacy of documentation must be clearly established before a survey of patient records is initiated. The more precisely the patient entry criteria are defined, the better is the chance that a meaningful analysis and interpretation of the data will be obtained. A clinical survey may be either retrospective or prospective; in this book, however, a clinical trial is defined as being prospective.

TYPES OF BIAS

List of Sackett

An excellent list was assembled by Sackett (1979) and is reproduced in Table 5.1. Below is an elaboration of a number of specific biases. A discussion of publication bias is presented in Chapter 106.

Other Biases

Selection Bias

Physicians may recruit patients for clinical trials in ways that bias the data. Patients available for inclusion may differ markedly from others with the disease and affect the extrapolatability of the data.

Information Bias

The information patients provide to physicians (or others) is heavily biased by their own beliefs and values. This may be random and not influence a clinical trial, but if a major event is common to the group (e.g., a contaminated landfill is discovered nearby) it may influence their perceptions of preexisting symptoms that occurred (even prior to their moving to the area).

Observer Bias

The objectivity of physicians or others who measure the magnitude of patient responses varies greatly, even for tests with objective endpoints. A systematic increase observed by physician A may yield results different from those obtained by physician B. Alternatively, a single physician may measure tests differently for different types of patients. Both inter- and intraobserver variability should be assessed in clinical trials.

Interviewer Bias

Interviewer bias is one of the most well-known and obvious sources of bias in clinical trials in which interviews are conducted, particularly when interviews are used in measuring endpoints that determine the clinical trial's outcome. The expectations of the interviewer often influence how information is recorded.

Interviewer dress, manner of asking questions, accent, and many other characteristics often influence respondent's answers to questions. These factors should be standardized, insofar as possible.

Use of Nonvalidated Instruments

The use of nonvalidated instruments is extremely widespread in clinical trials. The results of surveys and questionnaires are published routinely in medical and other journals without any evidence of their validity presented. This raises potential problems because many physicians, health professionals, psychologists, sociologists, and others apparently may not fully understand the ease of introducing marked biases into a survey or interview.

Active Control Bias

Smith (1989) presents a different type of example than that given in ''4g'' in Sackett's table. He reports a much higher cure rate for a new antifungal medicine when compared with an active medicine than when compared with placebo. This is part of the reasoning behind questioning clinical trial designs using active medicine controls without a placebo treatment group.

AVOIDING BIAS AND CONFOUNDING

The best way to avoid bias and confounding is to be aware of them in advance of designing and conducting a clinical trial. Bias may be minimized by considering

TABLE 5.1 *Sources of bias*

1. ***In reading up on the field***
   a. *The biases of rhetoric.* Any of several techniques used to convince the reader without appealing to reason, e.g., Good (1962).
   b. *The all's well literature bias.* Scientific or professional societies may publish reports or editorials that omit or play down controversies or disparate results, e.g., the debate on "control" and the complications of diabetes, well shown in editorials in the *New England Journal of Medicine* (Cahill et al., 1976; Ingelfinger, 1977).
   c. *One-sided reference bias.* Authors may restrict their references to only those works that support their position; a literature review with a single starting point risks confinement to a single side of the issue, e.g., Hamilton *et al.* (1963), Platt (1963).
   d. *Positive results bias.* Authors are more likely to submit, and editors accept, positive than null results, e.g., multiple personal experiences.
   e. *Hot stuff bias.* When a topic is hot, neither investigators nor editors may be able to resist the temptation to publish additional results, no matter how preliminary or shaky, e.g., recent publications concerning medication compliance.

2. ***In specifying and selecting the study sample***
   a. *Popularity bias.* The admission of patients to some practices, institutions or procedures (sugery, autopsy) is influenced by the interest stirred up by the presenting condition and its possible causes, e.g., White (1953).
   b. *Centripetal bias.* The reputations of certain clinicians and institutions cause individuals with specific disorders or exposures to gravitate toward them, e.g., the striking rate of posterior fossa cerebral aneurysms reported from the University of Western Ontario.
   c. *Referral filter bias.* As a group of ill persons is referred from primary to secondary to tertiary care, the concentration of rare causes, multiple diagnoses, and "hopeless cases" may increase, e.g., secondary hypertension at the Cleveland Clinic (Gifford, 1969).
   d. *Diagnostic access bias.* Individuals differ in their geographic, temporal and economic access to the diagnostic procedures that label them as having a given disease, e.g., Anderson and Andersen (1972).
   e. *Diagnostic suspicion bias.* A knowledge of the subject's prior exposure to a putative cause (ethnicity, taking a certain drug, having a second disorder, being exposed in an epidemic) may influence both the intensity and the outcome of the diagnostic process; e.g., the possibility that rubber workers were victims of this bias was studied by Fox and White (1976).
   f. *Unmasking (detection signal) bias.* An innocent exposure may become suspect if, rather than causing a disease, it causes a sign or symptom that precipitates a search for the disease, e.g., the current controversy over postmenopausal estrogens and cancer of the endometrium.
   g. *Mimicry bias.* An innocent exposure may become suspect if, rather than causing a disease, it causes a (benign) disorder that resembles the disease, e.g., Morrison *et al.* (1977).
   h. *Previous opinion bias.* The tactics and results of a previous diagnostic process on a patient, if known, may affect the tactics and results of a subsequent diagnostic process on the same patient, e.g., multiple personal experiences with referred hypertensive patients.
   i. *Wrong sample size bias.* Samples that are too small can prove nothing; samples that are too large can prove anything.
   j. *Admission rate (Berkson) bias.* If hospitalization rates differ for different exposure disease groups, the relation between exposure and disease will become distorted in hospital-based studies (Berkson, 1946; Roberts *et al.*, 1978).
   k. *Prevalence–incidence (Neyman) bias.* A late look at those exposed (or affected) early will miss fatal and other short episodes plus mild or "silent" cases and cases in which evidence of exposure disappears with disease onset (Neyman, 1955).
   l. *Diagnostic vogue bias.* The same illness may receive different diagnostic labels at different points in space or time, e.g., British "bronchitis" versus North American "emphysema" (Fletcher *et al*, 1964).
   m. *Diagnostic purity bias.* When "pure" diagnostic groups exclude comorbidity, they may become nonrepresentative.
   n. *Procedure selection bias.* Certain clinical procedures may be preferentially offered to those who are poor risks, e.g., selection of patients for "medical" versus "surgical" therapy (Feinstein, 1977, p. 76).
   o. *Missing clinical data bias.* Missing clinical data may be missing because they are normal, negative, never measured, or measured but never recorded.
   p. *Noncontemporaneous control bias.* Secular changes in definitions, exposures, diagnoses, diseases, and treatments may render noncontemporaneous controls noncomparable, e.g., Feinstein (1977, pp. 94–104).
   q. *Starting time bias.* The failure to identify a common starting time for exposure or illness may lead to systematic misclassification, e.g., Feinstein (1977, pp. 89–104).
   r. *Unacceptable disease bias.* When disorders are socially unacceptable (V.D., suicide, insanity), they tend to be underreported.
   s. *Migrator bias.* Migrants may differ systematically from those who stay home, e.g., Kruger and Moriyama (1967).
   t. *Membership bias.* Membership in a group (the employed, joggers, etc.) may imply a degree of health that differs systematically from that of the general population, e.g., exercise and recurrent myocardial infarction (Rechnitzer *et al*, 1972).
   u. *Nonrespondent bias.* Nonrespondents (or "late comers") from a specified sample may exhibit exposures or outcomes that differ from those of respondents (or "early comers"), e.g., cigarette smokers (Seltzer *et al.*, 1974).
   v. *Volunteer bias.* Volunteers or "early comers" from a specified sample may exhibit exposures or outcomes (they tend to be healthier) that differ from those of nonvolunteers or "late comers," e.g., volunteers for screening (Shapiro *et al.*, 1971).

3. ***In executing the experimental maneuver (or exposure)***
   a. *Contamination bias.* In an experiment, when members of the control group inadvertently receive the experimental maneuver, the difference in outcomes between experimental and control patients may be systematically reduced, e.g., recent drug trials involving aspirin.
   b. *Withdrawal bias.* Patients who are withdrawn from an experiment may differ systematically from those who remain, e.g., in a neurosurgical trial of surgical versus medical therapy of cerebrovascular disease, patients who died or "stroked-out" during surgery were withdrawn as "unavailable for follow-up" and excluded from early analyses.
   c. *Compliance bias.* In experiments requiring patient adherence to therapy, issues of efficacy become confounded with those of compliance; e.g., it is the high-risk coronary patients who quit exercise programs (Oldridge *et al.*, 1978).
   d. *Therapeutic personality bias.* When treatment is not "blind," the therapist's convictions about efficacy may systematically influence both outcomes (positive personality) and their measurement (desire for positive results).
   e. *Bogus control bias.* When patients who are allocated to an experimental maneuver die or sicken before or during its administration and are omitted or reallocated to the control group, the experimental maneuver will appear spuriously superior.

(*continued*)

TABLE 5.1 (*Continued*)

4. In measuring exposures and outcomes

a. *Insensitive measure bias.* When outcome measures are incapable of detecting clinically significant changes or differences, type II errors occur.

b. *Underlying cause bias (rumination bias).* Patients may ruminate about possible causes for their illnesses and thus exhibit recall of prior exposures different from controls, e.g., Sartwell (1974) (see also the *Recall bias: 4k*).

c. *End-digit preference bias.* In converting analog to digital data, observers may record some terminal digits with an unusual frequency, e.g., a notorious problem in the measurement of blood pressure (Rose *et al.*, 1964).

d. *Apprehension bias.* Certain measures (pulse, blood pressure) may alter systematically from their usual levels when the subject is apprehensive, e.g., blood pressure during medical interviews (McKegney and Williams, 1967).

e. *Unacceptability bias.* Measurements that hurt, embarrass, or invade privacy may be systematically refused or evaded.

f. *Obsequiousness bias.* Subjects may systematically alter questionnaire responses in the direction they perceive desired by the investigator.

g. *Expectation bias.* Observers may systematically err in measuring and recording observations so that they concur with prior expectations, e.g., house officers tend to report "normal" fetal heart rates (Day *et al.*, 1968).

h. *Substitution game.* The substitution of a risk factor that has not been established as causal for its associated outcome (Yerushalmy, 1966).

i. *Family information bias.* The flow of family information about exposure and illness is stimulated by, and directed to, a new case in its midst, e.g., different family histories of arthritis from affected and unaffected sibs (Schull and Cobb, 1969).

j. *Exposure suspicion bias.* A knowledge of the subject's disease status may influence both the intensity and outcome of a search for exposure to the putative cause, e.g., Sartwell (1974).

k. *Recall bias.* Questions about specific exposures may be asked several times of cases but only once of controls (see also the *Underlying cause bias: 4b*).

l. *Attention bias.* Study subjects may systematically alter their behavior when they know they are being observed, e.g., Hawthorne revisited.

m. *Instrument bias.* Defects in the calibration or maintenance of measurement instruments may lead to systematic deviations from true values.

5. In analyzing the data

a. *Post hoc significance bias.* When decision levels or "tails" for α and β are selected *after* the data have been examined, conclusions may be biased.

b. *Data dredging bias (looking for the pony).* When data are reviewed for all possible associations without prior hypothesis, the results are suitable for hypothesis-forming activities only.

c. *Scale degradation bias.* The degradation and collapsing of measurement scales tend to obscure differences between groups under comparison.

d. *Tidying-up bias.* The exclusion of outliers or other untidy results cannot be justified on statistical grounds and may lead to bias, e.g., Murphy (1976, p. 250).

e. *Repeated peeks bias.* Repeated peeks at accumulating data in a randomized trial are not dependent and may lead to inappropriate termination.

6. In interpreting the analysis

a. *Mistaken identity bias.* In compliance trials, strategies directed toward improving the patient's compliance may, instead or in addition, cause the treating clinician to prescribe more vigorously; the effect on achievement of the treatment goal may be misinterpreted, e.g., Sackett (1976).

b. *Cognitive dissonance bias.* The belief in a given mechanism may increase rather than decrease in the face of contradictory evidence, e.g., Sackett (1980).

c. *Magnitude bias.* In interpreting a finding, the selection of a scale of measurement may markedly affect the interpretation, e.g., $1,000,000 may also be 0.0003% of the national budget (Murphy, 1976, p. 249).

d. *Significance bias.* The confusion of statistical significance, on the one hand, with biologic or clinical or health care significance, on the other hand, can lead to fruitless studies and useless conclusions, e.g., Feinstein (1977, p. 258).

e. *Correlation bias.* Equating correlation with causation leads to errors of both kinds, e.g., Hill (1971, pp. 309–320).

f. *Underexhaustion bias.* The failure to exhaust the hypothesis space may lead to authoritarian rather than authoritarive interpretation, e.g., Murphy (1976, p. 258).

Modified from Sackett (1979) with permission.

and weighing all therapeutic alternatives and using objective criteria established in advance. Having sufficient time to extirpate most biases is important, because a clinical trial assembled hurriedly virtually always includes some flaws resulting from biases.

Confounding Variables

These variables affect the patients' disease or condition and are associated statistically with the medicine or treatment being evaluated. In studying whether cigarette smoking causes lung cancer in a case-control study, drinking alcohol would be a confounding factor. It would be associated with lung cancer because people who smoke cigarettes are more likely to drink than nonsmokers.

Confounding may be examined by subgroup analyses after a clinical trial is completed and may be minimized by stratification or matching techniques in advance (e.g., severe disease patients are randomized separately from mild disease patients).

Confounding may occur in many aspects of a clinical trial including the trial's outcome, patient's disease status, and interactions among medicines. For example, there is often an uneven loss of patients in different treatment groups within a clinical trial. To identify the confounding factors compare those patients lost to follow-up with those not lost to follow-up and determine the direction of bias. If patients with severe disease do not improve and drop out of a trial and those with mild disease improve and remain, then the results are biased toward falsely high efficacy of the treatment. On the other hand, patients with mild disease may get better and then see no reason to remain in the clinical trial and drop out, whereas those with more severe disease remain, hoping for improvement. The results in this case are biased toward falsely low efficacy of the treatment, and both sets of results are confounded by disease severity.

CHAPTER 6

Classification and Description of Phases I, II, and III Clinical Trial Designs

INTRODUCTION

The present classification of clinical trial designs listed in Table 6.1 is only one of several that could be created. This chapter describes clinical trial designs for Phases I, II, and III. Chapter 7 describes designs for Phase IV, although there are circumstances in which one of these designs is used in Phase IV and Phase IV designs are used in Phases I to III. (For definitions of phases I, II, III, and IV, see the terminology section at the beginning of the book.)

PROSPECTIVE VERSUS RETROSPECTIVE CLINICAL TRIALS

There are three possible types of clinical trials, in terms of the period of time evaluated: prospective, retro-

TABLE 6.1 *Classification of Phases I to III clinical trials described in this chapter*

A. Prospective versus retrospective
B. Single group of patients
C. Two groups of patients
    1. Parallel cross-sectional
    2. Parallel longitudinal
    3. Crossover
    4. Matched pair
    5. Historical controls
    6. Sequential
D. Multiple groups of patients
E. Clinical trial designs for evaluating prophylactic activity
F. Design variations
    1. Withdrawal of treatment trials
    2. Single-patient clinical trials
    3. Chart review trials
    4. Factorial designs
    5. Novel clinical trial designs based on variation in informed consent or randomization
        a. Prerandomization method
        b. Double-consent prerandomization method
        c. Deferred consent process
        d. Two-tiered consent process
G. Run-in period designs
    1. Placebo run-in
    2. Compliance run-in
    3. No-treatment run-in
    4. Combination type of run-in
    5. Dose ascension[a]
H. Other trial designs that attempt to avoid ethical problems
    1. Fail-safe designs
    2. Dose-response designs
    3. Alternative designs
I. Designs in specific therapeutic areas or modalities[a]
    1. Oncology
    2. Surgery
    3. Antibiotics
    4. Medical devices
    5. Pharmacokinetics
    6. Compassionate plea

[a] These topics are discussed in other chapters.

spective, or a combination of both approaches within the same clinical trial (Fig. 6.1). Numerous references show how retrospective trials often lead to false conclusions. This occurs because effects may be blamed on the wrong causes, the correct probabilities may be poorly understood, and many biases plus confounding factors may enter the clinical trial, which can be neither purged nor fully understood. Unless there are strong reasons to the contrary, clinical trials should use a prospective design whenever possible.

SINGLE GROUP OF PATIENTS

In some open-label or single-blind clinical trials, all patients are treated with the same medicine throughout the study. Criteria may be established to change patients from one medicine to another or to allow for dosage reductions (e.g., for adverse reactions) or dosage increases (e.g., for lack of toxicity or lack of optimal improvement). Thus, a single homogeneous group of patients at the start of a clinical trial may

complete the trial as a heterogeneous group of patients because each was treated with a different dosing regimen.

Study designs utilizing historical controls could be considered as either a single group of patients or two groups of patients. In this book, studies using historical controls are discussed as designs with two groups of patients.

TWO GROUPS OF PATIENTS

Cross-Sectional versus Longitudinal Trials

Definitions

Cross-sectional trials are usually short-term trials in which a cross section of the patient population of interest is evaluated for a period of up to 10 weeks. Longer cross-sectional trials are possible, but are less common. Patients are usually placed into one of two or more treatment groups and data obtained from each group are compared (Fig. 6.2).

Longitudinal trials are usually long-term clinical trials conducted for several months or longer. Placebos and active medicine controls are seldom used although a "usual care" or "no treatment" group may be included as a control group. Patients' data are generally compared with their own baseline to identify changes. If a control group is included in the clinical trial, then a between-group comparison is conducted as well. Although most longitudinal trials are long-term, a longitudinal trial may also last over a short period. A single bronchodilator used by patients four times over the course of a day to look at serial forced expiratory volume in 1 second (FEV_1) values is an example of a longitudinal trial.

Use of Cross-Sectional and Longitudinal Trials

Most efficacy and safety assessments of investigational medicines are conducted in short-term cross-sectional trials, but a few long-term longitudinal trials are often conducted as well, primarily during late Phase II and during Phase III. Many epidemiological population studies conducted during Phase IV are longitudinal studies. These include the famous Framingham study and many large cohort studies of patients followed for more than a year.

Ideally, more clinical trials should be longitudinal, but this approach is often impractical and most trials are cross-sectional instead. One of the dangers of conducting cross-sectional trials is illustrated thus: If a cross-sectional trial was conducted in Miami, Florida, to study what languages are spoken, the data would

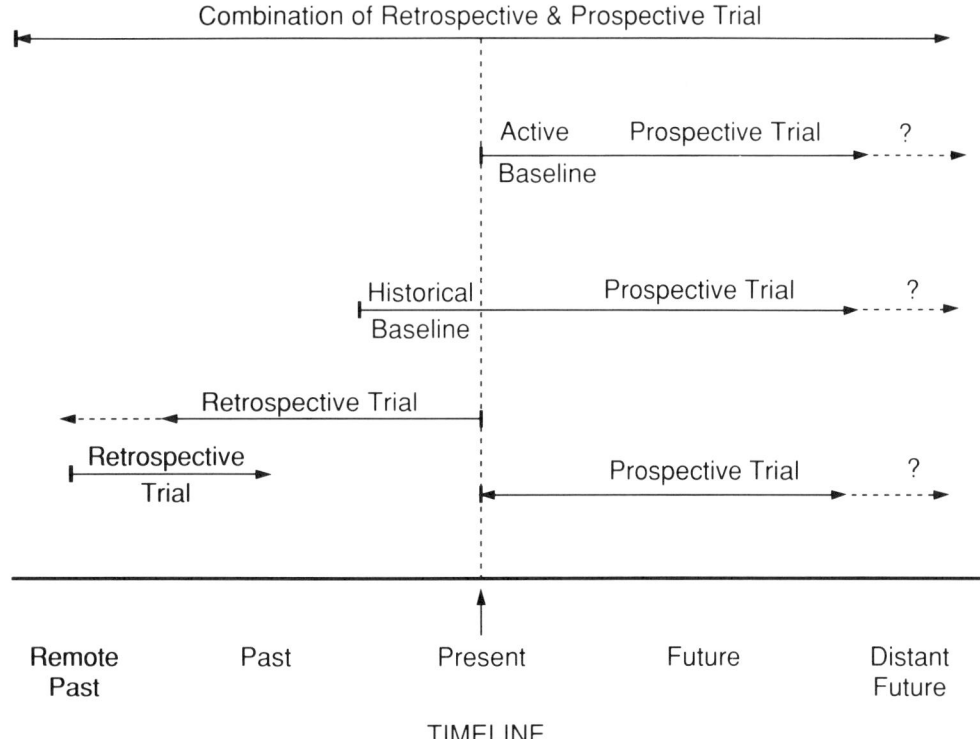

Combination of Retrospective & Prospective Trial

Active
Prospective Trial
?
Baseline

Historical
Prospective Trial
?
Baseline

Retrospective Trial

Retrospective
Trial
Prospective Trial
?

| Remote Past | Past | Present | Future | Distant Future |

TIMELINE

FIG. 6.1 Clinical trial time line illustrating various types of retrospective and prospective trials.

suggest that most people speak Spanish during childhood and Yiddish during old age.

Parallel Designs

The two most common designs utilizing two groups of patients are the parallel (noncrossover) and crossover designs. The parallel design is applicable to most experimental situations. It is "robust" (i.e., tolerant) to many kinds of problems that can occur in clinical trials (e.g., missed visits, missing data). In the parallel design, patients are randomized to one of two treatment groups and usually receive the assigned treatment during the entire trial. The treatments assigned to the two groups differ. Each group generally receives either trial medicine or placebo, one of two different trial medicines, or one of two doses of the same trial medicines. Two placebo medications could also be evaluated. One variation of the parallel design is for each group to receive alternating (and escalating) doses of the same drug. Some of the possible variations of a parallel design are shown in Fig. 6.3.

Crossover Designs

In the crossover design, each patient receives both treatments being compared in the clinical trial. If one of the treatments is placebo, then the effect of the trial medicine may be expressed as the difference between

responses to the two treatments. The variability of data obtained with this design is less than that associated with those obtained with the parallel design (i.e., within-patient differences are used to assess treatment differences in a crossover trial, whereas between-patient differences are used to assess treatment differences in a parallel design). Because of its increased sensitivity and smaller variability, the crossover design requires fewer patients than does the parallel design to detect the same effect. For the same sample size, the parallel design is less sensitive in detecting differences between two treatment groups than is the crossover design. The analysis of data obtained with a crossover design is adversely affected by patient dropouts and missing data (i.e., the analysis is not as "robust" as with a parallel design).

Requirements for Using Crossover Designs

In order to use a crossover design, the patient must have a stable (usually chronic) disease during both treatment periods, and a similar baseline condition must be present at the start of each of the two treatment periods. It is obvious that if the patient's baseline differs markedly at the start of each treatment, then it is impossible to compare the two treatment effects accurately. Not only must the baselines be similar, there must not be any carryover (i.e., residual) effects (even psychological ones) after either treatment. This means

Cross-Sectional Trial

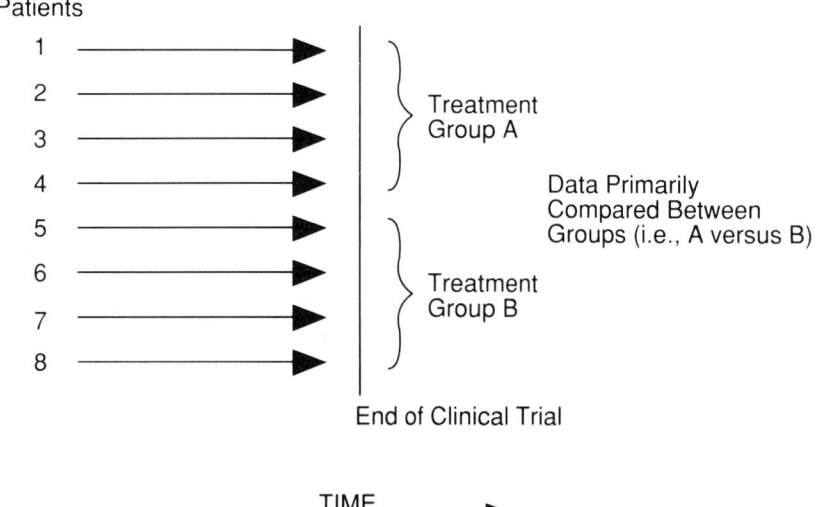

Longitudinal Trial

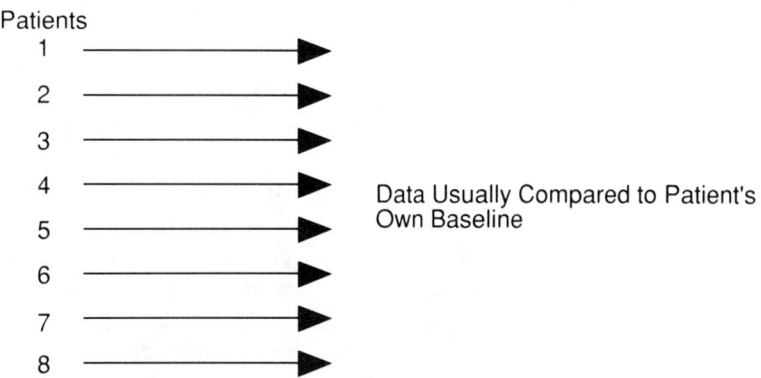

FIG. 6.2 Schematic illustrating characteristics of cross-sectional clinical trials (*above*) and longitudinal trials (*below*). Whereas cross-sectional trials are measured in terms of days or weeks (usually not more than 10 weeks), longitudinal trials are usually measured in terms of months or years.

that the disease manifestations should revert to the same baseline and that the effect of the treatment should disappear when either treatment is stopped. See Table 6.2.

Carryover Effect

One of the major reasons that this design is not used more frequently is that a carryover effect is noted after many medicines are stopped. The test for carryover effects may not be adequately sensitive to confirm the absence of this phenomenon. Thus, the data obtained with a crossover design may be challenged even when no carryover is observed. An additional reason why this design is not used more often is that many chronic diseases vary in their intensity or in frequency and number of episodes; thus, similar baselines are not likely to occur. The crossover design is also well suited to bioavailability trials. A period of at least ten half-lives is usually allowed between the two periods of the crossover.

TABLE 6.2 *Requirements and desirable attributes for use of crossover clinical trial designs*

1. Adequate number of patients enrolled to detect clinically significant within-patient difference
2. Objective measurements are possible to assess
3. Relatively stable chronic disease is being evaluated, or volunteers are enrolled
4. Patient groups start at the same baseline values of major parameters
5. Patient groups return to their baseline values between treatments
6. No period effect [i.e., patients respond better (or worse) to the first treatment received] observed
7. No physical or psychological carryover effects are present in the second treatment period that cannot be readily and convincingly eliminated (e.g., the first 2 weeks of each treatment are ignored for efficacy)
8. Appropriate statistical analyses are conducted
9. Each period of the crossover is of sufficient duration to provide convincing data
10. Patients are willing to enter a clinical trial that is twice as long as needed to demonstrate efficacy[a]

[a] This occurs because each half of the clinical trial must be of sufficient length to provide convincing data of adequate duration.

1. COMMON PARALLEL DESIGNS

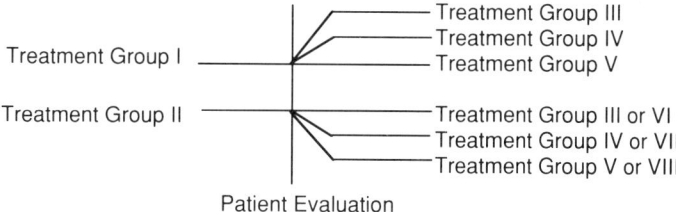

2. TWO PART PARALLEL TRIAL

3. PARALLEL DESIGN WITH PLACEBO INITIATION

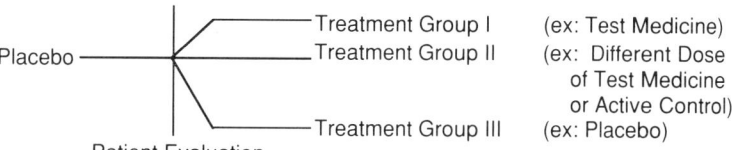

4. INTRODUCTION OF PLACEBO DURING TREATMENT

Treatment Group I	Placebo	Treatment Group I
Treatment Group II	Placebo	Treatment Group II
Treatment Group III	Placebo	Treatment Group III

5. MULTIPLE DOSES WITHIN EACH TREATMENT GROUP

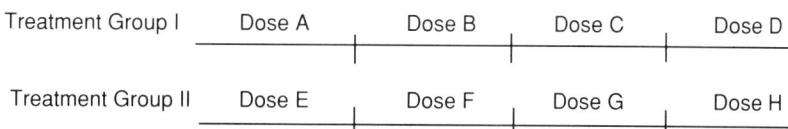

6. PARALLEL EVALUATION OF A COMBINATION MEDICINE

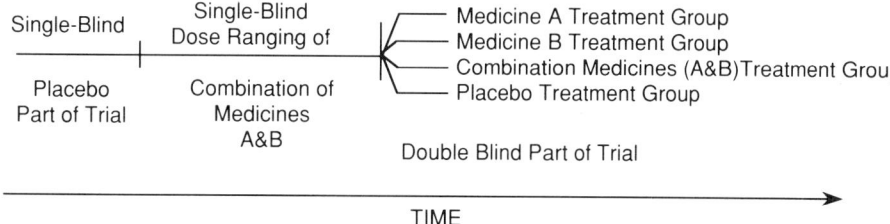

TIME

FIG. 6.3 Selected schemata for treatment periods of parallel clinical trials. Baselines are not illustrated, and time is along the abscissa. Unless indicated, each part may be conducted in either a single-blind or double-blind manner. In *schemata 1 to 4,* each treatment group may constitute a different dose or medicine. In *schema 3,* the placebo trial may be conducted at the end of the trial. In *schema 4,* the placebo trial may be conducted at an announced or unannounced time during the treatment and for a specified or unspecified duration. In *schema 5,* each dose is of a fixed or variable length, and doses may be given in an ascending or random order. One or more of the doses in each treatment group may be a placebo, or each of the two treatment groups could be subdivided into two or more subgroups (e.g., medicine and placebo) at each dose period.

TABLE 6.3 *Selected diseases or conditions in which crossover clinical trials may be conducted*

1. Migraine
2. Epilepsy
3. Narcolepsy
4. Glaucoma
5. Chronic diarrhea
6. Chronic pain
7. Chronic headache (e.g., tension headache)
8. Angina
9. Insomnia
10. Ankylosing spondylitis

Carryover effects may be either physical or psychological effects observed during the second part of the clinical trial. Carryover effects can be influenced not only by the first treatment, but also by what occurs during the crossover part of the trial.

Diseases Suitable for Evaluation Using a Crossover Design

A selected number of diseases that are suitable for evaluation using a crossover design are listed in Table 6.3. Depending on patient responses and return to baseline, clinical trials in any of these diseases may fail and the second part of the crossover may be invalid.

Period Effect

The order of the two treatments in a crossover design is usually randomized so that half the patients receive treatment A in period 1 and treatment B in period 2, whereas the other half receive treatment B and then treatment A. It is possible in an open-label crossover design for one treatment to be an "observation" and not a medicine or placebo.

When Should the Crossover Occur?

In designing a crossover trial, it must be determined whether the change from one treatment period to another will be time-dependent (e.g., after 10 weeks on treatment A all patients will be switched to the second treatment), or whether it will depend on the condition of the patient's disease state. The former practice is usually preferable. Another issue is whether or not to inform the patient at the time when their treatments are switched. It is not necessary to do this if the patient has been generally apprised of this event in the informed consent.

Multiple Crossovers

A "double-crossover" design refers to a clinical trial in which each group of patients receives each treatment twice during the trial. Three or more crossovers are also possible in a trial. Figure 6.4 illustrates a number of variations of the crossover design. The extra-period design attempts to avoid one of the major problems of the crossover design, i.e., the presence of residual effects.

If the data are examined at the end of the first treatment period, and the difference between treatment groups is highly significant, then it may not be ethically permissible to continue the clinical trial (see section on early trial discontinuation).

Attempting to Save a Flawed Crossover Clinical Trial

Many crossover clinical trials that are carefully designed do not achieve all of the required elements during their conduct. The most common problem is that patients do not return to their original baseline after the first treatment is stopped. If the clinical trial is continued nonetheless, it becomes impossible to use the data from the second part of the trial. Many investigators naively continue with the second part of their crossover, as if the return to baseline were unimportant. Interestingly, some prestigious journals are willing to publish flawed data from such clinical trials. The only acceptable option after completion of the crossover, in this case, is to view the first part of the clinical trial as a parallel design and to compare the data of the two groups. This approach is invariably unsatisfactory because fewer patients were originally enrolled in each treatment group than would have been enrolled if the clinical trial were initially designed as a parallel trial.

An alternative approach is to delay initiating the second part of the crossover until patients have returned to their original baseline. This may be done by extending the baseline or washout period between the two parts of the crossover until patients' responses recur at or near their original level (i.e., baseline).

Failure to do this can lead to regression to the mean becoming a problem. Patients with higher baselines usually change more on treatment than those with lower baselines, and patients who are most severely abnormal usually show greater improvement and change than those with a lesser degree of abnormality. This problem was seen in the literature in the case of Timolol (Stellar et al., 1984). The failure of patients to return to baseline between treatments in this clinical trial means that data from the second period are invalid and may not be used. The fact that these results were published in a highly respected journal is more of a comment on the current quality of clinical trial reports in the literature than a criticism of that particular journal. Several of the problems discussed in this section are illustrated in Fig. 6.5.

1. SINGLE CROSSOVER WITH NO INTERVENING BASELINE
(i.e., No Medicine -free Interval)

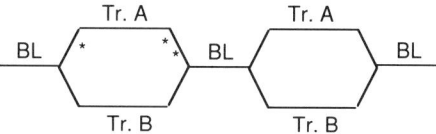

2. SINGLE CROSSOVER WITH INTERVENING BASELINE

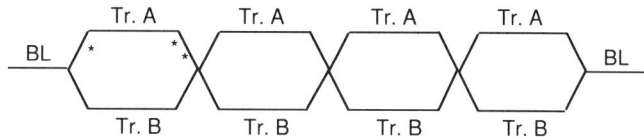

3. DOUBLE CROSSOVER WITHOUT INTERVENING BASELINE

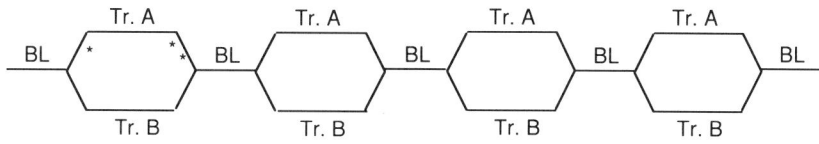

4. DOUBLE CROSSOVER WITH INTERVENING BASELINES

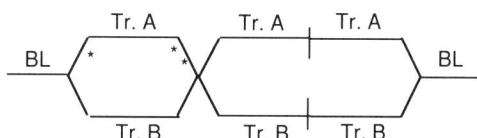

5. EXTRA PERIOD CROSSOVER

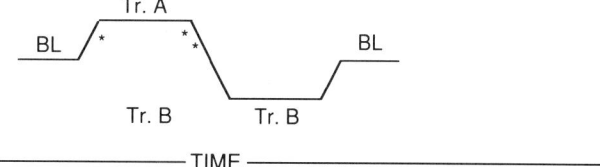

6. OPEN-LABEL CROSSOVER WITHOUT RANDOMIZATION

FIG. 6.4 Selected schemata for crossover trials. *Schemata 1 to 5* may be open-label, single-blind, or double-blind. BL, baseline; Tr.A, treatment A; Tr.B, treatment B. *, Dose ascension part of each period. **, Dose taper part of each period. All baselines that occur after treatment has been initiated include washout of medicine. In *schema 1*, there is usually a brief washout period between treatments A and B. Although the change from one treatment to another in all schemata is shown as being time-dependent, it is possible that this change may be dependent on the condition of the patient's disease state.

A. Invalid Initiation of a Crossover Trial Illustrating Regression to the Mean.

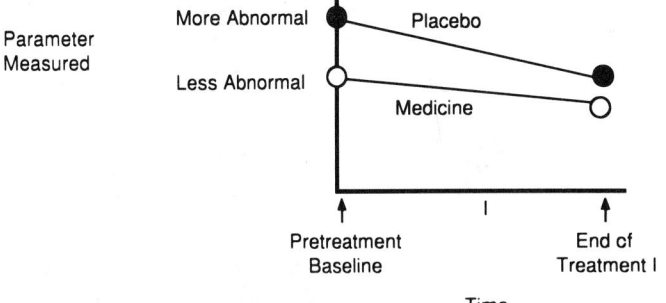

B. Invalid Initiation of Second Part of a Crossover Trial Because Patients Start Treatments I and II From Different Baselines.

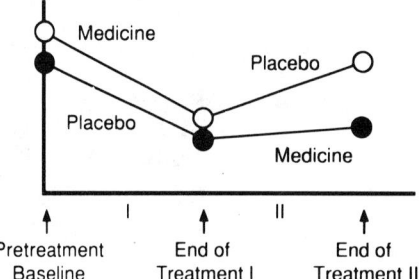

C. Valid Crossover Trial Illustrating a Period Effect.

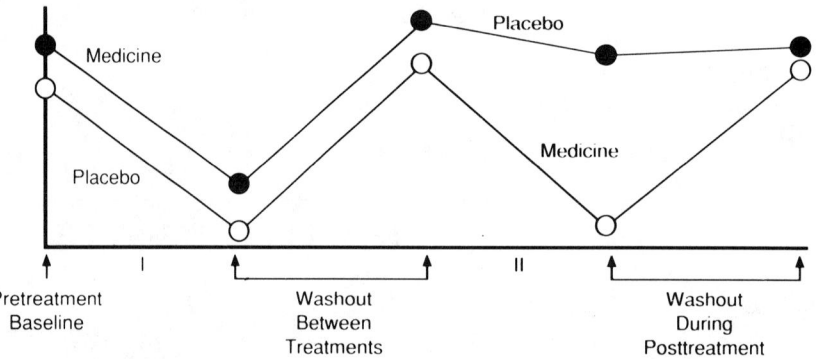

D. Ideal Data Collected During a Crossover Trial.

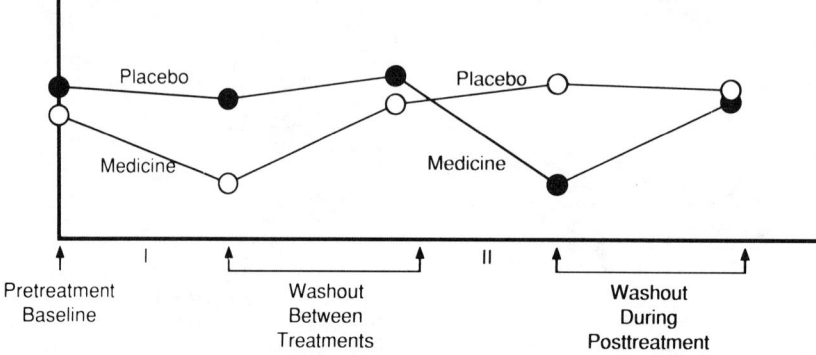

FIG. 6.5 Examples of types of data obtained from crossover trials. In **A** there is a significant difference between the two groups at baseline, which precludes the trial from yielding valid data, unless each group returned to its original baseline before the start of the second treatment. In **B** the treatments were initiated before the groups returned to their original baseline. **C** illustrates a well-conducted trial with both a period effect during the first treatment and a medicine effect during the second treatment period. **D** illustrates a perfect example of a crossover trial. I and II identify treatment periods.

Disadvantages of Crossover Designs

It is difficult to interpret either the efficacy or safety of a medicine if patients have a disease whose natural course waxes and wanes. If concomitant medicines or other treatments are used in an uncontrolled manner, it may be impossible to evaluate the effect of a test medicine.

Matched-Pair Designs

Two other clinical trial designs using two groups of patients are matched pairs and historical controls. Neither of these designs is as scientifically and statistically reliable as the parallel and crossover designs, although there can be certain exceptions. Both matched pairs and historical controls were used more frequently in the past.

The matched-pairs design is a type of parallel design in which pairs of patients who are "identical" in respect to all relevant factors are identified. One patient is randomized to receive treatment A and the other to receive treatment B. This method is more applicable to acute medicine trials than to chronic ones. Because of the difficulty of identifying well-matched pairs, this technique is difficult to use if recruitment proceeds slowly, but if all patients begin a medicine trial at approximately the same time, this technique becomes easier to implement. The matched-pairs design can also be implemented within one individual; in this case, one arm, eye, or foot receives one treatment, and the other arm, eye, or foot receives the other treatment. One major problem with this design, however, is that all relevant factors may not be known.

Historical Controls

With the historical control design, all patients receive the same clinical trial medicine treatment. The control group is composed of similar patients who were previously treated, sometimes by different investigators. The weakness of this method is that it is almost impossible to have an adequately controlled historical group and to have known all the relevant information required. Even if the historical trial included the same patients as in the active treatment part of the trial, major differences might still be present. Using the same patients, however, would add a degree of credibility to the study, but no randomization would have been performed, and significant investigator or patient bias could easily have entered the trial (e.g., differences may have arisen through changes in diagnostic criteria, personnel treating the patient, or concomitant therapy).

Data used from a historically controlled group may be limited to information on the natural history of the disease, or to information on effects of active therapy.

Types of Historical Controls

1. Data based on surveys of patients or data bases.
2. Data based on information obtained in a similar group of patients (treated or untreated).
3. Data obtained in the same patients. Even in this situation, environmental or other conditions may be quite different from those present originally.

Sources of Historical Control Data

Historical control data may be derived from the literature, from previous clinical trials, from registries that have systematically collected data from defined groups of patients, from patients' medical charts, or from a centralized and possibly computerized data bank within a large institution. This latter technique for obtaining patient information is one means of improving the quality of historical controls. If adequate data are retained from completed clinical trials, they will help to surmount one of the major problems of this type of trial, i.e., lack of sufficient information to confirm that patients in the two groups are comparable.

Improving the Validity of Historical Controls

Another method of improving the validity for the use of historical controls is to include two control patients for each test patient and to analyze for differences between patients. It is preferable to use unpublished data for historical controls, since there is a well-known bias towards publishing positive data. The case for using historical controls in certain situations was presented by Lasagna (1982). The inclusion of historical controls (i.e., clinical experience) is frowned on in current medical research, and data obtained are seldom accepted as definitive. The degree to which historical controls in a trial design are accepted depends in large measure on their objectivity.

A Few Examples of Misleading Historical Control Trials

1. Intra-arterial infusions of chemotherapy for metastatic colorectal carcinoma of the liver was reported to be superior to standard chemotherapy in several historical control studies with over 1,000 patients. A randomized controlled trial did not show any benefit of the new treatment (Grage and Zelen, 1982).
2. Portocaval shunt operations for portal hypertension were reported positive in 24 of 32 (75%) uncon-

TABLE 6.4 *Advantages of historical controls*

1. Need fewer patients in a clinical trial because an active control group is not included
2. Easier to recruit patients in a clinical trial because a current control group (e.g., one given placebo) is not included
3. Fewer ethical issues arise
4. Usually less expensive

TABLE 6.6 *Clinical trials in which use of historical controls could be considered*

1. If natural history of the disease is well characterized
2. If natural history of the disease is relatively stable over time
3. If major ethical or practical difficulties would occur if a randomized prospective clinical trial were to be conducted
4. If only a few patients are available to evaluate in a prospective clinical trial (e.g., for a rare orphan disease)
5. If a pilot evaluation is seeking a rapid means to identify whether a specific hypothesis is valid
6. If an established data base is available
7. If a major treatment effect is likely to be observed when compared with alternative therapy
8. If patients received precisely defined treatment in the past
9. If important prognostic aspects of the disease are the same
10. If standard treatment is highly ineffective

trolled studies, in 10 of 15 (67%) studies using nonrandomized controls, and in 0 of 6 randomized studies (Grace et al., 1966).

Diehl and Perry (1986) carefully compared data obtained in historically controlled trials and randomized controlled trials. Large differences between the two types of data were evident and indicated that historical controlled data are not generally valid. Byar et al. (1976) also reached this conclusion. Tables 6.4 and 6.5 list advantages and disadvantages of historical control trials. Table 6.6 indicates when this design could be considered and Table 6.7 describes steps to improve the value of historical controls.

Sequential Designs

A novel clinical trial design that has not been widely used to date is called *sequential design and analysis*. Sequential designs are variations of parallel trials in which patients are assigned to receive one of two treatments. Figure 6.6 shows the results of a hypothetical double-blind clinical trial to illustrate the use of sequential analysis. Each patient in this trial would have received simultaneous treatment with a new and standard topical steroid on different lesions (e.g., drug A

on one limb and drug B on the contralateral limb) for a period of time. After each patient completes the protocol, a choice is made by the investigator (based on various criteria) as to which of the two steroids was preferable or whether it was impossible to discern a distinction in efficacy. For every preference for the new steroid, one mark in a vertical direction is made in the figure, and for each preference for the standard steroid, one mark in the horizontal direction is made. No marks are placed on the figure when a choice cannot be made between the two treatments. Patients are entered into the study until one of the three boundaries illustrated in the figure is reached. In the case illustrated, 33 preferences were made before a decision was reached (i.e., that the new topical steroid was superior to the standard medicine). The graph does not indicate the number of patients in whom no distinction between the two treatments was made. The major emphasis of sequential design and analysis is focused on the time at which sampling in a clinical trial should be stopped.

Data from sequential trials can be analyzed in an open manner, as described above, or analysis may be done in a double-blind manner. In the latter case, treatments may be identified as A and B, so that both patients and investigators remain blind until one of the boundaries is crossed.

TABLE 6.5 *Disadvantages of historical controls[a]*

1. Patients may have been monitored less intensively than in clinical trials using concurrent controls
2. Historical control groups are less likely to be as clearly defined in terms of inclusion criteria than those in prospective randomized controlled clinical trials
3. Responses are often more difficult to quantify and often do not contain a sufficient amount of information
4. Criteria of responses may differ between groups
5. Results often do not convince the medical community
6. Many biases are usually present and at least some of them are difficult to identify
7. Statistical tests are not easily applied to the data
8. The longer the historical period being studied, the larger (usually) are the number and magnitude of differences (e.g., in referral patterns, clinical endpoints, environment, use of equipment, diagnostic tests, measurement of risk factors)
9. Accepted medical practice changes over time and a historical environment may bear little resemblance to current medical environments

[a] These indicate the types of factors that could be responsible for differences between the two groups, other than the major treatment received.

Characteristics of a Clinical Trial Necessary for Sequential Analysis

The major requirements for using this design are (1) rapid evaluability of patients, (2) simple trial design,

TABLE 6.7 *Steps to improve the value of historical controls*

1. Train the data collectors carefully
2. Hire a contract group to visit each site (a single group collecting data at multiple sites should introduce less variability)
3. Use multiple controls for each patient of interest
4. Use multiple chart reviewers to collect the data

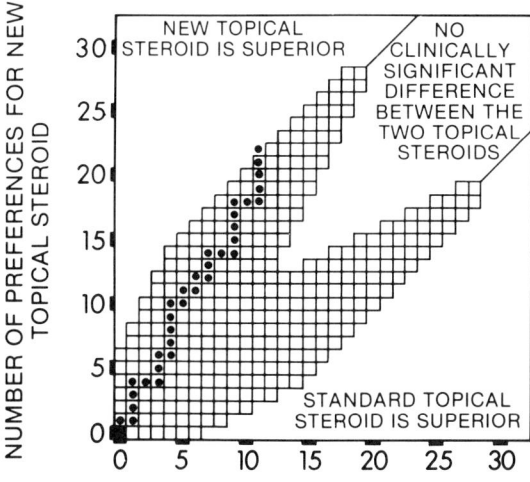

FIG. 6.6 Illustration of sequential design procedure. (Reprinted by permission of Futura Publishing Co. from Rodda, 1974.)

(3) clear endpoint, and (4) limited hypothesis to be tested. Figs. 6.7 and 6.8 illustrate characteristics of this method.

Advantages and Disadvantages

The major advantages of a sequential analysis design are that fewer patients may be needed to complete the clinical trial than with a fixed sample size. The design is convenient to implement and is cost effective if the trial has appropriate characteristics.

The negative aspect of this methodology is that it is not suitable for most clinical trials, since a trial must have a number of characteristics for this design to be appropriate, including simple trial design, limited scope of hypotheses, and rapid evaluability of effects (i.e., the results of the trial must be able to be determined in a short time interval). Planning budgets, packaging medicines, and other practical aspects of the clinical trial are more difficult administratively with this design, and data for different sites cannot be pooled even if the same protocol is followed at all sites. An additional negative aspect is that if the two therapies being evaluated are comparable in their efficacy, this technique may require more patients than would be required in a conventional medicine trial design. The reader is referred to Rodda (1974) and Thompson (1980) for more details on this technique.

Group Sequential Design

Another type of sequential design is the group sequential approach. In this design, a number of patients are entered and studied. An interim analysis of the data

is then conducted, and if the results are significant or if the treatment groups are totally alike, then the clinical trial is stopped. If there is a difference between the two groups that is nonsignificant (statistically), then a second group of patients is enrolled, and the same type of randomization is used as was employed for the original group.

Play-the-Winner Design

A third type of sequential trial design is the "play-the-winner" design. If patients are entered into a trial in specific blocks (e.g., 20 patients at a time), then patients in the second and subsequent blocks are assigned to treatment groups as data are generated in the trial. In this "play-the-winner" design, there may be 20 patients in the first group studied, 10 on placebo and 10 on active medicine. If positive data (preferably, "all-or-none" responses are determined) are found in 8 of 10 on active medicine and in 4 of 10 on placebo, the assignment of treatments to the second group of 20 patients will overplay the winner and put 15 patients on active medicine and only 5 patients on placebo. Because of the relatively recent introduction and unproven validity and acceptance of this method, this approach should be reviewed thoroughly with a statistician before it is adopted as a clinical trial design. This design provides several potential advantages: (1) fewer patients are needed to complete a trial with a highly effective medicine than for a trial with a fixed sample size, (2) if only a few patients with a particular disease or problem are available, then this design may offer a significant advantage over more traditional trial designs, (3) there is a savings in the cost of the trial, and (4) a more rapid answer may be reached about a supposedly superior therapy.

MULTIPLE GROUPS OF PATIENTS

Although many variations of clinical trial design are possible using multiple groups (i.e., more than two), the vast majority are based on the two main concepts described above, parallel and crossover designs.

Latin Square Design

A well-known type of crossover design involves the use of the Latin square (Table 6.8). In this "complete-crossover" design, each group of patients receives each treatment, but in a random order. In addition, the design is balanced in that each treatment is given first to one group, second to one group, third to one group, etc. for the number of groups included in the design. An example of this is shown below. This permits each

TABLE 6.8 *Latin square design*

Group	Treatment period			
	1	2	3	4
I	A	B	C	D
II	B	D	A	C
III	C	A	D	B
IV	D	C	B	A

patient to serve as his or her own control. A period of time usually elapses between successive parts of the clinical trial to allow for any carryover effects from prior treatment to disappear and to establish a new baseline.

In a relatively large Latin square design, ten groups received ten different treatments (Carruthers and Bailey, 1987). The treatments may be administered at daily or weekly intervals. In an incomplete Latin square, each group does not receive all of the treatments, or each treatment is not used at each period. Even in a complete Latin square only a few of the possible sequences of treatments are used. The major criterion is that each treatment is tested before and after each of the others, which requires the same number of sequences (i.e., groups) as the number of treatments.

Subgroups

When a decision is made to select the number of groups of patients in a clinical trial design, the opportunity also exists to form a number of subgroups. For example, two doses of a trial medicine plus placebo may be evaluated in a parallel trial. Each of the three groups may be subdivided on the basis of gender or disease severity or other characteristics. Many imaginative and useful variations are possible in the formation of subgroups. One potential "trap" is to establish a large number of subgroups with too few patients in each to yield meaningful statistical analyses.

Use of Pilot Groups

If the results of a clinical trial are difficult to anticipate, and one does not wish to expose a substantial number of patients to the risks of toxicity from a particular medicine or dose, it may then be appropriate to use a pilot group of patients. The pilot group would consist of a small number of patients who are given the medicine (or dose) before the larger group is exposed. The pilot group could remain in the vanguard and test each higher dose of a new medicine, with the larger group(s) following after initial assurance of relative safety has been obtained.

CLINICAL TRIAL DESIGNS FOR EVALUATING PROPHYLACTIC ACTIVITY

When Are Patients Treated?

Patients may be treated with a medicine either *before* they have been exposed to a disease causing organism (e.g., diphtheria) or *after* [e.g., acquired immunodeficiency syndrome (AIDS)]. If treatment is after exposure, then the progression of disease signs and symptoms in patients may be measured. For patients being treated with a medicine to decrease mortality in a clinical trial that also has a placebo and/or an active medicine group, actuarial life tables of survival may be used to evaluate efficacy. Vaccines are often tested in field trials in which large groups of volunteers are given, for example, one of three treatments. These may be dose A or B of a real vaccine, or a sham injection.

Challenge Tests

Each treatment group may be pretreated with the medicine assigned (or placebo) and subsequently challenged with an agent that causes symptoms (e.g., castor oil may be given to induce diarrhea, citric acid may be given to induce cough). The ability of the test medicine to prevent the symptom is a measure of the medicine's efficacy.

Chronic Illnesses

Patients with episodic chronic illness may be entered into prophylactic trials. They are treated either with different medicines, doses, or dosing schedules or with placebo, or given no treatment; the time until reinfestation or recurrence of symptoms is evaluated.

Prodromal Period Treatment

Patients may be treated during a prodromal period to prevent a medical problem. The difficulty with this type of clinical trial design is that it is usually difficult, if not impossible, to prove that the patient was really in a prodromal phase and that it was not a false prodrome. If the clinical trial involves viral prodromes (e.g., prior to herpes labialis), it may be possible for patients who know that they are in a prodromal period to culture themselves just prior to treatment. This would provide the necessary verification. Otherwise, the lack of the disease's appearance could either represent significant efficacy of the medicine or a false-positive prodromal period.

DESIGN VARIATIONS

Withdrawal of Treatment Trials

In clinical trials in which test medicines are added to already present regimens (i.e., add-on trials), it is sometimes of interest to withdraw concomitant medicines. The purpose is primarily to determine if patients may be treated with the new medicine as a monotherapy, or whether combination treatment is required. General rules must be established in the protocol to determine the basis on which withdrawal will occur. Parameters should include (1) time since last dosage change or addition of last medicine (e.g., at least 3 months must have elapsed since the patient was given the test medicine), (2) stability of the patient as determined by clinical and laboratory parameters, and (3) an assessment that the patient was medically able to accept the withdrawal. Withdrawal of medicine may be made in either fixed increments (33% reduction each week for 3 weeks), total cessation of medicine, or steps (e.g., 66% reduction at once and reevaluation in 1 month before the final 33% reduction is made). It is important that these procedures be conducted in a double-blind manner. This approach was used in a clinical trial by Leppik et al. (1986).

Single-Patient Clinical Trials

There are important differences between case studies and patient trials in which there is an *n* of one person. There has recently been increased interest in single patient clinical trials; Chapter 38 presents information on this topic.

Chart Review Trials

Chart review trials are by definition retrospective. They therefore have all of the limitations, described elsewhere, of retrospective trials. Nonetheless, there are often sound reasons to conduct such clinical trials and they can provide important information. These reasons include (1) the medicine is no longer on the market because of toxicity, (2) too few patients exist to conduct an adequate clinical trial, (3) the resources to conduct a prospective clinical trial are greater than anyone is willing to provide, and (4) the clinical methods used are no longer followed because of changes in technique or ethics.

A protocol is prepared of exactly what will be done at each step and data collection forms are also prepared. If it is uncertain whether the review will be successful in obtaining the data desired, or other difficulties are anticipated, a pilot trial may be conducted.

A chart review may be combined with physician or patient interviews, but if this is contemplated, then careful clinical trial design is essential to avoid recall and other types of bias that may readily occur. This should be discussed with a knowledgable statistician.

Methods used to select specific hospitals and to select patient charts for review must be carefully considered. Haphazard approaches (i.e., arbitrarily chosen hospitals or patient charts) are not acceptable as randomized approaches. If *all* charts that meet certain criteria will be evaluated, it is unnecessary to have a randomized method, but if only a selection will be evaluated, the specific charts chosen should be based on tables of random numbers or a computer-generated code. Reviewing only charts that are readily available is usually an unacceptable method because of potential biases that may enter the study.

Independent reviewers or contractors should be enlisted to read the charts and extract the data. People with a vested interest in the clinical trial or its outcome should not be the ones to extract data. Quality checks and audits of their work are important. Quality may be enhanced if there are multiple sources of the same information (e.g., laboratory reports, physician notes, nursing notes, occupational therapy reports). Also, multiple chart reviewers will enhance the quality of data collected (Haley et al., 1980).

Prepare a checklist of data to obtain from each chart, as well as a log book of pertinent observations and events.

Factorial Designs

The most simple factorial design is referred to as a 2 × 2 complete balanced factorial design. There are two treatments (i.e., A and B). Patients are assigned to treatment randomly so that there is an equal probability of their being in one of four groups (i.e., no A, plus B; A plus B; A and no B; no A and no B). A 2 × 2 (2^2) factorial design is shown in Table 6.9 and a 2 × 2 × 2 (i.e., 2^3) in Table 6.10. Sanderson et al. (1984) describe a 2 × 2 × 2 × 3 factorial design with

TABLE 6.9 *A 2 × 2 completely balanced factorial design*

Treatment A	Treatment B		
	Present +	Absent −	Total patients
Present +	Group 1 + + (n)	Group 3 + − (n)	2n
Absent −	Group 2 − + (n)	Group 4 − − (n)	2n
Total patients	2n	2n	4n

n, number of patients in each cell.

TABLE 6.10 *A two-by-two-by-two completely balanced factorial design*

Group	Treatments received		
	A	B	C
1	+	+	+
2	+	+	−
3	+	−	+
4	+	−	−
5	−	+	+
6	−	+	−
7	−	−	+
8	−	−	−

24 separate combinations of formulations and process variables evaluated.

Factorial designs may be considered when it is possible to give the treatments together without modification (i.e., they do not interfere with each other or potentiate each other's toxicity). A number of clinical trials involving cancer therapy are suitable for factorial designs (Byar and Piantadosi, 1985).

NOVEL CLINICAL TRIAL DESIGNS BASED ON VARIATIONS IN INFORMED CONSENT OR RANDOMIZATION

Numerous authors have approached the topic of clinical trial design from a philosophical or ethical perspective. They have raised questions about or objections to the manner in which or the point in time at which patients are asked to give an informed consent or are randomized to treatment. A number of variations to the timing of the usual approaches have been proposed.

Prerandomization Method

Zelen (1979) proposed a novel approach for clinical trials that compare a new treatment with standard treatment. He suggested that patients who were prerandomized to the standard therapy *not* be required to give informed consent and not be informed that they were enrolled in a clinical trial. The other group of patients who were prerandomized to the investigational therapy would be required to provide informed consent.

This model was strongly criticized for many reasons that will not be repeated here (see Ellenberg, 1984, for numerous references). Ellenberg (1984) stated that no major clinical trial was conducted using this method.

Double-Consent Prerandomized Method

This model, also proposed by Zelen (1982), is a variation of the method described above. The major differ-

ence is that patients in both treatment groups provide informed consent. This design requires more patients to achieve the same power than conventional methods, but this method also facilitates patient enrollment (at least in theory and sometimes in practice).

Ellenberg (1984) presents persuasive arguments against this approach based on science, ethics, and practical grounds. She reviewed experience with the method in large cancer clinical trials and concludes that this method "should be considered a last-resort measure." The author agrees, but there may be very special situations in which it may be ideal.

Another point of interest is that in the prerandomization method, patients assigned to the investigational group can cross over to the standard therapy, but the other group does not have this option. In the double-consent prerandomization method, both groups can cross over to the other treatment. This raises additional statistical issues of whether to analyze data by treatment received or by intention-to-treat. If the treatment received analysis is used, people who crossed over may differ in a major way from those who did not, and the comparability of the two groups may be seriously affected. In the intention-to-treat approach, major problems result because two different treatments were received in each group, although they are compared as single treatment groups.

The author also objects to the open nature of the clinical trials that use these designs. While there are a few occasions when open-label trials are permissible, they rarely provide strong or convincing data.

Deferred Consent Process

In emergency situations it is usually impossible to obtain a nonpressured informed consent to test a method or treatment that is only used or is to be tested in a medical crisis. Under these circumstances patients may be debriefed and an informed consent requested a certain period of time after the treatment is given. If this procedure is contemplated, then rigorous Ethics Committee/Institutional Review Board (IRB) surveillance is necessary, possibly involving a patient representative (e.g., religious leader, ethicist) not associated with the clinical trial.

Two-Tiered Consent Process

In the situation described above for a treatment that lasts for more than 24 or 48 hours, two approaches may be considered. First, adhere to the above model and obtain a full informed consent at 24 to 48 hours from the patient or family. Second, obtain an abbreviated informed consent from the patient or family at the original time of crisis that might be oral and not

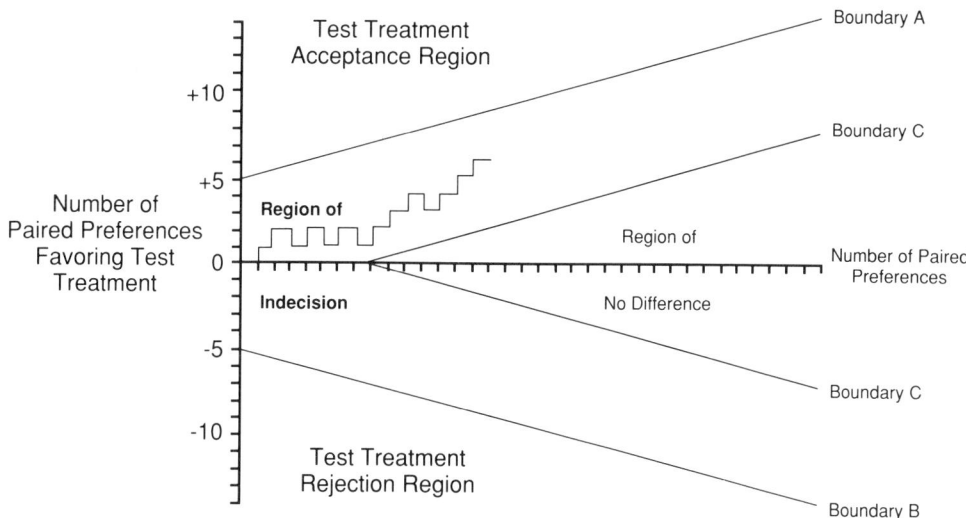

FIG. 6.7 Trial continues until observed number of preferences (ignoring ties) crosses a boundary line. The test treatment is considered superior to the control treatment if boundary line A is crossed, inferior to the control treatment if boundary B is crossed, and equal to the control treatment if boundary C is crossed. The C boundary lines are deleted in trials designed to continue until the test treatment is declared superior or inferior to the control treatment. (Reprinted from Meinert, 1986, with permission of Oxford University Press.)

written. Then, 1 or 2 days later, obtain a full informed consent as described in the first approach.

Run-In Period Designs

Placebo Run-In

In some clinical trials it is important to eliminate patients who are placebo responders or noncompliers.

This is particularly relevant during Phase II clinical trials when the goal is to evaluate the true activity of the medicine. Large placebo effects or noncompliant patients both tend to obscure the true activity of a medicine, making it more difficult to detect. During Phase III trials, however, the goals are to evaluate the activity and safety of a medicine under normal use conditions. Thus, it is not appropriate to exclude placebo responders or noncompliers during Phase III clinical trials.

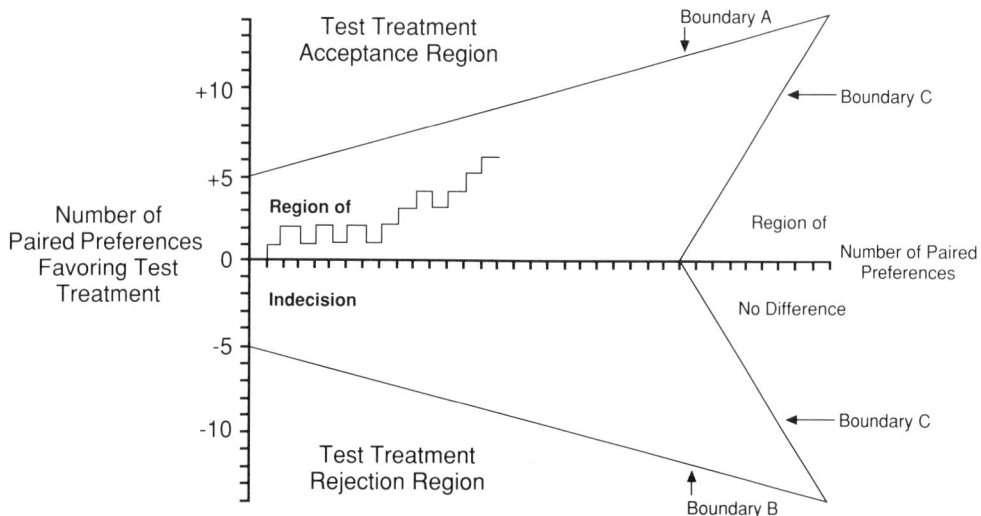

FIG. 6.8 Trial continues until observed number of preferences (ignoring ties) crosses a boundary line. The test treatment is considered superior to the control treatment if boundary line A is crossed, inferior to the control treatment if boundary B is crossed, and equal to the control treatment if boundary C is crossed. (Reprinted from Meinert, 1986, with permission of Oxford University Press.)

Placebo periods may also be used, either as run-in or at other times during a clinical trial, to determine the magnitude of response to the placebo. These may be analyzed on a within-patient or within-group basis during Phases II or III.

Compliance Run-In

The compliance run-in method is discussed in Chapter 15.

No-Treatment Run-In

Another type of run-in may include a period of no treatment, possibly as a baseline. An example of a placebo run-in following a no-treatment period is described by Harrison et al. (1984), and a run-in to assess compliance and eliminate noncompliant patients was used in the Physician and Health Study that evaluated aspirin and beta carotene (The Steering Committee of the Physicians' Health Study Research Group, 1988).

TRIAL DESIGNS THAT SPECIFICALLY ATTEMPT TO AVOID ETHICAL PROBLEMS

There are limited alternatives to consider when it is not ethically acceptable to maintain patients on placebo medication in a clinical trial. The use of an active medicine may be used as a control, but this approach has significant drawbacks, which are discussed in several chapters.

Fail-Safe Designs

A different clinical trial design that incorporates both trial medicine and placebo in a double blind trial but avoids the ethical dilemma of maintaining seriously ill patients on placebo is to incorporate relatively frequent examinations into the protocol with unequivocal criteria for defining clinical improvement and deterioration. In this design, any patient who is observed at the first examination (while on a medicine) to be worse than at baseline is called a treatment failure and is discontinued from the clinical trial. Any patient who has not shown clinical improvement according to defined criteria by the second (or third) examination is likewise called a treatment failure and is discontinued from further trial treatment. The advantage of this approach is that patients receiving placebo who deteriorate at first or fail to show improvement by a specific date will be removed from the trial and can be given alternative

treatment. This study design has been approved by various Ethics Committees/IRBs as having a sound ethical basis in situations in which routine use of a placebo is not acceptable.

Concentration–Response Designs

Two approaches to using concentration–response designs may be described. In the first, all patients are given fixed doses or dose ranges of a medicine and their plasma concentrations are determined, usually at a steady-state. These values are plotted either individually or as a few strata versus the clinical response obtained to determine whether a relationship exists.

In the second approach, patients are titrated with various doses of a medicine until a predefined plasma concentration is achieved. Clinical responses are assessed at that point. Both of these approaches may only be used for a select group of medicines (e.g., theophylline). The concentration-response concept cannot be applied generally for a large number of reasons; for example, a medicine may cause an irreversible response, or a medicine may act by depleting tissues of a substance that cannot be rapidly synthesized.

Dose-Response Designs

An alternative clinical trial design to consider in situations in which an Ethics Committee/IRB will not accept a placebo control trial is a dose-response evaluation. In this situation, a dose that is close to the threshold for activity is evaluated as well as one or two (or more) higher doses that would generate a dose-response relationship. This design has the potential advantages of satisfying Ethics Committees/IRBs that no placebo is used and of meeting regulatory requirements when use of a placebo would be desirable but not mandatory.

The dose-response trial should not be confused with a dose-titration trial. In the former, separate groups of patients usually receive different doses of the same medicine (e.g., group A receives 10 mg/day, group B receives 50 mg/day, and group C receives 100 mg/day), whereas patients on the trial medicine in the latter design may all receive doses from 10 to 100 mg/day depending on their responses, adverse reactions, or other factors. Placebo or active medicine control groups may be used in either design. A combination of both the dose-response and dose-titration design is possible. In the combination design, patients are titrated within specified dose ranges (e.g., group A receives 10–40 mg/day, group B receives 50–90 mg/day, and group C receives 100–150 mg/day).

Obtaining Dose-Response Relationships

Medicines Given by Infusion

Dose-response relationships for infused medicines may be based on increasing the concentration of medicine and keeping the time of infusion constant. Another approach is to use the same concentration of medicine and to lengthen the duration of infusion. A third approach is to either compare a bolus with infused medicine or to compare different combinations of boluses plus infusion.

Medicines Given Orally

It is possible to hold the concentration or amount of a dry dose constant and to vary the number of days patients receive treatment. This approach is particularly relevant for anticancer medicines given on different schedules. Different toxicities and different efficacies may be observed as either the duration of dosing or magnitude of the dose increases. An abbreviated three-dimensional checkerboard approach for evaluating schedules (i.e., matrix of number of doses, versus magnitude of each dose, versus time between cycles), is often used to identify the best treatment, in terms of efficacy and safety. A systematic approach is needed to evaluate schedules because a single schedule that initially seems effective may not represent the schedule with greatest efficacy and least toxicity.

Designs with Escape Clauses or Rescue Treatments

To avoid ethical problems, numerous protocols are designed with escape clauses. This would include the fail-safe design described above as well as other designs. For example, a clinical trial evaluating herpes genitalis in pregnant women might state that if a viral culture becomes positive, a cesarean section will be performed. Use of rescue medication may be recommended or required if a patient has a medical problem (e.g., experiences pain that requires treatment in a trial in which the patient may receive medicine or placebo).

Establishing Treatment Groups Based on Compliance

Compare efficacy results in patients with high and low compliance in taking their medicine. Then, because you may have biased groups of patients, in a second part of the clinical trial (or in a new trial) expose all patients the same way to the medicine (i.e., when the degree of compliance is controlled and is nearly identical for all patients). Attempt to show that both high and low compliers based on the first trial (or part of the trial) can react the same way to the test medicine. If this is confirmed, then one could conclude that the patient groups were comparable and that differences observed in the first part of the clinical trial were real and were based on differences in compliance. Moreover, if both statistically significant and clinically significant differences are present in efficacy data of the two compliance groups, it supports the concept that the medicine is active. The low compliance group may be considered as a near-placebo group because those patients are not ingesting sufficient quantities of medicines to elicit a maximal therapeutic response.

Alternative Designs

Other designs such as the sequential design should also be considered in situations in which the Ethics Committee/IRB raises various ethical concerns. If strong ethical reservations persist about conducting a given clinical trial, then it may be useful to consider a pilot trial to obtain data that may indicate whether or not the trial design would be acceptable from an ethical perspective.

Comparison with Nonmedicine Therapy

Patients receiving medicine may be compared with others who are receiving (1) no treatment, (2) surgical treatment, (3) medical devices, or other therapies (e.g., physical therapy, acupuncture).

CHAPTER 7

Classification and Description of Phase IV Postmarketing Study Designs

BROAD CATEGORIES OF CLINICAL STUDIES CONDUCTED DURING PHASE IV

Phase IV studies include much more than just postmarketing surveillance and other types of pharmacoepidemiology studies. Marketing-oriented seeding trials, comparison trials, and clinically oriented trials to learn more about a medicine are also part of Phase

IV. This latter group of trials includes those to evaluate (1) mechanism-of-action, (2) fine points of the safety profile, (3) quality of life, and (4) questions that arose during Phases I to III. Almost any type of clinical study or trial may be conducted during Phase IV. This chapter focuses on postmarketing surveillance and other pharmacoepidemiology studies. Marketing-oriented trials are discussed in Chapter 51 and clinically oriented trials similar to those conducted in Phases I to III follow the same principles described elsewhere in the book.

PURPOSES OF CLINICAL STUDIES CONDUCTED DURING PHASE IV

Purposes of clinical trials and studies conducted during Phase IV are to:

1. Address questions that arose during Phases I–III, but that have not yet been completely answered or adequately addressed. These clinical trials include comparison trials with other drugs, cost-effectiveness studies, quality of life trials, mechanism-of-action trials, and trials that explore specific hypotheses. Evaluations of new indications, routes of administration, and dosage forms are carried out in Phases I–III (usually conducted primarily as Phase II trials) and not in Phase IV.
2. Continue clinical trials initiated but not completed during Phase III.
3. Investigate interactions of a new medicine.
4. Expose more patients to the new medicine to confirm its efficacy.
5. Expose more patients to the new medicine to confirm and better understand its safety (e.g., delayed effects, prolonged use effects). Quantitate rates of known adverse reactions. Evaluate the medicine in patient populations (e.g., children, pregnant women, nursing mothers, elderly, immunosuppressed) not previously exposed or not exposed in sufficient numbers to the new medicine.
6. Determine if results obtained at tertiary care and excellent hospitals during Phases I–III can be confirmed in other hospitals as well as when the medicine is used by a large number of new physicians.
7. Evaluate whether any rare but serious adverse reactions occur.
8. Discover new indications that are then explored and developed in Phases II and III. These discoveries may occur through serendipity or via informal tests by private clinicians.
9. Evaluate the pattern of a medicine's utilization in a specific or general population.
10. Study the clinical characteristics of overdosage and the means of counteracting this problem.
11. Assess the costs of adverse reactions to various sectors of society and develop the means to meet these costs.

In sum, the primary goals of pharmacoepidemiology are to discover previously unknown adverse reactions caused by medicines to describe specific risk factors and to estimate the frequency of medicine-related ad-

verse reactions. This information is used to assess the benefit-to-risk relationship for a medicine, to decrease risks to patients, and ultimately to improve the quality of medical treatment. The field of pharmacoepidemiology addresses broad therapeutic questions that cannot easily be addressed in Phases I–III clinical studies, or in other Phase IV studies.

CATEGORIES OF PHASE IV STUDIES

The world of Phase IV studies is divided into five categories in this book, as follows:

1. *Descriptive studies.* Provide information on pattern of disease occurrence in populations according to demographic and prognostic characteristics. Data used are routinely collected epidemiologic intelligence (Table 7.1) which is analyzed to identify the occurrence of rare adverse reactions or to generate an hypothesis. Passive monitoring of events and reports is an important method for collecting data included in descriptive studies.
2. *Cross-sectional studies.* Also called *surveys or prevalence studies*, these usually involve a statistically based random sampling of a target population. Data are classified according to reported exposure to medicines and observed outcomes. Results pertain to a single point in time, and this type of study is therefore like a snapshot in time. If this study is conducted retrospectively, it may be unclear whether exposure truly preceded the outcome.
3. *Case-control studies.* Case-control studies are always retrospective. Cases have the disease and controls do not. Data are collected by looking backward in time to determine differences between the two groups in the past. Each case is matched for specific confounding factors (e.g., age, sex) with one or more controls. Multiple controls are used to increase the efficiency of matching for each case included, especially because it is difficult, if not impossible, to identify a single control that has all factors. Cases could also have some, but not all factors. It is sometimes difficult to find appropriate controls (e.g., for psychotic pa-

TABLE 7.1 *Sources of epidemiological intelligence to raise "red flags" or generate hypotheses*

1. Case reports published in the medical literature
2. Spontaneous adverse reaction reports received by a pharmaceutical manufacturer (i.e., field reports)
3. Spontaneous adverse reaction reports received by a regulatory authority
4. Data from observational or controlled studies reported to or conducted by the manufacturer

tients), and information obtained is often incomplete and subject to recall bias.

4. *Cohort studies.* A cohort is a group that is exposed, and followed forward to a point in time when its members are evaluated retrospectively to look for differences in the frequency of one or more outcomes from a control unexposed group. If the case and controls both come from the same study population, the results of the study are more easily validated. It is important to determine that both cases and controls are free of disease (i.e., the outcome) at the start of the observation period.

5. *Controlled clinical studies and trials.* These experimental studies with controlled assignments are described throughout this book.

COMPARISON OF INVESTIGATIONAL MEDICINE AND POSTMARKETING SURVEILLANCE PROTOCOLS

In theory there are no differences between the elements included in a clinical trial protocol (i.e., Phases I, II, III) and the elements in postmarketing surveillance studies. In practice, some elements are usually more abbreviated and others are more developed.

Elements that are often abbreviated in Phase IV protocols include: background, inclusion criteria, and methods of statistical analysis to be used. Elements that are often more fully described in Phase IV protocols include: steps to take in reporting adverse reactions, roles and responsibilities of one or more coordinating centers, data processing, steps to address in loss of patients to follow-up, and procedures of data validation.

DESCRIPTIVE STUDIES CONDUCTED DURING PHASE IV

The primary use of passive monitoring studies is for assurance of safety and/or early detection of rare but clinically important adverse reactions.

Although not "technically" a form of study at all, monitoring for signals of adverse medicine events during wide use of a medicine represents the backbone of epidemiology, including pharmacoepidemiology. Known as "epidemiological intelligence," this approach deploys a wide spectrum of "sentinel" devices in an attempt to elicit from the background incidence of disease unusual clusters, increases in incidence, or unexpected or inexplicable phenomena. For adverse reactions attributable to medications, such monitoring consists of ongoing solicitation of "news" about problem cases in medical practices in which practitioners suspect that a medicine may have caused a problem.

This takes the form of solicitation of pharmaceutical sales representatives on their "detailing" visits, solicitation by the Food and Drug Administration (FDA) through its *FDA Drug Bulletin* (and by the Department of Health in the United Kingdom), requests for examples of unexpected medicine-associated events by specialty groups (e.g., the medicine-induced ocular side effects registry), and, of course, spontaneously reported associations by concerned practitioners to the manufacturer, a regulatory authority, United States Pharmacopeia (USP), or, if unusual enough, through the published literature as an article, case report, or letter to the editor.

Spontaneous Adverse Reaction Reports

The three steps that must occur before the medical community receives information on a spontaneous adverse reaction are (1) the adverse reaction must be detected, (2) the adverse reaction must be attributed to the medicine, and (3) the adverse reaction must be reported. Reporting may occur to a regulatory authority (e.g., Form 1639 in the United States, Yellow Card in the United Kingdom), to the manufacturer, or to the medical community (e.g., in a published medical report).

There are many reasons why physicians present adverse reaction reports (Table 7.2). Given that these data are a valuable source of new information, although they can result in the overgeneration of hypotheses, it is relevant to attempt to improve the reporting of valid data. One approach is to encourage hospitals to develop their own systems for obtaining these data. Hospital physicians could be encouraged to dictate coded summaries of adverse reactions into permanent medical records that could be later abstracted in a systematic way.

Benefits of Spontaneous Adverse Reaction Reports

Spontaneous adverse reaction reports:

1. Provide an early recognition of actual or potential problems

TABLE 7.2 *Selected reasons why physicians report adverse reactions*

1. Ethical responsibility
2. Legal obligation
3. Guilt feelings
4. Professional reward
5. Inadvertently, when reporting other data
6. Peer pressure
7. Request of a sales representative

2. Provide a continuous monitoring system of a medicine's use by various patient populations
3. Are able to compare adverse reaction profiles of medicines within a therapeutic class
4. May characterize iatrogenic syndromes and identify predisposing factors (e.g., age, dose, sex).

Limitations of Spontaneous Adverse Reaction Reports

Spontaneous adverse reaction reports:

1. Rely on physicians to make a clinical diagnosis of a medicine's toxicity and to establish causality
2. Underreport suspected adverse reactions, which leads to bias, particularly in estimating incidence
3. Are not suitable for detecting adverse reactions with high background rates in the population.

Case Reports

One or a few patients are usually described in detail in a case report submitted as a manuscript for publication, report to a regulatory authority, or report to a pharmaceutical company. Case reports may discuss adverse reactions or benefits. This method usually serves as a sentinel of potentially important events. A careful review of original papers in major medical journals found that 38% of all research reports consist of case reports (Fletcher and Fletcher, 1979). Although they can be biased or invalid, these reports are a valuable source of information on rare events.

Case Series

A report on a group of patients exposed to a medicine or who had an adverse reaction (i.e., a case series) often contains information on the incidence and prognosis of an adverse reaction. The lack of a true control group limits the value of any interpretation of data from a case series.

OBSERVATIONAL STUDIES CONDUCTED DURING PHASE IV

Medicine development and evaluation in Phase IV do not always require, nor is it always appropriate to conduct, randomized clinical trials. There are clinical situations in which it is either unethical, undesirable, or unnecessary to conduct double-blind, randomized, controlled trials. In these situations, it is often possible to conduct observational studies to determine the outcome of medicine treatment. Observational studies record specific events that are occurring in a defined population without any intervention by the researcher.

Differences between Experimental and Nonexperimental (i.e., Observational) Studies

Nonexperimental studies include most of the studies performed in the field of pharmacoepidemiology and usually measure medicine safety in routine use. Utilizing experimental studies to address most epidemiological issues would incur enormous expenses. Another reason to use nonexperimental methods to answer epidemiological questions is that it is ethically unacceptable to expose people to toxic medicines or conditions resulting from natural, industrial, or other human-caused disasters or situations (e.g., radiation exposure resulting from a nuclear weapons explosion).

Nonexperimental epidemiological studies differ from clinical trials in that the former (1) generally observe medical or health outcomes without actually intervening in patient encounters; (2) usually involve more patients (often over 1,000); (3) study situations in which patients receive medicines through normal prescribing practices; and (4) follow patients who are treated according to routine clinical practice, often over long periods of time. Approval of the study protocol by an ethics committee and the obtaining of patient informed consents are not always required and may be inappropriate in some cases, since it would compromise the basis and assumptions of the observational approach. In some cases approval is indirect (e.g., Medicaid Administration) and individual patient consent may not be obtained. Figure 7.1 illustrates some differences between an observational study and an experimental trial.

Brief Historical Background of Observational Studies

On the basis of extensive public debate and detailed evaluations of the limitations of the "epidemiologic intelligence" approach, the Joint Commission on Prescription Drug Use (Melmon, 1980) recommended that more active postmarketing surveillance (observational cohort or case-control studies be instituted (perhaps even mandated) for all major new medicines. The commission also emphasized the usefulness of large-population observational studies for developing new hypotheses and uncovering serendipitous discoveries about medicines. These are two important areas that (like detecting adverse reactions) are not expected to be compromised by the biases of nonblinded techniques. Nonetheless, numerous other biases are present (e.g., biases of patient selection, different treatment regimens, lack of standardized evaluation criteria) when nonblinded techniques are used.

Observational studies to explore efficacy have the greatest potential to provide useful clinical data when

A. Observational Study

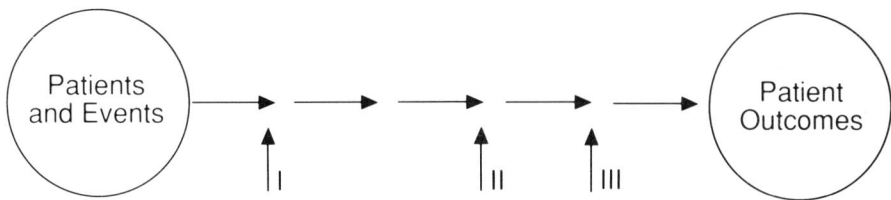

Investigator observes at times I, II, III.
Investigator does not interfere with events.

B. Clinical Trial

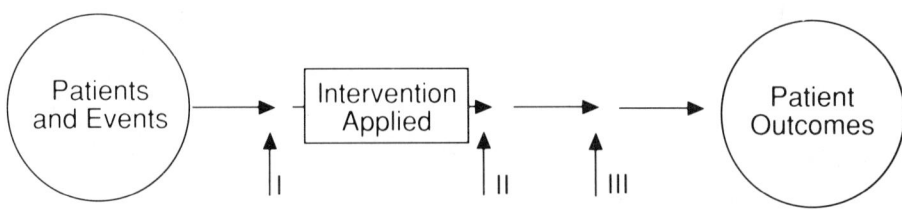

Investigator observes effects of intervention at times
II and III after interfering with events, and compares
with baseline (I).

FIG. 7.1 Some of the most important differences between an observational study and clinical trial. In panel A, time points I, II, and III are earlier (i.e., intermediate) patient outcomes and the circle represents the final patient outcome(s) measured. In panel B, time points II and III are the earlier outcomes measured.

the desired effects of the medicine are opposite to the inherent tendencies and trends within the study. Examples of this occur when a medicine (1) saves patient lives that would be lost if no treatment were provided, (2) arouses a patient from a coma, (3) provides immunological protection against a common disease such as measles, or (4) provides prophylactic protection in well-characterized medical situations. Observational studies are most often used in Phase IV postmarketing surveillance to evaluate medicine safety. Observational Phase IV studies to explore medicine efficacy further are described by Strom et al. (1983).

Despite the recommendations of the Joint Commission on Prescription Drug Use, experience with large observational studies for monitoring medicine safety has not been entirely satisfactory. An FDA review of three major postmarketing studies (cimetidine, cyclobenzaprine, and prazocin), which included from 7,607 to 22,653 people, concluded that the studies did not reveal any adverse reactions to these medicines that were not previously known. But physician case reports that were spontaneously submitted ("epidemiologic intelligence") provided information on new adverse reactions for two of these three medicines (Rossi et al., 1983). Lasagna (1983) commented on this

report with sobering statistics indicating that rare adverse reactions (one event in 10,000 or more patients) will almost never be observed with formal Phase IV studies, which for logistic and/or financial reasons rarely involve even 10,000 patients. Lasagna concluded that spontaneous physician reports will remain an important source of information about previously unknown benefits and risks of marketed medicines.

Choosing between Cohort or Case-Control Methods

The choice of either the cohort or case-control study methodology is dependent on the amount of medicine use and whether the suspected events occur frequently or rarely. For rare (but identifiable) events of a frequently used medicine, the case-control methodology is superior, whereas for more frequent events of a less frequently or rarely used medicine, the cohort methodology is better. If both medicine use and the event being studied are frequent, then either method will be adequate, but if both medicine use and the event studied are rare, then neither method will work well.

If the cost, logistics, and feasibility of case-control and cohort designs are comparable, the cohort method is preferable because of the biases inherent in the case-control method. When use of a newly approved medicine is to be monitored for early detection of adverse reactions, the prospective cohort method may be more practical, i.e., in the formation of a patient registry.

Cohort Studies

A cohort is a population or group of patients or healthy people who are followed over time. These individuals share common attributes relevant to the research question being evaluated. For example, the cohort could be 1,000 patients who have experienced their first episode of back pain but have no objective neurological defects. The cohort study is similar to clinical trials except that patients are not randomly assigned to a specific treatment or group prior to the study. One type of cohort study involves two (or more) groups of people [with one major difference (exposure) between them] without a disease who are followed forward in time and examined for the incidence of the disease. The Framingham, Massachusetts cardiovascular disease study is an example of a public health cohort study. Cohort studies may be either prospective, retrospective (historical), or a combination of both. The control group (i.e., control cohort) may be defined to be similar to the study cohort, except for the exposure being studied, or data obtained in the general population may be used as control.

Steps in Conducting a Prospective Cohort Study

1. People at risk are identified.
2. Two (or more) similar groups are formed.
3. One group is exposed to the test treatment.
4. The occurrence of disease or other endpoint is measured in each group.
5. Rates of outcome are compared with respect to exposure.

Large prospective cohort studies (Fig. 7.2) were more popular in the early 1980s than they are today. The major reasons why they have lost favor are summarized in Table 7.3. A synopsis of these studies (as well as a primer on postmarketing surveillance) is presented by Hagler et al. (1987).

TABLE 7.3 *Disadvantages of ad hoc pharmacoepidemiological studies*

1. Only a single major question or hypothesis may be addressed in most studies
2. A large amount of time is required to conduct them
3. The cost is expensive
4. It is difficult to address rare events

Steps in Conducting a Retrospective Cohort Study

1. A group of diseased or exposed individuals is identified.
2. A group of nonexposed control individuals is identified.
3. The occurrence of one or more factors is evaluated and an association sought with the exposed group.

Example: The principles of a retrospective cohort study are outlined in Fig. 7.3. A group of women with breast cancer is identified as a cohort and a group of women at risk for breast cancer is the control group. A retrospective examination determines the number exposed to estrogens. The degree of exposure and confounding factors are also evaluated.

Steps in Conducting a Retrospective Case-Control Study

1. Cases are chosen.
2. Controls are identified. Two or even more control groups are desirable.
3. Each group's data are evaluated for certain exposures that occurred in the past.
4. A positive association is sought between one or more exposures that are more common in the cases than in the controls. The exposure rate of the cases is compared with the exposure rate of the controls.

The principles of a retrospective case-control study are outlined in Fig. 7.4, and the advantages and disadvantages of the case-control design are listed in Tables 7.4 and 7.5. Mayes et al. (1988) collected 56 topics with contradictory results in case controls. They proposed using the principles of clinical trials to develop appropriate standards for case-control research. The author agrees.

There are several rules that apply to the proper choice of a control, but these are not considered here. It should be pointed out that a process requiring recall is highly susceptible to problems of scientifically unacceptable bias, both subtle and obvious. The inter-

TABLE 7.4 *Advantages of the case-control design study*

1. Well suited to rare diseases or to those diseases with a long latency period[a]
2. Existing medical records may occasionally be used
3. Relatively inexpensive to conduct
4. Relatively rapid to initiate and conduct
5. Allows evaluation of multiple causes of a disease
6. Less involvement and effort for patients than in cohort or controlled studies

[a] This is true because the few ''one in a million'' cases are already identified.

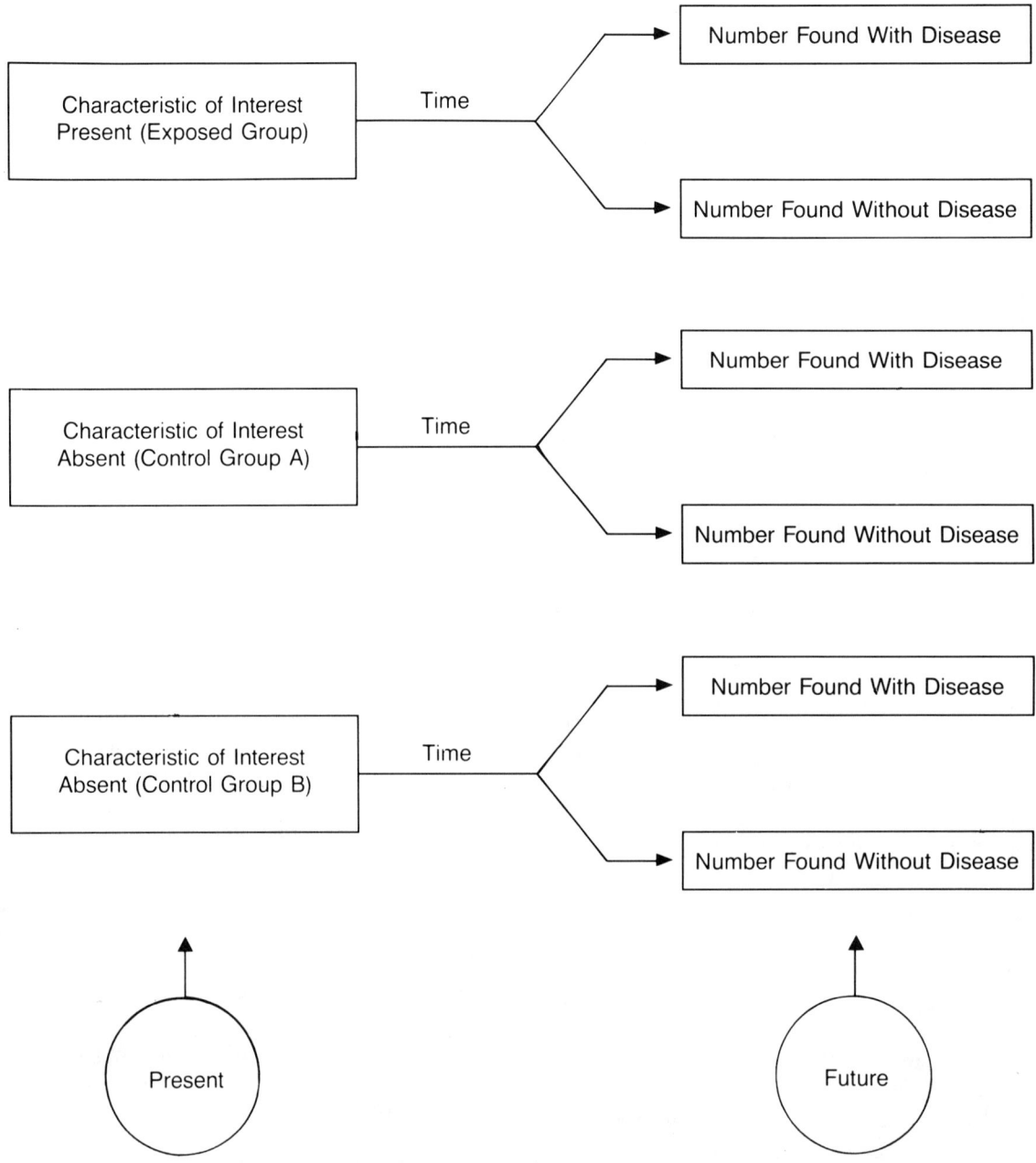

FIG. 7.2 Schematic of a prospective cohort study. Control group B is not essential. The disease rate in the exposed group is compared with that in the unexposed group(s).

TABLE 7.5 *Selected disadvantages of the case-control design study*

1. Relies on patient recall of data or on medical records for information on past exposure to medicines
2. Validation of data is either difficult or impossible
3. Control of extraneous variables is difficult
4. Patients in the two groups may be quite different, even if each patient serves as his or her own control

ested reader is referred to the epidemiological literature for additional methodological details. It is recommended that expert epidemiological counsel be obtained before case-control studies are initiated.

The application of this methodology in the pharmaceutical area involves assembly of a population exposed to a medicine or class of medicines and a comparable population that has not been exposed. The study may be designed either to generate or to test a hypothesis. The target outcome or dependent variable must be determined at the outset, prior to initiation of

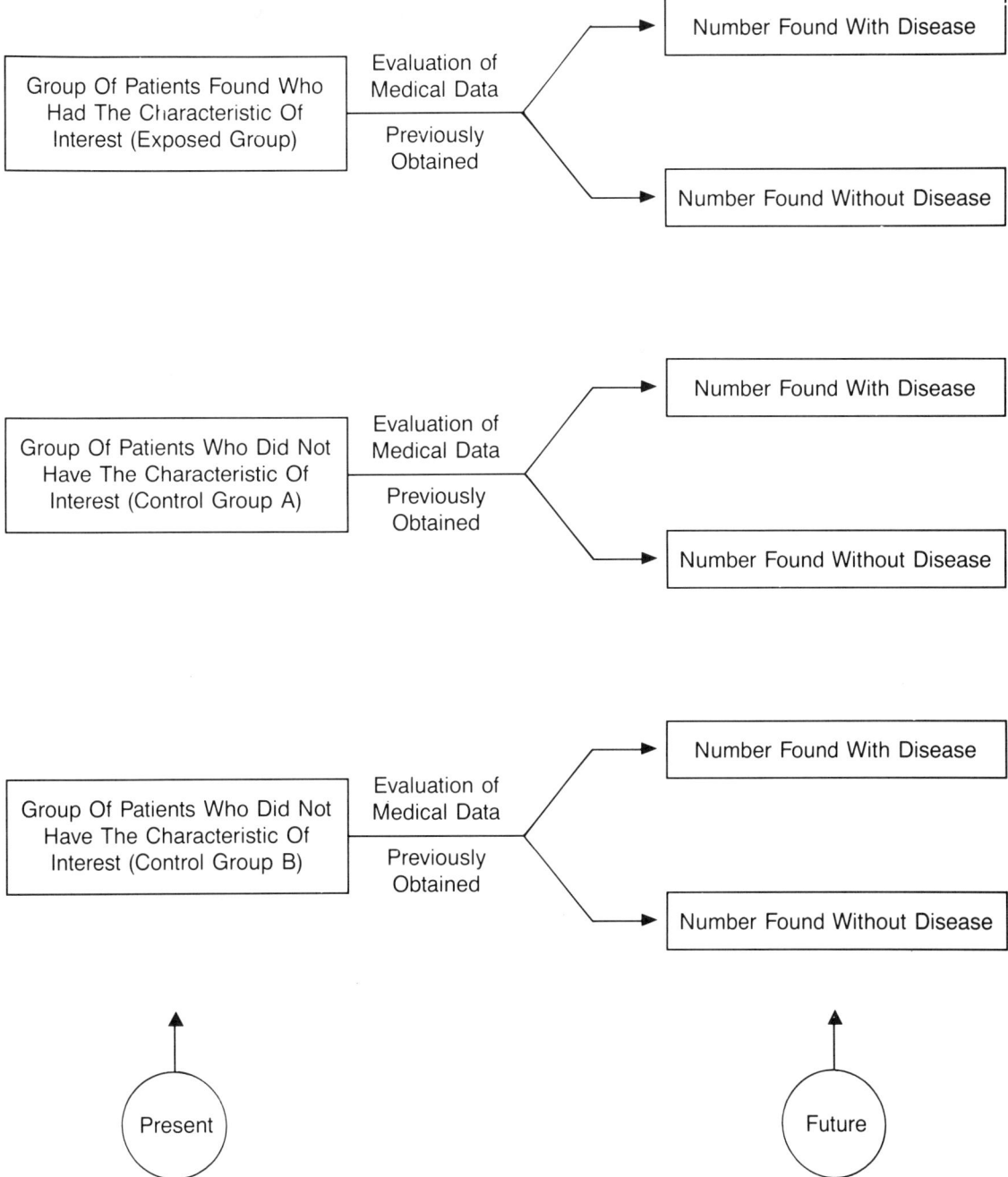

FIG. 7.3 Schematic of a retrospective cohort study. Control group B is not essential, but additional control groups may be included.

the study. The outcome events (e.g., specific disease, death, adverse reactions, specific benefits) become the numerator of an incidence rate that is calculated. The size of the cohort is usually the denominator of the fraction. Outcomes are compiled in both populations, and the rates are compared. Unusual or unexpected results may be evaluated in additional studies.

It is not mandatory to have a comparison or control group, but the data will be far less convincing if no comparison group is used. The more control groups used to compare with the test cohort, the more convincing the data will be. Each control cohort should be as similar as possible to the test cohort, but the control cohorts should differ among themselves in separate and important aspects. Cohorts are a useful method for conducting a long-term longitudinal study. In long-term trials, the importance of follow-up to prevent losses of patients cannot be overstressed.

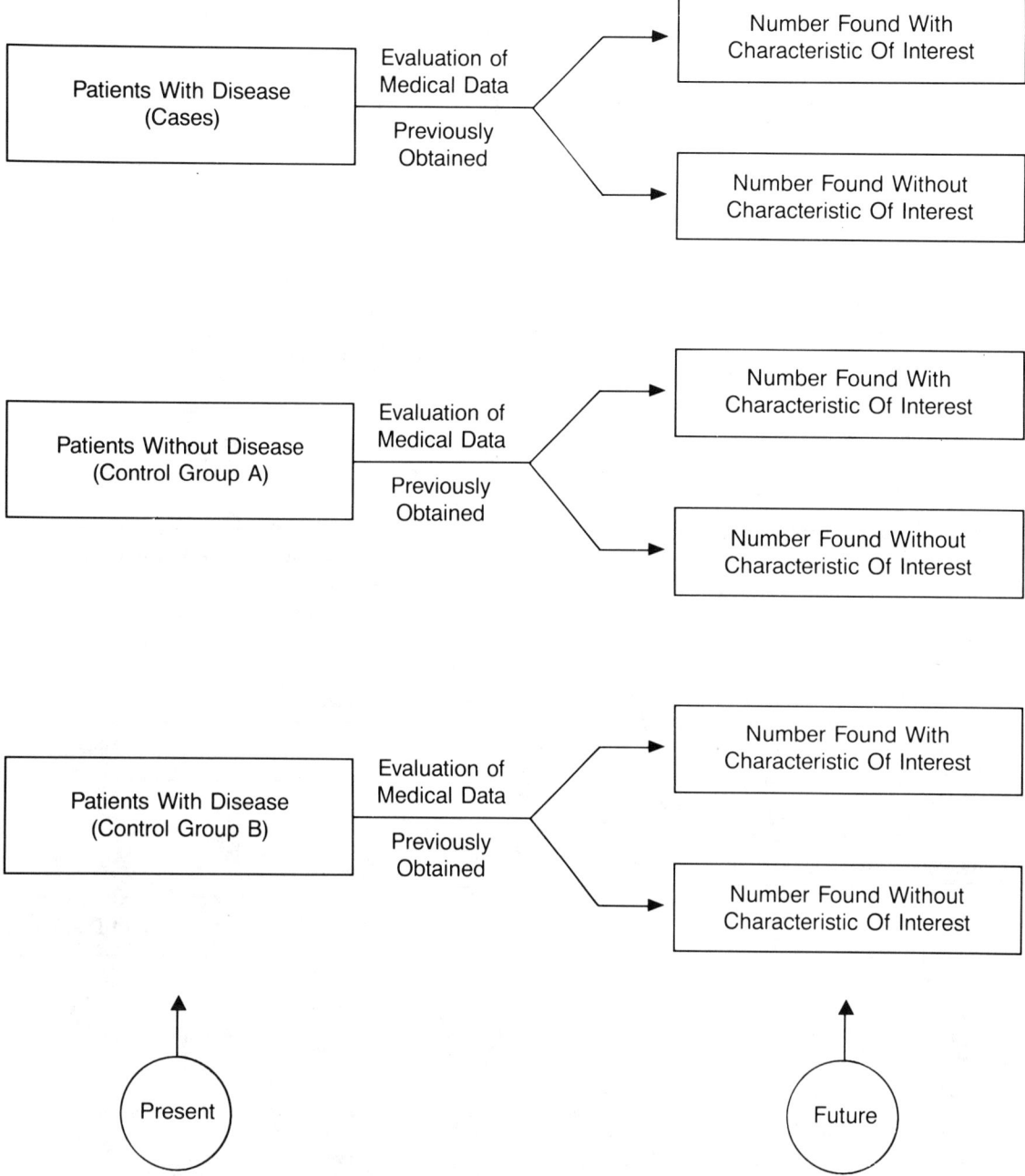

FIG. 7.4 Schematic of a retrospective case-control study. Control group B is not essential, but additional control groups may be included. The exposure rate of the cases is compared to that of the controls.

Case–Control Studies

In this type of study, a group of cases and a group of controls are chosen, or a matched patient is located for each "case" patient. Cases and controls are equivalent in all relevant factors except for the disease that only the case patient (or group) has. The investigator then looks back in time to learn what important differences existed between the two patients or the two groups, especially in terms of exposure. Such historical investigation may provide valuable information as to why the case patient(s) developed a particular disease.

For this method to be most effective, all cases with the disease in a defined population should be included in the study. The controls should be chosen from the same defined population such that they would qualify as case patients if they had the disease. Two examples of defined population are (1) all persons seen at a given clinic or clinics and (2) all persons within a given geographical area. The case group may represent the entire population of patients who have the disease, or they may be a subset of the entire population.

Primary Goal of Observational Studies

Because spontaneously reported adverse reactions do not provide sufficient data for sophisticated analysis and interpretation or to test hypotheses, observational studies were developed to fill this need.

The goal of observational studies is to obtain the same conclusion that would have been achieved if a well-controlled trial had been conducted. To move toward this goal it is important that a protocol be designed prospectively in which the collection and flow of data are identified. In larger studies an advisory board may be appointed to oversee the study's conduct and interpretation. This board may be composed of members from academia, the coordinating center, and the pharmaceutical sponsor (see Chapter 17 on Data Review Committees).

Endpoints of Observational Studies

The types of endpoints used in observational studies to determine if a medicine causes organ impairment or adverse reactions are:

1. Hospitalizations attributable to a medicine
2. A significant increase in a laboratory measure during hospitalization
3. An increase in a laboratory analyte by a specific amount or percent over baseline over a predetermined period (e.g., 1 year on medicine therapy)
4. Death.

ISSUES IN OBSERVATIONAL STUDIES

Validity of Case-Controlled and Cohort Studies

This issue is indirectly addressed throughout this section and in Chapter 43 on validation. Esdaile and Horwitz (1986) present guidelines for evaluating the validity of these studies.

Choice of Sites and Patients

This topic can be addressed by answering a series of questions. Should only academic sites be selected for the study? If so, then the practices of general medicine may be missed and this could be an important source of data to measure. Is it preferable to use a sample of patients at each site observed or all patients that meet specific criteria (e.g., age over X years and have had a prescription from date 1 to date 2)?

Medical Intervention

To what degree (if any) should intervention in medical practice be allowed in an observational study? For example, could a laboratory test be requested that was deemed important for the study or for the patient? In the former case (for the study) the answer is clearly no, or it could not be an observational study. In the latter case (for the patient) this would possibly change medical practice, even if it could provide extremely valuable data. A compromise would be achieved by prompting the physician to maintain good medical records, so that data would be listed if they were obtained. Alternatively, sites could be selected for the study where good records are kept and good medical treatment occurs. Ethical standards of appropriate medical care must always be maintained.

Definitions and Usages of Case-Controlled and Cohort Studies

Greenland and Morgenstern (1988) describe a major definitional issue of whether the distinction between case-control and cohort is in reasoning from cause to effect in a cohort study and from effect to cause in a case-control study as proposed by Kramer and Boivin (1987), or whether the key distinction "is that a case-control study involves gathering data on only a subset of the source population. In a cohort study, risk factor and incidence data are obtained on all source population members in order to estimate effects of the factors on incidence."

EXPERIMENTAL STUDY DESIGNS

The epidemiological designation for experimental studies is appropriate when those studies involve large populations and/or address public health rates and issues. In general, experimental epidemiological studies utilize prospective designed protocols and are of three basic types.

Clinical Studies

Clinical studies are the traditional prospective Phase-III-type disease treatment studies described in detail in this book, but in the present context, they address "epidemiological" questions or issues such as the ability to reduce transmission rates of infectious disease through treatment of a segment of the community. In such studies, outcomes are often measured at the population level (in terms of attack rates) as well as at the individual level. An interesting variation of this approach is the so-called risk factor reduction study in which the study measures nontraditional outcomes rather than the disease parameters usually monitored in clinical studies.

Field Trials

Field trials involve the evaluation of large-scale field studies of medicines, vaccines, or other biologicals for the prevention or management of disease. These studies usually require more patients than clinical studies and are conducted at the patients' homes, schools, workplaces, or central locations. They often use observational approaches but are considered experimental designs inasmuch as they actively select persons who will or will not be exposed to treatment.

Community Intervention Studies

Community intervention studies are essentially field studies in which one or more entire communities may be involved (Morgenstern and Bursic, 1982). In a strict sense, the community intervention study requires that the entire community be exposed, since results are compared to control communities in which the treatment was not implemented. Examples of community intervention studies include analysis of the effects of water fluoridation and evaluation of the presence of paramedical rescue teams in a given community.

LARGE, AUTOMATED, MULTIPURPOSE DATA BASES

Large, automated, multipurpose data bases are systems with a linkage of two or more sets of medical records. The medical records that are linked contain previously collected data on many exposures to medicines, medical outcomes, and potential covariables.

Purposes

These data bases may be used for:

1. Hypothesis-testing studies.
2. Hypothesis-generating studies, also known as fishing expeditions.
3. Incidence estimation studies relating to clinical safety of medicines. A numerator and denominator of one or more adverse reactions are estimated.

Certain types of questions are particularly well suited to address using large data bases. For example, the issue may be to find and evaluate all users of medicine X over the last 10 years and their hospitalizations. To address this question using a large, automated, multipurpose data base information is needed of several

TABLE 7.6 *Characteristics of an ideal data base*

1. The population is well defined
2. Contains records of all inpatient and outpatient medicines prescribed
3. Contains records of all hospitalizations
4. Contains records on all relevant variables
5. All deaths are recorded
6. Original records are readily available and accessible
7. Expertise is available to assist with data searches
8. Each patient is identified by a unique number

types. An ideal data base has data on:

1. A well-defined population.
2. All medicines available.
3. All hospitalization diagnoses.
4. All deaths.
5. All important covariates for patients (e.g., alcohol use, cigarette use, oral contraceptive use, lifestyle).

Unique patient identifiers are used and original records are available to confirm (i.e., validate) data. Characteristics of an ideal data base are listed in Table 7.6, criteria to use in judging a large data base are in Table 7.7, and data included in large data bases are in Table 7.8. The reasons why large, automated, multipurpose data bases are created and details of their funding and maintenance are provided in Chapter 120 and in the references quoted in that chapter.

Advantages

1. *Flexibility.* Large data bases include information on all medicines and diseases of members and are organized in such a way that groups can be formed on the basis of common exposure or event experience. They are also organized so that individual patient histories can be reviewed, and they allow many kinds of hypotheses to be tested.
2. *Speed.* Speed results from the computerized nature of the data base. Another aspect of speed re-

TABLE 7.7 *Criteria to use in judging a large data base*

1. Completeness of the data base: to what degree does it capture all patient exposures to medicines and hospitalizations?
2. Adequacy of the patient identifiers
3. Review of original medical records to confirm patient diagnosis
4. Stability of the patient population, rather than high turnover
5. Relatively large number of the type of patient desired in the data base (e.g., older patients who will have a high incidence of cancer, younger patients who will have a higher incidence of birth defects than old patients)
6. Use of the medicine of choice by the group, rather than being restricted by the formulary (e.g., the medicine may not be in the formulary or the medicine may have a limited duration of use)
7. Confirmatory laboratory tests

TABLE 7.8 *Data that are often included in a large, automated data base*[a]

A. Patient demographics
   1. Code for name
   2. Date of birth
   3. Sex (i.e., gender)
   4. Dates of coverage
   5. Race
B. Medicine data
   1. Generic name of medicine(s) prescribed
   2. Manufacturer's name of each
   3. Date(s) dispensed and number of refills
   4. Dose dispensed
   5. Amount of medicine dispensed
C. Events data
   1. Hospital discharge/diagnoses using a code (e.g., ICD-9)
   2. Deaths
   3. Outpatient diagnostic code (i.e., reason for the medical visit)
   4. Outpatient text notes (this information field is usually limited)
   5. Laboratory orders
   6. Laboratory results
   7. Outpatient procedure
D. Other medical data
   1. Surveys of members of group in data base conducted by the group
   2. Medical history completed on entry into the group
E. Original medical record

[a] Information in categories A to C must be present and linkable.

lates to the ability to reach an initial impression about a problem rapidly, i.e., it is easy to determine how many patients have the disease of interest, medicine of interest, and both. This decreases the number of actual medical records that must be reviewed.

3. *Cost efficiency.* This advantage results from the above two points. A single data base allows many different studies to be conducted, which is more cost effective than building a separate data base for each separate study, as is done in ad hoc pharmacoepidemiological studies. Staff personnel required to conduct the study is reduced. It is also possible to stop a study before a large investment is made (e.g., if it is learned that the proposed study is not feasible to conduct using the specific data base).

4. *Large numbers.* The number of patients with data in many of these data bases is large. This allows much larger studies to be conducted than are possible with either clinical studies or ad hoc pharmacoepidemiological studies. In many cases the entire population of an area or group is enrolled.

5. *Timing of events.* The knowledge of when the medicine was prescribed and when the adverse reaction occurred allows determination of the latent period to be made.

6. *Recall biases.* This problem is not present because patient interviews are not conducted. On the other hand someone decided what information to put in the data base and what information to leave out.

7. *Trend analyses.* May be done by comparing present and past experiences.

8. *Multiple projects.* Because of the nature of the data base many projects may be conducted simultaneously.

9. *Comparison of hospitals.* For data bases in which multiple hospitals are involved, it is easy to compare data between them.

10. *Decision making.* Such data bases are useful in reaching clinical decisions, particularly on issues involving risks.

Inappropriate Uses

It is not recommended to use multipurpose data bases in the following situations:

1. *Complicated patients.* This includes patients with multiple medicines and/or multiple diagnoses; they often introduce many confounding variables into the assessment. Many older patients would fit this category.

2. *Interactions between medicines.* Many factors influence medicine interactions and unless the incidence of the interaction is relatively great, a survey using such a data base is unlikely to reveal the presence of an interaction between medicines.

3. *Continuous outcomes.* This includes frequently measured clinical or laboratory outcomes (e.g., blood pressure, forced vital capacity). In most patients, these data are not routinely collected on a frequent basis. Moreover, the group of patients in which the data are frequently collected are a special group in terms of their pharmaceutical use and clinical treatments (e.g., blood levels of phenytoin will be measured more frequently in patients with unstable seizures and epileptic problems than in those who are more stable).

4. *Dietary factors.* These are rarely measured for patients and incorporated in the large data base.

5. *Compliance issues.* One of the only means of assessing compliance with large data bases is to measure the number and frequency of medicine refills based on the number of days or weeks of medicine dispensed. The appropriateness of refills is assessed.

6. *Nonserious medical events.* These are defined as medical events that do not force a medical contact to be made and therefore medical records are not consistently obtained and entered in the data base. Nonserious is a term that refers to the patient's assessment, and some of these are undoubtedly clinically serious from a physician's perspective.

Nonetheless, reports on these events would not systematically find their way into the data base.

7. *When medical review is impossible.* The most conservative approach to using large multipurpose data bases is to insist on the ability to confirm data in patients' original medical records. Some authors do not believe that this is necessary if the data base has been previously validated.

8. *Insufficient amounts of types of data.* It is desirable for data to exist at multiple levels in the data base. If only one level of data is present, or if insufficient amounts of data exist, then searches are compromised or impossible. The levels include (1) discharge abstracts from the hospital, (2) individual patient identifiers, (3) enrollment or registry file for each patient, plus (4) linkages to pharmacy records and other medical data.

9. *Sensitive medical areas.* In the case of acquired immunodeficiency syndrome (AIDS), the privacy of patient data might be extremely important to protect.

Disadvantages

1. They are not appropriate for all situations (see previous section), particularly if necessary data or linkages to other data bases are not present.

2. Pattern recognition as a tool for understanding the data is difficult to use. It is not easy to focus on patterns if only a small number of patients of interest are found.

3. The large numbers of patients and events contained in such a data base do not guarantee more accurate or precise results. Although random errors may become less important than in studies utilizing smaller data sets, the variations in data quality and confounding factors found in a large, automated, multipurpose data base may have a great impact on the outcomes and conclusions of a study.

4. Unless data (particularly diagnoses) are confirmed (i.e., validated) in the original records, unreliable results will be obtained. Computer-generated findings must be confirmed for accuracy. Patient diagnoses must be confirmed because keypunch operators may easily enter a wrong code for a diagnosis. It is easier to confirm a fracture than it is to confirm a gastrointestinal bleed or other diagnosis based on a physician's judgment.

5. Population of patients entered in the data base may be atypical of the entire patient population.

6. Data may contain many biases, deliberate reporting of certain problems by physicians, sloppy record keeping by the hospital, impact of diagnosis-related groups (DRGs) on patient diagnoses

and discharge rates, and patients who do not interact with the health care system or who are not considered.

7. Certain outcomes (e.g., quality of life) may be quite important, but are not incorporated in the data base.

8. Research is usually near or at the bottom of the list of possible uses and priorities for large data bases in the minds of their administrators, as well as technical experts. Also, administrators of large data bases may change professional positions, and the quality of data in these data bases often changes as an administrator tightens or loosens the quality and standards used. This creates other problems.

9. Linkages are not easy to obtain between large data bases. It takes a great deal of time and effort to create relevant linkages, especially to the degree necessary to conduct research.

Data Bases and Pharmacoepidemiological Studies

Certain prerequisites must be satisfied before a large, automated, multipurpose data base is chosen for a pharmacoepidemiological study:

1. Experienced investigators.
2. Sufficient funding.
3. Data in machine-readable form that may be accessed by the computer.
4. Linkages of hospital diagnostic data to patient numbers. This raises issues of confidentiality. Other linkages (e.g., to hospital's pharmacy records) are desirable.
5. Sufficient quality of data to achieve adequate predictive power.
6. Methods must be used to ensure patient confidentiality in the research activities.

Large, automated, multipurpose data bases may be used in many different ways, depending on the requirements of the project and the characteristics of the data base. One typical problem is to evaluate the hypothesis that medicine A causes a high incidence of adverse reaction B. The approach used would include the following steps.

1. Identify all patients who have taken medicine A, based on prescriptions given and patient name or number.
2. Develop one or preferably more appropriate control groups for these data (e.g., patients with the disease who have not taken medicine A).
3. Check all of the hospitalizations of these patients and analyze them for adverse reactions of interest.
4. Use standard methods to validate the diagnoses, analyze the data, and evaluate the hypotheses.

TABLE 7.9 *Strengths and weaknesses of a clinical data base obtained from treated patients[a]*

A. Strengths
  1. Better generalizability (i.e., extrapolatability) exists because patients are more typical of the patient population than those in a clinical trial
  2. There are lower costs to address a clinical question than funding a new clinical trial
  3. There is rapid accessibility to data that facilitate research
  4. Numerous related questions may also be addressed as an adjunct to clinical trials
  5. No ethical issues arise because data are already present
  6. Compliance of patients was according to normal conditions
  7. Investigator bias tends to be minimal
  8. Changes in patients' outcomes over a long time period may be assessed
  9. Patients may be identified for possible enrollment in a randomized controlled trial
  10. Population-based disease incidence or mortality may be evaluated
  11. Information on the natural history of a disease and prognostic factors may be obtained
B. Weaknesses
  1. Biases may result from a patient population that is not randomly distributed in terms of disease characteristics, prognostic factors, or other aspects
  2. Biases may result from various conditions under which patients were treated
  3. Legal and ethical issues arise in terms of who has access to the data base, who owns the data, and how the data may be used
  4. The validity of data in the data base must be ensured for the questions posed, but this is not always practical or possible
  5. Many methodological issues can arise that would affect the results of any study (e.g., missing data, various definitions, changes in treatment over time, biases in assigning treatments)

[a] The Mayo Clinic is an example.

5. Evaluate potentially confounding factors (e.g., what does the disease itself do).

The more clear the clinical endpoint being evaluated the more likely it is that this approach will be successful. If the endpoints involve determining reasons (e.g., why were specific patients prescribed specific medicines), it will be necessary to go to the data.

The usefulness of large, automated, multipurpose data bases has been increasingly appreciated and documented during the 1980s (anonymous, Lancet 1989a; Faich and Stadel, 1989; Jick and Walker, 1989; Strom and Carson, 1989).

Records of Patients

Patients enter or leave any health group or organization that has a large data base on a more or less continuous basis. It is therefore essential to know each patient's dates of entry and exit to know who was in the group at any particular time. Depending on the hypothesis or question being addressed, it may be unwise to include patients who just entered a plan with those who were in it for a long period or with those who have left. Strengths and weaknesses of a clinical data base obtained from treated patients are listed in Table 7.9.

Record Linkage

The key to record linkage is a common number or code in each pair of data bases being linked. Future progress in the ability to answer important Phase IV questions with large data bases depends to a large degree on increasing the number of links between data bases.

TABLE 7.10 *Advantages and disadvantages of epidemiological study designs[a]*

Study design	Advantages	Disadvantages
Randomized clinical trial (experimental study)	Most convincing design Only design that controls for unknown or unmeasurable confounders	Most expensive Artificial Logistically most difficult Ethical objections
Cohort study	Can study multiple outcomes Can study uncommon exposures Selection bias less likely Unbiased exposure data Incidence data available	Possibly biased outcome data More expensive If done prospectively, may take years to complete
Case-control study	Can study multiple exposures Can study uncommon diseases Logistically easier and faster Less expensive	Control selection problematic Possibly biased exposure data
Analyses of secular trends	Can provide rapid answers	No control of confounding
Case series	Easy quantitation of incidence	No control group, so cannot be used for hypothesis testing
Case reports	Cheap and easy method for generating hypotheses	Cannot be used for hypothesis testing

[a] Reprinted from Strom (1989) with permission of Churchill Livingstone.

OTHER COMPUTERIZED APPROACHES TO POSTMARKETING SURVEILLANCE

1. *Computerized general medical practices.* Data from medical practices may be aggregated into a large computerized data base suitable for postmarketing surveillance studies (Hall et al., 1988).
2. *Pharmacy-based prescription drug histories.* In countries where each patient usually obtains medicines from the same pharmacy, it is theoretically possible to evaluate some medicine-induced adverse reactions that would be treated by another medicine (Petri et al., 1988). This method has serious drawbacks in its current proposed form, and whether it will ever be of value is uncertain.
3. *Linking retail chain pharmacies.* A number of chain pharmacies may be approached to have their retail stores participate in a study whereby each enrolls individual patients. Careful planning can result in rapid recruitment within a short time period. The Upjohn Company used this approach to obtain data on 10,000 minoxidil (Rogaine) users within a 12-month period (Keith Borden, personal communication).
4. *Linking nursing home pharmacies.* A data base may be aggregated from nursing homes to address effects of medicines specifically in the elderly.
5. *Vital statistics.* National data bases of mortality data may be used to monitor results of interventions. These data bases are less commonly used to generate or substantiate hypotheses about adverse reactions.

A number of other methods and variations of conducting Phase IV studies are described by Stephens (1985a), and a summary of advantages and disadvantages of various epidemiological study designs is given in Table 7.10.

MEDICAL RECORD ABSTRACTION STUDIES

One type of Phase IV study involves review of the medical records of a patient who has received a specific treatment. Using a previously prepared form, important data are abstracted that may be analyzed at a later date. This type of study may obtain data on a specific use of a medicine.

CHAPTER 8

Controls Used in Clinical Trials

DEFINITIONS OF CONTROLS IN CLINICAL TRIALS

There are several ways of defining "controls" in clinical trials. Two definitions are used in this book, one specific and one broad. In the specific definition, "control" refers to the group of patients who receive a treatment used for comparison with the trial medicine. Examples include placebo control, active medicine control, and historical control groups.

The broad definition of control relates to the adherence of the clinical trial to a tightly designed protocol. The purpose of this control is to reduce the variability of many factors and biases that might influence the trial. One of the factors that could be designed tightly would be the number and nature of comparison groups of patients.

When many factors are tightly designed the clinical trial is referred to as controlled or well-controlled.

DIFFERENCES BETWEEN A CONTROLLED AND WELL-CONTROLLED CLINICAL TRIAL

There is no consensus on this question; it is apparent that the meaning of "well" must be determined. The preferred implication is that the clinical trial contains state-of-the art controls for studying the specific disease. Thus, "well" is relative and will change over time. It is impossible to give an absolute difference between a controlled and a well-controlled clinical trial.

Does Well-Controlled always Mean Double-Blind?

The answer to this question is "no." Double-blind is only one feature of a well-controlled clinical trial; others include the adequacy of the group(s) used as controls. There are many occasions when a clinical trial is double-blind in name only, because investigators and/or patients are aware of their treatment. Although some of these trials are referred to as well-controlled, they really are not. Some well-controlled clinical trials are retrospective and not prospective. In this case, it would be improper to describe the clinical trial as double-blind.

Whether a clinical trial is well controlled or not is primarily determined in the trial design. It is often impossible to describe a clinical trial accurately as well-controlled until it is completed and an assessment is made that the controls were generally appropriate and that most biases were controlled.

A controlled clinical trial using the broad context of the term is one in which at least some of the elements of the trial design are relatively fixed and are not allowed to vary. The broad concept implies, however, that a trial is neither controlled nor uncontrolled. The greater the number of factors of the trial design that are specified and the more tightly they are delineated, the greater is the control that is built into the trial. In a ''well-controlled'' Phase II study, there traditionally is tight control on most of the important factors that are expected to vary. Since almost all aspects of a trial design may affect the degree to which a trial is controlled, careful thought is required to evaluate which trial design to choose and how tightly to control each aspect of that design. The final trial design chosen is the basic framework or organization of the entire trial, and it should be established only after comprehensive discussions with statisticians, experienced colleagues, and investigators.

Controlled clinical trials of medicines do not always require the use of a placebo or active medicine control group. For example, two groups of patients may be given the same fixed dose of a test medicine with an additional factor (e.g., surgery, concomitant medicine) that acts to help control the trial design.

Add-On Clinical Trials and Nonmedicine Treatments

If patients cannot be taken off their present medicines, then the clinical trial may be designed as an ''add-on'' evaluation of the test medicine. Under those circumstances, controlling the study requires that the name, dose, reason for use, and effectiveness of each concomitant medicine be strictly documented and monitored. Another concern in the control of many clinical trials is the presence of nonmedicine treatment modalities such as individual (or group) psychotherapy or other psychological therapies for testing many medicines that are acting on the central nervous system, or the heat, manipulation, braces, exercises, bed rest, and physiotherapy that are used concomitantly with medication to treat back pain. The presence of nonmedi-

cine modalities may be ignored or either loosely or tightly controlled in the protocol of a medicine trial.

Number of Personnel Interacting with Patients

An example of a relatively minor factor that may be controlled is the number of physicians seen by a patient. In any clinical trial in which more than one physician is involved, it is usually considered optimal to have each patient see the same physician at each visit. The same consideration applies to other trial personnel. Evans (1979) has demonstrated, however, that this is not essential to control in all clinical situations.

TYPES AND NUMBERS OF CONTROL GROUPS

In any clinical trial it is important to control the makeup of the groups of patients being evaluated. The inclusion criteria are the major means by which these groups are made more (or less) homogeneous. The assumption is usually made that the greater the similarity between the groups, the more likely it will be that any differences found in the data from a well-controlled clinical trial are caused by the trial medicine and not by chance or other factors. In choosing the type(s) of individuals who will constitute the control group, it may be important to specify whether patients with the same (or related) disease, random volunteers, healthy medical students, blood donors, nearby laboratory technicians, professional personnel, or others are to be included in the trial. Types of control groups are summarized in Table 8.1.

Multiple Control Groups

The use of multiple control groups (using the specific definition of control) may be the optimal means in some clinical trials to solve the problem of establishing the most suitable control group. This solution may be especially relevant for clinical trials to which large amounts of resources are being devoted to achieve the trial objectives. If, for example, a medicine is being evaluated in patients with a given disease who undergo

TABLE 8.1 *Types of control groups in medicine trials*

1. Concurrent use of placebo
2. Concurrent use of an active medication
3. Concurrent use of no-treatment
4. Concurrent use of a different dose of the same medicine
5. Concurrent use of usual care
6. Historical comparison of data obtained in the same patients on no therapy, the same therapy, or different therapy
7. Historical comparison of data obtained in other patients on no therapy, the same therapy, or different therapy

surgery, it may be necessary to have both a control group with the same disease who are not undergoing surgery and a control group without the disease who are undergoing the same surgery. The use of two (or more) control groups in a clinical trial should be considered if the additional groups will add valuable or essential information. There is a possibility, however, that adding unnecessary control groups in a trial may yield equivocal data and raise additional questions.

Other Control Groups

Another possible control group to include in a trial could be a "no-treatment" observational group, although this approach is not commonly followed in Phase I, II, or III clinical trials of medicines. The no-treatment control group fails to account for the pill-giving ritual and any effects that this event may have on efficacy. A group receiving a low dose of a trial medicine may act as a control group in a design in which a dose-response relationship is being established (see Chapter 94). A usual treatment group has also been included as a control in numerous trials. The principle to follow in establishing a control group is that the control patient population should be as identical to the test treatment population as possible.

Number of Active Medicine and Placebo Control Treatment Groups

When a new medicine is being evaluated, it is often important to incorporate an active medicine and/or a placebo medication as controls into the clinical trial design. A well-established standard medicine (active medicine) may be used as a control in addition to, or in place of, a placebo control group. Active medicine controls such as the use of aspirin in evaluating new analgesics and antiinflammatory agents are an accepted tradition in some areas of medicine development. Before an active control may be incorporated into a pivotal clinical trial design, however, it must be unequivocally demonstrated that the active medicine actually does work (i.e., is active) and is generally accepted to work. This latter point is especially relevant when pivotal trials on investigational medicines are submitted to regulatory bodies, and these agencies must be willing to accept an active medicine's inclusion into the study. The counterargument is that if the active medicine does not work, at least in the clinical trial, then the test medicine may be statistically and clinically superior; this difference gives credence to the evaluated efficacy of the test medicine. Moreover, incorporating an active medicine of questionable efficacy allows a clinical trial to take place when ethics would preclude the use of a placebo group (e.g., in certain types of cancers).

As a general principle, placebo-controlled clinical trials of medicines are preferable to active medicine-controlled trials. If both an active medicine and placebo may be incorporated into a single trial design, then this design is preferable in almost all cases to either the inclusion of an active medicine or placebo control alone. The case against using an active medicine as a control without a separate placebo group was presented by Temple (1982).

In nonpivotal clinical trials of medicines, the investigator or clinical scientist need not have the same constraints about including an active medicine without placebo. The same comments, however, apply to how the results of the trial will be viewed in the medical community. That reception will depend on the quality and nature of the results obtained as well as on the disease being studied. It is not considered ethical to compare a new investigational trial medicine as monotherapy with placebo in certain diseases (e.g., epilepsy). In the case of evaluating a new antiepileptic medicine, add-on trials are often performed with a trial medicine versus placebo. After a new medicine has demonstrated efficacy, then future studies may be designed in which concomitant medicines are removed one at a time (perhaps at 2- to 4-month intervals) to arrive at the point where the new medicine is evaluated as monotherapy.

Basis for Choosing the Active Control Medicine

The basis for choosing a particular medicine for the active control group varies among clinical trials. Some of the most common reasons are listed in Table 8.2. An active medicine may be chosen in some cases to allow the test medicine to perform better and demonstrate significant statistical and clinical advantages.

TABLE 8.2 Basis for choosing a particular active medicine for the control group[a]

1. Established standard medicine to treat the disease studied
2. A new-generation medicine used to treat the disease studied
3. The medicine that is the market leader
4. The medicine that causes the most adverse reactions
5. The medicine that causes a specific adverse reaction
6. A medicine that has the most similar (or different) chemical structure as the test medicine
7. A medicine that is available in the same dosage form as the test medicine
8. The medicine with the greatest variability in a given efficacy or pharmacokinetic parameter
9. A medicine recommended by one or more regulatory authorities
10. A medicine used by other sponsors as an active medicine control
11. A medicine made by the same company that makes the test medicines
12. A medicine not made by the same company that makes the test medicine

[a] Two or more of these factors may be most important for the final decision.

CONTROLS USED IN CLINICAL TRIALS

The terms *controls* and *control group* are used so often in association with clinical trials that they sometimes appear to be permanently connected. This section examines several facets of the word *control*. As a part of speech the term is both a verb (*to control*) and an adjective (the *control* group). Controls may be viewed as "in," "on," "of," "by," and "for" clinical trials.

Control Groups "in" Clinical Trials

In addition to the test medicine or treatment, clinical trials often include one or more control (i.e., comparison) groups. The control group may receive placebo, no treatment, "usual" (i.e., unspecified by protocol) treatment, an active medicine, or a very low dose of the test medicine. (This is the "specific definition" given earlier.)

Controls "on" Clinical Trials

The major groups that exert controls on clinical trials are sponsors, investigators, ethics committees, and regulatory authorities. Under some conditions one (or more) of these groups will be dominant in their influence on the design or conduct of a specific clinical trial. The only groups always involved in clinical trials are investigators and Ethics Committees/Institutional Review Boards (IRBs). For investigational medicine trials, regulatory authorities are also always involved.

Controls "of" Clinical Trials

The types of controls used in clinical trials include historical controls, case-controls, concomitant control groups, or no controls. Also, single-blind, double-blind, or triple-blind controls may be used. Each of these types of controls are discussed elsewhere in this and other chapters.

Controls Used "by" Groups Involved in Clinical Trials

Certain controls refer to the general standards and approaches used by the group(s) that are monitoring the clinical trial and developing the strategy.

Controls "for" Clinical Trials

Controls "for" clinical trials refers to the methods used to ensure the quality of the results, including the careful monitoring of a clinical trial and also the auditing of the results (see Chapters 62 and 63).

PLACEBO CONTROL GROUPS

Reasons to Include a Placebo Treatment Group in a Clinical Trial

The placebo group:

1. Controls for the psychological aspects of being in a clinical trial
2. Helps control for adverse events being attributed to a medicine when they result from spontaneous changes in the disease or from other causes
3. Enables randomization and blinding procedures to be used, although placebo is not required for their use
4. Allows a stronger interpretation of data to be reached; thereby the clinical trial may have a stronger effect on medical practice.

Finally, if an active medicine but not placebo is used in a clinical trial, there is no statistical test to demonstrate that active medicine was effective, regardless of the effect observed. This is because any change observed may have been a placebo effect.

Conditions for the Ethical Inclusion of a Placebo Treatment

Various medical conditions enable a placebo treatment group to be included in a clinical trial:

1. No standard treatment exists.
2. Standard treatment is ineffective or unproven to be effective.
3. Standard treatment is inappropriate for the particular clinical trial.
4. Placebo has been reported to be relatively effective in treating the disease or condition.
5. The disease is mild and lack of treatment is not considered to be medically important.
6. The placebo is given as add-on treatment to an already existing regimen that is not sufficient to treat patients.
7. Allowing concomitant treatment shown to be effective (e.g., antacids for peptic ulcers) on an as-needed basis. The amount of concomitant medicine used is one measure of efficacy in these clinical trials.
8. If the disease process is characterized by frequent spontaneous exacerbations and remissions (e.g., peptic ulcer).
9. "Escape clauses" or points are designed into the protocol.

Other clinical trial designs with placebo exist, but some are controversial and also the use of some depends on regulatory authorities or Ethics Committees in the specific areas concerned. If alternative therapy is available, it is necessary to convince the Ethics Committee/IRB that it is ethical to include a placebo. Some clinical trials are conducted in therapeutic areas in which one does not traditionally consider a placebo to be ethical (e.g., evaluating an oral contraceptive). A placebo could be included, even in contraceptive trials, however, if the women entering the trial desire to become pregnant and are willing to take placebo.

Alternatives to Traditional Placebo Designs

Several clinical trial designs may be considered when neither a two-arm comparison versus placebo nor a two-arm comparison versus an active medicine is desired. Other examples are given in Ch. 6.

1. Compare two (or more) doses of the test medicine with each other and possibly with an active medicine.
2. Use an extremely low dose of the test medicine, plus a dose believed to be effective, in a two-arm clinical trial. A third arm (e.g., active control) could be added. The purpose of this design is to use a subtherapeutic dose that would satisfy the Ethics Committee/IRB and also enable a statistically and clinically significant difference to be observed.
3. Use a fail-safe protocol in which patients are given either placebo or an active medicine, but are taken off their therapy if any deterioration in their status occurs at a later date. In this design, patients are evaluated at appropriate intervals. This design may be considered even in relatively severe diseases in which a placebo group is rarely included (e.g., ulcerative colitis).
4. Rescue-medicine protocol. Patients on placebo or active medicine may take a rescue medicine (e.g., nitroglycerine for angina, antacids for ulcers) as needed. The number of patients using rescue medicine and the amount of concomitant medicines are compared as an outcome measure of effectiveness.

RESPONSES TO THERAPY OBSERVED WITH CONTROLLED VERSUS UNCONTROLLED TRIAL DESIGNS

It has been generally shown that uncontrolled open-label clinical trials yield a greater percentage of positive results (i.e., the therapy is found to be effective) than do well-controlled double-blind trials. The magnitude of the difference in efficacy between controlled and uncontrolled trials is often quite substantial.

Trials with Historical Controls

Sacks, et al. (1982) reported that 44 of 56 historically controlled clinical trials (79%) found that the experi-

mental therapy was better than the control regimen, whereas only 10 of 50 randomized controlled trials (20%) reached a similar positive conclusion. Within a single therapy, the reason for the difference in response between the randomized and historical controlled trials was found to be centered in the control groups. Patients in the historical control group generally did worse than those in the randomized control group. The authors suggested that biases in patient selection may weight the outcomes of historical control trials in favor of the experimental therapy. The major problem with randomized trials is that they often have an inadequate number of patients.

The same authors evaluated historical and randomized controls in clinical trials of six therapies that were evaluated by both methods (Sacks et al., 1983). They observed that 84% of historical controls reported that the therapy was effective and only 11% of the randomized controlled trials evaluating the same therapy demonstrated positive responses.

Selected advantages of historical control trials are shown in Table 8.3. See Lasagna (1982) for additional discussions.

Controlled versus Uncontrolled Trials in Medicine

Psychiatric Trials

A review of 72 psychiatric clinical trials of medicines reported that an 83% rate of positive findings was obtained in open-label trials and a 25% positive rate was obtained in controlled trials (Foulds, 1958). The mean number of schizophrenic patients who were given chlorpromazine and improved was 60% in 23 single-blind trials and 38% in 12 double-blind trials (Glick and Margolis, 1962).

Antidepressant clinical trials reported over a 5-year period (1958 to 1963) were evaluated by Wechsler et al. (1965). They showed that patients in 57% of 30 trials without controls had a mean improvement of 65% or greater, but only 29% of 22 trials with a placebo control group had a mean of 65% or greater improvement (Wechsler et al., 1965). It is of interest that 49% of 55 clinical trials with an active medicine control reported a mean of 65% or greater improvement. This is con-

TABLE 8.3 *Selected advantages of historical control trials*

1. No ethical issues arise about the propriety of randomizing patients
2. Cooperation of fewer patients is required
3. Clinical trials are easier to conduct
4. Patients do not have to provide informed consent in most cases[a]
5. Clinical trials are less expensive
6. Fewer recruitment issues arise

[a] Patients receiving the test medicine in a prospective clinical trial (using historical controls) must provide informed consent.

sistent with the belief that an active-medicine-controlled trial is often not a true control. A larger comparison of controlled or uncontrolled trials with depressed patients (Smith et al., 1969) confirmed the observation of Wechsler et al. Smith et al. found that 58% of 220 trials without controls reported 70% or more of patients improved, whereas only 33% of 98 trials that were controlled and blinded yielded a 70% or greater improvement.

Other Therapeutic Areas

A review of 72 uncontrolled clinical trials on the effectiveness of medicines in treating alcoholism showed that 95% claimed success, whereas only 1 of 17 controlled trials (6%) claimed success (Viamontes, 1972). In pediatrics, Sinclair (1966) classified clinical trials for treatment of respiratory distress syndrome on the basis of whether controls were used. It was reported that 89% of 19 trials without controls reported therapeutic success, but only 50% of 18 trials with controls were positive.

Rheumatoid Arthritis

Within a group of 24 uncontrolled clinical trials evaluating indomethacin in patients with rheumatoid arthritis, it was found that when investigators primarily based efficacy on subjective evaluations, 62% of the trials demonstrated good or excellent responses. When investigators used some objective evaluations, only 25% of the trials demonstrated good or excellent responses (O'Brien, 1968). He also reported that controlled clinical trials were less likely to yield positive data than were uncontrolled trials. This same result was shown for trials evaluating effects of antihistamines and the common cold (West et al., 1975).

Methodological Issues

One approach to comparing outcomes of controlled versus uncontrolled clinical trials is to list all of the controlled trials separately from the uncontrolled ones and to compare their results. This is what was done in the above evaluations of the literature. They clearly showed that the rate of positive outcomes is much greater in uncontrolled trials. A similar approach to the issue is to obtain all of the trials on a specific topic and to sort them by outcome. Then, negative and positive trials can be viewed as to the number or percentage that are either controlled and uncontrolled.

Diethylstilbestrol

Chalmers (1974) followed this process for 13 clinical trials conducted on diethylstilbestrol between 1946 and 1955. Seven of the trials (which included a total of 2,464 patients) resulted in enthusiastic conclusions, and none of these trials used active controls. Two of the seven trials, however, did use historical controls. Six other trials (which included a total of 2,617 patients) were conducted and showed that diethylstilbestrol was ineffective. All six of these clinical trials used controls, and three were conducted double blind. The interpretation of this analysis strongly supports the conclusion that controlled trials are less likely to provide positive data. Nonetheless, there are several types of situations in which use of uncontrolled trials may be useful and justified. This is especially so when the outcomes of the trial are unknown or may be unexpected (e.g., surveillance of safety data).

Controlled versus Uncontrolled Trials in Surgery

An evaluation was made of all surgical and medical clinical trials reported in 16 specialty journals in cardiology in 1971 (Spodick, 1973). It was found that nine of 21 reports of medical therapy were controlled to some degree. On the other hand, none of the 49 surgical reports involved the use of controls. The author of this report primarily blamed the journal editors who accepted and published the surgical trials for perpetuating this double standard. He strongly admonished journal editors to utilize comparable standards for reporting all results.

It is the author's impression that the ratio of controlled surgical trials has increased since that time. This is supported by an evaluation of the neurosurgical literature by Haines (1983). He evaluated 51 clinical trials according to the method of Chalmers et al. (1981) and found "a weak trend toward improvement of the quality score in recent years." He concluded, however, that "few, if any, major neurosurgical questions have been answered by clinical trials." He found that trials in which a statistician was involved had higher scores (i.e., higher quality) than did other trials and recommended this practice. Generally similar results were reported by Sundaresan et al. (1981) in evaluating 53 neurosurgical trials. They observed that the majority of the trials in their sample had an inadequate sample size.

It was reported that 75% of surgeons who conducted 32 uncontrolled clinical trials of portacaval shunt operations for portal hypertension were markedly enthusiastic (Grace et al., 1966). None of the six reports of well-controlled trials were markedly enthusiastic, although three of the six obtained data that were supportive of the operation (Gilbert et al., 1977a, presented the original data plus two additional trials reported to them by the original authors). Gilbert et al. (1977b) stated that in their review of 107 surgical trials, less well-controlled trials tended to give innovative surgeries a higher rate of success than did well-controlled trials.

CHAPTER 9

Sample Size and Number of Parts of a Clinical Trial

SAMPLE SIZE

The number of patients required for a clinical trial (sample size) refers to the number of patients who finish a trial rather than the number who enter. Thus, in planning a clinical trial the definition of a "completed" patient is important to establish, as is the expected rate of patient dropouts and discontinuers. An important result may fail to be detected if too few patients complete a trial.

Another problem that may occur if too few patients complete a clinical trial is that a false-positive result may occur. Although a false-positive result may occur in all trials, the chances of its happening are higher when fewer patients are enrolled than intended. Numerous biases and errors in a clinical trial may be minimized by increasing the number of patients entered until adequate power is obtained.

Types of Sample Sizes to Establish

There are two main types of sample size to consider: fixed and sequential. When a fixed sample size is used in a clinical trial, the number of patients in each group may be fixed (1) at a defined number, (2) within a narrow or broad range, (3) by a minimum number, or (4) by a maximum number. In a sequential trial design, the final number of patients enrolled will depend on analyses performed throughout the trial. In this design, a significant result can be obtained more rapidly and

probably with fewer patients than with a fixed sample, provided that there is a real difference to be detected.

Multiple Sample Sizes within a Single Clinical Trial

If multiple objectives (e.g., both safety and efficacy) are included in a clinical trial, then each will probably require a different sample size. The larger the expected difference in magnitude of the effect between medicine and placebo or between two medicines, the smaller is the sample size that will be required to detect this difference. Thus, a clinical trial generally requires larger sample sizes to demonstrate the smaller differences expected in safety parameters between a medicine and placebo and smaller sample sizes to demonstrate the larger differences expected in efficacy parameters. On the other hand, the smaller variability in data obtained (e.g., with vital signs) may mitigate against the requirement for larger sample sizes to show smaller differences. When multiple sample sizes are computed, the most reasonable one should be utilized. This often requires compromises and an ordering of the most important objectives to be addressed.

HOW SAMPLE SIZES ARE ESTABLISHED

Equal versus Unequal Sample Sizes

Clinically experienced investigators used to estimate the number of patients to include in a clinical trial based on their judgment and clinical expertise. These "guesstimates" of sample size are absolutely invalid and scientifically unacceptable for controlled clinical trials, no matter how experienced the guessers. This same process of guessing sample size occurs in most preclinical experiments conducted today, although there are strong reasons why these scientists should also involve statisticians or more statistical principles in determining sample size for their experiments. For all trials, the required sample size is usually determined by statisticians on the basis of (1) the magnitude of the effect expected (or desired), (2) the variability (often estimated) of the variables being analyzed, and (3) the desired probability (power) of observing that effect with a defined significance level. A power of 80% (0.8) is usually chosen as adequate for most controlled trials, although some groups prefer to use a higher power. Examples of power curves are shown in Fig. 9.1.

In determining sample size, one must address the consideration of establishing a suitable ratio of patients between the two (or among three or more) treatment groups. There are basically two choices: either using equal-size samples in all treatment groups or using un-equal- but proportional-size groups (e.g., using a 2:1 ratio that assigns 12 patients to receive medicine X and 6 to receive placebo). The general rule to follow is that groups of equal size are preferable from a statistical perspective for clinical trials, although not all statisticians would require equal-size groups in all situations. An advantage of using equal-size treatment groups is that the clinical trial gains in power. Losses

of power are not great, however, and may be acceptable if the ratios are no more than 2 or 3 to 1. A disadvantage of using equal-size groups is that more information may be gained on patient responses to a new medicine if unequal-size groups are used and more patients receive the trial medicine.

Some statisticians advocate that all patients should have an equal chance of receiving a clinical trial medicine and thus would assign patients in a trial with a high- and low-dose group and placebo group in the ratio of 1:1:2 (i.e., twice the number on placebo as in either of the other groups). From a practical and often ethical point of view, patients are usually more willing to enroll in a medicine trial when the chance of their receiving active medicine is greatest. Thus, this particular apportionment of patients would make the clinical trial more difficult to initiate than an equal distribution of patients among groups, or an apportionment in favor of the medicine group. The relative importance of the patient's feelings in determining the ratio of group size in a trial relates to a large degree on the particular disease studied and the severity of its symptomatology. A patient with severe chronic pain will be less willing to enter a trial in which the chances of getting placebo are 50% than one in which the chances are about 10%.

The magnitude of the placebo effect that will be observed in a clinical trial is useful to know while planning the trial. The magnitude of the placebo response impacts greatly on sample size and often represents the difference between a clinical trial that demonstrates an effect and a trial that does not. The mag-

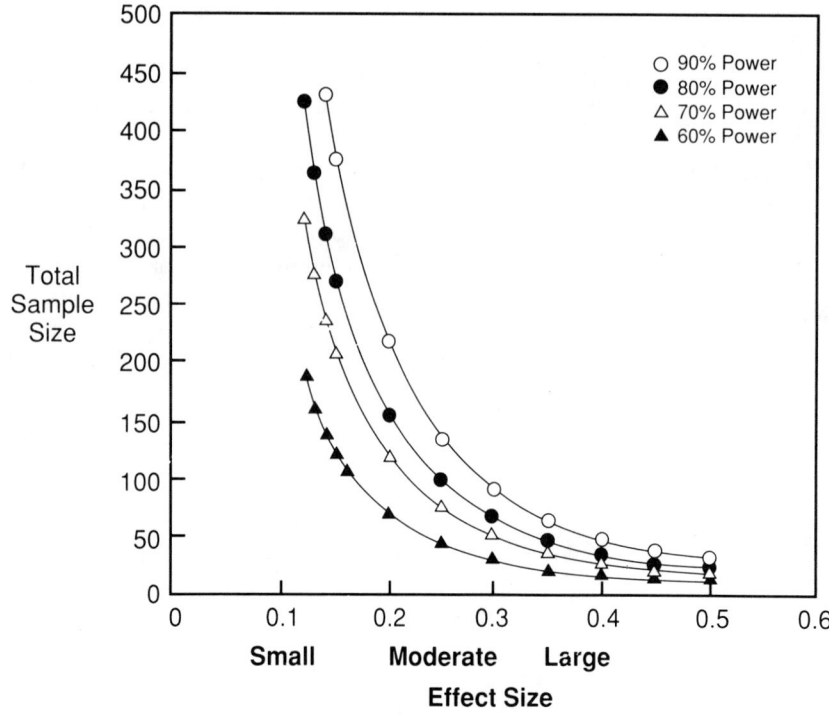

FIG. 9.1 Power curves show sample size needed to obtain various levels of power for various levels of effect size, 5% one-tailed test. (Reprinted from Kraemer, 1986, with permission of J. B. Lippincott.)

nitude of the placebo effect was estimated to be about 35% in most clinical trials (Beecher, 1961, 1962) regardless of therapeutic area; there is widespread support in the literature for this value. On the other hand, the actual magnitude of placebo responses reported in the literature varies over an enormous range (even for double-blinded clinical trials), almost totally independently of therapeutic area. Many factors are responsible for this variation, which is observed even when objective endpoints and measures are used. Use of subjective endpoints and measures does not mean that a large placebo response will be obtained, but it appears to facilitate that finding.

Nomograms

A linear nomogram was presented by Day and Graham (1989) to help calculate sample size for two to five parallel groups of patients.

Trials to Show Equivalence

Calculating the number of patients to enroll in active medicine controlled trials presents special problems. The goal of the trial is to demonstrate equivalence of outcomes, but there are no good statistical tests that can establish equivalence of two treatments. Makuch and Johnson (1986, 1989) discuss this issue and present an approach to use. Very large numbers of patients are usually needed to establish with a high degree of confidence that two treatments have comparable efficacy.

NUMBER OF PARTS OF A CLINICAL TRIAL

If two or more clinical trial designs are included within one protocol, then the trial may be said to have two (or more) parts. Even with only one trial design, there may be two (or more) parts if different patient populations are treated in each part.

Dependent Parts of a Clinical Trial

There are a number of possibilities to consider in determining the number of parts to incorporate into a clinical trial. These parts may be essentially independent, or they may be dependent on each other. A protocol with dependent parts means that a decision must be reached or an evaluation made after the first part has been completed (or has reached a certain point in the protocol) about whether to proceed, or on what basis to proceed, with the next part. It is also possible that specific aspects of the trial design in the second part cannot be finalized until data from the first part are available and analyzed [e.g., an ED_{50} (dose that elicits 50% of the total response) may have to be calculated after part 1 of a trial is completed so that this dose may be given to patients in part 2].

When planning the protocol design, one must decide if significant decisions are to be incorporated into a protocol. If they are, it must be clearly defined who will be making each decision, that is, whether it will be the sponsor, the investigator, or both. It should also be specified if decisions will be made on the basis of blinded or unblinded data and what criteria will be used in reaching the decision.

Independent Parts of a Clinical Trial

Two or more parts of a clinical trial are specified in advance of its initiation. For example, if a given medicine is evaluated in patients with two different diseases using the same protocol design, the medicine may be studied in patients with disease A in part A and disease B in part B. Another example occurs when a pilot and well-controlled trial are both incorporated into one protocol rather than separated into two distinct protocols.

Incorporating Decisions About Trial Designs Into a Protocol

There are two opposite positions that are often taken about how to incorporate major decisions affecting clinical trial design into a protocol. Most investigators and individuals who design trials prefer that a protocol have a clearly defined problem that can be addressed in a clearly defined manner and limit the protocol to that evaluation. According to this viewpoint, any decision that must be made during a trial to define or modify the design requires a new protocol.

The opposite position allows for decisions to be incorporated at specific points in the protocol, which will then permit continuation of the clinical trial with a modification not fully defined at the outset of the trial. The logical extension of this latter approach, however, is a protocol that allows more and more decisions and modifications of design during the clinical trial and it becomes progressively more vague at the outset exactly what will be done at each step of the trial. One variation of this approach is to define the criteria for all modifications to the protocol in advance. Obviously, the Ethics Committee/Institutional Review Board, regulatory bodies, and other groups that must approve the trial will act to prevent extreme examples of allowing unspecified changes in a protocol to occur during a trial.

Conclusions

The number of distinct parts of a clinical trial must be determined in advance even if progression between subsequent parts of the study is "automatic" and does not require any decisions to be made. Since there are many possibilities of which types of trials may be combined into a single protocol, practical and realistic guidelines, as well as the established guidelines of a sponsoring institution (for sponsored trials), must be followed in determining the number and types of parts of a trial.

Randomization Procedures

BACKGROUND

Randomization is a technique to ensure that statistical significance tests may be used in a valid manner. Randomization is not a method to ensure that there is an equal distribution of characteristics between treatment groups. To achieve that goal it is necessary to stratify patients into groups (e.g., males or females, intense or mild pain), each of which is then randomized independently. Alternatively, the method of minimization may be used. Randomization is the process by which patients in a clinical trial are "randomly" assigned to receive one of the treatments being evaluated. Randomization is used to reduce bias in assigning patients to treatment and is usually implemented through a randomization code that assigns patients to different treatments. In a two-period crossover trial, a randomization code usually determines the order by which patients receive treatments. In a Latin-square design with three or more periods, a randomization code is also used to determine the order in which patients receive treatments. Patients may be randomized to different treatment groups in open-label, single-blind, or double-blind trials, but its use is most important in double-blind trials. It is in double-blind trials that a suitable process of randomization is essential to determine how well the blind will be maintained and, in part, how the results of the trial will be viewed and judged.

Simply using an alternating ABABAB order for assigning patients to one of two treatment groups (coded A and B) is not acceptable for double-blind clinical trials. Other unacceptable methods of patient randomization are listed in Table 10.1. The investigator will tend to develop biases that one treatment is preferable, and patients may be purposely placed in one group or the other by the investigator. Also, if the trial code is broken for one patient, then it is effectively broken for all patients.

Advantages and Limitations

Advantages of using randomization in a controlled trial include the following:

1. Randomization procedures attempt to decrease the effect of interjecting one's own biases (either known or unknown) in assigning patients to treatment groups. They should minimize the differences in relevant characteristics of the groups receiving treatment in a parallel design.
2. Randomization permits certain statistical methods to be used with the resulting data.
3. Randomization allows for blinding of the patient and the investigator in the sense that if the blind is broken for one patient, it is not broken for all.
4. Randomization procedures are the current norm for demonstrating efficacy and safety of investigational medicines.

Two limitations of using randomization in a clinical trial are these:

1. The randomization procedure alone often will not adequately eliminate the differences between the treatment groups. If baseline values were widely

TABLE 10.1 *Examples of unacceptable methods of patient randomization to treatment groups*

1. Alternate assignments (e.g., every other patient entered is assigned to one group)
2. Alternate day assignments (e.g., patients entered on even number days enter one arm of the trial and patients entered on odd number days enter the other arm)
3. Birthday assignments (e.g., certain months or days are used as the basis of patient assignment)
4. Coin tosses (i.e., coin is flipped once for each patient; those for which the result is heads are assigned to one group, and those for which the result is tails are assigned to the other)
5. Card drawn by the investigator (e.g., odd cards and queens are assigned to one group, even cards, jacks, and kings are assigned to the other)
6. Initials of patients (e.g., first names beginning A to K are assigned to one group and L to Z are assigned to the other group)[a]

[a] For three (or more) groups a slightly modified division may be made.

divergent between the two treatment groups, it could create a major problem for the interpretation of the results. If there was a characteristic known to have a bearing on the outcome of the clinical trial that was not found to be equal in the two groups studied, then an interpretation of the results obtained might be seriously challenged. For example, if a medicine is being evaluated for prevention of myocardial infarction in patients with heart disease and the risk factors for having a myocardial infarction were not evenly divided between the two groups chosen by randomization procedures, then an interpretation of the results might be seriously questioned. Randomization will not ensure an equal distribution of risk factors or other relevant patient characteristics to each treatment group. There is a technique called stratification that can minimize the probability of obtaining an unequal distribution of important patient or disease characteristics between groups. The pros and cons of stratification are discussed later in this chapter.

2. Incorporating an appropriate randomization process into a clinical trial may be complex or difficult to administer and thus pose practical problems that will have to be considered and solved in advance.

At What Stage in a Clinical Trial Should Randomization Be Performed?

In designing the protocol it is apparent that patients should generally be randomized after screening is completed. Otherwise, numerous data collection form packages may be started for patients who do not complete and pass screening tests. Patients should also sign the informed consent form before they are considered enrolled in the trial and may be randomized to treatment.

The major choice in randomizing patients is whether to do it at the start or at the end of an active baseline. The advantage of waiting until a baseline is completed before randomizing patients is that any adverse events that arise during this baseline period are then not attributed to a specific treatment. This may prevent an investigational medicine from unnecessary and unfounded criticism because a patient randomized to receive treatment with the medicine had a serious adverse event during baseline, which according to intention-to-treat principles is associated with the medicine (even though the patient never received any medicine). The time at which patients are randomized to treatment may be quite different from the time at which they are considered to be enrolled in the clinical trial, and also may be fixed by the protocol.

There are many methods used to randomize patients. The basic types of randomization are (1) simple randomization, (2) block randomization, (3) systematic randomization, (4) stratification, and (5) minimization.

SIMPLE RANDOMIZATION

Simple randomization is a procedure that uses a code to assign all patients to receive one of two (or more) different medicine treatments at the start of the trial (i.e., prior to treatment). This code is usually generated prior to the initiation of the trial and usually assigns treatments based on the order of patients admitted to the trial.

In clinical trials in which the same patients receive progressively higher doses of a trial medicine at each visit, as in some Phase I single-dose trials, it may be advantageous to carry out a new randomization at each clinic visit (dosing period) for patients to receive either the trial medicine or placebo. Alternatively, the original randomization of patients to treatment groups could be maintained throughout the trial. One advantage of conducting a new randomization of patients prior to each dosing is that it may minimize the psychological apprehension of volunteers who had experienced adverse reactions and believe that they have received the active trial medicine. Another advantage is that a larger number of patients will be exposed to the test medicine. One disadvantage, however, is that the pharmacokinetic data obtained will not be as complete, since each patient may receive different doses of a medicine or different numbers of doses. Another disadvantage will be that interpretation of dose–response data will be more difficult.

BLOCK RANDOMIZATION

In the block randomization method, a block size (e.g., 4, 8, or 20 patients) is chosen, and the number of patients assigned to each treatment is proportional (1:1, 2:1, 3:1) within the block size chosen. For example, if a block size of eight is chosen and there are two treatments, then for every block of eight patients entered, if a balanced block (equal numbers of patients are assigned to each treatment) is used, four will receive one treatment and four will receive the other. It follows that the block size chosen should be divisible by the total number of treatments (e.g., for three treatments, block sizes of 6, 9, and 18 are possible). The main advantage of using a block randomization is that if the clinical trial does not enroll the full number of patients expected, there will still be an equal or approximately equal number of patients in each treatment group for a balanced block and proportional numbers of patients in each group for a proportional block randomization.

A variation on the block randomization is to use blocks of variable size, although there are not many instances when this precaution would be necessary. The first block is sometimes larger than subsequent blocks, especially if it is believed that the investigator will attempt to "second guess" the assignment of patients to treatment. A block size of two is not used (except for matched pairs), since only two possibilities exist for randomizing patients to treatment A or B (i.e., AB and BA). If a block size of four is chosen, then there are six possible choices for randomizing patients in balanced blocks of four patients: ABAB, AABB, ABBA, BABA, BBAA, and BAAB. As the block size increases, the number of possible combinations of creating a balanced or proportional block increases.

It is advisable to use block randomization in clinical trials instead of simple randomization. The one exception is when it is known with certainty that all patients desired to be enrolled will be enrolled. This often occurs in Phase I dose-tolerance or pharmacokinetic trials in which all patients or volunteers start the trial at one time.

SYSTEMATIC RANDOMIZATION

In systematic randomization, patients are assigned to receive treatment based on (1) a random order in the first block, whose pattern is then repeated in all subsequent blocks; or by (2) a sequential assignment to treatment. Two examples of this latter approach are when alternate treatments are assigned to patients as they are enrolled in a clinical trial and when every *n*th patient receives a different treatment.

STRATIFICATION

It is quite common to assign patients to treatment groups, based on their sex, age, weight, race, intensity of disease, disease risks, or any other relevant prognostic variable that is expected to have an important influence on the outcome of the clinical trial. Assignment of patients to groups based on a relevant factor is termed stratification. Although patients may be stratified on the basis of several factors, the resulting increase in the number of strata obtained and decrease in stratum size limit the number of factors that may be used with this method. Thus, patients are stratified based on the smallest number of characteristics possible. Within each stratum, patients are randomized to receive one of the clinical trial treatments.

Stratification is more important with small sample sizes since the need for this technique usually decreases to a degree in clinical trials with an extremely large sample size. One problem of stratification is that it creates additional administration to deal with, beyond that imposed by other types of randomization. It may also divide a clinical trial of two groups into a trial of several smaller groups if the outcome of the data is not consistent in the subgroups and cannot be combined. Stratification may be performed either prospectively or retrospectively in regard to the time of conducting the clinical trial. If it is performed prospectively, then one usually cannot also use stratification at the end of the trial (using subgroup analyses) to balance treatment groups. If stratification is only performed retrospectively, then it involves subgroup analysis, which is a topic that has strong proponents and critics.

MINIMIZATION

An interesting variation of the randomization process is a technique termed minimization (Taves, 1974). Minimization is a sophisticated form of stratification. In stratification, only one or a few factors believed to have a significant impact on the results are used to construct similar groups, whereas in minimization all known factors that might possibly have an important effect on treatment outcome are generally included. The goal of this technique (as well as stratification) is to minimize the differences in makeup of the two (or more) treatment groups at the outset of the clinical trial. Parameters may be weighted differently to give selected ones more importance. This process can be most effectively utilized if patients are entered slowly or in groups. Clinical examples of the use of minimization are illustrated in two trials by Weintraub et al. (1980, 1983).

In the process of minimization the first X number of patients (e.g., 20) entered in a clinical trial are randomly assigned to treatment groups by simple or block randomization methods. At that time the characteristics of all patients in each group are assessed. Each subsequent patient who is to be randomized is assigned to that group where the total difference from the other groups is minimized. A central site or individual maintains these data and must be available during all times when patients may be entered. The person at the central site usually has a simple computer program that indicates which assignment would minimize the differences in prespecified variables among treatment groups. He or she assigns a code for each patient based on patient characteristics and informs the investigator, or other person at the site of the code's identity.

OTHER VARIATIONS OF RANDOMIZATION PROCEDURES

There are instances in which one does not wish to have a particular patient group overrepresented in the clinical trial. Instead of stratifying patients to balance the treatment groups, it may be a useful ploy to introduce a quota system. In this method, a specific group (e.g., patients over a specified age) is restricted to a specific percentage of the total trial sample. Thus, one subgroup cannot be overrepresented in the total sample beyond the desires of the protocol's authors.

An alternative to using minimization when there are many prognostic factors to control is to obtain an overall clinical index of risk factors. Patients can then be grouped (i.e., stratified) into two (high- and low-risk scores), three (high-, middle-, and low-index scores), or another number of different treatment groups. The possibility still exists, however, that one or more of the prognostic factors will not be evenly distributed among the groups.

Other variations of the traditional randomized clinical studies are occasionally proposed (e.g., Zelen, 1979). Zelen proposed a means to compare new and standard treatments whereby one-half of the patients choose between the new treatment and the standard treatment. The other half of the patients receive the standard treatment. It usually takes a number of years before the medical community evaluates and accepts the merits of new approaches. The trend in clinical trial methodology over the last 25 years has been towards including more appropriate control groups and objective approaches to developing trial designs.

Another variation on the theme of randomization concerns the nature and size of the unit that is being randomized. Although this unit is the individual patient in most clinical trials, there are occasions on which it may be more practical to randomize treatments by hospital, investigators, communities, large geographical areas, school, clinic, worksite, household, or other factors. This approach may be considered for trials conducted in developing countries with limited resources. In such cases, entire geographical areas may be randomized. This approach, however, may severely con-

found treatment with centers (geographical areas) and hamper the interpretation of statistical tests. Another approach has entire treatment centers arbitrarily assigned to one group, especially when one treatment requires the use of expensive or rare equipment that is not widely distributed. There are obvious disadvantages to this technique, but this method may allow useful trials to be conducted when more traditional randomization schemes are not practical.

An innovative method for assigning patients to provider teams in hospitals was proposed (Cargill et al., 1986) as a means of conducting research on medical care. The Cargill method is being used at three hospitals. The authors describe a long history of this type of practice (e.g., Cook County Hospital in Chicago assigned every fifth medical case and every fourth surgical case to homeopathic physicians during the 1880s). Various types of research questions that may be appropriately addressed using this type of patient assignment are mentioned.

OBTAINING AND USING RANDOMIZATION CODES

The process that is usually followed to obtain and use a randomization code is shown in Fig. 61.4. The randomization procedures should be developed and the codes generated by individuals trained in statistics who have adequate resources for obtaining the necessary codes. Numerous questions relating to group size and stratification should be discussed with statisticians, and all elements in the clinical trial design clarified prior to the request for a randomization code(s). The method by which the investigator assigns patients to treatment (i.e., does he call the monitor or a central office, or does giving the appropriate bottle with the patient's number assign the proper treatment, etc.) must be determined and clearly specified prior to initiation of the study. If the monitor(s) is to remain blind to patient randomization, then the code that is generated must be delivered to other trial personnel or to individuals who will package the medicine, whether at the investigator's site or at the sponsoring institution.

Investigators conducting unsponsored trials and sponsors of clinical trials should keep randomization codes in two separate places, in case one set is lost or inaccessible when needed. The codes may be maintained by the statisticians who generated them to help ensure that the trial's blind is not broken. If they are printed on double or triple tamper-proof labels that are placed on the patient's data collection form, then the investigator has easy access to the code if it must be broken. Whatever method is used, the integrity of the codes should be confirmed at the conclusion of the clinical trial.

Identification Codes to Maintain Patients' Anonymity Throughout a Clinical Trial

In some clinical trials in which data collection is to be done on two or more occasions (e.g., pretest and post-test) there may be a need to maintain patient anonymity with an investigator and to link each of the patient's replies. A satisfactory solution is for the patients to generate their own code.

A simple example of a code generated by the patient was a five-component one used with school children (i.e., first letter of the: middle name, month of birth, gender, street name, and mother's first name). Damrosch (1986) proposed an eight-component code based on the (1) first letter of mother's first name, (2) first letter of father's first name, (3) number of older brothers, (4) number of older sisters, (5) whether the patients first name began with a letter in the first or second half of the alphabet, (6) first letter of birth month, (7) whether patient was born in an even numbered year, and (8) first letter of patient's middle name.

CHAPTER 11

Screening, Baseline, Treatment, and Posttreatment Periods

The various periods of a single clinical trial are defined as *screening, baseline, treatment*, and *posttreatment* periods. One variation is to combine screening and baseline as a pretreatment period. Another variation is to divide treatment into dose ascension, dose maintenance, and dose taper. A washout period of current medicines could also be included as a separate part of the pretreatment or treatment period. The actual designation and duration of the periods are defined by the clinical trial protocol.

SCREENING PERIOD

Purpose and Types of Screens

A screen is an evaluation of potential patients to determine their eligibility to enter a clinical trial. This evaluation may be entirely based on an interview or review of medical records, but in almost all prospective clinical trials, a series of tests (e.g., physical examination, laboratory evaluations) are conducted.

Screens may also be conducted in stages so that only patients who pass an initial verbal screen are evaluated with more time-consuming and expensive tests.

An initial screen is often conducted by telephone or medical record review prior to the first clinic visit. This may be performed with a prepared form that addresses the most salient points of inclusion and exclusion, which helps to "screen" many patients who do not meet the inclusion criteria. Pharmacy records may also be "screened" in some instances (e.g., in nursing homes) to find suitable patients. A relatively straightforward approach of conducting this initial screen is to list all inclusion (and exclusion) criteria that can be requested by telephone or evaluated in medical records as a series of questions on a preprinted form.

Presenting Data on Number of Patients Screened

When the number of patients "screened" is described, it must be clarified whether this number refers to the patients "interviewed" or to the number tested and examined to determine their suitability for the clinical trial. In some trials, additional numbers are presented, such as the number of patients who constituted the total pool of potential patients and the number of those who were eligible for the trial but did not consent to take part.

Transition from Screen to Baseline

The time that may elapse between the completion of screen and onset of baseline (or treatment period) is usually specified in the protocol. If an "excessive" time elapses between screen and baseline, and certain entry criteria (primarily clinical signs and symptoms) have changed, it is possible to allow a modified screen to be used for reevaluating potential patients who had already been screened.

Screening Tests

The specific tests that may be conducted during the screening period are usually listed in a time and events schedule. See Chapter 24. The time period during which a screening examination may be conducted is usually indicated in the protocol (e.g., 2 to 6 days prior to initiation of baseline). Results of all relevant screening tests should be obtained and reviewed (if at all possible) prior to formally initiating the baseline or treatment period. Patients have been admitted to the treatment (or baseline) period in many clinical trials while the results of some of their screening (or baseline) tests were still pending. If important abnormal results (e.g., laboratory data) are noted after the patient has already entered the trial, and the patient is allowed to continue with treatment, the entry criteria will probably be breached. In addition to this "technical" problem, a serious medical and ethical problem may develop if a patient was already treated with the trial medicine and developed a severe adverse reaction that could have been prevented.

Double-Screen Technique

A commonly used method to eliminate patients who do not meet strict and specific inclusion criteria is to repeat the battery of screening tests one or more times. This procedure decreases the chance of false-positive results arising in the parameters tested as a result of normal patient variation after patients are randomized to treatment. A double screen confirms that patients' values are within specific limits over a defined period of time. The relative stability of values measured during the screen may be applied to laboratory, other safety, or efficacy parameters.

BASELINE PERIODS

The baseline period is used to obtain measurements that will determine whether the clinical trial groups are comparable at the start of treatment and also to provide values (in some trials) against which treatment values may be compared. Baseline periods are not required in all protocols, and the screening period may function as a baseline in some trials, that is, the data obtained during screening may serve as baseline values for comparison with treatment values. Patients are usually randomized to one of the treatment groups at the end of the screening period or baseline.

Types of Baselines

Baselines may be active, historical, or both. Active baselines refer to a time period when data are collected after the protocol has been initiated, whereas historical baselines utilize data (often collected during screen) that were generated, though not necessarily recorded, before the patient entered the protocol.

When Do Baselines Occur?

The baseline period does not always follow the screening period. If an active baseline is incorporated into the study design, then it usually follows the screening period and formal admission of the patient into the clinical trial. When historical baselines are to be obtained, then this baseline period may actually precede or overlap the screening period. The protocol should clearly define the time limits of each of these periods and their relationship to each other.

Baselines are not restricted to pretreatment assessments. Baselines may be interspersed during a clinical trial, such as between different doses of the same medicine, between the two periods of a two-period crossover, or between successive periods of a Latin-square design trial. Utilizing multiple baselines in a trial has the advantage that carryover (residual) effects may be more easily investigated.

How Long Should a Baseline Last?

Numerous factors must be considered in determining the length of a baseline period. These factors relate to the nature of the disease, characteristics of the patients and medicine(s), location and setting of the clinical trial, and available resources. One must determine whether any time may elapse between termination of baseline and start of the treatment period. It is the author's view that this would be a poor practice in most trials.

What Data Constitute the Baseline?

At least two sets of measurements should be obtained during baseline (whenever possible) to optimize the validity of the data and calculate its variability for comparing baseline data with those obtained during treatment within a group or for comparing baseline values between groups. If more than one baseline value is obtained in a specific test, there is the question of whether all values should be averaged or whether only specific values (e.g., the last two or three) should be averaged, or possibly only the most recent (last) value should be used. These are all relevant concerns to address prior to initiating a clinical trial, although it may be necessary to conduct or utilize data from a pilot trial in order to obtain a sound basis for reaching a decision on this issue.

It may be impossible to obtain all necessary information on a patient during baseline (e.g., if the treatment must start before it is possible to obtain either important laboratory data or various measures of a disease needed to assess the patient's suitability for enrollment based on the inclusion criteria). This situation often occurs when one wants to initiate treatment rapidly in patients with an acute disease. Patients are therefore sometimes entered before their eligibility is fully assessed. Various alternatives for dealing with this potential problem should be addressed in the protocol or by providing verbal or written instructions to the investigator. For example, the entry criteria could be adjusted prior to the clinical trial to allow for this possibility. Alternatively, patients who are later found not to fit the protocol's entry criteria could be dropped or possibly enter an open-label or single-blind trial that is conducted simultaneously.

Choosing Control Values for Patients with a Continually Changing Baseline

Imagine that a new medicine is being tested in alcoholics for its effect in diminishing the intensity and duration of withdrawal symptoms. Patients enter the clinical trial when they have high blood alcohol levels. After 12 hours patients are in a state of withdrawal, just prior to receiving the test medicine. After 4 to 6 days patients are becoming "normal." One day before their release they become stressed by the prospect of reentering their milieu, possibly because they are without work and without a home. The difficult question in this clinical trial is: What control values should be used for psychomotor tests given to assess improvement in the relevant parameters?

The major choice in this example is between using patients as their own control and choosing a separate control group. If patients are used as their own control, one must determine when during the clinical trial, or how long afterwards, they should be tested. Values in a test obtained shortly prior to giving patients the medicine cannot constitute a true baseline, and there is no truly stable period during treatment in which to obtain a true baseline. If a control group is included, should they be normal volunteers matched by age or should they be former alcoholics who are (confirmed) not drinking? Should patients be matched according to quantity of alcohol imbibed, degree of impairment, or disease? There are no clear answers to these types of dilemmas, but this is a case in which a baseline may actually be obtained in patients after their participation in the clinical trial is completed.

Extended Baseline

An extended baseline is one that is prolonged by a set period or until a specified event occurs. If the extended baseline is between two legs of a crossover, the baseline is extended so that a patient's values for one or more parameters returns to the original baseline level. Alternatively, the baseline may be extended at the outset of a clinical trial if a patient's values for one or more parameters have not yet achieved a certain level. The maximum time of extension allowed should be indicated in the protocol.

TREATMENT PERIODS

Establishing the length of the treatment period requires careful consideration of many factors. The primary factors relate to the objective(s) of the clinical trial. Other important factors include previous medicine experience with the trial medicine, toxicological data, stability and variability of the disease, phase of medicine evaluation, and the intended duration of medicine use in the general patient population that may be given the medicine.

Number of Evaluations

The frequency of outpatient visits (or inpatient evaluations) during the treatment period is usually an issue that is evaluated in planning a clinical trial. Many factors will influence the decision of when patient visits (evaluations) are scheduled and whether the visits are to be equally or unequally spaced throughout the treatment period. In general, visits are often scheduled more frequently at the start of a trial and less often as the trial progresses. Each trial will have different factors to consider in determining the appropriate number of patient visits, but the additional time, cost, and energy that each visit entails must be considered for patient, staff, and investigator in addition to consideration of the value of the additional data that will be generated. It is often convenient to schedule patient visits in even multiples of days, weeks, or months (e.g., every 2 weeks for four visits, then every 4 weeks for the remaining visits).

Endpoints Measured

An important aspect of treatment that is related to clinical trial design concerns the endpoint chosen for use in a trial or treatment. The endpoint is usually merely alluded to in the trial objectives in terms of assessing the efficacy and/or safety of the treatment even when specific tests are identified.

If medicine effects on safety parameters are the major objectives of the clinical trial, then a decision should be reached in the planning stage as to whether the termination of the trial is defined as (1) the point at which adverse reactions begin to appear or (2) the point at which adverse reactions become more marked and medicine intolerance appears. Another alternative is to test the safety of doses that have been, or are expected to be, tested for efficacy in other trials. A pharmacological, laboratory, or clinical endpoint or a combination of these may be used in a trial. Other aspects related to medicine treatment, including dosage and adverse reactions, are dealt with in other chapters of this section.

Dose Ascension and Dose Taper Periods

The dose ascension and dose taper periods of a clinical trial (when present) are considered part of the treatment period during evaluation or consideration of safety. When efficacy is evaluated, the dose ascension and dose taper periods may or may not be considered part of the treatment period. Although the decision is based on the half-life of the medicine, duration of treatment, mechanism of the medicine, and trial design, the general rule is to exclude this period from the efficacy analysis if it is reasonable and possible to do so, but to indicate this decision in the protocol.

POSTTREATMENT PERIOD

Purpose

Posttreatment refers to the time after the trial medicine has been discontinued. The major purposes of a posttreatment period are to check for any withdrawal effects and to ensure the patient's safety. The posttreatment period may also be useful to study residual effects of treatment. In evaluating the need for a posttreatment period in a clinical trial of a medicine (as well as its duration), one may consider (1) previous experience with the medicine in similar patient populations, (2) whether the medicine dosage is being tapered slowly or abruptly stopped, (3) the clinical status of the patients, (4) whether patients are in a secure and/or con-

trolled environment, and (5) the pharmacokinetic characteristics of the medicine.

Methods of Conducting a Posttreatment Evaluation

Clinic visits to conduct posttreatment evaluations may be scheduled as part of a clinical protocol. This is particularly relevant if withdrawal effects are expected or if the clinical trial is particularly designed to evaluate the return of original symptoms and signs of disease (e.g., how long does it take them to recur?). Ad hoc scheduled clinic appointments may be made. Another possibility is to assess one or more particular clinical endpoints at annual clinic visits.

Duration of a Posttreatment Period

The posttreatment period may last for a fixed number of days (or weeks or months) after treatment is completed, or it may last until a predetermined date is reached. In the latter case, each patient may have a different length of posttreatment evaluation. Either one or several posttreatment clinic visits may be scheduled for all patients, and the return of specified (or all) parameters to their original baselines may be required. It is important to schedule a clinic visit at a time when virtually all of the medicine has been eliminated from the patient's body (five or more half-lives) and any expected withdrawal reactions will have had a chance to occur.

The posttreatment evaluation and data collection may be conducted by telephone in appropriate trials or under selected conditions (e.g., if the patient has moved away from the area).

Use of the Term Follow-Up

The term *follow-up* is used in different ways depending on the type of clinical trial described. If the study evaluated a surgical procedure rather than a medicine, then the postsurgical period is usually described as follow-up. In the case of therapeutic or Phase I medicine trials, as described in this book, follow-up is used synonymously with posttreatment. In studies in which a medicine (or vaccine) is given for prophylactic protection, follow-up is the period of time after the medicine (or vaccine) is given, during which contact is maintained with the patient. This definition is also used in many cases in which diet, exercise, or some other factor is altered in an attempt to reduce a known risk factor for a given disease. The distinction among the above usages of the term ''follow-up'' is that in a therapeutic medicine trial it is usually a short period of minor importance to the trial objectives, whereas in many surgical, prophylaxis, and risk-factor reduction trials it is usually an extremely important part of the trial, in which critical data are obtained that address the trial objectives.

CHAPTER 12

Patient Populations, Clinical Trial Environment, and the Placebo Effect

CHOOSING A PATIENT POPULATION

Numerous questions must be addressed in determining the general makeup of patients who will enter a clinical study. Some of these are addressed in the following sections.

Total Number of Patients and Sites

Will normal volunteers or patients with a specific disease be most suitable? What total number of patients should be enrolled to address the clinical trial objectives adequately? Is it likely that the required number of patients can be enrolled at one site, or will a multicenter trial (two or more sites) be required? Those questions are generally discussed with statisticians, and the power of detecting clinically meaningful treatment differences should be evaluated.

Inpatients versus Outpatients

Should the study be conducted with inpatients (patients kept in a hospital or clinic setting), outpatients, or both? In some studies, patients are entered and studied as inpatients and then continue the clinical trial on an outpatient basis. In other trials, outpatients enter the hospital (or clinic) one or more times for various periods and, after discharge, return to their outpatient status. Another alternative is to enroll both inpatients and outpatients in a trial, although this approach may have significant drawbacks for interpreting the data obtained.

Use of Alternate or Replacement Patients

Should some patients be enrolled as alternates at the start of a medicine trial? "Alternate" patients are defined as those patients who complete the screen and usually the baseline periods and are ready to be enrolled in the treatment period. Alternate patients may enter the trial without delay if they are housed nearby in the event one or more of the enrolled patients does not arrive at the trial site at the scheduled time, does not pass the screen (or baseline) examination, or must be discontinued for any reason once the clinical trial has begun. "Replacement" patients refers to patients who have not completed the screen or baseline even though they might have been recruited prior to the dropout of the patient they have replaced.

It may be relevant to measure or assess the expectations of patients entering a medicine trial. It has been shown in a double-blind study of two antiinflammatory medicines plus placebo that treatment outcomes were related in part to patient expectations (Berry et al., 1980).

Conducting a Clinical Trial in Nonresponders

Although it is usually desirable to avoid a large number of nonresponders in a clinical trial, there are occasions when they should be or must be sought. A relatively toxic medicine for a poorly treated condition (e.g., severe psoriasis) should initially be tested in Phase II for efficacy and safety in nonresponders. If the medicine possesses adequate safety, it may then be tested for efficacy in more responsive patients, based on enhanced benefit-to-risk considerations (i.e., lesser risks than originally thought possible). A similar situation is the use of terminal cancer patients to test Phase I safety, i.e., to determine the maximally tolerated dose.

Another case in which nonresponders are desired is when a medicine acts by a mechanism of action different from other medicines used to treat the disease. A group of nonresponders to traditionally used medicines would be of great interest to evaluate with the new agent. A stronger clinical trial design could be created by having all purported nonresponders treated with standard medicine initially. Only confirmed nonresponders would be assigned to one of two or more treatment groups.

Less Commonly Used Patient Populations

There are occasions when less commonly used patient populations may provide more valuable information or are more easily recruited. Some of these populations include (1) nursing home residents, (2) twins, (3) military recruits, and (4) patients in military hospitals.

Obtaining a Medical History

Sufficient time should be allocated to obtain a relatively complete medical history. Rushing through this step of the screening examination may result in failure to uncover important information. When historical data are of particular importance, patients' families may be interviewed or, preferably in most situations, hospitals or physicians' offices may be contacted for corroborative or additional information. To improve patient recall of previously used medicines, it is useful to have a pill board prepared. Many patients who are unable to remember names of medicines they have taken have no trouble identifying them by visual inspection.

PHASE I TRIALS

Types of Subjects Enrolled in Phase I Trials

Four major types of subjects are enrolled in Phase I trials:

1. Normal male volunteers are the most commonly used group in Phase I clinical trials. Occasionally, postmenopausal normal women or normal women with either tubal ligations or other acceptable means of preventing conception are enrolled.
2. Patients who are severely ill with the disease to be treated are used in clinical trials when it is unethical to expose normal volunteers to the test medicine. This is because of expected toxicity of the medicine (e.g., anticancer treatments).
3. Patients with the target disease who are stable and generally healthy are sometimes used to evaluate pharmacokinetics (e.g., for antiepileptics) or safety (e.g., for antiarrhythmics). This is particularly important if the pharmacokinetic profile is expected to differ between normals and patients.
4. Surrogate patients who are severely ill, but do not have the targeted disease, may be evaluated in Phase I clinical trials. An example would be when patients with acquired immunodeficiency syndrome (AIDS) who do not have *Pneumocystis carinii* pneumonia (PCP) are enrolled to test a new anti-PCP medicine in Phase I.

When Should Patients and Not Volunteers Be Enrolled in Phase I Clinical Trials?

There are four major categories of reasons for enrolling patients rather than volunteers in clinical trials: ethical, regulatory, pharmacokinetic, and other types. Ethical reasons require the use of patients when the medicine is too toxic (or potentially toxic) to expose normal volunteers. This includes most new medicines tested in Phase I anticancer, antiarrhythmic, and anti-AIDS clinical trials. Regulatory authorities in some countries (e.g., Germany) prohibit the enrollment of patients in initial clinical trials if it is ethical to use volunteers. Some regulatory authorities have required that initial clinical trials of disease-modifying antiarthritis medicines be conducted in patients, even though the investigators and Ethics Committees/Institutional Review Boards (IRBs) were willing to enroll volunteers. The third category (i.e., pharmacokinetics) applies when patients are known or suspected of having altered metabolism or absorption. A well-known example is that of epileptic patients who have induced microsomal enzymes as a result of other concomitant antiepileptic medicines. The last group of reasons would include those of scientific or medical interest.

Use of Volunteers or Patients

The first question to address is whether normal volunteers (usually males and possibly postmenopausal women or those with a tubal ligation) or patients are to be enrolled. If patients are to be enrolled, should they (1) be in a state of remission, (2) have stable disease, or (3) be in the midst of an acute episode? Patients must also be described in terms of disease severity and specific symptoms.

Use of Prisoners

Numerous Phase I medicine trials were often conducted on prisoners, prior to 1970, but this practice is infrequently followed in the United States today. The major reason that prisoners are no longer allowed to participate in clinical trials is that it is believed that they are not able to provide a freely given informed consent. There are individuals who believe that the "loss" of this population for medicine trials represented both a gain and loss for these prisoners and our society because of benefits that this population gained from participation in these trials (Lasagna, 1977; Shubin, 1981). In addition, the relative safety of virtually all medicines tested meant that few individuals experienced long-term adverse reactions to the trials.

Use of Patients

Most Phase I clinical trials are currently performed with normal volunteers. There is, however, a growing belief that patients may sometimes be appropriate to use in Phase I trials to test new medicines for safety (Weissman, 1981). This may be especially useful if patients metabolize medicines differently than do normal volunteers. For example, epileptic patients who are currently receiving microsomal enzyme-inducing medicines may metabolize a new medicine differently than will a normal volunteer. Another example in which patients may be used for Phase I trials relates

to the use of medicines with expected toxicity, such as evaluating the safety of new anticancer medicines that are potentially toxic. In this situation it is usually not ethically acceptable to enroll normal volunteers in a Phase I trial.

Factors to consider in determining whether to use patients or volunteers depend on whether the investigator will be able to complete the clinical trial more rapidly, efficiently, safely, ethically, and cost-effectively and also obtain more reliable information with patients or volunteers.

Mandatory Use of Patients in Phase I Clinical Trials

There are a number of diseases for which it is mandatory to enroll patients instead of normal volunteers in Phase I clinical trials. The most well-known examples are for medicines to treat cancer, arrhythmias, and any other disease in which the investigational medicine is expected (or is likely) to possess toxicity unacceptable for exposure to volunteers (e.g., disease modifying agents for treating patients with severe arthritis). Thus, the crucial point is not that there is something special about cancer, arrhythmias, or other diseases when patients are enrolled in Phase I trials, but that the medicines used to treat these diseases are relatively toxic.

Variations of Phase I Clinical Trial Designs

It may be preferable in some Phase I clinical trials to expose a larger number of patients or volunteers to a maximally tolerated dose than to lower doses. This has the advantage that more information may be obtained on the specific dose or doses that are of greatest interest. If a trial has two treatment periods, then a smaller group of patients may be enrolled in the first period, in which a maximally tolerated dose is deter-

TABLE 12.1 *Volunteers in Phase I clinical trials: characteristics of single vs. multiple groups*

Single group	Multiple groups
1. Enhanced basis for comparison of effects from week to week	1. More accurate measurement of reaction(s) to individual doses are possible
2. More reliable kinetic data	2. Preferable if the medicine has a long half-life
3. Convenient	3. Less convenient
4. Less expensive	4. More expensive
5. More rapid for most medicines	5. More rapid completion of the clinical trial for medicines with long half-lives
6. May assess cumulative effects if desired	6. Carryover effect of medicine on the subsequent baseline is not a problem

mined. A larger number of patients are then enrolled in the second treatment period, in which they receive a dose based on the results obtained in the first period.

A Phase I rising single-dose clinical trial may expose one group of patients (or volunteers) to each dose evaluated, or a new group of patients may be enrolled to receive each dose. There are numerous advantages and disadvantages of each approach (Table 12.1).

TYPES OF EFFICACY TARGETS

In evaluating the efficacy (or safety) of a new or established medicine, the precise target(s) for evaluation should be identified. Possible types of targets for evaluation of efficacy include the following:

1. Clinical parameters. These include symptoms and signs of the primary or coexisting disease.
2. Clinical tests. Abnormalities present are determined by tests used to measure or study the disease or a manifestation of the disease.
3. Disease abnormality. This may include a biochemical defect attributable to the primary or coexisting disease, an anatomical lesion attributable to the primary or coexisting disease, or any other abnormality attributable to the primary or coexisting disease.

The term *coexisting disease* is used to include risk factors. The clinical trial may evaluate treatment of an active disease or risk factor, diagnosis of the disease state, or prophylactic treatment to prevent a disease from occurring. The major variables chosen to evaluate efficacy (or safety) are often indicated in the design section of a protocol. Parameters that provide objective measurements of medicine efficacy are almost always preferable to subjective measures of response, although it is often reasonable to include both types of measurements. When no objective or even semiobjective measurements are available, then subjective measurements must be used. A double-blind controlled design will provide some degree of control and assurance that results obtained with subjective data will be reproducible and interpretations will be meaningful.

Choosing Efficacy Targets

As a general principle, one should not employ any methodology that is not well documented and/or widely accepted as providing valid data. In particular, measurement of the major indicator of efficacy should utilize validated procedures. It may be relevant to determine the scientific basis for the proposed methods, since many widely used tests have never been adequately validated.

In choosing the correct tests to include in a clinical

protocol, both the specificity and sensitivity of the tests should be evaluated. A specific methodology detects a signal for the desired event and does not detect signals for other events. Specificity refers to the probability of correctly diagnosing a negative case as negative. Specificity in a test is lacking if a positive result occurs when it should be negative. This is a false-positive result. Sensitivity refers to the probability of correctly diagnosing a positive case as positive. Sensitivity in tests is lacking if a negative result occurs when it should be positive. This is a false-negative result. A methodology with high sensitivity, therefore, has the ability to detect a small change in the magnitude of the signal measured.

Amount of Detail to Provide in a Protocol

It may be important to specifically indicate details in the protocol that are related to tests used. The details may be given in either the protocol or an appendix and may vary from model numbers of specific equipment used to paper speed of the recording paper [e.g., for electrocardiogram (ECG) recordings]. The amount of relevant detail to include for each test must be determined. If multiple tests are included in a clinical trial, their order of use may be controlled or scheduled in a fixed (or random) order, and the time allowed between the tests specified. The number of repeat measurements should be determined and indicated for each test (at least on the data collection forms). It may be important to document whether responses to a test remain constant in the absence of any medicine, since a major error would be introduced if normal changes in a test score were inappropriately ascribed to a medicine.

In discussing the nature of measurements as part of the clinical trial design, measurements that relate to meeting the trial's objective will be emphasized. For example, the exact time of day that a medicine (given once daily) is administered is usually not specified in the design section of most protocols; however, that time could be critical if the trial is primarily concerned with diurnal rhythms and is designed to evaluate the effects of a medicine given at 8 P.M. versus those effects measured when it is given at 8 A.M.

HOW THE PATIENTS' ENVIRONMENT AFFECTS THE CLINICAL TRIAL'S OUTCOME

If patients have to be hospitalized to test a new agent, this may have a moderate or strong influence on the characteristics and nature of the patients' disease. Many (if not most) diseases treated in outpatients will appear to change in nature or severity when outpatients are hospitalized. This has been demonstrated for patients with various forms of epilepsy (Riley et al., 1981). In addition, responses to pain and pain thresholds appear to differ between clinical and laboratory settings (American Medical Association, 1983). Data obtained at an early stage of a medicine's development in a setting where the disease process is altered from the patient's usual environment may not yield a valid impression of the trial medicine's true potential efficacy.

If pertinent efficacy measurements may be obtained in outpatient clinical trials while the patient is at home (e.g., blood pressure measurements, number of bowel movements and consistency of stool), then more choices of suitable trial designs will be available. Many factors (e.g., patient reliability, adequate measuring devices) have to be considered before this type of data collection is endorsed.

Contact Reactions among Patients

In many clinical trials it is important to keep patients separated from each other, either in a waiting room or in a treatment room. In the waiting room, some patients have been found to exchange information that has adversely affected compliance or cooperation of other patients, or even the clinical trial itself. In some rare cases, patients have been caught sharing medicines. This has usually occurred because of their desire to have a better chance of receiving the active medicine. Patients who are kept waiting may become upset and cooperate less with the staff and their requests.

In Phase I clinical trials, volunteers are often housed in a single large room or are allowed to socialize freely in a single large room after receiving medication. Although there are benefits from this type of relatively open environment, there may be severe drawbacks if one patient experiences an unpleasant reaction (e.g., syncope, ataxia, emesis) in the presence of others. This occurrence tends to encourage others (consciously or not) to have the same experience. The inclusion of volunteers on placebo is one means of preventing this type of reaction from causing an entire program to be delayed, while the suspected "adverse reaction" is probed in depth. The same type of adverse reaction might readily occur if the temperature in the room was too high, or if patients had insufficient sleep the night before.

Types of Clinical Artificiality That Influence the Evaluation of Efficacy in Clinical Trials

Artificiality is defined as the type and degree of difference between routine medical practice and a clinical trial. Five types of clinical artificiality in clinical trials are defined:

1. Patients with a disease are treated in the usual manner with few protocol requirements.
2. Patients with a disease are treated as outpatients in a clinic or in another usual medical care environment, following a protocol.
3. Patients with a disease are treated as inpatients in a hospital or as outpatients in a laboratory environment.
4. Patients with a disease in remission are given a substance that either provokes their disease or mimics one aspect of it (e.g., allergen-induced bronchospasm in atopic patients to evaluate antiasthmatic effects).
5. Volunteers without a disease (i.e., at least without any disease that could influence the clinical trial) are given a substance that mimics one or more aspects of a disease in a laboratory environment (e.g., castor oil to elicit diarrhea).

Results obtained in multiple clinical trials may differ because of the nature of the physical environment in which the trials were conducted as well as from disparities in the patient populations treated (Blackburn, 1984).

DEFINING CLINICALLY SIGNIFICANT ACTIVITY OF THE TEST TREATMENT

In establishing the standard(s) for defining medicine activity, the differences between statistical and clinical significance must be considered. Statistical significance may be precisely defined. Clinical significance is a subjective parameter. For evaluating the usefulness of a new medicine, clinical significance is applied to the minimal difference between two treatments that would affect a clinician's judgment of how to treat patients with the same or a similar problem. Although the difference between two treatments that is considered clinically significant will not be the same among physicians, these differences generally tend to cluster around a specific figure or range.

The degree or magnitude of change in efficacy parameters that will be considered to represent a true clinical improvement should be established in the planning phase of a clinical trial. An efficacy test that demonstrates a 10% change after medicine treatment may be statistically significant, but a change of 50% may be required for the results to be clinically significant (clinically meaningful). Statistically significant changes in many parameters used to evaluate safety are not always clinically significant. For example, a statistically significant change in heart rate of 4 beats per minute, either within or outside the normal range, will almost never be clinically significant. In some cases, however, such minor changes may indicate an effect that should be evaluated in greater detail or closely monitored in future studies.

Clinical Equivalence

A clinical trial may be designed to show equivalence, i.e., the same effect may be sought for a new medicine and standard therapy. In this type of trial, the definition of clinical significance may be based on establishing a minimal intragroup difference from baseline, or it may be based on whether both treatments yielded the same magnitude and type of effect. Neither of these data, however, would be as convincing as those demonstrating a true difference between treatment groups.

PLACEBO EFFECT

Definitions and Uses of a Placebo

The term *placebo* is generally used to refer to (1) medication taken, (2) effect observed, or (3) control group of patients. As medication, it is "blank" (i.e., without any active medicine) and is given to some or all patients one or more times during a study. The term placebo is also used to describe the "placebo effect" that is elicited by the placebo medicine or is caused by the influence of nontrial medicine or nontreatment factors, usually on efficacy measures. The "placebo group" refers to a control (comparison) group in a clinical trial made up of those patients who were given a placebo medication. Placebos are used in medicine trials to control for major sources of misleading data: (1) prejudice on the part of the investigator and/or (2) patient, and (3) spontaneous alterations and variations that occur during treatment and are related to the disease studied or to other factors. Prejudices may be based on psychological and emotional factors that enter a trial plus physical effects that are related to receiving medication.

Types of Placebo

Several types of placebo responses are observed in clinical trials, based primarily on the number of placebo responders and the magnitude of their response. The placebo effect may be observed in all patients, or it may only be present in a subset of the total number studied. The magnitude of the placebo response may be either 0 or 100% in a specific parameter (e.g., when a placebo affords either no pain relief or complete pain relief), but usually the placebo effect is noted as a relative change between 0 and 100% (e.g., 20% decrease in the number of anginal attacks). The placebo response is a major factor that must be considered when evaluating analgesics, antidepressants, and many other types of medicines. Substantial clinical data have been obtained in recent years indicating that most disease states may be significantly affected by placebo medication. It is important to note that the placebo response may increase or decrease over time.

It is commonly accepted that a small or moderate placebo effect will be present in most medicine trials conducted in conscious individuals. Although a variety of approaches exist to control or diminish the placebo effect, in some cases the placebo effect is ignored in developing a trial design. Either a separate placebo group or a placebo treatment period for all patients may be incorporated into the trial design to evaluate and/or control for the placebo effect.

Placebo Run-In Technique

Certain techniques may be used to exclude those patients from a clinical trial in whom a large placebo response is anticipated. For example, all patients could be given a placebo medication (single or double blind) for a fixed period, after which they would be tested; any patients who improved by more than a specified amount would be excluded from further participation in the trial. This technique may not only eliminate placebo responders from a study but, if a pill count is also performed during this period, may sometimes eliminate noncompliant patients as well. Any procedure for excluding placebo responders from a trial introduces a bias that would generally make this practice inappropriate during Phase III. In Phase III studies, a medicine is evaluated in a general population with a given disease, and "all" types of responders and patients that satisfy entry criteria should receive the medicine to develop more clearly the full spectrum of the medicine's safety and efficacy profile. The bias that is introduced by excluding placebo responders, however, may be acceptable in a Phase II clinical trial, in which the primary objective is to determine if the medicine possesses the desired activity. Minimizing the placebo effect in Phase II is desirable, since it allows the medicine's efficacy to be more clearly assessed.

Evaluating the Magnitude of the Placebo Response

The magnitude of the placebo response may be determined by evaluating the response of patients in a double-blind clinical trial to placebo and an active trial medicine. Another approach to evaluating the magnitude of the placebo response is to compare the results of an active trial medicine in an open-label trial with results obtained in a double-blind trial utilizing the same design. The assumption made in this comparison is that if more individuals respond to a medicine (or respond better) in an open-label trial than in a double-blind trial, then at least part of the difference is attributable to a placebo effect, which in turn may reflect greater expectations of patients who enter the open-label trial.

Other approaches for evaluating or controlling placebo responses are to interject a placebo treatment at an unannounced time(s) in the protocol. This could occur at the start or termination of the clinical trial or at intermittent points during the trial depending on the nature of the medicine and trial design. In this situation, both patients and investigator are informed that each patient will receive active medicine and placebo, but they are not told when each will be administered or if several placebo periods will be introduced. Information on the length of each placebo period could also be withheld from the investigator and patient if this were considered ethical by the relevant Ethics Committee/IRB. A discussion of placebo control groups may be found in Chapter 8.

DURATION OF CLINICAL EVALUATION

Duration of Patient Treatment

The duration of each patient's treatment in a clinical trial may be (1) fixed (e.g., 2 hours, days, weeks, or years); (2) variable (e.g., the study lasts until a specified measure of efficacy returns to normal, 12 to 18 weeks); (3) indefinite (e.g., ongoing treatment of chronic disease); or (4) unspecified. The type and length of duration chosen for the trial should almost always be indicated in the protocol. Types of duration are listed in Table 12.2.

The duration that is established for treating patients in a clinical trial is often dependent on the expected or established therapeutic use of the medicine as well as the extent of toxicological data. Many trials have a duration that parallels the duration of the disease or exposure to an external factor (e.g., prophylactic study of an antimalarial in people visiting a specific country for a defined period of time). The terms acute, subacute, subchronic, and chronic are often used to describe the duration of medicine therapy as well as the duration of diseases. Their definitions vary to some degree among diseases and among clinicians. Therefore, these terms should be clearly defined in any protocols in which they are used.

Uses of Acute Clinical Trials

Acute clinical trials are often used for acute diseases or for chronic diseases with acute episodes, and chronic trials are often used to study chronic diseases. Nonetheless, even in testing medicines for a chronic disease, there are occasions when an acute trial design is preferable. Some common reasons are:

1. To evaluate bioavailability and the pharmacokinetics in patients with the disease who may be expected to absorb, distribute, metabolize, or excrete the medicine differently from the normal population (e.g., in epileptic patients receiving medicines that induce hepatic microsomal enzymes) or in a subset of patients with a "specific" problem (e.g., patients with renal impairment).
2. To evaluate the acute effect of a medicine on a specific test in patients, such as studying acute electroencephalographic (EEG) effects caused by a new antiepileptic medicine.
3. To avoid a placebo effect that is observed in chronic studies. For example, the relatively marked placebo effect observed in chronic medicine trials in patients with angina is primarily absent in acute medicine trials (Redwood et al., 1971).

Duration of a Clinical Trial

In addition to establishing the duration of a patient's treatment, it may also be important to establish the duration of the entire clinical trial. An important consideration relating to a trial's total duration is the pattern in which patients are entered into a trial. Examples of enrollment patterns include those in which (1) all patients start a clinical trial at the same time, (2) defined groups of patients start a trial at fixed times, (3) different numbers of patients start a trial at fixed times, (4) variable dates are used for patient entry and trial initiation, (5) no specific dates are used, and patients enter the trial as they are enrolled, or (6) another pattern of patient enrollment is established.

A target date for completion of a clinical trial is usually established at the outset. There are a wide variety of reasons, however, why this date is commonly not achieved, and it requires a great deal of planning, effort, and even luck in most cases to achieve the established goals.

TABLE 12.2 Types of "duration" of a clinical trial[a]

1. Period of time allowed for patient enrollment
2. Period of time for an individual to participate in a clinical trial
3. Period of time for an entire clinical trial to be conducted
4. Period of time for number three, plus the time necessary for data processing, statistical analysis reports, and a final medical report or publication to be prepared

[a] Any or all of the durations may be unspecified in a clinical protocol or plan. For example, number 1 above could be stated to last until X patients are enrolled; number 2 could last until patients recover or have a Y percent change in a specified parameter; number 3 could last until all patients are enrolled and treated; and number 4 is usually unspecified, except in clinical plans.

CHAPTER 13

Patient Recruitment

MAJOR SOURCES OF PATIENT RECRUITMENT

A series of questions are asked as patients are contacted about enrolling in a clinical trial. Figure 13.1 is a flow chart presenting these questions in the order they are considered, and also shows the general sources used to recruit patients.

Although patients are often recruited for clinical trials from the medical practice of the investigator, there are numerous occasions when this is either not possible or is not the sole source of patient recruitment. A series of articles dealing with recruitment of patients from various other sources was published in *Circulation* (Agras and Bradford, 1982). These articles discuss the advantages and disadvantages of using the sources of patient recruitment listed in Table 13.1. Another discussion of recruitment in a large multicenter trial presented data from the National Cooperative Gallstone Study (Croke, 1979).

LASAGNA'S LAW: THE CENTRAL ISSUE IN PATIENT RECRUITMENT

The overly optimistic projection of available numbers of patients to enroll that are made in almost all clinical

TABLE 13.1 *Sources of patient recruitment*[a]

1. Government employees (e.g., military)
2. Private industry (e.g., clinics in large industries)
3. Medical referrals from professional colleagues (i.e., from direct contact)
4. Referrals from clinical laboratories
5. Mass media strategies (via newspaper or radio advertisements)
6. Mass mailings
7. Community screening (e.g., health fairs)
8. Participants in other clinical studies
9. Blood banks (blood donors)
10. Local advertisements (notices on bulletin boards)
11. Other sources

[a] Other than through the investigator's own practice or through unsolicited visits by patients to the investigator.

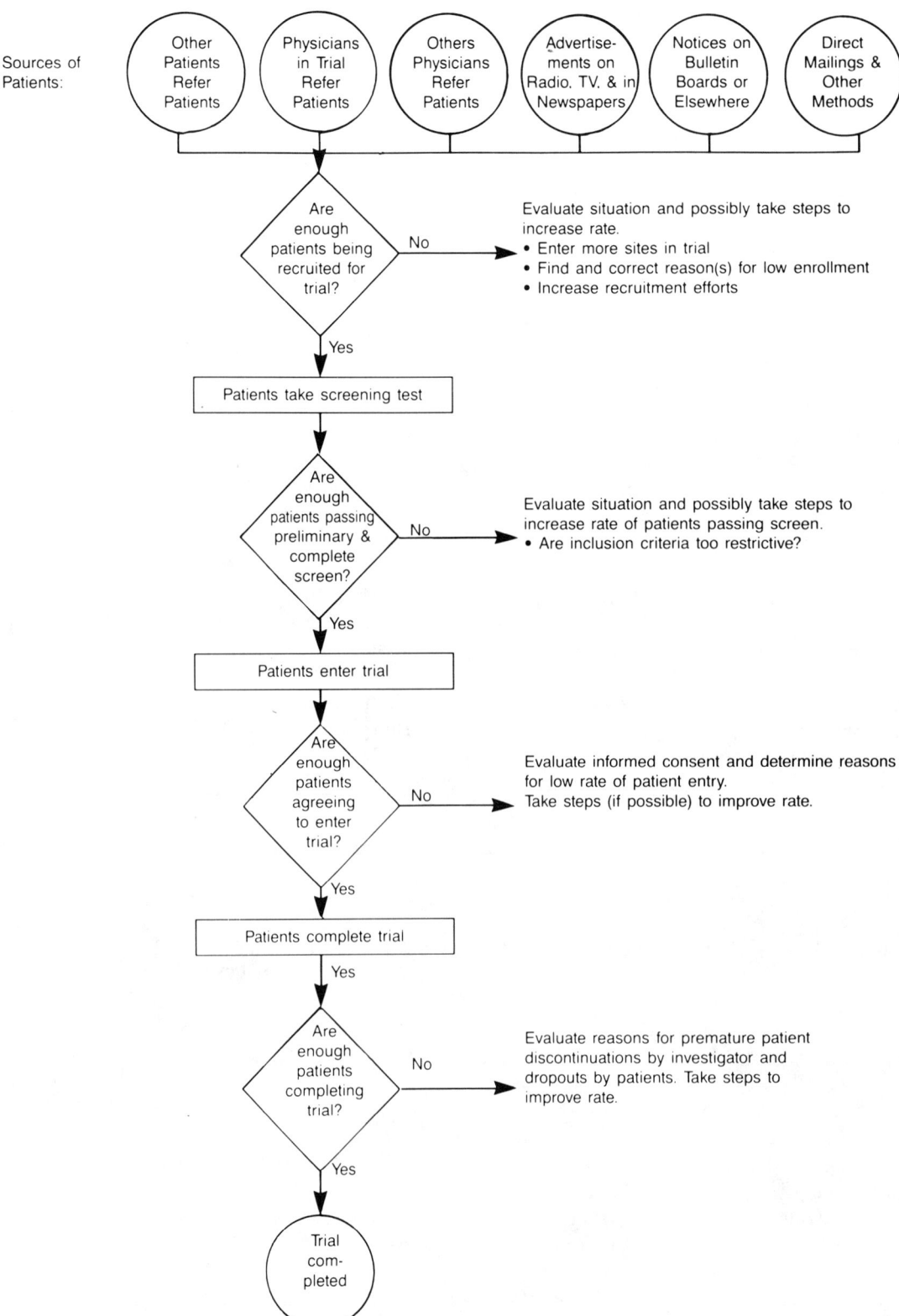

FIG. 13.1 Patient recruitment and participation in a clinical trial. (Reprinted from Spilker, 1989a, with permission of Raven Press.)

trials is so widespread and well known that a general principle known as Lasagna's law'' (Fig. 13.2) has evolved. Most investigators and sponsors know this effect to be true from their own experience, but few groups have systematically evaluated this issue. Williford et al. (1987) found that in eight of nine multicenter trials conducted within the Veterans Administration Cooperative Studies Program, the original recruitment projections were overrated.

It is an accepted generalization that in most clinical situations patient recruitment becomes progressively easier as the admission criteria of the study ease. This was confirmed when Croke (1979) observed that the ability of ten centers to recruit volunteers was increased by loosening the criteria of admission into the clinical trial. This change had a far greater impact on the enrollment rate of patients than did any of the other methods used to increase patient enrollment at the different sites. Other discussions of patient recruitment are found in the following references: Agras and Marshall (1979), Prout (1979), Schoenberger (1979), and Benedict (1979). A list of some factors that influence patient recruitment is presented in Table 13.2.

The trend described by Lasagna's law occurs primarily because admission criteria prevent many patients from enrolling that the investigator initially considered as viable candidates for the trial. Other reasons may relate to naiveté, not reading the protocol carefully, and ignoring relevant factors (e.g., degree of pa-

TABLE 13.2 *Selected factors that influence patient recruitment*[a]

1. Source of patient referral: medical sources, other clinical studies, clinical laboratories, blood banks
2. Number of patients contacted via letter, telephone, or direct approach using mass mailing, mass media, friends, advertisements, or other methods
3. Specific place where mass screening occurs: at workplace, educational facility, social group, community location, or elsewhere
4. Socioeconomic composition of the patient pool
5. Resources of time, personnel, and money available to devote to this effort
6. Location of the study site relative to patients' home or work[b]
7. Degree of concern that patients have for their disease
8. Nature of the appeal to patients to enroll in the study[c]
9. Specific requirements and demands of the study (e.g., in terms of difficult or disagreeable tests)
10. Amount of remuneration or other benefits (e.g., meals, transportation) given to patients

[a] Most inclusion and exclusion criteria are not considered in this table, but these criteria have a major impact on patient recruitment.
[b] Use of outreach programs and flexible schedules for clinic visits may improve recruitment.
[c] Presenting benefits in a positive approach and concentrating on personal motives of the patients may improve recruitment.

tient interest in the treatment being tested). Lasagna's law may be countered in several ways, most of which involve modifying the admission criteria. One must determine, however, whether the admission criteria can be modified without affecting the trial's integrity.

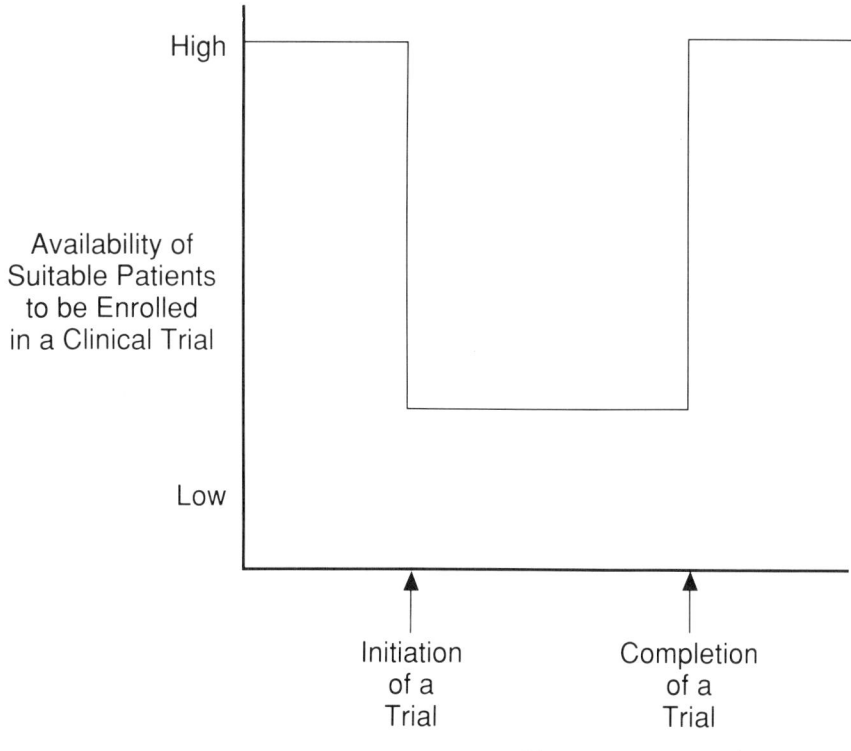

FIG. 13.2 Lasagna's law.

SPECIAL POPULATIONS TO CONSIDER WHEN RECRUITING FOR CLINICAL TRIALS

Probably the best single source of information and experience on patient recruitment comes from the previously mentioned December, 1982 issue of *Circulation* (Agras and Bradford, 1982). These articles summarize experiences of patient recruitment at many lipid research clinics that participated in a very large clinical trial. Separate groups referred and screened for entry into the trial included occupational groups (e.g., government employees, private industry) and patients referred from private medical practices, clinical laboratories, community screening, other clinical trials, and blood banks. Experiences with mass mailings and mass media strategies are also described. A surgical trial's recruitment experiences are described by Buchwald et al. (1987), and a valuable literature summary and annotated bibliography of recruitment experiences in clinical trials is presented by Hunninghake et al. (1987).

In addition to the above-mentioned groups, other patient populations that could be considered are mentioned below.

Military Recruits or Military Patients

Military hospitals and facilities contain groups of patients who are seldom used in clinical trials. These patients are often a good source for recruitment, especially if they are located in an area where a particular disease is prevalent. For example, military personnel may be tested or screened for tropical diseases after they return to their home country from a country where tropical diseases are prevalent. Military recruits may be used as a cohort during their training, particularly when it is important to have relative control on factors such as diet, exercise, and lifestyle.

Island Populations

Groups of people who are living on isolated islands may represent an ideal group for a clinical trial if a prophylaxis or treatment study is to be conducted on a prevalent disease. Some of the prophylactic clinical trials on NIX (permethrin) were conducted in this environment (Dr. John Delehanty, personal communication).

Health Maintenance Organizations and Other Health Groups

Health Maintenance Organizations are sometimes an excellent source of patients for selected trials. Various other similar groups (e.g., Preferred Provider Organizations) also could be considered.

Private Practice Physicians

Private practice physicians may be approached to determine their interest in becoming individual investigators for a clinical trial. Alternatively, these physicians may be grouped into regions in which they act as investigators or sources for patient referrals to regional hospitals. One of the most difficult problems to address is the fear on the part of referring physicians of losing their patients and the economic benefits derived from their treatment. This must be seriously considered prior to approaching physicians in private practice to refer patients for a trial.

Prisoners

Prisoners are no longer a suitable source of volunteers or patients because of issues of informed consent. Nonetheless, there may be special circumstances under which prisoners could participate in a clinical trial. These must be discussed with an Ethics Committee/IRB.

PRESENTING DATA ON PATIENT RECRUITMENT

The steps used for patient recruitment may be described in numerous ways in a report or paper. Common methods include tables, graphs, or algorithms. Some of the ways of expressing recruitment include:

1. Patients enrolled as a percent of those screened.
2. As a list of successive categories (see Table 13.3). A list of the major reasons why patients do not progress from step to step would be extremely helpful in interpreting data, as would a comparison of demographic and prognostic criteria of each group. This latter category of information is impractical to obtain for each separate subgroup that does not enter the trial, but could be obtained for the combined group of patients from point 2 in Table 13.3 until points 8 or 10, when patients are officially said to enter the trial. A list of such reasons are presented and discussed by Calimlim and Weintraub (1981). If these categories are of importance to the investigators, then a patient log should be designed to collect the data.
3. As a graph of time (abscissa) versus cumulative number (or percent) of patients enrolled (ordinate). The projected enrollment plan should be drawn as well as a plot of the actual enrollment. Thus, it is possible at a glance to assess how well enrollment is progressing and whether changes in

TABLE 13.3 *Categories of patients that may be described prior to entry into a clinical trial[a]*

1. Patients potentially available for entry into a clinical trial (i.e., the total pool of patients in a given area)
2. Patients available for initial verbal screening (e.g., many patients are unavailable for a variety of reasons)
3. Patients preliminarily excluded because of failure to meet basic inclusion criteria
4. Patients available for initial interview and screening tests (e.g., some patients are unavailable for a variety of reasons)
5. Patients available for interview and informed consent discussion (e.g., some patients are not suitable because of language problems, personality traits unsuited to a clinical trial, physical impairments, mental impairments, severe allergies)
6. Patients who pass screening tests who are offered informed consent (e.g., others are rejected for a variety of reasons)
7. Patients consenting to enter the clinical trial
8. Patients signing informed consents
9. Patients who enter the active baseline period of a clinical trial
10. Patients who receive treatment in a clinical trial

[a] Entry into a clinical trial may be defined as the time of signing the informed consent (point 8), entry into an active baseline (point 9), or as the moment when treatment is initiated (point 10). Each of these may be appropriate in different clinical trials.

the methods of recruitment (indicated by an arrow under the abscissa) led to changes in actual recruitment.
4. In terms of costs of the efforts needed to enroll each patient.
5. In terms of prevalence of the disease (e.g., one-third of all patients with the rare disease X in the United States were enrolled in the clinical trial).
6. In terms of goals or quotas for each center.

PATTERNS OF PATIENT ENROLLMENT

1. All patients may be enrolled at one time (e.g., in pharmacokinetic trials).
2. Patients may be enrolled on an ad hoc basis until a fixed date occurs.
3. Patients may be enrolled on an ad hoc basis until a fixed number are enrolled either at the site or at all sites combined.
4. Patients may be enrolled in prespecified groups (e.g., eight patients in group 1 followed by eight patients in group 2, and so on).

HOW TO INCREASE RECRUITMENT OF PATIENTS

Stepwise Approach

The most important answer to this issue is to develop a strategy that involves multiple stages. If initial efforts fail to enroll sufficient numbers of patients, then further efforts should be rapidly implemented. If the reason(s) for low enrollment can be determined, then

specific efforts should be directed toward their amelioration.

The initial step is to determine whether the central problem relates to (1) patients, (2) investigators, (3) protocol requirements, (4) other factors, or (5) a combination of two or more of these factors. The next step is to identify the specific causes as well as possible solutions.

It is generally useful to develop (prior to the clinical trial) a series of alternative techniques to attempt to increase enrollment if the rate of patient enrollment becomes a problem. Lists of some of these techniques are presented in Tables 13.4 and 13.5. If these techniques are not successful, then it may be necessary to decrease the number of patients in the trial. The new number chosen should be reached in collaboration with a statistician. Although a lowering of the required sample size is usually accompanied by a decrease in the power of the statistical tests used, it is sometimes possible to decrease the sample size without compromising these values. For example, consideration of a secondary hypothesis may be dropped, or different statistical tests may be found to be more appropriate tools to analyze the data.

Financial Incentives for Patients

There may be a temptation in some Phase II and III clinical trials to encourage patients to enroll in the trial

TABLE 13.4 *Selected techniques for investigators to increase patient recruitment*

1. Loosen the inclusion/exclusion criteria[a]
2. Loosen the demands of the protocol (e.g., eliminate some or all disagreeable tests)
3. Speak informally to additional colleagues directly or by telephone to request referrals
4. Speak at formal or informal professional meetings and request referrals
5. Write letters to colleagues and request referrals
6. Put notices in places where colleagues and/or patients may notice
7. Print leaflets and distribute directly to potential patients
8. Advertise in local or regional sources (newspapers, TV, radio)
9. Contact patients directly at health fairs or by radio and TV appearances (for large multicenter studies with widespread relevance)
10. Add additional sites to the study[a]
11. Increase or initiate payment or other benefits to patients (e.g., include payment for transportation and/or meals)
12. Increase the time of the study's duration[a]
13. Hire additional personnel to help recruit patients
14. Conduct additional chart reviews and/or reviews of pharmacy records (e.g., in a nursing home)
15. Add a continuation protocol so that patients may continue to receive a medicine if they have demonstrated clinical improvement in the study[a]
16. Determine which techniques are working best at sites with high recruitment rates and utilize those techniques at sites with lower recruitment rates

[a] This should be evaluated with a statistician and may require Ethics Committee/Institutional Review Board (IRB) approval.

TABLE 13.5 *Methods and approaches to enhance patient enrollment in clinical trials*[a]

1. Determine what is motivating patients to enter (as well as not to enter) a clinical trial and attempt to address patient needs

2. Inform referring physicians that their patients may receive medical treatment not otherwise available

3. Determine if inadequate patient enrollment relates primarily to patients, investigators, protocol, facilities, or other factors

4. Place signs about the clinical trial in places where both physicians and potential patients may see them

5. Ask the investigator's staff to review hospital admissions or clinic appointments to seek potential patients

6. Modify the inclusion criteria after determining which changes would not affect the clinical trial and yet would increase patient enrollment

7. Increase the number of trial sites in a multicenter clinical trial

8. Have a major well-respected expert come to a site with low enrollment and encourage physicians to refer or enter patients into the clinical trial

9. Provide a tour of the clinic for prospective patients and answer their questions

10. Devote more time to recruitment and give it a higher priority in terms of efforts

11. Attempt to find populations of patients that may be accessed (e.g., see section on other patient populations)

12. Provide funds to a hospital for supporting meetings, dinners, or texts, to be allocated at the hospital's (or investigator's) discretion

13. Increase financial incentives for investigators or patients to improve recruitment

14. Contact sources of other patient populations

15. Simplify the protocol in those areas in which patients or investigators complain

16. Increase the duration of the recruitment period

17. Provide more feedback to referring physicians about the clinical trial and the status of the patients they have referred or will refer

[a] Many are implemented through investigators too. See Table 13.4 for other methods.

by offering overly generous benefits. It is the author's view that neither money nor other nonmedical inducements should be given to patients so that their primary motivation to enroll in a trial is for any monetary "reward" that may be offered. This view must be modified for Phase I clinical trials and for bioavailability and selected other trials, in which financial benefit is accepted as the primary motivating factor for many volunteers rather than the desire to help medical research. Patients with most chronic diseases usually enroll in a trial out of a strong desire to receive an effective treatment for their medical disease. This desire is also shared by many other patients who participate in clinical trials.

Modifying Investigator Views about Enrollment

Methods to increase patient enrollment are not solely directed toward finding populations of suitable patients. Sometimes the investigators must be convinced of the importance and reasonableness of entering certain types of patients. Reasons for low patient enrollment that relate to the views of the investigator are discussed by Taylor K. M. et al. (1984). Some of the types of reasons they advanced plus others are listed in Table 13.6.

Modifying Investigator Motivation about Enrollment

The motivation of investigators and their staff must be carefully considered, as well as the motivation of physicians that an investigator counts on for referrals. For example, if the residents and other house staff have incentives (e.g., less work) to discharge patients as soon as possible, then enrolling them in a clinical trial will slow the patient turnover for the house staff. Thus, the house staff would be reluctant to encourage their patients to enroll in a clinical trial. If it is possible for these patients to be transferred to a special ward, the house staff may develop an entirely different attitude

TABLE 13.6 *Selected reasons why some physicians are reluctant to enter patients in clinical trials*

A physician may have discomfort with the:

1. Inclusion of a placebo
2. Size of the group given placebo
3. Randomization process
4. Informed consent procedures
5. Restricted eligibility requirements
6. Excessive time required to care for patients
7. Administrative requirements of completing data collection forms
8. Interference with the usual patient-physician relationship
9. Perceived conflicts between care offered patients in usual treatment versus that required by protocol
10. Insurance issues that prevent or make it difficult for some groups of patients (e.g., those in a Health Maintenance Organization) to enter certain hospitals and receive insurance coverage[a]
11. Level of financial reimbursement may seem inadequate
12. Overall value of the trial (e.g., additional information may have been obtained since the trial started, preference for one treatment)

A physician may experience a change in his or her:

1. Personal life (e.g., new children, marriage, divorce)
2. Commitments to other clinical trials
3. Commitments to other activities or projects as a result of a promotion, new responsibilities, or new interests
4. Plans for vacation or upcoming sabbatical

[a] Some insurance-related issues are discussed by Wood (1989).

about the clinical trial. Physicians may be contacted for referrals through grand rounds, signs on bulletin boards, notices in the house staff lounge, and personal contact.

Inform investigators in a multicenter trial of how well they themselves are doing compared with other investigators. Encourage friendly competition among investigators to enroll patients, but be careful that their enthusiasm does not lead to enrolling ineligible patients.

Modifying Patient Motivation about Enrollment

The method to counter low patient enrollment may be as simple as providing patients a modest stipend for meals and transportation. Costs for patients' expenses may not be as simple as providing money for meals and transportation. Wood (1989) describes several of the extremely large costs that patients and their insurance companies are asked to pay in some academically sponsored clinical trials. A more complex approach is to modify the protocol to simplify demands on patients and having the protocol reapproved by the Ethics Committees/IRBs at each site (for multicenter trials).

Advertising for Patients

Types of Advertising

Advertising for patients ranges from placing discreet notes in a medical clinic to paid advertisements on radio and television and in newspapers. Some advertisements are presented in the media as a public service or even as news. Numerous investigators and study coordinators have found that advertising often boosts patient contacts and usually enrollment. The tone of advertising varies from objective factual statements to more forward solicitation of patients. Advertising has often made the difference between a successful and unsuccessful clinical trial.

Press Releases

Another type of advertising is to issue one or more press releases about a clinical trial that either is about to begin or is already underway. Newspapers and other media that carry the story as a news item are often used to boost enrollment. A potential problem with this approach is that what is actually printed or reported is often quite different from the material originally in the press release furnished to the media.

Issues

The major questions regarding advertisement as a means of increasing recruitment are (1) is the advertisement conducted in an ethical manner? (2) does it lead to enrollment of the types of patients desired? (3) is it initiated during the clinical trial or from its outset? If advertising is initiated after a clinical trial is in progress, a different population of patients could be enrolled yielding results different from those that would be obtained from patients enrolled before the trial was initiated. Thus, the data of the two groups (i.e., patients enrolled via advertisements versus others) should be analyzed separately and compared prior to being pooled and combined.

Solicited versus Nonsolicited Patients

One must consider not only *which* patient populations to seek (e.g., current military, veterans, mental institutions), but also *how* to attract them. The population of patients obtained by advertisements of various types may be called a solicited patient group. These patients may differ significantly from traditionally referred patients, called a nonsolicited group. Krupnick et al. (1986) evaluated 14 published reports of clinical trials in which comparisons were made between solicited and nonsolicited patients. In eight of these trials, the comparisons were made within the same trial and in six of these trials the comparisons were between different trials. The results were not conclusive, but they suggested that the populations could be similar in response to treatment if patients were carefully screened and chosen for enrollment.

RECRUITMENT THAT IS "TOO SUCCESSFUL"

Recruitment can be "too successful," meaning that there are more patients wishing to enter a clinical trial than can be handled with available resources. If the patient supply is expected to remain high, then the number of patients entering the trial every day (week or month) may be budgeted. If, however, the patient supply is only temporarily high (e.g., students are expected to return home from school), then an attempt should be made to increase or adjust the resources to handle the temporarily increased patient load. There are limits to how many additional patients may be enrolled into virtually all clinical trials within a given time period. The quality of a trial will undoubtedly suffer if an excessive number of patients are either rushed through a trial or dealt with more superficially than is appropriate.

FEEDBACK TO PROFESSIONALS ABOUT REFERRALS

When patient recruitment has utilized referrals from other physicians, there are a number of additional issues that must be considered. Investigators should provide relevant clinical trial data and information about the patient to colleagues who have referred patients for the investigator's trial. This can be done on one or more occasions, depending on the length and nature of the trial, and usually takes the form of a letter or possibly a telephone call. This practice should be followed as a matter of professional courtesy as well as a part of the ethical responsibility of temporarily caring for another physician's patient. If the trial has a clinically significant effect on the disease for which the patient was being treated by the referring physician, then a detailed account of all clinically relevant events and data should be communicated to the original physician.

EFFECTS OF CHANGING RECRUITMENT DURING A CLINICAL TRIAL

There is a spectrum of possible outcomes when patient recruitment methods are changed while a clinical trial is in progress. At one extreme, patients may be enrolled who differ in one or more significant characteristics or prognostic factors, yielding different results. At the other extreme, no differences between the patients may be observed. Changes in recruitment that may occur in long-term clinical trials are summarized in Table 13.7.

When patient recruitment practices are modified during a clinical trial, it is important to analyze the data obtained separately for the two groups prior to pooling them to ensure that the data are comparable. The precise methods used must be established by statisticians.

TABLE 13.7 *Selected effects that may occur in clinical trials conducted over a protracted period*

1. Recruitment methods may change and a different type of patient may be enrolled (e.g., in demographics, in prognostic criteria)
2. Previously unacceptable patients may be enrolled because of investigator and staff frustration over low enrollment
3. Diagnostic criteria may be applied differently to newly enrolled patients
4. The conduct of the clinical trial may change in minor or major ways

UNETHICAL RECRUITMENT PRACTICES

Using Influence over the Volunteer as a Coercive Tactic

An investigator who encourages his staff or students to enroll in a clinical trial is using coercion, whether or not this is intended. Teachers of psychology often coerce their students to participate in clinical trials. A pharmaceutical company that requests junior level people to enroll in clinical trials is also using coercion.

Using Money as a Coercive Tactic

Paying patients more than a reasonable amount of money to defray incidental costs (e.g., food, transportation, baby sitters) is unethical in Phase II and III trials because it introduces an element of coercion and makes it unclear whether patients may remain in a clinical trial for the money when it is in their best interests to drop out. Patients may also distort their true feelings in answering questions and report fewer adverse events if they fear being discontinued from a clinical trial that is going to pay them money they need. These events could affect the type of data obtained and the interpretation of results.

"DISAPPEARANCE" OF PATIENTS WITH SPECIFIC DISEASES

Recruitment of patients for evaluation of a new antiulcer medicine was not a problem for sponsors with investigational medicines to test in the mid-1970s, but by the late 1980s finding enough patients to study became a major issue. Most patients with ulcers are being well maintained on regimens using one of several available medicines. Thus, patients usually have little motivation or need to enter a clinical trial to evaluate a new therapy that does not offer hope of a significant advantage. Physicians have little motivation to refer such patients for a clinical trial of yet another antihistamine (either H-1 or H-2). The same situation has occurred for several other therapeutic areas as well. This is clearly a positive event for society if a medicine is introduced on the market that adequately treats most patients with a particular disease. Nonetheless, sponsors must often attempt to find populations of patients or methods of recruitment that address this issue. Some of the approaches are to eschew tertiary care centers and to approach primary practitioners, to approach Health Maintenance Organizations, and to conduct clinical trials in other countries.

CHAPTER 14

Dosing Schedule

CHOOSING A STARTING DOSE TO TEST A NEW MEDICINE

The choice of a starting dose for the initial study of a new medicine in humans is based on several factors. These include the ED_{50} (the effective dose that elicits 50% of the total response) of the most sensitive animal species, a comparison of the medicine's potency and activity with the potency and activity of known standards that have a similar mechanism of action, LD_{50} (the dose that kills 50% of the test animals; median lethal dose) values in various species, available pharmacokinetic data of blood levels obtained in animals, and information on the medicine's expected absorption, distribution, metabolism, and excretion. After a conservative dose is found that is expected to represent the threshold of the dose–response relationship in humans, a fraction of that dose is chosen as the starting dose. The fractions used by most investigators generally range between one-half and $\frac{1}{10}$ of the expected threshold dose for human efficacy. Some investigators choose a starting dose based solely on the use of a fraction of the threshold dose that caused an adverse reaction or positive effect in the most sensitive animal model tested.

In Oncology Trials

In cancer research it had been customary to initiate Phase I human clinical studies of anticancer medicines at one-third of the lowest dose (per square meter) that caused reversible toxicity in the most sensitive large animal species (dog or monkey) (Penta et al., 1979), although some authors believe that toxicology data in normal and tumor-bearing mice should also have been considered (Goldsmith et al., 1975). Retrospective analysis of preclinical and clinical data for a large number of compounds indicates that $\frac{1}{10}$ mouse LD_{10} (on a body surface basis) should provide a safe starting dose for Phase I clinical trials. This starting dose is both safe and efficient in that the minimal number of Fibonacci escalation steps (see next section for details) is required to achieve the maximally tolerated dose

(Rozencweig et al., 1981). Current accepted practice at the National Cancer Institute is to utilize rodent lethality studies to derive the human starting dose and large animal toxicology results to predict those toxicities that may be encountered in initial clinical trials.

Using Area under the Curve (AUC) Measurements

Several investigators have utilized AUC measurements to guide Phase I clinical trial dose escalation in oncology trials (Collins et al., 1986; EORTC Pharmacokinetics and Metabolism Group, 1987). This approach is based on the concept that the multiple of concentration versus time is a more representative measure of exposure to medicine than is the dose. The concentration multiplied by time of the human maximally tolerated dose, divided by concentration multiplied by time at the LD_{10} dose, in mice is closer to unity than is the simple ratio of doses, which ignores any pharmacokinetic differences between the species. Collins et al. (1986) have modified the Fibonacci scheme to accelerate the testing of anticancer medicines by eliminating several steps.

The methods described above attempt to provide a margin of safety in case a hypersensitive reaction or unexpected effect is manifested by a patient. A survey of scientists in academic and industrial institutions was conducted to compare their views on the conduct of initial medicine trials in humans (Blackwell, 1972a). It would be interesting to determine how these views have changed (if at all) over the intervening years.

Choosing a Dose Range for the Initial Phase I Clinical Trials

Dose evaluation in Phase I is intended to uncover toxic effects and helps define the therapeutic index. The starting dose is chosen as described. The upper dose evaluated in the United States is usually that dose that reaches the upper limit of patient tolerance. This limit may be approached by choosing doses believed to surpass the upper dose limit. Some protocols describe this limit and indicate that the trial should be terminated when patients do not tolerate the medicine's dosage. Alternatively, a conservative and safe upper dose limit may be evaluated and then a further limit may be studied if doses up to the initial ceiling are found to be safe.

In the other basic approach to choosing a dose range for initial Phase I clinical trials, volunteers are titrated up to the blood concentration of medicine expected to demonstrate efficacy in Phase II trials. This means that the primary objective of the initial clinical trial(s) is for both pharmacokinetics and safety, whereas the first approach described is primarily a dose-ranging toler-

ance trial (i.e., safety) and is only secondarily focused on pharmacokinetics.

CHOOSING DOSE INCREMENTS

The increments between increasing doses of the same medicine should reflect a consistent pattern in terms of absolute or percentage increments. If doses of 50, 100, 200, 400, and 800 mg are tested in a clinical trial, then the next dose to be given should not be 900 mg but either 1,200 or 1,600 mg. If the adverse reactions observed at the 800-mg dose warrant, then the next dose may be adjusted downward to 1,000 mg. Dose increments in animals and in in vitro studies tend to

TABLE 14.1 *Various options to consider in developing a dosing schedule for the different periods of a clinical trial protocol*

A. Frequency of dosing
 1. Fixed intervals (e.g., q.i.d., t.i.d., b.i.d., q.d., q.o.d.)
 2. Variable intervals (e.g., p.r.n., titrating to a given effect or blood level)
 3. Combination of above
B. Medicines allowed between screen and dose ascension[a]
 1. Take patients off all medicines
 2. Take patients off specifically designated medicines or classes of medicines
 3. Allow specific medicines or a specific number of medicines to be taken
 4. Switch all patients to a standard medicine
 5. Allow patients to continue taking any or all medicines they were previously taking
C. Dose ascension[b]
 1. None, start the trial medicine at a maintenance dose
 2. Use a loading dose, then decrease dose to maintenance level
 3. Use a fixed dosage ascension for all patients
 4. Use a variable dosage ascension based on established criteria. Either the amount of the dosage, the time of administration, or both may be varied
 5. Taper a concomitant medicine during dose ascension of the trial medicine
D. Dose maintenance[c]
 1. A fixed number of doses or dose ranges allowed. Doses may not be changed during the maintenance period of the clinical trial
 2. Doses may be raised during this period for lack of an adequate therapeutic effect or for other reasons
 3. Doses may be lowered for adverse reactions, laboratory abnormalities, or other reasons
 4. Doses may be subsequently raised or lowered after an initial dosage change
E. Dose taper and discontinuation
 1. Dosage stopped without taper
 2. Fixed dosage taper schedule used for all patients
 3. Variable dosage taper schedule is based on established criteria or clinical judgment
 4. Trial medicine is tapered as another medicine is added
 5. Trial medicine is tapered after another medicine is added

[a] The doses and durations associated with each step must be specified.
[b] In several of these procedures, dose ascension may be performed in a fixed number of steps, or the number of possible steps may vary between patients. See Fig. 14.1 for an illustration of alternative methods for dose ascension.
[c] The frequency of allowable dose changes must be specified for any of these four choices (e.g., one change may be made per week or per trial or without limit).

increase in a logarithmic manner (e.g., x, $10x$, $100x$, $1,000x$ or x, $3.3x$, $10x$, $33x$, $100x$), but doses in humans usually increase arithmetically by (1) equal amounts (e.g., x, $2x$, $3x$, $4x$, $5x$), (2) approximately equal percentages (e.g., x, $2x$, $4x$, $8x$, $16x$), or (3) according to a specific formula (e.g., the modified Fibonacci dose escalation scheme of x, $2x$, $3.3x$, $5x$, $7x$, $9x$, $12x$, and $16x$; Penta et al., 1979). An alternative is to use 100% increments until the first hint of toxicity is observed and then to use the modified Fibonacci scheme or another plan with decreased increments of dose escalation. In some cases it is necessary to round doses up or down to match the strength to available tablets or capsules. There are numerous options to consider in planning dose ascension, maintenance, and withdrawal as well as the frequency of dosing. Some of these are shown in Tables 14.1 and 14.2, and alternatives to use in dose ascension are shown in Fig. 14.1.

1. Rapid (R) Gradual (G) or Slow (S) Dose Ascension

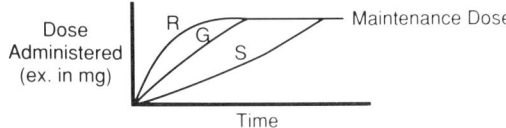

2. Loading Dose(s) Followed By Maintenance Doses

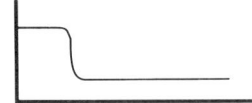

3. No Dose Ascension

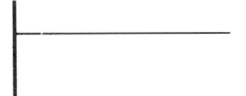

4. Stepwise Ascension

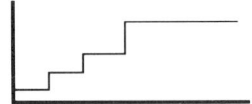

5. Ascension of Trial Medicine as Another Medicine is Tapered

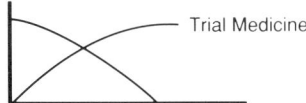

6. Ascension of Trial Medicine Followed by Taper of Another Medicine

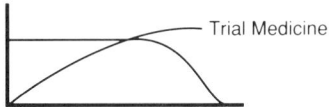

7. Combination of Above Methods

8. Temporary or Permanent Decreases in Doses During Ascension

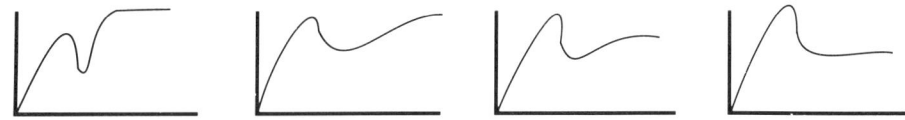

FIG. 14.1 Options available for dose ascension with a new or established medicine. Dose taper may follow the same schemata as those presented for dose ascension. Each *graph* has the same ordinate (dose administered) and abscissa (time). In the example of stepwise ascension, the number of steps may be variable or fixed, and the time between steps may be variable or fixed. In options 5 and 6, the dose ascension of the new medicine may follow any of the dose ascensions shown in options 1 to 4. Dose ascension is also referred to as the run-in period.

TABLE 14.2 *Options for choosing fixed and/or flexible dosages[a]*

1. Fixed/unchanging. Dosage held constant at a fixed level (e.g., 100 mg/day for 5 days) or within a specified range (e.g., 10–20 mg/day for 5 days) for entire clinical trial
2. Fixed/changing. Dosage held constant at a fixed level (e.g., 5 mg/day for the first week, 10 mg/day for the second week, and 30 mg/day for the third and fourth weeks) or within a specified range (e.g., 5–10 mg/day for the first week, 20–40 mg/day for the second week) with increasing and/or decreasing levels
3. Flexible. Dosage changes according to the patient's needs (e.g., dose may be titrated to achieve and maintain a given clinical endpoint or laboratory effect such as blood level); an upper and lower dose limit are usually provided
4. Fixed/flexible[b]. Dosage fixed for initial and/or earlier administrations, but with an option for the investigator to individualize dosage according to patient needs after a certain point is reached in the protocol. Dosage changes may be based on time, number of doses given, amount of medicine given, toxicity, or therapeutic effect. The optional (i.e., flexible) dosages may be (1) limited to one or a set number or range of doses chosen according to specific criteria or (2) limited to a set amount or range (or other measure), (3) limited or specified by other criteria, or (4) not specifically limited at all
5. Flexible/fixed[b]. Dosages are flexible in the initial phases of the protocol, often until a specific effect or blood level is achieved, and then the dosage is fixed for the remainder of the clinical trial

[a] These options refer to one group being treated with a trial medicine. Different groups may be treated in the same manner with different doses or dose ranges of the trial medicine to create a dose–response relationship.
[b] Variations of these options are possible using a third part (e.g., a fixed/flexible/fixed schedule or other criteria in choosing trial doses).

FACTORS INVOLVED IN DEVELOPING DOSAGE SCHEDULES

The dosage form and route of administration to be used have a major impact on the dosage schedule developed. The choice of these variables is generally determined at an early phase of the clinical trial's conceptualization and is sometimes related to the trial's objectives (e.g., comparing effects of an i.v. and oral form of a medicine). The topics of dosage form and route of administration are presented in Chapters 18 and 19, respectively.

Fixed versus Variable Dosing Schedules

It is pertinent to determine whether to study a fixed or variable dose(s) of the trial medicine. If a substantial amount of information is available about the trial medicine, then using fixed doses rather than a dose range(s) offers a number of advantages. If, however, a new medicine is being initially evaluated for efficacy, then it may be preferable to use variable doses. This is because insufficient data exist on a new medicine that could be used to choose the most appropriate fixed doses to study, and using dose ranges allows for flexibility in evaluating more doses.

Dose-Ranging Trials

The goals of a dose-ranging trial are to identify the:

1. Maximally tolerated dose (i.e., the top or plateau of the dose–response relationship in terms of safety)
2. Minimally effective dose (i.e., the threshold of the dose–response relationship in terms of efficacy)
3. Effective dose range for maintenance therapy (i.e., the range of doses demonstrating both efficacy and safety over the duration of time desired)
4. Starting dose to initiate treatment. This dose may or may not be the same as the minimally effective dose and may be within or below the effective dose range
5. Rate of dose ascension
6. Rate of dose taper and withdrawal.

Both the maximally tolerated dose and minimally effective dose may be defined in terms of single doses or multiple doses. Examples of dose-ranging trials in Phase I are listed in Table 14.3.

Dose Ascension

During Phases I and IIa, it is important to gradually increase the amount of medicine given to a patient. The exact definition of "gradually" must be determined for each medicine and for each patient population receiving it. Rapid escalation of the administered dose may lead to severe adverse events that could terminate the development of a promising new medicine. Kleinbloesem et al. (1987) demonstrated that slower dose ascension of nifedipine decreased or eliminated the serious hemodynamic adverse events that were observed with a more rapid ascension.

Establishing the Optimal Dose of a New Medicine for Clinical Trials

Selected approaches to follow in Phase I to shorten the time for conducting clinical trials is shown in Table 14.4. One goal of Phase I is to know the peak of the dose response prior to initiating Phase II clinical trials. In Phase II pilot trials, it is important to titrate patients up to the maximally tolerated dose or slightly below and look for evidence of efficacy. If patients are unable to tolerate that dose, progressively lower doses must be tested. Determine the peak dose tolerated and whether satisfactory efficacy occurs based on clinical trial objectives and the definition of a responder. If satisfactory efficacy occurs, then subsequent clinical trials may investigate if efficacy is observed at lower doses, or with doses spaced further apart.

No evidence of efficacy (or insufficient efficacy)

TABLE 14.3 *Types of dose ranging in Phase I clinical trials*

Type of trial	Type of dosing	Method of trial	Objective
One single dose per patient	Fixed	Gradual increase in doses, using new population for each dose	Establish upper limit or range of dose tolerance
Multiple single-doses per patient	Fixed	Same as above, but in the same population	Establish upper limit or range of dose tolerance for single doses
Multiple doses per patient for 3 to 7 days	Fixed	Each group receives a fixed dose	Establish upper limit or range of dose tolerance for multiple doses given over 3 to 7 days
	Titrated	Each group is titrated to their fixed level, or all patients are titrated to their maximally tolerated dose	
	Variable	Each group receives either fixed or titrated doses, but can be adjusted upwards or downwards depending on responses	
Multiple doses per patient for 1 to 4 weeks	Fixed, titrated, or variable	Same as above	Establish upper limit or range of dose tolerance for multiple doses given over 1 to 4 weeks

may be observed at peak responses tested in pilot Phase II trials. This could occur because patients are able to tolerate much higher doses than the volunteers used in Phase I clinical trials. If that outcome can be anticipated in advance, then patients rather than volunteers should be included in at least some Phase I clinical trials to determine their maximum tolerated dose. If this is not done and the tolerance of patients is discovered in a Phase II clinical trial, then it will be necessary to conduct a new Phase I clinical trial to identify patients' true maximal tolerated dose.

The correct dosing schedule should be established during Phase IIa for all but a few medicines. The major exception is for anticancer medicines, since so many different dosing schedules are possible and identifying the best schedule often takes many years. Standard

TABLE 14.4 *Methods to shorten the time of Phase I clinical trials[a]*

1. Start the clinical trial at a larger dose. This is most easily done in a second Phase I trial[b]
2. Use a more rapid escalation of doses than the modified Fibonacci scheme
3. Use fewer patients per dose. This step is particularly relevant for anticancer trials in which patients are often studied sequentially rather than simultaneously
4. Test fewer dosing schedules for anticancer medicines[c]
5. Conduct fewer duplicative clinical trials

[a] A slower dose escalation minimizes patient risk for toxicity, but for anticancer medicines, a single Phase I clinical trial may take from 1 to 2 years to complete, can exhaust the pool of available patients, ends up treating most with subtherapeutic doses, and requires an excessive number of dose levels.
[b] For example, use 100% dose escalations until any biological effect is observed, then use 50% dose escalations until toxicity is first observed, and then use 33% dose escalations. The modified Fibonacci scheme usually requires too many steps to reach the maximally tolerated dose. Oncologists tend to use percent increases instead of amounts of medicine (e.g., 200 mg) to express increments between doses.
[c] Dosing schedules (e.g., weekly ×3, daily ×3, single dose every 3 weeks) are changed to alter and hopefully decrease toxicity. They have little to do with efficacy of anticancer medicines.

textbooks on anticancer methodology discuss this issue in detail.

Expressing Dosages

Dosages may be specified on the basis of a patient's (1) weight (e.g., mg/kg), (2) size (e.g., mg/m² of body surface area), (3) result of a laboratory test (e.g., creatinine clearance), or (4) other characteristics of the patient. Doses are often given in milligrams per kilogram instead of a total number of milligrams (1) for newly tested medicines with steep dose–response curves, (2) when safety and/or efficacy are not well defined, or (3) if toxicity (or efficacy) has been found to be directly proportional to the dose per body weight. The general options of utilizing fixed or flexible dosages are shown in Table 14.2. Dosage regimens (schedules) are based on both the quantity of the dose and the intervals chosen for medicine administration, i.e., a dosing regimen includes a measure of both quantity and time.

Dosing Schedules for a Safety Trial

For most clinical trials a plan for frequency of dosing, dose ascension, taper, and withdrawal must be based on previous clinical experience, pharmacokinetics, and relevant preclinical data. In a safety study, patients may be dosed either to intolerance or to a dose expected to yield a therapeutic effect or prespecified blood level or range. It is usually valuable in at least one Phase I clinical trial to increase the dose of a new medicine to the point at which clinically significant adverse reactions appear. This provides information on the upper limits of safety and indicates a dose range in which efficacy studies may be conducted. A list of many of the parameters used in selecting medicine dosages is given in Chapter 16.

Developing a Strategy for Determining a Dosing Schedule

The particular clinical trial being designed may be part of a larger plan to develop a new medicine or to explore a specific clinical area through a number of trials. If this is so, then the goals of the clinical program as they relate to dosage (e.g., b.i.d. or q.d. dosing; narrow or broad dose ranges) must be kept in mind as one proceeds from trial to trial, developing clinical data that one hopes will support the established goals. For example, in order to maximize the chances of demonstrating efficacy, it may be prudent to dose patients four times a day initially even though the goal of the clinical program may be eventually to dose patients twice a day.

Another part of the strategy should be to determine the lowest maintenance dose that can be used. This is important to establish because that dose will generally be safer for patients than a higher one. More attention has been paid to this topic in recent years because it was found that traditionally used doses for certain medicines were greater than those required for efficacy (e.g., hydrochlorothiazide, captopril). This may result from many factors, such as the desire in early clinical trials to demonstrate efficacy as rapidly as possible, thus testing a high dose. Also, because less severely ill patients are often treated with marketed medicines, the doses necessary to elicit sufficient efficacy usually decrease.

Describing a Dosing Schedule

Many descriptions of dosing are vague. Instructions to take a medicine three times a day could mean every 8 hours, three times arbitrarily chosen during working hours, or at meal times. Instructions to take a dose with meals could mean five doses to someone who eats five times a day, or one dose to someone who only has one meal a day.

It may be relevant to note in a protocol whether the dosages of the trial medicine are given in terms of salt or free base and also whether the medicine(s) should be ingested in a fixed relationship to meals or with a certain amount of fluids. Phase I studies often specify the amount of water to be used for ingesting each oral dose (often 200 to 400 ml) and the relationship of medicine dosing to meals. These factors are not generally indicated in Phase II and III protocols unless the medicine is (1) known or believed to cause local irritation, (2) not adequately dissolved without ingestion of an

appropriate volume of fluid, or (3) affected by some or all foods (e.g., tetracyclines are bound by dairy products).

After the dosage schedule has been determined, it must be clearly presented in the protocol. A few sample table headings that could be adapted or modified are shown for single-dose clinical trials in Table 14.5 and for multiple-dose trials in Table 14.6. Many additional tables of dosing schedules are presented in *Presentation of Clinical Data* (Spilker and Schoenfelder, 1990). One of the most important principles is that dosing decisions should usually be based on clinical endpoints rather than pharmacokinetic ones.

Factors to Consider in Developing a Dosing Schedule for Anticancer Medicines

Some of the factors to consider in developing a dosing schedule for an anticancer medicine are listed in Table 14.7 and some examples are listed in Table 14.8. It is often difficult to know how to balance the amount of resources devoted to evaluating efficacy and safety for a single dosage schedule in depth versus spreading available resources to evaluate many possible dosage schedules. A sampling of different types of schedules is often tried in an attempt to find the optimal method of administering the medicine.

TABLE 14.5 *Sample tables of dosage regimens for acute single dose medicine studies*

Study day	Patient group code[a]	Dosing period no.[b]	Active group (N = 12)	Placebo (P) group (N = 6)	Total active dose (mg)
1	A	1	1 × 200 mg + 5 P	6 P	200
4	B	2	2 × 200 mg + 4 P	6 P	400
8	A	3	3 × 200 mg + 3 P	6 P	600
11	B	4	4 × 200 mg + 2 P	6 P	800
15	A	5	5 × 200 mg + 1 P	6 P	1000
18	B	6	6 × 200 mg + 0 P	6 P	1200

Dose period	Placebo group (N = 6) (no. of placebo capsules)	0.5 mg	1.0 mg	4.0 mg	8.0 mg	Placebo capsules (no.)	Total dose (mg)
1	4	1	0	0	0	3	0.5
2	4	0	1	0	0	3	1.0
3	4	0	2	0	0	2	2.0
4	4	0	0	1	0	3	4.0
5	4	0	0	2	0	2	8.0
6	4	0	0	0	2	2	16.0

[a] A and B are two separate groups of patients.
[b] The time between dosing periods may be specified in terms of a fixed time, the minimum or maximum time allowed, or a range of times.

TABLE 14.6 *Sample tables of dosage regimens for multidose medicine studies*

Day of trial	Placebo group (tablets)	Low-dose group					High-dose group				
		75-mg tablets	150-mg tablets	P[a]	Total (mg/dose)	Total (mg/day)	75-mg tablets	150-mg tablets	P	Total (mg/dose)	Total (mg/day)
1	3	1	0	2	75	300	0	1	2	150	600
2–5	3	0	1	2	150	600	0	2	1	300	1200
6–10	3	1	1	1	225	900	0	3	0	450	1800

Daily time of dosing (days 1–21)		No. of capsules to be taken			Total (mg/day)	
Elapsed time (hr)	Actual time (hr)	Placebo (P) group (N = 12)	Active medicine		Low dose	High dose
			Low dose (N = 12)	High dose (N = 12)		
0	8–10 A.M.	2 P	1–5 mg + 1 P	2–5 mg	20	40
4	12–2 P.M.	2 P	1–5 mg + 1 P	2–5 mg		
8	4–6 P.M.	2 P	1–5 mg + 1 P	2–5 mg		
12	8–10 P.M.	2 P	1–5 mg + 1 P	2–5 mg		

Weight of patient (kg)	Total dose of trial medicine (mg) for three groups of patients in each of the 9 weeks of study[b]								
	1	2	3	4	5	6	7	8	9
10–19.9	50 (50)	100 (100)	100 (100)	150 (50, 100)	150 (50, 100)	200 (200)	200 (200)	100 (100)	0
20–39.9	100 (100)	150 (50, 100)	150 (50, 100)	200 (200)	200 (200)	300 (100, 200)	300 (100, 200)	150 (50, 100)	0
40–60	150 (50, 100)	200 (100, 100)	200 (100, 100)	300 (100, 200)	300 (100, 200)	400 (200, 200)	400 (200, 200)	200 (200)	0

[a] P, placebo.
[b] The tablet sizes required for each dose are in parentheses (tablets are assumed to be available in 50, 100, and 200 mg). Placebos are used to make up two tablets per dose.

Adjusting Dosages during a Clinical Trial

Dosage adjustments are often described in a protocol in various tables (e.g., Table 14.6). Many examples are given in *Presentation of Clinical Data* (Spilker and Schoenfelder, 1990). These adjustments are based on a number of factors that may be used in clinical trials when specific adjustments are unspecified or are general.

1. Safety parameters (e.g., laboratory analyses, adverse reactions, clinical signs, electrocardiograms).
2. Efficacy parameters.
3. Blood level of parent medicine.
4. Pharmacokinetic parameters.
5. Patient characteristics (e.g., sex, age, weight, size).

Dosing Variations

Some of the less common approaches to dosing are to dose patients every other day (e.g., with steroids) or to use drug holidays. With some anti-Parkinson's disease medicines patients take medicine during the week but not on weekends. Another common variation is for patients to take most (or all) of their medicine at bedtime.

TABLE 14.7 *Factors to consider in developing a dosing schedule for anticancer medicines*

1. Injection versus infusion
2. Duration of injection (e.g., bolus, 30 seconds)
3. Duration of infusion
4. Concentration of infusion
5. Number of injections per day or per week
6. Time between injections
7. Number of injections in a cycle
8. Time between cycles
9. Number of cycles in a treatment

TABLE 14.8 *Selected types of dosing schedules for anticancer medicines[a]*

Frequency[b]

1. Weekly for 3 to 6 weeks
2. Daily for 3 days, every 3 to 4 weeks
3. Daily for 5 days, every 3 to 4 weeks
4. Single dose, every 3 to 4 weeks
5. Continuous intravenous infusion of 24 hours, up to 120 hours

[a] Many cycle variations are possible and just about everything imaginable is in fact used.
[b] This cycle is often repeated after 3 to 4 weeks, which provides sufficient time for the patient's bone marrow to recover.

WITHDRAWAL OF THERAPY

The most conservative method of evaluating withdrawal of an investigational medicine is to gradually remove it over a period of time. If no problems are observed with this type of taper, a more rapid withdrawal, and also a sudden withdrawal may be evaluated under carefully controlled conditions during late Phase II or Phase III. It is important to evaluate whether the withdrawal elicits symptoms related to a withdrawal phenomenon resulting from the medicine or from a rebound effect of disease symptoms. The time until return of symptoms of the disease is also important to assess.

MODIFYING DOSING SCHEDULES

Approaches

There are two general approaches for developing dosing schedules for a clinical protocol. The first approach is to establish the dosing schedule to be used on the assumption that each patient behaves as an ideal patient and that no complications will occur that require modification of the dose. The second approach is to provide information that describes what the investigator and patient should do when everything is not proceeding according to the protocol plan and dosage modifications are required. The first aspect was discussed in the chapters on choosing a clinical trial design, and the second is briefly reviewed in this section.

Modifications Allowed by Protocol

Modifications or variations of dosing that are permitted by protocol could be included in the type of table illustrated in Tables 14.5 and 14.6. Examples of situations that might require dosage modification include adverse reactions, abnormal laboratory or clinical examinations, blood or urine trial medicine levels outside an acceptable range, exacerbation of the disease, remission of the disease, missed appointments, and missed doses. It is impossible to describe fully each of these potential problems in a protocol. The protocol should describe whether dose changes are acceptable and, if so, whether fixed dose increments (or ranges) or unrestricted dose adjustments may be used and whether any restrictions will be imposed on the total number or frequency of dose adjustments. The general or specific criteria that the investigator must follow to alter the dose of the trial medicine are usually stated in the protocol.

Concomitant Medicines

In some cases, dose adjustments must be made in the prescription of concomitant medications rather than in the dose of the trial medicine. Criteria for dose adjustments of concomitant medications must also be established. See Table 14.9 for a list of some of the options used to control dosages and use of concomitant medicines during a clinical trial. For example, in the area of epilepsy, blood levels of concomitant antiepileptic medicines are often monitored. If these levels fall outside the normal therapeutic range (or possibly change by a specific percentage from the baseline value but still remain within the therapeutic range), it may be desirable to adjust the dose to try to bring the blood level within the normal range. Laboratory data, however, are not infallible, and a repeated determination to confirm the accuracy of the abnormality is often important to obtain. In the case of an abnormal value, the need to repeat the test may be specified in the protocol. A further complication may ensue if an abnormal laboratory value is reported in an outpatient trial after the patient has returned home and the patient lives a great distance from the trial site. The patient may be requested to go to another laboratory to have the required test performed. This situation may also

TABLE 14.9 *Options for controlling concomitant medicines during the clinical trial*

1. No medicines other than the study medicine may be used for any reason
2. Other medicines are permitted only to treat adverse reactions
3. All patients must continue their specific antidisease medicine(s) at their initial (fixed) dose
4. Same option as 3, but the concomitant medicine's dose may be adjusted by the investigator according to criteria described in the protocol
5. Same option as 3, but the concomitant medicine's dose may be self-adjusted by the patient according to general (or specific) criteria
6. Patients may be given one (or more) medicine from a list of standard antidisease medicines if it is necessary for them to receive adjunctive treatment
7. Medications used prior to the clinical trial to treat other diseases or problems will be permitted during the trial, and the dosages used (may not) vary
8. Concomitant medicines are allowed to treat the disease being studied, but no concomitant medicines may be used to treat other diseases
9. In the case of a disease exacerbation or in the case of a medical emergency unrelated to the disease, other medicines may be used, and the patient may remain in the trial
10. No restriction on other medicine therapies will be made either for the trial disease or for other diseases
11. Use of nonprescription medicines may (may not) be restricted; any restrictions must be specified
12. Certain combinations (or variations) of the above options may be specified, including qualifications of the frequency, per-dose amount of medicine, total daily (weekly) dose amount, or other factors

be resolved by establishing criteria based on whether the abnormal blood level value of the medicine is accompanied by adverse reactions (presumably from too high a blood level) or seizure exacerbations in studies on antiepileptic medicines (presumably from too low a blood level). If either of these clinical observations is made, then dosage adjustments would occur immediately, without a requirement to confirm the blood level abnormality.

How Can One Conserve Rare Supplies of a Medicine during Initial Phase I Human Trials?

The major procedure recommended to conserve a medicine is based on the principle that patients can usually tolerate a higher single dose of medicine than multiple smaller doses. One can potentially conserve medicine supply in Phase I by giving patients a low single dose, followed by washout, and subsequently giving the same patients multiple doses of the same strength previously received. This process is repeated in the same patients or in a separate group at each dosage level. This procedure is particularly well suited where acute adverse reactions occur at much higher doses than when a low dose is repeated several times.

Other methods to conserve medicine are to have a small number (the vanguard group) of patients take a higher dose of medicine before a larger group of patients. It is also possible to use fewer patients in a clinical trial, to use maximally acceptable dosing strength increments, and, simply to stay below the maximally tolerated dose in the initial clinical trial. Finally, make up the fewest dosage strengths possible,

since each requires a great deal of compound for technical development activities (e.g., formulation development, stability testing).

How Can One Conserve Rare Supplies of a Medicine during Phase II and Phase III Clinical Trials?

The major procedures recommended to conserve supplies of a medicine during Phases II and III (in addition to those relevant ones listed above) are:

1. Do not order as much overage as usual in terms of amount of bulk medicine to be made into capsules or other dosage forms.
2. Do not design clinical trials with fixed doses per patient group, but titrate patients from low doses to high based on their tolerance (i.e., safety) and responses (i.e., efficacy).
3. Do not put as many extra capsules or tablets into each container.
4. Do not ship each investigator more than a few (if any) extra containers of medicine.
5. Ensure that any glass vials or bottles are packed extremely carefully. Take any other steps necessary to ensure delivery of medicine and impress on investigators the fact that medicine supplies are scarce.
6. Repackage the unused bottles that are returned to the sponsor after the trial is completed. This practice may not be followed for all types of medicines.
7. Transfer unused bottles from one site to another in a multicenter clinical trial.

CHAPTER 15

Methods of Assessing and Improving Patient Compliance in Clinical Trials

IMPORTANCE OF ASSESSING COMPLIANCE

The term *compliance* is generally used in clinical trials to describe the adherence of patients to taking their medicines as prescribed. *Patient compliance* means a great deal more than merely "the patients took their medicines as directed." Other types of adherence may be described. In addition, the compliance of several different groups of people (e.g., investigators, sponsors) involved with a clinical trial may be described.

Assessment of compliance often enables individuals to determine whether a negative clinical trial resulted from an inactive medicine or from a failure of patients to take their medicine. To assess the efficacy and safety of a medicine under various conditions, patients must take the medicine as prescribed. Negative results of a clinical trial could also relate to either a failure of an investigator to follow adequately (i.e., comply with) a protocol or a failure of the medicine to work. Compliance of both patients and investigators should be measured and evaluated before the results of a clinical trial are interpreted. Compliance by investigators is only briefly discussed in this chapter.

POTENTIAL RAMIFICATIONS OF POOR PATIENT COMPLIANCE

Poor compliance that is undetected in a clinical trial may result in (1) invalid results and (2) in a medicine that is actually effective for certain populations (under certain conditions) being labeled as ineffective. A number of reasons for poor patient compliance are listed in Table 15.1. Positive data regarding a medicine's effectiveness obtained in compliant patients should not be extrapolated to noncompliant patients. The opposite situation of extrapolating ineffective data obtained in noncompliant patients to compliant patients may also be inappropriate. Data obtained in a mixed population of both compliant and noncompliant patients may not be appropriate to extrapolate to a single patient. Thus, dosage recommendations in package inserts that are based on patients with an average rate of compliance may be inappropriate for patients who take full doses, and definitely will be inappropriate for noncompliant patients. Another ramification of poor patient compliance is that excess medicine from the clinical trial is available to patients after their participation is completed. This potential health hazard is aggravated by the already large number of partially consumed medicines available in most households.

When physicians observe that a medicine is ineffective and they are unaware of a patient's noncompliance, they often inappropriately increase the dose in an attempt to improve efficacy. This occurs during both clinical trials and treatment. Figure 15.1 is an example of this (Case 3). Numerous studies have attempted to identify compliers and noncompliers based on personality traits and behavior (Davis, 1968; Schwartz and Griffin, 1986), but the results of such studies are mixed and universal generalizations have not emerged. Some patient behaviors required for compliance are listed in Table 15.2.

TABLE 15.1 *Selected reasons for poor patient compliance*

A. Disease-related reasons
 1. Few symptoms present (e.g., mild hypertension)
 2. Terminal illness known to patient, particularly when accompanied by physical debilitation
B. Patient-related reasons
 1. Forgetfulness
 2. Lack of complete belief in the value of the treatment
 3. Poor taste of the medicine
 4. Size of the medicine tablets or capsules
 5. Cost of therapy
 6. Adverse reactions
 7. Safety containers
 8. Mental illness
 9. Lack of understanding of terms used (e.g., take with meals may mean before, during, or after meals)
 10. Anger at, or dissatisfaction with, investigator or his or her staff
 11. Incomplete understanding of how to be compliant with the protocol
C. Clinical trial- or medical practice-related reasons
 1. Number of pills required to ingest at each dosing
 2. Number of times a day the medicine must be taken
 3. Large number of medicines prescribed
 4. Medicine regimens that tend to be confusing or complex
 5. Requirements of protocol may be too painful, stressful, or demanding
 6. Long duration of therapy
D. Investigator-related reasons
 1. Long time period from referral to appointment
 2. Patient is kept waiting a long time by the investigator
 3. Failure of physician to keep appointment
 4. Poor physician–patient relationship[a]

[a] See Table 15.7.

TABLE 15.2 *Patient behaviors required for compliance in an outpatient clinical practice*

1. Visit physician or clinic
2. Answer questions about their medical history honestly
3. Cooperate in testing, particularly when a voluntary effort is requested (e.g., forced expiratory volume in 1 second)
4. Allow required tests to be performed
5. Purchase or obtain medicines prescribed
6. Take medicines as prescribed in terms of doses and timing
7. Adhere to appointment schedule
8. Adhere to advice or requests regarding diet, exercise, relaxation, or other aspects of behavior

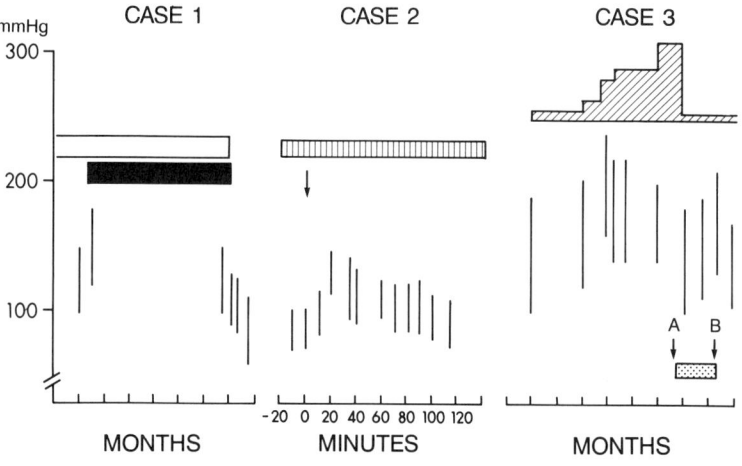

FIG. 15.1 Difficulties in interpreting drug adverse reactions, illustrated from hypertension. **Case 1**, hypertension unresponsive to clonidine (solid bar), but relieved by withdrawing oral contraceptive (open bar). **Case 2**, interaction in a normal subject given small doses of debrisoquin continuously, with a single 50 mg oral dose of phenylephrine (↓). **Case 3**, a patient-doctor interaction: up to A the patient was not taking the bethanidine tablets (dosage, prescribed from hospital, 40 mg/day rising to 300 mg/day, diagonal hatch lines). At A an admonition was given. At B the general practitioner agreed to withdraw diethylpropion (horizontal hatch lines); bethanidine now 30 mg/day. Reprinted from Vere (1976) with permission.

TYPES OF COMPLIANCE

For ease of discussion, the types of compliance in a clinical trial are categorized by their primary relation to patients, sponsors, or investigators. Compliance issues could also be described in terms of problems of omission (e.g., failure to take medicine, to file a regulatory document, or to report an adverse reaction) or commission (e.g., overdose, inappropriate self-medication, not adhering to protocol requirements by doing something differently).

Patient Compliance and Noncompliance

Patients must comply with the investigator's instructions by taking the recommended number of medicines at the correct times, coming to the clinic as directed, being cooperative and honest with the staff who are conducting the study, and adhering to all other aspects of the study (e.g., avoiding the forbidden concomitant medicines, following the recommended diet, following the prescribed exercise program). Additionally, in some clinical trials patients must fill prescriptions. It is usually assumed that patients who ingest their medicine as prescribed are also compliant with other aspects of a protocol, but this is certainly not always the case.

Patients who are noncompliant with the protocol often withdraw from a clinical trial. If patients from different treatment groups withdraw from a clinical trial at variable rates, results may be affected, especially in longitudinal studies.

Although noncompliance is at the opposite end of a spectrum from compliance, both are relative concepts. In some clinical trials, patients may be (or must be) discontinued because of noncompliance. Although there are pros and cons to this practice, it should not be done during Phase III clinical trials. If it is to be done during a Phase II clinical trial, a standard of noncompliance should be defined, before the trial starts, that will be used as a basis for patient discontinuation. The standard may contain any one or more of the following concepts: (1) fewer than X% tablets used, based on pill counts or medication bottle openings; (2) tablets missed for Y days, based on patient history or medication bottle openings; (3) blood levels below Z; (4) poor attitude and cooperation with staff; (5) missing two or more consecutive clinic visits without an excellent excuse; (6) use of prohibited medicines; or (7) failure to cooperate in a specified manner. Several patterns of noncompliance are described by Urquhart (1989).

Sponsor Compliance

Sponsors of clinical trials must adhere to regulatory compliance. This involves many steps and processes including producing an Investigational New Drug Application (IND); submitting the protocol (for clinical trials conducted in the United States) to the Food and Drug Administration (FDA); ensuring that the investigator has had the protocol approved by the Ethics Committee or Institutional Review Board (IRB); and adhering to Good Manufacturing Practices, Good Laboratory Practices, and Good Clinical Practices regulations. Other regulations affecting the sponsor's adherence to a protocol may also apply (e.g., reporting of adverse reactions).

Investigator Compliance in Clinical Trials and Medical Practice

Investigators must comply with numerous aspects of a clinical protocol. These include submitting the protocol to their Ethics Committee or IRB and providing periodic updates and an end-of-clinical-trial report, adhering to agreements made through negotiations with sponsors (and vice versa), adhering to details of the protocol in treating patients, and adhering to administrative responsibilities (e.g., reporting adverse reactions, completing data collection forms).

In private medical practice, clinicians may not comply with the manufacturers' advice in the package labeling about using a medicine.

WHY AND HOW PATIENTS DO NOT COMPLY WITH CLINICAL TRIAL REQUIREMENTS

There are many reasons why patients may not comply with the requirements of a protocol. These may relate to the characteristics of the trial design, trial medicine, individual patient's personality, relationships with study personnel, or other factors. Some of these reasons are listed in Table 15.1.

The quality of most outpatient studies is enhanced by incorporating a test or tests for compliance in the protocol. A compliance test with follow-up questioning of noncompliant patients may uncover a reason for diminished compliance that could be addressed in a protocol amendment (or new protocol). The revised protocol would enable data to be collected that would have a greater chance of meeting the objectives of the clinical trial.

Information on why protocol compliance was inadequate might assist in the interpretation of the data. A number of the ways in which patients fail to comply with a clinical trial are listed in Table 15.3. These illustrations of decreased compliance are broadly divided into those related to the trial medicine and those related to other aspects of the trial.

TABLE 15.3 *Selected ways in which patients fail to comply with a protocol*

A. Noncompliance primarily related to the clinical trial medicine
 1. Patients do not fill their prescriptions for medicine
 2. Patients do not take the medicine as directed; patients take
   a. Too few doses per day, but at the correct times
   b. Too few doses per day and at irregular times
   c. Irregular numbers of doses per day
   d. Correct number of doses per day, but at incorrect fixed times (i.e., in relation to meals or over too short a period)
   e. Too many doses on some days
   f. Irregular number of tablets per dose
   g. No doses on some days and a correct or incorrect pattern on other days
 3. Patients may prematurely discontinue the medicine (this is especially significant if antibiotics or some other classes of medicines are prematurely stopped)
 4. Patients place the medicine in their "cheek" (for inpatient studies) and then discard the dosage (or otherwise improperly ingest the medication)
B. Noncompliance unrelated to the clinical trial medicine
 1. Patients may not adhere to the clinic visit schedule, may not contact the clinic as directed (e.g., for adverse reactions), or may fail to bring their medicines, diaries, or biological samples (e.g., urine) to clinic
 2. Patients may not properly complete patient diaries or other materials
 3. Patients may not maintain a diet, exercise program, or other outpatient aspect of the clinical trial

TABLE 15.4 *Tests for compliance*

A. Direct methods
 1. Observation of patient taking medicine
 2. Measure the levels of a medicine or metabolite in biological fluids (e.g., blood, urine)
 3. Measure the presence of a biological marker attached to placebo or medicine
 4. Conduct unannounced spot checks on patients at their homes to obtain a biological fluid or sample
 5. Measure clinic attendance and count the number of missed and canceled appointments
 6. Screen urine or blood samples for medicines prohibited by protocol (e.g., caffeine and nicotine, if relevant)
B. Indirect methods
 1. Question the patient at the outset of a clinical trial
 2. Assess patients' compliance based on their clinical response
 3. Conduct pill counts of trial and possibly other medicines
 4. Use electronic counters
 5. Determine the number of prescriptions filled and also refilled at pharmacies (i.e., the total quantity of medicine dispensed is calculated)
 6. Question the patient verbally or via questionnaire during treatment
 7. Use medication monitors (i.e., mechanical dispensers)
 8. Measure physiological markers
 9. Evaluate patient diaries for completeness and compliance with instructions
 10. Assess children's compliance through a school nurse or teacher

DIRECT METHODS TO MEASURE AND EVALUATE PATIENT COMPLIANCE

Patient compliance with taking medicines may be assessed directly (i.e., proof of a certain degree of compliance) or indirectly. Indirect methods depend on patient reports or on data that could be modified, if desired, by the patient. A summary of these methods is given in Table 15.4.

Observation

Probably the most direct method to assess compliance is to observe patients taking their medication. This approach would be limited to a few inpatient trials or those outpatient trials where patients are required to come to a clinic to receive medicine each time it is to be taken. Even in those situations, some patients are not compliant. For example, they may "cheek" their medicine or merely pretend to put it in their mouths. If this is suspected it may be possible to assay directly blood or urine samples for the medicine, a metabolite, or an added marker.

Biological Markers

Markers are sometimes added as a means of determining compliance when assays are unavailable to measure the level of medicine or its metabolites present in a plasma or urine sample. Markers are also considered for clinical trials in which a placebo is used. The marker that is added must be (1) nontoxic at the doses added, (2) chemically stable in biological fluids, (3) easily detected at levels used by methods that are sensitive and specific, and (4) biologically inert. It is also important that absorption and kinetic parameters are similar to those of the medicine with which it is combined. The marker should be unaffected by food or other medicines used and the patient should be unaware of its use. Riboflavin may be added as a marker to both placebo and medicine. It is eliminated in the urine and fluoresces when exposed to ultraviolet light. If the medicine is excreted or eliminated via the urine, then fluorescing agents may be used as markers and urine samples collected for evaluation. Biological markers include quinine, phenol red, sodium bromide, phenobarbital, and digoxin.

Levels in Biological Fluids

When medicines have a long half-life, arbitrarily defined as greater than 24 hours, their presence in a biological fluid does not confirm compliance, since recent doses may have been skipped. A medicine with a short half-life may be ingested by a patient shortly before going to a clinic and thus its presence in blood or urine does not confirm compliance. In fact, the presence of a medicine, its metabolite, or a marker in blood or urine only confirms that one or a few doses have been taken within a limited time period, whose length is determined by the half-life of the medicine, metabolite, or marker measured.

The interpretation of medicine levels in biological samples may be viewed in either qualitative or quantitative terms. In qualitative terms, the test result is scored as present or absent, and in quantitative terms, the precise level is measured and evaluated. In evaluating the quantitative levels of medicine and comparing different patients, it is important that each patient have ingested his or her most recent dose at the same time interval prior to the taking of the biological sample.

A problem may arise in interpreting blood level data if the clinical trial test medicine has a short half-life. For example, consider three patients who took their medicine at the same time on the day of their clinic visit: one patient had not taken the medicine since his or her last clinic visit, the second patient had only taken the medicine for the day preceding the present visit, and the third had taken all of the prescribed medicine. The problem would be that all three patients might have the same blood level recorded on the day of the clinic visit, and the data would therefore be misleading in terms of measuring patient compliance.

Other biological samples have been used to assess compliance in selected cases. These include secretion of a medicine into sweat (collected with absorbent pads), saliva samples, and breath samples.

Coefficient of Variation

Other obstacles to direct measurement of compliance include variations in a medicine's metabolism and dose-response relationships. These issues also make single determinations of blood levels uncertain indicators of compliance. Leppik et al. (1979) proposed a coefficient of variation as a method to overcome these problems in epileptic patients treated with phenytoin. A problem with this measurement is that if patients consistently take one-half or other fractions of their prescribed dose, they will have a low coefficient of variation, which implies a high degree of compliance. Another potential problem is that this method can only test medicine taking events for a few half-lives prior to the time of sampling.

Spot Checks on Patients

If it is believed that outpatients are compliant for a short period prior to their clinic visit, but may not be compliant at other times, it is often possible to conduct spot checks on some or all patients in the clinical trial. Using this method, a member of the clinical team makes unannounced visits to patients at their homes sometime between clinic visits. This clinician or nurse collects a blood, urine, or other biological sample in which the amount of study medicine is measured. This method represents a potential invasion of privacy and must be carefully discussed with patients prior to their enrollment in the clinical trial. The agreement of patients to this procedure of spot checking should be part of the informed consent. This technique is only feasible if patients live relatively close to the clinical trial site and resources are available to visit patients and collect samples.

One variation on this method is for a nurse to visit patients after they call to make an appointment. While it provides patients greater opportunity to cheat (i.e., increase their compliance prior to the visit) it is uncertain that this would occur.

Clinic Attendance

If compliance is assessed in terms of clinic attendance, then examining the records of clinic attendance is a direct method to assess patient compliance.

INDIRECT METHODS TO MEASURE AND EVALUATE PATIENT COMPLIANCE

Numerous indirect measures of patient compliance exist. The extrapolation of acceptable compliance from data gathered with some of these methods may be unwarranted.

Questioning the Patient at the Outset of a Clinical Trial

Patients may be asked at the outset of a clinical trial whether they intend to be compliant (e.g., ask patients if they are willing to take the medicine as directed). An affirmative response to this question should be one of the inclusion criteria in almost any clinical trial. Any patient answering "no" should not be enrolled or should be discontinued, except for extenuating circumstances (e.g., psychosis, parents to ensure compliance).

Assessment Based on Clinical Response

The patient is assumed to be compliant if he or she improves on the active treatment, or does not improve on placebo.

Pill Counts

The most commonly used measure of compliance apart from direct questioning is probably that of the pill count. The actual number of tablets or capsules in the medicine container used by the patient are counted at each (or selected) clinic visits, and the expected number to be used is also determined. The ratio of actual pill use divided by expected pill use (multiplied by 100) gives a figure that may be referred to as percent compliance. Any refills obtained by the patient must be considered in calculating the actual number of pills used, and any changes in the dose prescribed must be considered in calculating the expected number of pills to be used. Care must be used in determining these figures, since patients often switch medicines between bottles (e.g., a "purse" bottle may be created by the patient), which could affect the numbers counted. Some protocols are written to exclude some or all of a patient's data from analysis if the patient's percent compliance falls below a defined level and to discontinue patients who are unable to offer a satisfactory explanation of their failure to comply adequately with the clinical trial.

If the patient does not bring his or her medications to the clinic or office visit, a definite plan should have been evolved to deal with the situation. The patient may be asked to count the number of pills at home and to telephone the information to the investigator, but this is not a wholly satisfactory method since it alerts the patient to the attention paid to pill counts and may make the patient feel that he or she is being watched too closely. In fact, all pill counts should be conducted out of the patient's sight. Another alternative is to omit performing the pill count in question and to give special attention to the pill count at the next visit. This option is reasonable if there are several pill counts scheduled during the clinical trial, but if the instance in question represented the only pill count in the trial, then requesting the patient to return to the clinic the next day or having a member of the clinical trial team visit the patient's home should be considered. Mailing medicines to patients or to the trial site is not generally advocated except when absolutely necessary and under carefully controlled conditions.

The method of pill counting has been validated in some clinical trials (Cromer et al., 1989), but other recent publications have been highly critical of this approach (Rudd et al., 1989; Pullar et al., 1989). The value of pill counts undoubtedly depends on the particular clinical trial and group of patients enrolled; they cannot be assumed to be an accurate reflection of patient compliance. It is expected that the use of this method will decrease in the future.

Electronic Counters

Electronic counters in the tops of specially prepared medicine bottles have been developed that record the exact day, hour, and minute each time the bottle of medicine is opened or used (Cheung et al., 1988a,b; Kass et al., 1984, 1986; Spector et al., 1986; Cramer et al., 1989). This method may demonstrate that patients open the container the correct number of times or either too few or too many. It also can demonstrate whether patients take their medicines at correct intervals. Despite the inability to know with certainty that patients have ingested the correct dose of medicine each time the bottle is opened, this is probably the best method to measure compliance in most outpatient trials. Selected advantages and disadvantages are listed in Table 15.5.

Pharmacy Refills

Pharmacy records demonstrate whether patients fill and refill their prescriptions at appropriate intervals. When this method is available, it may be valuable, since most patients do not purposely try to fool pharmacists. On the other hand, some people stockpile medicines, especially those they obtain at no cost or low cost. Obtaining refills of medicine according to a set schedule does not ensure ingestion of those medicines on schedule.

Questioning the Patient during Treatment

Physicians question patients informally about whether the patient remembers to take medicines as prescribed, and the physician believes the patient's compliance to be acceptable. The most simple and open approach to measuring compliance is to ask the patient a direct question such as "Are you taking all of your medicine?" or "Have you missed taking any of your medicine?" or, somewhat indirectly and possibly in a less threatening manner, "Are you having any difficulty remembering to take your medicine?"

TABLE 15.5 *Selected advantages and disadvantages of assessing compliance with electronic medication counters*

A. Advantages
 1. Precise data are obtained
 2. Data are easily quantifiable and expressed
 3. Provides the most accurate compliance data possible in numerous situations (e.g., medicine has a very short or very long half-life)
B. Disadvantages
 1. Patients may purposely fool the system if they desire (e.g., open lid an excessively large or small number of times)
 2. Patients may inadvertently invalidate the data (e.g., put medicine in other containers, check contents frequently, remove extra medicine for later dosing)
 3. The approach is expensive and therefore often impractical for large clinical trials
 4. The approach is an indirect measure in that it does not ensure ingestion of an appropriate number of tablets at the time the bottle is opened

Medication Monitors

Medicine bottles containing either the precise number of pills for a daily dose or a standard number of pills may be placed into a mechanical device, sometimes called a "medication monitor." In inpatient studies, the patient may be advised to operate this machine to obtain medication but is not informed that the number of bottles is being monitored. The number of bottles of trial medicine dispensed to a patient may be easily determined, although it is a separate question whether all doses of the trial medicine dispensed were actually ingested.

Physiological Markers

In certain clinical trials, physiological markers provide an indication of the degree of patient compliance. A well-known example is that of measuring heart rate in patients receiving β-adrenergic receptor-blocking medicines. If the heart rate is not in the expected range, and the patient is receiving a dose shown to decrease heart rate, then this is indirect evidence of a lack of compliance, if there were no other reasonable explanations for the "elevated" heart rate.

Patient Diaries

Another means of estimating compliance is by evaluating patient diaries. Both the frequency (i.e., the number of times an entry was made compared to the number of times an entry should have been made) and the quality of the entries may be evaluated. The quality of the entry might be judged by whether the clinical trial medicine was taken as scheduled and whether all requested information was filled out (e.g., daily evaluations of the patient's pain).

Assessment through a School Nurse

A child's container of medicine is collected from the school where it is kept, and the school nurse is questioned about the child's compliance.

Each of the indirect methods described may be misleading, and direct methods should also be used when possible to confirm findings. Numerous examples are referenced by Pearson (1982). Under certain circumstances, each of the indirect methods may yield accurate data. The validity of results obtained by these measures depends on such factors as disease severity, degree of hope for improvement, and cultural and social factors in the population.

REASONS FOR POOR PATIENT COMPLIANCE

Number of Doses per Day

It has long been believed that compliance decreases with the number of doses required per day. This hypothesis was recently proved (Pullar et al., 1988).

Disease Severity

Another factor that affects patient compliance is disease severity. This often affects patient's motivation to comply with a clinical trial. Patients with mild forms of a disease tend to comply less than patients with moderate and moderately severe disease. Patients with extremely severe or even terminal disease usually comply less than the moderate group (Fig. 15.2). This may be because those with severe disease are depressed and have lost hope or the physical ability to take care of themselves appropriately. The actual shape of this curve varies greatly for different diseases. For example, in hypertension the curve illustrated would be appropriate for a large group of patients, but for eczema or cancer, even "mild" cases would lead to high levels of compliance. The shape of this curve for a single patient also depends, in part, on personality factors of the patient, as well as the patient's values, culture, religion, and previous experiences with the disease and medical establishment.

A patient's motivation often depends on the severity of his disease, how the disease affects his quality of life, and how he or she views the anticipated benefits (and costs) of the clinical trial. Another factor for assessing compliance in severely ill patients is how well

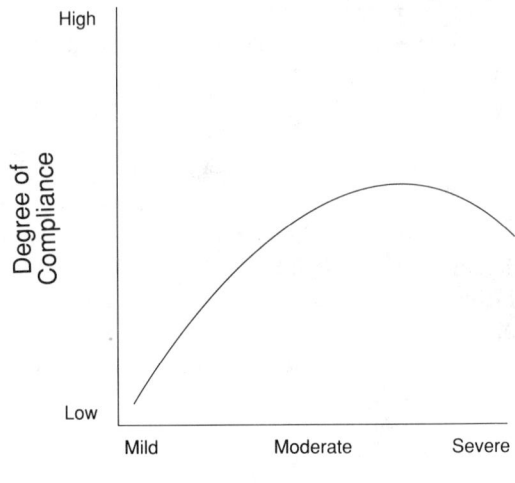

FIG. 15.2 Generalized relationships between a patient's degree of compliance and severity of disease.

they are physically able to comply with a clinical trial (e.g., to open child-proof caps). Patients with a mild treatable skin disease will generally be more compliant than for a mild or even moderately severe disease without symptoms or external manifestations (e.g., hypertension).

Other Reasons

Other reasons for poor patient compliance relate to requests made of them that they consider unfair, unclear, made with too short notice, too expensive, too inconvenient, or made without discussion with them. Poor relationships with medical professionals is sometimes a major factor in compliance. Adverse reactions that the patient wishes to avoid are another problem. Some patients' compliance decreases after they run out of pills. Sackett and Snow (1979) reported that patients kept about 75% of clinic appointments they made for themselves, but only about 50% of the appointments made for them.

The degree of noncompliance clearly varies enormously from trial to trial. Authors who have reviewed compliance data in the literature have documented noncompliance ranging from about 15 to 93% (Blackwell, 1972b; Greenberg, 1984). Part of this variation may be explained by differences in definitions used, methods used to measure compliance, severity of disease, and treatments used.

Compliance has been found to be unrelated to a patient's income, social class, occupation, or educational background (Peck and King, 1982).

WHEN SHOULD MEDICATION COMPLIANCE BE MEASURED?

1. *Phase I.* There is little need to measure compliance in most Phase I acute safety or pharmacokinetic clinical trials. Medicines are often given directly to volunteers by staff who observe the ingestion or injection, and compliance is seldom an issue in single dose or short-term clinical trials. For chronic Phase I clinical trials, compliance may be more of an issue.
2. *Phase IIa.* During pilot efficacy trials it may be extremely valuable to assess patient compliance, particularly if unexpectedly poor activity occurs. Patient interviews concerning compliance may be more valuable than merely assessing it in objective terms.
3. *Phase IIb.* It is almost always important to have an assessment of compliance during these clinical trials. The degree to which this factor should be evaluated must be judged for each clinical trial.
4. *Phase III.* The value of obtaining data on compli-

ance greatly varies and must be judged for each clinical trial.
5. *Phase IV.* It is not generally possible to assess compliance during observational studies. Compliance is generally impossible to assess in retrospective Phase IV studies and not practical in most prospective studies, but exceptions do occur.

HOW TO CHOOSE A METHOD TO EVALUATE PATIENT COMPLIANCE

To obtain accurate compliance data, the manner in which compliance is assessed may be more important than the specific methods used. Physicians or others who do not behave in an empathetic manner or who ask questions about compliance in a negative tone may not only obtain false data, but may encourage some patients to alter their degree of adherence to the clinical trial's requirements. Nonthreatening questions about the patient's compliance should be created and included in the protocol to help ensure that everyone associated with the clinical trial uses the same wording in eliciting information. A description of the empathetic tone to be used should also be included.

In some clinical trials it is so important that patients receive medicine that it should always be given by the staff. There is no question about patient compliance in these trials, although there could be questions about staff compliance. If patients are to medicate themselves, the relative importance of their compliance should determine which method(s) are chosen to evaluate it. The amount of resources available to evaluate compliance will determine whether it is possible to use medication bottles with electronic counters or whether it is necessary to rely on pill counts. The nature of the protocol will determine whether audits of pharmacy records can be used to measure refills. If that method is desirable but impractical to use, it may be possible to modify a protocol ahead of time to allow that method to be used.

Overall, a review of the pros and cons of each method for a particular clinical trial will indicate which methods should be used and how the methods should be modified to provide the best compliance data possible. One of the golden rules of measuring compliance is that a combination of methods is most effective, especially since most methods are extremely easy to implement (e.g., general probe, patient diary, pill count).

DESIGNING CLINICAL TRIALS TO MEASURE COMPLIANCE

Assessing compliance is rarely the primary objective in a clinical trial, but it is often one of the secondary ones. Compliance is rarely a major objective for in-patient trials because patients have less control over medicine intake, diet, and exercise as compared with patients in outpatient trials. Compliance may be the primary objective when a sponsor wants to determine whether compliance is enhanced by switching medicine regimens (e.g., comparing twice-a-day and four-times-a-day regimens, comparing capsules with suppositories).

If a clinical trial is designed primarily to evaluate compliance, it is critical to determine the basis for enrolling patients. Patients with the highest rates of compliance are those with the greatest motivation. Many of these patients can be identified in advance. If this is done and a select group of patients is chosen for the clinical trial, the representativeness of the groups must be assessed carefully, as well as the ability to extrapolate the trial's results to other patients.

Types of clinical trials that could be conducted to measure compliance include:

1. Crossover or parallel trials with two formulations of the same medicine (e.g., uncoated tablet with a bitter taste and a film-coated tablet in which the bitter taste is masked).
2. Crossover or parallel trials with two packages of the same medicine (e.g., blister pack and screw top bottle, bottles with and without a child-resistant cap).
3. Crossover or parallel trials with capsules (or tablets) of two different colors.
4. Crossover or parallel trials with capsules (or tablets) of two different sizes.
5. Parallel trials with and without a patient package insert.
6. Parallel trials with and without frequent encouragement of professional staff to comply with the medicine regimen.
7. Crossover or parallel trials with two (or more) dosing regimens (e.g., twice a day versus three times a day, medicine holiday versus none).

Compliance Run-In Technique

If patient compliance during a clinical trial is deemed particularly important or even critical, then a run-in period of X days or weeks may be included in the trial. Only patients with a satisfactory rate of compliance are then randomized to enter the true clinical trial. This approach is similar to that used to eliminate placebo responders from trials in which a large placebo effect is anticipated. Just as the "Placebo Run-In Technique" is appropriate to use for Phase II but not Phase III clinical trials, the "Compliance Run-In Technique" is also appropriate to use for Phase II, but not Phase III clinical trials.

Electronic Monitors of Compliance

Electronic monitors of container openings have become more sophisticated in recent years and the Medication Event Monitor Systems (MEMS, Aprex Corp., Freemont, CA) have been widely studied (Cramer et al., 1989). The goal for the Medication Event Monitor Systems is that it may help explain apparent failure of a regimen because of variable compliance. This goal is only an ideal, because this system is, at best, an indirect method of assessing compliance. One drawback of the system is that if each dose consists of two tablets, it is impossible to know the number of tablets actually taken. Other drawbacks of this system are that a patient may transfer some or all medicine to another container or may lay pills on a counter ahead of time. Table 15.5 summarizes selected advantages and disadvantages of electronic medication counters. A system under development for monitoring use of oral contraceptive pills has the advantage of using sensors to count the number of pills removed from a ring device for each dose (Potter, 1991). Nonetheless, for most outpatient trials this method offers a more reliable measure of compliance than virtually all others. It may also be used to monitor use of rescue or concomitant medicine in addition to, or instead of, the clinical trial medications. An important issue is whether the additional validity of the data obtained is sufficient justification for the cost.

Cheung et al. (1988a,b) describe a different electronic system of tracking compliance based on the principle used in the Medication Event Monitor Systems system (i.e., each opening is recorded). Cheung reported that their system overestimated compliance, but to a lesser degree than did pill counts. Eyedrop monitors and nebulizer monitors based on the same principle also are available. These devices log the exact amount of liquid medicine dispersed (Kass et al., 1984, 1986; Spector et al., 1986).

METHODS TO IMPROVE COMPLIANCE

Improving Patient Compliance

Give the Medicine to Patients Directly

The best approach to ensure total patient compliance is for the clinical trial staff to give the medicine(s) to patients. This is appropriate for depot injections and medicines with long half-lives, or if the patient lives within a reasonable distance of the clinic and can arrange to come for the medicine.

Demonstration and Practice of Techniques

For any medicine or therapy that involves techniques to self-administer the treatment that are not familiar to the patient, it is necessary to demonstrate the techniques and to have the patient practice. This approach is routinely followed when diabetic patients are first taught to inject themselves. Other methods that require practice are the use of inhalers and nasal insufflation. The compliance of patients who are uncomfortable or unfamiliar with a technique can be enhanced by practice with nonjudgmental professional staff.

Instructions

Another aspect of education that affects compliance relates to the nature of verbal instructions given patients. Simple instructions have a better chance of being understood and followed than do more complex or less clear instructions. Even for college graduates or those with advanced degrees, the KISS rule applies (i.e., Keep It Short and Simple). Asking patients to repeat what they are told helps ensure that the message transmitted is received accurately. Providing written instructions is a further tool that enhances the verbal message and assists patients' accurate recall of the verbal instructions. Details that cannot easily be remembered (e.g., dosing information, telephone numbers, names of contacts, instructions for completing patient diaries) may be provided on paper. In addition, some professional groups have prepared videos about taking medicines that can be shown to groups of patients in a clinic.

Clear labeling of medicine containers and appropriate packaging will enhance compliance in studies in which label instructions are unclear or packages are inconvenient to use (e.g., too large, too difficult to open).

Summary of Methods

Methods to enhance patient compliance are summarized in Table 15.6, have been reviewed elsewhere (Peck and King, 1982), and are listed below in a modified form. Few of these methods have been systematically assessed, and most represent a common-sense approach.

1. *Ask patients why they did not take their medicines.* Although the reasons offered may be only excuses and not necessarily true, they should be sought and taken seriously. Patients may be asked about compliance in a diary rather than in conversation. Patients may be noncompliant for reasons related to the clinical trial's outcome (e.g., cure obtained, no cure obtained, adverse reactions) or personal factors (e.g., forgetfulness, anger with staff, anger with demands of trial). A discussion about the topic may encourage patients to take their compliance more seriously and to improve their degree of adherence.

2. *Improve the physician–patient interaction.* Many facets of this relationship have an important effect on

TABLE 15.6 *Methods of improving compliance[a]*

1. Review the definition of compliance. Does missing one pill over 1 month mean the patient is defined as noncompliant? Measures should be relative
2. Simplify the demands of the protocol on patients
3. Simplify the instructions of how to follow the protocol or how to take the medicine
4. Minimize the number and duration of unpleasant or painful tests
5. Maintain relatively frequent contact with patients, especially at emotionally or physically difficult periods for the patient; contact the patient before scheduled visits
6. Allow for flexible dosing regimens to deal with adverse reactions, toxicity, and unanticipated situations
7. Provide the patient with appropriate information on the clinical trial and strive for a positive physician–patient relationship[b]
8. Avoid making the patient feel guilty about poor compliance and provide positive feedback to all patients
9. Establish a therapeutic goal in conjunction with the patient and assess the patient's progress towards that goal
10. Plan patient visits at a mutually convenient time and ensure that the patient has a minimal delay in waiting to see the physician or staff
11. Allow for and encourage patients to participate in their own care (e.g., with self-monitoring of their disease and treatment)
12. Involve the patient's spouse, family, or support group in the clinical trial
13. Prepare informational materials in the language that the patient speaks
14. Prepare pictorial instructions for patients who are not literate

[a] This table does not include a number of methods described in the text, or used in general medical practice, in which different factors must be considered and different techniques exist to improve compliance (e.g., switching patients to a different medicine or manipulating factors that are not permitted in most protocols).
[b] See Table 15.7.

a patient's compliance. A number of ways to enhance this relationship and patient compliance are listed in Table 15.7.

3. *Create fear about consequences of noncompliance.* The impact on patient compliance through use of fear-arousing messages is uncertain. This method has (at best) only limited (if any) usefulness in clinical trials.

4. *Educate patients about their disease(s).* The importance of educating interested patients about their disease is clear from an ethical perspective, but education's effect on compliance is not yet known and may not always be positive. There are reports of both enhanced compliance (Norell, 1979) and no effect (Pye et al., 1988) after educational interventions. Videotapes may be prepared to encourage patients to enroll in a trial as well as to adhere to assigned dosing schedules.

5. *Provide written instructions.* Written instructions have been found to be effective in increasing compliance for short-term therapy. For long-term therapy this approach does not necessarily elicit the same benefit. The instruction sheet should be reviewed with patients, not merely handed to them. Patients have been known to take all of their pills for the entire day early in the morning because they are planning to be away

from home; others take all their pills for a week at one time because they are afraid of forgetting to take them later.

6. *Use special medicine packaging*. This is a valuable method of improving compliance in clinical trials. This improvement is achieved by reducing or eliminating confusion about dose schedules, and by making medicines easier to remove from containers. This may involve using easy opening bottles or blister packs in which dates and times are printed on the foil.

7. *Tailor reminders to patients*. Patients can be reminded about when to take their medicines through simple cues (e.g., notes put on a refrigerator or bathroom mirror, telephone calls from relatives or friends, alarms that ring at preset intervals). In long-term clinical trials as well as in private practice, a reminder to refill a prescription may be sent prior to the expected date of need. This must be carefully considered and, preferably, discussed with patients, since they may resent this method. Automatic telephone calls with computerized voice reminders represent a similar method that may annoy patients rather than improve their compliance.

8. *Allow patients to schedule their own appointments*. In some clinical trials it may be possible to do this, within limits; the method has been shown to work.

9. *Self-monitoring*. Providing calendars or cards to be checked off may remind those patients who are noncompliant because of forgetfulness. This method will not improve the compliance of those who are noncompliant for other reasons.

10. *Rewards*. Patients may be given tokens for complying with medicine taking and other aspects of a clinical trial. Tokens may be exchanged for desired rewards (e.g., a trip to town). This approach is only appropriate for some selected patients (e.g., patients in institutions) and is primarily applicable to medical practice. The use of rewards in clinical trials is almost always inappropriate.

An additional approach is to simplify the therapeutic regimen. Although this is usually a possibility in med-

TABLE 15.7 *Selected methods to enhance compliance through improving the physician–patient relationship*

1. Have patients see the same physician at each visit
2. Educate physicians about the importance of being sympathetic and caring with patients
3. Provide positive feedback to patients about their performance
4. Interview patients about what aspects of a clinical trial they object to or what aspects interfere with their full compliance; discuss these situations and remedy them insofar as possible
5. Negotiate how the patient will take medicines if it is difficult to arrange a suitable schedule (e.g., take the medicine after school versus during school)
6. Prepare patients for expected adverse reactions so that they do not become upset and discontinue therapy when the reactions occur

ical practice, it has limited applicability in a clinical trial. Appointments should be scheduled at times that are convenient for the patient, and patients should be encouraged to participate in their own care, in clinical trials as well as in medical practice. Having a parent, friend, spouse, or other person (e.g., pharmacist) take an active role in ensuring medicine compliance has been shown to be effective, especially for patients who live alone or are known to be somewhat noncompliant.

A behaviorally oriented strategy (i.e., providing blood pressure measuring equipment to hypertensive patients known to be noncompliant) enhanced compliance (Haynes et al., 1976), but several biases may have accounted for the improvements in compliance observed.

To dispel any doubts about the importance of trial design to compliance, imagine the following trial. Patients are required to take two huge (size zero) capsules six times per day, every 4 hours around the clock. Capsules are dispensed in childproof containers and patients must complete their diaries three times a day. Every 3 days, for 6 weeks, patients must attend clinic. In the clinic they undergo a rigorous 8-hour period of forms, tests, and blood draws and are questioned about adverse reactions every 20 minutes. This hypothetical scenario could be continued, but it makes the point that in many cases the compliance of both patients and investigators is a function of the clinical trial's design. Clearly, compliance could be improved in this hypothetical trial by careful attention to the clinical trial's design, particularly by minimizing its complexity and requirements.

Assessing and Improving Investigator Compliance

Monitoring a clinical trial and evaluating the conduct of its investigators and staff is the best way to ensure that personnel are complying with the trial in the many ways required. Deviations should be discussed with the investigator, who should also be involved in planning modifications. Issues that are not readily resolved should be discussed with senior executives at the sponsoring institution. In some situations creative solutions must be found. For example, one investigator was suspected of avoiding his responsibilities because he was not completing data collection forms. But when the situation was explored, he was found to be simply overworked. The solution reached was to have him hire an assistant for the duration of the clinical trial whose job included filling out the data collection forms.

Investigator compliance can also be assessed by evaluating audits conducted by sponsors or regulatory authorities. In private practice, the reports of adverse reactions reaching the manufacturer or published in the literature should indicate whether the medicine is being used correctly (i.e., as labeled). Physicians who are noncompliant with a medicine's labeling may observe a higher incidence or different nature of adverse reactions.

Activities by Sponsors to Enhance Compliance in a Clinical Trial

Sponsors may enhance compliance by writing a protocol in a logical sequence that makes sense to physicians and patients. Complex, unnatural, or unusual dosing regimens, tests, or other activities in a clinical trial will diminish compliance by both physicians and patients. For example, if 16 hours of tests are scheduled on a single day, if patients are awakened during the night to answer questions about adverse reactions, if patients are starved unnecessarily, or are otherwise harassed, patient noncompliance and dropouts will result.

The preparing and dispensing of medicine varies enormously between clinical trials and certainly affects compliance. A patient given a large glass jar containing a month's supply of medicine to take four times a day will comply less (on average) than one given four separate weekly blister packs on which each day's dose is labeled. Alternatively, a calendar pack (similar to the oral contraceptive packages) could be used to package the medicine for a whole month.

INTERPRETING DATA ON COMPLIANCE

Electronic monitors may help interpret clinical trial results. For example, an excess number of medicine bottle openings associated in time with adverse reactions may be related to an overdose, and too few bottle openings associated in time with adverse reactions may be related to an underdose and withdrawal effects or to reemergence of disease symptoms.

In clinical trials with a test medicine and active control but no placebo, data may be analyzed separately for the groups of high versus the groups of low compliers. If efficacy is found to be greater in both groups of high compliers than in the comparable groups of low compliers, the validity of the clinical trial can probably be substantiated and both treatments can be assessed as effective.

If compliance is less than expected, it may be necessary to examine the data and question patients to determine if the problem is primarily with the clinical trial design (e.g., too arduous), the medicine (e.g., poor tasting), clinical response (e.g., improvement, lack of improvement), patient (e.g., personality, motivation to be in the trial), or some other factor.

In clinical trials with a placebo control, the rela-

tionship of efficacy versus degree of compliance should be assessed for both the active medicine and placebo. These results allow one to determine the degree of patient compliance necessary to obtain full efficacy.

SHOULD NONCOMPLIANT PATIENTS BE DISCONTINUED FROM A CLINICAL TRIAL?

Yes, if it is a Phase II clinical trial and if it is important to determine that a medicine is effective. Poor compliers may yield poor efficacy data, which will confound the results and lead to an incorrect conclusion about a medicine. If poor compliers are discontinued from a clinical trial, their data still *must* be included in the safety analyses. Their data should probably also be included in the efficacy analysis (under intention-to-treat principles) for the time they were in the clinical trial. Do not use "last observation carried forward" methods of statistics for patients discontinued for noncompliance because this could greatly bias and influence the outcome.

If one accepts the principle of eliminating poorly compliant patients from a clinical trial, it becomes necessary to establish a critical level of compliance and a method(s) for measuring it. The standard or cut-off level of compliance will depend on the disease and its severity and on the medicine's characteristics, value, and rate of use. Overall, the level that is considered reasonable must be established before the start of the clinical trial. The ultimate answer must involve clinical judgment and should be discussed by a group of appropriate individuals.

No, if a Phase III clinical trial is involved, because the objective of Phase III trials is to evaluate a medicine under conditions of essentially normal use. Eliminating patients who are poor compliers could skew results and result in the loss of important information.

A number of clinical trial reports have stated that a medicine is more effective with compliant patients than with noncompliant patients (Noseworthy, 1988). This has also been observed with patients treated with placebo (see Table 15.8). These observations raise the

TABLE 15.8 *Five-year mortality in patients given clofibrate or placebo according to cumulative compliance with protocol prescription*[a]

Compliance	Clofibrate		Placebo	
	No.	% Mortality	No.	% Mortality
Less than 80%	357	24.6 ± 2.3	882	28.2 ± 1.5
Greater than 80%	708	15.0 ± 1.3	1,813	15.1 ± 0.8
Total	1,065	18.2 ± 1.2	2,695	19.4 ± 0.8

[a] From Coronary Drug Project Research Group (1980). The differences between the two groups of compliers was found to be statistically significant for both clofibrate and placebo.

question of whether noncompliant patients differ from compliant patients in substantial ways that affect mortality, and suggest a number of subgroup analyses that may be conducted.

CONCLUSION

Compliance of a single patient or group is rarely an all-or-none phenomenon; instead it may be expressed as a percentage varying from 0 to 100. It should be measured in all well-controlled clinical trials, particularly during Phase II. Prior to their initiation, clinical trials conducted during other phases should also be examined to determine the value of assessing compliance. Thought should be given while designing the protocol for a clinical trial to attaining as high a level of compliance as possible. The ideal method of measuring compliance is not yet available, but the use of multiple methods will yield reasonable data for most clinical trials. When compliance is measured, data for over-compliers should be compared with data for under-compliers. The interpretation and extrapolation of data must consider these results. In Phase II well-controlled clinical trials, efforts may be made to exclude non-compliers from entering, but this should not be done in Phase III clinical trials. Data from noncompliant patients should not be omitted from most statistical analyses in a clinical trial.

The discussion in this chapter was based on the assumption that it is desirable to have as high a degree of patient compliance as possible. Although this assumption is not being questioned in most trials, partial compliance is usually sufficient to evaluate a medicine's efficacy. If compliance was poor, this fact should be apparent and can then be factored into the data analysis and interpretation of the results.

Additional discussions on patient compliance are found in articles by Blackwell (1972b), Hussar (1980), Pearson (1982), and Peck and King (1982), and in the book *Patient Compliance in Medical Practice and Clinical Trials* (Cramer and Spilker, 1991).

CHAPTER 16

Pharmacokinetic Principles

Pharmacokinetics concentrates on describing the absorption, distribution, metabolism, and excretion of a medicine. This chapter is not intended as a review of pharmacokinetics but rather is a brief nonmathematical synopsis of some pharmacokinetic principles that an investigator should consider in developing a clinical trial design. An attempt is made to emphasize practical considerations.

The pharmacokinetic behavior of a new medicine is usually determined in animals before the medicine is tested in humans. Additional tests in animals usually progress at the same time that a clinical program evaluating the medicine is developing. There are often important differences between pharmacokinetic results obtained in humans and laboratory animals, which emphasizes the relevance of pharmacokinetic trials performed in humans.

PHARMACOKINETIC PARAMETERS AND PRINCIPLES

A number of pharmacokinetic parameters evaluated in humans are discussed, and a few examples of cases in which these parameters have had a significant outcome on the results of clinical trials are provided. The pa-

rameters to be described include those used to choose a medicine-dosing regimen (Table 16.1). These parameters are often evaluated in clinical trials designed specifically to characterize and understand the pharmacokinetic profile of a medicine. It should be stressed that at least several of the parameters listed in Table 16.1 must be considered in selecting a medicine dosage or dosing regimen. A number of the most important pharmacokinetic parameters described below are illustrated in Fig. 16.1.

Bioavailability

Bioavailability of an orally administered medicine describes the net result of all processes from oral ingestion of the drug to the appearance of the medicine in the systemic circulation (availability of the medicine in the systemic circulation following absorption from various parts of the gastrointestinal tract). The term *bioavailability* is sometimes used to describe both the amount and rate of medicine present in the systemic circulation, but the amount of medicine present is the more commonly described parameter. Bioavailability is usually expressed as a percent of the dose administered that is available within the body intact (unmetabolized) compared with an appropriate reference.

TABLE 16.1 *Selected parameters used to choose medicine dosages and regimens*

A. Parameters related to the medicine's pharmacokinetics and pharmacological characteristics
1. Peak blood levels[a]
2. Time to peak concentration
3. Duration of blood concentration[a]
4. Duration of biological effects
5. Medicine half-life
6. Bioavailability
7. Accumulation
8. Microsomal enzyme induction
9. Distribution characteristics
10. Plasma protein binding
11. Metabolism
12. Excretion
13. Synergism
14. Medicine interactions
15. Tachyphylaxis
16. Tolerance
B. Parameters related to the patient's characteristics
1. Age
2. Sex
3. Weight
4. Race or ethnic background
5. Geographical location
6. Severity of disease
7. Concomitant medicines
8. Concurrent diseases
9. Other inclusion criteria (e.g., smokers versus nonsmokers, food intake)

[a] Usually determined in plasma or serum.

The bioavailability data of an oral dosage form may be compared with the same medicine administered i.v. (absolute bioavailability) or compared with a standard oral dosage form or solution (relative bioavailability). Many factors (e.g., food, disease, age, other medicines) can enhance or diminish the degree of a medi-

TABLE 16.2 *Factors influencing absorption of oral medicines into the systemic circulation*

1. Physical–chemical properties of the medicine (e.g., solubility in stomach and small intestine, molecular size, type of molecule, crystal form)
2. Formulation used (e.g., characteristics of excipients, amount of pressure under which a tablet is compressed, range of particle sizes, enteric or other coating of tablet)
3. Gastrointestinal contents (e.g., presence of food or other medicines)
4. Gastrointestinal characteristics (e.g., gastric pH and emptying time, metabolic activity of the intestinal surface, intestinal emptying time, gastrointestinal secretions, disease)
5. Gastrointestinal flora (e.g., bacteria in the gut)
6. Hormonal secretions into the gastrointestinal system
7. Activity of the autonomic nervous system
8. Metabolic state of the patient (e.g., malnourishment)
9. Pathological diseases (e.g., malabsorption diseases)
10. First-pass phenomenon in the liver
11. Biliary flow
12. Other factors

cine's bioavailability, and these factors must be controlled in a clinical trial in which bioavailability is measured (Table 16.2). The three main factors to evaluate in a bioavailability trial are (1) peak plasma concentration, (2) time to peak plasma concentration, and (3) area under the plasma concentration-versus-time curve (see Fig. 16.2). The means by which a different formulation of the same medicine can affect these parameters is shown in Fig. 16.2. In this example, the rate of absorption for formulation B is slower, as reflected by the greater time required to reach the peak plasma concentration. Nonetheless, the extent of the two dosage forms absorbed is the same, as reflected by equivalent areas under the curve. The

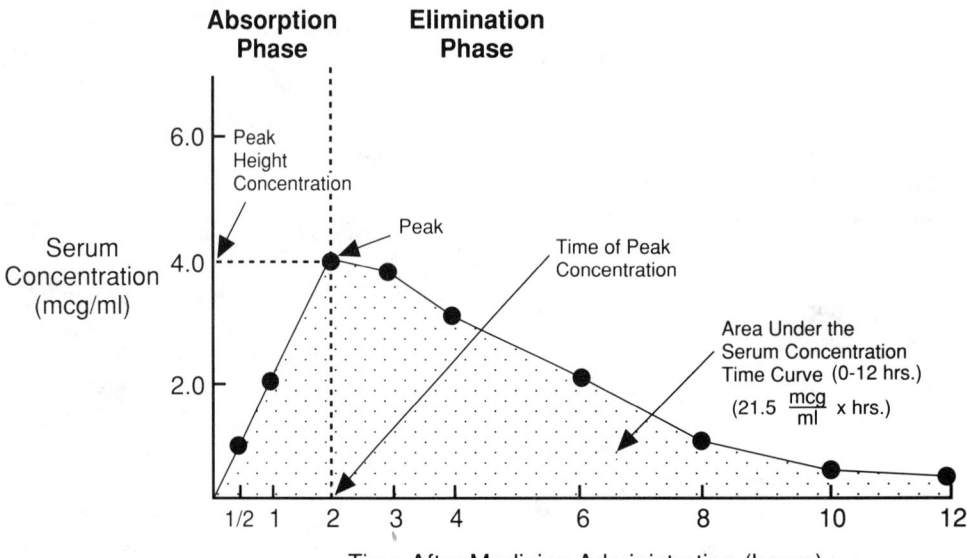

FIG. 16.1 Serum concentration–time curve following a single dose of a medicine, illustrating a number of basic pharmacokinetic concepts. (Reprinted by permission of American Pharmaceutical Association from Dittert and DiSanto, 1973.)

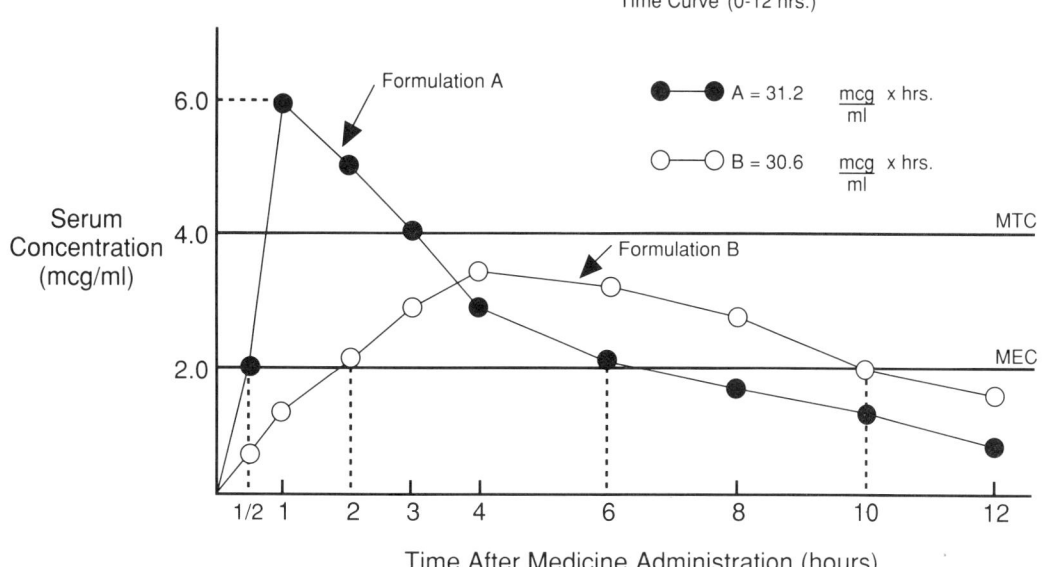

FIG. 16.2 Serum concentration–time curves for two different formulations of the same medicine given at the same dose. The relationship of the curves to the minimum toxic concentration (MTC) and the minimum effective concentration (MEC) is shown. (Reprinted by permission of American Pharmaceutical Association from Dittert and DiSanto, 1973.)

biological advantage of formulation B is that the maximum blood level remains below that which causes toxicity.

Peak Blood Levels

If a peak blood level above a certain value is associated with a high incidence of medicine toxicity (e.g., phenytoin levels above 20 μg/ml), then this level should be avoided through periodic monitoring. There are numerous other reasons why it is desirable to monitor trial medicine levels in plasma and other physiological fluids. Some of the reasons are listed in Table 16.3. Simulations of expected peak plasma levels based on relevant pharmacokinetic models made prior to the clinical trial are useful in selecting an appropriate dosage regimen to avoid undesirable plasma levels (Figs. 16.3 and 16.4). It is difficult to include consideration of all potentially important factors in developing this mathematical model, since many of the factors that can influence blood levels are difficult to quantitate (e.g., medicine interactions, elevated or decreased liver microsomal enzymes). Actual multiple-dose trials are even more useful.

Time to Steady-State Concentration

The time to reach steady-state concentration is solely influenced by the medicine's half-life. For example,

50% of the steady state is reached in one half-life, whereas 90% of the steady state is reached in 3.3 half-lives (Fig. 16.5). If the time to reach steady-state concentration is relatively long (e.g., several days or longer), then a loading dose of a medicine may be useful. If the time to steady-state concentration is quite short (because of a short half-life) and the medicine is rapidly eliminated, then a controlled-release (long-acting) formulation may be developed.

TABLE 16.3 *Reasons for measuring trial medicine concentration in plasma and/or other biological fluids*

1. Evaluate medicine bioavailability and kinetics under different conditions
2. Measure patient compliance
3. Determine presence and degree of tolerance
4. Evaluate and quantify a clinical impression of underdosage or overdosage
5. Help to differentiate between the causes of an adverse reaction that could be caused by the patient's disease or the trial medicine
6. Establish suitable dosage schedules
7. Provide a guideline for when multiple medicines will be given and when medicine interactions are probable
8. Provide a baseline when long-term treatment in a chronic disease is initiated
9. Evaluate errors in dosing
10. Evaluate different responses due to genetic factors
11. Evaluate whether the medicine has a plasma range at which beneficial clinical effects are observed
12. Monitor the course of patients who are experiencing adverse reactions and/or an overdose
13. Other reasons

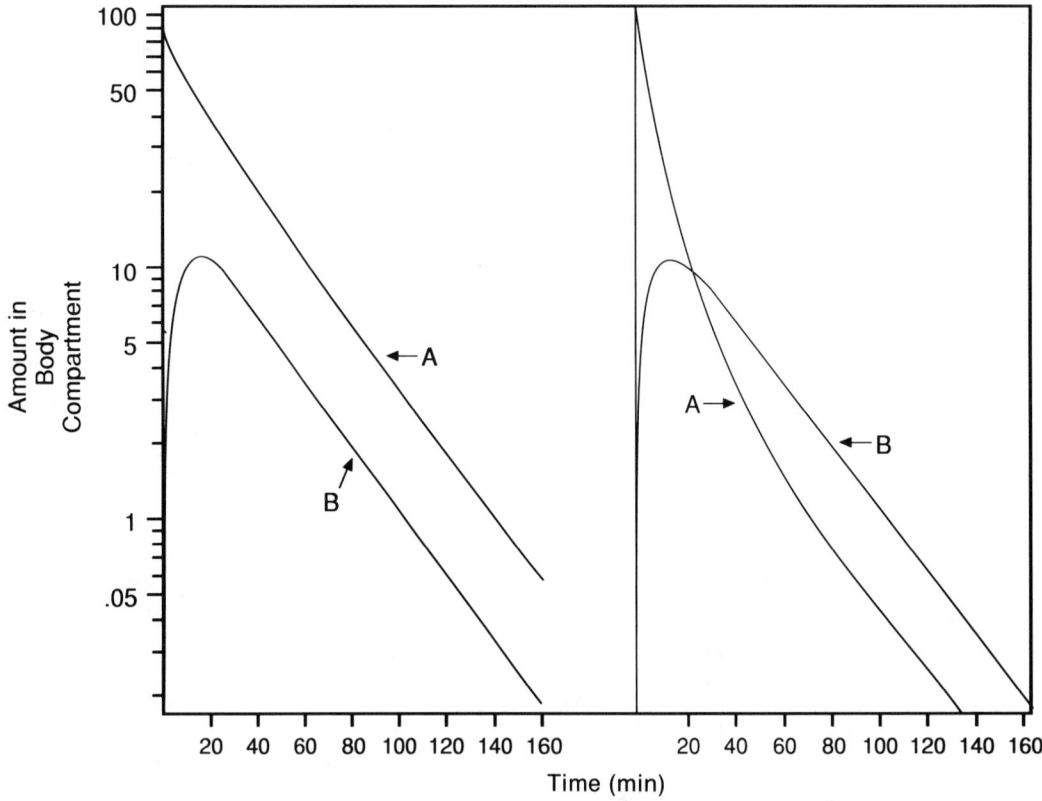

FIG. 16.3 Semilogarithmic plots of the amounts of medicine in the central (*A*) and peripheral (*B*) body compartments as a function of time following the intravenous administration of two medicines. Characteristics of a two-compartment model are shown, but each medicine has different distribution characteristics.

Duration of Blood Concentration

The duration of an adequate (above a minimum therapeutic concentration) blood concentration of a medicine is an important factor in determining the frequency at which to administer the doses (see Fig. 16.2).

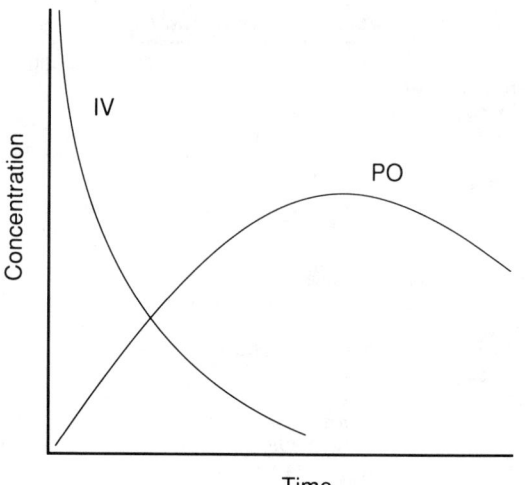

FIG. 16.4 General plots of the medicine's concentration in blood when given intravenously and orally.

Duration of Biological Effects

For some medicines there is no direct correlation between medicine plasma concentration and biological response to the medicine. The duration of a medicine's presence in the plasma may be relatively short, but the biological effect elicited may be prolonged. In this situation, less frequent medicine administration can be utilized. Figure 16.6 illustrates how neutral and ionizable medicines distribute through the body.

Medicine Half-Life

Half-life is the time for half of the medicine to have disappeared from the blood serum or plasma (see Fig. 16.1). The half-life of a medicine is the sole determinant of the time necessary for steady-state concentrations to be reached on chronic dosing. Dosage interval considerations are most often based on half-life values, although they may be based on the duration of the biological half-life, or safety considerations. For example, diazepam has a half-life of over 30 hours, but small doses are usually given two or three times a day to reduce sedation.

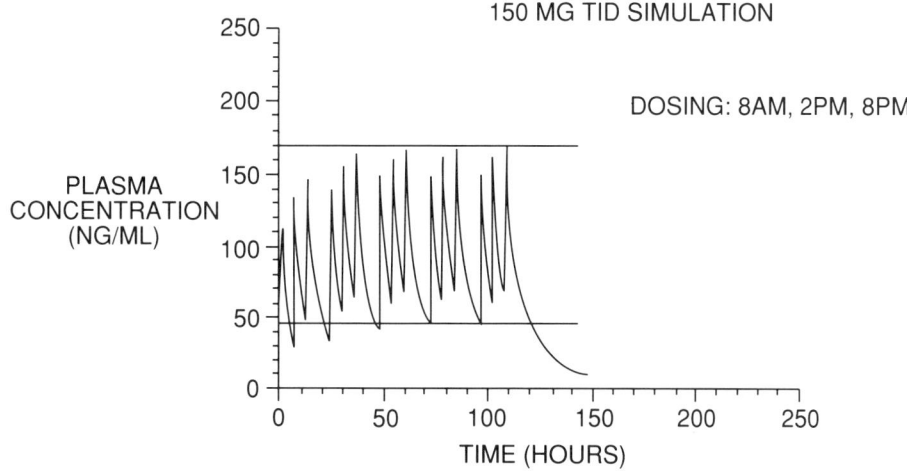

150 MG TID SIMULATION

DOSING: 8AM, 2PM, 8PM

FIG. 16.5 Repetitive doses lead to a steady-state concentration after about 4 to 5 half-lives. Curves such as these may be modeled prior to clinical trials, as well as plotted from actual data.

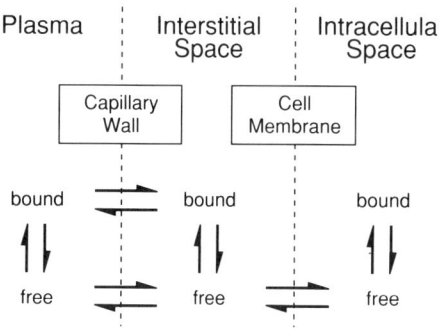

A. Neutral Medicines

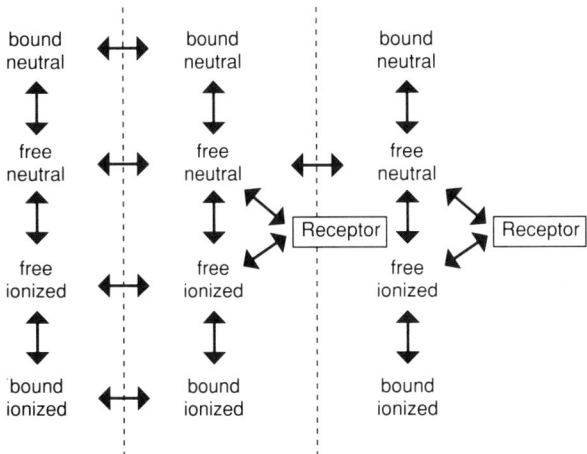

B. Ionizable Medicines

FIG. 16.6 How a medicine changes its form as it is distributed to and from plasma and interstitial and intracellular spaces.

Accumulation

Accumulation refers to the buildup or increased levels of a medicine in the body on multiple medicine administrations. The potential for accumulation must be carefully considered in medicines with long half-lives or whenever the second dose is given while a significant fraction of the first dose is still present in the body.

Time for Plasma Levels to Return to Baseline

When a patient whose medicine concentration in plasma is at steady state stops taking a medicine, the concentration eventually falls to zero. The concentration-versus-time curve of this decline is the opposite of the curve for the medicine's accumulation: it falls to 50% of the steady-state value in 1 half-life, to 10% of the steady-state value in 3.3 half-lives, and is essentially gone by 5 to 7 half-lives.

Microsomal Enzyme Induction

When certain trial or concomitant medicines are given chronically (e.g., phenobarbital, phenytoin), there is usually an increased level of microsomal enzymes in the liver. These enzymes metabolize a number of other medicines and thus increase their rate of elimination from the body. Therefore, a given dose of a medicine that is metabolized by the induced microsomal enzymes may exert less of an effect than anticipated. This issue is especially important in testing new antiepileptic medicines, since most patients will be taking medicines that have caused enzyme induction. It must also be remembered that a medicine that induces microsomal enzymes may also increase its own rate of metabolism, thus reducing its own pharmacological (i.e., therapeutic) effect. This generally occurs, however, only after a period of about 3 to 10 days, when the microsomal enzymes have been induced.

Distribution Characteristics

The rate and pattern of medicine uptake into various body tissues can affect the selectivity and duration of medicine action (Fig. 16.6). For example, barbiturates rapidly leave the systemic circulation and enter fat tissues, from which they are slowly released. Different barbiturates have different affinities for fat tissues and differ in their distribution characteristics. These characteristics affect the size and frequency of doses to use in clinical trials.

Plasma Protein Binding

Many medicines interact reversibly with plasma proteins such as albumin. Because the unbound or "free" concentration of a medicine generally correlates with pharmacological responses, any alteration in binding (especially for highly bound [i.e., >90%] medicines) can affect therapeutic and/or toxic effects of a medicine. Hypoalbuminemia or concomitant administration of other medicines that are highly protein bound (which would compete for binding sites) could elevate the "free" concentrations of the medicine of interest. It may be necessary to consider these factors in protocol design and in establishing patient inclusion criteria.

Metabolism and Excretion

These topics are too enormous in scope to be summarized in a short space. Readers are referred to standard pharmacology and pharmacokinetic textbooks and references for information on these topics and for the myriad of ways in which they may influence medicine trial design. Major routes of excretion for medicines involve the kidneys and biliary system. The following routes are usually of minor significance: lungs, skin, saliva, hair, intestines, gastric secretions, and milk. Patients with altered liver function can be expected to metabolize medicines normally metabolized by the liver differently from individuals with normal

livers. This difference may have significant clinical consequences. Likewise, patients with altered renal function will excrete medicines (normally excreted in urine) differently from normals. The altered blood levels of a medicine or duration of tissue levels in patients with abnormal renal function may yield clinical effects significantly different from those observed in a population of patients with normal renal function. Pathological conditions such as hypo- and hyperthyroidism or malnutrition states also affect metabolism of many medicines, as do environmental chemicals and diet (Conney et al., 1977).

Promedicine

Promedicines are medicines that are designed to improve the delivery of an active medicine to its site of action. Promedicines are converted inside the body into active medicines (Fig. 16.7). A promedicine may be developed because it can be absorbed whereas the medicine cannot. For example, bitotalol is a promedicine in which the ester groups on the catechol part of the molecule protect the molecule from degradation in the gastrointestinal tract. After the molecule is absorbed the esterases cleave the ester bonds releasing the ester and liberating the parent molecule. Other reasons to develop a promedicine might be to achieve better solubility for an i.v. medicine, less toxicity, longer duration of action, better control of dose, patent protection, or enhanced stability.

Promedicines may be biologically and clinically active or inactive on their own. However, a promedicine almost always leads to the same biological and clinical effects as the medicine itself. One exception is for Ritmos-Elle, a promedicine of ajmaline (an antiarrhythmic medicine) because Ritmos-Elle has some different pharmacological properties than ajmaline (Spilker, et al., 1975b).

Tolerance

Individuals may show tolerance to a medicine (i.e., a decreased response or pharmacologic effect of a medicine resulting from previous exposure to that medicine) and may require a greater dose to yield an equivalent effect. Tolerance may be viewed as developing

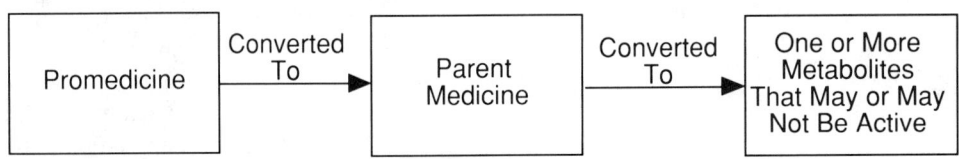

FIG. 16.7 Relationship of a promedicine, parent medicine, and metabolites. One or more metabolites may be reconverted to the parent medicine. It is also possible, in theory, for small amounts of a promedicine to be converted directly to metabolites.

through either of two mechanisms. In one mechanism, the medicine concentration at the receptors will have decreased as a result of diminished medicine absorption, increased medicine elimination, altered binding of a medicine, or other factors. The other mechanism involves a diminution of the medicine's effects once it has reached the target tissue.

Acute tolerance, in which a progressively decreased effect is observed on repeated dosing, is known as tachyphylaxis. This is an example of tolerance occurring at the cellular site of a medicine's effect. This effect may be easily demonstrated with repeated i.v. doses of many sympathomimetic medicines.

If a medicine is known to cause tolerance, then this must be considered in developing the clinical trial design, particularly with regard to frequency of dosing, amount of medicine per dose, duration of the trial, concomitant medicines, frequency of patient evaluation, and other factors.

One of the most well-known examples of tolerance to the clinical effects of a medicine is that of tolerance to nitroglycerin. A recent editorial in *Lancet* (Anonymous, *Lancet*, 1988b) quoted an article about nitroglycerin tolerance from nearly a century ago in *JAMA* (Anonymous, 1898). The author reported that munitions workers placed nitroglycerin on their hatbands when away from work to maintain their "immunity" from headaches. Tolerance to nitroglycerin was therefore well known for many years when transdermal patches were developed. These patches were not thought to elicit this problem; however, rapid tolerance to transdermal nitroglycerin patches was observed after marketing (Jordan et al., 1986; Anonymous, *Lancet* 1988b). Intermittent dosing of patients with these patches was subsequently found to prevent tolerance (Cowan et al., 1987).

Other well-known examples of tolerance to medicines include tolerance to the analgesic effects of morphine, and to the hemodynamic effects of hydralazine in patients with heart failure.

Plasma or Serum Level Half-Life versus Biological Half-Life

Most medicines remain effective while their plasma concentration is above a certain level. The time for the concentration to fall to 50% of the peak value is the plasma half-life ($t_{1/2}$) of the drug. The dosing schedule is usually related to a medicine's plasma half-life. For most medicines the shorter the half-life, the more often the medicine must be given. Developing sustained release or other long-duration formulations is usually an attempt to prolong the absorption of the formulation and, thus, the medicine's activity.

Another category of medicine half-life is the duration of its biological (i.e., pharmacological or clinical) ef-

fect. For many medicines the clinical half-life and plasma half-life are similar, but for some medicines there is a large difference. Medicines that bind irreversibly to enzymes (e.g., irreversible cholinesterase inhibitors) have a prolonged clinical effect. The clinical effect of a medicine that acts by depleting a chemical that is slowly synthesized (e.g., reserpine) lasts long after the medicine is eliminated. Other medicines affect enzymes and are then eliminated, but their effect persists long after elimination. For example, the anti-platelet-aggregation effect of aspirin results from inhibition of the enzyme cyclooxygenase. A medicine whose action persists after it is eliminated from the body requires a different consideration when establishing a dosage schedule than one whose effect persists only while the plasma level is above a certain value.

SELECTED MATHEMATICAL MODELS USING PHARMACOKINETIC DATA

After limited pharmacokinetic data are available (e.g., rate of absorption and elimination and a constant for the volume of distribution) on a new medicine, it is usually possible to simulate expected steady-state plasma concentrations under other conditions (e.g., using multiple doses). It may be possible to simulate certain pharmacological responses after information on blood levels and pharmacological responses is available (e.g., one may simulate the time necessary for 90% recovery from neuromuscular paralysis induced by a neuromuscular blocking medicine).

Models have been developed that consider the body as consisting of one, two, or more compartments for understanding how a medicine is distributed. A two-compartment model (see Fig. 16.3) of rapidly equilibrating tissues (generally plasma and high perfused organs such as the liver or kidney) or of more slowly equilibrating tissues is often used to study the effects of many medicines, although a single homogeneous compartment (one-compartment model) is used for some medicines.

Models are also used to determine the type of kinetics involved in the elimination of a medicine. Commonly used models allow mathematical description of the time course of medicine levels under various dosing conditions. This description permits one to make predictions about both optimal amount and rate of medicine dosing.

MEDICINE INTERACTIONS, COMPARABILITY, AND COMPATIBILITY

Two or more medicines may interact in a myriad of ways and at various stages of medicine administration, action, metabolism, and excretion. The effects of the interaction may lead to (1) a synergism of beneficial effects, (2) decreased therapeutic effects, (3) toxic adverse reactions, (4) unusual or complex effects that defy easy categorization, or (5) any other net result. A few common mechanisms that are involved in medicine interactions include (1) medicine incompatibility on administration, (2) induction of hepatic microsomal enzymes by one medicine that affects the metabolism of another, and (3) renal effects of one medicine that alter the elimination of another.

If medicine interactions in a clinical trial are anticipated, then there are measures that can be followed either to prevent or minimize their impact. If the interactions are expected to occur during the absorption stages, then the times of administration of the two (or more) medicines may be staggered. The same approach may be followed for preventing problems of incompatible solutions of i.v. or other parenteral liquids. Two medicines should never be placed together in the same syringe or physiological solution unless well-documented compatibility tests have been performed. If the anticipated medicine interactions are expected to occur after the absorption phase and to arise from physiological effects that will cause adverse reactions, then an alternative medicine(s), dose, or dosage regimen should be sought whenever possible

to avoid or minimize the problem. If these procedures are not possible, then appropriate laboratory and clinical monitoring of the patient should be considered.

Determining which Interactions to Evaluate

Basic types of interactions are shown in Fig. 16.8. Of the almost unlimited numbers of specific interactions that could be evaluated, a few are obvious choices for consideration.

1. Interactions with medicines commonly used by patients who would be likely to take the test medicine.
2. Interactions with medicines of similar chemical structures.
3. Interactions with medicines for which adverse reactions are observed that are proved or hypothesized to be the result of an interaction.
4. Interactions with concomitant medicines that are known to have a narrow therapeutic index.

Reactions may differ for enantiomers of a medicine (Jamali et al., 1989). This issue is becoming much more important as a basis of possibly selecting a single form of a molecular structure (i.e., with a specific sterochemical nature) for development.

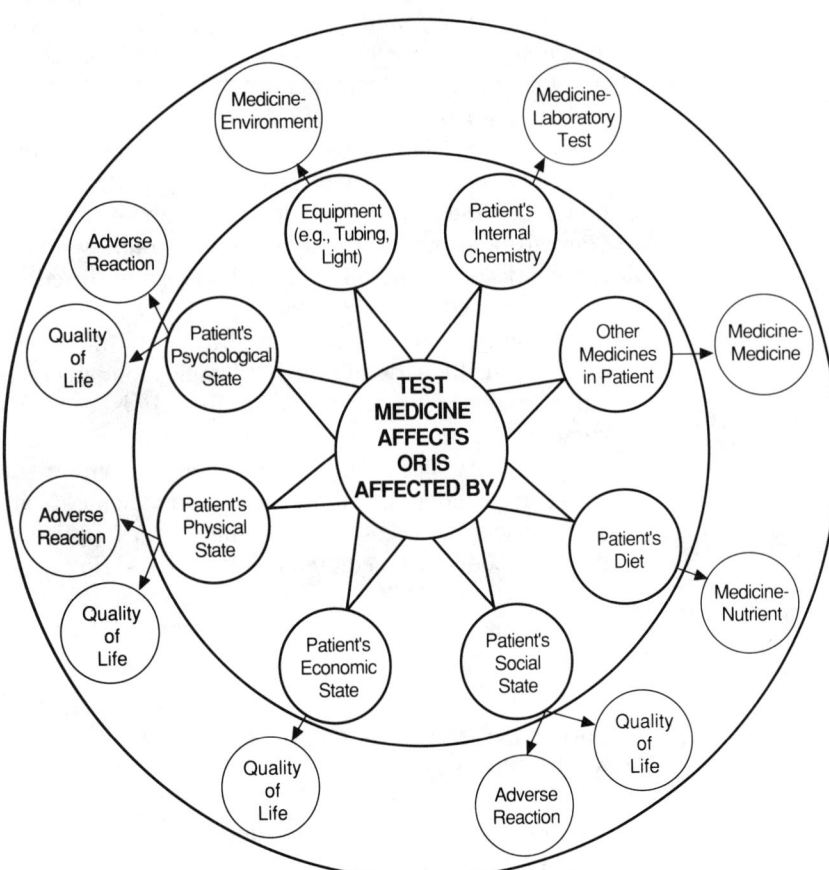

FIG. 16.8 Schematic illustrating various types of medicine interactions in the outer circle and factors that affect it in the inner circle.

Designs for Medicine Interaction Trials

At least two dose levels of the test medicine should be evaluated alone and in combination with the purportedly interacting medicine. Doses chosen should be clinically appropriate, but as different as practical. Patients on the first medicine may be given progressively higher doses of the second medicine. This may be done by assigning patients placed on a fixed dose of medicine A to receive three different maximal doses of medicine B or by titrating all patients on the first fixed dose of medicine A to a predetermined ceiling dose of medicine B. Pharmacokinetics should be evaluated at each dose level. The timing of the two doses should be clinically relevant and chosen to achieve peak levels of both at a similar point in time.

Comparability Trials

Comparability trials compare clinical effects of two medicines manufactured or prepared by different methods (e.g., by an older versus a new method) to ensure comparable clinical responses. These trials are particularly important for assessing biotechnology products manufactured in two identical facilities or when a minor (or major) change in manufacturing has occurred. If a bioequivalence clinical trial includes clinical measurements, then it too may be described as a comparability clinical trial.

It is most relevant to conduct a comparability trial when one is comparing a newly made versus older medicine (i.e., evaluating the impact of age), original medicine versus modified medicine (e.g., comparing two formulations or salts), medicine synthesized by two manufacturers or two plants of a single manufacturer. Some of the questions to consider in designing the trial are (1) should a placebo arm be used? (2) What endpoints should be measured? and (3) Can the duration of the trial be shortened?

Comparability versus Compatibility Trials

Comparability trials should not be confused with compatibility studies. Compatibility studies are conducted to ensure that solutions of the medicine may be mixed with blood and intravenous solutions without any problems. Compatibility studies also confirm that the medicine does not interact with intravenous or other tubing through which solutions pass, and that it does not interact with the container (e.g., glass, polypropylene) in which it is kept, or other materials that it may contact (e.g., rubber stopper, Teflon liners).

CHAPTER 17

Data Review Committees

OTHER NAMES FOR DATA REVIEW COMMITTEES

Data Review Committees have also been referred to as Data Monitoring Boards, Policy Advisory Boards, External Safety Committees, Operations Committees, Quality Assurance Committees, Policy Committees, Safety and Efficacy Monitoring Committees, or other similar names. Each of these committees may deal with the same or different functions. In some clinical trials the functions they fulfill are handled by an overall Trial Steering Committee, or by other groups.

COMMITTEE FUNCTIONS

The specific function(s) of a Data Review Committee should always be clearly defined (insofar as possible) prior to initiating a clinical trial. A Data Review Committee usually reviews accumulating data to detect evidence of early dramatic benefit or harm for patients while a clinical trial is in progress. This function may include review of only safety data or only efficacy data, or it may include both. The specific question(s) the committee is often asked to address include:

1. Should a clinical trial be stopped as soon as it is demonstrated that the test treatment is statistically

and clinically significantly better than placebo or the alternative treatment? Guidelines should be established in advance for the statistically significant difference at each stage when the data are to be examined. It is also appropriate to ask what specific changes from baseline or differences between groups would constitute a clinically significant difference. Magnitudes of change in specific endpoints and levels of significance must be established that will be convincing to the vast majority of clinicians who will be interested in and potentially affected by the results of the clinical trial. If the trial is stopped before the data are sufficiently significant clinically, the trial may have been conducted in vain.

2. Should a clinical trial be stopped as soon as it is demonstrated that the test treatment has no chance of being statistically and clinically significantly better than placebo or the alternative treatment?

3. Should a clinical trial be stopped as soon as it is demonstrated that safety considerations indicate a benefit-to-risk ratio in favor of discontinuing the test medication?

4. Do certain types of patients belong in a clinical trial?

Numerous other questions often arise during a clinical trial that are addressed by a Data Review Com-

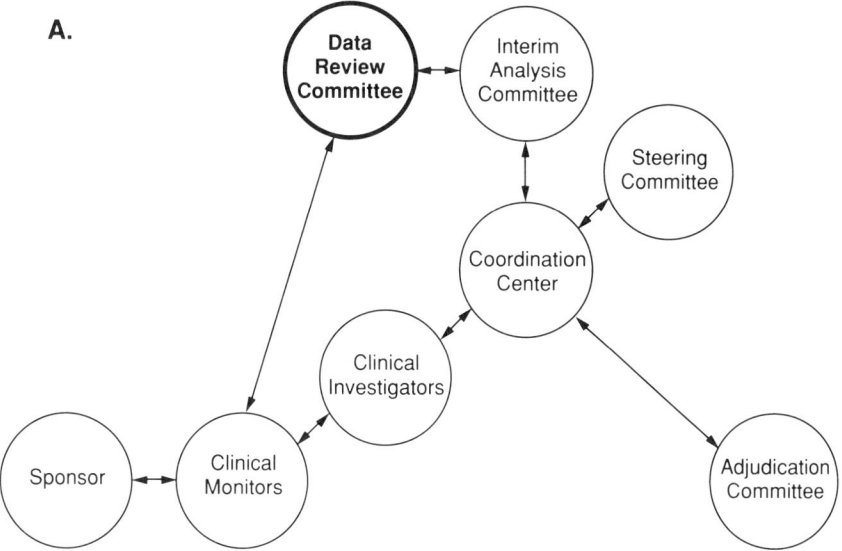

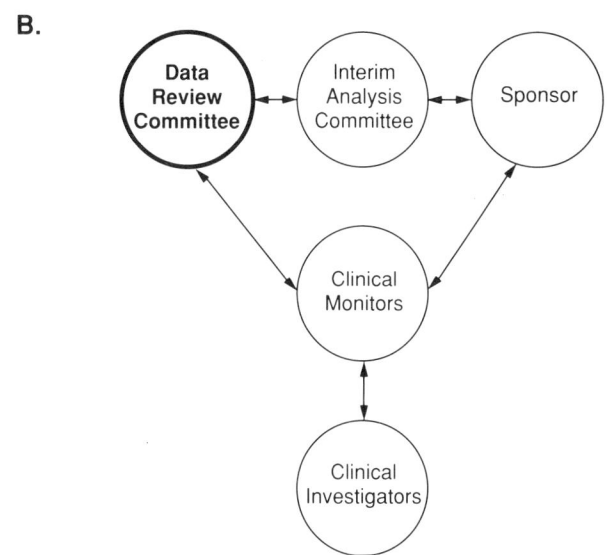

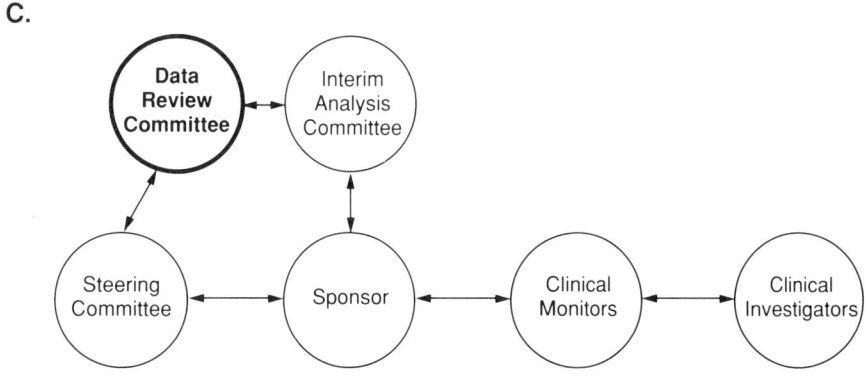

FIG. 17.1. Three representative models of how a Data Review Committee may interact with other groups in a clinical trial. Numerous variations are possible.

mittee. The experiences of one such committee have been described by DeMets et al. (1982). The issues dealt with by that committee included (1) the problem of multiple outcome variables, (2) the decision of whether to extend the recruitment period to attain the targeted sample size, and (3) the problem of monitoring patient survival with a time lag (known or unknown) in the reporting. These issues may be dealt with by multiple committees connected with a clinical trial, rather than by a Data Review Committee.

Committees to discuss these and related clinical trial questions have been created more often in recent years. The major outcome choices of their data review are usually to (1) continue the clinical trial unchanged, (2) modify the protocol, or (3) terminate the trial. Three models of how these committees may interact with other groups in a clinical trial are shown in Fig. 17.1.

COMMITTEE MEMBERSHIP

Affiliation of Members

There are three general approaches to determining the membership of Data Review Committees. The first is to appoint or invite participation from individuals who are outside the sponsoring organization of the clinical trial. This approach usually enhances the credibility of the group if and when they make a public statement. If it is deemed politically important to have experts on this committee who have impeccable credentials, then those chosen should not be affiliated with the sponsor in any manner (e.g., as consultant, as investigator). This will prevent any conflict of interest issues from arising.

The second approach is to appoint members from inside the institution sponsoring the clinical trial. This approach makes sense if the clinical trial is not expected to be in the political limelight and the sponsor regards this committee primarily as an additional safeguard for the patients' welfare or as an assistant in making important decisions. Members chosen for the committee should not be directly affiliated with the clinical trial, although they may be department heads of groups associated with the trial. Lastly, a combination of membership of both sponsors' representatives and outsiders may be assembled to serve on a Data Review Committee.

Number of Members

There are no guiding rules as to the most appropriate number of members on a Data Review Committee, except that each relevant discipline and constituency should be represented. Size generally is within the range of 3 to 12 members, although 4 to 6 members would appear to be an ideal size for most trials. In addition to one or more statisticians and clinicians, it is usually important to include ethicists on the committee. Epidemiologists and scientists from other disciplines are also represented when relevant.

Qualifications of Members

Qualifications for membership include (1) expertise in the field one represents on the committee, (2) experience in randomized controlled trials, (3) integrity, (4) common sense, and (5) knowledge of statistical principles. Another qualification in most cases is independence from the direct ability to influence the clinical trial. The balance between a conservative or risk-taking personality in each committee member is one of the most critical factors determining how the group will function. Depending on the number of members it may not be necessary for each of them to be familiar with statistical principles and randomized controlled trial methodologies.

WHEN SHOULD A CLINICAL TRIAL INCLUDE A DATA REVIEW COMMITTEE?

Interim Analyses

A Data Review Committee should be considered if one or more interim analyses are to be conducted to address any of the questions posed above under "Committee Functions," and it is desired to have a group of independent experts evaluate the data. If credibility of the clinical trial and its results is considered to be an actual or potential issue, then additional emphasis should be given to the possibility of constituting a Data Review Committee. In other words, the stakes of the outcome must be considered in determining the need for this committee.

For a Safety Review

Even if no interim analyses are planned, it may be relevant to have a Data Review Committee to review safety aspects of the clinical trial at appropriate times. These reviews may focus on such questions as whether the number of serious adverse events experienced is acceptable for the trial to continue. Including a Data Review Committee in a clinical trial in which lives may be saved is generally much more relevant than in a trial in which treatment merely makes patients feel a bit better.

If Important Political or Medical Ramifications Exist

A Data Review Committee is also desirable when long-term mortality or significant morbidity is being studied.

An alternative to the committee would be to establish rules governing the outcome of the interim analyses. If a clinical trial has important national or regional ramifications, then either formal interim analysis rules, a Data Review Committee, or both may be ethically required.

OPERATIONS OF A DATA REVIEW COMMITTEE

Scheduling of Meetings

Given the busy schedules of most professionals who might join a Data Review Committee, it makes sense to schedule meetings as long in advance as reasonable. Members should know that ad hoc meetings may also be held to discuss important events. It makes sense for most groups to meet after clinical trial milestones are achieved (e.g., 25%, 50%, 75% of the trial completed), but this approach to scheduling may be difficult to achieve. Alternatively, the committee could meet every 6 to 12 months.

Blind versus Open Statistical Analysis of Data

A group of statisticians, usually from the sponsoring organization, analyzes the interim data and provides summary results to the committee. These statisticians are not members of the Data Review Committee in most cases, and may also be kept blind to the identity of treatments (e.g., data may be indentified as treatment A or B). Whichever specific procedures and operations are to be followed by each group involved in the data analysis and data review, the details should be clearly specified in the trial's protocol.

Scope of Data To Be Given to the Committee

The scope of data that the committee are to receive must be established. Data generally include baseline data, safety data, efficacy data, quality assurance data, projections of recruitment, and times to milestones.

Blind versus Open Committee Review of Data

Treatment group data may be reviewed and analyzed by the Data Review Committee in either a blind or open manner. In blind analysis, each treatment is identified with code letters (e.g., treatment A, treatment B), masking the identity of groups receiving placebo (or active control) and the active test medicine. The choice of approach to reviewing data should be discussed at the initial meeting of the committee. Alternatively, the groups organizing the clinical trial may make this determination. If there is any doubt on this issue, then adhering to an examination of blind data is preferable.

The reasons a Data Review Committee should not be blind to the data they evaluate are:

1. Special or unanticipated issues or problems may occur in preparing reports if the committee is kept blind.
2. Reviewing data blind implies that decision making is symmetrical, i.e., the committee will reach the same conclusion if treatment A is better than B, or vice versa, whereas this is often untrue.
3. Integration of results with other information about the investigational treatment is more difficult.
4. Consideration of data from other sources is difficult.

Committee Output

The output of the committee may include the following:

1. A statement to the clinical trial's organizers and/or sponsors after each meeting that there is, or is not, a reason to stop the trial.
2. An ad hoc report to federal authorities (if relevant).
3. Reports prepared for relevant groups about concerns regarding quality of the data, the clinical trial's conduct, or relating to the trials continuation.
4. A report to the Ethics Committee(s)/Institutional Review Board(s) [IRB(s)] on an annual basis.
5. Any other appropriate statement. If the clinical trial is terminated the reasons for this decision must be stated.

The committee's operations must be conducted in a confidential manner and without leaks to outsiders. Even inadvertent disclosures through "body language" at open meetings could have significant repercussions.

STOPPING RULES FOR TERMINATING A CLINICAL TRIAL

In attempting to identify how great a difference between treatments is sufficient to justify stopping a trial, Meier (1979) described a framework (Fig. 17.2) that may be used as a starting point for Data Review Committees. His framework describes "a maximum acceptable difference" in the treatment effects such that it would be inappropriate to deny patients that much benefit because of societal interest in continuing the clinical trial to obtain useful information. He also describes a "least interesting difference" such that a difference of that magnitude or greater would be sufficient to justify a decision in favor of the winning therapy. The stopping rule is stated "Should the range

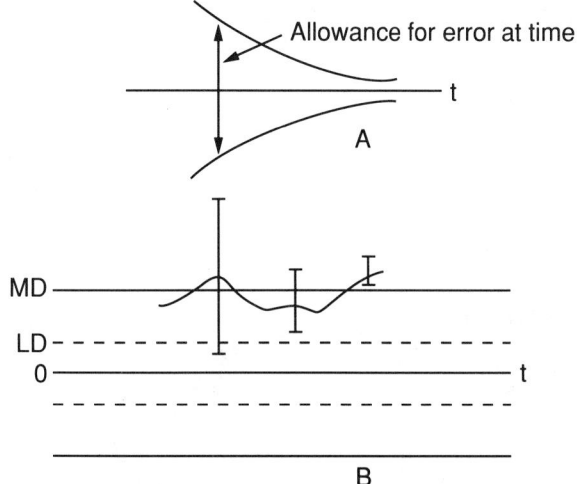

FIG. 17.2. Framework for conceptualizing stopping rules for a clinical trial. **A:** Allowance for error in the estimate of difference in outcome between two treatments as function of time. **B:** Estimated difference in outcome as a function of time. Vertical bars represent the allowance for error. MD, maximum acceptable difference; LD, least interesting difference. (Reprinted from Meier, 1979, with permission.)

of uncertainty (error) ever show that we are clearly outside the maximum acceptable difference, we have gone too far and we must stop, because we now judge that further experimenting would be abusive.'' This stopping rule is illustrated in Fig. 17.2. It is a quite reasonable rule, provided that the Data Review Committee can agree on the definitions of the two boundaries for the specific clinical trial.

Other stopping rules have been proposed (see discussion by Meier, 1980; Gordon Lan and Friedman, 1986; Armitage, 1989). It is essential to consider how great a difference in effects for either safety or efficacy parameters is required to demonstrate clear clinical significance and to make the data convincing to clinicians. Several of the proposed stopping rules focus on statistical levels of significance, which may not indicate that the data are also clinically significant. An example of a clinical trial that was stopped early with data that were convincing to physicians is the Beta-Blocker Heart Attack Trial (De Mets et al., 1984). An example of a clinical trial that was stopped early in which the data were not convincing to many physicians is the University Group Diabetes Program (UGDP) trial. Choi et al. (1985) and Fleming and Watelet (1989) discuss stopping rules for trials in which treatment differences are small and are not likely to become significant even if additional data are collected.

Selected Reasons to Proceed with Ongoing Trials

Among the reasons that should be considered before terminating a clinical trial are the following:

1. One should complete what has been started.
2. A different conclusion might result.
3. Greater acceptance of the data will occur.
4. The clinical trial is unique and it may never be possible to repeat it.
5. No harm will occur to control patients.
6. More data on various endpoints will be collected.

Efficacy versus Safety Rules

Stopping rules based on efficacy parameters can be specified more precisely than rules based on safety parameters. Efficacy-based rules may be specified in advance of the clinical trial, but rules based on safety parameters are more difficult to specify in advance. Safety rules also are more judgmental.

Future clinical trials will probably be more likely to include Data Review Committees than do those today, particularly in large trials and when significant ethical issues exist.

CHAPTER 18

Dosage Forms and Formulations

MEDICINE FORMULATIONS

In the majority of clinical studies, both the form of the medicine to be studied and route of administration are known prior to development of the clinical trial design, and these factors are not raised as issues to be evaluated. Nonetheless, there are instances when either the forms of the medicines or routes of administration are the major focus of the clinical trial (e.g., comparison of two different dosage forms or two different routes of administration). It is also possible that the pros and cons of each form (or route) that could be used must be considered prior to a determination of the most appropriate choice. A description of possible forms of medicines and routes of administration is presented in this and the following chapter.

The different forms of a medicine shown in Table 18.1 are briefly described below, and a few considerations relating to their use in clinical trials are presented. Most of these forms contain a wide variety of additives or vehicles called excipients [e.g., lubricants, disintegrants, antioxidants, binders, diluents, buffers, surfactants, antibacterials (Table 18.2)]. Some of these additives may cause allergic responses in some individuals, and this factor must be considered in the clin-

ical testing of the medicine. The conversion of raw materials into compounds that are formulated into medicines that may degrade (Fig. 18.1) involves many processes and aspects not discussed in this chapter.

Formulating a placebo for controlled studies may pose pharmaceutical problems for some of these medicine forms. (Table 25.1 lists many factors in a placebo that must be matched to the trial medicine.) The preparation of a placebo should be initiated early in the process of medicine development.

The comments below are generally brief and limited in scope. Additional information is presented in *Remington's Pharmaceutical Sciences* (Gennaro, 1990), *Modern Pharmaceutics* (Banker and Rhodes, 1989), *The Theory and Practice of Industrial Pharmacy* (Lachman et al., 1986), and in numerous other sources.

FORMS OF MEDICINES THAT MAY BE TAKEN ORALLY

Tablets

Tablets are solid forms of a medicine that are usually prepared by compression and are the most common

TABLE 18.1 *Forms of medicines*

A. Forms of medicines that may be administered via the mouth
  1. Tablet
  2. Capsule
  3. Solution
  4. Suspension
  5. Emulsion
  6. Aerosol
  7. Gas
  8. Whips
  9. Syrups
  10. Elixirs
  11. Spirits
  12. Gums
B. Other forms of medicines that may be used topically or placed in natural orifices in the body
  1. Powder
  2. Ointment
  3. Cream
  4. Gel
  5. Lotion
  6. Paste
  7. Suppository
  8. Transdermal patch
  9. Sponge
  10. Enemas
  11. Tinctures
  12. Shampoos
  13. Liniments
  14. Douches
  15. Irrigants
  16. Pessaries
C. Long-acting dosage forms
  1. Sustained action
  2. Prolonged release
  3. Repeat action
  4. Depot
D. Injectables
  1. Solid implants
  2. Solutions
  3. Suspensions
  4. Emulsions
  5. Vegetable oils

form of medicines sold. Tablets may be coated or uncoated. If coated, they may be film coated to aid in swallowing, give a cosmetically acceptable appearance, and also to protect the medicine from rapid dissolution. Enteric coating is one type of film coating that prevents a tablet from dissolving in the acid medium of the stomach. The tablet is thus absorbed in the intestines and not in the stomach. Tablets may also be sugar coated, which masks objectionable odors or tastes and protects the medicine from many interactions (e.g., the sugar coating serves as an antioxidant). Sugar coating is a more time consuming process than is film coating. Layered tablets contain two or three different layers in each tablet. Press-coated tablets have a core tablet that is surrounded by a different material (i.e., it is a tablet within a tablet).

Active ingredients released from tablets may be absorbed under the tongue (e.g., sublingual nitroglycerin) or in the buccal cavity. These two routes of administration are useful for medicines that would otherwise be extensively metabolized in the liver in a "first-pass effect," and the sublingual route can achieve rapid absorption of a medicine (e.g., nitroglycerin). The onset and duration of various nitrate formulations are shown in Fig. 18.2. Tablets may be chewable (e.g., aspirin has been sold in a gum form) or effervescent (e.g., Alka

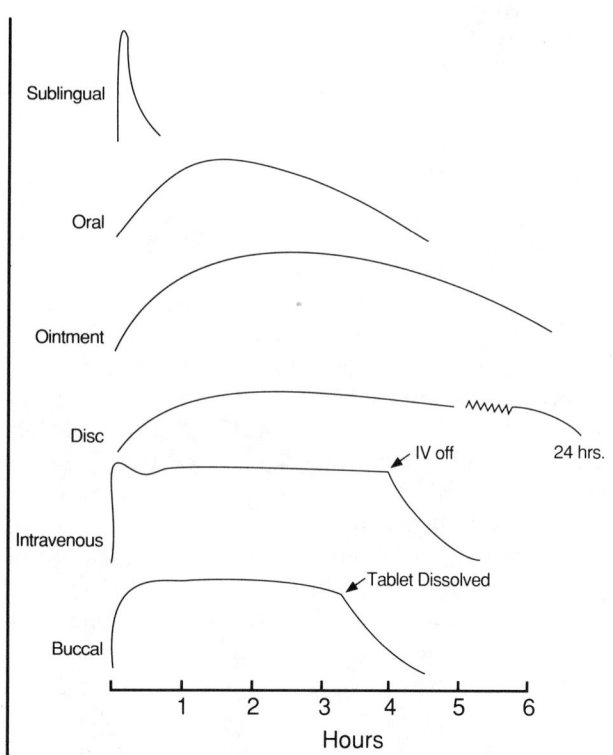

FIG. 18.2 Nitrate delivery systems. This schematic demonstrates the average time to onset and duration of action for the various nitrate formulations. (Reprinted from Abrams, 1983, with permission of the *American Journal of Medicine.*)

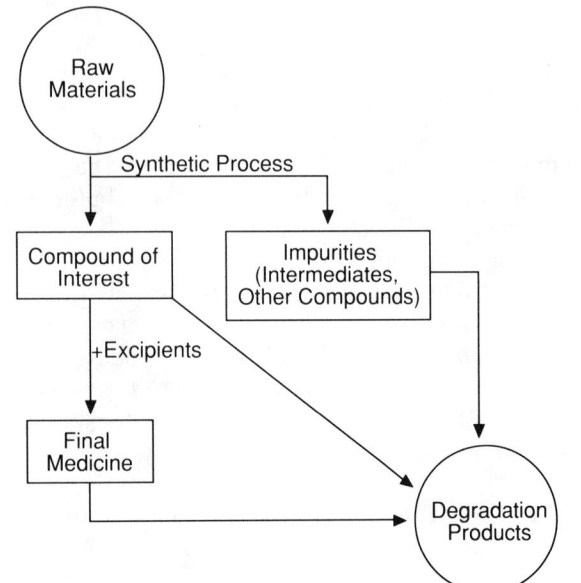

FIG. 18.1 The various processes by which degradation products and impurities arise from raw materials.

TABLE 18.2 *Types of excipients (with examples)[a]*

1. Absorbents (e.g., petrolatum and lanolin alcohols, white wax)
2. Acidifying agents (e.g., citric acid, fumaric acid, malic acid)
3. Adsorbents (e.g., magnesium aluminum silicate, magnesium carbonate, powdered cellulose)
4. Alkalizing agents (e.g., potassium citrate, sodium bicarbonate, sodium citrate)
5. Anesthetics, local (e.g., benzyl alcohol)
6. Antiadherents (e.g., magnesium stearate)
7. Antiadhesives (e.g., talc)
8. Anticaking agents (e.g., colloidal silicon dioxide, talc, tribasic calcium phosphate)
9. Antibacterials (e.g., chlorhexidine, phenylmercuric acid)
10. Antifungals (e.g., mineral oil, potassium sorbate, propylene glycol)
11. Antimicrobial preservatives (e.g., benzalkonium chloride benzyl alcohol, methylparaben, sorbic acid)
12. Antioxidants (e.g., ascorbic acid, citric acid, sodium metabisulfite)
13. Antiseptics (e.g., benzalkonium chloride, benzyl alcohol, phenylmercuric nitrate)
14. Bacteriostatics (e.g., benzoic acid, butylparaben, sodium benzoate)
15. Binders, tablet (e.g., acacia, alginic acid, dextrin, gelatin, hydroxyethyl cellulose, povidone)
16. Buffering agents (e.g., citric acid, sodium bicarbonate, sodium citrate)
17. Bulking agents (e.g., mannitol)
18. Chelating agents (e.g., edetic acid and edetates)
19. Clarifying agents (e.g., bentonite)
20. Cleaner–polishers of capsules (e.g., sodium chloride)
21. Coating agents (e.g., carnauba wax, gelatin, methylcellulose)
22. Color extenders (e.g., dextrose, pregelatinized starch)
23. Demulcents (e.g., glycerin, sucrose)
24. Denaturants (e.g., diethyl phthalate)
25. Dessicants (e.g., calcium sulfate)
26. Detergents (e.g., benzalkonium chloride, cetrimide, sodium lauryl sulfate)
27. Diluents (e.g., calcium phosphate, dextrose, lactose, mannitol, sodium chloride, starch, sucrose)
28. Direct compression excipients (e.g., dibasic calcium phosphate, dextrose, magnesium carbonate)
29. Disinfectants, local (e.g., isopropol alcohol, propylene glycol)
30. Disintegrants (e.g., alginic acid, magnesium aluminium silicate, starch)
31. Dispersing agents (e.g., lecithin, polyoxyethylene castor oil derivatives)
32. Emollients (e.g., carnauba wax, lecithin, petrolatum)
33. Emulsifying agents (e.g., acacia, calcium stearate, emulsifying wax, lecithin, sodium lauryl sulfate)
34. Expectorants (e.g., potassium citrate)
35. Fillers, tablet (e.g., mannitol, tribasic calcium phosphate)
36. Film formers (e.g., hydroxyethyl cellulose, hydroxypropyl methylcellulose, polymethacrylates)
37. Filters (e.g., magnesium carbonate)
38. Flavoring agents (e.g., fumaric acid, glucose, malic acid)
39. Flavoring stabilizers (e.g., carboxymethylcellulose calcium, dextrose)
40. Foaming agents (e.g., poloxamer)
41. Gelling agents (e.g., bentonite, poloxamer)
42. Glidants (e.g., colloidal silicon dioxide, magnesium stearate, starch)
43. Granulating agents (e.g., hydroxypropyl cellulose, sucrose)
44. Humectants (e.g., glycerin, lecithin, mineral oil and lanolin alcohols, propylene glycol)
45. Lubricants (e.g., calcium stearate, glycerin, magnesium stearate, mineral oil, talc)
46. Milling aids (e.g., calcium stearate)
47. Ointment bases (e.g., hydroxypropyl methylcellulose, lanolin, petrolatum, polyethylene glycol, yellow wax)
48. Oleaginous vehicles (e.g., corn oil, cottonseed oil, ethyl oleate, mineral oil, peanut oil, sesame oil)
49. Plasticizing agents (e.g., citric acid, glycerin, propylene glycol)
50. Polishers (e.g., carnauba wax, sodium chloride)
51. Preservatives (e.g., alcohol, benzalkonium chloride, benzyl alcohol, glycerin, mineral oil, propylparaben, sodium benzoate)
52. Propellants (e.g., butane, carbon dioxide, dichlorodifluoromethane, isobutane)
53. Protectives (e.g., acacia, petrolatum, titanium dioxide)
54. Solubilizing agents (e.g., acacia, emulsifying wax, glyceryl monostearate, lanolin alcohols, stearic acid)
55. Solvents (e.g., benzyl alcohol, corn oil, glycerin, mineral oil, propylene glycol)
56. Stabilizers (e.g., bentonite, dextrin, glyceryl monostearate, white wax)
57. Stiffening agents (e.g., cetyl alcohol, hydrogenated castor oil, paraffin)
58. Suppository bases (e.g., polyethylene glycol, white wax)
59. Surfactants (e.g., docusate sodium, lecithin, sorbitan esters)
60. Suspending agents (e.g., carbomer, gelatin, guar gum, kaolin)
61. Sweetening agents (e.g., dextrose, mannitol, sorbitol, xylitol)
62. Thickening agents (e.g., carboxymethylcellulose sodium, dextrin, magnesium aluminum silicate, zinc stearate)
63. Thixotropics (e.g., magnesium aluminum silicate)
64. Timed-release agents (e.g., carnauba wax, stearyl alcohol, zein)
65. Tonicity agents (e.g., glycerin, mannitol, sodium chloride)
66. Ultraviolet absorbers (e.g., titanium dioxide)
67. Viscosity-controlling agents (e.g., bentonite, calcium stearate)
68. Viscosity-increasing agents (e.g., acacia, carbomer, gelatin)
69. Waxes (e.g., emulsifying, microcrystalline, paraffin)
70. Wetting agents (e.g., benzalkonium chloride, lecithin, sodium lauryl sulfate)

[a] A few examples are compounds used in the manufacture of medicines and are not strictly excipients.

Seltzer contains sodium bicarbonate and citric acid and releases CO_2 when placed in water) or prepared as lozenges (candy-like forms of a medicine) that dissolve slowly and maintain contact with the oral cavity and are especially useful in treating pediatric patients. Some examples of medicine classes put into lozenges (also called pastilles or troches) are antibiotics, local anesthetics, antitussives, analgesics, and deconges-tants. A final type of tablet is one that disperses when placed in solution or on the tongue.

Disadvantages of tablets are that they require more excipients than do capsules or other dry forms of medicines. The types of excipients that may be required in tablets include lubricants (e.g., magnesium oxide) to keep the medicine powder from sticking to the manufacturing punches, binding agents or gums (e.g., sucrose, gum acacia) to hold the tablet together, and disintegrants (e.g., starch, cellulose) to facilitate disintegration of the tablet in the gastrointestinal tract. Each excipient placed in a tablet may influence the bioavailability of a medicine.

Capsules

Capsules may be composed of hard or soft gelatin, although hard gelatin capsules are more common. Soft gelatin capsules are generally used to contain a medicine in the liquid form. Capsules may be enteric coated for the same reasons as tablets. Capsules are filled with loose powders, granules, beads, lightly compressed plugs, or even tablets. Tablets are sometimes placed inside opaque capsules to double blind an investigational medicine. The outside covering may be clear, semiclear, or opaque. One of their advantages is that many patients find them easier to swallow than tablets. For pediatric trials it may be desirable to open a capsule and sprinkle the granules on food.

Disadvantages of capsules are that they (1) are often more expensive than tablets to produce, (2) may require too large an empty capsule shell to include all medicine required, and (3) are slower to manufacture than are tablets.

Medicines in Phase I trials are usually made in capsules since less pharmaceutical development work and less expense are required to produce capsules rather than tablets. One exception to this generalization is when the dry material is so fluffy that it cannot be placed easily into capsules.

Solutions

Solutions are mixtures that are formed by dissolving a solid, liquid, or gas homogeneously in a liquid. Solutions are especially useful for pediatric and some geriatric oral medicines and are the most common form of all parenteral medicines. Potential problems must be considered in relation to solubility, stability, irritation to tissues, compatibility with preservatives, and other factors. Freeze drying is a process used for solutions and colloidal solutions. Freeze-dried forms of medicines are generally reconstituted shortly prior to use.

Suspensions

Suspensions are usually formed when the preparation of a solution is not possible. Suspensions are finely divided solids mixed or dispersed in a solid, liquid, or gas; the term is mainly applied to solids dispersed in liquids. A stable suspension that does not have to be shaken has advantages over suspensions in which settling occurs. Potential problems must be considered in

relation to taste, odor, aftertaste, color, stability, compatibility with preservatives, and other factors.

Suspensions are often developed in addition to a solid dosage form. Suspensions are particularly useful for children, geriatric patients, and patients who have difficulty swallowing. In cases of poisonings, an antidote given as a suspension begins to act more rapidly than does a solid dosage form.

Emulsions

Emulsions are mixtures of two immiscible liquids, one of which is uniformly dispersed throughout the other. Emulsions are usually oil in water or water in oil. They may be applied topically, or given orally or parenterally. There are extremely few emulsions used parenterally. A 10% intravenous (i.v.) fat emulsion (Intralipid 10%) is an example of one such product and is used for parenteral nutrition.

Aerosols and Sprays

Aerosols are pressurized containers with a valve and have been used to administer medicines both orally (into the mouth and lungs) and topically. Many medicines have been placed in aerosol containers for treating numerous cutaneous or systemic diseases (e.g., asthma). They contain two major ingredients, the medicine (with excipients) and the propellant, which forces the medicine out of the container when the valve is pressed open.

The advantages of aerosols include ease and rapidity of use, protection of the contents from contamination by air, moisture, and light, and the ability to deliver "precisely" measured doses with metered valves. Disadvantages include the presence of fluorocarbon propellants (in some aerosols), which may cause environmental problems related to their effects on ozone, possible allergic and toxic reactions to some propellants, and generally high cost.

The types of aerosol products available may be described as (1) fine space sprays of small particles of the active medicine, (2) surface-coating sprays, which use larger particle sizes to cover the surface with a film, and (3) aerated sprays, which dispense various foams and creams, although this latter type is not used orally. Aerosols may be used to deliver either liquids or small particles of solids. Pump sprays and the intermittent positive-pressure breathing apparatus are other methods of delivering inhalationally applied medicines. Examples include bronchodilators given by aerosol.

Sprays differ from aerosols in several ways. Sprays are not maintained under pressure and are delivered from a container by human power squeezing a bottle or pressing a pump or plunger. A variable delivery occurs with sprays, whereas aerosols that deliver prescription medicines usually are constructed to deliver a fixed amount each time the nozzle is squeezed. Sprays are usually housed in plastic or glass containers whereas aerosols are usually kept in metal containers. Various sprays containing topical antibacterials are commercially available.

Gases

Gases are usually given by mouth but may also be administered via the nasal cavity. General anesthetics are the most common type of medicine given in this form and are supplied as gases (e.g., nitrous oxide) or as liquids that volatilize (e.g., halothane).

Whips

Whips are a newer dosage form resembling whipped cream or shaving cream. They are particularly useful in pediatric situations because the whip does not fall off a spoon and because ingredients that mask the medicine's taste can be incorporated. A metered valve can be inserted on a pressurized container to dispense a fixed amount of medicine. An alternative method to dispense medicine is to put a syringe on top of the container and press down on the valve until the syringe fills to the desired level. This syringe (without needle) may be placed into a patient's cheek and the contents dispensed.

Syrups, Elixirs, and Spirits

Syrups are aqueous sugar solutions that contain a dissolved medicine. They are most often used for pediatric and sometimes geriatric patients. Elixirs contain ethanol in addition to sugar, whereas spirits contain ethanol and not sugar.

Gums, Lozenges, and Troches

Gums may contain chicle, lozenges are sugar based, and troches are chewable.

FORMS OF MEDICINES THAT MAY BE USED TOPICALLY OR PLACED IN NATURAL ORIFICES

Powders

Powders are most often packaged in sprinkling cans, aerosols, and jars. Powders and crushed tablets may be mixed with foods (e.g., applesauce) for administration to children. Advantages of powders include flexibility in preparation (compounding with excipients) and generally good chemical stability.

Powders are useful in certain applications, including foot powders, powders for decubitous ulcers, dental powders, douche powders, dusting powders (applied to the skin for various hygienic purposes), and insufflation. Insufflation describes the delivery of powder directly into the lungs (e.g., the Spinhaler turbo-inhaler is used to deliver micronized cromolyn sodium powder to lungs). The drawbacks of powders often include (1) poor adhesiveness to the skin, (2) that they are time consuming to prepare and package, (3) difficulty of patients obtaining equal doses, especially if the powder is affected by humidity, is hygroscopic, or is fluffy, and (4) unsuitability to medicines that have an unpleasant odor or taste.

Ointments, Creams, and Gels

Ointments, creams, and gels are semisolid formulations. Ointments are generally translucent, creams are usually opaque white, and gels have a clarity that ranges from clear to a translucence similar to that of petrolatum. The term "cream" has been used both for oil-in-water emulsions and for water-in-oil emulsions, although the former are more prevalent. Ointments are high-viscosity suspensions of the active medicine(s) in a vehicle.

One limitation of these formulations is the difficulty encountered in delivering a precise dose with commercially available products. There are a number of techniques used to measure the dose of medicine delivered from a jar or tube containing ointment, cream, or gel. Probably the best method is to weigh the tube or other container before and after either one or several applications. It is understood, however, that not all of the medicine expressed from the tube or removed from the jar or other container will have been applied to the target lesion. Another system to calculate the dose is to measure the length of the ribbon squeezed from a tube (e.g., this system is used with nitroglycerin 2% ointment). A third approach is to measure the area covered with the medication and to express the dose as the amount of medicine required to cover a defined area, but this latter method is the least reliable of the three described to define dosage. It is often preferable to prepare unit-of-use foil packs or other units that contain precise amounts of medicine. This presupposes, however, that the contents of one (or more packs) will contain the appropriate quantity of medicine for all patients and for all lesions.

Lotions

Lotions are usually liquid suspensions that are used externally on the body. The decision to develop a lotion usually depends on the intended use (e.g., shampoo, special skin treatment). In preparing medicine dosages for clinical trials, it may be useful to consider unit-dose containers, each having a fixed amount of lotion to apply. An alternative means of measuring the dose is to weigh containers before and after treatment(s).

Pastes

Pastes are stiff semisolid mixtures of powders (e.g., starch, zinc oxide, talc) dispersed in petrolatum as a base (i.e., an ointment) intended for use on the skin. Pastes are often used to treat oozing and moist lesions such as burns and open wounds, where pastes absorb serous fluids and secretions. They adhere well to the skin and form an opaque layer. Pastes may be thick and therefore serve as a protective coating for the lesions on which they are applied. Pastes may be removed with a vegetable or mineral oil. Examples of pastes are zinc oxide paste and those used by outdoor athletes on their face to prevent windburn.

Suppositories

These solid forms are usually placed in the rectum, where they melt and deliver medicine that is absorbed through mucus membranes. Suppositories are also placed in the vagina and, albeit rarely, in the urethra. Local effects occur within 30 minutes and usually last for at least 4 hours. This form is also used to elicit systemic effects. In the formulation of suppositories, special attention is concentrated on achieving the optimum size, shape, hardness, melting characteristics, and bioavailability. Under situations in which an individual has difficulty swallowing, suppositories may be given orally for patients to suck in order to deliver a medicine.

This form was used by ancient Egyptians, Greeks, and Romans, and today suppositories are more widely used in some countries than others. In the United States, this form is most widely used for pediatric and geriatric patients. In pediatrics, suppositories are used to treat emesis and other conditions. The adult population mainly uses this form to treat hemorrhoids and constipation, but suppositories are suitable as a carrier for many classes of medicines.

Transdermal Patches

Transdermal patches are developed to avoid the first-pass effect, increase patient compliance, and achieve a longer half-life. Medicines to be placed in a reservoir inside the patch must cross the skin barrier and not cause sensitization. A simple model of a transdermal patch has three layers (i.e., release liner, medicine reservoir, and system backing), whereas more sophisticated models have two additional layers (i.e., a rate-controlling membrane and a contact adhesive) between the reservoir and release liner.

A Phase I program to evaluate a transdermal patch is often more complex and involves more clinical trials than those for most conventional medicines. These trials are necessary to address questions of (1) where the patch should be placed on the body, (2) what are the release characteristics of the medicines, (3) what size patch is optimal, and (4) should dosages be adjusted through the number of patches placed simultaneously, or through different amounts of medicine placed in a single size patch or in different-sized patches? If tolerance develops in Phase II trials, it is pertinent to evaluate whether release may be completed in less than 24 hours and tolerance avoided.

Transdermal patches have recently been introduced for the gradual absorption of nitrates in patients with angina and for scopolamine to prevent motion sickness. Other examples include transdermal estrogen as a replacement therapy and Catapres for treatment of hypertension. Transdermal patches for nitroglycerin vary widely in dose (2.5 to 15 mg) and size (3.3 to 32 cm^2) in the United States. These patches are often effective if worn on the body for 10 to 12 hours daily, though they rapidly become ineffective when used around-the-clock. The use of this dosage form will probably expand in the future as a means of obtaining constant but low level of medicine delivery over a prolonged period.

Sponges and Pessaries

Sponges impregnated with medicines are currently being used for contraception. A disposable vaginal polyurethane sponge with nonoxynol-9 is now sold over the counter in the United States. Wax and polymer pessaries are used intravaginally to provide controlled release prostaglandin E2 that acts on the cervix to help induce labor. One advantage is that the pessary may be removed if the uterus is overstimulated, however, removal is sometimes difficult.

Enemas, Tinctures, Shampoos, Liniments, and Douches

Enemas are given rectally. Tinctures are alcohol based and often contain topical antibacterials. Shampoos are surfactants usually applied to the scalp. Liniments and rubs are usually nonaqueous. Douches are usually applied vaginally.

OTHER FORMS OF MEDICINES

Depot

In a depot form of a medicine, a sustained release occurs. Some depots (e.g., medroxyprogesterone, fluphenazine) have effects whose duration is measured in weeks. Depot medicines are placed inside body tissues or cavities for prolonged periods. The depot acts as a reservoir from which the medicine is slowly leeched over an extended period at a relatively constant rate. There are a variety of physical–chemical means whereby release of the medicine from the depot may be delayed and controlled. Examples of depots include depot injections given intramuscularly (e.g., procaine penicillin G, medroxyprogesterone acetate suspension) and subcutaneously (e.g., protamine zinc insulin), and implants that are professionally placed (e.g., Progestosert®). Silicon rubber (Silastic) inserts that contain medicines have been more widely used in recent years. Medicines are either sealed inside an inner cavity or may be made as part of the inert Silastic matrix itself, from which it diffuses. Silastic has been formed into many shapes, including tubes, membranous sacs, rings, and other shapes. There is wide speculation that implants will be used more widely in the future to provide medicine release close to the target organ.

EXCIPIENTS

A few inactive ingredients (excipients) are listed below, along with their purpose(s). A more complete list plus examples is given in Table 18.2.

Binder. Improve compression characteristics of powder mixtures or granulations.

Disintegration materials. Help the tablet break up after it has been ingested.
Lubricants. Help the materials flow during the product's manufacture and prevent tablet presses from binding up.
Preservatives. Help prevent bacterial destruction of the materials.
Flavorings. Provide desirable flavors, while masking any unpleasant tastes present.
Coloring agents. Allow medicine identification and enhance marketability.
Wetting agents. Used for extremely fluffy compounds that are difficult to compress into tablets.

LONG-ACTING DOSAGE FORMS

Long-acting dosage forms have been referred to by many names, including controlled release, timed release, delayed release, modified release, and extended release, plus the three names used in this section: sustained release, prolonged release, and repeated release. There are occasions when it is desirable to release the medicine from the formulation over an extended period to provide an adequate medicine level during the entire sleep or waking period (e.g., to maintain sleep, an antibacterial effect, or many other effects) or at other times when the medicine used does not have the desired duration of effect. There are various types of long-acting dosage forms and various techniques of formulating these products. Three types of long-acting dosage forms are:

1. Sustained release. The medicine is absorbed and acts the same pharmacologically as the usual single dose, but its effect continues for a longer period, and constant medicine levels in blood are maintained (see Fig. 18.3).

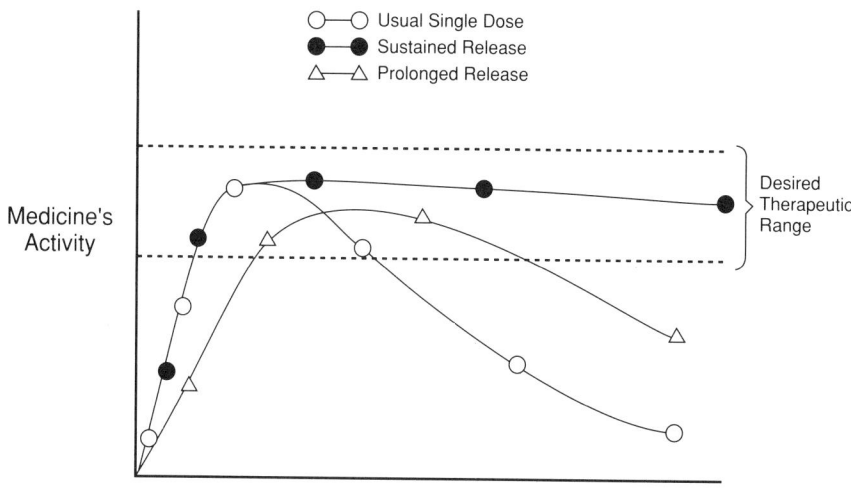

- ○—○ Usual Single Dose
- ●—● Sustained Release
- △—△ Prolonged Release

Medicine's Activity

Desired Therapeutic Range

Time

FIG. 18.3 Two types of hypothetical long-acting formulations of a single medicine (sustained release and prolonged release) compared with activity over time of a single dose of the same medicine. (Reprinted by permission of Philadelphia College of Pharmacy and Science from Gennaro, 1990.)

2. Prolonged release. The medicine is absorbed somewhat less rapidly and for a longer period than the usual single dose, and its total duration of effect is greater than that provided by the single dose, although constant medicine levels in blood are not necessarily maintained (see Fig. 18.3).
3. Repeat release. The medicine is manufactured to have a usual dose absorbed at two different times (e.g., by placing an enteric-coated tablet inside a regular tablet).

Various authors (Chien, 1983; Madan, 1985; Longer and Robinson, 1985; Li et al., 1987; Krowczynski, 1987) have defined these and other similar terms in a variety of ways (e.g., from general to specific, based on kinetics, blood levels, or therapeutic effects).

The most difficult form of the above three types to prepare is the true sustained-action dosage form, and this is rarely achieved. Several different manufacturing methods are used to prepare sustained- and prolonged-release dosage forms. These include the use of (1) tablets with slow-release cores, (2) capsules containing coated slow-release beads, (3) multilayered tablets, (4) porous inert carriers or (5) ion-exchange resins to complex medicines, and (6) tablets compressed from different types of granules (e.g., coated and uncoated) that provide release at different times.

Sustained release of parenteral medicines may be attained through the use of relatively insoluble salts or esters of the active parent molecule. Vehicles may be chosen for use from which the active medicine is slowly absorbed. Newer techniques for creating long-acting liquids have begun to provide new medicines with this property, and there are many novel ideas being evaluated for new forms of medicine delivery (Merz et al., 1983). A good review of medicine delivery systems is presented by Bondi and Pope (1987).

Types of Coatings Put on Medicines

Tablets are coated for one or more of the reasons given in Table 18.3. There are three major methods of coating.

1. *Enteric coating.* Tablets containing ingredients that are inactivated by gastric pH or that cause gastric irritation are coated to prevent dissolution in the stomach. The tablet passes to the small intestines where the altered pH breaks down the coating and the tablet dissolves.
2. *Film coating.* A thin layer of a solvent is usually applied to a tablet. It provides a thinner coat than does a sugar coating and thus does not mask tastes as well.
3. *Sugar coating.* A generally thick layer of sugar or sorbitol and color is created that is particularly useful to mask unpleasant odors and tastes.

Racemic Mixtures versus Stereoselective Medicines

Most physicians who prescribe medicines and most investigators who study medicines are unaware of whether the medicine they are using or studying is a racemic mixture of the isomers or contains stereoselective forms. This is hardly surprising when no literature source describes medicines this way (Drayer, 1987) and even the pharmacokinetic literature does not adequately describe this aspect (Ariëns and Wuis, 1987).

TABLE 18.3 *Reasons for coating a tablet*

1. Improve appearance
2. Mask an unpleasant taste
3. Enhance a neutral taste
4. Mask odor
5. Decrease gastrointestinal irritation
6. Deliver tablet to site of absorption
7. Delay disintegration and absorption
8. Eliminate irritation in mouth
9. Prevent interactions between components
10. Enhance a tablet's identity
11. Improve ability to swallow a tablet

CHAPTER 19

Routes of Administration

INTRODUCTION

Routes of medicine administration may be considered
as being of two types—*enteral* and *parenteral*. The
enteral routes place the medicine directly into the gastrointestinal tract by oral, sublingual, buccal, or rectal
administration. All other routes, including topical
routes, may be defined as parenteral, although topical
routes are not commonly described as a parenteral
route of applying medicines.

Routes of medicine administration may also be divided into one of four general categories: (1) oral, (2)
topical, (3) injected into the body or placed under the
skin, or (4) placed into a natural orifice in the body
other than the mouth. Examples of routes that are included in these four broad categories are presented in
Table19.1. The choice of a particular route to use in
most studies is usually evident to the author of a protocol, but there are occasions when a choice among
several routes is possible. Each route of administration
has a number of potential and actual advantages and
disadvantages. There are also considerations that
should be familiar to individuals using these routes. A
number of these factors are described in the sections
that follow.

ROUTES OF ADMINISTRATION IN WHICH MEDICINES ARE PLACED INTO A NATURAL ORIFICE IN THE BODY, INCLUDING ORAL ROUTES OF ADMINISTRATION

Medicines placed into a natural orifice exert local effects and in many instances systemic effects as well.
The possibility of systemic effects occurring when
local effects are desired or of local effects occurring
when systemic effects are desired should be considered.

For routes of administration in which the medicine
is taken *orally* or placed into an orifice other than the
mouth, clear instructions about the correct application
of the medicine must be provided. Many cases are
known of oral pediatric drops for ear infections being
placed into the ear, and vice versa (ear drops being
swallowed). Errors in medicine utilization are especially prevalent when a medicine form is being used in
a nontraditional manner (e.g., suppositories that are
taken by the buccal route).

Many patients are not familiar with terms such as
sublingual (under the tongue), buccal (between the
cheek and gingiva), otic, and numerous others. A clear
description of each of these nontraditional (i.e., non-

oral) uses should be discussed with patients, and instructions may also be written and given to patients. Demonstrations are often useful to illustrate selected techniques of medicine use (e.g., how to use an inhaler or aerosol for asthma). Some medicines must be placed by physicians into body orifices (e.g., medicated intrauterine devices such as Progestasert). Numerous medicines have been given by the buccal route (Anonymous, 1987).

Inhalational Routes of Administration

The *inhalational route* via mouth or nose is used for medicines that are in a gaseous state (e.g., anesthetic gases) and for liquids and solids (via aerosols). Both the liquid and solid particles are so small that they remain suspended in air as they are inhaled into the lungs. In general, the smaller the particle size, the further the particles travel before depositing along the tracheopulmonary tree. There is less of a tendency for smaller particles to sediment at the upper end of the pulmonary system, where they are inhaled. When patients inspire a large volume of air, the velocity of the air moving into the respiratory tract is greater, forcing

TABLE 19.1 *Routes of administration*

A. Oral routes
  1. Oral
  2. Inhalational[a]
  3. Sublingual
  4. Buccal
B. Placed into a natural orifice in the body other than the mouth
  1. Intranasal
  2. Intraauricular
  3. Rectal
  4. Intravaginal
  5. Intrauterine
  6. Intraurethral
C. Injected into the body or placed under the skin
  1. Intravenous
  2. Subcutaneous
  3. Intramuscular
  4. Intraarterial
  5. Intradermal
  6. Intralesional
  7. Epidural[b]
  8. Intrathecal[c]
  9. Intracisternal
  10. Intracardiac
  11. Intraventricular
  12. Intraocular
  13. Intraperitoneal
  14. Intravitreally
D. Topical routes
  1. Cutaneous
  2. Transdermal[d]
  3. Ophthalmic

[a] This route is usually via the mouth, although the nose may be used.
[b] This route is also referred to as peridural and extradural.
[c] This route is also referred to as subarachnoid.
[d] This route is also referred to as transcutaneous and percutaneous.

all particles to go further into the tracheopulmonary tree before they are deposited. Thus, aerosols of mixed particle size will cause less consistent pharmacological responses than will those of a more uniform size. Also, smaller-size particles are generally deposited closest to the alveolar membranes, from which they will be absorbed more rapidly into the circulation. Finally, patients should be instructed to inhale with a strong effort when they use an aerosol to deliver a medicine.

Significant systemic absorption occurs with many medicines given by inhalational techniques, which use small particles. Although pressurized and nonpressurized aerosols have been used to deliver numerous medicines into the systemic circulation, this approach has not been widely used.

ROUTES OF ADMINISTRATION IN WHICH MEDICINES ARE INJECTED INTO THE BODY OR PLACED UNDER THE SKIN

General Considerations

Most injected routes of administration place the medicine directly or indirectly into the systemic circulation. In a number of these routes, however, the medicine exerts a local effect, and most of the medicine does not enter the systemic circulation (e.g., intrathecal, intraventricular, intraocular, intracisternal). Certain routes of administration may exert both local and systemic effects depending on the characteristics of the medicine and excipients (e.g., subcutaneous, percutaneous, and rectal).

Choosing a Parenteral Route

The choice of a particular parenteral route will depend on the required time to onset of action, the required site of action, and the characteristics of the fluid, among other factors.

The need for a rapid onset of action usually requires that an *intravenous* (i.v.) route be used, although at a certain stage of cardiopulmonary resuscitation, the need for a rapid effect may require the use of an intracardiac injection. The required site of action may influence the choice of route of administration [e.g., certain radiopaque dyes are given intraarterially near the site being evaluated; streptokinase is sometimes given experimentally into the coronary arteries close to coronary vessel occlusion during a myocardial infarction to (it is hoped) cause lysis of the thrombus and reestablish coronary blood flow].

The characteristics of the fluid (i.e., clinical trial medicine) to be injected will influence which parenteral routes of administration are possible to consider. The compatibility of the fluid used must be evaluated with other fluids (e.g., saline, dextrose, Ringer's–lactate) that the medicine may be combined with for administration to the patient.

When Are Parenteral Routes Preferred?

There are certain clinical situations in which a parenteral route of administration is preferred to other possible routes. These include the following:

1. When the amount of medicine given to a patient must be precisely controlled (e.g., in many pharmacokinetic studies), it is preferable to use a parenteral (usually i.v.) route of administration.
2. When the "first-pass effect" of a medicine going through the liver must be avoided, a parenteral route of administration is usually chosen, although a sublingual route or dermal patch will also avoid the "first-pass effect."
3. When one requires complete assurance that an uncooperative patient has actually received the medicine and has not "cheeked" it or otherwise rejected it (e.g., via emesis).
4. When patients are in a stupor, coma, or otherwise unable to take a medicine orally.
5. When large volumes (i.e., more than a liter) of fluid are injected in peritoneal dialysis, hyperalimentation, fluid replacement, and other conditions. Medicines given in large volumes require special consideration of fluid balance in the patients receiving the large volumes.

Intravenous Route

The *i.v. route* is the most common means to introduce a medicine directly into the systemic circulation. It has the following advantages:

1. Rapid onset of effect.
2. Usefulness in situations of poor gastrointestinal absorption.
3. Avoidance of tissue irritation if present with intramuscular or other routes (e.g., nitrogen mustard).
4. More precise control of levels of medicine than with other routes, especially for toxic medicines, when the levels must be kept within narrow limits.
5. Ability to administer large volumes over time by a slow infusion.
6. Ability to administer medicines at a constant rate over a long period of time.

It also suffers from these disadvantages:

1. Higher incidence of anaphylactic reactions than with many other routes.
2. Possibility of infection or phlebitis at site of injection.

3. Greater pain to patients than with many other routes.
4. Possibility that embolic phenomena may occur, either air embolism or vascular clot as a result of damage to the vascular wall.
5. Impossibility of removing or lavaging medicine after it is given except by dialysis.
6. Inconvenience in many situations.
7. Possibility that rapid injection rates may cause severe adverse reactions.

For i.v. fluids it must be determined how the dose will be given (i.e., by bolus or slow injection, intermittent or constant infusion, or by constant drip) and whether special equipment will be used to control and monitor the flow. Medicines with short half-lives are usually given by a constant drip or infusion technique. All i.v. fluids given immediately subsequent to an i.v. drug must be evaluated for their compatibility with the trial medicine. Suspensions are not given i.v. because of the possibility of blocking the capillaries.

When an intravenous medicine from a vial or ampule is to be given in a bag of solution (e.g., saline, dextrose in water, Ringer's) there are two options. The exact amount of medicine needed is measured and placed in the bag of solution; all of the bag's contents are then given to the patient. This approach is not usually followed. The more common method in hospitals is to place all of a medicine from a vial or ampule in the bag and adjust the rate of infusion and amount of solution given the patient.

Constant Infusion

Numerous practical problems may occur with *constant infusions,* particularly if the site or staff is not familiar with this approach. Potential problems include (1) extravasation, (2) pump problems, (3) people changing rates of infusion, (4) pharmacy not ready with the follow-up bag of solution, and (5) nurses not starting follow-up bags promptly. By anticipating these problems, most of them may be avoided.

Subcutaneous Route

Medicines given by the *subcutaneous route* are forced into spaces between connective tissues, as with intramuscular injections. Vasoconstrictors and medicines that cause local irritation should not be given subcutaneously under usual circumstances, since inflammation, abscess formation, or even tissue necrosis may result. When daily or even more frequent subcutaneous injections are made, the sites of injection should be continuously changed to prevent local complications. Fluids given subcutaneously must have an appropriate tonicity to prevent pain, and fluids given into the central nervous system must be pure and sterile to prevent neurotoxicity and infection. Care must be taken to prevent injection of the medicine directly into veins.

The absorption of medicines from a subcutaneous route is influenced by blood flow to the area, as with intramuscular injections. The rate of absorption may be retarded by cooling the local area to cause vasoconstriction, adding epinephrine to the solution for the same purpose (e.g., with local anesthetics), decreasing blood flow with a tourniquet, or immobilizing the area. The opposite effect may be achieved with the enzyme hyaluronidase, which breaks down mucopolysaccharides of the connective tissue matrix and allows the injected solution to spread over a larger area and thus increase its rate of absorption.

In addition to fluids, solid forms of medicines may be given subcutaneously. This has been done with compressed pellets of testosterone placed under the skin, which are absorbed at a relatively constant rate over a long period.

Intramuscular Route

The *intramuscular route* is frequently used for medicines dissolved in oily vehicles or for those in a microcrystalline formulation that are poorly soluble in water (e.g., procaine penicillin G). Advantages include rapid absorption in many cases, often in under 30 minutes. Other advantages of the intramuscular route include the opportunity to inject a relatively large amount of solution and a reduction in pain and local irritation compared with subcutaneous injections. Complications include infections and nerve damage. The latter usually results from the choice of an incorrect site for injection.

Although the time to peak medicine concentration is often on the order of 1 to 2 hour, depot preparations given intramuscularly are absorbed extremely slowly. Numerous physical–chemical properties of the material given intramuscularly will affect the rate of absorption from the site within the muscle (e.g., ionization of the medicine, lipid solubility, osmolality of the solution, volume given). The primary sites used for intramuscular injections are the gluteal (buttocks), deltoid (upper arm), and vastus lateralis (lateral thigh) muscles. The rate of drug absorption and the peak medicine levels obtained will often differ between different sites used for intramuscular injections. This is related to differences in blood flow among muscle groups (Evans et al., 1975). The site chosen for an intramuscular injection may be a critical factor in whether or not the medicine exhibits a therapeutic effect (Schwartz et al., 1974).

Intraarterial Route

Intraarterial injections usually require a surgical "cutdown" procedure before they can be given. This route requires highly skilled individuals to prevent a variety of potentially serious complications, including thrombosis formation, arterial spasm, and the possibility of loss of blood supply distal to the site of injection. Its uses include injection of radiopaque contrast media and selected antineoplastic agents. A totally implantable pump is sometimes placed in patients who receive intraarterial infusions of chemotherapy (Niederhuber et al. 1984), or hepatic arterial perfusion scintigraphy (Ziessman et al., 1984).

Intradermal Route

Intradermal injections are often used with allergy-testing materials used for diagnosis of types of allergies or for evaluating improvement after treatment. Small volumes (0.05 ml) of isotonic solutions are usually used and are placed into the skin so that a small wheal is formed (a small circumscribed transitory area of edema of the skin). If a wheal is not raised, then the injection has probably been given subcutaneously and must be repeated at another site or at a later time.

Intralesional Route

Intralesional administration is used for several medicine groups, of which corticosteroids are the most common. This route is often chosen when topical agents either lack adequate potency or do not satisfactorily penetrate the epidermal skin barrier. Medicines given by this route may be used on their own or as an adjunct to topically applied medicines as therapy for many diseases. Long-term use of intralesional injections may cause systemic effects to occur (Amene, 1983).

Intrathecal and Epidural Routes

Intrathecal injections of medicines (in isotonic fluids) are also referred to as subarachnoid injections. Medicines are placed in the cerebrospinal fluid in the subarachnoid space inside the spinal canal. Injections are often made between lumbar vertebrae 2 and 5. This route is used for numerous purposes, including induction of spinal anesthesia and treatment of leukemic foci in the central nervous system. The term "spinal" injection is colloquial for a subarachnoid injection.

Epidural injections are also referred to as peridural and extradural injections. Medicines are injected into the space surrounding the dura mater but within the spinal canal. Both caudal and lumbar approaches are used. Intraspinal is a general term referring to subarachnoid and epidural routes together.

Intraventricular, Intraperitoneal, Intrapleural, and Intracardiac Routes

For *intraventricular injections,* an indwelling catheter may be used with a reservoir to provide chemotherapeutic drugs to patients when the blood–brain barrier is intact. This system provides high local concentrations plus low systemic medicine levels.

The *intraperitoneal route* is rarely used in humans but has been used to administer anticancer drugs for abdominal ascitic tumors. An implantable medication system has been used to deliver insulin intraperitoneally (Saudek et al., 1989). Patients receiving continuous ambulatory peritoneal dialysis have been given intraperitoneal acyclovir (Burgess and Gill, 1990). *Intrapleural instillations* of tetracycline have been used to decrease the rate of recurrence for spontaneous pneumothorax (Light et al., 1990). *Intracardiac injections* are for the most part used only during emergency cardiopulmonary resuscitation attempts. These injections may be made through an open or closed chest.

TOPICAL ROUTES OF ADMINISTRATION

When using a *topical route* in a clinical trial, many design factors arise that are hard to control. Such potential problems are a major reason why double-blind well-controlled trials are less common in dermatology than in many other areas of medicine. A number of these considerations, which, again, are difficult to control adequately, are the following:

1. Where on the body surface will the medicine be applied? Should mucus membranes be avoided? Even on the skin surface, the absorption of a medicine varies enormously between different sites and depends on clinical conditions (e.g., approximately 1% of topical hydrocortisone penetrates normal human skin on the forearm, but only one-seventh as much will penetrate the skin through the plantar foot arch, and 42 times as much will penetrate through scrotal skin; hydration of the skin increases absorption of hydrocortisone by about four- or fivefold; inflammation also markedly increases the skin penetration of hydrocortisone and most other topically applied medicines).

2. Will the medicine be absorbed into the systemic circulation, and if so, what are the consequences for the patient and for the study?

3. How will the amount of medicine dispensed be measured (e.g., length of a ribbon, size of skin covered, weight of medicine container before and after application)?

4. If a percutaneous route is used (i.e., absorption of medicine occurs through unbroken skin) with rubbing of an ointment or other form of medicine, how will the rubbing be quantitated and controlled in terms of pressure and duration?

5. How will the effect of the medicine be measured (e.g., by a clinical scale of several gradations, biopsy results, other techniques)?

6. At which of the following sites is the medicine presumed (or known) to act: skin surface, stratum corneum, viable epidermis and upper dermis, glands, and/or systemically?

7. How will the clinical trial be controlled, since clinical lesions vary markedly in intensity of symptoms and appearance from site to site within one patient as well as between patients? Although it is desirable for each patient to serve as his or her own control (e.g., by treating lesions on each arm or leg with different medicines), it is often difficult to quantitate different lesions accurately in one individual, though this often must be done.

8. Numerous other factors must be considered (e.g., vehicle used, appropriate form of medicine).

9. May a simultaneous crossover clinical trial design be used? In this design one part of the body serves as the control and the symmetrical part as test site. This approach may be used for evaluating topically applied medicines placed on the back, chest, forearm, wrist, and legs and in the eyes.

PART II

Developing and Writing Clinical Protocols

I never did anything worth doing by accident; nor did any of my inventions come by accident; they came by work.

—Thomas Alva Edison

The language of truth is unadorned and always simple.

—Marcellinus Ammianus (Roman historian, 4th century A.D.*)*

CHAPTER 20

Formulating an Approach to Developing a Protocol

INTRODUCTION

A protocol is the written mechanism that describes how the clinical trial design will be implemented. There is no single approach that all individuals follow in developing a protocol for medicine trials. Furthermore, the same individual will follow different approaches in developing different protocols. Nonetheless, there are a number of principles that are usually adhered to and a general approach that is often followed, although many variations are possible. The chapters in Section II describe this general approach and are presented with the assumption that individuals will generally need (or desire) to modify the proposed order of steps in preparing specific protocols to make this approach work more effectively for them. The stages or steps presented in Table 20.1 represent a sequence of activities that may be modified or reordered to meet the requirements of specific situations effectively. Many specific types of clinical trials exist, which are described and discussed in Section III.

One may begin to write a clinical protocol after many discussions among numerous individuals. Alternatively, the writing of a protocol may represent the initial groundbreaking in a new clinical area, and one can only rely on his or her previous experience without a background of recent discussions. The clinical trial may be modest in scope and conducted at one site, or it may be scheduled for several years and encompass many sites. Whatever the size of the projected trial, and regardless of how much prior preparation has been done by the individual responsible for the protocol, many steps must be considered. A thesis of this book is that the development of most protocols usually follows a similar series of steps, even though protocols are written in a highly diverse manner and are applied in different areas of medicine. It is assumed that a protocol is a self-contained document and does not need to refer to other protocols or texts for content.

FACTORS AND STEPS

The procedures to be followed in developing a protocol have been arbitrarily divided into the 17 points (items 2–18) listed in Table 20.1. Each of the topics is the focus of a separate chapter in Section II. The individual who is writing the protocol is also generally engaged

TABLE 20.1 *Issues to consider in developing and writing clinical protocols after the trial design is chosen*[a]

1. Formulating an approach to developing a protocol
2. Establishing criteria for patient inclusion
3. Identifying, choosing, and evaluating efficacy parameters
4. Identifying and choosing safety parameters
5. Developing time and events schedules
6. Preparing, packaging, and dispensing of clinical trial medications
7. Collecting adverse event and adverse reaction data in clinical trials
8. Informed consent and Ethics Committee/Institutional Review Board processes
9. Remote data entry
10. Preparing the introduction
11. Standardizing information across protocols
12. Patient refusers, nonqualifiers, dropouts, dropins, and discontinuers
13. Regulatory, patent, and legal considerations
14. Ethical considerations and issues
15. Completing and reviewing the initial draft
16. Improving the quality of a protocol
17. Preparing data collection forms
18. Instructions for patients, investigators, and trial personnel

[a] Each of these topics is addressed in a separate chapter in this section.

in numerous other activities designed to initiate the protocol. A number of these activities are being considered or conducted at the same time that the protocol is being written. Many of these activities (e.g., interviewing potential investigators) are discussed in Section IV of this book.

MEDICAL TRAINING OF AUTHORS

It is widely believed that a first-hand clinical appreciation of the disease being evaluated helps the author of a protocol to choose the most appropriate clinical trial design in order to address the objectives and the optimal parameters for measuring the anticipated clinical changes. For this reason, there is a potential problem when trained scientists prepare protocols rather than medically trained individuals, since members of the former group lack clinical experience. Collaboration between a scientist and a clinician in the protocol development process, however, can almost always resolve any clinical trial design issues that arise.

STYLE

The style used in writing clinical protocols depends on the skills and personality of the person writing the protocol as well as the requirements (if any) of the institution at which the clinical trial will be conducted, the requirements of the sponsor (if any), and other factors. Thus, there may be stylistic constraints placed on the individual who is in the process of developing a clinical protocol. The presence and nature of any stylistic requirements should be determined before the writing phase commences.

The most obvious differences in style relate to whether the author (1) is terse or verbose, (2) is simple and clear, or complex and vague, and (3) describes all contingencies and possibilities that may arise or only mention events that definitely will arise.

CHAPTER 21

Establishing Criteria for Patient Inclusion

INTRODUCTION

Inclusion versus Exclusion

This chapter describes the various criteria that can be used for patient *inclusion* and *exclusion*. Inclusion criteria constitute the definition of patient characteristics required for entry into a clinical trial and may generally be used for patient exclusion as well as inclusion, since most criteria (e.g., age range of 18–65 years) establish both inclusion (18–65 years) and exclusion (lower than 18 or above 65 years) groupings. The single term inclusion is usually used in a general sense throughout this book to include the concept of exclusion as well.

Narrow versus Broad Limits

If the limits for patient entry are set too broadly, then a heterogeneous group of patients may be enrolled which may create a problem when the data generated are inadequate to address the clinical trial objectives. Under circumstances in which an excessively heterogeneous group of patients is enrolled, the interpretation and relevance of the trial may be questioned. Conversely, if the limits of patient entry are set too narrowly, then it may be impossible to obtain an adequate number of patients to conduct the trial. In addition, it may be difficult to compare data from such a population with data generated from a broader population (i.e., interpretation of the data may not be relevant for general clinical situations).

The advantage of using relatively "tight" entry criteria is that the clinical trial will be conducted with a more homogeneous population. This factor will often provide more meaningful data and interpretations, especially for Phase II controlled studies. Many of the criteria used to determine patient inclusion are listed in Table 21.1. These criteria have been arbitrarily divided into four groups: (1) characteristics of patients, (2) characteristics of the disease and its treatment, (3) environmental and other factors, and (4) results of screening examinations.

Choosing Criteria and Documenting Adherence

In determining the criteria to be used for patient inclusion, it is important to exclude those patients for whom the clinical trial will create unacceptable clinical risks. If patients with a given disease, state, or attribute are to be excluded from a trial, then it is important to determine the procedures used to exclude these patients. For example, if all patients with a given disease are to be excluded from a trial, it may be sufficient for

TABLE 21.1 *Factors to consider as criteria for patient inclusion*[a]

A. Characteristics of patients
  1. Sex
  2. Age
  3. Weight
  4. Education
  5. Race and/or ethnic background
  6. Social and economic status
  7. Pregnancy and lactation
  8. Use of tobacco; ingestion of caffeine and/or alcohol
  9. Abuse of alcohol or drugs
  10. Diet and nutritional status
  11. Physiological limitations and genetic history
  12. Surgical or anatomical limitations
  13. Hypersensitivity to a clinical trial medicine or test
  14. Other medicine and nonmedicine allergies
  15. Emotional limitations
B. Characteristics of the disease and its treatment
  1. Disease being evaluated
  2. Concomitant medicines
  3. Previous medicine and nonmedicine treatment
  4. Washout period of nontrial medicines or nonmedicine treatments
  5. History of other diseases
  6. Present clinical status
  7. Previous hospitalizations
C. Environmental and other factors
  1. Patient recruitment and cooperation
  2. Participation in another clinical trial
  3. Participation in another part of this clinical trial or in any other clinical trial using this study medicine
  4. Institutional or environmental status
  5. Occupation
  6. Geographical location
  7. Litigation and disability
D. Results of screening examinations

[a] This term is used to encompass criteria used for exclusion as well.

the investigator to question all prospective participants as to whether they presently have the given disease. An additional question that may be posed by the investigator is whether the patient has ever had the disease. A further step is to request that a laboratory or other test be performed to document that the patient does not have the disease. The degree of documentation required for patients to enter the clinical trial may be set at whatever standard is deemed appropriate to ensure that patients in the trial do not have the excluded disease. The criteria established in most of the categories discussed in this chapter may be (1) ascertained by patient history as recounted by the patient or as noted in medical records, (2) observed by the investigator, (3) documented by scores on tests, or (4) confirmed by other professionals using clinical judgment. It may be important for key tests to be performed by independent investigators, laboratories, or groups to prevent bias from entering into critical measurements that affect patient inclusion. Inclusion criteria should be designed to eliminate (insofar as possible) hard-core nonresponders with the disease being evaluated. If this is not done, then no matter how well the clinical trial is designed and conducted in a large number of hard-core nonresponders, the data obtained may actually represent a false-negative result.

CHARACTERISTICS OF PATIENTS

The first group of specific inclusion criteria to be discussed relates to characteristics of patients (Table 21.1).

Sex

Certain clinical trials are limited to patients of one sex by their objectives (e.g., prostate or ovarian evaluations). Women of child-bearing potential must be excluded from almost all clinical trials of investigational medicines until appropriate reproductive and teratological studies have been performed. Many Phase I trials, therefore, exclude all women. Inclusion criteria usually indicate which classes of women of non-child-bearing potential may be enrolled (i.e., women who are postmenopausal and/or those who have had a hysterectomy and/or those who have had a tubal ligation). In pediatric trials, girls are often excluded once they have reached the menarche.

Age

The ranges of patients' ages have been arbitrarily grouped into three categories: children (until age of majority), adults, and elderly. Ensure that the upper age limit is not set below the age of most patients with the disease.

Children

A frequently discussed and debated question relates to the acceptable lower age limits for patients who are included in a medicine trial. Establishing a lower age limit depends on many factors such as the nature of the disease, adequacy of available treatment(s), evaluation of the trial medicine's safety and efficacy, guidelines of pediatric committees, and the views of the various ethics and administrative committees that must approve the protocol. If separate pediatric trials are being planned, then the investigator should review the various guidelines for conducting medicine trials in children prior to writing the protocol (Food and Drug Administration, 1974, 1977a; American Academy of Pediatrics Committee on Drugs, 1977; Ryan, 1977; Working Party on Ethics of Research in Children—British Paediatric Association, 1980). With parental or legal guardian consent, minors below the age of 18 may be included in medicine trials. Children from the age of about 7 to their majority (legal adult age) must give their "assent" (usually verbal and in the presence of a witness) to participate in a clinical trial. In addition, the investigator must obtain the informed consent from the child's parent(s) or legal guardian.

Elderly

It has been well known for many years that neonates, infants, and children respond to certain medicines differently than adults, primarily because of pharmacokinetic differences. Now there is increasing information indicating that older individuals also respond to some medicines differently than younger adults. The impact of these findings on the testing of investigational medicines is that early clinical trials usually exclude older individuals as well as children. Older individuals are gradually included in clinical trials as a medicine's safety is more firmly understood and established. Separate trials targeted to the elderly age group are also performed on both investigational and marketed medicines. Definitions of elderly patients based solely on age are arbitrary and do not consider that chronological age and physiological age are often quite different in any one patient or within a group of patients.

Why Is Increased Attention Focused on Clinical Trials in the Elderly?

In recent years, more attention has been directed towards the evaluation of medicine effects in the older

population as a result of the following:

1. An increased number of older people in society and projections for a steadily increasing percentage of older patients in the population.
2. A disproportionately high use of medicines in the older population.
3. An increased frequency of adverse reactions in the older population.
4. Differences in pharmacokinetics, pathology, and receptor sensitivity and/or density plus impaired homeostasis.

Which Medicines Should Be Evaluated in the Elderly?

Medicines that are particularly important to evaluate in the geriatric population are those that (1) are widely used in the elderly, (2) affect the central nervous system, (3) have a low therapeutic ratio (i.e., the minimal dose that elicits clinically significant adverse reactions divided by the minimal dose that elicits a clinically significant beneficial effect), especially if the medicine is eliminated via the kidneys or if there is a hepatic "first-pass" effect, and those that (4) change the body's homeostatic mechanisms (e.g., in hypertension).

Date at which a Patient's Age Is Established for a Protocol

It may be relevant to indicate the specific point in the clinical trial at which the age criterion applies. For instance, in a trial with age inclusion of 16 to 70 years, an investigator may call the monitor and state that he has two prospective patients, one who was 70 last week and another who will be 16 midway through the clinical trial. It is desirable to have one standard to apply to all such situations. One valid standard is to specify that all patients must meet the entry criteria on the day that they officially enter the clinical trial, whether this is defined to be at screen, start of baseline, or treatment. Some leniency may be applied to the upper but not to the lower age limit.

Weight

In clinical trials in which the patient's weight is of major interest, a detailed description of acceptable patient weight characteristics and history must be specified. Those characteristics would probably be utilized for efficacy determinations and are not discussed in this book. In trials that do not focus on weight characteristics, it may be necessary or prudent to exclude patients who fall outside general weight limits. In many clinical trials, however, no guidelines or inclusion criteria need be presented. In trials of new investigational medicines, general prudence has often dictated that patients be relatively close (possibly $\pm 10\%$) to an ideal or average weight. As experience with a new medicine increases, this requirement is generally loosened to $\pm 15\%$ or $\pm 20\%$ and then eliminated entirely. The concept of ideal weight has been criticized (Knapp, 1983), and it is preferable to exclude only extremely thin or obese patients, and not to focus on including individuals near their ideal weight.

There may be reasons (relating to medicine metabolism or the ability of the investigator or patient to perform certain examinations or tests adequately) to exclude individuals of excessively high or low weights from a clinical trial. Individuals of certain weights outside the normal range may be required, however, in other trials such as those designed to evaluate questions relating to metabolism. The conditions under which a patient's weight is measured may be specified (e.g., noontime, prior to meal, in socks, after voiding).

In certain protocols, height may be viewed as a factor to be used in stratifying patients or considered in a manner similar to (or in addition to) weight. It is also possible to specify the maximal weight loss (or gain) that may have occurred over the last X months. The minimum skinfold thickness may be specified.

Education

Although a patient's education is not specifically addressed in the inclusion criteria of most protocols, there are clinical trials in which a patient's education may be a significant factor. To evaluate the effect of an investigational medicine on a complex series of sophisticated psychological tests, it may be appropriate to include a criterion relating to the patients' education (e.g., being high school graduates). One variation of this criterion is to require patients to have an education equivalent to that of a high school graduate.

It is also possible that a clinical trial objective may relate to evaluating patients with different educational levels. Thus, a predetermined number of patients may be required with specified levels of education. One example of this approach is in evaluating the comprehension and usefulness of patient package inserts in individuals with different levels of education.

Race or Ethnic Background

In certain clinical areas, such as in dermatology, the question of race may be important. In measuring the flare reaction to injected histamine, for example, it may be appropriate to limit a clinical trial to white individuals or to those blacks with pale-colored skin.

In other clinical trials, the question of race may be the central focus of the trials. For example, several trials have evaluated the responses of white and black individuals to antihypertensive medications. In this type of trial, entry criteria may be established to include specific numbers of patients of each race. Another area in which race is important is in evaluating diseases that are more (or less) prevalent in a given race (e.g., sickle cell anemia in blacks).

The ethnic background of patients may also be relevant in clinical trials in which a similar control population is desired. For example, many patients with the disease thalassemia are individuals whose families originate from the Mediterranean area around Greece or Italy. It may be relevant to require that the control population also have the same ancestry as the trial group.

Social and Economic Status

The marital status of the patient may be used as a selection factor for some clinical trials (i.e., single, married, divorced, or widowed), although this is not a common criterion. In addition, the patient's income or economic status is only rarely included, although certain diseases and types of drug abuse are more common in specific social or economic groups. Social class is measured differently in different countries, and numerous clinical trials have used this factor as a primary criterion by which to rank and compare outcomes (see Chapter 87 for specific references).

Pregnancy and Lactation

Most clinical trials exclude women who are pregnant or lactating. The name of a specific urine or blood test to be used for confirming the lack of pregnancy is often indicated in the protocol. The protocol might contain a sample waiver of pregnancy form in the appendix if women of child-bearing potential are to be included in the clinical trial. An example of such a form is shown in Chapter 27. If the length of the trial warrants, a second or even multiple repetitions of the pregnancy test may be included.

Information is sometimes presented in the protocol indicating the steps to be followed if a female patient becomes pregnant. These steps will probably include immediate discontinuation of the trial treatment, medical supervision and examinations during the course of pregnancy, and evaluation of the newborn infant.

Specific clinical trials may be conducted in women who are pregnant or lactating. Defining the limits of inclusion criteria for such trials requires extremely careful and cautious consideration of the patients to be studied and the objectives of the trial. Ethical considerations must be carefully evaluated.

Ingestion of Tobacco, Caffeine, or Alcohol

Patients who smoke tobacco may be excluded from clinical trials for a variety of reasons such as interference with ward procedures for inpatient trials, possible or demonstrated interactions of tobacco with the trial medicine, interactions with diagnostic or other tests, and the desire to control as many factors as possible that might influence results obtained in the trial. One of the most well-studied areas of interaction between smoking and medicines involves altered metabolism of medicines in patients who smoke (Conney et al., 1977). Caffeine-containing drinks such as coffee, tea, and certain sodas may also have an influence on the adverse reactions noted with the trial medicine because of their stimulant effect and the variable amounts that patients use. These beverages also may affect performance on certain efficacy tests. Chocolates contain xanthines, and their consumption by trial patients may also be regulated. During the clinical trial, the quantities of caffeine-containing drinks consumed can only be controlled to a variable degree if the trial is conducted in outpatients but may be controlled to a more significant degree if inpatients are used.

Alcohol consumption is often regulated (i.e., an attempt is made to control the amount of alcohol consumed) in many or even in most clinical trials. If this is an especially important factor to control, then periodic blood alcohol levels may be measured, or an inpatient trial may be considered. Nonetheless, it remains a difficult (if not impossible task) to control this factor fully, even in patients who do not abuse alcohol.

Abuse of Alcohol, Drugs, or Medicines

One general definition of licit medicine abuse is when a patient uses more than the recommended dose, uses the recommended dose for longer than the recommended period, or uses prescription medicines that have not been therapeutically recommended and are not indicated. Abuse of alcohol or illicit drugs by patients entering a clinical trial is undesirable for numerous reasons, including a decreased reliability of the patient in following the protocol, increased possibility for medicine interactions, and increased difficulty in clarifying adverse events.

A history of drug, medicine, or alcohol abuse is important to probe for in the entry criteria. An important consideration in this regard is whether a positive history that is more than 6 (12, 18, or a more appropriate number) months in the past should be a basis for patient

exclusion. Clinical trials dealing with diseases having a high incidence in alcoholics (e.g., cirrhosis or pancreatitis) may have more lax entry criteria concerning alcohol abuse. Inpatient trials in alcohol abusers will provide more supervision of patients and may circumvent at least some of the potential problems that might be encountered in an outpatient trial (i.e., patients consuming alcohol during the trial).

A potentially highly effective method of identifying drug abusers is to screen their urine for licit or illicit drugs. This approach, however, has a number of major limitations. Screens must be able to determine each specific drug of interest. The screens are usually expensive and both false positives and false negatives are common; also the standardization of such screens among laboratories is at a far lower level than for routine blood or urine tests (Davis et al., 1988).

It is a simple matter to write an exclusion criterion that excludes patients who abuse either licit or illicit drugs. It is a difficult matter, however, to know whether such individuals have, in fact, actually been excluded. After a definition of abuse has been established, a patient history, laboratory tests for evaluating liver function, and a urine drug screen are among the few methods or tests available to ensure that such individuals are truly excluded from the clinical trial. These methods, however, are not completely effective.

Diet and Nutritional Status

There are many variations in a patient's diet or nutritional status that may be desired as either an inclusion or exclusion criterion. No attempt will be made to list all possible variations except to state that in developing a protocol it may be relevant to address this issue.

Types of Interactions

Bioavailability, biological activity, medicine elimination, and toxicity of many medicines are known to be affected by food in general and by specific nutrients and chemicals. Clinically important medicine–nutrient interactions have been reported for numerous combinations of medicines and specific nutrients. Many lists are available of the most common medicine–nutrient interactions observed. The interactions may lead to effects primarily on the nutrient (e.g., folate deficiency caused by phenytoin) or the medicine. In the former situation, medicines may affect nutrition through effects on taste, appetite, intestinal motility, and the absorption, metabolism, and excretion of nutrients.

The dividing line between medicine–medicine interactions and medicine–nutrient interactions is not always clear. For example, minerals and vitamins that are self-prescribed may be considered as either nutrients or medicines, depending on the dose taken, the need for a dietary supplement, and other factors. These substances sometimes interfere with medicine absorption (e.g., iron salts reduce absorption of tetracycline).

How Foods Affect Medicines

Food or specific nutrients may interfere with the actions of a medicine by numerous mechanisms such as altering the absorption of oral medicines and therefore the bioavailability of a medicine by affecting gastrointestinal pH, secretions, osmolality, motility, and transit time. Food may also alter the ionization, stability, and solubility of a medicine or form a complex with a medicine in the gastrointestinal tract. The net effect of food on medicine bioavailability cannot be predicted on a theoretical basis but must be determined through clinical experience and evaluation. Food may affect a medicine's metabolism (e.g., through enzyme induction or inhibition) or excretion (e.g., by altering urine pH). An active substance in food may exert an agonistic or antagonistic pharmacological effect on a medicine. Some of the well-known examples of food affecting medicines are (1) the divalent metal ions (primarily calcium) contained in dairy products, which can combine with tetracycline to form complexes that are poorly absorbed, (2) charcoal-broiled meat, which accelerates the oxidation of phenacetin, and (3) the normal deactivation of pressor amines such as tyramine by hepatic monoamine oxidase being blocked by the class of medicines known as monoamine oxidase inhibitors. When patients receiving monoamine oxidase inhibitors (usually for depression) ingest tyramine-containing foods, a fatal increase in blood pressure sometimes occurs in susceptible individuals.

When some medicines (e.g., lithium) are given with food, the absorption of the medicine increases. This is usually because food delays gastric emptying or increases gastrointestinal transit times. These delays allow the medicine to have a longer time of contact with the site(s) of absorption and permits more complete dissolution of the medicine.

Patient Diets and Nutritional Status

Patients who enter clinical trials may be receiving special diets for medical reasons (e.g., low sodium, low glucose) that may be adversely affected by certain medicines (e.g., those with high sodium or glucose contents). If the diet of a patient changes during a clinical trial, it may have an influence on the therapeutic outcome (e.g., if a patient's diet changes during a trial evaluating a hypolipidemic medicine). The state of a patient's nutritional status may be important to qualify, since malnutrition and its associated deficiency disorders and diseases may affect medicine activity and pharmacokinetics in multiple ways.

Physiological Limitations and Genetic History

The criterion of physiological limitations refers to the use of results of certain tests as a basis of patient inclusion (exclusion). One methodology for implementing this concept is to include (exclude) patients when results of their physiological tests are within or outside established limits. This particular criterion overlaps with that describing clinical characteristics of the trial disease, laboratory examinations, and other sections as well.

A genetic history can be used to concentrate on a patient's condition that is desired to be included as the focus of a clinical trial or as a characteristic to be excluded. There are genetic disorders known to affect medicine responses (e.g., G6PD deficiency, porphyrias, hemoglobinopathies), and patients with these conditions are often excluded from clinical trials in which adverse reactions would be predicted or anticipated on the basis of these genetic defects.

Surgical or Anatomical Considerations

It is relatively common to exclude patients who have had surgery within a specified period. Additionally, patients may be included (or excluded) because of anatomical characteristics (e.g., patients without a spleen or other organ). Anatomical limitations may be related to the disease being studied (e.g., amputation in diabetic patients, blindness caused by a specific disease) or to the patient's characteristics (e.g., body surface area above or below a given range).

Emotional Limitations

Patients with clinically significant emotional problems or retardation are often excluded from clinical trials unless the trial is designed specifically to include them. These groups usually require special consideration in obtaining informed consent and eliciting acceptable cooperation. Specific *DSM-III* categories (American Psychiatric Association, 1980) or other standard classification systems may be used to exclude (or include) certain groups of patients (e.g., those with organic brain syndrome).

Patients who have active suicidal tendencies are virtually always excluded from studies, although this is not always listed in the exclusion criteria. If a psychotropic medicine is being evaluated, it is usually relevant to specify this exclusion criterion in the protocol.

Hypersensitivity to a Trial Medicine or Test

Hypersensitivity is a standard exclusion criterion that is included in most clinical trials. Patients with a higher risk of having a serious adverse reaction because of the likelihood of being hypersensitive to a trial medicine should be excluded. In addition, many clinical tests use chemicals or medicines, and these agents may also be a source of hypersensitivity reactions.

The investigator must probe for a history of hypersensitivity or allergic reactions to medicines chemically related to the trial medicine. Common chemical ''relatives'' are sometimes listed in the protocol or appendix to assist the investigator in obtaining this history.

Other Medicine and Nonmedicine Allergies

Known allergies to medicines other than the trial medicine(s) and to nonmedicine materials may be relevant factors to insert as an inclusion criterion. Individuals with numerous allergies may or may not be desirable patients to enroll in a medicine trial.

CHARACTERISTICS OF THE DISEASE AND ITS TREATMENT

The following inclusion criteria relate to characteristics of the disease and its treatment.

Disease Being Evaluated

The disease under study probably provides the most important entry criterion or group of criteria for clinical trials involving patients as opposed to trials that involve normal volunteers. In defining the presence of a disease, one may focus on the basic lesion or the primary or secondary clinical features. For example, the basic lesion in myelogenous leukemia is the presence of immature leukocytes, and the primary clinical features include fever, enlarged spleen, and anemia. Secondary clinical features include weakness and infections.

Establishing How the Diagnosis Will Be Established

The specific (or general) diagnosis of the disease being evaluated will almost invariably be stated in the inclusion criteria, as will the basis on which the diagnosis is to be made. Determine whether there are standard sources of diagnostic criteria that can be utilized, such as guidelines promulgated by societies or national or international organizations. Two examples are the *Primer on the Rheumatic Diseases* (Schumacher et al, 1988), which is prepared by a committee of the American Rheumatism Association of the Arthritis Foundation, and the *DSM-III,* which is prepared by the American Psychiatric Association (1980). Consider whether laboratory tests are mandatory, helpful, or not helpful in establishing the patient's diagnosis. The intensity or severity of the disease may be relevant for entry criteria, as may be the duration of the disease.

If there are specific tests that will be used to evaluate the primary or secondary characteristics of the disease being studied, then these tests should be utilized, if possible, to screen patients for the desired effect or response and to establish a baseline. Some of the qualifications of the stated disease that may be described in the inclusion criteria are listed in Table 21.2. These qualifications will probably be used for purposes of both inclusion and exclusion.

Concomitant Medicines

There are two major aspects to the issue of concomitant medicines in a clinical trial. The first aspect is to

TABLE 21.2 *Selected qualifications to use for diseases described in the inclusion or exclusion criteria*[a]

1. No qualifications presented
2. Disease present (or diagnosed) for at least ____ months (years)
3. Previous hospitalization for this disease is (is not) required
4. The duration of hospitalization was no longer than (at least) ____ days (weeks)
5. The number of hospitalizations was more (less) than ____ during the last ____ weeks (months, years)
6. The disease is clinically stable (unstable)
7. A diagnosis of this disease has been previously made
8. The following characteristics are present at this time: ____, ____
9. Specific laboratory values measured at screen (and/or during the preceding ____ weeks) were above (or below, or between) ____ units
10. The disease is presently clinically characterized by the following signs and/or symptoms: ____, ____ with the following intensity ____, ____
11. The disease has been characterized as ____ with the following specific methods: ____, ____ within the last ____ months (years)
12. The patient has been diagnosed with ____, ____ tests (e.g., biopsy), within the last ____ months (years)
13. The patient has been treated (or not treated) presently (previously) with the following medicine(s) ____ at the following dose (dose range) ____, or nonmedicine modalities with the following characteristics: ____, ____
14. The patient did (did not) respond to the medicine (nonmedicine) treatment described above, with the following results ____

---

[a] Each disease described may be general (e.g., renal disease) or specific (e.g., glomerulonephritis).

determine which concomitant medicines are (or are not) permitted at the outset of the clinical trial. This issue is related to inclusion criteria and is discussed in this chapter. The other aspect relates to which concomitant medicines are (or are not) permitted during the conduct of the medicine trial. This latter question is discussed in Chapter 14.

It is generally desired to exclude patients using specific medicines or classes of medicines when an adverse interaction between medicines may occur. When it is important to eliminate the possibility of all interactions between medicines then no concomitant medicines should be allowed in the clinical trial. This is generally the case for pharmacokinetic trials, Phase I safety trials, and a number of Phase II efficacy trials. Allowing concomitant medicines in a trial increases the possibility of medicine interactions confounding the results obtained, but it may be ethically unacceptable to evaluate the trial medicine as monotherapy.

If a patient is taking a concomitant medicine that is allowed by protocol, the minimum length of time should be specified that each accepted medicine or class of medicines must have been taken without dosage changes prior to entry into the clinical trial. This precaution is necessary to ensure that patients are in a steady-state condition when initiating treatment with the trial medicine.

Required Concomitant Medicine

If the trial objective is to evaluate the effects of a test medicine in patients already receiving a specific medicine, then the inclusion criteria must reflect this as well as the parameters of the concomitant medicine that will be controlled. Parameters that may be controlled include the name (generic or trade name) of the medicine, dosage(s) permitted, frequency of dosing, duration of treatment, adverse reactions allowed (or required), and blood levels. The term "required" is emphasized, since a number of medicine trials are designed to evaluate the effect of one medicine on adverse reactions caused by a different (concomitant) medicine (e.g., to treat emesis caused by *cis*-platinum or other chemotherapeutic drugs). Table 21.3 lists several variations of the criteria that may be established to delineate the types of concomitant medicines that either may or may not be allowed in a clinical trial. Combinations of these criteria are also possible to specify in the inclusion section of the protocol.

Combination Medicines

If any concomitant medicines are allowed at the outset of a clinical trial, then a policy for dealing with combination medicines should be considered. For example, if patients may receive one medicine from a specified category or list as a concomitant medicine, it must

TABLE 21.3 *Options for describing concomitant medicines in the inclusion criteria[a]*

1. Patients may not take any medicines at the time of entry into the clinical trial[b] (e.g., in many pharmacokinetic trials and in trials of acute analgesia)
2. Patients may take specific antidisease medicines. The number of medicines and dose ranges may be specified, as may acceptable blood levels (e.g., in epilepsy, since it is not generally considered ethically acceptable to evaluate a newly developed medicine as monotherapy)
3. Patients may take any number of medicines to treat their disease. Dosages may or may not be specified (e.g., in some Phase III and most Phase IV clinical trials, in which medicines are being evaluated under "normal use" conditions)
4. Patients may take any number of medicines for other diseases but not for the disease being treated with the trial medicine (this option is commonly used in many medicine trials)
5. Patients may not take medicines to treat other diseases but must take a specific medicine or medicines to treat the disease being tested with the trial medicine (in clinical trials in which specific medicine interactions are being evaluated)
6. Patients may take medicines without any restrictions on the number, purpose, or dosage regimens (in a long-term clinical trial such as the Framingham study)
7. Qualifications for nonprescription medicines may be described separately from those for prescription medicines (when nonprescription medicines may cause interactions with trial medicines or may influence the results noted with ethical trial medicines)
8. Certain combinations (or variations) of the above options may be specified

[a] The length of the medicine-free period should be specified for medicines that have been stopped prior to entry into the clinical trial. It may be relevant to specify different medicine-free periods for different classes of medicines or for specific medicines.
[b] Patients should be carefully questioned about this point, since many patients state that they are not taking medicines when they are using oral contraceptives or a variety of over-the-counter (OTC) medicines on an occasional or chronic basis, such as laxatives, mild analgesics, and vitamins.

be determined how to classify the patient who is taking one combination medicine. It may be desired to treat a combination medicine as either one or two medicines (or more, depending on the specific combination). If some combinations but not others are acceptable, then a specific listing of acceptable medicines may be appropriate. For concomitant medicines that are commonly given by more than one route of administration (e.g., corticosteroids), it may be relevant to specify separate criteria for each route (e.g., "No systemic corticosteroids may be used for 7 days, and no topical steroids may be used for 24 hours prior to the baseline").

Which Disease Is Being Treated?

It is important to clarify whether a concomitant medicine may be taken to treat the disease or problem being studied, or whether the concomitant medicine is limited to treating other diseases the patient may have. A clinical trial may become unacceptably complicated if a patient continues to take a concomitant medicine to treat an unrelated disease and that medicine also has an effect on the disease being studied. This situation could occur when diazepam is being used by a patient to treat anxiety and the patient enters a study evaluating muscle spasm. Diazepam will affect muscle spasm as well as anxiety. This type of potential problem should be considered and resolved prior to the initiation of a clinical trial.

Previous Medicine and Nonmedicine Treatment

There are often appropriate reasons to include or exclude patients from a clinical trial who have been treated previously with certain medicines or nonmedicine treatment (e.g., radiation therapy in patients with cancer). The various nonmedicine or medicine treatments that may affect the trial should be evaluated and a decision reached about whether to enroll patients who have ever been treated (or treated within some number of preceding weeks or months) with specific therapies.

Washout Period of Nontrial Medicines or Nonmedicine Treatments

Whenever patients are being taken off one treatment and a different one is being initiated, a period of time must elapse to eliminate or minimize the influence of the original medicine or treatment on the subsequent treatment. This interval is referred to as the washout or medicine-free period. The plasma half-life of a medicine is a useful tool to determine how long it will require for almost all of a medicine to be removed from the patient's body. A period of five half-lives is usually adequate to allow for biological removal of the medicine. The half-life of a medicine in normal individuals, however, may be significantly prolonged in some patients (e.g., those with renal or liver disease) or shortened in other patients (e.g., those with induced microsomal enzymes in the liver). Another factor to consider is the duration of the biological effects of a medicine. For example, the biological effects of reserpine on catecholamine depletion persist for a much longer period than the reserpine itself remains in the body.

Carryover Effect

The possible carryover or residual effect of a medicine must be considered in determining an adequate washout period. In this situation, the effects of a previous treatment persist beyond the time of the medicine's known biological activity. This carryover effect must be considered not only prior to initiating a clinical trial but also between successive parts of the trial, such as when a crossover design is used. If it is considered possible or likely for a carryover effect to occur, then a baseline period inserted between the two periods of a crossover will provide additional baseline measurements and also allow for an adequate washout period prior to initiation of the second part of the trial.

When a Medicine-Free Period Is Unacceptable

Once an optimal period of time has been determined for the medicine's washout period, it may not be clinically possible or acceptable to apply this time as a requirement for patient inclusion in the protocol. Many patients with numerous diseases cannot tolerate the necessary medicine-free period required for an adequate washout of a medicine. For example, many patients with Parkinson's disease cannot be completely taken off L-DOPA for an adequate period to become medicine-free prior to being tested with another medicine.

One approach to this problem is to taper the concomitant medicine gradually until it is removed and then to add the trial medicine. A second solution is to add the test medicine in a gradually ascending dose at the same time (or before) the original medication is tapered. Thus, after a certain time period, patients will be completely weaned from their original medicine and will be receiving the trial medicine. This latter approach has disadvantages in that it does not allow baseline measurements to be obtained during a medicine-free period and allows for medicine interactions to occur.

Another approach to this problem is to decrease the optimal medicine-free period to an acceptable duration that will allow sufficient numbers of patients to be enrolled. Data obtained from patients with a shortened washout period may be analyzed separately from those with an acceptable washout period.

History of Other Diseases

A history of diseases other than the one(s) being studied may be considered as an entrance criterion in some clinical trials. Certain patients should be excluded from a trial because of safety considerations. For example, in the early stages of testing a new medicine that affects the central nervous system, patients with a history of epilepsy may be excluded to prevent the possibility of the medicine precipitating seizures. Apart from safety, the presence of certain diseases (e.g., renal failure) in patients may affect the quality and type of data obtained with a trial medicine. Data obtained in patients with renal failure or serious cardiovascular disease could adversely prejudice results of a clinical trial and give a new medicine an undeserved "bad reputation."

Once sufficient information and experience with a new medicine's use are obtained, however, then adequate provisions and precautions may be made for evaluating the medicine in patients with various diseases. Thus, individuals with many specific diseases are generally excluded from early clinical trials of a new medicine's investigation until adequate data are obtained on how various types of patients are affected by the trial medicine. The history of other diseases may be qualified by whether patients have required hospitalization for one or more specific diseases. The means of qualifying previous hospitalizations is discussed in the following section.

Previous Hospitalizations

Previous hospitalizations for a specific disease may be used as a general measure or indicator of a certain level of disease severity that may be relevant for the entrance criteria. The parameter of prior hospitalizations may be used to exclude some, but not all, patients with a specific disease. The duration of hospitalization also may be indirectly related to severity of disease and thus be used to qualify the criterion describing hospitalization [e.g., patients with a history of psychiatric disease requiring hospitalization within the last X number of months (years) will be excluded if the hospitalization lasted for Y number or more days].

Present Clinical Status

Patients with clinically unstable acute or chronic diseases unrelated to the clinical trial disease are usually not acceptable for entry into a trial. Even patients with stable chronic diseases unrelated to the trial disease are often excluded from a trial, especially in Phase II.

For certain diseases or types of disease that are the focus of the clinical trial, it is not always straightforward to define which patients may be included. One approach to this issue is to state that patients with a certain disease must be excluded:

1. If they have been hospitalized for this disease within the last _____ months (years).
2. If they require treatment with _____ .
3. If their disease has recurred more than _____ times in the past _____ months (years).
4. If their disease was originally diagnosed more than _____ months (years) ago.
5. If their disease is of an intensity more than or equal to _____ (describe a degree of intensity on a standard test, measure, or scale).

If patients with a relatively normal medical examination (except for the clinical trial disease) are desired, one may simply exclude all patients who presently have any clinically significant cardiovascular, renal, pulmonary, or other specified category of disease. Various qualifications of this type of statement may be made (e.g., only specific diseases may be excluded instead of types or classes of diseases).

ENVIRONMENTAL AND OTHER FACTORS

The following inclusion criteria relate to environmental and other factors.

Patient Recruitment and Cooperation

If specific recruiting practices or specific sites for recruitment are to be used, information on patient recruitment may be incorporated into the protocol. Examples might include a provision that patients live within X miles or Y hours by car of the clinical trial site. Another possible specification is that only patients who work in a given place or attend a specific school or clinic may be enrolled in the protocol. Also, the possible solicitation of patients by advertisements or by referrals from other professionals may be discussed.

Patients who are not likely to cooperate in a clinical trial because of their mental status or other factors may be excluded. Determining the degree of future cooperation in advance for the entire course of a trial is virtually impossible for most (if not all) patients, but categories of patient types may be described that are expected to include a high percentage of noncooperative patients. Although patients in these categories may be excluded from the trial, the value of this type of exercise is questionable. A more detailed discussion of patient recruitment is given in Chapter 13.

Participation in Another Medicine Trial

Some patients enroll in as many medicine trials as they can for financial gain, to obtain temporary housing, or for other motives that are questionable. This is especially common in Phase I clinical trials. In Phase I trials (and often in Phase II trials), it is therefore usually advisable to exclude any patient who has participated in another medicine trial within a specific period (e.g., 3 months). This is primarily to minimize the chance of any carryover effect from the preceding trial, especially when the preceding trial involved an investigational medicine, a large proportion of the clinical pharmacology of which is unknown.

Participation in Another Part of the Same Trial or in any Other Trial Using the Same Trial Medicine

It may be relevant to exclude patients who have participated in another part of the same clinical trial or in other trials conducted with the same medicine. The pros and cons of each alternative relating to this point should be discussed among the individuals responsible for the protocol.

Institutional or Environmental Status

There are occasions when specific types of patient populations are desired. Sometimes these patient groups live in a particular type of institution, and the specific catchment areas that are (or are not) acceptable may be specified. Certain clinical trials are conducted with patients who reside in institutions or nursing homes or who constitute a specific population (e.g., patients visited by a public health nurse). This may be an important or relevant factor in a number of protocols, especially those utilizing psychiatric populations, chronic care facilities, or debilitated populations.

In an outpatient psychiatric trial, it may be desired to limit patient enrollment to any (or all) of the following catchment areas: office of a private practitioner, clinic of a general hospital, community mental health center, or other type of psychiatric clinic. Some studies use both inpatients and outpatients.

Occupation

It may be important to exclude patients engaged in occupations involving the use of dangerous machinery (including driving a car) from certain clinical trials. This is especially relevant when it is expected that sedation or disorientation could result from use of the trial medicines.

Other occupations may be relevant to identify as a specific inclusion criterion, especially if the clinical trial is conducted to address a question as it relates to workers (or patients) within a specified work group (e.g., farmers exposed to specific pesticides). Numerous occupations are associated with specific diseases (see Chapter 87).

Geographical Location

In relation to patient inclusion, geographical location generally refers to the place where the patient lives or works. Clinical trials may be limited to those patients who reside within a specified neighborhood or area in order to evaluate differences with another area. Trials

may also be undertaken to evaluate patients who have lived in the same area for different periods of time.

Litigation and Disability

Some diseases are associated with a high incidence of litigation, such as cervical pain or back pain resulting from trauma. When there may be secondary gain to the patient if he or she does not improve with treatment, the beneficial effects of a medicine may be compromised or completely unobserved if a patient with pending litigation is entered into a clinical trial. Thus, criteria of patient inclusion are sometimes established that consider workman's compensation, disability benefits, and whether or not any litigation related to the disease is pending. In addition, a consultation with an attorney about the disease may be sufficient grounds to render the patient unacceptable for admission to the trial.

RESULTS OF SCREENING EXAMINATIONS

Physical Examinations

Most patients receive a physical examination prior to entry into a clinical trial. The inclusion criteria may list specific findings that either are not acceptable for entry (e.g., nystagmus, absent deep tendon reflexes) or are mandatory (e.g., specific skin lesions of defined size and severity). Another approach is to state generally that the results obtained must be clinically acceptable to the investigator.

A routine physical examination includes a neurological examination and measurement of vital signs. Nonetheless, protocols often discuss vital signs as if they were a separate event. Any aspect of the physical examination, such as the neurological examination, that is of particular relevance to the clinical trial may also be listed separately in the inclusion criteria. The details of how thoroughly the investigator is to conduct each of the screening examinations are usually indicated in the protocol and described in detail in data collection forms.

Laboratory Examinations

Screening examinations generally include safety evaluations that are also conducted during or after treatment, such as the electrocardiogram (ECG), electroencephalogram (EEG), and ophthalmological and laboratory examinations. Criteria for patient exclusion based on abnormalities in the hematological, blood chemistry, urinalysis, or other related tests may be specific (e.g., white blood cell count over 9,000/mm³) or general (e.g., "results must be clinically acceptable to the investigator").

The number of laboratory and other tests requested in the screening examinations will depend on both past experiences with the test medicine(s) and expectations of potential problems. The tests requested should be adequate to include baseline values of important safety tests for each patient. As experience with a medicine develops, the need for extensive clinical laboratory studies gradually decreases, although the need to monitor a specific laboratory test(s) may increase. A list of the most commonly utilized laboratory tests is presented in Chapter 23.

Values in Normal Volunteers

Many normal volunteers will not have all clinical laboratory results within "normal limits." Thus, a rigid adherence to a criterion that insists that all laboratory values must be within normal (i.e., reference) limits will undoubtedly lead to a variety of problems with patient enrollment. Repeating laboratory tests in patients whose initial results were abnormal will often demonstrate that the repeated value is now within the reference range, although values of other tests that were originally within the reference range may have "crept" outside in the interim. Repeating baseline laboratory measures, both at the start and throughout a clinical trial provides a better perspective than relying on one set of data and is also one means of minimizing difficulties with variations in the data obtained. The author agrees with Joubert, Rivera-Calimlim, and Lasagna (1975) that a reasonable approach to obtaining "normal" individuals lies between the extremes of absolute rigidity and totally lax entry criteria.

Use of the Term *Normal* in Describing Inclusion Criteria

The use of the term *normal* has little real meaning except as it is defined for one or more parameters or is applied as a general term. The misuse of the word normal is observed not only in relation to laboratory values, but also in regard to patient psychiatric history. Halbreich et al. (1989) reported that 16.5% of 121 normal volunteers met criteria for diagnoses of current mental disorders, and of the 104 without current diagnosis, 36% had past histories and 39% had family histories of mental illness. Extrapolating data obtained in normal volunteers to patients may prove to be a difficult endeavor.

Sackett (1978) showed that the percent of people with at least one laboratory or other abnormality increases markedly as the number of tests increases. With one test it is 5% and with five tests it is 23%. This increases to 64% with 20 tests and 99.4% with 100 tests.

Must All Patients Meet All Inclusion Criteria to Enter a Clinical Trial?

The answer to this question appears to be a firm "yes." Or is it? The true answer is "it depends." In theory, all patients who enter a clinical trial must meet all inclusion criteria. This will be virtually impossible to achieve if the criteria are set too narrowly for a clinical trial. In all clinical trials some inclusion criteria are more important to meet than others. Some are particularly important because of regulations, ethics, patient safety, or for other reasons. Their relative importance should be indicated to and discussed with investigators. A few criteria may be bent a bit (e.g., upper age limit, an acceptable range of a laboratory analyte), but others must be rigidly consistent.

CHAPTER 22

Identifying, Choosing, and Evaluating Efficacy Parameters

TYPES OF EFFICACY CRITERIA

General Considerations

Although it is impossible to provide specific details in this chapter, a number of general considerations and principles of efficacy criteria are discussed. The major efficacy measure(s) for most diseases is usually well established, but one must evaluate which tests will provide the most definitive data within the limits of the resources available to the clinical trial. For example, it might be desirable to obtain computerized tomography scans in a particular trial but only financially possible to perform a clinical examination. It is almost always preferable to include direct validated measures rather than indirect measures of efficacy, whether they

have been validated or not. If no direct efficacy measures are available to use in a clinical trial, then indirect measures must be used.

Types of Criteria to Measure Efficacy

Various types of criteria may be used to measure efficacy (or safety) parameters.

1. Presence or absence (i.e., existence) criteria. This refers to a symptom, sign, lesion, or other manifestation of a disease that is either present or not. Criteria or operational definitions may be established to define the existence of the effect.
2. Graded or scaled criteria. This refers both to scales of the types shown in Table 22.1 and to visual an-

TABLE 22.1 *Examples of grading systems used in clinical scales*

A. 1 = Not at all ____
   2 = Very little ____
   3 = A little ____
   4 = Mildly ____
   5 = Moderately ____
   6 = Quite a bit ____
   7 = Distinctly ____
   8 = Markedly ____
   9 = Extremely ____
B. 0 = Not assessed
   1 = Normal, not at all ____
   2 = Borderline ____
   3 = Mildly ____
   4 = Moderately ____
   5 = Markedly ____
   6 = Severely ____
   7 = Among the most severely ____
C. 0 = Absent
   1 = Slightly present or a suspicion of its presence
   2 = Clearly noticable but mild and occurs not more than ____ per ____
   3 = Clearly present and occurs from ____ to ____ times per ____
   4 = Definitely present and frequent
   5 = Continuous and gross
D. 0 = Absent
   1 = Rarely present (occurs less than ____ times per ____)
   2 = Occasionally present (occurs ____ to ____ times per ____)
   3 = Often present (occurs ____ to ____ times per ____)
   4 = Always or almost always present (occurs more than ____ times per ____ or continually)

TABLE 22.2 *Types of endpoints used to measure efficacy of a medicine in clinical trials*

1. Time for an important parameter to improve by a fixed percent (e.g., 75%, 100%)
2. Time to recurrence of symptoms after treatment is stopped (e.g., return to 50% or 75% of baseline)
3. Time to a new episode of disease while treatment continues
4. Degree of recurrence of symptoms after treatment is stopped
5. Duration of improvement while on maintenance therapy
6. Magnitude of improvement noted at a fixed time (e.g., 1 week or month) after therapy is initiated
7. Any calculated parameter related to efficacy that is calculated from parameters measured[a] (e.g., ejection fraction, integrated area under the curve, dp/dt of left ventricular end diastolic pressure)
8. Any subjective parameter of improvement
9. Any quality of life domain or component

[a] Any of the endpoints listed could be used for the calculated parameter.

alog scales. Graded scales can be applied to subjective as well as to objective clinical symptoms and signs. A number of scales have become well established in clinical medicine (e.g., cardiac murmurs are graded from 0 to 6, neurological reflexes are graded from 0 to 4).

3. Relative change criteria. These criteria refer to measurements in specific tests that provide direct or indirect indications of efficacy.
4. Global criteria. This category involves the overall evaluation of a patient's disease or change in disease (e.g., severity of disease, global improvement). The individual factors that this aggregate evaluation is based on may or may not be specified. Specific (or general) criteria or a scoring system may also be developed to rate each of the factors.

One must determine the pros and cons of each efficacy measure incorporated into the study. The potential value of data obtained from each efficacy test added to the clinical trial must be evaluated against the increase it will elicit in time requirements, personal efforts, financial costs, and additional complexity of the trial. At some point in virtually all clinical trials, adding tests becomes counterproductive, and the trial becomes inefficient. Types of endpoints used to measure efficacy are listed in Table 22.2.

Types of Preventive Therapy

Most clinical trials assess one or more therapies for treating a disease, syndrome, or condition. Fewer clinical trials assess prevention therapy (or diagnosis). Brief descriptions of three types of preventive therapy are presented.

Type 1. Preventive of disease occurrence. Therapy prevents patients from contracting the disease. This is the purpose of many vaccines (e.g., tetanus, diphtheria, pertussis). Vaccines are usually given to volunteers prior to any direct threat of disease, but they may be given after a presumptive threat has been experienced (e.g., a puncture wound that may lead to tetanus).

Type 2. Preventive of episodes of disease. Therapy is given to patients so that the number, duration, or severity of disease episodes are decreased. This type of preventive therapy is used with many medicines given to patients with chronic diseases (e.g., asthma, epilepsy).

Type 3. Prevention of progression of the patient's underlying disease. Medicines may delay or prevent disease progression. This occurs with medicines used to prevent more serious sequelae of the disease in patients who are either asymptomatic (e.g., lowering blood pressure in hypertensive patients, decreasing lipids in patients with hyperlipidemias) or symptomatic [e.g., decreasing blood sugar in diabetic patients, treating mildly and moderately symptomatic patients who are human immunodeficiency virus (HIV)-positive with zidovudine to slow the progression of acquired immunodeficiency syndrome (AIDS)].

Risk Factors

Risk factors for a disease are often used as clinical endpoints in clinical trials. They may be used to define subpopulations of patients with a disease, including those who may benefit from a particular treatment. Risk factors also serve to identify an individual's risk and are often used as a prognostic factor to stratify patients entering a clinical trial.

TYPES OF DATA: NOMINAL, ORDINAL, INTERVAL, AND RATIO

Four numerical types of data are described and defined as four levels.

Nominal Data (Level One)

Data are grouped into mutually exclusive classes (or categories) with names, but no order, so that all patients or objects in one class are equivalent in relation to the class attribute. Examples include patients classified by sex, blood type, or vital status. Patients' diagnoses may also be characterized into a (generally) small number of classes. Classes may be assigned codes on data collection forms to assist in data processing (e.g., males equal A and females equal B).

Ordinal Data (Level Two)

Data are grouped into classes (or categories) with names that are used to indicate an order or rank. Intervals of the spectrum used are not strictly quantifiable. An example of an ordinal scale is: 1, *continuously;* 2, *frequently;* 3, *sometimes;* 4, *rarely;* and 5, *never.* Although there is an order in this example, the distance between consecutive categories or classes of the scale is either unequal or unknown. Specific examples would include patient attitudes, radiological rating scales of deterioration in osteoarthritis, degree of pain, and ability to walk unassisted. Common categories used in ordinal scales include terms such as higher, more, better, lower, less, and worse. Forrest and Andersen (1986) describe five types of ordinal scales and also discuss briefly the statistical evaluation of data obtained from ordinal scales. MacKenzie and Charlson (1986), and Forrest and Andersen (1986) describe useful standards and problems associated with ordinal scales. Guyatt et al. (1987) and Jaeschke et al. (1990) compared two types of ordinal scales (visual analog and Likert scales) and found comparable responsiveness.

Interval Data (Level Three)

Data are grouped into continuous classes (or categories) with names (e.g., four degrees, five degrees, six degrees) that are ordered in size or magnitude and have

equal intervals between them. The zero point may be placed arbitrarily and does not necessarily mean that the property measured is absent. For example, a temperature of zero degrees (either Celsius or Fahrenheit) does not mean no temperature (i.e., absolute zero). Other examples include the intelligence quotient, weight, number of cigarettes smoked per day, and degrees of range of motion.

Ratio Data (Level Four)

Data are grouped into classes (or categories) with names that are ordered in size or magnitude and have equal intervals between them. The zero is set at true (i.e., absolute) zero. Examples include number of medicines, age of patients in years, temperature in Kelvin units, speed in kilometers per hour.

Use of These Data

Data of any one level may be statistically or clinically used at a lower, but not higher level. For example, everyone's age may be known precisely (i.e., ratio data), but when the data are described it is possible to categorize age as 0 to 15, 16 to 30, 31 to 45, 46 to 60, and 61 to 75 (interval data), or 15 to 44, 45 to 65, and above 65 (ordinal data), or as adult and children (nominal data). Different types of statistical tests applied to each of these levels are discussed in statistical textbooks. A list of desirable characteristics of any test is presented in Table 22.3, and a figurative description of using tests to measure either static or dynamic states is shown in Fig. 22.1.

Combining Numbers to Create a Relationship

Any two numbers (e.g., A and B) may be compared in at least eight different ways. Each of these ways

TABLE 22.3 *Desirable characteristics of scales, tests, and measures*

1. Easy to administer
2. Rapid to administer
3. Little or no training necessary to administer
4. Easy to interpret
5. Rapid to interpret
6. Little or no training necessary to interpret
7. Sensitive to changes elicited by medicines of interest
8. Insensitive to efforts brought about by treatments that might interfere with the test
9. Low rate of false-positive responses
10. Low rate of false-negative responses
11. May be used multiple times without a training effect
12. Results are reproducible
13. Results are valid
14. Interpretation is correlated with other clinical parameters of interest

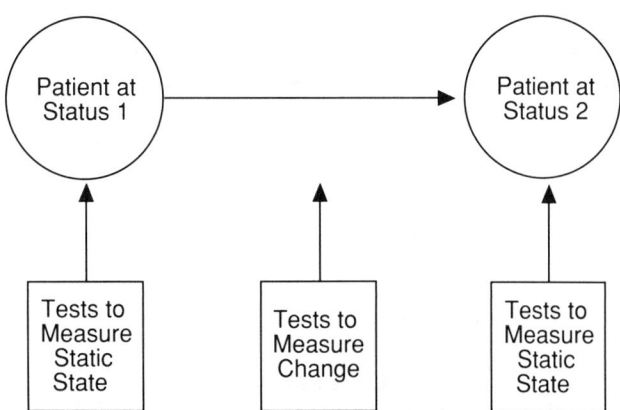

FIG. 22.1 Differences between tests that measure a patient's static or dynamic state. Tests may also measure patients at two or more static states to demonstrate (i.e., measure) change. Some types of states are not sensitive to changes caused by medicines (e.g., intelligence quotient).

may be illustrated or presented using a wide variety of formats (Table 22.4).

CLINICAL SCALES, VISUAL ANALOG SCALES, PATIENT DIARIES, AND DRAWINGS

Clinical Scales

Clinical scales may be developed if no satisfactory efficacy measures exist. Scales may be established to describe subjective or semiobjective parameters in a fixed number of categories (usually from three to seven). The most common type of scale is a variation of the scale describing a parameter or question for which the response is *normal* or *not present* (score = 0), *mild* (score = 1), *moderate* (score = 2), *severe*

TABLE 22.4 *Methods of establishing relationships between two numbers[a]*

1.	$\dfrac{A}{B}$	Ratio
2.	$\dfrac{B}{A}$	Ratio
3.	A minus B	Incremental change
4.	B minus A	Incremental change
5.	$\dfrac{A-B}{B}$	Proportionate change
6.	$\dfrac{B-A}{A}$	Proportionate change
7.	$\dfrac{A-B}{B} \times 100$	Percent change
8.	$\dfrac{B-A}{A} \times 100$	Percent change

[a] The reference point to be used for a comparison may be obtained from baseline, placebo, or an old value.

(score = 3), or *extremely severe* (score = 4). Other variations are shown in Table 22.1. The individual scores from a number of separate categories are often added to derive a total composite score. One of the most important clinical scales used to measure efficacy is the clinical global impressions (CGI) scale. This scale provides a measure of the overall improvement or deterioration of a patient's condition and is completed by the investigator or the patient. It may also be used to evaluate safety and is described in more detail in the following chapter. Discussions on developing scales are found in Jaeschke and Guyatt, 1990, and Hulley and Cummings, 1988.

Visual Analog Scales

Another approach to the issue of developing efficacy measures when satisfactory ones do not exist is to develop a visual analog scale. Visual analog scales have been widely used in recent years to provide quantitative measures of subjective ratings. They are frequently used to measure the intensity of pain or quality of the patient's mood at a particular time. These scales may also be used to document changes over time when they are used on multiple occasions. Specific examples of parameters measured with visual analog scales include stress, anxiety, itch, hunger, alertness, and depression. Subjective ratings of clinical improvements (or deterioration) or the value of a specified treatment may also be measured with a visual analog scale.

Visual analog scales may be created to have patients evaluate a parameter between two fixed points that may be arbitrarily defined (e.g., 0–10, 1–100, "not at all"–"extremely") along a straight line with or without gradations or on a round dial (with or without gradation). A few examples are illustrated in Fig. 22.2. Other types of visual analog scales are illustrated in *Presentation of Clinical Data* (Spilker and Schoenfelder, 1990). It is preferable to use a validated visual analog scale in a medicine trial unless the trial is specifically designed to evaluate the validity of the scale. Certain parameters (e.g., pain) have been shown to be reliably measured with these scales. Sriwatanakul et al. (1983) evaluated five different visual analog scales to measure pain and observed that graded linear horizontal scales were more reliable and also were preferred by more patients than were the other scales they tested. In addition, they concluded that the visual analog scales yielded more accurate and more sensitive information on pain intensity than did descriptive pain scales.

Choosing Anchor Terms

In deciding on the types of terms or words to use as anchors at each end of the visual analog scale it is

1.

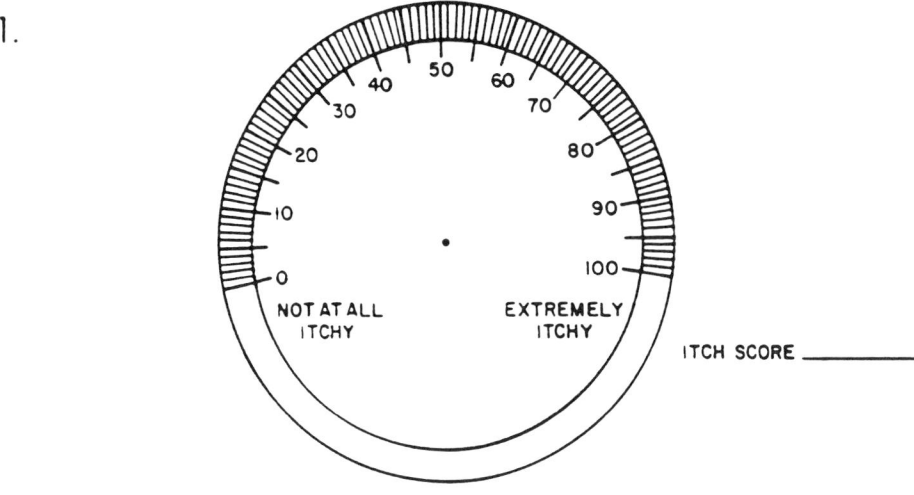

2.

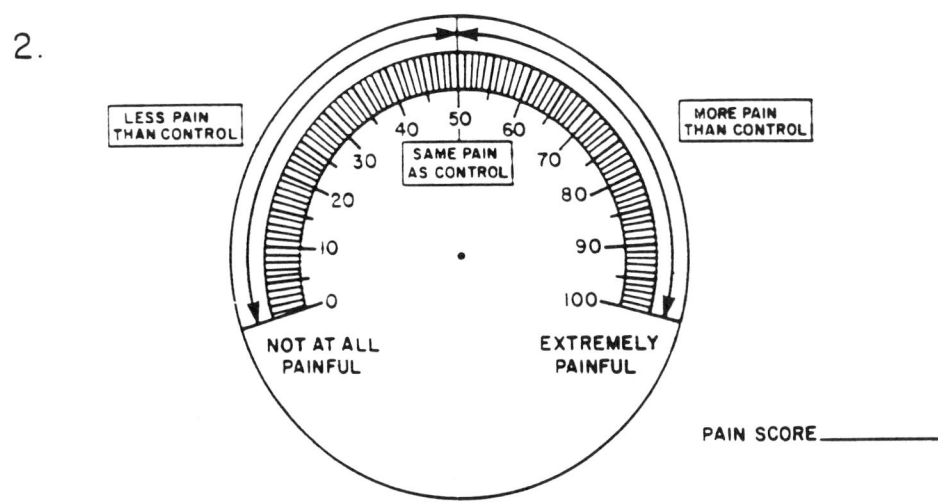

3.

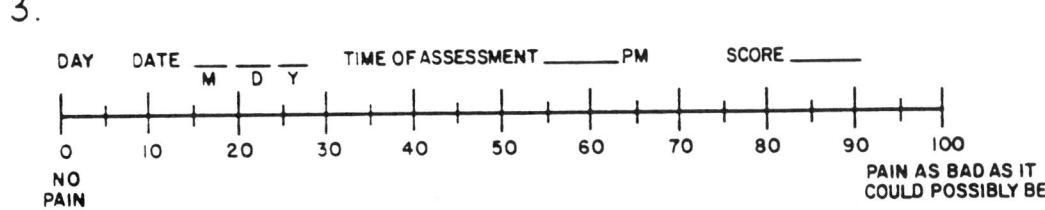

FIG. 22.2 Examples of visual analog scales.

necessary to decide between emotive terms (e.g., *very annoying*), sensory terms (e.g., *difficult to swallow, hard to speak*), and quantitative terms (e.g., *much better, no reduction*). Specific words or terms may not apply to all patients. It is generally desirable to use scales so that most patients initially cluster at one end and can demonstrate great change during a clinical trial. If one end of a scale says *"the worst pain I've ever experienced"* and the other end says *"absolutely no pain,"* most chronic pain patients will tend to be in the middle of the scale and may not demonstrate as

much change as they would on a scale stating *"severe pain"* at one end and *"almost no pain"* at the other.

Patient Diaries

Another potential source of efficacy data in certain clinical trials is patient diaries. Data obtained from patient diaries provide the most important efficacy data in outpatient evaluations of antidiarrheal medicines (stool number and consistency) and antiepileptic medicines (number and type of seizure occurrences). If diaries are used by patients, then the diaries should be supplied by the investigator or sponsor to ensure that each patient addresses similar questions and completes them in a similar manner. Instructions for using diaries should be reviewed with patients and, ideally, should be printed in the diary itself.

Patient diaries are reasonable to consider if patients collect data at least every other day (or daily) so that they do not forget to complete the diary. Patients could be instructed to keep the diary next to their bed or in their kitchen. Data from the diary must also be collected by the investigator on a relatively frequent basis (e.g., weekly, biweekly). The more important and objective the data collected (e.g., a migraine attack, an epileptic seizure), the more likely it is that patients will record data accurately. The more subjective the data (e.g., intensity of leg pain at night) the less accurate the results will probably be. A checklist may be presented for the patient to mark. This usually facilitates its completion by the patients, as well as data processing and analysis. Electronic diaries using small computers have also been developed and used (Dahlström and Eckernas, 1991).

Drawings

Drawings or figures may be utilized as a technique to collect data on efficacy, safety, or medical history. Patients may be requested to either fill in drawings, prepare drawings, or write something themselves. An example of the fill-in approach is the *McGill Pain Questionnaire,* in which patients are asked to indicate on both front and back drawings of a person exactly where their pain is located (Melzack, 1975). See figures in Chapter 36. Serial drawings provide data on the effects of their therapy or course of disease. Many visual and ophthalmological tests involve the patient interpreting a visual design. An example in which patients are asked to provide written material is in Parkinson's disease, in which samples of the patient's handwriting over time are often used as one indicator for evaluating therapy. Psychiatric evaluations of a patient's psychological state are sometimes based on interpretations of drawings prepared by the patient.

INDEXES OF EFFICACY

An index could be developed for each patient when evaluating a disease for which great variability in clinical signs and symptoms exists between patients. For example, it is difficult to enroll sufficient numbers of patients with scleroderma in a clinical trial when focusing on a single symptom, but if an index is used then many more patients may be enrolled.

Four types of efficacy indexes may be created. These are indexes for (1) individual patients, (2) individual clinical trials, (3) individual medicines, and (4) for a specified disease.

Individual Patients

Patients with multisystem diseases (e.g., systemic lupus erythematosus, scleroderma, irritable bowel syndrome, severe debilitation) may have their own spectrum of clinical signs and symptoms. If an index score can be created for each patient in a clinical trial, it should make assessment more appropriate and accurate. One means to do this is for the patient, with or without the physician's assistance, to identify and rate on a list the severity and importance of each symptom and sign associated with the disease. This is done prior to the start of a clinical trial. A fixed number of the most important signs and symptoms for each patient could be chosen and combined to create an index. Alternatively, all symptoms that are rated at a prespecified severity and frequency could be combined to create the index. The index is then used during the clinical trial to evaluate treatment.

It is possible that a relative weighting of each symptom rated during the clinical trial could also be developed. The symptoms could either be weighted according to their importance to the patient or merely averaged to create a single overall index for each patient. The weighting of the most important symptoms should be done by the patients, who would thus incorporate their own knowledge of their disease into the assessment of treatment in a clinical trial. A clinical trial of highly dissimilar patients with a similar type of problem (e.g., physical debility resulting from trauma) could therefore yield highly meaningful data using individual scales and overall indexes on a per patient basis.

Individual Clinical Trials

Academic investigators may wish to create a special index for a single clinical trial, depending on the nature of their patient population. On the other hand, this index would not have been validated and results might not be widely accepted. Pharmaceutical companies and government sponsors are less likely to create an efficacy index for a single clinical trial, but that option does exist.

Individual Medicines

The advantage of creating a single efficacy index for all Phase II and III clinical trials conducted with a single medicine is that the data will be more convincing to regulatory authorities and practicing physicians. Any question of improperly creating or using an index would be removed, particularly if the rationale for creating the index is sound and the index is composed of parameters known to be relevant and important for measuring the disease. For example, a medicine that has a small or moderate effect on each of the major parameters usually measured in patients with rheumatoid arthritis (e.g., morning stiffness, ring size, range of motion), might be best evaluated against other standard medicines and placebo using a composite index of all major parameters. This composite index could be weighted or unweighted but should be used in all clinical trials with the new medicine.

Index for a Disease

All of the above considerations should be included when evaluating the possibility of proposing, validating, and using an index for a particular disease.

CHOOSING EFFICACY PARAMETERS TO MEASURE

Types of Endpoints that May Be Evaluated

In choosing efficacy parameters to evaluate in a clinical program it is especially beneficial if the parameters chosen can demonstrate endpoints related to:

1. Objective measurements that are validated and accepted to represent appropriate criteria of efficacy. Some subjective measurements may also be relevant to include as parameters.
2. Reduced progression or even reversal of the disease process (e.g., reduction of the number, area, or severity of lesions; reduction of the number, severity, or other manifestations of disease episodes; increased number of cured lesions; decreased duration of disease).
3. Improved quality of life. This aspect is becoming increasingly important to measure. Both quantitative and nonquantitative parameters are available to evaluate this endpoint. Some are more objective (e.g., number of days worked in a given period), while others are more subjective. It is possible to use standard questionnaires for some diseases being studied, standard measures of daily living and functioning interviews, or even just a few questions that assess those aspects that are of primary importance to the patient.
4. Reduced mortality in those trials in which this parameter has relevance.
5. Clinical global impression of both the physician and patient.
6. Reduced number or severity of risk factors.

7. Improved symptomatology of the patient.
8. Biochemical measures that assess the underlying state of the disease.
9. Direct visualization and measure of the lesion (e.g., in ulcer disease, in arterial blockage).

Identifying the Best Parameter(s) to Measure

To identify the parameters that are best able to measure these attributes it may be desirable to convene a panel of experts and/or general practitioners. Debating the pros and cons of available parameters will indicate:

1. The parameters that are most important for influencing physicians' decisions to switch to a new medicine therapy. How do the physicians rank these in importance?
2. The combination of parameters that is most practical and makes the most sense to measure in a trial.
3. The hard objective (i.e., quantitative) parameters that provide less information than soft-objective or subjective parameters. For example, the erythrocyte sedimentation rate is a precisely quantitated laboratory value measured in many trials conducted in arthritis patients, although it is subject to daily variation within a single patient. It provides less information on patient response than does the "softer" measure of morning stiffness.
4. How much of a change in the parameters would be clinically significant. Also, how much of a change in the parameters would be sufficient for these physicians to switch therapy in some (or most) of their patients?

Time to Observe Effects

Some parameters require a long period to illustrate changes (e.g., wall thickness in congestive heart failure). One must examine more rapidly changing parameters in shorter-term trials. Parameters for acute trials must be able to demonstrate effects of the trial within the time period studied. Other types of parameters are listed in Chapter 82.

Multiple Approaches

Utilizing multiple approaches usually provides the most convincing data of a medicine's efficacy, assuming that the most accepted parameters of efficacy are included. Including parameters at different levels of organization (e.g., biochemical, pathological, pharmacological, physiological, symptomatic, objective clinical), assists the process of extrapolating data to other patients. The relative importance of the various parameters should be established prior to the trial and indicated in the protocol. In some situations, what is measured is not the true endpoint of the medicine.

Presenting Data

In some diseases the major efficacy parameter to measure is clear. For example, in patients with essential hypertension, blood pressure is measured. However, even in this disease with an objective endpoint there are multiple means of presenting the data (e.g., initial fall of blood pressure over X weeks, maintained blood pressure loss for Y months, maintained normal pressure for Z months). The choice of one of these or other formats for presenting data depends on the trial's objectives and should be determined, if possible, prior to the trial. For postmyocardial infarction patients who are to be treated with a medicine to prevent reinfarction or sudden death the choice of parameters to measure is much more complex. One may measure the number of deaths at one year, ventricular function either invasively with dyes or noninvasively, clinical endpoints relating to quality of life, or others. *Presentation of Clinical Data,* (Spilker and Schoenfelder, 1990) illustrates many methods useful for data presentation.

ESTABLISHING EFFICACY OF A NEW MEDICINE

To demonstrate that a new medicine (medicine A) has improved efficacy over standard medicine therapy used to treat a disease, several areas may be explored. Clear-cut advantages of medicine A over available medicines could be in terms of (1) time to onset of effect, (2) magnitude of effect, or (3) duration of effect. There are also other means by which greater efficacy may be objectively or subjectively demonstrated. A few of these include: (1) study of different and more relevant parameters; (2) reduction in the number, severity, or duration of subsequent episodes of the disease; (3) improved quality of life; and (4) a decreased rate of relapse after therapy is discontinued.

Indirect Contributors to a Medicine's Efficacy

There are numerous aspects of the profile of a new medicine that may indirectly contribute to its efficacy but are not efficacy measures per se. Examples of this would be any characteristic of the medicine that leads to increased patient compliance (e.g., lower cost, better taste, decreased number of tablets per dose, decreased number of doses per day).

It is important to evaluate efficacy data for a new medicine to assess critically whether or not efficacy has been demonstrated and full-scale medicine development should continue or be initiated. This usually occurs sometime during Phase II. The methods used to establish efficacy must be the most relevant ones or a mistaken conclusion may be drawn. If individual patient histories are used there must be adequate controls. If measurements are compared with baseline (or other approaches used) then statisticians must confirm that the conclusions reached are appropriate. If different forms of the medicine are being developed then a different risk-to-benefit assessment must be made for each.

Dose–Response Relationships

In interpreting data when two medicines are being compared to determine which has the greater efficacy, the data may be relatively clear-cut, but still yield a mistaken view. For example, dose–response curves are often expressed using percent values of the effect measured (to 100%) on the ordinate. Two medicines will each reach 100% regardless of the response they cause. Figure 22.3 shows that medicine A is less potent than medicine B, but its effect (i.e., activity) is greater. In some cases a misleading interpretation of clinical efficacy is obtained, when information on only relative potency is presented without information on relative activity. A recent book of a conference's proceedings on dose-response relationships discusses numerous topics of importance (Lasagna et al., 1989).

Relapse Rates

The measurement of relapse rates is especially relevant for medicines that are not intended to be used permanently. Relapse rates are also relevant for measuring effects of medicines in diseases marked by discrete episodes. One therapeutic area in which relapse rates have been evaluated is in peptic ulcer disease. It is important to note that objective observations through endoscopes and not patient symptoms were used as a clinical endpoint in establishing whether a patient had relapsed. Endoscopic examinations were scheduled to occur at periodic times after the treatment was discontinued. The basic trial design used in these evaluations is the initial administration of medicines that heal their ulcers to ulcer patients. A healing rate (percent of patients whose ulcers heal within a certain time) is then determined. At that point, this treatment is discontinued and the recurrence rate of endoscopically proven ulcers is determined over a fixed time interval (Fig. 22.4).

This evaluation of both ulcer healing and recurrence

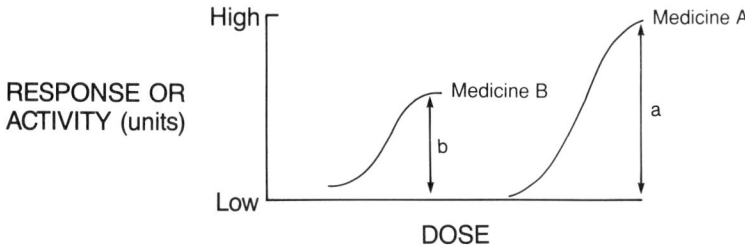

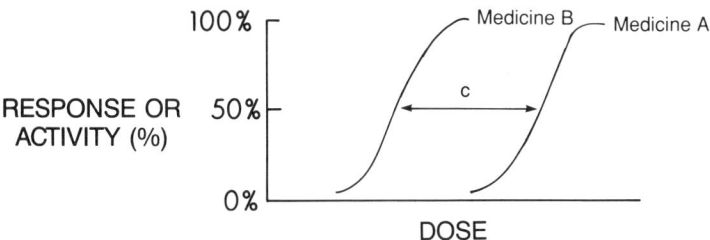

FIG. 22.3 Measuring activity and potency of medicines through use of dose–response curves. In the **upper graph** the activity of each medicine is noted by the *vertical arrow*. In the **lower graph** the comparative potency is shown by the *horizontal arrow*, such that at 50% response medicine B is more potent than medicine A by the magnitude c.

yields several interesting possibilities. The medicine with the highest rate of cure may also have a high rate of ulcer recurrence. Thus, the percent of patients who can be successfully treated for a given period and then remain disease free may be greater for a medicine with a smaller initial cure rate. If the safety and pharmacokinetic profiles of medicines A and B are identical, then the "most effective" medicine would be medicine B for most patients.

A relevant comparison is to subtract the number of patients who relapsed from the number of patients cured to determine the number of patients with long-term cures, presumably resulting from the initial treatment. The numbers can be converted to percent of initial patients treated and two or more medicines may be compared. This comparison can become highly complex if retreatment of patients with these medicines yields different types of curves or if the safety or pharmacokinetic profiles of the medicines differ to a degree that is clinically important.

OTHER FACTORS RELATING TO EFFICACY

Practical Pointers

Many efficacy measures yield less objective data than one would ideally like to obtain. Subjective measures often depend on clinical evaluation or examination of the patient or on the investigator's interpretation of the patient's statements. Under these circumstances, it is generally desirable to have the same investigator perform the nonobjective measures throughout the clinical trial.

It is also advisable for certain tests to be performed at the same time of day throughout the clinical trial. Whenever possible, key efficacy parameters should be measured at the times of both peak and trough blood levels. Most investigators are aware that cortisol levels (and certain other hormones) vary during the day and that the time of their collection must be specified and controlled. Many nonobjective or objective tests also vary or tend to vary during the day, sometimes in a predictable manner (e.g., morning stiffness in arthritis patients), and these tests should be performed at the same time(s) of day throughout the trial.

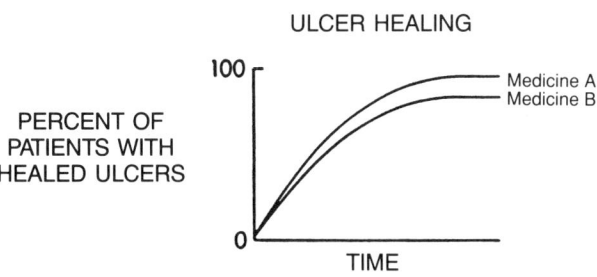

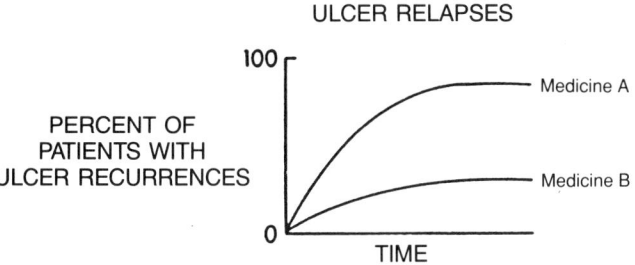

FIG. 22.4 Hypothetical rates of ulcer healing for two medicines **(upper graph)** and recurrence of disease (i.e., relapses) after medicine treatment is discontinued for the same two medicines **(lower graph)**.

Factors Affecting Efficacy

The results of efficacy (or other) tests can be affected on occasion by extraneous factors that may easily be controlled. Examples include the physical position a patient is placed in for taking a test, having the patient relax (or exercise) for a given period of time prior to starting a test, having patients empty their bladders before a lengthy test, starting a test just prior or subsequent to mealtime, and conducting a test at various times of day during the course of the clinical trial. Many of these factors may be outlined or discussed in instructions that the investigator and/or patient follows. Efficacy (and safety) tests should not be required more often during a clinical trial than necessary (and realistic) to accomplish the trial objectives. The schedule should be arranged to cause the minimum hardship or harassment to the patient and investigator.

Interrater Checks

It is sometimes relevant to enumerate the different individuals in the protocol who are permitted to perform certain tests for either one or for all patients. The qualifications of individuals conducting efficacy (or safety) tests in terms of degrees, certification, or training may be relevant to specify. Interrater reliability may be measured prior to the clinical trial to confirm the validity of having more than one individual conduct certain tests in which individual technique, bias, or experience may be a factor.

Quality of Life

The quality of life is an important parameter to consider in some clinical trials. The relative values of the use of objective and/or subjective criteria are discussed by von Kerekjarto (1982). This topic is presented in detail in Chapters 52 and 97.

An Endpoint Is not an Endpoint Is not an Endpoint: Evolution of an Endpoint

Blood pressure is a stable endpoint that has been measured for decades in clinical trials. Or is this not true? Clearly, this first sentence has to be qualified. Blood pressure was measured in the 1940s and 1950s with patients usually in the seated *or* lying position. In the 1960s and 1970s it became important not only to specify the position of the patient, but to obtain recordings with the patient in seated, lying, and erect positions. It also became important to repeat the measurements on three separate occasions before the diagnosis of hypertension was applied and treatment with medicines initiated.

Toward the mid- to late-1980s it became evident that single measurements (like snapshots) were insufficient to judge a medicine's overall effect on the patient's hypertension throughout the day and night. Multiple measurements (like a motion picture) were necessary to assess nighttime and daytime effects fully, particularly those values taken when the patient was outside the clinic where measurements were traditionally made. Blood pressure measurements in patients while they are ambulatory, or even exercising, have sometimes been added to the requirements for a complete assessment of the mild or moderately hypertensive patient (White, 1989).

Another aspect of the evolution of endpoints relates to the equipment used to obtain the measurements. Blood pressure instruments have gone through a relatively rapid stage of development over the last decade. These developments have aided the evolution of the parameter, as described above, by making it possible to obtain 24-hour continuous measurements in a relatively unobtrusive manner.

Comparable discussions could be made for electrocardiograms and for numerous laboratory tests (e.g., for cholesterol). Telemetry techniques, although available for over 20 years, are now being used more widely in clinical trials and medicine.

CHAPTER 23

Identifying and Choosing Safety Parameters

OVERALL APPROACH TO ASSESSING SAFETY

Choosing Safety Parameters

Choosing the appropriate safety parameters for a clinical trial depends on a number of factors. A selected list of examinations and tests commonly used to assess the safety of medicines is given in Table 23.1. The majority of these tests will not be conducted in most medicine trials. An assessment of the quantity and quality of prior experience and previous data obtained with the medicine is essential to enable one to decide which specific safety tests to incorporate in a medicine trial. The choice of safety parameters requires both data in areas where there are indications of potential (or actual) safety problems to monitor and also additional experience and data with a new medicine. Until a sufficient body of safety data has accumulated, more laboratory parameters of safety are generally included than will be needed at a later date. The nature of the clinical trial and efficacy tests used may dictate that certain safety parameters should or should not be included (e.g., in testing a new anticancer medicine, it may be necessary to perform a bone marrow biopsy and smear to confirm the lack of toxicity, and in assessing an agent in anesthetized patients, the appropriate tests to ensure the patient's safety while under anesthesia must be performed). If, on the basis of preclinical pharmacological or toxicological data, any toxicity is either anticipated or considered possible, then

TABLE 23.1 *Selected list of examinations and tests used to evaluate safety*

A. Clinical examinations
   1. Physical
   2. Vital signs (usually considered as part of the physical examination)
   3. Height and weight (state of dress is usually specified, e.g., in socks)
   4. Neurological or other specialized clinical examinations
B. Clinical laboratory examinations
   1. Hematology (see Table 23.2)
   2. Clinical chemistry (see Table 23.2)
   3. Urinalysis (see Table 23.2)
   4. Virology (viral cultures or viral serology)
   5. Immunology or immunochemistry (e.g., immunoglobins, complement)
   6. Serology (e.g., VDRL)
   7. Microbiology (including bacteriology and mycology)
   8. Parasitology (e.g., stool for ova and protozoa)
   9. Pulmonary function tests (e.g., arterial blood gas)
   10. Other biological tests (e.g., endocrine, toxicology screen)
   11. Stool for occult blood (specify hemoccult or guaiac method)
   12. Skin tests for immunologic competence[a]
   13. Medicine screen (usually in urine) for detection of illegal or non-protocol-approved medicines
   14. Bone marrow examination
   15. Gonadal function (e.g., sperm count, sperm motility)
   16. Genetics studies (e.g., evaluate chromosomal integrity)
   17. Stool analysis using in vivo dialysis[b]
C. Probe for adverse reactions
D. Psychological and psychiatric tests and examinations
   1. Psychometric and performance examinations[c]
   2. Behavioral rating scales[d]
   3. Dependence liability
E. Examinations requiring specialized equipment (selected examples)
   1. Audiometry
   2. Electrocardiogram (ECG)
   3. Electroencephalogram (EEG)
   4. Electromyography (EMG)
   5. Stress test
   6. Endoscopy
   7. Computed tomography (CT) scans
   8. Ophthalmological examination[e]
   9. Ultrasound
   10. X-rays
   11. Others

[a] Examples are *Candida albicans*, tricophyton, and dinitrochlorobenzene.
[b] Wrong et al. (1965).
[c] See Table 23.8.
[d] See Tables 23.6 and 23.7.
[e] See Table 23.4.

an attempt should be made to evaluate patients for those possible problems. The anticipated use(s) of a medicine will also influence which safety parameters are chosen for evaluation (e.g., ophthalmological tests would be included for medicines intended for ocular use).

Measuring Safety Parameters

After specific safety parameters are chosen, it is necessary to determine how thorough an evaluation of each parameter should be conducted. It is also possible that different types of examinations would be suitable at different points of a clinical trial. For example, a physical examination may be specified to include more or fewer measurements or facets, and a complete examination may not be necessary or even suitable during some periods of the clinical trial.

Vital signs may be measured with the patient in a supine, seated, and/or erect position. Both supine and erect positions are usually used if orthostatic changes are being evaluated. The need for such data will depend on the situation, but the position of the patient for this examination, as well as the period of time desired for stabilization, should be noted in the protocol.

Parameters that Measure either Safety or Efficacy

Certain parameters may be viewed as being either safety or efficacy parameters. The electroencephalogram (EEG) is an example, although there is some controversy as to its true adequacy as an efficacy parameter. Blood pressure is another. Nonetheless, it is important to establish clearly in the protocol whether each parameter is being incorporated in the protocol for safety or efficacy evaluations (or possibly both). Almost any safety parameter can be used for measuring efficacy.

Appropriateness of Each Parameter for the Clinical Trial and Patient

There are four categories of appropriateness of safety tests used in clinical trials:

1. *Appropriate for patients, but not necessary for the clinical trial.* All of these tests should be included in the clinical trial. They indirectly benefit the trial because they may be monitored for progress or trends or they may simply ensure that patients are receiving appropriate care.
2. *Appropriate for the clinical trial, but not necessary for the patients.* These tests should be included in the clinical trial if they do not place the patient at unacceptable risk or discomfort. If any tests are deemed unethical in the context of the trial and the patients enrolled, then they should be excluded.
3. *Appropriate for both patients and the clinical trial.* All of these tests should be included in the clinical trial.
4. *Appropriate for neither patients nor the clinical trial.* All of these tests should be identified and excluded from the clinical trial.

LABORATORY EXAMINATIONS

Precautions

Clinical laboratory parameters must be specified individually in the protocol. Abbreviations such as "SMA-6" or "SMA-12" are rarely acceptable (unless each component is specified), since different laboratories include different tests in their "SMA-6" (or "SMA-12") battery, and using these abbreviations without an explanation will adversely affect the clarity of the protocol and possibly lead to the collection of data on different parameters at different sites. Other precautions to consider prior to initiating a clinical trial are to decide if (1) severely abnormal results should be routinely confirmed, (2) samples should be divided and sent to two separate laboratories when specified abnormalities are determined, (3) additional tests should be routinely requested if specified abnormalities are observed, (4) medical consultants should examine patients whenever severe abnormalities are observed, and (5) aliquots of known concentrations of standard medicines should be sent to laboratories for confirmatory measurements and interlaboratory evaluation.

Summary of Tests

Common dermatological tests are shown in Table 23.5; ophthalmological tests are shown in Table 23.4. Note that any of these tests could be utilized as measures of efficacy if they addressed the clinical trial objectives. Selected pointers are given in Table 23.3. Specific tests that may be used in hematology, clinical chemistry, and urinalysis are shown in Table 23.2, adult and pediatric behavioral rating scales in Tables 23.6 and 23.7, and psychometric and performance tests in Table 23.8.

TABLE 23.2 *Hematology, clinical chemistry, and urinalysis parameters usually evaluated during the development of a new medicine*

A. Hematology
1. Red blood cell (RBC) count
2. Hemoglobin
3. Hematocrit
4. White blood cell (WBC) count and differential
5. Platelet estimate or platelet count
6. Red blood cell indices (MCV, MCH, MCHC)[a]
7. Prothrombin (PT), partial thromboplastin time (PTT)
8. Reticulocytes
9. Fibrinogen
10. Any additional tests suggested by previous data

B. Clinical chemistry
1. Albumin
2. Albumin/globulin ratio
3. Alkaline phosphatase (and/or its isoenzymes)
4. Amylase
5. Bilirubin, total and direct
6. Bicarbonate (carbon dioxide)
7. BUN/creatinine ratio
8. Calcium
9. Chloride
10. Cholesterol (and/or a lipid panel)
11. Creatinine
12. Creatine phosphokinase (CPK)
13. γ-Glutamyl transferase (GGT)
14. Globulin
15. Glucose, nonfasting or fasting
16. Glucose-6-phosphate dehydrogenase (G6PD)
17. Glutamate oxalacetic transaminase (SGOT), now frequently referred to as aspartate aminotransferase (AST)
18. Glutamate pyruvate transaminase (SGPT), now frequently referred to as alanine aminotransferase (ALT)
19. Iron (and/or other related parameters such as ferritin, total iron binding capacity)
20. Lactic acid dehydrogenase, total (LDH, and/or its isoenzymes)

21. Inorganic phosphorus
22. Potassium
23. Sodium
24. Total iron binding capacity (TIBC)
25. Total protein
26. Triglycerides
27. Urea nitrogen (BUN)
28. Uric acid

C. Hormones and/or other chemical substances in blood

D. Urinalysis[b]
1. Appearance and color
2. Specific gravity
3. Acetone
4. Protein
5. Glucose
6. pH
7. Bile
8. Urobilinogen
9. Occult blood
10. Microscopic evaluation of sediment
   a. Red blood cells (number per high-power field)
   b. White blood cells (number per high-power field)
   c. Casts (describe and give number per high- or low-power field)
   d. Crystals (describe and give number per high-power field)
   e. Bacteria (generally rated as few, many, or loaded)
   f. Epithelial cells (number per low-power field)

E. Other urine tests sometimes evaluated
1. Creatinine (actual values are preferable to estimated values)
2. Electrolytes (usually sodium, potassium, and chloride)
3. Protein
4. Specific hormones or chemicals
5. Twenty-four-hour collections for specific evaluations

[a] MCH, mean corpuscular hemoglobin = hemoglobin divided by RBC count; MCHC, mean corpuscular hemoglobin concentration = hemoglobin divided by hematocrit; MCV, mean corpuscular volume = hematocrit divided by RCB count.

[b] Sample codes used to quantify several parameters in the urinalysis are the following. Protein, glucose, ketones, bilirubin: 0, none or negative; 0.5, trace or positive (qualitative); 1, + or 1+; 2, + + or 2+; 3, + + + or 3+; 4, + + + + or 4+. Epithelial cells, crystal, WBC, RBC, casts: 0, none or negative; 0.5, rare, occasional, few present, trace (1–5); 1, several, mild (6–10); 2, moderate (11–25); 3, many, much (26–50); 4, loaded, severe (>50). Bacteria: 0, none or negative; 0.5, rare, trace, occasional, few, several (1–10); 1, mild (11–50); 2, moderate (51–75); 3, many, numerous (76–100); 4, loaded, severe (>100).

TABLE 23.3 *Selected pointers relating to laboratory data*

1. Ask the laboratory to maintain assayed samples that are of particular importance; if questions arise as to the accuracy of results it might be possible to retest the original samples.
2. If laboratory problems are anticipated, divide the initial (and subsequent) samples and send them to two different laboratories, or to the same laboratory at two different times
3. If laboratory samples for a complete blood count are going to remain unexamined for a long period of time (e.g., sample obtained on Sunday), prepare a fresh smear so that a comparison may be made with one made 24 or more hours later, because abnormalities may occur when a sample lies around even when it is kept at an appropriate temperature

Choosing Laboratory Tests

There is no standardized series of laboratory parameters that are evaluated in all clinical trials, nor is there one standard that is applied to medicines in Phases I, II, or III. There are, however, loose standards and general guidelines for laboratory tests that are performed at each stage of clinical development.

Tests in Phase I

In Phase I clinical trials, there is the greatest need to obtain a wide variety of laboratory evaluations as part of developing the safety profile on a new medicine. This entails an evaluation of the basic hematology, clinical chemistry, and urinalysis parameters (Table 23.2). There will never be 100% agreement among investigators and/or clinical scientists as to which specific tests constitute a "basic" workup.

Tests in Phases II and III

The total number of normal laboratory values that is sufficient to collect on a new medicine to demonstrate safety is impossible to specify. Numerous factors must be considered, such as the toxicological profile on other safety parameters and the expected use of the medicine in patients. It is important to determine if a medicine is to be used topically or parenterally, whether it is to be used in generally healthy patients or in seriously ill patients, whether it is a "me-too" medicine or a totally novel medicine chemically, and whether it will be life saving or provide a minimal therapeutic effect. The number of laboratory tests performed usually decreases as an investigational medicine moves closer to the market, but one or more tests may be added to the list in Table 23.2 and studied in great detail.

Tests in Medical Practice

The ordering of laboratory tests in medical practice (as opposed to Phases I to II clinical trials) is extremely inefficient and often irrational (Wong and Lincoln, 1983). This suggests the need in some clinical situations to develop logical protocols and algorithms for physicians to follow in ordering tests, particularly when the most appropriate tests are changing (e.g., in hepatitis), in therapeutic areas in which an excessive number of tests are often ordered (e.g., thyroid tests), or when hospitals have developed their own approaches to diagnosis (e.g., use of cardiac isoenzymes in diagnosing a myocardial infarction). This approach has been adopted over the last two decades for patients admitted to hospitals with certain diagnoses, such as Rule Out Myocardial Infarction, Transient Ischemic Attacks, or Stroke.

Less Commonly Used Methods

Evaluations of virtually any biological fluid, tissue, or sense (taste, smell, hearing, sight, and touch) can be conducted to ascertain the safety of a medicine. Captopril has been reported to affect taste in some patients (Coulter, 1988), and there are many other examples involving medicine-induced effects on one of the five senses. The choice of tests will depend on experiences with the medicine and suspicions about possible problems. Hair analysis is a relevant test to detect the qualitative presence of certain toxic metals in individuals occupationally or otherwise exposed to heavy metals (Obrusnik, 1986; Kono et al., 1990). Medicines may also be reviewed for teratogenic potential, drug dependence, and carcinogenicity (Folb, 1980).

Identifying the Most Important Laboratory Analytes to Monitor in a Clinical Trial

A choice often must be made among the numerous laboratory analytes that could be measured in a clinical trial. This choice is based on (1) past experience with the treatment(s) being evaluated, (2) therapeutic area, (3) cost of the tests, (4) convenience of obtaining data, (5) resources available, (6) state-of-the-art concepts of the data's importance, and (7) the ability of data obtained to convince both regulators and medical practitioners. To arrive at a decision, given these and other factors, may be difficult. Bull et al. (1986) described a method called consensus analysis that can identify which tests respond most to disease activity. Their method was applied to rheumatoid arthritis, but could be applied to other diseases that do not have a specific etiological cause or measurable pathophysiological process.

Uses of Specific Laboratory Tests to Discover, Confirm, and/or Exclude a Disease

Some tests can confirm the diagnosis of a disease (e.g., tissue histology from bronchoscopic biopsy to confirm lung cancer), but cannot be used to exclude the disease or to discover the disease in routine screening. Other tests can be used both to confirm and to exclude the diagnosis of a disease (e.g., glucose tolerance test for diabetes mellitus), but are too inconvenient to be used to discover the disease in routine screening. The uses of each laboratory test to discover, confirm, or exclude a disease must be known before a test is simply added to a clinical trial protocol. This ensures that the test is appropriate in the context of the clinical trial or other purpose for which it is being used.

Hematology

A basis hematology evaluation usually includes determination of hemoglobin, hematocrit, red blood cell (RBC) count, white blood cell (WBC) count, RBC indices [mean corpuscular hemoglobin (MCH), mean corpuscular hemoglobin concentration (MCHC), and mean corpuscular volume (MCV)], and platelets. Either a platelet estimate or platelet count may be obtained. The former measurement is less expensive and usually suffices to demonstrate a lack of medicine effect unless there is a previous indication or current expectation of a possible effect on platelets. The white blood cell differential count is usually not required as part of a basic hematological workup unless a specific parameter of the differential count is being evaluated. Nonetheless, a white blood cell differential count is often obtained in Phase I and generally provides useful information. Other hematological parameters (some of which are indicated in Table 23.2) are not usually obtained unless there is a specific reason to do so. As experience with medicine develops, there is a progressively diminishing need for monitoring the parameters shown to be normal.

Clinical Chemistry

A measurement of renal function (creatinine and/or BUN) is an "essential" test for most clinical studies, as is the inclusion of at least one liver function test (SGOT, SGPT, LDH, CPK, GGT, and/or alkaline phosphatase). The specific tests chosen to be included in a study are somewhat dependent on both the in-

vestigator's and/or clinical scientist's experiences and the characteristics of the medicine. Other important parameters to measure include serum electrolytes and at least some of the tests listed in Table 23.2.

Medicine Levels in Plasma

Medicine levels may also be measured in a clinical trial. Medicine levels are usually part of a pharmacokinetic analysis but also provide important safety data. This information would be particularly relevant in cases of suspected or actual medicine overdosage, medicine interactions, to correlate medicine levels with toxic events, or in other situations (see Chapter 16). It must be clarified whether free levels of the medicine or the salt will be measured by the laboratory.

Total Blood that May Be Taken from Patients

The total amount of blood that may be taken from a patient in most medicine trials should be limited to one unit (about 460 ml) per 8-week period. This figure represents the standard practice followed in blood banking, where an individual may donate 1 unit of blood every 8 weeks.

Urinalysis

Most clinical laboratories have established a standard battery of tests that includes most or all of the basic parameters listed in Table 23.2. If a dipstick is used to test the urine for several parameters, it is useful to use one that measures occult blood, even if a microscopic examination will count the number of red blood cells per high-power field. The means of obtaining the specimen should be indicated (i.e., normal voiding sample, clean catch, midstream, catheterization, suprapubic tap, or cystoscopy), especially in clinical trials in which an antibiotic (or other relevant medicine) is being tested.

It is usually unnecessary to obtain a microscopic examination on all urinalyses unless there are reasons to believe that important information and data may be lost. This is particularly true after it has been demonstrated that the test treatment does not affect the parameters measured in the microscopic evaluation of urine.

Urine Screens

A urine screen can be used to confirm generally that patients being screened or entering the baseline period of the clinical trial are not using illicit drugs or medicines contraindicated in the protocol. It can also be used on a scheduled or random basis during the study to confirm that patients are not using illicit or unacceptable drugs. The urine screen is limited in that it is unable to detect positive compliance with the protocol and only measures certain aspects of compliance failure. If a urine test will be conducted at unannounced times in the clinical trial, then this point must be mentioned in the informed consent.

The number of drugs tested in the urine screen is generally determined individually for each clinical trial, since there is a wide variety of possible drugs that may be measured. The choice of drugs to screen will be based on their relative importance for the trial plus the cost and reliability of the methodology. Results of urine screens are usually best viewed in qualitative (i.e., present or absent) rather than quantitative terms. The identification of specific drugs in a patient's urine may help in explaining unusual adverse reactions, laboratory abnormalities, or other events. Urine screens may detect the presence of the trial medicine. If the urine screen is able to detect the presence of the trial medicine, and this is reported as an unknown drug that is present or as a false–positive for another drug, then it could essentially unblind a double-blind clinical trial. To prevent this situation from occurring, data from urine screens may be reported to a nonblinded monitor rather than to the investigator. If a sample of the trial medicine is put in urine at a physiological concentration and sent to the laboratory, the possibility of cross reactivity with known medicines may be assessed prior to initiation of the trial.

Type of Container to Be Used

The specific type of container used to collect blood or urine samples is sometimes indicated in a protocol, especially if a special anticoagulant or additive is required or if other specific conditions of sample collection and handling are required. It is generally not necessary to provide this information for commonly requested laboratory tests.

Use of International System Units

Although the international system of laboratory analyte units is almost universally agreed upon, many people in the United States resist using it. Typically, these are physicians (and others) who desire to retain the system with which they were trained, which makes more sense to them. Numerous anecdotal reports state that some hospitals in the United States are giving up on international units and returning to their older system.

Identifying New Diagnostic Laboratory Tests

Numerous laboratory tests are periodically proposed as aids in the diagnosis of disease states. The standards that must be met before a new test is accepted are extremely high, particularly in terms of calculating the rates of false-positive and false-negative results. Nirenberg and Feinstein (1988) proposed a five-phase process leading up to acceptance of a new diagnostic test. They discuss lessons learned from the rejected dexamethasone suppression test. Other laboratory diagnostic tests that have not been widely endorsed (in recent years) include alpha feto-protein and carcinogenic embryonic antigen. The process of validation is described elsewhere (Chapter 43).

Ophthalmological Examination

Various parts of the ophthalmological examination are shown in Table 23.4. The most important single ophthalmological test to evaluate patients for the presence of chronic medicine-induced toxicity is the slit-lamp examination. Specific types of medicines with a known potential for ocular toxicity may require that special attention be directed to other examinations shown in Table 23.4 (e.g., the possibility of nystagmus with certain anticonvulsants). Most medicines that are to be taken systemically require at least some evidence of ocular safety prior to approval for marketing. Hawkins (1988) discusses the selection of controls for clinical trials in ophthalmology.

Dermatological Examinations

A few selected safety measurements and tests for a specialized dermatological examination are listed in Table 23.5.

TABLE 23.4 *Procedures and tests performed in an ophthalmological examination*

1. Ophthalmological history (attention is paid to patient and family history plus patient's diseases and medicines used)
2. Visual acuity (Snellen chart) corrected (i.e., with glasses if present)
3. External ocular examination (i.e., check for inflammation, ptosis, nystagmus, tearing, proptosis, and other abnormalities)
4. Extraocular muscle testing
5. Pupil size and evaluation (in darkened room with intense illumination)
6. Slit-lamp biomicroscopy (with dilated pupils)
7. Tonometry (Goldmann applanation tonometer and/or American Optical noncontact tonometer)
8. Ophthalmoscopy with fundus photographs (with dilated pupils)
9. Visual field testing and color vision testing
10. Gonioscopy[a]
11. Lacrimation[a] (Schirmer test)

[a] These tests are of minimal value in determining medicine toxicity and are not recommended for routine inclusion in ophthalmological examination to detect medicine-induced toxicity.

TABLE 23.5 *Selected examples of safety measurements and tests for a specialized dermatological examination*

1. Biopsy
2. Erythema at site of lesion
3. Absorption of medications systemically (e.g., blood levels)
4. Signs and symptoms of absorption
5. Interactions with standard treatment (e.g., ultraviolet light)

SPECIFIC ISSUES

Using a Central Laboratory for Conducting Some or All Tests

For multicenter trials, it is often possible to have all laboratory tests conducted at each individual site, or to use a central laboratory. A third possibility is that some tests may be conducted by each site's laboratory and other tests conducted at a central laboratory. A fourth possibility is to offer each site the option of using their own laboratory or a central one.

These options should be carefully evaluated before a choice is made. Advantages of a central laboratory are that it offers (1) a single procedure for conducting tests, (2) a single set of reference values, and (3) a better control on data reporting (e.g., a "panic value" or "critical limits" may be used for reporting the value to the coordinating center or company, Kost, 1990). Disadvantages include the fact that stat (i.e., immediate) results are difficult to obtain and the possibility that samples may not reach the central laboratory in adequate condition. Specialized tests (e.g., hormone levels, levels of a medicine and its metabolites) generally are conducted most efficiently at a central site. The added costs and administrative efforts of evaluating samples at a central site are often critical factors in reaching a decision on whether a central laboratory will be used.

Using a Single Center to Interpret Selected Safety Data

Many tests of safety parameters often have a strong subjective component to their interpretation. Examples include electroencephalograms, fundoscopic pictures of the eye, pathological slides, and X-rays. In many cases the results of these, or other tests, are important for (1) patient enrollment (i.e., does the patient pass the inclusion criteria?), (2) assignment to a strata for randomization (e.g., is the severity of a symptom above or below a given point?), (3) determination of whether a patient may remain in a clinical trial, (4) assessment of the treatment's efficacy, or (5) assessment of the treatment's benefit-to-risk ratio.

If large numbers of tests are to be read and interpreted, or if a great degree of standardization and consistency in reading is important, then using a single reading center makes sense. At a central site it is possible for two individuals to read and interpret results. If this is done, then the same two individuals should be involved in interpreting all data received at the central center. A third reviewer may be used to arbitrate any disagreements in interpretation. Readers should also be blind to the treatment group of all patients whose results they interpret.

Handling Samples

Details of how biological samples may be most efficiently and appropriately handled must be determined for each clinical trial. Nonetheless, there are some general principles and also tips that can be mentioned. The major principle is to simplify the process and minimize the number of different people who obtain, handle, and transport laboratory specimens. The laboratory printout of results should include the times that the sample was drawn and analyzed.

Listing Laboratory Analytes on Data Collection Forms

Data collection forms or screens for remote data entry should list laboratory analytes in the same order that the laboratory lists them on their reports. This will create difficulties for multicentered trials because some sites' laboratories will list them in a different order. Nonetheless, except for trials with more than 10, 20, or (?) sites, effort should be made to follow this practice. An alternative is to use the laboratory printout as the data collection form. This avoids transcription errors.

Dealing with Frozen Samples

Laboratory specimens that are to be frozen should be frozen on their side, then stored erect. Any thawing and refreezing that occurs may then be readily detected (Fig. 23.1). Because of the potential for samples to deteriorate if they are stored for a long period, it may be advisable to send one or more standards to each site to be frozen, stored, and shipped with the other samples.

Problems in Laboratories in Offices of Individual or Groups of Physicians

Sponsors should be cautious about the quality of the laboratories in private offices used for hematology, clinical chemistry, microbiology, or urinalysis testing. There is no federal regulation of office laboratories and only three states in the United States (Idaho, Penn-

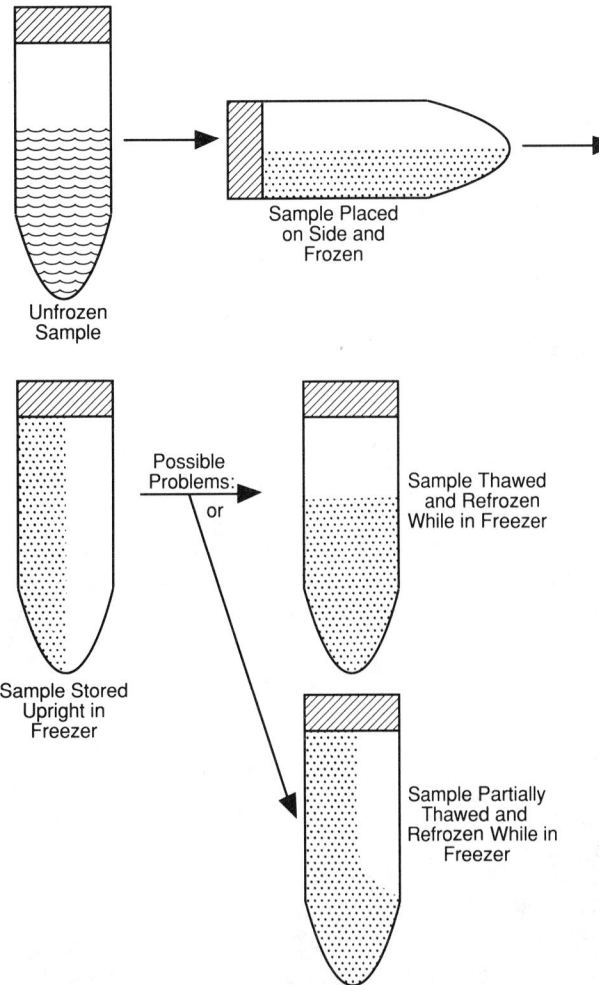

FIG. 23.1 Method of freezing samples that readily demonstrates if partial or complete thawing has occurred.

cilities. Ten drug-spiked urine samples were sent quarterly (i.e., 40 samples per year) to each laboratory for identification. Their study covered data obtained between 1973 and 1981. They found that the percent of laboratories with an acceptable performance was 9% for barbiturates, 0% for amphetamines, 50% for methadone, 9% for cocaine, 15% for codeine, and 8% for morphine (Hansen, et al., 1985).

IMPAIRMENT OF DRIVING

A Consensus Development Panel (1985) from the Research Technology Branch of the National Institute on Drug Abuse published their results on numerous aspects of this issue. Although few medicines have been evaluated for effects on driving performance, the importance of such tests is growing. Particular attention has been given to ethanol in the past, but evaluation of illicit drugs and medicines affecting the central nervous system are currently of particular interest. Epidemiological data suggest that apart from ethanol and cannabis, the medicines most likely to be associated with impaired driving are antihistamines and sedative–hypnotics (Consensus Development Panel, 1985). Currently available methods to assess driving impairment (e.g., cognitive function tests, motor function tests, driving simulators) all have serious drawbacks and do not adequately assess most drivers who may have been awake for 16 hours and are now driving somewhere. The Consensus Development Panel also discussed problems in interpreting data obtained in various tests.

PROCEDURES TO COUNTERACT ABNORMAL LABORATORY OBSERVATIONS

In evaluating the safety of medicines using laboratory or other tests, it is important to develop data that will establish the nature and magnitude of any issue or problem (real or potential) that arises with abnormal laboratory data. Data obtained must also measure the strength of the association between the medicine and event noted or of the serial trends that are observed. While this information is being collected, the alternative courses of action in dealing with the issue or problem can be developed and evaluated. These countermeasures may take the form of (1) periodic monitoring [e.g., prothrombin (PT) or partial thromboplastin time (PTT) times for patients receiving anticoagulants], (2) cessation of medicine treatment, (3) decreasing the dose or changing the dose schedule, (4) initiating countertreatment (e.g., antiarrhythmic medicines may be used to treat arrhythmias induced by a test medicine), (5) specific antidotes may be used to counter or reverse medicine effects (e.g., neostigmine may be used to reverse the neuromuscular block-

sylvania, and Wyoming) have comprehensive regulations (Crawley et al., 1986). These authors report that many problems in office laboratories that existed in Idaho before their regulations were greatly improved when the offices were assessed after the regulations. These problems included (1) lack of quality control in testing procedures, (2) lack of knowledge about quality control, (3) lack of adequate procedure manuals, (4) lack of preventive maintenance, (5) lack of knowledge about laboratory safety, (6) errors in proficiency testing conducted during onsite visits, and (7) inability to understand and retain information about quality assurance guidelines.

Problems in Major Laboratories

Unfortunately, the problems in laboratory quality described above are not localized to laboratories in physicians' private offices. The Centers for Disease Control (CDC) reported on an evaluation of the quality of 13 laboratories that serve 262 methadone treatment fa-ade caused by nondepolarizing types of neuromuscular blocking medicines), (6) increasing surveillance of the patient, or (7) various other alternatives.

DEATHS IN CLINICAL TRIALS

Determining the cause of deaths in clinical trials is extremely important, but this goal is often difficult or impossible to achieve. Investigators should be prepared to present reasons to family members to convince them of the importance of conducting an autopsy. The autopsy should include examination of the brain, whenever possible.

Any history of drug or alcohol abuse by a patient should trigger a request for appropriate blood and urine tests. Blood samples should always be taken to assess the levels of test medicines and any concomitant medicines used. The medicine containers should always be analyzed to confirm their contents. This usually entails sending these medicines to their manufacturer.

The circumstances surrounding the patient's death should be as well documented as possible, including a description of all possible influences of the clinical trial procedures on the death, even influences that are clearly independent of the medicine(s) being tested. Even procedures in a clinical trial apparently unrelated to a patient's death might have contributed to the death in some way. For example, these procedures could include (1) the requirement for excessive physical exertion, (2) prolonged periods of psychologically difficult testing that lead to extreme fatigue, or (3) giving patients many (e.g., 30) large capsules to ingest per day that lead to choking or aspiration.

Evaluation of the data surrounding the death by physicians who are unassociated with the clinical trial lends additional credibility to the report and conclusions. Physician biases probably will strongly influence their decision regarding the association of a patient's death with the clinical trial, and this factor must be considered in interpreting their report. This is particularly true for developing survival curves in cancer or other often fatal diseases, when deaths unrelated to the disease or to the treatment are excluded from the analysis. The topic of deaths in clinical trials is discussed in more detail by Haynes (1988).

BEHAVIORAL RATING SCALES, PERFORMANCE, PERSONALITY, AND DISABILITY TESTS

A number of behavioral rating scales and psychometric and performance tests, listed in Tables 23.6 to 23.8, are briefly described below. Since many of these scales and tests may be used to evaluate safety as well as efficacy, they are included in this chapter. The following comments on the tests provide only a few highlights; readers who are interested in more details are advised to obtain additional information before choosing the tests that appear most relevant to be included in their particular protocol. Additional information may be obtained from the *ECDEU Assessment Manual for Psychopharmacology* (Guy, 1976), which was the source for many of the details listed in this section, *Mental Measurements Yearbook* (Buros, 1972), and psychiatrists, professional associations, and other sources. The two-volume *Mental Measurements Year-*

TABLE 23.6 *Adult behavioral rating scales[a]*

Scale	Scale rated by		
	Professional		Patient
1. Anxiety Status Inventory (ASI)	X		
2. Beck Depression Inventory (Beck)			X
3. Brief Psychiatric Rating Scale (BPRS)	X		
4. Carroll Depression Scale			X
5. Clinical Global Impression (CGI)	X	or	X
6. Clyde Mood Scale			X
7. Covi Anxiety Scale	X		
8. Crichton Geriatric Rating Scale	X		
9. Depression Status Inventory (DSI)	X		
10. Hamilton Anxiety Scale (HAMA)	X		
11. Hamilton Depression Scale (HAMD)	X		
12. Hopkins Symptom Checklist (HSCL)			X
13. Inpatient Multidimensional Psychiatric Scale (IMPS)	X		
14. Nurses Observation Scale for Inpatient Evaluation (NOSIE)	X		
15. Plutchik Geriatric Rating Scale (PLUT)	X		
16. Profile of Mood States (POMS)			X
17. Sandoz Clinical Assessment—Geriatric	X		
18. Self-Report Symptom Inventory (SCL-90)			X
19. Wittenborn Psychiatric Rating Scale (WITT)	X		
20. Zung Self-Rating Anxiety Scale (SAS)			X
21. Zung Self-Rating Depression Scale (SDS)			X

[a] Standard abbreviations are used (See *ECDEU Assessment Manual for Psychopharmacology*, Guy, 1976). Additional tests are described in *Mental Measurements Yearbook* (Buros, 1972).

book contains numerous references and critiques of many of these and other related tests.

These scales may be used either as part of a clinical trial or as major endpoints in an efficacy trial. In this chapter they are described as a means of obtaining ancillary data on psychological factors in a clinical trial. If these scales are used to demonstrate efficacy, it is mandatory to include only those scales known to be valid.

Unless otherwise noted, all of the adult and children's behavioral scales are given once pretreatment and at least once posttreatment. Investigators may schedule additional evaluations with these tests, but this is usually not done at less than weekly or biweekly intervals. Many tests provide data on both a total score and subtest (factor) scores. The specific subscale factors used for certain tests are listed. The times given to complete tests are subject to significant variation depending on the anxiety and characteristics of the patient and/or the experience of the professional. The times listed do not include either scoring or preliminary and/or necessary observations of the patient. Within each of the following three subheadings (Adult Behavioral Rating Scales, Pediatric Behavioral Rating Scales, and Performance Tests), tests are presented in alphabetical order. A few additional personality and physical disability tests are discussed at the end of this chapter.

Adult Behavioral Rating Scales

Anxiety Status Inventory. The Anxiety Status Inventory (ASI) scale is the professional-rated version of the Zung Self-Rating Anxiety Scale (SAS). Both tests (ASI and SAS) contain 20 items, each with a four-point scale, and are designed for use in adults diagnosed as having anxiety neurosis. Both assess anxiety as a clinical disorder rather than a "feeling state." The tests rate either the present time or the average status of the patient during the week preceding the evaluation. The ASI takes up to 15 to 20 minutes to complete and gives two scores: state anxiety and trait anxiety.

Beck Depression Inventory. The Beck Depression Inventory (Beck) test may be used to measure the depth of depression as a rapid screen for depressed patients. It is a self-rating scale of 21 items (13 in a shortened form), with each item rated on a four-point scale. It measures the immediate present and has been used in antidepressant medicine trials. The original 21-item scale can be completed in about 10 minutes and the test is able to discriminate between anxiety and depression. No subtests are present in the Beck.

Brief Psychiatric Rating Scale. The Brief Psychiatric Rating Scale (BPRS) is used primarily in adult inpatients to evaluate treatment response in medicine trials and in nonmedicine clinical treatment, but it is also used in some outpatient trials. Abbreviated instructions are printed on the form. Ratings are based on observations of patients. Originally developed for psychopharmacologic research, this test contains 18 symptoms, each rated on a seven-point severity scale. It requires approximately 20 minutes to complete and rates the period of time since the last test. If the test is being used for the first time, it rates the previous week. Five separate subscales are obtained: anxiety–depression, anergia, thought disturbance, activation, and hostility–suspiciousness.

Carroll Rating Scale for Depression. The Carroll Rating Scale for depression (52-item self-rating scale) is scored with yes or no answers by patients. It was designed to match closely the information content and specific items included in the Hamilton rating scale. It has been validated by comparisons with both the Hamilton Depression Scale (HAMD) and Beck and requires approximately 20 minutes to complete. Seventeen components of depression are measured.

Clinical Global Impressions. Although the ECDEU *Assessment Manual for Psychopharmacology* (Guy, 1976) provides a formal test for the Clinical Global Impression (CGI) Scale, numerous investigators have modified the three major questions as well as the scales used in order to fit this test to their own clinical trials. The three questions, which may be applied in almost all Phase II and Phase III clinical trials, are:

1. Severity of illness. "Considering your total clinical experience with this particular population, how mentally ill (the investigator may substitute a more appropriate term if this is not applicable) is the patient at this time?"
2. Global improvement. "Rate total improvement, whether or not in your judgment it is due entirely to medicine treatment."
3. Efficacy index. "Rate this item on the basis of medicine effect only." This utilizes a rating of both efficacy and adverse reactions and divides the efficacy score by the adverse reaction score to form a ratio ("efficacy index").

Severity of illness is the only one of these three rated pretreatment. All three questions may be rated posttreatment, and additional ratings are possible during a clinical trial. The CGI measure, which is widely used in all types of medicine trials, is generally well accepted.

A scale of two to nine gradations is usually used for questions 1 and 2, although five or so gradations are probably most common. A typical five-point scale for question 2 would be that the patient is rated as 1 (much worse), 2 (minimally worse), 3 (unchanged), 4 (minimally improved), or 5 (markedly improved).

Clyde Mood Scale. The Clyde Mood Scale test may be used as either a self-rated or observer-rated scale. It contains 48 items to measure mood and has been shown to be sensitive to medicine effects. The test takes 5 to 15 minutes to complete and measures the immediate present in a patient or normal individual. The test gives six scores: friendly, aggressive, clear-thinking, sleepy, unhappy, and dizzy.

Covi Anxiety Scale. The Covi Anxiety Scale is a global observer's rating scale of patient anxiety. There are three items that are each rated on a 0-to-5 scale. The test is simple to use and requires only a few minutes to complete.

Crichton Geriatric Rating Scale. The Crichton Geriatric Rating Scale test measures the level of behavioral function in elderly psychiatric patients using a five-point scale on 11 items. It rates either the present or the period within the last week and takes 5 to 10 minutes to complete.

Depression Status Inventory. The Depression Status Inventory (DSI) scale is the professional's version of the Zung Self-Rating Depression Scale (SDS). Each of the two scales (DSI and SDS) consists of the same 20 items rated on a four-point scale and is applied to adults with depressive symptomatology. The DSI is completed by the professional, and the SDS is completed by the patient. Both tests take about 5 to 10 minutes to complete. The DSI rates either the present situation or the last week prior to the test, and a total score is obtained.

Hamilton Anxiety Scale. The Hamilton Anxiety (HAMA) scale was designed to be used in adult patients who already have a diagnosis of anxiety neurosis rather than for making a diagnosis of anxiety in patients who have other problems. The test contains 14 items, each with a five-point scale, and is completed by a physician or psychologist. The test emphasizes the patient's subjective state. The two subscales determined are somatic anxiety and psychic anxiety.

Hamilton Depression Scale. The HAMD is one of the most widely used tests to evaluate the severity of depressive illness quantitatively in adults. The most widely used form of this test contains 21 items covering a broad range of symptomatology, with a three- to five-point scale for most items. The minimum time required to complete this test is usually 10 to 20 minutes, and it requires a skilled interviewer. Either the present time or the period within the last week is rated. Six sub-scales are obtained in the HAMD: anxiety/somatization, weight, cognitive disturbance, diurnal variation, retardation, and sleep disturbance.

Hopkins Symptom Checklist. The Hopkins Symptom Checklist (HSCL) is a scale that has been used to measure the presence and intensity of various symptoms in outpatient neurotic patients. It is a 58-item self-rating scale and has generally been replaced by the Self-Report Symptom Inventory (SCL-90). It measures the symptoms during the past week and requires approximately 20 minutes to complete. There are five subtests: somatization, obsessive–compulsive, interpersonal sensitivity, depression, and anxiety.

Inpatient Multidimensional Psychiatric Scale. The Inpatient Multidimensional Psychiatric Scale (IMPS) is used to measure psychotic syndromes in hospitalized adults capable of being interviewed. The 89 items are rated on the basis of a psychiatric interview. This test has been well validated and requires 10 to 15 minutes following a 35- to 45-minute interview. There are ten scores: excitement, hostile belligerence, paranoid projection, grandiose expansiveness, perceptual distortions, anxious intropunitiveness, retardation and apathy, disorientation, motor disturbances, and conceptual disorganization.

Nurses Observation Scale for Inpatient Evaluation. The Nurses Observation Scale for Inpatient Evaluation (NOSIE) (30-item test) is used by nursing personnel to rate a patient's behavior on the ward, with a five-point scale for each item. This test is widely used and is well accepted for adult inpatients. The test, which rates the most recent 3 days, is relatively easy to use and requires 3 to 5 minutes to complete. A revised NOSIE was validated in over 600 chronic schizophrenic patients aged 26 to 74 years. This test has also been validated in mentally retarded patients and gives seven scores: social competence, social interest, personal neatness, irritability, manifest psychosis, retardation, and total score.

Plutchik Geriatric Rating Scale. The Plutchik Geriatric Rating Scale (PLUT) (31-item test) is designed to measure the degree of geriatric functioning in terms of both physical and social aspects. The three-point scale for each item is completed on the basis of direct observation of the patient's behavior and takes 5 to 10 minutes to complete. The subscales measure overall dysfunction, aggressive behavior, sleep disturbance, social isolation, sensory impairment, work and activities, and motor impairment.

Profile of Mood States. Profile of Mood States (POMS) self-rating scale is used in both normals and psychiatric outpatients to evaluate feelings, affect, and mood. It has been widely used in medicine trials. The 65 adjectives included in this test may be used to rate the present and/or previous week. This test requires from 5 to 10 minutes to complete and provides scores for six subtests: tension–anxiety, depression–dejection, anxiety–hostility, vigor, fatigue, and confusion.

Sandoz Clinical Assessment—Geriatric. The Sandoz Clinical Assessment—Geriatric (SCAG) test measures 18 individual symptoms plus a global rating using a seven-point scale similar to those used in the Brief Psychiatric Rating Scale. It measures the present period or that within the last week, requires about 10 to 15 minutes to complete, and does not contain subtests.

Self-Report Symptom Inventory. Each of the 90 items in the SCL-90 uses a five-point scale of distress. It was designed as a general measure of symptomatology for use by adult psychiatric outpatients in either a research or clinical setting. It rates either the present or previous week. It requires about 15 minutes for the patient to complete this form and about 5 minutes for a technician to verify identifying information. This test is sensitive to medicine effects and may be used with inpatients. Nine subscales are measured: somatization, obsessive–compulsive, interpersonal sensitivity, depression, anxiety, anger–hostility, phobic anxiety, paranoid ideation, and psychoticism.

Wittenborn Psychiatric Rating Scale. The ECDEU version [Wittenborn Psychiatric Rating Scale (WITT)] is a 17-item test shortened from the original 72-item test. All but one item use a four-point scale, and the test takes 5 to 10 minutes to complete. It is used in both in- and outpatients and rates either the present or previous week. This test is not intended to make diagnoses but to reflect changes within one patient and to provide a basis for comparing different patients. This test provides descriptive, as opposed to etiological or prognostic, information on patients and includes the following subscales: anxiety, somatic–hysterical, obsessive–compulsive–phobic, depressive retardation, excitement, and paranoia.

Zung Self-Rating Anxiety Scale. The SAS test requires approximately 5 to 10 minutes to complete. See Anxiety Status Inventory for details.

Zung Self-Rating Depression Scale. The SDS test requires approximately 5 to 10 minutes to complete. See *Depression Status Inventory,* above, for details.

Pediatric Behavioral Rating and Diagnostic Scales

Many of the behavioral rating scales described for adults are not suitable for use in the pediatric population. Special tests have been designed, and a number of pediatric behavioral rating scales are presented in Table 23.7. General comments on these tests are presented below. A further description of rating scales used in pediatric medicine trials is given in the *ECDEU Assessment Manual For Psychopharmacology* by Conners (1976). His article is a practical guide to identifying appropriate scales for a particular situation. Conners discusses the two broad approaches of many pediatric rating scales as either "rating current behaviors, symptoms or states; or . . . describing basic traits, dispositions, and personality characteristics." The choice of one of these two approaches depends in part on the purpose of using a scale in a medicine trial. Three general purposes have been suggested for using a behavioral test (prediction, measurement of change, and classification). The choice of one of these three purposes usually implies that one of the two specific approaches implicit in the pediatric behavioral scales will be more appropriate:

1. To be able to predict something about a patient, choose a scale that rates basic traits.
2. To measure change in a patient, choose a scale that rates current symptoms.
3. To assess a patient's classification, choose a scale that rates either basic traits or current symptoms, depending on the purpose of the classification.

The type of patient population and the desired format of the test to be used in a clinical trial also influence the particular scale(s) chosen.

Conners (1976) reviewed six different scales (tests) for teachers and recommended two for use in medicine trials (Devereux and Conners). Information on all six scales is available in his article. Three scales are described for parents to complete, and two of these are mentioned below (Devereux Child Behavior Rating Scale and the Conners Parent Questionnaire). A small number of child psychiatry rating scales are available. Conners briefly described a few and stated that the scale reported by Davis et al. (1969) for use in retarded children was sensitive to medicine treatment. A scale

TABLE 23.7 *Pediatric behavioral rating and diagnostic scales*[a]

1. Children's Behavior Inventory (CBI)
2. Children's Diagnostic Classification (CDC)
3. Children's Diagnostic Scale (CDS)
4. Children's Psychiatric Rating Scale (CPRS)
5. Clinical Global Impression (CGI)
6. Conners Parent Questionnaire (PQ)
7. Conners Parent–Teacher Questionnaire (PTQ)
8. Conners Teacher Questionnaire (TQ)
9. Devereux Child Behavior Rating Scale
10. Devereux Elementary School Behavior Rating Scale
11. Dosage Record and Treatment Emergent Symptoms (DOTES)
12. Stereotyped Behavior in Retarded[b]

[a] Additional tests are described in *Mental Measurements Yearbook* (Buros, 1972).
[b] This test is described by Davis et al. (1969).

that can be used in a wide variety of pediatric inpatients is the Children's Behavior Inventory.

Children's Behavior Inventory. The Children's Behavior Inventory (CBI) is a 139-item, two-point (yes–no) scale to record maladaptive behavior in children aged 1 to 15 years. Relatively little training is needed to administer this test. It is easily used by nurses, teachers, graduate students, psychologists, and others. This test usually requires at least 2 hours of observation of the child, but better reliability is achieved if behavior is observed over an 8-hour period. Nine subtest scores are provided: anger–hostility, conceptual dysfunctioning, fear and worry, incongruous behavior, incongruous ideation, lethargy–dejection, perceptual dysfunctioning, physical complaints, and self-deprecation.

Children's Diagnostic Classification. Children's Diagnostic Classification (CDC) test may be used instead of the Children's Psychiatric Rating Scale (CPRS) to arrive at a diagnosis. This differs from the CPRS in that it is highly directed and leads the observer to a diagnosis. It rates the current status of the child and may be used at pretreatment and/or the termination of the clinical trial.

Children's Diagnostic Scale. The Children's Diagnostic Scale (CDS) is used in children up to 15 years of age to assist in the diagnosis and classification of the child's condition. It contains 13 items, eight of which have a seven-point scale. The others are specific diagnostic questions. It measures current status only and is mainly used at the start of a study, although it may be used at the termination of the study as well.

Children's Psychiatric Rating Scale. The CPRS is a comprehensive scale to assess a wide range of psychopathologies in children up to age 15. It contains 63 items, with a seven-point scale derived from the Brief Psychiatric Rating Scale (BPRS). This test rates 28 items by direct observation of the child, based on behavior expressed during the interview, and rates other items based on the child's reports of events that occurred either over the preceding week or that occurred during the interview. Scores of 15 separate clusters of the rated items are provided as well as the overall score.

Clinical Global Impression. See adult behavioral rating scale description of the CGI.

Conners Parent Questionnaire. Conners Parent Questionnaire (PQ) is a 94-item checklist of symptoms that evaluates common behavior disorders using a four-point scale in children up to 15 years of age and takes 15 to 20 minutes to complete. It is used once

pretreatment and may be repeated but is often replaced after the first use by the 11-item Conners Parent–Teacher Questionnaire (PTQ). There are eight subscales: conduct problem, anxiety, impulsive–hyperactive, learning problem, psychosomatic, perfectionism, antisocial, and muscular tension.

Conners Parent–Teacher Questionnaire. See descriptions above for Conners Parent Questionnaire and below for the Conners Teacher Questionnaire (TQ). The PTQ is used in conjunction with either the PQ to TQ and yields a total score only (i.e., no subscales are given). The PTQ takes about 5 minutes to complete and is not used pretreatment.

Conners Teacher Questionnaire. The TQ form was designed to obtain teacher evaluations of children up to age 15 in terms of their interactions with peers and their ability to cope with the school environment and requirements. There are 41 items, and the first 39 have a four-point scale. Question 40 deals with the teacher's evaluation of the child's severity of illness, and question 41 deals with global improvement in four different areas. This test is used once at pretreatment and as needed afterwards. It takes about 15 minutes to complete and covers either the present or any interval period up to 1 month. A shorter 11-item PTQ is often used after the initial use of the 41-item TQ. Teachers require some instruction in the use of this test. The five subscales included are conduct, inattentive–passive, tension–anxiety, hyperactivity, and social ability.

Devereux Child Behavior Rating Scale. The Devereux Child Behavior Rating Scale contains 97 items and is similar to the Devereux Teacher Scale. It is used for emotionally disturbed and mentally retarded children aged 8 to 12 years. Besides being easy to use, this scale is well researched and discussed in the literature. It requires 10 to 20 minutes to complete by clinicians, child care workers, parents, or others and gives 17 scores. There is a Devereux Adolescent Behavior Rating Scale for children from ages 13 to 18.

Devereux Elementary School Behavior Rating Scale. The Devereux Elementary School Behavior Rating Scale is a widely used test incorporating 47 items that have a high test–retest reliability. It uses a checklist format and is easy to use (requires 10 min). There are 11 factor scores and three item scores. Conners (1976) believes that this might be the test of choice for teachers to complete in many medicine trials.

Stereotyped Behavior in Retarded. The Stereotyped Behavior in Retarded test (Davis et al., 1969) has been reported to be sensitive to medicine treatment in retarded and severely disturbed inpatients.

Psychometric and Performance Tests

The psychometric and performance tests presented in Table 23.8 may be grouped as being applicable for use in either children or adults. In children, the tests measure intellect (GOOD, Porteus Mazes, WISC, Peabody), achievement (WRAT), and motor performance (vigilance tests, reaction time). There are other tests that may be used to measure learning, although many of these tests utilize equipment and are not described. All of these tests (unless otherwise noted) are given once pretreatment, at least once posttreatment, and at additional times if desired by the investigator. The contribution of learning in the scores obtained at second and third testings is usually unknown. The methods used to motivate patients to perform to the best of their ability in all tests should be standardized and reported.

Bender–Gestalt Test. The Bender–Gestalt is a nonverbal performance test in which the individual copies a design shown on a card. It is often used to identify a problem of visual perception and/or motor performance or minimal brain dysfunction in children.

The scoring used for children (age 4 or 5–11 years) differs from that used for adults (age 15–adult). This test measures perceptual maturity, possible neurological impairment, and emotional adjustment in children. It measures maturation, intelligence, psychological disturbance, and cortical impairment in adults. The test requires 10 minutes to complete. Scores may fluctuate from test to test and thus must be cautiously interpreted.

Conceptual Clustering Memory Test. For the Conceptual Clustering Memory Test, patients are given a list of 24 specific words from a number of different categories such as birds, cars, or types of drinks. The words are presented one at a time over 2 minutes, after which patients are asked to recall as many of the specific words as possible. The test measures the total

recall as well as the degree to which words of a specific category (e.g., birds) are recalled from the cluster of words given in that category (e.g., crow, dove, pigeon).

Digital Symbol Substitution Test. A subtest of the Wechsler Adult Intelligence Scale (WAIS), the Digital Symbol Substitution test measures sensory–motor integration and learning relationships of symbols. It has been used in many psychopharmacological studies. Patients are given different forms of this test at each session. The test requires the patient to match as many of 100 symbols to their respective numerals, found in a code key, as possible within 60 seconds.

Embedded Figures Test. For the Embedded Figures Test, patients are shown a complex design and must identify as quickly as possible a simple figure that is "embedded" within the design. Twenty-four embedded figures are included, and a maximum of 3 minutes is allowed for each one.

Frostig Developmental test of Visual Perception. The Frostig Developmental Test of Visual Perception (FROST) measures the development of perceptual skills in children from 4 to 8 years of age or in older children with learning difficulties. It may be administered individually (requires 30–45 minutes) or to groups (requires 40–60 minutes).

Goodenough–Harris Figure-Drawing Test. The Goodenough–Harris Figure-Drawing Test is a brief (10–15 minute) easy to use test for children 4 to 15 years of age to measure intellectual maturity.

Peabody Picture Vocabulary Test. The Peabody Picture Vocabulary Test is a rapid 10–15-minute intelligence test for children aged 2.5 to 18 years that is useful when there is inadequate time to give the WISC.

TABLE 23.8 *Psychometric and performance tests*[a]

Test	Adults	Children
1. Bender–Gestalt Test	X	X
2. Conceptual Clustering Memory Test	X	X
3. Digital Symbol Substitution Test	X	X
4. Embedded Figures Test	X	X
5. Frostig Development Test of Visual Perception		X
6. Goodenough–Harris Figure-Drawing Test (GOOD)		X
7. Peabody Picture Vocabulary Test		X
8. Porteus Mazes	X	X
9. Reaction Time	X	X
10. Vigilance Tests	X	X
11. Wechsler Adult Intelligence Scale (WAIS)	X	
12. Wechsler Intelligence Scale for Children (WISC)		X
13. Wechsler Memory Scale (WMEN)	X	X
14. Wide Range Achievement Test (WRAT)		X

[a] Additional tests are described in *Mental Measurements Yearbook* (Buros, 1972).

Porteus Mazes. The Porteus Mazes is a nonverbal test that has been shown to be sensitive to medicine effects in both children (over 3 years) and adults. The test has three series of mazes to prevent score improvement on retesting with the same test. It requires about 25 minutes and provides both a qualitative and quantitative score.

Reaction Time. There are many different tests used to measure reaction time. These tests measure the period of time between the presentation of a stimulus to a patient and the onset of the resulting response. The signal is usually a visual or auditory stimulus, and the onset of a motor reaction, such as the lifting of a finger, arm, or leg or the pressing of a buzzer, is used to measure the speed of response.

In simple reaction times, a stimulus is presented that always requires the same response, even if the nature of the stimulus changes. A complex reaction time requires the patient to respond to some stimuli but not to others.

Vigilance Tests. Numerous tests have been designed to measure vigilance. In these tests, patients are requested to respond in some manner to certain stimuli or occurrences but not to others. The stimuli may be controlled to present minimally perceived signals that require vigilance on the part of the patient.

Wechsler Adult Intelligence Scale. The WAIS consists of 11 subtests—six verbal tests and five performance tests. This provides an age-related IQ in adults from 16 to 75 years of age, i.e., the test measures intelligence of the person in relation to his age group and not to the entire population. It may be used either as an initial assessment or as a tool to measure change. The test, which takes 40 to 60 minutes to complete, provides 13 scores in verbal and performance categories plus a total score.

Wechsler Intelligence Scale for Children. The Wechsler Intelligence Scale for Children (WISC) was extensively revised in 1974, and it became the WISC-R, which requires 40 to 60 minutes to complete. This widely used scale in children from 6 to 16 years of age may be used for either screening or baseline data or as a measure of change. There is a "preschool and primary scale of intelligence" version that may be used in children from 4 to 6½ years of age (requires 50–75 minutes). The WISC-R has six verbal and six performance subtests.

Wechsler Memory Scale. The Wechsler Memory (WMEM) Scale is a brief test that is used to measure memory deficits. There are two forms of the test, and they are generally alternated to avoid a training effect in children taking the test on two or more occasions.

Wide Range Achievement Test. The Wide Range Achievement Test (WRAT) is used in children from age 5 years to adults in college. It assesses basic skills in reading, spelling, and mathematics. It is simple, easy to administer, and requires 20 to 30 minutes to complete.

Personality Tests

In addition to the above behavioral and performance tests, there are a number of well-known tests of personality that may provide useful information in a clinical study. The most well known of these tests is the Minnesota Multiphasic Personality Inventory (MMPI). This test consists of 550 affirmative statements to which a true or false reponse is given and requires about 1 hour to complete. It is given to adults over the age of 16 and is scored for ten scales: depression, hysteria, hypochondriasis, psychopathic deviate, masculinity–feminity, paranoia, hypomania, schizophrenia, psychasthenia, and social introversion.

Disability Tests

When medicines are tested in geriatric or other patients who have a significant degree of disability, it is useful to ensure that medicine-induced changes do not affect their ability to function at their usual level of activity. This information is usually obtained by evaluating adverse reactions and physical examinations. However, there are tests that directly measure and/or assess the patients' activities of daily living. These tests can provide an estimate of change that may not be specifically noted on evaluating adverse reactions or physical examinations. Some of these tests include the Northwestern (University) Disability Test and the Activities of Daily Living Test.

The Northwestern Disability Test measures the patient's ability to walk, dress himself or herself, eat, perform personal hygiene, and speak. Each of these categories is scaled with five to ten explicit gradations that are described in reasonable detail (e.g., grade 4 for walking: sometimes walks alone. Walks short distances with ease; walking outdoors is difficult but often done without help; rarely walks longer distances alone).

The Activities of Daily Living Test is often modified from study to study. A representative example includes six activities (walking, sitting, standing, putting on shoes and socks, getting into or out of a chair or car, and sleeping) that are each graded on a five-point scale. Grade 1 is normal, i.e., able to perform the activity without limitation, impairment, or discomfort. Grades 2, 3, and 4 represent mild, moderate, and severe impairment and/or discomfort, and grade 5 indicates that the patient is unable to perform the activity.

CHAPTER 24

Developing Time and Events Schedules

GENERAL ORGANIZATION OF TIME AND EVENTS SCHEDULES

Categories of Items to Include

Time and events schedules (or charts) are synopses of all planned events that will transpire during a clinical trial, although the information and categories incorporated into these schedules may either be highly specific or general. Table 24.1 lists many of the common categories included in the "events" part of the schedule, and Table 24.2 lists the various table headings and descriptions of "time" that are often used. A sample time and events schedule is shown in Table 24.3. This was the schedule used in a double-blind add-on crossover clinical trial of cinromide (an agent tested for antiepileptic activity) versus placebo (Spilker et al., 1983).

Levels of the Clinical Trial to Include

The time and events chart should be organized to present a complete profile of the overall clinical trial. In many trials it will be advantageous to construct a second, more detailed time and events chart in which one part of the trial can be more fully delineated. This is usually presented as a separate schedule. An alternative form of the time and events schedule is to list events that will occur at each hour, day, or week of the study as opposed to putting them in a chart (Table 24.3). Other examples are shown in two books by Spilker and Schoenfelder (1990, 1991).

Time(s) of Dosing

In determining the frequency of medicine dosing and the intervals between doses, it is often appropriate to choose conditions that are similar to those under which the medicine will eventually be used. For example, if the trial medicine is intended to be given four times a day (q.i.d.), then a dosing schedule and time and events chart can be prepared to indicate that patients are to be dosed at equal intervals during the waking period (e.g., 7 A.M., noon, 5 P.M. and 10 P.M.) rather than every 6 hours around the clock. This would not apply to certain medicines (e.g., some antibiotics), when around-the-clock dosing is desired. Likewise, medicines given two or three times a day in a clinical trial can be ingested at times that will mimic eventual clinical use rather than being given at equal intervals throughout a 24-hour day. This approach yields information that is more relevant to the eventual clinical use of the medicine than would information obtained from equally spaced doses, which would significantly differ from those of the intended use.

Alternative Methods of Data Collection

It is sometimes possible to collect information via telephone conversations with patients or even via the mail.

TABLE 24.1 *Selected events that may be included in a time and events schedule*[a]

1. Clinic (physician) visit
2. Screening interview
3. Informed consent
4. Medical history
5. Physical examination (complete)
6. Physical examination (abbreviated)[b]
7. Vital signs and weight (single test at each time point that is marked)
8. Vital signs and weight (multiple tests at each time point that is marked)
9. Neurological or other specialized examinations
10. Clinical laboratory battery (each test, such as hematology, clinical chemistry, and urinalysis, may but need not be listed separately)
11. Biological samples of trial medicine (usually collected in blood or urine)[c]
12. Biological samples of concomitant medicines
13. Admit patient to research facility
14. Randomize patient to treatment group
15. Adverse reaction probe
16. Electrocardiogram (ECG)(12-lead)[d]
17. ECG (lead II)
18. ECG (24-hour Holter monitor)
19. Other safety measurements
20. All efficacy measurements (usually listed separately)
21. Medicine administration
22. Dosage record of the study medicine
23. Dosage record of concomitant medicines
24. Pill count or other compliance check(s)
25. Nurse's evaluation
26. Patient's global evaluation
27. Physician's global evaluation of disease severity
28. Physician's global evaluation of improvement
29. Release from research facility
30. Clinical trial discontinuation record
31. Patient discharged from clinical trial

[a] Footnotes may be used to qualify or detail any notations. The categories used to denote time are shown in Table 24.2, and a sample schedule is shown in Table 24.3. It may be relevant to indicate when many of these procedures and tests will be conducted relative to meals, expected peaks and troughs of blood levels, or other factors.
[b] This may be described and defined in the text or in a footnote. Both categories of physical examination may be listed in the time and events schedule, as with ECGs.
[c] Samples should be obtained at times of peak, trough, or at multiple time points on the medicine concentration curve.
[d] It is often useful to obtain an ECG at the time of peak plasma levels in addition to pre- and posttreatment, when blood levels of the trial medicine would generally be low or absent.

Under carefully designed conditions, this type of data collection may replace visits to the clinic and may be noted by different symbols or by footnotes in the time and events schedule.

DEFINING PERIODS AND TIMES OF A TIME AND EVENTS SCHEDULE

Numbering the Periods of a Clinical Trial

The various periods of a clinical trial may be denoted as screen, baseline, treatment, and posttreatment, but various other terms are also used (Table 24.2). The manner in which the duration of each trial is divided and described varies. A trial may be numbered se-

TABLE 24.2 *Possible headings and subheadings for the time component in time and events tables*

A. Possible major study period headings
  1. Screen[a]
  2. Baseline[b]
  3. Dose ascension
  4. Treatment[c]
  5. Taper
  6. Posttreatment (follow-up)
  7. Dose period 1 to n[d]
  8. Optional visit(s)
  9. Extended baseline[f]

B. Possible subheadings for each of the study periods
Day, hour, and/or minute specified from 0 (or 1) to n for entire study or from 0 (or 1) to n for each period of the study.[e] Other variations of specifying the time in a study are possible.

[a] Negative numbers may be used when convenient, e.g., screen may occur during days -7 to -1, baseline from days 1 to 10, treatment from days 11 to 30, and follow-up from days 31 to 35.
[b] Also referred to as the "stabilization phase" of a clinical trial.
[c] Also referred to as the "maintenance phase" of a clinical trial.
[d] Each dose period may represent a new dose, a new group of patients who are dosed, or a different period of the clinical trial.
[e] Subheadings of year, month, and/or week may also be used. See text for a discussion of the use of "0" times.
[f] This variation may be used if it will allow for specific measurements or parameters to return to a given value or range of values (e.g., between the two legs of a crossover trial). It also may be used for other specific reasons.

quentially from the start of screen (day 1) through to day n for posttreatment. One alternative is to begin each new period of a clinical trial as day 1 (day 1 of baseline, day 1 of treatment, etc.). In this latter example, the maximum duration or range of time that can elapse between the last day of one period and the first day of the following period should be established and indicated in the protocol. A third alternative is to number the time allotted to screen as day $-X$ to day -1 and to begin baseline on day 1 and continue numbering the days sequentially through treatment and posttreatment. Other possible methods of numbering the weeks, days, or hours of a study are possible.

Defining Day "0"

In some clinical trials there is notation of a day "0." If so, it must be made clear whether day "0" represents a full 24 hours or possibly an instant through which the trial passes as it goes from day -1 to day 1. Day 0 may also be a variable part of a 24-hour day rather than a complete day, depending on when day 1 begins. For example, patients may complete their screen or baseline on day 0 and start treatment on day 1, which begins immediately after screen or baseline. The designation of time must be clarified when patients are given their first dose (possibly in the clinic) immediately after the completion of screen or baseline. The principle described for day 0 also applies to hour 0 or week 0. It is the author's view that there are certain clinical trials in which inclusion of a day 0 or hour 0 is appropriate (e.g., if screen and/or baseline will be initiated and completed in 1 day, and the following part of the trial will begin the next day). When a "0" time is included in a trial, it is imperative that it be clearly defined.

When Does Each Clinical Trial Day Begin?

It is often relevant to consider whether each day of the clinical trial begins (1) at 12:01 A.M., (2) at another fixed time of day, or (3) at a different time for each patient (which is then fixed), depending on when each patient reaches a certain point in the protocol. For example, a patient may complete his or her screen examination in the morning or afternoon and immediately begin medicine treatment. Day 1 may be defined as beginning with this treatment. Another possibility is for medicine treatment to be withheld for all patients until the day after the screen (or baseline) examinations in order to start dosing all patients at the same time on day 1. If a patient takes some of the first day's doses at the end of screen, either the numbering of days will be variable from patient to patient or different patients will take a different number of doses on day 1 in order to have day 2 begin at 12:01 A.M.

Numbering the Hours, Days, or Weeks of a Clinical Trial

The numbering of days will probably not pose any significant problems in a long-term clinical trial, but in a trial in which important measurements are made during the first few days of the trial or several times during day 1, it is generally mandatory to apply the same definition of day 1 to all patients. There are many situations that may arise in which the numbering of days (hours) may become quite complex, and complications in the numbering system may develop. If one patient requires a longer washout of preexisting medicines than another patient before entering the trial, or if patients may remain in screen (or baseline) until they qualify to enter the baseline (or treatment), the acceptable lengths of each period as well as its numbering must be specified.

Another aspect of numbering in a clinical trial arises in the association of clinic visits and trial weeks or months. The clinic visit may always occur at the start, middle, or end of each specified week, or it may occur at any time during each specified week. Each of these possibilities is commonly used. There is no preferred method in the author's view, but consistency and clarification are necessary goals in writing the protocol. The numbering of trial weeks (or months) may have a

TABLE 24.3 Clinical trial time and events schedule

Event	Weeks:	Screen	Period 1 baseline A 2	4[a]	Period 2 treatment A 5	6	7	9	12	15	16[b]	Period 3 baseline B 17	18	20[a]	Period 4 treatment B 21	22	23	25	28	31	32[b]	Period 5 follow-up 33	36
Admission criteria		X																					
Informed consent		X																					
Medical/seizure history		X																					
Physical exam		X								X										X			
Neurological exam		X								X										X			
Investigator's assessment		X	X	X	X	X	X	X	X	X		X	X	X	X	X	X	X	X	X		X	X
Vital signs		X	X	X	X	X	X	X	X	X		X	X	X	X	X	X	X	X	X		X	X
Electrocardiogram (ECG)		X								X										X			X
Electroencephalogram (EEG)		X								X										X			
Laboratory																							
Hematology		X		X			X		X	X			X			X			X	X			X
Blood Chemistry		X		X			X	X		X			X			X		X		X			X
Urinalysis		X		X			X			X			X			X				X			X
Pregnancy test (when applicable)		X		X						X			X							X			X
AED plasma levels[c]		X	X	X			X	X	X	X	X	X	X	X		X	X	X	X			X	X
Adverse reactions		X	X	X	X	X	X	X	X	X	X	X	X	X	X	X	X	X	X	X	X	X	X
Dosage record		X	X	X	X	X	X	X	X	X	X	X	X	X	X	X	X	X	X	X	X	X	X
Seizure record		X	X	X	X	X	X	X	X	X	X	X	X	X	X	X	X	X	X	X	X	X	X
Physician's global evaluation										X										X			
Study discontinuation record																							X

[a] Dosage ascension of test medication initiated. Week numbers refer to end of week.
[b] Dosage taper/discontinuation of test medication.
[c] AED, antiepileptic medicine.

significant impact on how much medicine is to be dispensed at each clinic visit and how data collection forms may best be organized and prepared.

Associating Theoretical Times with Actual Dates

A time and events schedule of theoretical times (e.g., day 1 to x, week 1 to y, or month 1 to z) is usually written in a protocol since the exact dates that the clinical trial will be conducted are usually unknown when the protocol is written. The theoretical dates must be associated with real times (e.g., August 4–17, July–November) prior to initiation of the trial. If all patients start a protocol at different times, then this process must be individualized for each patient. Clinical trials may be quite flexible in this regard (e.g., patients may come to clinic each month at a "convenient" time) or quite rigid (e.g., unless patients arrive at a certain time on a certain day, the value of the data obtained will be compromised or lost entirely). In the latter case, the timing of the trial must be established after consideration of weekends, holidays, vacations, availability of staff and necessary equipment, plus other factors required to conduct the trial such as the scheduling of all necessary tests.

Flexible versus Rigid Schedules

Flexible schedules are usually appropriate in long-term outpatient trials in which patients are contacted to arrange a suitable time for visiting the clinic. With an intermediate schedule patients receive an appointment for their next clinic visit when they complete their current one, but this date may be subsequently modified (i.e., brought forward or delayed by a small amount of time). Patients are put on rigid schedules in most inpatient trials, in circadian rhythm trials, and many pharmacokinetic trials.

In clinical trials in which the initiation of medicine therapy is determined by the patient and not by the investigator (e.g., when certain symptoms or signs occur, the patient immediately begins medicine treatment), there will have to be special consideration given to devising an appropriate time and events schedule. Additional examples of time and event schedules are shown in *Data Collection Forms in Clinical Trials* (Spilker and Schoenfelder, 1991).

CHAPTER 25

Preparing, Packaging, and Dispensing of Clinical Trial Medications

OBTAINING AND PREPARING TRIAL MEDICINES

After the clinical trial design and dosing schedule have been developed, the optimal means of preparing, packaging, and dispensing the trial medicines may be determined.

The protocol does not generally include information on the procedures used to manufacture the trial medicine. Details are included (if relevant) that relate to the final preparation of the medicine, if any procedures have to be performed (e.g., medicine must be mixed or thawed), at or shortly prior to the time of its administration. Each of the ingredients in the formulation of trial medicines may be listed in protocols, as may a description of pertinent storage and handling information (e.g., if the medicine must be kept frozen).

Characteristics of Placebo

In specifying the characteristics of the placebo medications to be used, several factors may be considered.

These are indicated in Table 25.1. Placebos and active medicines should be similar in terms of all five senses—smell, taste, sight, feel, and sound. Sound is only applicable to aerosols and sprays. Since some dyes that color medicines may elicit adverse pulmonary responses, and a number of dyes used to color gelatin capsules, tablets, and solutions are not standard or accepted in all countries, this factor may be relevant to consider. The use of lactose in a placebo or active medicine may cause diarrhea and gastrointestinal distress in patients with lactose intolerance. If the clinical trial involves a group of patients among whom the expected incidence of lactose intolerance is anticipated to be higher than that in the general population, an alternate excipient for placebo and active medicine may be desired. If a solid form (tablet) of the active medicine has a distinct taste, then it and the matching placebo could both be coated to mask differences in taste. Another option might be to put the manufactured (marketed) medicine, either whole or ground up (if it is in tablet form), inside a capsule (usually opaque) and to use a matching placebo capsule. This technique has been successfully used but requires prior demonstra-

TABLE 25.1 *Factors to consider in establishing placebo characteristics[a]*

1. Overall visual appearance
2. Surface and internal color
3. Size
4. Shape
5. Taste on licking and chewing
6. Smell
7. Weight
8. Presence of dyes[b]
9. Presence of lactose[c]
10. Printing, scoring, or stamping on the surface
11. Finish of the surface
12. Surface and internal texture
13. Floating and dissolution characteristics
14. Viscosity
15. Sound[d]

[a] These characteristics of placebo medication are intended to be evaluated in comparison to the active medicine. The influence of placebo color on specific patient responses is discussed in the text. Not all of these factors will be relevant for all placebos.
[b] This factor may be important for patients who are susceptible to allergic reactions to specific dyes (e.g., yellow tartrazine dyes).
[c] This factor may be important for patients who are lactose intolerant.
[d] For aerosols and sprays.

tion of dissolution characteristics that meet U.S. Pharmacopeia (USP) standards and also a submission to regulatory authorities [i.e., Food and Drug Administration (FDA) in the United States].

Obtaining Medicines and Placebos

Clinical trial medicines and matching placebos may sometimes be obtained directly from the manufacturer. Printed markings on the medicine's surface must not be present if a placebo is to be used. Obtain placebos that are identical to the trial medicine in color, size, appearance, weight, taste, and even floating and dissolving characteristics (see Table 25.1). If placebos are not virtually identical to the active medicine, then the value of a trial is in jeopardy of being compromised.

Patient Responses to Colors of Placebo: A Basis for Choosing Placebo Color

Patients' responses to placebo have been reported to be sensitive to color, size, form, and number of placebos taken. For example, blue placebo capsules have been associated with sedative effects, red and yellow placebos were associated with stimulant effects, capsules were believed to be more potent than tablets, and larger capsules were perceived to be of a larger medicine strength (Jacobs and Nordan, 1979; Buckalew and Coffield, 1982a,b).

PACKAGING TRIAL MEDICINES

Numerous options to consider in choosing a method to package medicines are listed in Table 25.2.

TABLE 25.2 *Options to consider in determining the details of packaging clinical trial medicines*

1. Will the sponsor, investigator, pharmacist, independent contractor, or another group package the trial medicine?
2. When will the trial medicine be packaged relative to the shipping and starting dates of the trial?
3. Will trial medicine(s) be prepackaged by a sponsor or investigator prior to a trial or packaged from bulk supplies after a patient is screened and evaluated?
4. Will medicine packages be prepared for specific patients, and how will randomization codes be utilized in the packaging?
5. Should medicine containers be made of plastic or glass; should the color of the container be amber or clear; and, should the top be a screw cap or a child-resistant cap? Other relevant questions about the containers may be posed.
6. How much trial medicine should be put into each container to fulfill protocol requirements?
7. How much extra trial medicine should be put into each container to allow for missed or delayed appointments or other contingencies (as well as inserting a few extra tablets or capsules to make a pill count easier to conduct)?
8. Should a separate backup medication bottle be prepared for each patient in case of loss or damage to the original or in case of a missed or delayed appointment?
9. How many extra sets of medication should be packaged to allow for patient dropouts, broken bottles, and additional or replacement patients?
10. Should medicine be packaged by unit dose or unit of use?
11. Should patients be given the same number of capsules (tablets) at each dose during dose ascension?
12. If an active control is used that looks different from the trial medicine, or if different sized capsules will be used to make up certain doses of the trial medicine, how many different types of placebos will be necessary to maintain the blind, and how will the placebos be packaged?
13. If bottles are prepackaged, how should they be grouped for packaging and placement into cartons (e.g., should all bottles for one patient or for one treatment period be grouped together, or should another schema be utilized)?
14. Storage conditions of the medicines may require careful consideration for each point of their journey.
15. How will medicines be shipped to study sites?[a]

[a] See Chapter 30.

Involvement of a Pharmacist

Pharmacists may become involved in the packaging of medicines, particularly in academically oriented non-sponsored clinical trials. Packaging for each patient varies over a broad spectrum from single containers to complex packaging of double dummies, blister packs with printed times to be taken on the foil, or other variations. Randomization codes are used by pharmacists in the packaging and labeling of investigational medicines. To prevent bias, one pharmacist may place randomization codes in sealed envelopes, and then store the codes, in case it is necessary to break them. A second pharmacist is asked to check the codes against the medicines prepared to confirm the accuracy of the containers and codes, and a third pharmacist (who is kept blind to the randomization code) dispenses the medicines.

If a pharmacist at the clinical trial site is chosen to package trial medicines, confirm that the individual chosen has had prior experience with research protocols, especially if a complex packaging scheme is used. Also, determine the number of pharmacists that will be involved (and in what capacity) at each stage of the trial. Discuss with the relevant pharmacist how the randomization code will be utilized in packaging the medicine and what type(s) of dispensing container(s) may be used to maintain the integrity of the medicine. It is generally believed that the number of problems in conducting a clinical trial often increases when too many individuals are involved. The optimal number of individuals to be involved within the pharmacy should be determined (insofar as possible) prior to the trial.

Alternative Packaging Methods

In addition to rigid glass and plastic containers, flexible packaging materials are also used to package medicines. Flexible materials primarily include the use of thin plastic or cellulose films and aluminum foils. Films and laminates are used to make blister packs (push-through and peelable), strip packs, sachets, and other packages that can be used for unit-dose (contains one dose) packaging of solid or liquid medicines. In unit-of-use packaging, each package contains the proper amount of medication for one course of therapy (e.g., 20 tablets in a package labeled day 1 A.M., day 1 P.M., etc. to day 10).

Consequences of Improper Packaging

Improper packaging of a medicine can adversely affect a clinical trial in many ways:

1. If the package is permeable to moisture or gases, it may diminish the stability of a medicine or allow volatile components to be lost. Plastics are well known to be permeable to water vapor, volatile oils, flavorings, some components of creams, and glues used for attaching labels to the container.
2. If the components of the medicine container closure or seal interact with the medicine, then the medicine may leach out certain components from the container closure or seal, or an actual chemical reaction may occur. Teflon-lined closures are usually more inert than closures made of rubber.
3. The opposite phenomenon may occur if the seal, closure, or container absorbs certain chemicals from the medicine product.
4. Photosensitive medicines must be protected from light by the container, and it may also be necessary to keep the container in a dark place.

Consequences of Improper Handling of Medicines

Once the medicine package is opened, there are an entirely new group of potential problems that may adversely affect the clinical trial. Most of the potential problems that relate to trial medication will be directly or indirectly caused by inappropriate actions of individual patients (e.g., placing containers on a radiator, allowing excessive amounts of moisture or light to reach the medicine) and should not affect the entire clinical trial.

Choosing a Packaging Scheme

In determining the most appropriate packaging scheme, an intellectual trial-and-error exercise may be performed in which various possible problems that could occur during the clinical trial are considered. It will be useful to discuss the pros and cons of several alternative approaches before one is adopted. Some of the more common packaging schemes are presented in Table 25.3, and information that may be printed on

TABLE 25.3 *Common packaging schemes[a]*

1. Each dose for each patient is placed in a separate bottle
2. All doses for one patient for a given time period (day, week, month) are placed in a separate bottle
3. All doses for one patient for an entire clinical trial are placed in a separate bottle
4. Each patient is assigned (but not dispensed) a bottle or bottles of medication for the clinical trial, i.e., a bottle remains in a pharmacy or at another controlled site for the duration of the trial. Patients may obtain medicine from the pharmacy or from the nurse for an inpatient trial
5. Each patient receives additional medication in his or her bottle to allow for a missed or delayed appointment and/or to make a pill count to evaluate patient compliance easier to conduct
6. Each patient receives a backup bottle of medication for the clinical trial to allow for loss or damage to the original bottle or for a missed or delayed appointment
7. Each patient is given two bottles for a given time period or for the trial, and the patient takes an equal number of capsules (tablets) from each bottle every time a dose is taken
8. Each patient is given two bottles of two different dosage strengths of one medicine, and the patient takes medication as prescribed
9. Each patient is given or assigned two bottles for each dose. The entire contents of one pair of bottles are ingested at each dose
10. Bulk bottles are supplied to the investigator or pharmacist to be packaged into one of the above schemata
11. All bottles in an open-label clinical trial contain an identical number of capsules and label except for their code numbers. A calculated number of bottles are given to the patient at each visit to last until the next visit
12. Other variations of the above packaging schemata are possible

[a] Although these schemata are described for medicines put into bottles, medicines may be packaged in blister packs (push-through or peelable), paper envelopes, weekly or daily "medication sets," or other containers. Parenteral medicines are often packaged in ampules, multidose vials, prefilled syringes, minibags, or other containers for bolus injection or constant or intermittent infusion.

the labels is illustrated in Table 25.4. If the container is too small to accommodate a label with all required information, the following is sufficient for open-label trials: (1) proprietary name, (2) generic name, (3) lot or control number, and (4) name and place of business of manufacturer, packer, or distributor. All other required information must appear on the outer container or in a package insert.

In double-blind medicine trials with ascending doses, when it is not known how many doses will actually be used in the clinical trial, there is an option that may be useful in packaging individual-dose bottles. Both trial medicine and placebo are packaged, one bottle for each dose, by the sponsor in a double-blind fashion and sent to the investigator's site. Additional placebos are provided and subsequently added to each bottle prior to dosing at the investigator's site to provide the same total number of pills in each bottle. Thus, patients always receive the same number of pills at each dose. This technique has the advantage that one or more active (or placebo) pills may be removed from all containers to be used for the next dose and replaced

TABLE 25.4 *Information that may be placed on clinical trial medicine labels*[a]

1. Clinical trial name and medicine code number, lot (batch) number, formulation number, and form
2. Medicine name for open-label trial, plus active and inactive ingredients (including percent strengths of alcohol and all preservatives)
3. Patient number and group number
4. Clinical trial day, week, or month number (e.g., month 4 or week 5)
5. Proper name of the day, week, or month (e.g., April 2–17)
6. Dosing period number or test day number
7. Time of dosing (e.g., take one tablet at 8 A.M. and one at 8 P.M.)
8. Storage instructions
9. Dosing instructions, indications, and contraindications
10. Investigator's name and telephone number
11. Name and address of manufacturer or product license holder
12. Blank space for investigator or pharmacist to write on. The blanks may be for the patient's group, initials, name, number, and/or date or other data
13. Total number of tablets (capsules) in the container
14. Weight of medicine (both for each capsule and for the total net weight)
15. Volume of contents (e.g., total number of milliliters for a liquid)
16. Statement: "Caution, New Drug, Limited by Federal Law to Investigational Use Only." Other warnings or precautions may be listed
17. Date of expiration
18. Other information may be placed on clinical trial medicine labels

[a] A tear-off portion may be attached with the same (or different) information to place in the patient's data collection form, pharmacy book, or in another place. A third part of the label (attached to the second part) may be prepared with coded information identifying the contents of the bottle. This portion of the label could be opened and examined if the blind had to be broken for a medical emergency.

with placebos if the next dose to be given must be adjusted downwards or kept the same (assuming that the next series of medicine bottles to be used contained a higher dose). In this manner, the patient always receives the same total number of pills at each dose, which is generally preferable in double-blind studies.

Alternatively, one could prepackage all likely doses that would be anticipated to be used or initiate and conduct a new clinical trial to explore a selected portion of the entire dose range in more detail. Since these alternatives are both expensive and wasteful of medicine, a simple solution is to package all patients' medicine bottles at the trial site from bulk supplies. This solution, however, requires using an unblinded individual at the clinical trial site, whereas the first option described above avoids this necessity.

Labeling Packages

The expiration date of an investigational medicine is often not placed on the label, since the medicine would have to be returned to the sponsor or discarded if the expiration date were reached. If the data on expiration are maintained by the sponsor or manufacturer, then appropriate assays may be performed to extend the expiration date. It is desirable for all unused medicine to be returned to a sponsor to have complete accountability.

All ingredients must be listed on the label for products that are not taken by mouth (e.g., otics, topicals, injectables, and ophthalmics). The percent labeled strength must also be shown on labels for injectable medicines. Preservatives and alcohol plus their percent strength must always be shown.

It is important not to label bottles "Treatment A" or "Treatment B" in double-blind trials if the bottles are kept by blinded personnel. In a medical emergency, the code must be broken for one patient, and thus the entire clinical trial will be unblinded. Labeling bottles as "Treatment A," etc. also may serve to bias the investigator into believing that treatment A is either better or worse than treatment B and behaving differently towards different patients depending on which treatment they are receiving.

DISPENSING TRIAL MEDICINES

The same person who packages the trial medicine may dispense it, but this is usually not done. A number of common methods of dispensing and handling trial medicines are listed in Table 25.5. If the medicine is prepackaged with a tear-off portion of the label, then at the time that the medicine is dispensed, this portion may be placed either in the patient's data collection form or in another denoted place.

TABLE 25.5 *Common methods of dispensing and handling clinical trial medicines*

1. Investigator (or research coordinator under the supervision of the investigator) dispenses the trial medicines
2. Pharmacist dispenses the trial medicines
3. Nontrial medicines permitted by protocol are dispensed by investigator or trial pharmacist, or obtained independently by the patient
4. A log may be used by either the investigator or pharmacist to record the number of bottles (pills) dispensed and number of pills returned (see Fig. 25.1)
5. Returned medicines should be stored according to instructions given in the protocol. Prior to the return of the medicine to the sponsor, empty or partially filled containers may or may not be combined and the empty containers discarded
6. Returned medicines should be disposed of by the sponsor or appropriate individuals in accordance with Federal and other guidelines as specified in the protocol and/or in other documentation

TABLE 25.6 *Considerations for deciding whether clinical trial medicines should be dispensed by pharmacists or investigators*

1. Protocol requirements
2. Desires of sponsor (if the clinical trial is sponsored)
3. Desires of investigator
4. Availability and suitability of storage facilities
5. Location and convenience of storage facilities
6. Quality of security of the storage facilities
7. Experience of the pharmacists with conducting clinical trials
8. Availability of staff working with the investigator
9. Quantity of medicine to be dispensed
10. Proximity of the pharmacy to the investigator's clinic
11. How other sites in multicenter trials are planning to dispense medicines
12. Quality of the relationship and communications between the investigator and relevant pharmacists
13. Cost of pharmacy services to dispense medicines and ability to fund this service
14. Desire of the investigator and clinical trial staff to dispense medicines
15. Desire of the pharmacists to dispense medicines in the specific clinical trial

The tear-off portion of the label may contain duplicate information to that attached to the bottle or container as well as a third part to tear open in case of a medical emergency. The third part discloses the patient's treatment. If a pharmacy is involved in dispensing medicines, then a log book or other system should be used to keep relevant information on medicines dispensed. Figure 25.1 illustrates an example of one type of logbook form that may be used by a pharmacy.

ROLES OF DISPENSING PHARMACISTS IN CLINICAL TRIALS

Pharmacists may be involved with virtually any aspect or phase of a clinical trial. They may be well trained to be investigators, coinvestigators, monitors, study coordinators, or data processors, or to fulfill other functions. In some clinical trials pharmacists fulfill the roles most closely associated with their training—packaging and/or dispensing medicines. This section discusses the latter role of dispensing medicines.

Dispensing of Medicines by Pharmacists versus Investigators

Numerous clinical trials must deal with the issue of whether pharmacists or investigators should dispense medicines. When this issue arises there are various considerations (Table 25.6) that should facilitate a decision. Pharmacists should be interviewed in depth about their interest in dispensing medicines by the investigator, his or her staff, or a monitor from a sponsor, if the pharmacy is being considered as a dispensing site. The facilities should be carefully inspected and assessed.

In numerous clinical trials the nature of the medicine

dispensed (e.g., parenteral refrigerated supplies) may strongly suggest, if not require, that pharmacists dispense the medicine. If medicines must be prepared fresh on an as-needed basis, then it is usually important (or essential) for dispensing pharmacists to be included in the clinical trial.

Potential Problems with Investigator Dispensing of Medicines

A common reason why dispensing pharmacists are often included in clinical trials is because of various reports of investigational medicines being kept in investigators' desks, staff lounges, refrigerators specifically used for food, and other inappropriate sites. The exact prevalence of such substandard practices is unknown, but the fear of their occurrence, plus the irreparable harm that this could cause a major clinical trial, has led numerous trial designers to include provisions for competent, qualified, and experienced dispensing pharmacists.

Contact of Pharmacists by Investigators

Physicians conducting an academic (i.e., nonsponsored) clinical trial or a sponsored clinical trial should provide a list of patients enrolled to the pharmacist so that prescriptions for the investigational medicines are only filled for legitimate patients. Alternatively, the initial prescription presented at the pharmacy may be used to enter each patient's name on a clinical trial form created for that purpose, and kept at the pharmacy.

PROTOCOL NO: _____ TITLE OF TRIAL:

Patient Initials _____ Patient No. _____

Complete the following information and use a new line each time trial medication is dispensed or returned.

TREATMENT _____

Date Medicine Dispensed or Returned	7 Digit No. on Bottle (Or Other Code)	Quantity Dispensed (No. of Tablets)	Quantity Returned (No. of Tablets)	Initials of Pharmacist	Comments

FIG. 25.1 Sample pharmacy record indicating the type of information that could be maintained on all clinical trial patients.

Legal and Regulatory Responsibility for Dispensing Medicines

The FDA has stated that investigators have the responsibility for dispensing investigational medicines. This responsibility may be assigned to pharmacists. On the other hand, the Joint Committee on Hospital Accreditation and the American Society of Hospital Pharmacy both state that a pharmacy is responsible for medicines used in investigational trials. This potential conflict has not yet been addressed on a national basis in theory, and is addressed on an ad hoc basis in practice.

Inventory Control

Complete, clear, and accurate records must be maintained for all medicines dispensed. One or more special forms may be created to ensure that these goals are achieved. Separate records must be maintained for each medicine used in a single clinical trial, each dosage form and strength, and each location where medicines are stored. In addition to the size and number of containers dispensed, the name of the person who dispensed the medicine and the date it was dispensed should also be recorded.

An overall plan for inventory control should be created for each clinical trial, including the ordering, organizing, and dispensing of medicines. It may take significant effort and time to plan and organize inventory control, and this aspect of a clinical trial must not be rushed so that errors, or even a high likelihood of errors, may not result. If a central pharmacy has multiple satellite pharmacies involved in a clinical trial, then separate records must be maintained at each individual pharmacy. The accuracy of these records should be ensured by internal and external monitoring by the academic investigator's or sponsor's staff.

Blinding of Pharmacists

In double-blind trials it is usually important that the pharmacist who prepares a medicine not dispense it. This axiom fits the principle that a true double-blind trial includes blinding of all individuals who interact directly with patients. Unblinding of the actual pharmacist who dispenses the medicine raises the potential for him or her to provide undesired feedback to patients or investigators.

Providing Information about Medicines

Pharmacists are often asked about investigational medicines by both physicians and patients; for this reason they may prepare an information sheet. Patients in a clinical trial may ask the dispensing pharmacist questions that may or may not be best answered by the investigator. Pharmacists should refer patients to the investigator or clinical trial staff and discuss any questions or issues raised with the same personnel. Nonetheless, pharmacists have often established a degree of trust and a positive relationship with patients that facilitates the transmittal of information about medicines and its acceptance by patients.

Conducting Pill Counts

Pharmacists may be asked to count pills in containers returned by patients at each visit. This information is used to assess patient compliance, but several recent reports (Rudd et al., 1989; Pullar et al., 1989) have raised serious questions about whether it is possible to consider pill counts as a reliable measure of compliance. As pill counts are used less and less as a measure of compliance, this role will tend to disappear. See Chapter 15 for information on compliance.

ASSIGNING PATIENT NUMBERS

There are several methods of numbering patients in protocols, and the specific method used can provide information about the patient and assist in referring to patients and the data. In a multicenter clinical trial, for example, patients can be assigned numbers as in the following:

Method A
 1 to 30: Patient numbers reserved for site 1
 31 to 60: Patient numbers reserved for site 2
 61 to 90: Patient numbers reserved for site 3
 etc.

Method B
 101 to 130: Patient numbers reserved for site 1
 201 to 230: Patient numbers reserved for site 2
 301 to 330: Patient numbers reserved for site 3
 etc.

In method B, the specific site may be more easily identified than in method A as soon as the patient number is referenced. Another approach used is to assign codes to each site, such as letters, as in method C below:

Method C
 A1 to A30: Patient numbers reserved for site 1
 B1 to B30: Patient numbers reserved for site 2
 C1 to C30: Patient numbers reserved for site 3
 etc.

Method B is the most preferable of these three possibilities from the standpoint of data analysis and ease of communication.

It is desirable to be able to associate easily the name of each specific clinical trial site with a range of patient numbers assigned to that site regardless of the method used to assign patient numbers. Examples of common schemes used to assign specific patient numbers to specific sites for ease of recall include numbering the sites in order by listing the investigators' last names alphabetically or by listing the cities (or hospital names) of the investigators alphabetically. For instance, if a clinical trial is being conducted by three investigators (Drs. Brown, Jones, and Smith) it would be reasonable to assign patients numbers 100 to 199 to Dr. Brown, 200 to 299 to Dr. Jones, and 300 to 399 to Dr. Smith.

If the clinical trial is to be conducted at only one site, then it may be useful to number patients on the basis of the criteria used (if any) to assign them to groups. For example, patients may be assigned to two (or more) groups based on a characteristic of their disease, such as its severity, or based on a characteristic used to stratify patients, such as age, race, or weight.

Numbers could be assigned based on patient characteristics using either method B or C above.

Both site and patient or disease characteristics may be combined in assigning numbers. One example, shown below, used the first number to identify the site, the second for the disease intensity (1, mild; 2, moderate; 3, severe), and the last two for patient numbering. Many variations on these few examples are possible.

Method D

1101 to 1160: Patient numbers at site 1 with a mild intensity of disease.
1201 to 1260: Patient numbers at site 1 with a moderate intensity of disease.
1301 to 1360: Patient numbers at site 1 with a severe intensity of disease.
2101 to 2160: Patient numbers at site 2 with a mild intensity of disease.
2201 to 2260: Patient numbers at site 2 with a moderate intensity of disease.
2301 to 2360: Patient numbers at site 2 with a severe intensity of disease.
etc.

If there are more than ten sites in a clinical trial it is easiest to designate each site by a single-letter code for up to 26 sites. If there are above 26 sites, then a two-letter code may be used. This system is like Method C, although it could be expanded as follows:

Method E

A101–A140: Patient numbers on treatment 1 at site A
A201–A240: Patient numbers on treatment 2 at site A
B101–B130: Patient numbers on treatment 1 at site B
B201–B230: Patient numbers on treatment 2 at site B

CHAPTER 26

Collecting Adverse Event and Adverse Reaction Data in Clinical Trials

TYPES OF ADVERSE REACTIONS

Adverse reactions resulting from a medicine may result from intrinsic toxicity or they may be idiosyncratic. If related to the intrinsic toxicity, the adverse reactions are usually observed earlier in the medicine's development than if they are idiosyncratic. Adverse reactions may be classified into five broad types.

Type I Adverse Reactions: Resulting from an Excessive Dose

Two subtypes of adverse reactions resulting from an excessive dose of a medicine exist, intentional and unintentional overdoses. Examples of the latter include patients who receive an excessive dose because of their low weight or small size, or because they have characteristics (e.g., poor renal function, genetic disorder) that place them high on the dose–response curve for one or more adverse reactions.

Type II Adverse Reactions: Resulting from an Excessive Effect

A prolonged effect of a medicine can lead to that effect being classified as an adverse reaction. This may have been predicted in advance for some cases (e.g., a long-lasting barbiturate given for insomnia will cause fatigue the next morning). Alternatively, some examples are difficult to predict (e.g., a patient who is unable to metabolize a medicine completely, or at all, may experience prolonged effects).

Type III Adverse Reactions: Resulting from Interactions with Medicine or Other Factors

Interactions with medicines, food, or other factors (see Chapter 95) may or may not be predictable (i.e., part of a medicine's intrinsic toxicity).

Type IV Adverse Reactions: Idiosyncratic Effects

Idiosyncratic reactions include allergic and hypersensitive effects, and others with an immunological basis.

Many of these are rare and often are not observed until a new medicine has been used in large numbers of patients, which often occurs after marketing.

Type V Adverse Reactions: Administrative and Suggestive

Recent evidence has supported the often cited contention that mentioning the possibility of adverse reactions to patients in an informed consent may be viewed as a cause of adverse reactions (Myers et al., 1987; Levine, 1987).

ELICITING AND CATEGORIZING ADVERSE EVENTS AND REACTIONS

Adverse events were defined in the terminology section at the beginning of the book as the physical and psychological signs and symptoms of the patient that may or may not be related to the trial medicine, whereas *adverse reactions* are a subset where a relationship exists. Adverse reactions are either predictable or unpredictable, based on the known properties of the medicine. Operational definitions of each anticipated adverse reaction or at least of those most frequently expected in a clinical trial may be established prior to the trial. This would clarify the differences in definitions for adverse reactions that are similar in nature (sleepy, drowsy, fatigued) but that may be used differently by different investigators in a multicenter trial (or even in a trial conducted at one site). Adverse experiences are defined as the group of adverse reactions plus all other medical events that occur during the trial, such as illness or trauma, even though these latter events are generally believed to be unrelated to the trial medicine(s). Laboratory abnormalities are generally considered to lie within the definition given of adverse reactions but are sometimes treated as an independent class of abnormalities.

To Probe or Not To Probe for Adverse Events

A basic question to address in discussing the recording of adverse events is whether to probe for their presence or whether to record only those that are spontaneously reported. Spontaneously reported adverse reactions are of two basic types. In one type, patients are not given any instructions about reporting adverse reactions, and in the other type, patients are instructed to report any and all adverse events. Collecting only spontaneous reports has the disadvantage of probably underestimating the true incidence of adverse reactions, since many patients are reluctant to volunteer this information. Moreover, since patients differ in their willingness to volunteer information, collecting

adverse reactions in this manner introduces another source of variation into the clinical trial. This source of variation may be controlled by standardizing the means of probing for adverse reactions. If adverse reactions are to be probed for, then this probe may take place whenever certain events occur (e.g., dose changes) or at fixed points in the protocol (e.g., once per hour in a single-dose study).

Approaches to Probing for Adverse Events

Three approaches to probing for adverse events are described. In the first, the investigator reads a long list of possible adverse reactions, and the patient responds to those that are felt or experienced. This approach has a disadvantage in that it tends to elicit a greater number of adverse reactions than do the two other methods described below, because reading a list is suggestive to the patient and thus may magnify the true incidence of adverse reactions. A variation of this approach that has the same disadvantage is to have the patients read the list themselves and check off any adverse reactions that apply. Spilker and Kessler (1987) demonstrated that a group of normals report more symptoms in the previous 72 hours if they read a list than if they are asked to list the symptoms themselves. In some respects this is the background noise that exists in any clinical trial, except that for seriously ill patients the noise level is much greater.

In collecting adverse event data, investigators should generally report syndromes (e.g., congestive heart failure) rather than individual clinical signs (e.g., dyspnea, rales, cyanosis). Adverse events occurring secondary to other events (Fig. 26.1) should be identified by the primary cause (e.g., pain after endoscopy, dizziness after blood sampling). An adverse event that is a symptom being treated in a clinical trial must be extremely carefully evaluated to ensure it is not merely a change that is part of natural progression of disease (e.g., depression in a trial with an antidepressant, sneezing in a trial with an antihistamine). Collect all adverse events extremely carefully at baseline and during screen, because they represent the background

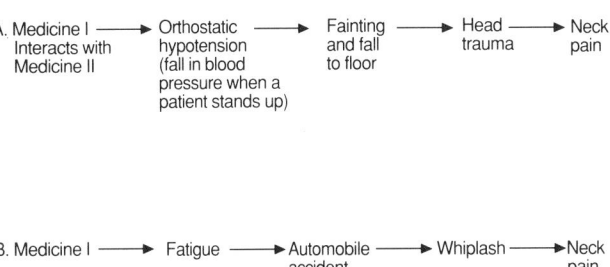

FIG 26.1 Identifying the adverse reaction in a chain of events. The medicine-induced adverse reaction may lead to other adverse events. (Reprinted from Spilker, 1989a, with permission of Raven Press.)

against which emergent or worsening signs are compared.

A second approach is for the investigator or patient to read an abbreviated list of the most commonly observed adverse reactions that have been associated with the clinical trial medicine.

It is the author's view that a third, or "neutral," approach to probing the patient about adverse events is the one that should most frequently be used. The presence of adverse reactions may be elicited using the same question for all patients, phrased in the same manner and tone at all times. This helps to ensure uniformity among patients and treatment periods. One straightforward means of achieving this goal is to formulate a simple question with minimal connotations that can be used as the initial question at all evaluation points in a clinical trial. An example of this type of simple question is: "How have you felt since your last clinic visit?" Another general question is: "Have you had any health problems since you were here last?"

The question "How do you feel?" is considered too general and a cliché and will rarely elicit as accurate a response as desired in all patients. Patients also tend to be more open about adverse reactions with nursing staff than with physicians unless the patients are carefully questioned or probed. This may in part reflect the patient's desire not to "disappoint" the physician with "bad news" about the medicine.

The general question used to probe for adverse reactions should be phrased to avoid direct reference to the clinical trial medicine. This is because patients often attribute adverse reactions to non-medicine-related events and may not associate their adverse reaction with a medicine. Thus, they may be reluctant to volunteer important information about signs and symptoms in responding to a question that directly relates to a medicine, such as "Have you had any problems caused by the medicine?" The period of time that is relevant for the physician to include in his or her questioning should be described in the protocol or data collection forms (i.e., is the probe intended to elicit those adverse reactions that are presently experienced or felt within the last X days or weeks or since the last probe).

Adverse reactions that have previously been reported by the patient should be probed each time a formal probe is conducted. This will allow their duration, intensity, and other characteristics to be followed in time. The degree to which this "reprobe" should be formalized must be determined by the individuals writing the protocol.

INTENSITY OF THE ADVERSE EVENT

If a positive response is elicited to the introductory question, the investigator should probe further to determine (1) the intensity of the symptom, (2) the time of onset, (3) its total duration, (4) whether the adverse reaction is still present, and (5) the frequency of its occurrence. The relationship of the adverse reaction to the clinical trial medicine or trial schedule should be probed (e.g., a headache may be caused by fasting that is part of the study schedule).

The intensity of the adverse reaction should be characterized and then classified into clearly defined categories. One system uses the terms *mild, moderate*, and *severe* for describing the intensity of the adverse reaction. The definitions of these terms and the relationship to the trial medicine may be described as follows:

1. *Mild.* The adverse reaction does not interfere in a significant manner with the patient's normal functioning level. It may be an annoyance.
2. *Moderate.* The adverse reaction produces some impairment of functioning but is not hazardous to health. It is uncomfortable or an embarrassment.
3. *Severe.* The adverse reaction produces significant impairment of functioning or incapacitation and is a definite hazard to the patient's health. This category includes adverse reactions that include or lead to (1) death or decreased life expectancy, (2) a life-threatening event, though acute and without permanent effect, (3) prolonged inability to resume usual life pattern, or (4) impairment of ability to adequately deal with future medical problems.

These three categories (mild, moderate, severe) are based on the investigator's clinical judgment, which in turn depends on consideration of various factors such as the patient's report, the physician's observations, and the physician's prior experience.

A different system for assessing the severity of adverse reactions was proposed by Ta!larida et al. (1979). They used seven categories for their assessments instead of the three described above.

RELATIONSHIP OF AN ADVERSE EVENT TO TRIAL MEDICINE

In evaluating whether an adverse reaction is related to a specific test medicine, there are three different approaches that may be taken. These methods (global introspection, algorithms, and formal logic) are described in more detail in Chapters 72 and 80. Six basic points that should be considered are:

1. Previous experience with the medicine and whether the adverse reaction is known to have occurred with the medicine.
2. Alternative explanations for the adverse reaction, such as the presence of other medicines, illness, new illness, nonmedicine therapies, diagnostic tests, procedures, or other confounding effects.

3. Timing of the events between administration of the medicine and the adverse reaction.
4. Medicine levels and evidence, if any, of overdosage.
5. Dechallenge, i.e., if the medicine dose was decreased or the medicine was stopped, what happened to the adverse reaction?
6. Rechallenge, i.e., what happened if the medicine was restarted after the adverse reaction had disappeared?

This information may be used to characterize the relationship of medicine and adverse reaction into one of any number of predetermined categories. Between three and five categories are usually used to describe the relationship of a medicine to an adverse reaction. An example of a three-category system is: (1) *probably related*, (2) *probably not related*, and (3) *unknown*. This last category may be used when there are insufficient data available to make a judgment about the first two categories. It may also be used when there is equally strong evidence pointing towards both of the other two possibilities.

Definitions are given below for a five-category system that may be used to classify the relationship between adverse reactions and medicine. These are adapted from Karch and Lasagna (1975).

1. *Definite*. A reaction that follows a reasonable temporal sequence from administration of the medicine or in which the medicine level has been established in body fluids or tissues; that follows a known or expected response pattern to the suspected medicine; and that is confirmed by improvement on stopping or reducing the dosage of the medicine, and reappearance of the reaction on repeated exposure (rechallenge).
2. *Probable*. A reaction that follows a reasonable temporal sequence from administration of the medicine; that follows a known or expected response pattern to the suspected medicine; that is confirmed by stopping or reducing the dosage of the medicine; and that could not be reasonably explained by the known characteristics of the patient's clinical state.
3. *Possible*. A reaction that follows a reasonable temporal sequence from administration of the medicine; that follows a known or expected response pattern to the suspected medicine; but that could readily have been produced by a number of other factors.
4. *Unknown*. Relationships for which no evaluation can be made.
5. *Not related*. A reaction for which sufficient information exists to indicate that the etiology is unrelated to the clinical trial medicine.

The three-category system is preferable in the author's view for Phase I and early Phase II studies, since it is usually unethical to rechallenge a patient with a medicine that has caused a suspected effect, especially if the effect was severe in intensity. Also, little information is available about a new medicine at this stage of development, and it is therefore difficult to know if the adverse reaction is typical of the medicine or has been previously observed. Although the three-point scale could theoretically be used in all phases of medicine development, the five-point scale provides a more complete description of adverse reactions that occur in studies conducted in late Phase II through Phase IV. There may be practical reasons, however, to utilize the same system throughout all phases of a medicine's development.

It is common for the nature, frequency, and/or intensity of adverse reactions to change significantly when the personnel reporting and evaluating them also changes. Blanc et al. (1979) have shown that trained investigators often disagree with each other on the relationship between a medicine and an adverse reaction. This factor may have a significant effect on the outcome of the clinical trial and supports the view that it is preferable to have a single investigator collect adverse reaction information on a single patient (and preferably on all patients) throughout a single trial.

Algorithms

A more sophisticated approach to the evaluation of adverse reactions has been proposed by one group of authors in three joint publications (Kramer et al., 1979; Hutchinson et al., 1979; Leventhal et al., 1979). The algorithms they propose are an attempt to relate more accurately the adverse reaction with the medicine as definite, probable, possible, or unlikely. It is the author's view that this approach, although elegant, is not practical in most clinical trials. Another scale, based on ten questions, was proposed by Naranjo et al. (1981) primarily for postmarketing surveillance and Phase III clinical trials. Their questions require a large body of information to be available about the trial medicine and thus are not particularly useful for Phases I and II studies. This topic is discussed further in Chapter 80.

After the information described above on adverse reactions is collected, the investigator must determine the treatment (if any) that will be initiated. The action taken by the investigator is generally one of those shown below.

Actions Taken by Investigators After Observing Adverse Events

Seven common steps (or lack of steps) are taken in response to adverse events:

TABLE 26.1 *Alternative actions (relating to a clinical trial) for severe adverse reactions*[a]

1. No further action is required
2. Notify the FDA or other regulatory authority
3. Notify the Ethics Committee/IRB (a sponsor may confirm with the investigator that this task has been performed)
4. Advise other investigators in a multicenter clinical trial
5. Advise other investigators working with the medicine but using other protocols
6. Revise the informed consent at all sites using the involved protocol or at all sites studying the medicine
7. Modify the involved protocol and submit it to the sponsor and Ethics Committees/IRBs for approval
8. Modify all protocols using the medicine and submit them to the sponsor and Ethics Committees/IRBs for approval
9. Initiate another clinical trial or trials to evaluate the questions raised
10. Suspend the trial at the site(s) using the involved protocol or at all sites studying the medicine
11. Discontinue the trial at the site(s) using the involved protocol or at all sites studying the medicine
12. Consult an expert or convene a panel of experts to discuss the problem and/or issues raised
13. Suspend further development of the medicine
14. Discontinue further development of the medicine

[a] Alternative actions to consider in treating the patient are discussed in the text.

1. None.
2. Increased surveillance of the patient to monitor the adverse event.
3. Counteractive medication or treatment.
4. Changing the dose of medicine in question.
5. Both 3 and 4.
6. Medicine administration is suspended.
7. Medicine administration is discontinued.
8. Other.

The possible approaches listed above relate to how the investigator treats the patient. The investigator must also notify his or her Ethics Committee/Institutional Review Board (IRB) and either the regulatory authority (for unsponsored trials) or the sponsor if serious adverse reactions are observed. Sponsors then have the responsibility of notifying the regulatory authority and of deciding whether the adverse reaction will have any influence on the conduct of the trial. There are several alternatives for sponsors (or investigators) to consider in this regard. These are listed in Table 26.1.

SAFTEE Forms

Other forms have been prepared to record "adverse health events." They are called Systematic Assessment for Treatment Emergent Events (SAFTEE) Form-GI (General Inquiry) and Form-SI (Systematic Inquiry). These forms are available from Jerome Levine, M.D. at University of Maryland, Maryland Psychiatric Research Center, P.O. Box 21247, Catonsville, MD 21228.

The following major items of information are solicited on each adverse event reported:

1. Date of onset (month and day are used if the event first occurred in the interval evaluated; if the event occurred prior to the interval evaluated, "00/00" is used).
2. Duration (recorded in days within the current assessment period).
3. Pattern (continuous, intermittent, or isolated).
4. Current status (ongoing problem or resolved, with or without sequelae).
5. Severity (five grades of intensity are used; this factor is assessed by the investigator through observation and/or the patient's report).
6. Functional impairment (five grades of impairment are used for describing the activities of daily living or of specific activities affected. This factor is assessed by the investigator through observation and/or the patient's report).
7. Contributory factors (one or more possible causes may be checked; seven possible causes plus "*other*" are listed).
8. Relationship of medicine to event [this category differs substantially from usual definitions; it is used to give the reason(s) why the investigator believes that the adverse reaction may be medicine related even if caused by a concomitant medicine: six categories plus "*other (specify)*" and "*not applicable*" are listed].
9. Action taken [seven possible actions plus "other (specify)" and "don't know" are listed].
10. Comments, descriptors, and additional specification (allows for text to be written into the form).

It is not possible to state at this time whether the SAFTEE forms will be widely used in clinical trials and replace previous measures of adverse reactions developed by the government: Dosage Record and Treatment Emergent Symptoms (DOTES), Treatment Emergent Symptom Scale (TESS), and Self-Rating Treatment Emergent Symptom Scale (STESS). It is the author's view that the SAFTEE forms appear to be preferable to the older government scales described.

MEASURES OF FREQUENCY

When indicating the frequency of occurrence of an adverse reaction, a disease or some other factor, a number of methods may be used.

1. *Counts.* This is the simplest approach and presents raw data. It is usually desirable to do this as the first presentation (but not the only one). A common presentation is to show a histogram of the number of cases (examples) per year.

2. *Cumulative incidence.* This approach typically presents the number of events during a specified period of months or years divided by the number of persons initially at risk. It applies to a fixed group (cohort). It may be used to illustrate the probability that a person will experience a specific event during a 5- (or other) year period.

3. *Incidence density.* Number of new occurrences of a disease in a population observed over a specified period of time divided by the total amount of person time (e.g., people years) experienced by members of the population during that period. This is also referred to as the hazard rate, and allows for observations in a dynamic population.

4. *Prevalence.* The frequency of a disease or event at a particular point in time. This is a snapshot of frequency relative to population or group size at a particular time (usually the present). Prevalence may be viewed over a period of time by comparison (e.g., the prevalence of disease X in the United States was A cases in Y population in 1930 and B cases in Z population in 1940). Each frequency measure can be associated with a confidence interval, and it is desirable that the interval be presented too, since its size depends on the particular situation measured.

5. *Incidence.* Rate of occurrence of something. Incidence is the number of specified events per specified group or population per specified time period. Two examples are:
   a. Number of new cases of disease X per 100,000 Americans per year.
   b. Number of new cases of adverse reaction "X" per 1,000 people taking the medicine.

Incidence requires both a numerator and denominator, and in presenting data both must be specified. Incidence rates refer to new cases of a disease or problem.

CHAPTER 27

Informed Consent and Ethics Committee/ Institutional Review Board Processes

INTRODUCTION

This chapter concentrates on the informed consent for participating in a clinical trial. (Consents are also given by patients whenever they are being diagnosed or treated by physicians or other health professionals.) Many clinical trial issues involve informed consents, and this chapter only addresses a selected number. Interested readers are referred to several fine monographs (Veatch, 1977; Barber, 1980; American Psychological Association, 1982; Levine, 1986) for additional details and discussions.

Informed consent may be defined as a patient's (1) being given adequate information about a clinical trial, (2) understanding and voluntarily accepting the terms of a clinical trial, and (3) agreeing to cooperate in its

conduct. The informed consent form (or simply an informed consent) presents information on which this concept is based and must be signed by the patient in the United States and some other countries. In some situations, this document may be replaced by a verbal discussion, with or without a signed statement that the patient agrees to enter the clinical trial. The patient must be a competent individual who can evaluate the benefit-to-risk concept. In other words, the patient should be able to choose his or her best alternative. It is the author's belief that it *is* possible to inform patients adequately about a clinical trial and that most patients with appropriate knowledge are capable of making a prudent choice.

No matter how well an informed consent is written and no matter how thoroughly a physician discusses

202

the trial's benefits and risks with a patient, a poorly designed clinical trial (with basic flaws or biases that will eventually make the data uninterpretable) is unethical to conduct. If a clinical trial is designed with too few patients to obtain acceptable power, then it is also unethical. Such trials are unethical primarily because they place the patients who are enrolled at risk unnecessarily. In addition, these clinical trials may raise needless questions that require additional trials to resolve.

ETHICAL AND REGULATORY REQUIREMENTS AND GUIDELINES

Many national, international, and professional guidelines and regulations describe and protect the patient's right to an informed consent before he or she may be given an experimental therapy. It is surprising to some people that almost all of these protections arose during the last 50 years. Before 1900 the only ethical guidelines for performing experimentation related to the physician's need to adhere to acceptable medical standards in designing and conducting a clinical trial. The issue of a patient's agreement was never addressed (Veatch, 1977). It may be argued, however, that there has always been an ethical responsibility on the part of a physician to adequately inform a patient who was enrolled in a clinical trial and received an experimental treatment and to obtain that patient's consent.

Major milestones for informed consents include the Nuremburg code (1949), which was an outcome of World War II; the Helsinki Doctrine of the World Medical Association (1964); and legislation in the United States regarding Institutional Review Boards (Volume 46 *Federal Register* 8975, January 27, 1981, 21 Code of Federal Regulations 56) and informed consent (45 FR 36390, May 30, 1980 21 CFR 50).

WHO OBTAINS THE INFORMED CONSENT?

The regulations governing informed consents do not cover many of the nuances relating to the individual who actually obtains the informed consent. For example, if a nurse, research coordinator, or other individual obtains the informed consent but is not able or qualified to discuss the details of the protocol or alternative treatments, then the signed consent form may not be legally valid if it is ever challenged. Variations on the traditional means of obtaining informed consents are discussed by Hassar and Weintraub (1976). They suggest that (1) holding a group meeting of patients, (2) testing patient comprehension, and (3) including relatives in discussions are among the techniques that can improve patient comprehension of the benefits and risks inherent in a trial.

When Is an Informed Consent Not Required?

United States regulations (Section 50.23) do not require an informed consent if (1) the patient is confronted by a life-threatening situation necessitating use of an investigational medicine, (2) the patient is unable to communicate and family members are not present or available, (3) there is insufficient time to obtain an informed consent, *and* (4) there is no alternative method of acceptable treatment available and therapy must be initiated rapidly.

ELEMENTS OF INFORMED CONSENT AND EXAMPLES

Each investigator should be familiar with his or her national guidelines on informed consent and procedures under which this obligation is conducted (for the United States, see Food and Drug Administration, 1981a; the regulations are summarized in Table 27.1). Investigators in other countries must familiarize themselves with the relevant laws. The protocol may state that the purpose of the clinical trial will be explained to the patient in the presence of a witness (plus the parent or legal guardian for pediatric trials) and an informed consent obtained.

Types and Elements

Although a witness is only required (in the United States) if the informed consent is obtained orally or in a summary written form, including a witness in the informed consent procedure is generally prudent. Elements to include are listed in Table 27.1, and a sample (generic) informed consent is shown in Fig. 27.1. A sample form used to obtain a pregnancy waiver from women of childbearing potential is illustrated in Fig. 27.2.

Examples of Statements That May Be Included

1. An infection or blood clot in the arm could possibly develop from the needle that will remain in your arm on days ___ and ___.
2. Your participation in this clinical trial will not result in any direct medical benefit to you personally.
3. During this ___ week clinical trial you will remain in the ___ hospital (medical school) for ___ consecutive ___ (e.g., Friday) nights and will remain there until approximately ___ P.M. on ___ (the next day), at which time you will be released. You are expected to return at ___ (time) every ___ and ___.

TABLE 27.1 *Elements of informed consent*

An informed consent must be written by the investigator, approved by the Institutional Review Board (IRB) (or Ethics Committee), signed by the subject (patient or volunteer) or authorized representative, and witnessed.

The points below must be included in all informed consents:
1. A statement that the study involves research, an explanation of the purpose of the research and the expected duration, a description of the procedures, and identification of any procedures that are experimental
2. A description of any reasonably foreseeable risks or discomforts to the patient
3. A description of the benefits to the patient or to others that may be expected from the research
4. A disclosure of appropriate alternative procedures or courses of treatment, if any, that might be advantageous to the patient
5. A statement describing the extent, if any, to which confidentiality of the records identifying the patient will be maintained and that FDA may inspect the records
6. For research involving more than minimal risk, an explanation as to whether any compensation will be paid, whether any medical treatments are available if injury occurs, and what those treatments are; information should also be provided on how further information about this study may be obtained
7. An explanation of whom to contact for answers to questions and whom to contact in the event of a research-related injury
8. A statement that participation is voluntary, that refusal to participate will involve no penalty or loss of benefits to which the patient is otherwise entitled, and that the patient may discontinue participation at any time without penalty

Additional elements of informed consent that must be present when appropriate:
1. A statement that the particular treatment or procedure may involve risks to the patient or to the fetus (if the patient is pregnant) that are currently unforeseeable
2. Anticipated circumstances under which the patient's participation may be terminated by the investigator
3. Any additional costs to the patient resulting from participation in the research
4. The consequences and procedures for withdrawing from the research
5. A statement that significant new findings (such as new hazards) developed during the research will be provided to the patient
6. The approximate number of patients who will be enrolled in the clinical trial

may be designated by Dr. ____ to assist or act in his or her behalf.
7. Because blood samples are being taken during this clinical trial, you should not volunteer to donate blood for at least 2 months after participation in this trial.
8. During this clinical trial your urine will be collected at random and unannounced times. It will be checked to confirm that you have not taken any medicines that are not allowed in the trial.
9. If we are unable to contact you directly during this clinical trial, we want to obtain your permission to contact your family, friends, employers, or other sources so that we may reach you to learn about your medical status.
10. You may be given a blank medication at random periods throughout this clinical trial and for durations that will not be told to you. This medication is called a placebo. Your chances of receiving a placebo are one in ____.
11. We would like to visit you at your home one time during this clinical trial in order to obtain a blood (urine or other) sample. We will (or will not) contact you prior to our visit.
12. This medicine has already been approved for marketing and is sold only with a doctor's prescription.
13. The purpose of this clinical trial is to gather information on the benefits and problems associated with this medicine.
14. This clinical trial is a continuation of the trial "[Protocol Title]" in which you previously participated. The purpose of the present trial is to evaluate long-term effects of ____ in patients who have benefited from this medicine. This trial will last for ____ months (years).

Additional Information That May Be Incorporated

Receiving a Placebo or Active Medicine

Discuss placebo medication and estimate the chances for any patient to receive a placebo. If the patient receives a placebo in the clinical trial, what are his or her possibilities of receiving the active medicine at a later date? If a patient receiving placebo may receive the active medicine after the "end" of the original trial, it must be clarified whether the "end" represents the termination of the patient's participation, the completion of all patients' participation, or the conclusion of the analysis of the data indicating that the medicine does in fact possess clinically significant efficacy. The distinction among these three time points for providing active medicine to patients may be several months or years and would have great significance for a patient who is considering enrollment in a long-term trial.

4. The estimated amount of radiation you will receive during this clinical trial from the radioactive medicine is ____ rads (total body dose). The following scale of radiation doses is provided for comparative purposes.

    One dental X-ray = 0.2 to 0.5 rads
    Fluoroscopic examination = 10 rads/min
    Abdominal X-rays (upper GI series) = 20 rads
    Normal chest X-ray = 0.01 to 0.05 rads
    Background radiation from natural sources = 0.1 to 0.5 rads/year

5. This clinical trial is to evaluate the medicine in a broad population of patients with ____ disease.
6. During this clinical trial you will be under the medical supervision of Dr. ____. Other professionals

Full Title of Protocol: _____

Name of Patient: _____

Date of Birth: _____ Age: _____ Sex: _____

Address: _____

Telephone: _____

1. *Purpose of the Trial*
   Medicine A is an experimental medicine developed by _____ Corporation and being evaluated for use in _____ disease. It has been tested extensively in animals to show this effect as well as to demonstrate that it is a safe medicine. Initial human trials, conducted in _____ normal volunteers, have demonstrated that Medicine A is generally safe at the doses that will be tested in this trial. At these doses, only mild adverse reactions (side effects) were observed. At _____ times higher doses, a number of other side effects were observed. This trial on Medicine A will last for _____ (days, weeks, months), and the purpose is to (1) evaluate its effectiveness in _____ _____ disease, (2) evaluate the tolerance of patients to therapeutic doses of Medicine A, and (3) study blood levels of the medicine. Two previous efficacy trials have demonstrated that Medicine A has been effective in _____ disease and was well tolerated.

   This trial has been approved by the _____ Medical University Institutional Review Board, which is an "Ethics Committee" charged by the U.S. Department of Health and Human Services to ensure that the rights of human subjects are protected. The trial is under the direction of Dr. _____ .

2. *Procedures to be Followed*
   In this trial you will be examined in these offices at _____ to _____ day (week, months) intervals over a total period of _____ days (weeks, months). During the trial you will have 2 to 4 samples of your blood taken for tests on Days _____ , _____ , _____ , and _____ , 2 urine tests on the same days, an electrocardiogram (ECG) on Days _____ and _____ , physical examinations on Days _____ and _____ , ophthalmological (eye) examinations on Days _____ and _____ , plus the following tests to measure your _____ disease: _____ (Days. . .), _____ (Days. . .) etc.

   This trial is a double-blind trial of _____ patients, lasting _____ weeks (months). The trial will compare Medicine A with a placebo. This means that you will not know whether the pill that you are given to take during the trial will be Medicine A or a pill that looks identical to Medicine A, but which is inactive. You will have to take this pill _____ times a day (at _____ , _____ , and _____ o'clock) and will not know whether you have received Medicine A or the placebo until after the trial is completed. The doctor and staff also will not know which of the two medicines you have been given. The identity of the pill can be determined immediately if any medical problem develops and it becomes important to learn which medicine you have been given.

   You will (will not) continue to take any other medicines you are presently taking to treat _____ , but you cannot change the dose of this other medicine during this trial.

FIG. 27.1 Sample sections to include in an informed consent. See text for additional statements that could be included.

Nonmedicines That May Affect the Clinical Trial

There are a variety of nonmedicine factors in many Phase II or III clinical trials that may have a marked influence on the outcome of a trial. Two such examples are the diet followed in a trial testing a lipid-lowering medicine and the amount of bed rest in patients receiving a medicine to modify acute back pain. If these factors are included in an informed consent or are personally discussed with patients at the start of a clinical trial, there is a reasonable chance that their inclusion may modify patient behavior, yet it may not be desired to standardize these nonmedicine treatments within the trial design. Under such conditions, investigators should be instructed how to approach these topics with patients in order to minimize the effect that patient-induced changes in diet, behavior, activity, or other factors will have on the trial as well as to minimize the variations that will occur between different sites.

Contact with the Trial Site

For clinical trials of long duration, the patient may be requested to maintain periodic (e.g., annual) contact with the clinic for a certain number of years even if he or she is no longer actively participating in the trial.

3. *Risks*

Medicine A is a new medicine and there is limited information available on its effects in humans. This medicine has been previously studied in _____ people and the most commonly observed adverse reactions at the doses you may receive were _____ , _____ , and _____ of _____ intensity. At higher doses, the following adverse reactions of _____ intensity were observed: _____ , _____ , and _____ . If these or other adverse reactions occur and become intolerable or severe the dose will be reduced or completely stopped.

There is a remote chance that you will experience an allergic reaction to the medicine, such as a skin rash, hives or possibly a more serious problem such as breathing difficulties or shock. It is not possible to predict in advance if any of these problems will develop, but if they do, you will be promptly treated.

Blood will be drawn at each clinic visit (a total of _____ blood drawings will be made over _____ months). The procedure of taking blood may cause local discomfort, bruising, swelling and rarely a local infection.

4. *Benefits*

The medicine is being studied as a potential treatment for _____ disease. It is therefore possible that it may improve your condition. Of course, this cannot be guaranteed or promised and you may not receive the experimental treatment.

Optional: If you do not receive the experimental treatment during this trial, then you will have an opportunity to receive this treatment within _____ months after this trial is completed.

5. *Alternative Treatments*

There are other medicines used to treat _____ disease. These drugs are: _____ , _____ , and _____ . If you wish, Dr. _____ will explain the benefits and risks of receiving treatment with any (or all) of these medicines. In addition to medicines, _____ disease may also be treated by the following non-medicine methods: _____ , _____ , and _____ . Dr. _____ will also discuss these treatments with you if you wish. You also have the alternative of not being treated. The possible consequences of this action can also be discussed with you.

6. *Confidentiality of the Records*

Your medical records that are related to this trial will be maintained in confidentiality. The sponsor (_____ Co.) may examine your medical records, as long as your name cannot be identified from these records.

Your records from this trial may be submitted by _____ Co. to the Food and Drug Administration (FDA), but your name will not be able to be identified from such records. No identity of any specific patient in this trial will be disclosed in any public reports or publications. The FDA has the right upon proper judicial order to review pertinent medical records and other data with your name identified. They are required by law, however, to handle this information in a confidential manner.

7. *If Problems Develop*

If any serious problems develop you will receive prompt and appropriate medical attention. It is agreed that the facilities of _____ Hospital will be made available to you. Reasonable medical treatment will be free when provided through the facilities of _____ Hospital. Financial compensation is not available for medical treatment elsewhere, loss of work, or other expenses.

FIG. 27.1 (Continued)

In the event that this contact is not maintained, the patient should be informed that the center reserves the right to locate the patient in order to determine his or her medical condition or vital status.

CHARACTERISTICS AND ISSUES OF INFORMED CONSENT

Several different types of informed consents, with different characteristics, will be discussed: (1) oral or written, (2) long or short, (3) concerned with pregnancy, and (4) obtained from the patients who will participate in the clinical trial or from another source (e.g., family member, court order, committee).

Oral versus Written Informed Consents

The clear distinction between totally verbal and totally written informed consents has been blurred in recent years. A signature may be given after an oral descrip-

8. *Financial Considerations*
   After participating in this trial, you will be given $ _____ . If you do not complete the trial then you will not receive this money. To help pay for your transportation and meals, you will also be given $ _____ per clinic visit.

   Optional:
   1. There will be no financial benefits to you or your family for participating in this trial.

   2. If you complete at least half of the _____ week (month) trial then you will receive one-half the usual amount of money (i.e., you will receive $ _____).

   3. If you do not complete the trial, payment will be prorated, based on the percent of the trial that you have completed.

9. *Obtaining Additional Information*
   You are encouraged to ask any questions that occur to you at this time or to ask questions at any time during your participation in the trial. You will be given a copy of this agreement for your own information. If you desire more information at a later date you may call _____ at _____ (during daytime hours) or _____ (at night).

10. *Basis of Participation*
    You are free to withdraw your consent to participate in this trial at any time. If you choose to do so, your rights to present or future medical care by Dr. _____ or at _____ Hospital will not be affected.

11. *Signature*
    I have read the above information and have had an opportunity to ask any questions and all of my questions have been answered. I consent to taking a medication called _____ . I fully understand that its use in humans is limited and that its safety and effectiveness have not been fully established and that there is a risk of adverse reactions to the medicine. I **have been given** a copy of this consent form.

    Signature _____ Date _____
                      (Patient)

    Signature _____ Date _____
         (Parent or Legal Guardian)

    I, the undersigned, have fully explained the relevant details of this trial to the patient named above and/or the person authorized to consent for the patient. I am qualified to perform this role.

    Signature _____ Print _____ Date _____
              (Investigator)   Name

    Signature _____ Print _____ Date _____
              (Witness)   Name

    Address of Witness _____

    (*Important Note:* For all women of child-bearing potential who are entering this trial include discussion of the Pregnancy Waiver Form and request agreement to its terms, signified by the patient's signature on the form).

FIG. 27.1 (Continued)

tion of the clinical trial and a signature may be omitted after a written paper is read. These two types of informed consent may be described as either oral or written.

In some countries and situations it is either impractical or it is not the established practice to obtain a written informed consent. An oral informed consent should always be witnessed by another person and the consent should be documented on paper with the patient's signature plus names, addresses, and signatures of the witness(es). The professional relationship of the witness to the person obtaining the informed consent may be relevant to state. The investigator should provide the patient with the same information, if possible, for an oral as for a written informed consent. Unfortunately, a completely oral informed consent may not involve witnesses, or signatures.

Some physicians feel strongly that oral informed consents are totally adequate and need not be replaced with written ones. Advocates of this position stress the individual and personal nature of the communication between physician and patient. They state that the appropriate and valid informed consent for each patient differs and should be customized individually by the physician. The author believes that these views provide an even stronger argument for using a written informed consent, in addition to any information the physician wishes to discuss verbally with the patient. The use of a written informed consent form ensures that each patient has received at least the standard (i.e., minimum) amount and type of information designed for all patients, which has been reviewed by an Ethics Committee. Moreover, a patient who has a copy of the written informed consent may easily review or study it at a later time when he or she is more relaxed or has more time or interest. Unfortunately, some investigators define written informed consent as having a patient read but not sign a written document, and others define it as having a patient's signature agreeing to enter the clinical trial based on a verbal request. Others do not provide a copy to patients.

In every country, the investigator is free to discuss the clinical trial with each patient in any terms that are appropriate. To obtain an informed consent *only* on the basis of an oral discussion does not assure anyone, except possibly the investigator, that the patient has been provided adequate information to arrive at a valid informed consent. There is a danger that the physician is "playing God" and imposing his or her own personal standards as to what information "He or She" will provide to each patient. The information, however, may or may not be sufficient or appropriate for the situation and needs of the individual patient. The author believes that this practice is unethical and that each patient entering a clinical trial is entitled to receive an acceptable minimal amount of information on a sheet of paper, even if no signature is obtained.

Written informed consents are being used more widely throughout the world, especially when the clinical trial is either directed from the United States or will be used as part of a regulatory submission in the United States.

Long versus Short Informed Consent Forms

The length of an informed consent is sometimes an issue. In the 1960s and early 1970s the difference between long and short forms primarily related to the amount and type of information presented on potential adverse reactions. There was a common belief that informed consent forms had to contain a description or at least a listing of all of the remotely possible adverse reactions and other negative consequences that could be imagined to occur in a clinical trial. Thus, a longer form would present extensive risk information, whereas it was only summarized in a shorter form. The sample informed consent shown in Fig. 27.1 is longer than the majority of such forms used. The inclusion of any of the specific points described above will make

the form even longer. Although this may seem to be excessively long, the information may be read at a leisurely pace by the patient. The patient will also be given a copy to refer to at a later time. Epstein and Lasagna (1969) reported that there was an inverse relationship between the length of the informed consent form and the comprehension of the form by the patients. They suggested that brief information be presented. The informed consents they compared, however, differed almost exclusively in the amount of information on risks that were presented by the medicine (aspirin, in their study). Also, only a brief statement of aspirin's common uses was included. Since there are new Federal regulations requiring the presentation of additional information to the patient, and since the present sample form does not overly emphasize the risks inherent in the hypothetical trial, the relatively long form is not considered to be a drawback to obtaining patient participation as long as the patient is able to understand the language used. The author agrees with Epstein and Lasagna that an excessive amount of peripheral risk information (e.g., all of the unusual adverse reactions reported for the medicine) is unwarranted. It is therefore no surprise that Epstein and Lasagna (1969) observed that patients were less willing to enroll in trials when presented with a longer informed consent. Federal regulations were not as clearly defined as they are today, and the required elements of an informed consent (Table 27.1) were not promulgated at the time of their study. When a long informed consent is written today, it is usually because some or all of these elements are described in more detail, not because less or more information on adverse reactions is being presented.

White et al. (1984) compared patient preferences for a long versus short informed consent form in chemotherapy trials. A majority of patients (51 of 75) preferred the longer form. Patients who initially were given the short form to read felt the information presented was adequate, but when they read the longer form, 65% of this group preferred the longer form. Increasing the amount of detail did not increase the patients' stress.

One of the best approaches to deciding how much information to present to patients is to determine the amount considered to be a lowest common denominator for all patients. This amount is then put in the written form and patients are encouraged (both verbally in discussion and in a written manner via the informed consent) to ask both general and specific questions about the clinical trial, definitions of any terms not understood, and their participation in it.

Pregnancy Waiver

Women of childbearing potential may not receive new investigational medicines until various teratogenicity and reproduction studies have been conducted in animals. Even then it is desirable that female patients not become pregnant while taking an investigational medicine. Because of this intention, a pregnancy waiver form is sometimes used. It may be considered either an addendum to the informed consent or as a separate informed consent. It is generally discussed and signed by the patient at the same time as the informed consent. The female patient (of childbearing potential) agrees either to abstain from sexual relations during the clinical trial or to use contraceptive methods that have been approved by the investigator. A sample form is shown in Fig. 27.2.

Consents Obtained from Special Groups of Patients

In numerous situations and patient populations it may be unacceptable or impossible to obtain an informed consent from the patient, and a parent, guardian,

judge, or close relative usually must provide it. Some of the groups who cannot provide an informed consent include: mentally incompetent patients, embryos, newborns, young children, patients in a coma, and potential organ donors. There is a growing body of opinion, however, stating that no one but the clinical trial participants themselves (if over 18 years) may provide consent, no matter how handicapped they are or whatever their degree of legal competence. The use of proxy consents is being challenged (Bicknell, 1989). A very different approach, using volunteer committees to provide informed consent for incompetent mentally disabled patients, is being evaluated (Sundram, 1988). It is controversial as to whether prisoners are able to provide an informed consent, but the general consensus at this time is that they are not.

Children above the age of approximately 7 years should be asked for their own assent, in addition to obtaining an informed consent from their parent(s) or guardian(s). Special considerations for obtaining in-

SAMPLE PREGNANCY WAIVER

For Females Only

The following procedures will be read and explained to all prospective trial patients of child-bearing potential:

(a) Patient is not known to be pregnant based upon results of the screening pregnancy test.

(b) Pregnancy tests will be administered at specified intervals (see protocol) during the trial and again at the end of the trial.

(c) Patients who are physiologically capable of becoming pregnant will voluntarily sign a statement (see below) indicating their intent not to become pregnant during the course of the trial, and they will agree to employ contraceptive methods acceptable to the investigator during the course of the trial period.

(d) Should a patient become pregnant during the trial, active drug treatment will be immediately discontinued. Monthly or bimonthly monitoring will be conducted by an obstetrician/gynecologist and pediatrician for up to two months following the end of pregnancy to assess the development of the fetus/infant.

VOLUNTARY STATEMENT OF INTENT TO AVOID PREGNANCY

I, _____ (print name) understand the above statements. Furthermore, I agree to attempt to avoid pregnancy while I am participating in this trial. Should I have sexual relations during this period, I will employ a contraceptive method that has been approved by my physician. I will immediately contact Dr. _____ if pregnancy is suspected. I am aware that I may decline to sign this statement and that my refusal to sign will have no effect on the further treatment of my disease at this clinic.

DATE _____ SIGNATURE _____
Patient

DATE _____ SIGNATURE _____
Witness

FIG. 27.2 Sample form that can be utilized as a pregnancy waiver for women of childbearing potential who enter a medicine trial. This form would be used in conjunction with the informed consent.

formed consents in children have been described (Pearn, 1984).

The question of competency is judged in legal terms. Models are available for physicians who desire assistance in determining a patient's competency (Drane, 1984; Spilker, 1987b). It was reported that the most common problem in recognizing incompetence was with previously competent patients who became transiently incapacitated during hospitalization (Munetz et al., 1985). Appelbaum and Grisso (1988) describe four related skills that are a legal prerequisite for establishing competency to consent to treatment: (1) communicating choices, (2) understanding relevant information, (3) appreciating the current situation and its consequences, and (4) manipulating information rationally.

Language Used

There is a wide variation in the quality and adequacy of written informed consents. One reason for this variation is that discussion of one or more elements may be missing. Another problem lies in the level of the language used. Modern word processing systems can help generate language suitable for any level of education. The proper level to use has been a subject of great debate for over a decade.

The comprehension level of language used in in-

formed consents should be tailored to the patient population. A study that will include patients with various levels of education should generally use language readily understood by at least 90% of the patients. Other patients may be coached and if desired an informal assessment of their degree of understanding may be conducted. Consent forms may be written in first, second, or third person style (e.g., I understand that I will be required to . . . , you will be required to. . . . , it is required that patients . . .). Informed consents may also combine different writing styles (i.e., first-, second-, and/or third-person descriptions) in different parts of the consent form. There is no single universally accepted rule as to which style is preferable. The overall language used and its connotations should neither be optimistic nor pessimistic about the patient's risks and potential benefits. Language should clearly indicate that the investigator cannot know or anticipate everything that may occur. The probability of the most significant risks for the patient should be discussed in easily understood terms and should avoid sophisticated scientific and legal terms. A number of general formats used to write informed consents are shown in Table 27.2.

Evaluating and Improving Patient's Understanding of Informed Consents

There is often a great difference between the readability of an informed consent form and the patient's understanding of it. The former may be assessed with standard scales, and the latter by testing the patient. Although the patient's understanding and recall of the words used may be readily tested, comprehension of the concepts involved (e.g. benefit-to-risk ratio) is difficult to measure even in controlled settings.

In certain situations it is often relevant to determine how well the patient has understood the contents of the informed consent, e.g., when the patient does not speak English as a native language or the patient appears to be confused or unclear about the study. Approaches vary from simple verbal questions (e.g., "Do you feel that you understand the contents of this document?") to extensive written tests to quantitate the degree of comprehension (Hassar and Weintraub, 1976; Howard et al., 1981; Riecken and Ravich, 1982; Benson et al., 1985; Irwin et al., 1985; Stanley et al., 1985). As expected, patients differ widely in their recall and understanding of a study. It may be useful to have the sample informed consent read by lay people to review it for comprehensibility. The group of lay people chosen should have the same educational background as the patient population to be tested.

It is ironic that patients entering a clinical trial with aspirin (or another commonly used medicine) will be informed in detail about many of aspirin's potential

TABLE 27.2 *Four alternative organizational formats used to prepare informed consents[a]*

A. Following the order of elements of informed consent specified by United States regulations[b]

B. 1. Purpose
2. Procedures
3. Risks
4. Benefits
5. Alternatives
6. Signatures

C. 1. Demographic information about patient (name, date of birth, sex, address, telephone number, social security number)
2. Brief history of the medicine's background and purpose of the present trial
3. Synopsis of the protocol
4. Statement of rights and details of the patient's agreement
5. Disposition and confidentiality of the records and data
6. Signatures and telephone numbers

D. 1. Research design (e.g., purpose of clinical trial, treatments studied, randomization and double-blind procedures if applicable)
2. Pros and cons of enrollment (e.g., risks, time commitments, discomforts, procedures, alternative treatments, benefits to the patient, benefits to society)
3. Convenant between investigator and patient (e.g., voluntary participation, confidentiality of records, limitations of medical liability)

[a] Alternatives B, C, and D would include information on all of the required elements listed in A, but would be organized differently.
[b] See Table 27.1.

TABLE 27.3 *Selected methods to increase the level of a patient's comprehension about a clinical trial*

A. Writing the informed consent form
1. Use words of one and two syllables whenever possible
2. Use short declarative sentences
3. Avoid legal phases
4. Follow a format that leads the patient logically through all parts of the clinical trial
5. Explain scientific terms and words in lay language (e.g., "test to look at brain waves" instead of EEG or electro-encephalogram)

B. Evaluating the informed consent form
1. Assess the readability with a standard scale (e.g., Flesch, Fry)
2. Assess the comprehension by having nontrial patients read and critique the form
3. Assess connotations of words used to ensure that patients are not misled

C. Counseling the patient
1. Review the overall nature of the clinical trial with each patient before they read the form
2. Have group question-and-answer sessions of several patients and supply background information
3. Have the patients keep the form for at least 12 to 24 hours before they are requested to sign
4. Repeat some or all aspects of the informed consent procedure during the trial
5. Have a patient advocate clarify issues with the patient

D. Other
1. Provide counseling to the patient's family who are instructed to discuss informed consent issues with patients
2. Divide the process into two parts, by which the second is done on a different day and confirms that the patient still desires (or is willing) to enroll and has no further questions
3. Have the patient explain the form to the investigator or another person to verify that the patient understands the nature of the clinical trial

adverse reactions, but the same patients treated in private practice are often advised to use aspirin with minimal or no other information provided. If it is considered important to improve the patient's understanding of the informed consent, it may be useful to utilize some of the methods in Table 27.3. Investigators must tell patients any relevant information that arises during the study that may affect the patient's informed consent and willingness to continue in the clinical trial.

ETHICS COMMITTEE/INSTITUTIONAL REVIEW BOARD REVIEW OF INFORMED CONSENTS

The Institutional Review Board (IRB) must review and approve an investigator's protocol and informed consent form in the United States before the study may be initiated. Other countries that have a comparable review group (i.e., an Ethics Committee) have different regulations. In the United States, the IRB must have at least five members including at least one physician and at least one who must be unaffiliated with the institution. An IRB may not be composed entirely of men or women of one profession, and at least one

member must be a nonscientist. Nonvoting consultants may be used. Experiences of Ethics Committees in the United Kingdom were reviewed by Wells and Griffin (1989).

IRBs may be institutional or independent. They may be formed on either a nonprofit or profit basis. They primarily consider the ethical acceptability of protocols and informed consent forms, along with other responsibilities (Table 27.4).

In reviewing the investigator's written informed consent form, the IRB must confirm that it includes all information required by law (see Table 27.1). The IRB may also view the informed consent in the context of one or both of the following questions:

1. Does this informed consent contain all of the information that most doctors in the community would provide to their patients under similar circumstances?
2. Does this informed consent contain all of the information that a patient would want to know who is considering enrollment in this clinical trial?

Depending on the nature of the clinical trial, the Ethics Committee/IRB may request the investigator to provide them with special updates that focus primarily on informed consent issues, in addition to periodic updates relating to the trial's conduct. For example, the Ethics Committee/IRB might require the investigator to include information or phrasing in the informed consent that the investigator believes would adversely affect patient enrollment. An agreement might be reached that the investigator would use the Ethics Committee/IRB's version for a specified period and maintain records on the effect, if any, that the informed consent had on patient enrollment.

In the United States the FDA may grant a waiver of local IRB approval of a treatment IND protocol. There is no requirement, however, that local IRBs not review the protocol. Protocols of both medical devices and biologicals (e.g., vaccines) that are regulated by the

TABLE 27.4 *Responsibilities of Institutional Review Boards*

1. Review and approve a clinical trial protocol and data collection forms to ensure that the patients or volunteers are not exposed to unnecessary or excessive risk
2. Review and approve informed consent forms
3. Receive periodic (e.g., annual) reports from the investigator
4. Receive reports from the investigator of any serious and unexpected adverse reactions or significant changes in the clinical trial
5. Investigate any relevant aspects of the clinical trial to ensure patient safety
6. Terminate the clinical trial if appropriate
7. Review and approve all significant modifications to the clinical protocol or its conduct
8. Maintain appropriate records of all correspondence regarding the clinical trial including minutes of meetings at which it is discussed

FDA must have IRB approval. The IRB maintains responsibility for the continuing review of the clinical study.

Physicians who maintain a private clinical practice or who work outside a formal institution often have access to an Ethics Committee/IRB. If they do not, they should determine how they may become associated with one. The obligations of an investigator towards the Ethics Committee/IRB should be well known by each investigator. These obligations include filing periodic reports, advising the Ethics Committee/IRB of any changes in the protocol, and advising them of any serious adverse reactions.

Other Review Committees

In certain institutions, investigators must have a protocol approved by more than one committee (e.g., Ethics Committee/IRB, Departmental Committee, and the Clinical Research Unit Committee that has responsibility for the site where the study will be conducted). A written copy of the Ethics Committee/IRB approval must be obtained by the investigator (and also by the sponsor for sponsored studies) before a protocol may be initiated. There are publications that have assessed the performance of Ethics Committees/IRBs (Gray et al., 1978) and evaluated both the consistency among different groups (Goldman and Katz, 1982) and their influence on research design (Allen and Waters, 1982). A general synopsis of their functions is included in a brief article by Brown (1979).

REVISING AN INFORMED CONSENT

Under certain circumstances it is necessary to prepare a new or revised informed consent for patients in a

TABLE 27.5 *Conditions under which a new or revised informed consent is often obtained*

1. Results of interim analyses demonstrate that some or all patients are at a greater clinical risk if they continue with their present treatment, but the clinical trial is not to be terminated early
2. Severe adverse reactions that are probably or definitely medicine-induced and that place some or all patients at greater clinical risk are observed
3. Significant beneficial effects of one treatment that place patients receiving the other treatment at a clinical disadvantage are observed in an interim analysis, but the clinical trial will not be terminated early
4. A decision is reached by the sponsor of an investigational medicine to discontinue future development of the medicine
5. Any of the statements in the informed consent have significantly altered since the statement was signed, and the alteration is believed to have a potential impact on the patients' well-being
6. A new investigator has replaced the original investigator
7. A major change in the site or its facilities has occurred that is believed to have a potential impact on the patients' well-being

clinical trial. Many of the reasons why a new (or revised) informed consent may be required are listed in Table 27.5. Informed consents are prepared by the investigator and not by the sponsor. The sponsor, however, will usually review the consent form to ensure that it satisfies Federal regulations.

INTERACTIONS OF THE GROUPS INVOLVED IN A CLINICAL TRIAL

Basic interactions between a sponsor, investigator, Ethics Committee/IRB, and patients are illustrated in Fig. 27.3. This figure shows that sponsors do not relate or interact with Ethics Committees/IRBs except through the investigator. Patients do not interact directly with either sponsors or Ethics Committee/IRBs.

Figure 27.3 simplifies the many interactions that occur in the ethical review of a clinical trial. Figure 27.4 illustrates numerous other groups that are often involved with informed consent issues. The investigator's academic department or clinical research unit at which the clinical trial is to be conducted often have separate ethical review committees from that of the institution (i.e., Ethics Committee/IRB). The potential for "Catch-22" situations and other problems to develop between the conflicting demands of different reviewing groups is real, but hopefully most issues will be readily resolved.

PERSPECTIVES OF THE DIFFERENT GROUPS

In addition to the interactions and reviews of an informed consent described above, each participant or group of participants has special perspectives. A few comments about the major participants in a clinical trial are presented below and a list of selected issues discussed in the literature is shown in Table 27.6.

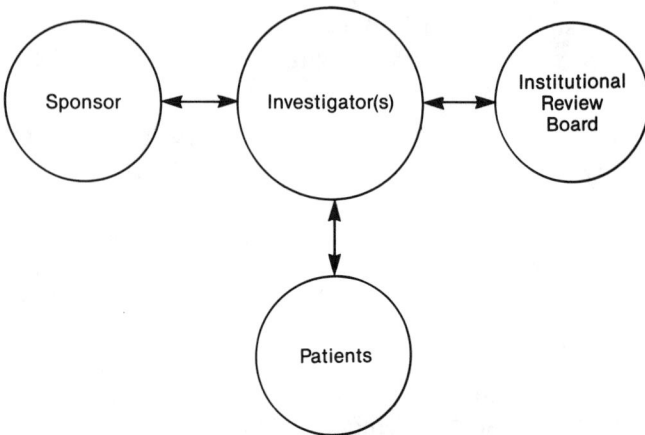

FIG. 27.3 General interactions between investigator(s), sponsor, Ethics Committee/IRB, and patients in a clinical trial.

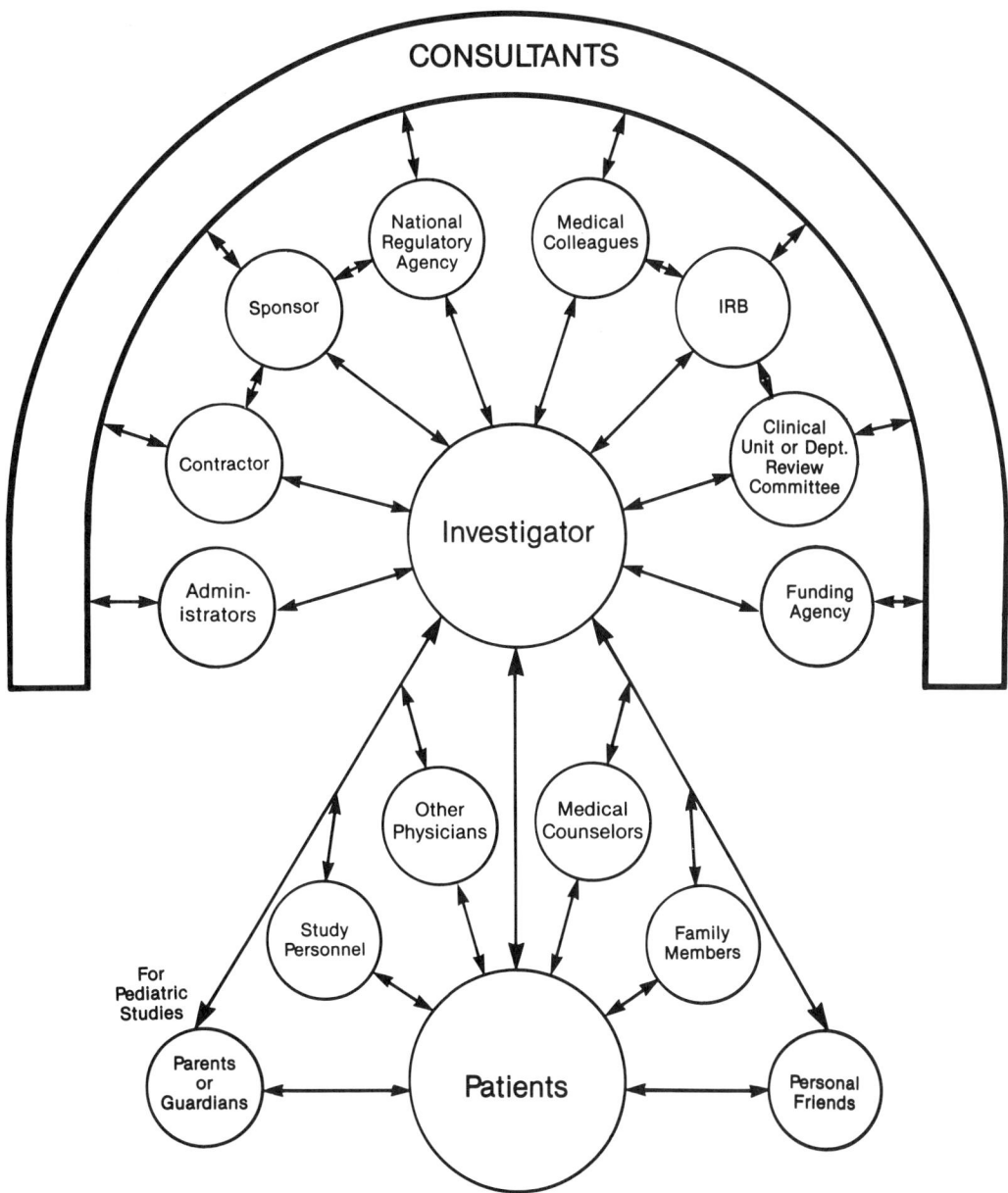

FIG. 27.4 Potential interactions in the ethical review of a clinical trial. Other interactions are possible, including those between any two or more of the six groups around patients. IRB, Ethics Committee/IRB.

Investigators

Investigators are often concerned about the procedures they will use to prepare and obtain the patient's informed consent. Depending on previous experience and current staff, the investigator may delegate some or even all of the responsibilities relating to informed consents. There are no laws preventing a nurse or other staff member from describing a clinical trial to a patient; however, the investigator should participate in discussions with the patient and sign the informed consent form. Although the procedures used to obtain an informed consent are generally similar within a clin-

ical trial they often vary widely from trial to trial, or sometimes from site to site within the same trial. An investigator should become alert to a potential problem if several patients refuse to sign the informed consent.

Sponsors

The clinical trial's sponsor wants the informed consent prepared by the investigator to meet all established regulatory standards, in part to minimize informed consent problems when the clinical trial is audited by regulatory authorities. Sponsors may help the investigator prepare informed consents by furnishing se-

TABLE 27.6 *Selected issues relating to informed consents[a]*

A. Patient-oriented issues
  1. How much information do patients really want about potential treatment risks?
  2. How does information on risks affect a patient's ability to make an informed decision?
  3. Does the amount of risk information given patients affect their medical outcome?
  4. Is any deception involved in the clinical trial? (See Chapter 64)
  5. How much time is given a patient to reach a decision about entering a clinical trial?
  6. How safe are Phase I clinical trials?
  7. What types of volunteers or patients enroll and participate in clinical trials?
  8. Does the patient understand the information presented?
  9. Should patients be tested to evaluate their understanding of the informed consent form?
  10. In what situations are patients coerced into enrolling in a clinical trial? This may be an issue for patients who reside in nursing homes or are visited by a public health nurse. It may also apply to students in the class of an academic psychologist or employees in a pharmaceutical company if they are asked to participate in a clinical trial
  11. Do patients always have the right to refuse treatment with psychotropic medicines?
  12. How may one test whether a patient is competent to give an informed consent?
  13. Should a verbal informed consent be obtained for information gathered from telephone interviews, and if so, how?
  14. Are prisoners able to provide an informed consent?
  15. Is the patient able to formulate and evaluate a benefit-to-risk concept? (See Chapter 99)
  16. Are patients being informed about changes in the benefit-to-risk ratio that arise during a clinical trial?
  17. Are patients informed about important risk information that arises after their clinical trial is completed and should be communicated to them?
  18. To what degree may a patient modify or alter an informed consent form? If this happens must the person who obtained the consent inform the physician in charge?
  19. What is the influence of describing adverse reactions in the consent form that a patient subsequently experiences as a probable result of suggestion?
  20. What alternative systems exist for obtaining informed consent?[b]
  21. How may patients be informed when only economic measures are being evaluated?

B. Investigator- and staff-oriented issues
  1. What are the effects of an investigator's emotions on the way they communicate information to their patients and obtain an informed consent?
  2. Do physicians adequately explain relevant information?
  3. Who should (or may) obtain a patient's informed consent?
  4. How may conflict-of-interest issues be resolved for physicians who have business ventures that will gain or lose in value based on the outcome of a specific clinical trial and want patients to complete the trial and not drop out?
  5. Can a physician avoid bias when asking patients to enroll in a clinical trial that will enhance his or her career?
  6. How may the potentially conflicting roles of a physician as therapist versus experimenter be resolved in enrolling patients?
  7. Should the investigator attempt to use a standard approach for obtaining informed consent from each patient or tailor the approach to each individual?
  8. What are the responsibilities of a physician's staff members if they believe a patient is not sufficiently informed?
  9. Can a physician be obligated to care for a patient without the physician's consent?

C. Informed consent form issues
  1. How may the contents of an informed consent influence a clinical trial?
  2. How much information should be presented in the form?
  3. At what comprehension level should the form be written? What are the ramifications if lawyers wish to impose a style that is difficult for patients to understand?
  4. In what format, tenses, and person should the form be written?
  5. Under which conditions should a witness be present for the discussion about a clinical trial and for signing the informed consent? Who may serve as a witness?
  6. Under which conditions should (or must) a new or revised informed consent be obtained?[c]
  7. Should the form contain information on how the investigator will benefit financially and in other ways from the study?

D. Ethics Committees/IRB issues
  1. Should Ethics Committees/IRBs adopt an active or passive role in reviewing protocols and influencing standards?
  2. What are the functions of Ethics Committees/IRBs and who are their members?
  3. How consistent are Ethics Committees/IRBs in their decisions?
  4. How may physicians have a protocol and informed consent reviewed if they have no direct access to an Ethics Committee/IRB?
  5. How may pharmaceutical companies have protocols and informed consents reviewed by an Ethics Committee/IRB if none are present at the clinical trial site and there are no national requirements for a review?[d]
  6. How do Ethics Committees/IRBs influence clinical trial design?
  7. What types of deception in study design may be condoned by an Ethics Committee/IRB, and on what basis is the deception condoned? (See Chapter 64)
  8. Should clinical trials without adequate power be approved, if it is considered that the power is too low?

E. Legal issues
  1. What laws apply if patients want access to, or a copy of, their clinical trial data?
  2. What protection do patients have against their data being revealed to others?
  3. What compensation and care do patients receive if any are injured in a clinical trial?
  4. What types of indemnification agreements may be entered into between sponsors, investigators, and institutions?
  5. Does the informed consent contain any language that waives (or appears to waive) any of the patient's legal rights?
  6. Is an informed consent valid if it is obtained by one of the investigator's staff (e.g., nurse, research coordinator)?
  7. What are the roles and values of patients' rights advocates?
  8. What is the degree of confidentiality of a patient's data in an epidemiological study?
  9. Should there be no-fault compensation for volunteers or patients injured in medical research?
  10. Under which conditions may a proxy informed consent be obtained for incompetent patients?
  11. Under which conditions may patients be forced to take medicines?
  12. How do laws regarding informed consents differ between countries?
  13. May parents withhold their consent for their teenage children to be treated medically?
  14. May a spouse sign an informed consent if the patient is competent, but currently unable to sign a form (e.g., while under anesthesia)?

[a] Many issues could be placed in two or more categories. Numerous references are available on each of these points.
[b] See Levine, 1986, pp. 105 and 106; Leikin, 1985; Matas et al., 1985; Abramson et al., 1986.
[c] See Table 27.5.
[d] See Faccini et al., 1984.

lected samples as well as by reviewing the investigator's draft. It is generally considered unacceptable for sponsors to prepare the informed consent that the investigator submits to the Ethics Committee/IRB for approval, although some sponsors allow this practice.

The sponsor must be sure that the Ethics Committee/IRB has approved the informed consent before the clinical trial begins and that the investigator has a signed form for each patient enrolled. A blank informed consent form should be placed in the sponsor's files. Figure 27.5 illustrates some of these interactions from a sponsor's perspective.

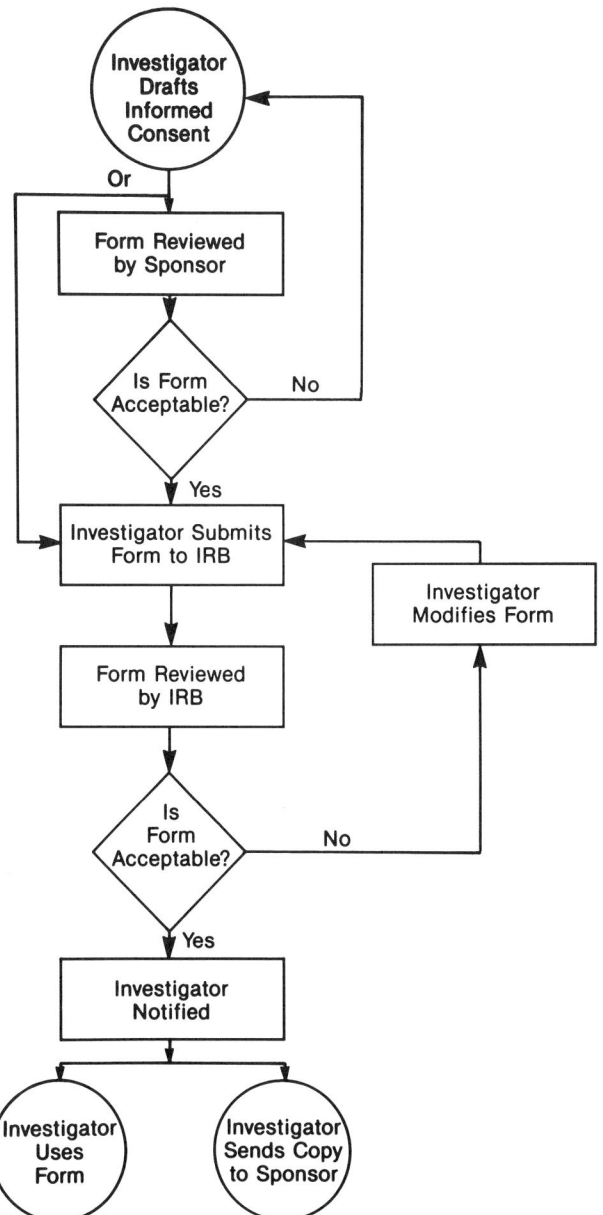

FIG. 27.5 Development and submittal of the informed consent by the investigator and review by the Ethics Committee/IRB. Sample informed consents, regulations, and elements to include may be furnished to the investigator by the sponsor.

Sponsors and investigators want to use an informed consent that does not adversely influence enrollment rates of patients. A negative influence has been reported (Epstein and Lasagna, 1969), especially when an informed consent accentuates the risks of a clinical trial and does not provide the balance of potential benefits.

Ethics Committees/IRBs

Many Ethics Committees/IRBs are in the position of having to "reinvent the wheel" each time they review an informed consent that raises new issues. Sometimes they debate issues without awareness of all relevant points of view. Ethics Committees/IRBs operate at different standards and consistency levels (Goldman and Katz, 1982), although one IRB reported a high degree of internal consistency over a several year period (Grodin et al., 1986). Ethics Committees/IRBs have the benefit of a journal (*IRB: A Review of Human Subjects Research*, edited by Robert J. Levine and published by The Hastings Center) to present issues, either as legal cases arise or in another format. These cases could be used to establish precedence and to provide additional points of view, which could be openly debated by other Ethics Committees/IRBs facing similar situations.

Some of the many important issues facing Ethics Committees/IRBs are listed in Table 27.6, and types of protocol changes requiring an Ethics Committee/IRB approval are listed in Table 27.7.

Patients

Summarizing the perspective of patients is more complex than summarizing those of the other groups: the makeup of patient populations, plus their motivation and behavior, varies greatly from trial to trial and within clinical trials as well. Normal healthy volun-

---

TABLE 27.7 *Protocol changes that must be submitted to an Ethics Committee/IRB for approval[a]*

1. An increase in medicine dosage or frequency of dosing or a change in the method of medicine administration; this generally includes any change in medicine formulation, since the bioavailability of the medicine may be affected
2. Significant increases in the number of patients to receive the clinical trial medicine; a 10% or greater increase is considered "significant" by some individuals
3. Use or inclusion of new groups of patients whose concurrent medical condition might significantly affect the scope and/or validity of the protocol
4. Use or inclusion of new groups of patients for whom special considerations are warranted in terms of care or other factors
5. Use or inclusion of new groups of patients whose concurrent therapy might confound clinical trial interpretation

[a] Each Ethics Committee/IRB may require submission of other protocol modifications for approval in addition to or in lieu of those listed in this table.

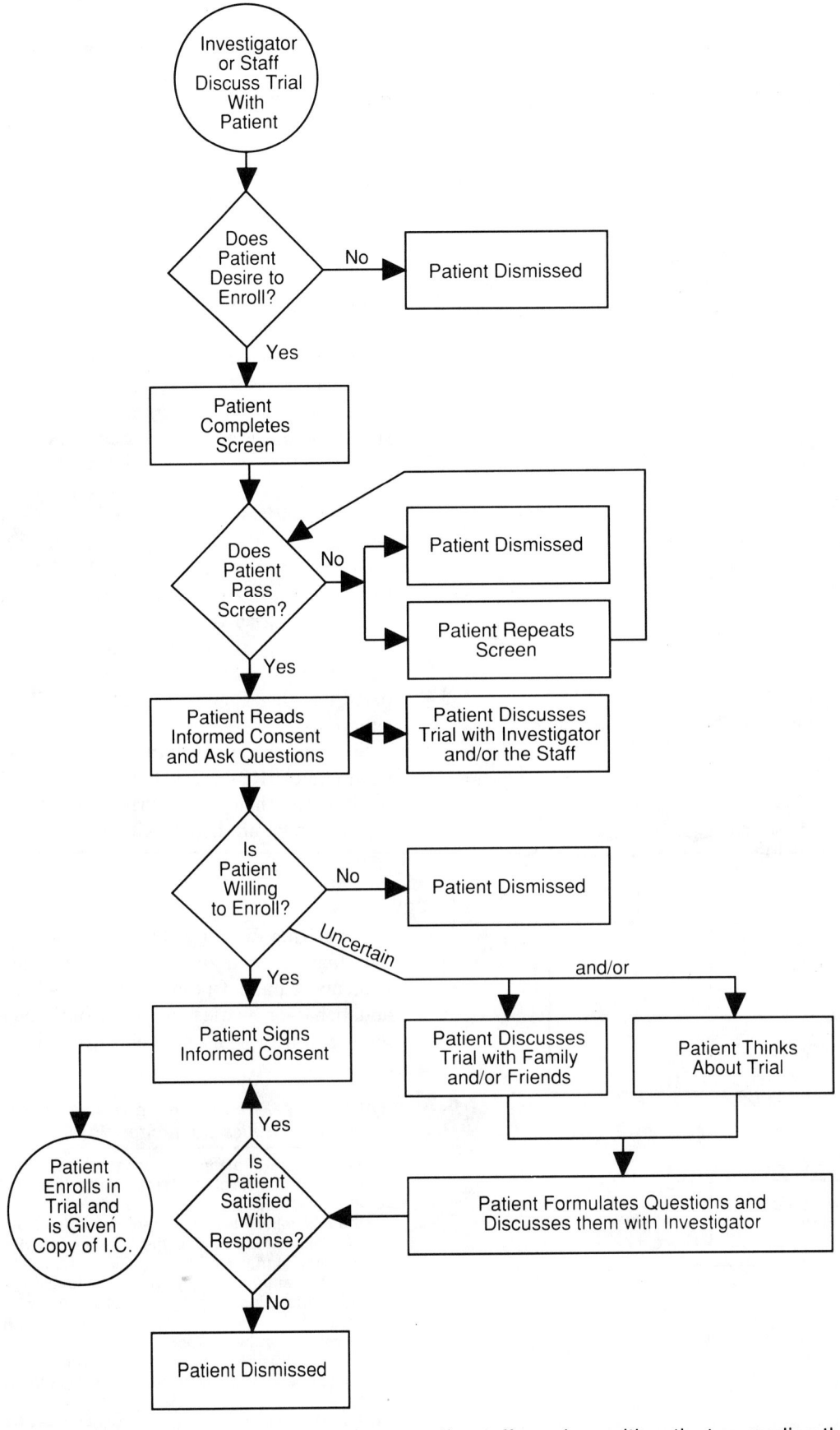

FIG. 27.6 Potential interactions of investigator and/or staff members with patients regarding the informed consent. The screen may be performed after the informed consent is signed. I.C., informed consent.

216

teers in Phase I clinical trials obviously have a different perspective about a trial than do patients who are mildly ill with a chronic illness or patients who are severely ill. In addition, a number of differing groups of patients deserve special consideration (e.g., see Table 27.8). A series of questions that are relevant for patients to ask before enrolling in a clinical trial and for evaluation have been presented (Nealon et al., 1985). The investigator–patient interaction process leading to the informed consent is illustrated in Fig. 27.6.

Patients Who Refuse to Sign Informed Consents

Using an informed consent may introduce bias into a clinical trial; this issue has not been adequately addressed in the literature. It was reported (Edlund et al., 1985) that psychotic patients who refused to sign an informed consent were generally more hostile than those who did sign. In addition, refusers were more likely to abuse alcohol and drugs. The literature reviewed by Edlund et al. (1985) revealed that only 4 of 232 studies evaluated presented characteristics of patients who refused to sign an informed consent form. These four papers were from epidemiological studies. Patients were interviewed on the eve of elective gynecological surgery about enrolling in a hypothetical trial. Those willing to sign an informed consent had less anxiety than those who refused (Antrobus, 1988). Another study (Dahan et al., 1986) reported that the age and sex distribution of patients who refused to sign an informed consent differed from those who did sign.

Refusal to sign might involve the patient's (1) religious or philosophical beliefs, (2) overestimating the magnitude of risks involved, (3) underestimating the likely or potential benefits of a trial, (4) dislike of the physician, staff, or facilities, (5) believing that protocol demands in terms of time or other commitments are excessive, (6) not fully understanding factors such as

TABLE 27.8 *Selected patient populations with special informed consent considerations[a]*

1. Mentally retarded patients
2. Psychotic patients
3. Severe trauma victims and medical emergency situations
4. Patients who are in a coma or are lethargic
5. Unborn embryos and fetuses
6. Newborn babies and infants
7. Children and adolescents
8. Prisoners
9. Pregnant and lactating women
10. Organ transplant donors and recipients

[a] These considerations (except for group 9) usually relate to the issue of competence or ability to provide an informed consent. Other groups such as students, employees, military, or police may be strongly encouraged (i.e., overinduced) to enter a clinical trial or they may be reluctant to refuse entry when asked.

the possibility of dropping out or of obtaining alternative treatment (7) being influenced by family or friends, or (8) believing the clinical trial will interfere with proper treatment. It is usually desirable to discuss or consider these and other clinical-trial-related issues before patients undergo time-consuming and possibly costly screening tests. If the informed consent has a significant effect on the makeup of patients who agree to enroll, the trial population will differ as a group from the intended patient population, which could compromise the extrapolatability of the data obtained to other populations of patients.

FUTURE ISSUES

Four issues are briefly mentioned below that may be more widely debated in the coming decade.

Surgical Consent

The routine consent forms required in the United States to perform a surgical operation are perfunctory documents that in reality do not ensure that any information appropriate for decision making has been provided. In most other countries the standards are the same or lower. The document is so poor that in one study conducted 2 to 5 days after surgery 27 of 100 patients were unaware of what organ was operated on and 44 of the same 100 patients were unaware of the exact nature of the surgery (Byrne et al., 1988).

Providing Information on Medical Disagreements

The possibility of providing information on clinical variability and disagreements has been discussed (Anonymous, *Lancet*, 1989b). This topic is not likely to become a popular cause because of the enormous complexity and the knowledge needed (often by experts) to understand the nuances needed to make the best decisions.

Obtaining Informed Consent in Emergency Situations

This topic has long been a difficult one to deal with because of the patients' stress and lack of time to discuss the alternatives at the very time that a rapid decision must be made. Traditional approaches, according to Grim et al. (1989), have been to (1) avoid clinical trials in emergencies, (2) omit the informed consent process, (3) obtain deferred consent, or (4) obtain customary consent. They propose a fifth possibility consisting of a two-step consent process that has more desirable characteristics than the other four procedures.

Informed Consent as a Source of Bias

There is no doubt that using an informed consent introduces bias into a clinical trial (Myers et al., 1987; Levine, 1987). There is no possibility of returning to pre-informed-consent days, but, as more investigators attempt to understand this bias better, it is hoped that they will study the means of diminishing its impact on a clinical trial.

Remote Data Entry

TYPES OF REMOTE DATA ENTRY

The term *remote data entry* generally conjures the image of clinical trial data transmission via computer and telephone line from an investigator's site to the sponsor. Although this is the most commonly discussed type of remote data entry, there are numerous other types, including transmission of laboratory data from laboratory to sponsor or investigator. Specialized tests may be conducted offsite, or data may be interpreted offsite, and results subsequently transmitted as desired. Attributes of a desirable remote data entry system are listed in Table 28.1, and protocol elements that may be included are listed in Table 28.2.

WHEN TO USE REMOTE DATA ENTRY

Although there is no right or wrong time to use remote data entry, its use is generally more advantageous in certain types of trials. These include (1) pivotal clinical trials, (2) trials with large amounts of data, (3) trials with both a moderately large number of sites and patients at each site, and (4) trials with seasonal data. Criteria suggesting that remote data entry should be considered are listed in Table 28.3.

Remote data entry tends to be impractical for clinical trials of long duration (i.e., over 1 year) because it ties up equipment and may not be cost effective. Trials with low volumes of data are also generally impractical for remote data entry. Even in these two cases, however, remote data entry might be considered after assessment of relevant issues.

PERSPECTIVES OF PROFESSIONALS AFFECTED

Monitor's Perspective

Electronic transmission of data from investigators to sponsors does not eliminate the need to monitor trials at the trial site. Although it is far better to assess the status of an ongoing clinical trial by reviewing data than by telephone contacts, the importance of direct contacts and visits cannot be underestimated. Nonetheless, a lower frequency of monitoring visits may be possible if data of acceptable quality are received by the sponsor at an acceptable rate, and telephone and other contacts indicate that no problems requiring a monitoring visit exist. Generally it is not necessary to monitor both paper and electronic data, although this often occurs.

In-house data processors may wonder about how remote data entry will affect them in terms of job security. Usually, it only means that data arrive at a sponsor's site somewhat faster and cleaner. The jobs of data processors are rarely, if ever, threatened.

TABLE 28.1 *Attributes of a desirable remote data entry system*

1. No vendor involvement is required
2. System is user friendly
3. Audit trails are present that are easy to use
4. Data are transferred to sponsor automatically
5. System is readily compatible with existing systems
6. System is relatively inexpensive
7. System allows an easy method of correcting errors to be used

TABLE 28.2 *Selected protocol elements that may be built into the remote data entry computer program*

1. Data collection forms
2. Patient entry criteria
3. Dosing schedules and acceptable modifications of dose
4. Patient visit schedules
5. Level of abnormal laboratory values that require a comment or action
6. Severity of adverse reactions or treatment that require notification of the sponsor
7. Adverse trends in laboratory or other values that require a comment or acknowledgment
8. Electronic mail for communication between site and sponsor

Investigator's Perspective

A company conducting clinical trials should only use remote data entry procedures when both the sponsor and the investigator desire it. Trying to convince a reluctant investigator to use this type of data transmittal is not an auspicious way to start a clinical trial. One approach that would be acceptable to most investigators who are not totally comfortable with computers (and even those who are) would be to hire a specialist to run and maintain the data entry and transmittal system. This method would free the investigator from that particular responsibility.

From the investigator's viewpoint it is redundant (in terms of time and resources) to rekey data that has come from the hospital's laboratory in a computerized format. Furthermore, investigators who are participating in medicine trials with several sponsors and are using remote data entry will need sufficient space to house multiple computer facilities. Cooperation between different sponsors resulting in a single system of computer equipment at one site would improve efficiency and decrease costs. This advance, however, does not appear to be forthcoming.

The cost of running a clinical trial increases if the data are to be sent by computer and telephone. These costs, as well as any incurred for hiring and training staff to operate and maintain the system, must be factored into the clinical trial budget. Investigators usu-

TABLE 28.3 *Factors that suggest remote data entry should be considered*

1. Trials are considered "fast track" (i.e., it is important for them to be conducted rapidly)
2. Trials are such that rapid decisions are needed
3. Medicine has particularly high commercial potential
4. Trials have a large patient enrollment
5. Multicenter trials are planned
6. Trials have a high volume of data suitable for remote entry (e.g., not an excessive amount of time or effort required by the site or sponsor)
7. Both the investigator and sponsor want to use remote data entry

ally delegate computer work to others, who then handle the technical issues and problems that arise.

It should be emphasized that serious adverse reactions are handled the same way, whether or not remote data entry is used; serious and unexpected adverse reactions should be telephoned to the sponsor. Patients are unaffected by remote data entry, except in rare cases.

HOW REMOTE DATA ENTRY FUNCTIONS

Security of a remote data entry is usually addressed by requiring a password to enter the computerized system. Additional passwords are required for the person who has gained access to enter data. Systems are created so that sponsors are unable to change data from their own computers during the trial. In telephone conversations with investigators, both must use the same password if they desire to enter the system simultaneously. Finally, data are stored in non-word-processing format.

Audit Trails

Remote data entry system should include audit trails. An audit trail should include the password identifier of the person making any changes, plus the date that the change is being made. The patient number, visit number, and variable being changed must be included, as well as the old and new values. The reason for the change should be given whenever possible.

Models of Data Flow Using Remote Data Entry

Figure 28.1 is a schematic representation of three models of data flow using remote data entry. In model A, both a hard copy and electronic copy of the data are available, whereas in model B only the electronic copy of the data exists. The electronic copy in model B serves both as the original data collection form and as the sponsor's copy. Model C differs from the others in that the individuals who send the data to the sponsor are actually from the sponsor (or a contractor) and are not the investigator or his or her staff. Model C requires more visits from sponsors, more time spent at sites, and therefore more monitoring. The advantage of this model is that data entry is performed by those monitors who are usually the most motivated to have data as pristine and accurate as possible. Their job evaluation is usually more closely related to the accuracy of the data than is the evaluation of the clinical trial coordinator or whoever else enters and transmits the data.

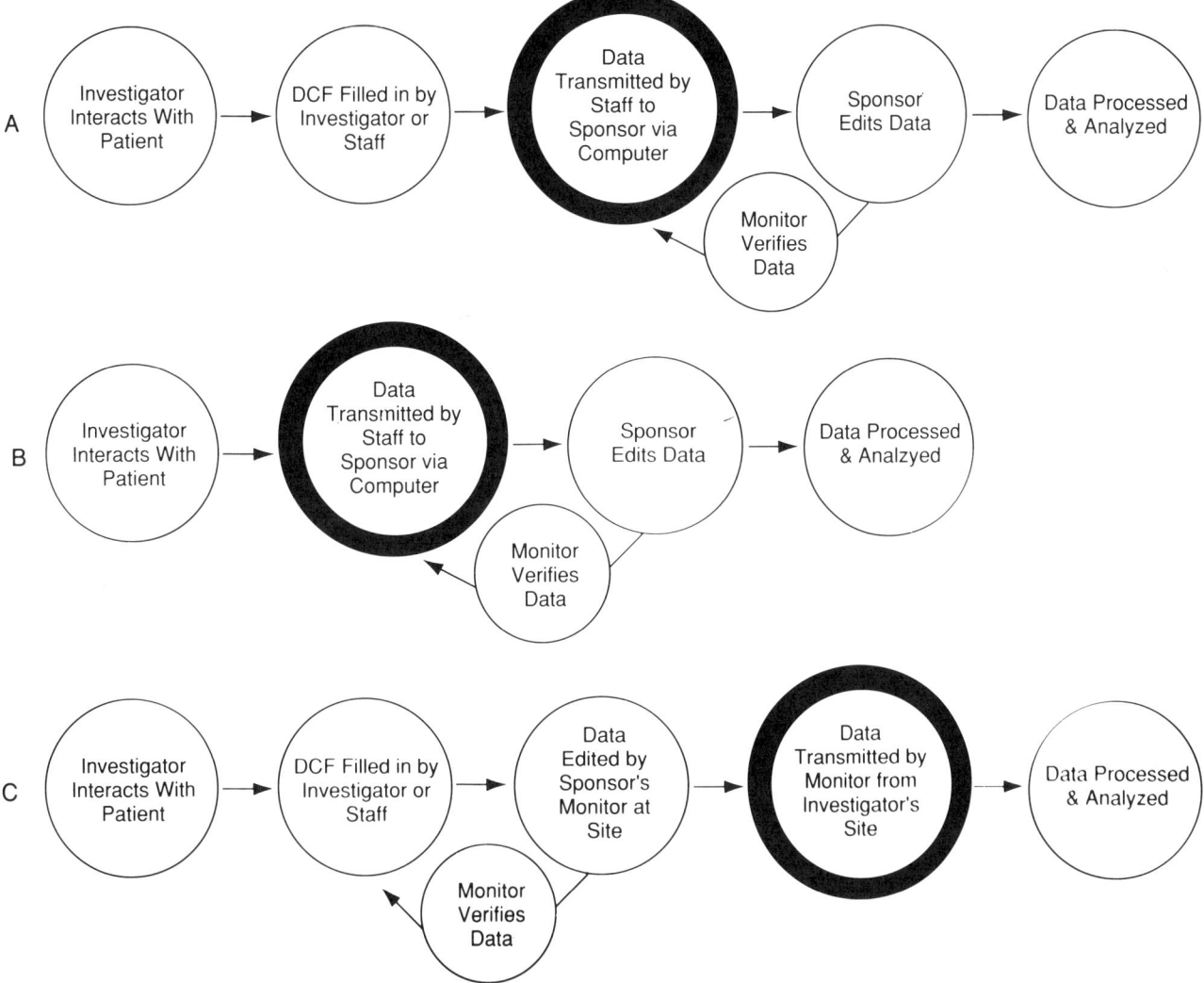

FIG. 28.1 Models of data flow using remote data entry. DCF, data collection form.

ADVANTAGES AND DISADVANTAGES

General advantages of remote data entry for different groups are listed in Tables 28.4 to 28.6 and practical pointers are listed in Table 28.7. Most remote data entry systems include a program that enables the computer to recognize when answers to a question (i.e., values on a data collection form) are unacceptable. When answers are typed into the system that lie outside accepted ranges, or are not understood by the

TABLE 28.4 *Advantages for the sponsor of using remote data entry*

1. Earlier availability of interim data for decision making
2. Earlier completion of final data base with reduction of key-punching and a savings in data comparisons of double-entered data
3. More rapid completion of clinical trial reports
4. More rapid completion of a regulatory submission
5. Savings in printing, shipping, and storing of hard copies of data collection forms
6. Rapid feedback on protocol problems

Modified from a talk by Dr. Lionel D. Edwards of Schering-Plough Corp., with permission.

TABLE 28.5 *Advantages for the monitor of using remote data entry*

1. Higher percentage of valid patients in the clinical trial
2. Rapid feedback on patient enrollment, adverse reactions, and clinical-trial-related issues
3. Ability to review completed data collection forms prior to visiting the site
4. Ability to have more productive site visits
5. Savings in time and expense of correcting multiple data collection forms at different sites
6. Less chance for data collection forms to get lost at the site, in the mail, or at the sponsor
7. Fewer problems of illegible entries, missing data, and missed abnormal results

Modified from a talk by Dr. Lionel Edwards of Schering-Plough Corp., with permission.

TABLE 28.6 *Advantages for the investigator of using remote data entry*

1. Remote data entry identifies and alerts staff about missing, inappropriate, or abnormal data
2. It identifies and alerts staff about desirable, undesirable, or abnormal trends
3. It simplifies the correction of data
4. It may provide an algorithm to assess the association between a medicine and an adverse reaction
5. It provides a hard copy on site for data sent (if desired)
6. It provides electronic storage on disk, plus a backup disk
7. It is a state-of-the-art system for those who enjoy using the latest techniques available
8. It allows nonvalid patients to be eliminated more rapidly from a trial

Modified from a talk by Dr. Lionel Edwards of Schering-Plough Corp., with permission.

computer, a signal (light or sound) is given. This method of alerting the data entry person to review the previous entry is a valuable means of saving time, both in data monitoring and in making corrections.

Technical problems can be substantial in a clinical trial using remote data entry, especially if the problems interfere with the trial's progress. Transmission line noise is one example. Other problems that may arise are listed in Table 28.8. Despite attempts to prevent technical problems, innumerable "gremlins" seem to inhabit electronic equipment and delight in causing problems at inopportune times.

Determining the precise costs of remote data entry is complex, requiring, first, a decision on which costs to include. If only hardware and software costs are considered, then remote data entry would cost more than a paper data collection method. If other costs related to the system are included, and time saved in processing the data is factored in, remote data entry may provide a savings of approximately 15 to 25%, according to informal analyses conducted by various experts in this field.

REGULATORY CONSIDERATIONS OF REMOTE DATA ENTRY

Regulatory authorities are willing to accept data from trials that use remote data entry techniques, provided

TABLE 28.7 *Practical pointers in developing and using remote data entry*

1. Develop a template to fit over the keyboard for data entry that identifies relevant functions to use in entering data
2. Use color monitors for ease of reading the screens
3. Use a single color for data areas that the investigator must complete and a different color or shade for other areas
4. Program a light to flash or buzzer to sound when errors are made in data entry
5. Use remote data entry for only some sites in a multicenter pilot trial; compare time and error rates in each group for every step of the process; compare overall costs

TABLE 28.8 *Selected problems that may arise in clinical trials with remote data entry*

A. Technical problems
 1. Changes to protocol are often difficult once the study is initiated
 2. Security may become an issue and is more complex than with other clinical trials
 3. Frequent updating of software is often required to improve the system
 4. Initial costs are usually significant
 5. Technical and compatibility problems may be a major problem, particularly outside the United States and between countries (e.g., telephone installation times, types of telephones available)
 6. The same modems cannot legally be used in all countries (e.g., United States and Germany)
 7. The quality of local telephone companies and their lines (e.g., transmission noise) vary greatly within some countries and between countries
 8. There may be multiple vendors responsible for hardware maintenance in some countries
 9. Backup of data at the investigator's site is essential
 10. It may be difficult to standardize various entry and transmission procedures unless identical equipment is provided to each site

B. Personnel problems
 1. There may be reluctance of some investigators, monitors, or sponsor's staff to utilize procedures
 2. There may be a lack of adequate training or available staff to serve as programmers, statisticians, and computer experts to establish, support, and maintain the system
 3. Training may present problems, particularly if staff turnover is high
 4. Backlogs of data may build up at transmitting sites

C. Political and administrative problems
 1. Governments may restrict the hardware that may be used (e.g., locally manufactured machines may be required)
 2. Some governments restrict the information that may be given to other governments and who has access to it
 3. Trade or commerce regulations and tariff barriers may be major issues
 4. Licenses to use telephone equipment may be restricted
 5. Issues of who owns the data (e.g., hospital, investigator, sponsor) may create problems in the submission of data to regulatory agencies

that data collection forms can be generated, audit trails exist, and supporting data are available for an audit conducted by the regulatory authority. The audit trail is extremely important from a regulatory perspective because it allows an individual to learn how the original data appeared and to follow their change over time through processing procedures or by intentional modifications. When a physician or other health professional sees a patient and then types results into a computer for remote data entry, there is no hard copy serving as a source document. The computer screen, with various fields to fill in, serves in the example given as source document, data collection form, and remote data entry. Although data collection forms are computer generated it is still important that the investigator sign them, as with hard copy forms.

PRACTICAL POINTERS

Careful planning is essential for a successful experience with remote data entry. Define what is desired from the experience and decide whether the goals are realistic, fit the time schedule and budget, and can be implemented. Equipment may be purchased or leased. Leasing is particularly valuable when a large number of computers are required for a relatively short period.

Changes to the format of individual computer screens for data collection should be done centrally and then given to all sites. Although small changes may be made by staff at each site, the "gremlins" that often appear in the equipment are more likely to create problems if changes are made at each site.

Software and hardware change rapidly, but older equipment may be satisfactory and it will be cheaper to run, will involve less training, often will be easier to repair, and will allow a group to start a trial faster. Newer programs and equipment should be evaluated for potential gains in an important area before they are adopted.

The flow of information between sponsor and investigator, or the movement of data at either site, may have to be modified to use remote data entry. The flow pattern often differs between groups and is specific to each sponsor. Data scrubbing may be done at the investigator's site or at the sponsor's. These aspects will lead a sponsor to choose a particular model of data flow (Fig. 28.1). The model chosen should allow the sponsor to achieve the "greatest byte for the least bucks."

Remote Trial Monitoring

The process of remote data entry must be clearly differentiated from remote trial monitoring. In the latter, the monitoring process is primarily or entirely conducted by receipt of frequent, even daily, electronic transmission of data sent to the sponsor. Data are sent more frequently using electronic transmission than for most cases of remote data entry using telephone or courier. The monitor must still visit the site to compare the data sent with the source documents.

CHAPTER 29

Preparing the Introduction

In writing a protocol's introduction, the purpose or intent of the clinical trial should be described as specifically as possible. Although the length of the introduction may vary from a single paragraph to many pages, it should be of minimal length to meet this goal sufficiently. Some of the possible specific goals for the introduction are to:

1. Present preclinical and clinical data on a new medicine that is being evaluated with the present protocol.
2. Present the background of a hypothesis that is being tested with the present protocol.
3. Present the background for a new methodology that is being evaluated or is being used to test a new medicine with the present protocol.

Adequate information must be presented on the safety, efficacy, and any other relevant aspects of the clinical trial medicine(s). Various points to consider for inclusion in an introduction are listed in Table 29.1.

TABLE 29.1 *Information that may be included in a protocol's introduction[a]*

1. Synopsis of the disease to be studied
2. Background of standard medicines or other current therapy used to treat the disease
3. Limitations of currently available medicines and/or other treatments
4. Background of the medicine(s) being studied in the present protocol:
   Chemistry
   Pharmacology
   Toxicology
   Pharmacokinetics
   Clinical safety
   Clinical efficacy
5. Rationale for the present trial
6. Other information

[a] Published (or unpublished) references that support the material presented should be included.

Standardizing Information Across Protocols

The term "boilerplate" refers to sections of information that are similar from protocol to protocol. Standardizing the format and content of these sections can save time for individuals who prepare numerous protocols. The term "standardization" does not mean that these parts of the protocol are identical in various protocols but that their format is often similar, and the material in the section can usually be easily modified to fit the specific nature of a new protocol. The various sections of the protocol that may be standardized are listed in Table 30.1. Several of these topics are discussed in other chapters within Section II. A summary of the processes of protocol preparation is given in Fig. 30.1.

PROTOCOL FORMAT

Title Page

There are many variations in the information presented on a title page. Table 30.2 presents a list of information that is usually present and sometimes present. Sponsors of clinical trials have usually established a preset format for the title page.

Table of Contents

A table of contents is an optional feature of a protocol, but it is often helpful, especially in longer protocols with distinct sections. A sample listing of possible items to include is shown in Fig. 30.2.

List of Abbreviations

If numerous abbreviations are used in the protocol, then it is useful to provide a listing. As a general rule, abbreviations should not be used at all or should be severely limited to a small number of commonly accepted ones.

References and Appendices

The need for references and appendices varies widely from trial to trial. Their usefulness in a protocol is dependent in part on the personal style of the individual writing the protocol as well as on the requirements of the sponsoring institution for sponsored clinical trials. There are few rules that can be used to evaluate the need for appendices, since styles and "accepted prac-

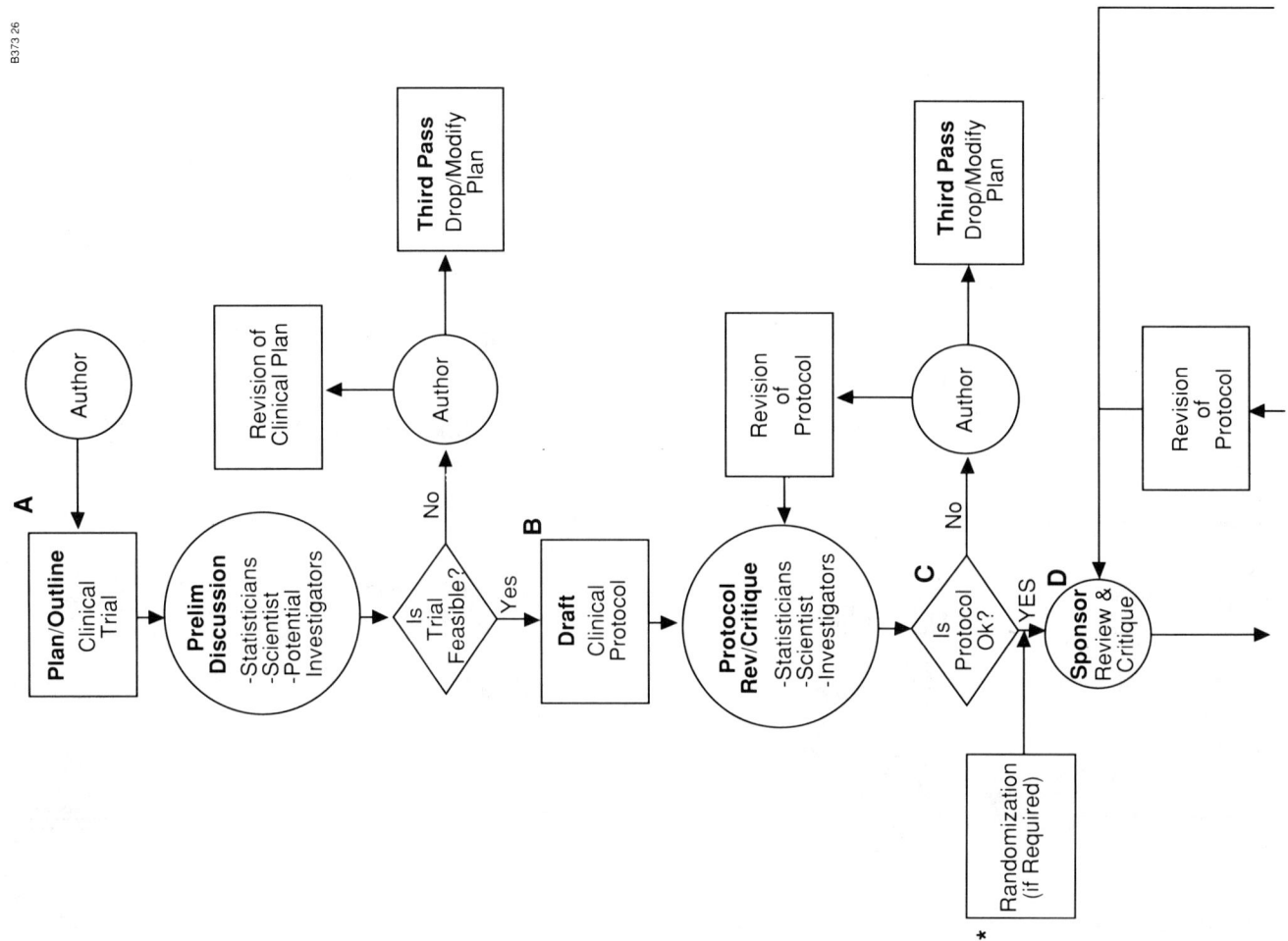

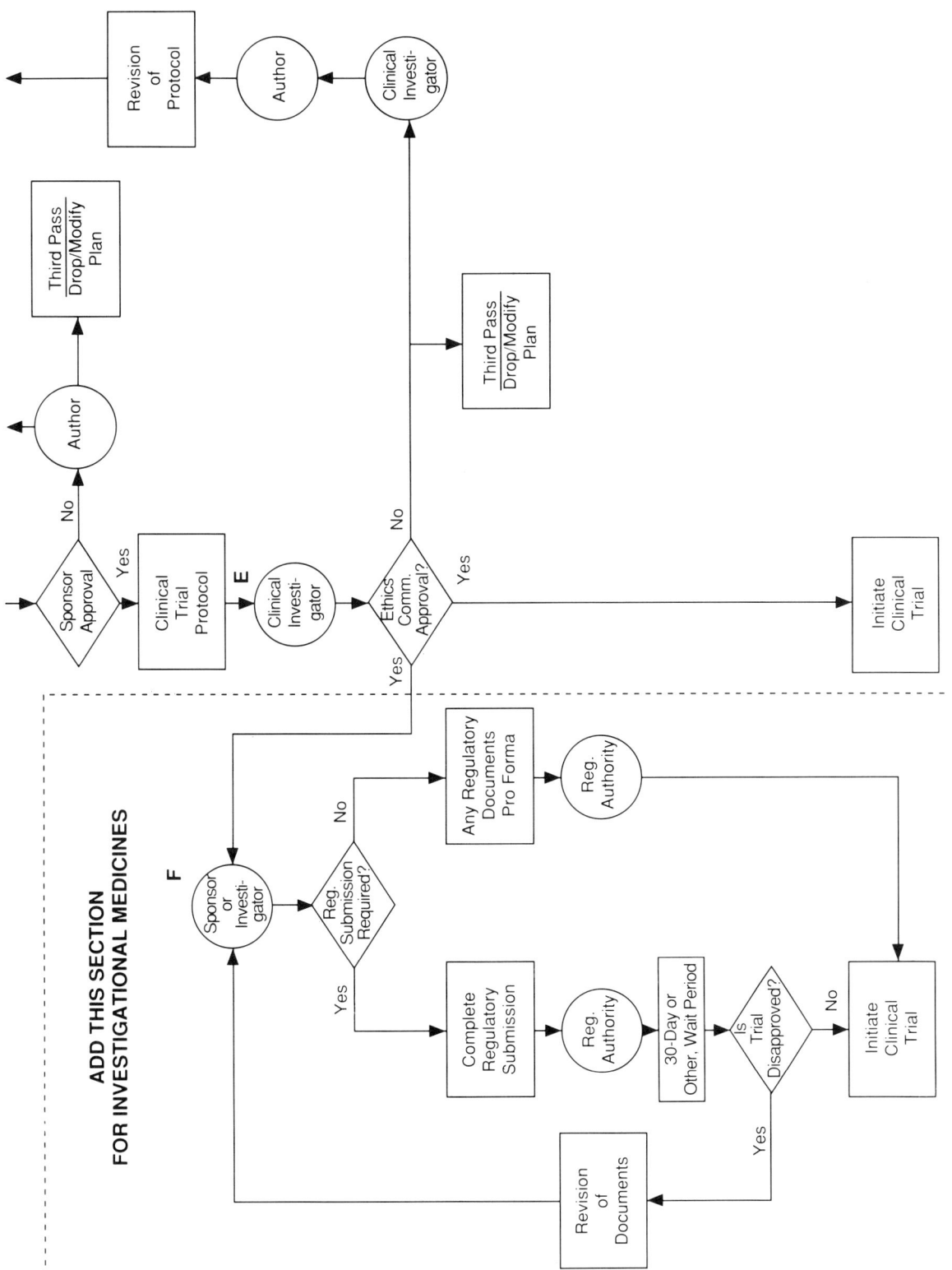

ADD THIS SECTION FOR INVESTIGATIONAL MEDICINES

FIG. 30.1 Processes involved in protocol development and approval for an investigational or marketed drug. The total process is arbitrarily divided into six stages. For unsponsored trials, stages C and D would be modified. For clinical trials using marketed medicines without need for regulatory documents, the last stage (F) would be omitted. Each Ethics Committee/IRB in a multicenter trial must approve any changes made to the protocol.

227

TABLE 30.1 *Protocol format, contents, and adminstrative elements that may be relatively standardized*

A. Protocol format
  1. Title page
  2. Table of contents
  3. List of abbreviations
  4. References and appendices

B. Protocol content
  1. Patient enrollment and duration of the clinical trial
  2. Location of trial site
  3. Factors to control within or outside the trial environment
  4. Shipping of medicines to and from the trial site
  5. Obtaining, handling, and shipping biological samples
  6. Defining the time of patient entry and completion
  7. Eliciting and categorizing adverse events
  8. Missed appointments
  9. Patients lost to follow-up
  10. Patient discontinuation, dropout, dropin, and refusers
  11. Early trial discontinuation
  12. Medical emergencies

C. Administrative elements
  1. Administrative responsibilities of the investigator
  2. Informed consent
  3. Institutional approval
  4. Confidentiality of data
  5. Collection and processing of data
  6. Publishing of data
  7. Monitoring the clinical trial
  8. Protocol amendments

tice'' differ so radically in this regard. Some individuals attempt to place all material suitable for an appendix into the data collection forms, whereas others prefer to include all tabular information and ''fine'' details of a protocol into an appendix. Table 30.3 lists numerous items that may be placed into appendices.

Material such as tables of male and female weights for dosing and/or other data needed to conduct the

TABLE 30.2 *Information listed on the title page of a protocol*

A. Usually present
  1. Title of clinical trial
  2. Name and address of investigator(s)
  3. Name and address of sponsor (if any)

B. Sometimes present
  1. Office and home telephone numbers of investigators
  2. Names of monitors
  3. Addresses and telephone numbers of monitors
  4. Date of issue of protocol
  5. Signatures of investigators plus date of signing
  6. Signatures and titles of individuals that have approved the protocol plus date of signing
  7. Signatures of monitors plus date of signing
  8. Specific information related to the trial medicine, such as IND number, NDA or PLA number, specific project or sponsor code numbers
  9. Phase (I, II, III, IV) of the clinical trial
  10. Person to contact in case of a medical emergency
  11. Statement of confidentiality
  12. Anticipated starting and completion dates for the clinical trial
  13. Other information

IND, Investigational New Drug; NDA, New Drug Application, PLA, Product License Application.

TABLE 30.3 *Information that may be included in the protocol's appendix[a]*

A. Patient information
  1. Sample copy of the informed consent
  2. Sample copy of the pregnancy waiver form
  3. Operational definitions to be used (e.g., for describing a patient's disease)
  4. Classifications to be used (e.g., diagnostic classifications)
  5. Instruction form to be given to or read to the patient

B. Clinical trial and other medicines
  1. Names and dosages of standard medicines (e.g., medicines that are acceptable for use by patients)
  2. Names of medicines chemically related to the trial medicine. Patients allergic to one of these medicines are often excluded from the trial to avoid a hypersensitivity reaction.
  3. Additional chemical, pharmacological, clinical, or other information
  4. Package insert(s), either actual (for marketed medicines) or tentative based on current information (for investigational medicines)
  5. Details of medicine preparation, packaging, and labeling
  6. Management of overdosage

C. Conduct of the clinical trial and tests used
  1. Types and details of equipment to be used in various tests
  2. Information about clinical, physiological, or pharmacological parameters (e.g., height and weight charts)
  3. Lists of specific laboratory parameters to be measured and other information related to these parameters (normal values)
  4. Details of efficacy parameters to be measured
  5. Details of how certain tests of efficacy and/or safety information will be performed
  6. Rating scales used for efficacy or safety parameters
  7. Description of how information on adverse reactions will be obtained
  8. Operational definitions of adverse reaction intensities and a description of how adverse reactions are to be related to clinical trial medicines (e.g., algorithms)
  9. How to collect, store, and handle biological samples containing trial and/or other medicines
  10. Description of assay procedures
  11. Samples of patient diaries, self-completion forms, or related material
  12. Other instructions for the investigator and/or research coordinator (e.g., procedures manual)

D. Data handling and statistics
  1. Randomization code for open-label or single-blind clinical trials
  2. Details of how certain calculations will be performed during the trial
  3. Details of statistical tests to be used to analyze the data
  4. Tables of random numbers or other mathematical information to be used in the trial
  5. Latin-square designs to be used for open-label or single-blind trials
  6. Sample data collection forms—either selected forms or the entire data collection form package

E. Management and administration of the clinical trial
  1. Glossary of terms
  2. Contractural agreement between investigator and sponsor
  3. Government regulations—printed as excerpts, in their entirety, or paraphrased
  4. Sample release form to obtain, and potentially use, photographs of the patient
  5. Any forms required by the sponsor, institution,[b] or Ethics Committee/IRB
  6. Other responsibilities of the investigator

[a] Many materials could be placed into more than one category. The five major categories listed were chosen to simplify the organization of this table.
[b] See Chapter 61.

Page

FIG. 30.2 Sample table of contents, indicating topics that may be included.

clinical trial should be readily available to personnel conducting the trial. These data may be placed either in the protocol or data collection forms and should not merely be referenced. Additional details of tests or procedures can be placed in appendices.

PROTOCOL CONTENT

Patient Enrollment and Duration of the Clinical Trial

Some protocols explicitly state the expected or desired rate of patient enrollment. Protocols may also include an anticipated starting and/or completion date. These points depend on many factors and often have to be modified both prior to a clinical trial and during its conduct. It is the author's opinion that indicating these projected time points serves little purpose in a protocol. Realistic dates and rate of patient enrollment can be best determined through discussion and an ongoing close collaboration of all people involved in the initiation and conduct of a trial.

Location of the Trial Site

Although most clinical trials are conducted at a hospital, laboratory, clinic, or professional office, trials may also be conducted at the patient's home (e.g., to evaluate intermittent positive-pressure breathing apparatus in patients with chronic obstructive lung disease), workplace, or other sites. More than one physical location may also be used to conduct a "one-site" study (e.g., an investigator with three offices). If so, it may be relevant to indicate which parts of the clinical trial are to be performed at each location or whether each location will serve as a "complete site."

Factors to Control Within or Outside the Trial Environment

It may be appropriate to control certain factors relating to the clinical trial environment (Table 30.4). Some concern the patient's behavior, and others the patient's environment. The quality and/or quantity of these factors may be controlled. The potential for caffeine-containing drinks, alcohol, or tobacco to affect the results of the trial should be considered. An attempt to control these factors may be made during the clinical trial as well as at the time of enrollment (i.e., limiting the inclusion criteria to patients with acceptable personal habits).

Shipping of Medicines To and From the Clinical Trial Site

Procedures on shipping medicine supplies to and from the trial site are not usually described in detail in a protocol. There are occasions, however, when a description of this activity is useful (e.g., for medicines that must be shipped in a frozen state). The address to which returned medicines should be sent after completion of the clinical trial is often listed in the protocol. General information on the documents that must accompany the shipment may also be included in the protocol. Other aspects of medicine shipments are included in the following section, which deals with the shipping of biological samples.

TABLE 30.4 *Selected factors within or outside the clinical trial environment that may be controlled by protocol*

1. Activity: type and amount[a]
2. Exercise: type and amount
3. Diet and availability of food and snacks between meals
4. Nutritional status
5. Fasting
6. Fluid intake
7. Conversation
8. Visual stimuli
9. Auditory stimuli
10. Tactile stimuli
11. Stress (may be controlled to some degree through the inclusion criteria)
12. Contact with other patients and number of patients per room
13. Size, design, and contents of the room in which the clinical trial is to be conducted and/or in which inpatients are housed
14. Number and nature[b] of personnel conducting the trial
15. Type and amount of tobacco, caffeine or other xanthine (e.g., chocolate), and/or alcohol use or consumption

[a] For example, how long are inpatients allowed or required to remain in bed.
[b] For example, age, sex, experience, formal training, personality, other commitments, and other factors may be relevant.

Obtaining, Handling, and Shipping Biological Samples

Various fluids or tissues (e.g., saliva, feces, cerebrospinal fluid, biopsy material) may be collected in clinical trials for later analysis of medicine levels or assessment of medicine effects. Instructions for collecting, processing, storing, and handling such samples may be explicitly described. These could include information on the (1) specific materials used to collect samples, (2) procedures and specific equipment used to process the samples (including model numbers or design characteristics of equipment if relevant), and (3) previous training of the individuals who will collect, handle, examine, or otherwise deal with the biological materials. Sample instructions are given in Tables 30.5 and 30.6.

In some clinical trials, a central laboratory will be used to analyze samples. Information on the packaging and shipping of samples may be listed (see Table 30.7) whenever biological samples are to be sent from the site of collection to another location.

Defining the Time of Patient Entry and Completion

It may be relevant to define the precise point at which a patient is formally entered into a clinical trial. Entry occurs at different points in various trials (e.g., at the start or completion of screen or baseline or at the start of treatment). It may be important to clarify this point

TABLE 30.5 *Sample instructions for collecting plasma samples containing medicine*

1. Thread needle into holder until secure
2. Insert tube into holder; push tube stopper onto needle until leading edge of stopper meets guideline on holder; tube will retract slightly
3. Apply tourniquet and prepare venipuncture site with an appropriate antiseptic
4. Place patient's arm in a downward position
5. Remove needle shield and perform venipuncture with the arm in downward position and tube stopper uppermost
6. Push tube to end of holder, puncturing diaphragm of stopper
7. Remove tourniquet as soon as blood begins to fill tube; do not allow contents of tube to contact stopper or the end of the needle during procedure
8. After the blood stops flowing into tube, immediately remove needle from vein, and apply pressure to puncture site with a dry sterile swab
9. Remove the tube from the holder
10. Gently invert the tube 8 to 10 times to mix the preservative with the blood; do not shake
11. Immediately place the tube in an ice water bath
12. Separate blood plasma and cells by using a refrigerated centrifuge
13. With disposable pipette and bulb, pipette all plasma into the appropriately labeled plastic test tube; allow enough space between plasma and the stopper cap to account for expansion during freezing
14. Freeze samples immediately, placing them horizontally, and store at $-15°C$ in an erect position until shipment
15. Complete the relevant data collection form

TABLE 30.6 *Sample instructions for patients and investigators for collecting 24-hour urine samples*

A. Patient instructions
1. Immediately after dosing, patients are to void and then collect all urine voided in both the 0- to 24-hour and 24- to 48-hour periods
2. Collect urine directly into the collection bottles provided; pooled samples should be refrigerated at all times except during collections

B. Investigator instructions
1. Measure the total volume of urine with a graduated cylinder immediately upon collection of 24-hour pooled samples; record results on the appropriate data collection form
2. Collect a 50-ml aliquot into a labeled urine sample bottle; freeze samples immediately and store at −15°C until shipment

to enable a clear determination to be made of the precise number of patients entered into a trial. In general, formal entrance into a trial occurs at the initiation of an active baseline or treatment.

It also is relevant to define the point at which a patient is considered a "complete" patient. This is important from the perspective of data analysis, since data from "complete" and "incomplete" patients are often analyzed separately. The time at which a patient is defined as complete often occurs at some point prior to the end of the clinical trial and may also be used as a criterion for replacing patients who have been prematurely discontinued or drop out (i.e., a protocol may state that patients who are discontinued by the investigator prior to a given week will be replaced).

TABLE 30.7 *Information on shipping biological samples*

1. *Package description.* Use styrofoam containers (____ × ____ × ____ cm) with minimum wall thickness of ____ cm
2. *Packing materials.* Fill to ____ % of volume and add ____ kg (pounds) of dry ice. Do not put filler material between samples and dry ice
3. *Labeling of package.* "Plasma (or other) samples, perishable, rush. Send to: ____."
4. *Contact with center (person) receiving the samples.* Notify site and contact ____ (person) 1 week (day) prior to shipping at telephone number ____.[a] Also contact this person just after the package is sent
5. *Shipping samples.* Use ____ carrier only,[b] and request their ____ service. Send sample either collect or prepaid
6. *Forms.* Ship plasma sample inventory form or sheet from each patient's data collection form
7. *Date of shipping.* Send the package only on a Monday, Tuesday, or Wednesday and no less than 3 days before a holiday
8. *Confirmation of receipt.* Determine how to confirm arrival and who will trace package if it does not arrive on time

[a] Inform this individual of the carrier used, the bill of lading number, and the time of day to expect arrival.
[b] Both the type of carrier (air, truck, boat) and the specific company may be specified.

Missed Appointments

When a patient does not keep a scheduled appointment, the missed tests may be either deleted and not made up or rescheduled, either as soon as possible or at a later and more convenient date. It is also possible to discontinue the patient from the clinical trial or to contact the monitor to discuss possible options. It is best to indicate the accepted procedure(s) in the protocol as well as the procedure to reintegrate the patient into the protocol schedule (i.e., when the tests scheduled at a patient's missed appointment are to be omitted as opposed to being rescheduled).

To minimize the occurrences of missed appointments, one may follow any or all of the following procedures: (1) give printed cards to patients with the date of their next visit when they complete one clinic visit, (2) contact the patient by telephone (or, less desirably, by letter) shortly (1 or 2 days) prior to the scheduled visit, and (3) provide transportation to the clinical trial site on the day of the appointment. In addition to these techniques, many of those described as methods to improve patient compliance may also have a role in decreasing the incidence of missed appointments.

Patients Lost to Follow-Up

In long-term clinical trials in which patients are being followed for a significant period, it is important to establish a system to maintain information on where patients live. This may require making periodic telephone calls or writing letters to patients. The question of how assiduously to search for patients who appear to be lost to follow-up must be addressed, as well as how to treat incomplete patient data. Large registries of mortality information and other sources may be utilized to search for missing patients if the need is present and resources are available. Tables 30.8 and 30.9 indicate a number of public and private agencies and businesses that may be contacted for information in addition to potential personal sources of information known to the patient, whose identity may be established by the in-

TABLE 30.8 *Agencies and organizations that provide information[a] on patients lost to follow-up*

1. State Department of Motor Vehicles
2. State vital records offices
3. Social Security Administration
4. Veterans Administration
5. Internal Revenue Service
6. National Academy of Sciences and the Medical Follow-up Agency
7. National Research Council
8. Equifax Services (McLean, VA)
9. Westat (Rockville, MD)

[a] The information provided either relates to the patient's present location or to medical data such as vital statistics. Some of these agencies will not supply information to the public.

TABLE 30.9 *General sources for obtaining information on patients lost to follow-up*

1. Employers
2. Relatives
3. Friends and acquaintances
4. Landlords
5. Former neighbors
6. Schools
7. Union office
8. Associations or clubs
9. Medical groups (e.g., Health Maintenance Organizations)
10. Criminal and traffic records
11. Occupation licensing records
12. Public utility records
13. Religious affiliations
14. Tax records
15. Voter registration
16. Birth and death records
17. Credit transactions
18. Insurance applications
19. Mortgages
20. Post office change of address forms
21. Private detectives

vestigator at the start of a clinical study (e.g., relatives, friends, employers). Additional information (e.g., social security number, driver's license number) that may be useful if a search has to be undertaken may also be requested. Middle-class patients are generally easier to locate than lower-class patients. Drug addicts are extremely difficult to locate. It should be decided in advance whether patients with a severe disease [e.g., acquired immunodeficiency syndrome (AIDS), cancer] who cannot be located will be considered dead or alive for statistical purposes.

Medical Emergencies

If treatments for trial medicine overdosage are known or are being developed, they may be outlined or discussed in an appendix to the protocol. For double-blind clinical trials in which patients may be receiving placebo or one of multiple medicines, a rapid means of breaking the blind must be devised. This may take the form of sealed information kept in the investigator's possession or coded labels that are placed in the data collection forms (e.g., as tear-off portions of the label attached to the medicine dispensed). Other forms of breaking the blind are possible, including direct contact with the monitor for sponsored clinical trials. Day and nighttime telephone numbers of monitors should be given to investigators. Patients participating in medicine trials may be given a wallet card with relevant medicine and trial information plus day and nighttime telephone numbers of the investigator(s) that can be used in case of emergencies.

The presence of standard resuscitation equipment (e.g., "crash cart") to be located at the clinical trial site may be specified, as well as details of any other emergency equipment deemed important. The pres-

ence of adequately trained staff to deal effectively with medical emergencies must be ascertained at pretrial site visits. This includes consideration of adequately trained staff coverage at all hours that inpatients are present at the trial site and the distance and time to a hospital if the trial will take place at a different type of facility.

ADMINISTRATIVE ELEMENTS

Administrative Responsibilities of the Investigator

The administrative responsibilities of an investigator for a clinical trial vary enormously between trials. A number of aspects of this function, however, are common to all trials. These and other aspects must be discussed prior to the trial by the investigator and sponsor (if any) or by the investigator and his or her colleagues who will assist with these responsibilities. Many of the responsibilities are listed in Table 30.10. One of these responsibilities includes the preparation of a final clinical trial report for the Ethics Committee/IRB and sponsor (if any). There may be various rules of the institutions involved regarding the format or content of this report. Information that is generally included in this report is listed in Table 30.11.

The investigator's final medical report is not sub-

TABLE 30.10 *Administrative responsibilities of investigators*

1. Create, or review and approve the protocol and data collection forms
2. Review the investigator's brochure (if any)
3. Prepare patient informed consent forms
4. Appropriate interactions with the Ethics Committee/IRB and other groups that must approve the protocol
5. Careful, complete, and legible record keeping on the patient's medical chart and data collection forms
6. Maintenance of "good clinical practices" according to institutional, Federal, and other regulatory guidelines
7. Periodic reporting to the Ethics Committee/IRB (and sponsor, if any) of the status of the clinical trial
8. Adherence to the protocol
9. Reporting of all serious adverse reactions or other events to the Ethics Committee/IRB, sponsor (if any), and appropriate regulatory authorities if no sponsor is involved
10. Preparation of a final trial report for the Ethics Committee/IRB and sponsor
11. Retention of either original or copied data collection forms according to Federal regulation[a]
12. Keeping all data related to the clinical trial accessible to monitors
13. Maintain accurate records of all medicines received and dispensed
14. Return all unused medicines to the sponsor (for sponsored trials)
15. Report any unusual and serious adverse reactions or deaths within 24 hours to the monitor or sponsor for sponsored trials or within the appropriate period to the regulatory authority and Ethics Committee/IRB for unsponsored trials

[a] For investigational medicines, this period is 2 years past the approval of a New Drug Application (NDA) or discontinuation of the investigational medicine.

TABLE 30.11 *Information to include in the investigator's final clinical trial report[a]*

1. Overall opinion and summary of experiences with the trial medicine, especially in terms of relevant safety and efficacy parameters, plus a comparison with standard medicines
2. Interpretation of laboratory test values outside the normal range
3. Description of any protocol deviations and the reasons for them
4. Discussion of specific experiences with each patient
5. Conclusions
6. Optional items to include in this report:
   a. Introduction and rationale of the trial
   b. Time and events schedule
   c. Dosage regimen
   d. Demographics of the patients
   e. Incidence of adverse reactions and adverse events
   f. Plasma or other medicine levels
   g. Any other data or comments that are considered relevant

[a] Usually sent to the Ethics Committee/IRB and sponsor (for sponsored trials) within _____ (e.g., 3 months) of trial termination. Some sponsors request the investigator's final trial report to be written before the trial's blind is broken.

mitted to regulatory authorities by the sponsor as part of a submission for a medicine's approval. This report allows the sponsor to determine, however, if the investigator's opinion of the clinical trial and the effects of the medicine(s) used differs from the sponsors. If this occurs, then monitors or other clinical personnel may wish to discuss the clinical trial's interpretation with the investigator.

Deaths

Investigators must perform a thorough evaluation of all circumstances associated with a patient's death. An autopsy should be conducted whenever possible. If the clinical trial is sponsored, the sponsor must be notified within 24 hours. The Ethics Committee/Institutional Review Board must also be notified. Sponsors notify regulatory agencies. For unsponsored clinical trials, the Ethics Committee/IRB can inform the investigator about pertinent regulations and responsibilities.

Confidentiality of Data

There are several types of confidentiality associated with clinical trials. Confidentiality relates to information supplied by the sponsor to the investigator and to the Ethics Committee/IRB plus information contained in the patient's medical record. Standard statements may be drafted to describe the confidentiality of patient data and information supplied to the investigator. These may be included in the protocol or put in a letter or statement that is sent by a sponsor to the investigator. If a letter is sent to the investigator, the letter will state that information supplied about a specific medicine must be kept confidential. A witnessed signature by the investigator may be requested, and if so,

it could be affixed to a copy of the letter, which is then returned to the sponsor. The sponsor may indicate in its letter some of the reasons for requesting confidentiality (e.g., to protect patent rights).

Confidentiality statements relating to patient information must be consistent with national regulations and with Ethics Committee/IRB and sponsor's policies. The rights of the sponsor to consult source documents such as electrocardiograms (ECGs), X-rays, laboratory reports, and workbooks in order to document or verify final data collection form entries (within reasonable institutional, regulatory, and ethical constraints) may be stated in the protocol and/or in the informed consent. These original data should have the patient's name removed and replaced with the patient's assigned number in the clinical trial and also the patient's initials, as a check that the patient's number has been transcribed correctly. Under certain conditions, the FDA has the right to see patient data with the patient's full name. This fact must be indicated in the informed consent in the United States. The rights of other appropriate regulatory authorities must be considered.

Collection and Processing of Data

Each protocol usually indicates how data will be collected, processed, and analyzed. In addition to the major procedures and approach that will be followed, the primary evaluations and statistical methods to be used may be indicated. Some protocols present this information in a general manner, whereas others are highly specific and detailed. The organization and content of this section of the protocol are generally discussed with the individuals who will be responsible for processing and analyzing the data.

The protocol should indicate which evaluations, if any, are to be performed during the conduct of the clinical trial and to what degree the data obtained will influence the trial design and completion of the trial. Any calculations or interim analyses that will be performed during the trial may be described in detail along with an indication of how the results will be used. A discussion on data analysis is presented in Section V.

Publishing of Data

Procedures relating to publication of clinical trial results are described in some protocols. If the trial is sponsored, the submission of a copy of the proposed publication (abstract or complete article) to the sponsor is usually requested a specific number of weeks prior to submission to the journal or society. If the study is multicentered, it may be appropriate to indicate whether a joint publication is planned or whether each site may publish its own data individually. Additional details relating to publication of articles should be reviewed at the roundtable meeting held prior to the trial's initiation (see Chapter 60 for a discussion about this meeting). Even if a monograph is planned to promulgate the data obtained, serious consideration should be given to publishing an article in a journal as well.

Monitoring the Clinical Trial

The general methods to be followed for monitoring a sponsored clinical trial should be defined, including whether monitoring will be conducted by the sponsor, an independent group, or representatives of a contract organization. A contract organization usually acts as a "middleman" between the sponsor and investigator (Chapter 58). Indicate that the monitoring will be conducted via periodic visits at the trial site and by telephone contact on a scheduled or "as-needed" basis. The nature of the monitor's function as well as the tasks that the monitor performs are not commonly detailed in a protocol. These aspects of the study are discussed more fully in Chapter 62.

CHAPTER 31

Patient Refusers, Nonqualifiers, Dropouts, Dropins, and Discontinuers

GROUPS OF PATIENTS ASSOCIATED WITH A CLINICAL TRIAL

A number of patients (designated *patient refusers*) usually decide on their own not to enter a clinical trial at one of several stages prior to its initiation. Alternatively, patients may be told that they do not qualify for a trial because of failure to meet one or more inclusion criteria (*nonqualified patients*). Other patients who enter a clinical trial decide themselves to drop out (*patient dropouts*) or are discontinued by the investigator before the trial is completed (*patient discontinuers*). In unusual circumstances, some patients switch their treatment group although they are unauthorized to do so (*patient dropins*). Those who complete a clinical trial are designated *patient completers*.

Figure 31.1 shows at what point during a clinical trial each group is formed. It is important to understand distinctions between these groups and their subsets, because the interpretation of a clinical trial's data and the extrapolation of a trial's results depends to some degree on how the characteristics of the patients who actually completed the trial compare with the characteristics of these other groups. In addition, it is often important to understand how the actual data obtained may have differed if the other groups had entered or remained in the clinical trial.

Patient refusers and dropouts are defined based on the patients' own decisions to not enter a trial or to not remain in one. Nonqualifiers and discontinued patients are defined based on the investigators' or staff's decisions not to allow the patients entry into a trial or not to allow patients to remain in a trial.

Patients Who are in Two or Three Different Groups

Although each of the six groups is described as a distinct entity, there are patients who may belong to two groups (e.g., a dropin who is later discontinued), and others whose situation is not clearly within one group or another (e.g., a patient who is thinking of dropping out and is encouraged to drop out by the investigator).

Two Venn diagrams illustrate some of these concepts (Figs. 31.2 and 31.3). Figure 31.2 shows one means of conceptualizing groups of patients prior to entry in a clinical trial. The degree to which each group becomes a smaller section of the larger one may influence the ability to extrapolate the data. Figure 31.3 refers to the time after a clinical trial is terminated.

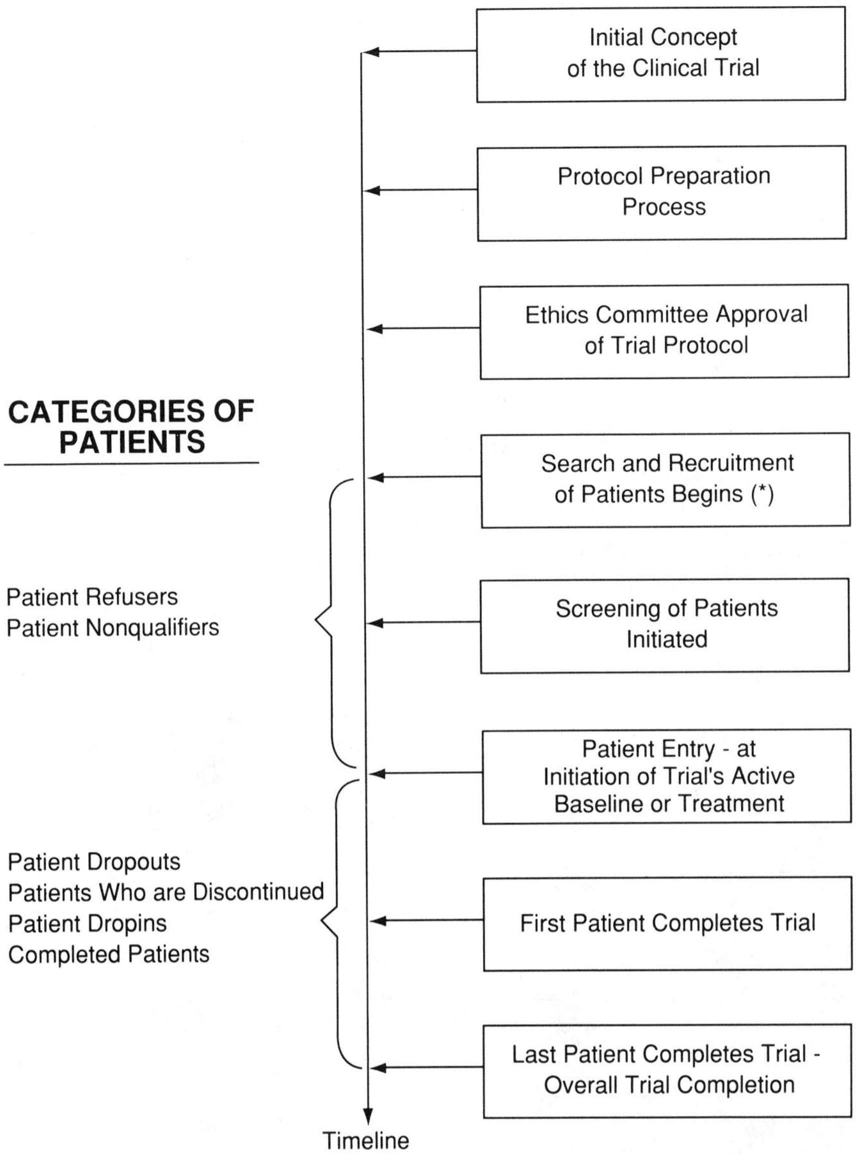

FIG. 31.1 A time line illustrating major events from the initial conceptualization of a clinical trial until the last patient completes the trial. Six categories of patients are defined during this period, two prior to patient entry and four after that point. The asterisk indicates an activity that is sometimes initiated prior to the one preceding it (i.e., prior to Ethics Committee/IRB approval of the protocol).

The overlapping circles show that some ambiguity may be present. For example, a patient who completes 20 weeks of a 25-week clinical trial may be defined as completing the trial. If during weeks 21 to 25 that patient drops out or is discontinued, then he or she should be considered as belonging to that category as well as being a completed patient. If the investigator is considering discontinuing a patient, but the patient decides to drop out of the clinical trial of his or her own volition after a discussion with the investigator, it is possible to include the patient in all three categories. It may be preferable to define this type of patient in the protocol as either a dropout or as someone who is discontinued.

Another term that may be used to describe this patient is *early completer*.

PATIENT REFUSERS

The category *patient refusers* includes all patients who refuse to enter a clinical trial prior to actually being enrolled. This may occur at any stage after the patient is contacted about a trial. The patient may or may not have expressed a willingness to be screened or to learn more about a trial. A subcategory of patients that could be defined is refusers who express no interest in joining

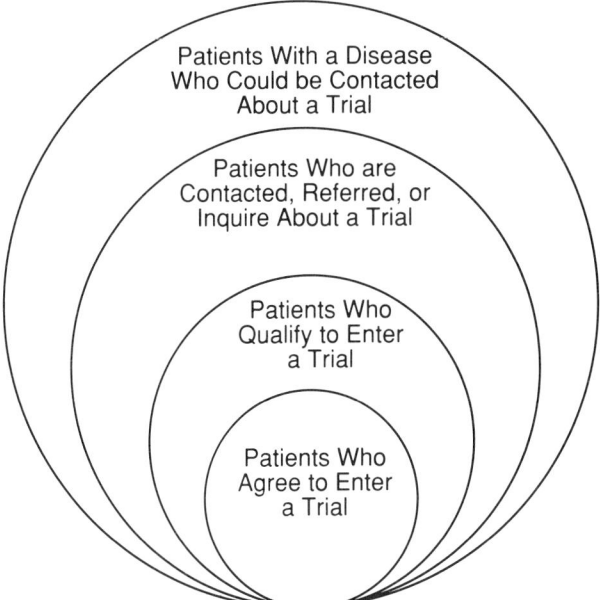

FIG. 31.2 Groups of patients prior to entry into a clinical trial. The Venn diagram illustrates successively smaller groups at separate stages prior to entry into a trial. One of the major issues is how each successive group of patients differs from the larger groups, and how those differences affect the ability to extrapolate data.

a clinical trial at the time of the initial contact. This would include patients who made an initial contact to gain information as well as those contacted by the investigator or his or her staff. Initial contacts by patients may occur as a result of advertisements (e.g., radio, television, newspapers), notices on bulletin boards, recommendations by friends, or information provided by health professionals not directly conducting the

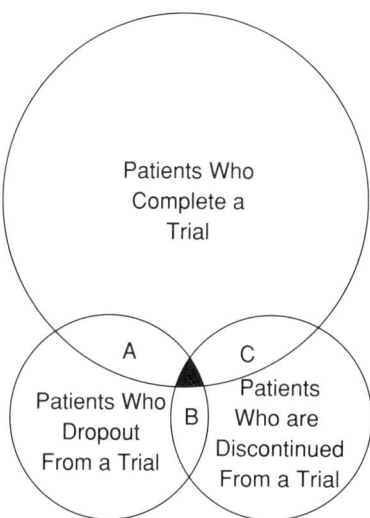

FIG. 31.3 Outcomes of patients who enter a clinical trial. Most patients fit one of the three categories, but some fit into two groups, labeled A, B, and C. A patient may theoretically fit all three categories (i.e., lie in the shaded area).

clinical trial. A different classification of refusers is presented by Allehoff et al. (1988).

Patient refusers who will not provide an informed consent to enter a trial after they have passed all of the screens comprise another subcategory of patient refusers. A suitable term for that subtype would be *nonconsenters*.

NONQUALIFIED PATIENTS

Many patients contacted about a clinical trial do not meet one or more inclusion criteria. This may be a simple matter for the investigator or staff to ascertain on the basis of a few questions (e.g., How old are you? How long have you had the disease? What medicines are you taking?). Alternatively, patients may have to undergo numerous long and complex screening tests before their failure to meet inclusion criteria is determined. This failure may be assessed on the basis of laboratory values, personal factors, factors related to their disease, or to any other inclusion criteria. All patients denied access to a clinical trial by the investigator and staff are defined as *nonqualifiers*.

Establishing the Time of Patient Enrollment

Those who qualify to enter a clinical trial, sign the informed consent, and either are randomized to treatment *or* enter the baseline period are said to have enrolled in (or entered) the trial. Patient enrollment for the purpose of data analysis may be considered as the moment they first receive or are given medication or treatment. The process of patient enrollment is shown in Fig. 31.4. Patients who leave a clinical trial after they have been enrolled but prior to completion are called either *dropouts* or *discontinuers*.

PATIENT DROPOUTS

Distinguishing Between Dropouts and Discontinuers

The category of patients who drop out of a clinical trial of their own volition (i.e., patient dropouts) should be differentiated in all trial documents from patients who are discontinued from a trial by the investigator. The failure to make this differentiation in most publications leads to mixing two usually quite different groups of patients and often creates difficulties in interpreting trial data.

The category of *patient dropouts* includes patients who leave a study for a wide variety of reasons, some of which are listed in Table 31.1. The general types of reasons patients have for dropping out should be indicated in a report to help readers of the report interpret the data. The major question to assess is whether

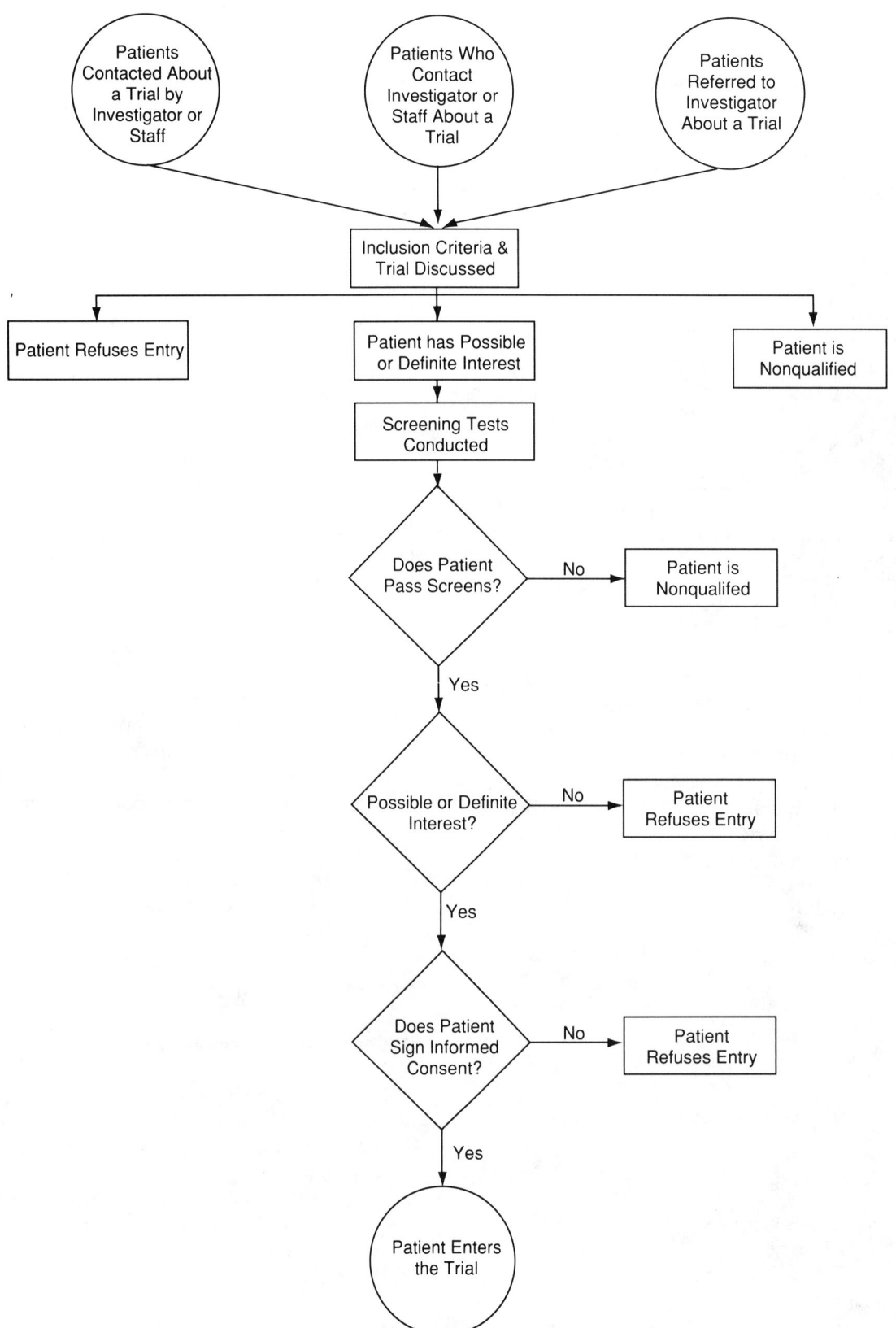

FIG. 31.4 Process of patient entry into a clinical trial, illustrating the points in this process at which patients refuse entry or are disqualified. Note that informed consent may be oral.

TABLE 31.1 *Selected reasons for patients dropping out of a clinical trial*

A. Disease-related reasons
  1. Patient is feeling improved and either does not understand the importance of remaining in a clinical trial or does not accept this as a valid reason to remain in the trial
  2. Patient's condition fails to improve or deteriorates and the patient feels unable (or unwilling) to remain in the clinical trial

B. Medicine-related reasons
  1. Patient experiences adverse reactions[a]
  2. The medicine has unpleasant properties (e.g., taste, odor)

C. Clinical-trial-related reasons
  1. The requirements of the clinical trial are too onerous
  2. Patient dislikes some member(s) of the clinical trial staff
  3. Patient loses interest
  4. Patient believes the clinical trial is too long
  5. Patient becomes upset with some aspect of the clinical trial and refuses to participate

D. Other reasons
  1. Patient's reasons are unknown because he or she does not return for scheduled visits, is totally inaccessible, and is considered lost to follow-up; methods utilized to locate these patients have failed
  2. Patient refuses to state reasons for dropping out
  3. Patient moves from the area
  4. Patient's family or friends encourage dropping out
  5. Patient's personal situation changes at work (e.g., more responsibility, more travel) or at home (e.g., marries) and patient has less time or motivation to participate
  6. Patient develops an intercurrent illness and is unable or unwilling to continue in a clinical trial[a]

[a] The assumption is that the investigator did not wish to discontinue the patient from the clinical trial.

the reasons were related to the medicine used, the clinical trial design, the disease, or other factors. The number of dropouts has been assessed in numerous large clinical trials. Even when the number of dropouts is the same in two treatment groups, the rates of dropout should be assessed. It is possible that most early dropouts were in the placebo group and late dropouts in the active medicine group. Probstfield et al. (1986) describe a successfully conducted program for recovering patient dropouts back into a clinical trial. Macera et al. (1988) present a method to analyze several mechanisms that could be responsible for patient dropouts.

PATIENT DISCONTINUERS

An investigator may discontinue a patient from a clinical trial for many reasons. If the investigator makes this decision, or if the decision reached is mutually agreed, then the patient should be considered categorized as a discontinuer rather than a dropout.

The most common reasons for discontinuation are nontrial-related adverse events or medicine-related adverse reactions. It may be medically prudent to discontinue a patient from a clinical trial even if a serious medical event is judged definitely not medicine-re-

lated. Another common reason for discontinuation is lack of acceptable cooperation with protocol requirements or with staff requests. A less common reason is lack of adequate compliance. If compliance is quantitatively assessed, a specific level may be required of all patients to maintain participation in the study. Patients who fail to maintain an adequate score on any test or in any evaluation may be deemed unsuitable to continue participating. Noncompliers may or may not be discontinued from a clinical trial even if their noncompliance is well documented. There are various pros and cons to this question. Some investigators, scientists, and statisticians believe that noncompliant individuals should not be discontinued from a trial, since the reason(s) for their noncompliance may relate to difficulties with the medicine. These reasons might include (1) patients' difficulty in swallowing a large cap-

TABLE 31.2 *Selected reasons for patients to be discontinued from a clinical trial by the investigator*

A. Patient-related reasons
  1. Failure to maintain a preset level of compliance with clinical trial medication
  2. Failure to maintain adequate compliance with one or more aspects of a clinical trial protocol
  3. Failure to cooperate adequately with the investigator or staff during clinical visits (e.g., poor voluntary effort in tests in which a good ventilatory effect is required)
  4. Failure to adhere adequately to protocol requirements within or outside the clinical environment
  5. Patient's disease deteriorates
  6. Patient experiences a serious adverse reaction in intensity or a specific one that requires discontinuation according to the protocol
  7. Patient no longer meets the criteria for continuation in the clinical trial
  8. Patient found not to meet the original entry requirements
  9. Use of a nonapproved medicine or treatment
  10. Abnormal laboratory values, either severely abnormal or including specific abnormalities that, according to protocol, require discontinuation
  11. Lack of efficacy of the treatment
  12. Improvement, resolution, or severe deterioration of disease being studied
  13. Deterioration of patient's medical condition unrelated to disease being studied
  14. Patient moved from area
  15. Failure of patient to return for an appointment or for a specified number of appointments
  16. Pregnancy (observation and follow-up procedures must be initiated)
  17. Any combination of the above
  18. Withdrawal of patient's informed consent
  19. Death

B. Clinical-trial-related reasons
  1. Clinical trial is terminated at a preset date and some patients are not completed
  2. Clinical trial is terminated prematurely because of unacceptable safety concerns of the medicine being tested; patients currently in the trial are deemed to have been discontinued
  3. Clinical trial is terminated prematurely because the benefits observed do not ethically permit the trial to continue

[a] The tests that should be performed in patients at the time of discontinuation (or as shortly thereafter as possible) should be detailed in the protocol.

TABLE 31.3 *Options concerning replacement of patients who discontinue treatment*

1. Do not replace any patients who discontinue treatment with the trial medicine
2. Replace all patients who do not complete the entire trial
3. Replace all patients who do not complete at least a defined portion of the trial (e.g., day X or part A)
4. Replace all patients who discontinue treatment for pre-specified reasons (e.g., protocol violations)
5. Replace all patients who discontinue treatment until a defined minimum number of completed patients is reached
6. Replace patients who discontinue treatment at the investigator's and/or monitor's discretion

(2) requiring a large number of pills to be ingested, or (3) the trial medicine having a bad odor. Nonetheless, data for discontinued noncompliers should be included in statistical analyses to prevent the suspicion or accusation that they were discontinued to avoid using their data. For intent-to-treat analyses their data must be included.

Patients who are currently participating in a clinical trial when it is prematurely terminated are another category of discontinued patients. Numerous reasons for patients to be discontinued are listed in Table 31.2.

If a patient is unable to take the trial medicine for valid reasons (e.g., unrelated medical problems), the length of time that a patient may discontinue taking the trial medicine and still remain in the trial should be indicated. Special precautions relating to sudden withdrawal of medication must be provided in the protocol.

In addition to describing reasons (i.e., criteria) for patient discontinuation in the protocol, the basis for replacement of discontinued patients should be discussed. One may intend to replace all or none of the patients who do not complete a trial or only those patients who do not complete the trial for specific reasons (e.g., for reasons unrelated to the trial). These and other options are listed in Table 31.3.

A specific list of all tests and procedures to be conducted at the time of patient discontinuation is usually determined prior to initiation of the trial and included in the protocol. Before patients are discontinued because of abnormal laboratory values, it is usually important to repeat the test to confirm the presence and magnitude of the abnormality. If relevant, biological samples (e.g., blood, urine) may be divided and sent to two different laboratories to confirm the abnormal results as well as to evaluate the reliability of the original laboratory. In monitoring the progress of the abnormal laboratory value and its return to normal, it may be useful to continue sending divided samples to two separate laboratories.

PATIENT DROPINS

Dropins are infrequently discussed in the medical literature and cannot occur in most clinical trials. A dropin is someone who takes a test medicine, even though he or she was not randomized to receive it and should not be taking the medicine as part of the trial. This usually occurs because of a patient's strong desire to receive the active medication and not to be randomized to the placebo group. Patients usually do not know with certainty if they are assigned to the placebo or active medicine group when they decide to drop in to the active treatment group.

Dropins in Over-the-Counter Medicine Trials

Dropins may readily occur in clinical trials that include over-the-counter medicines. Examples include aspirin and vitamin C, but few clinical trials that evaluate these medicines include an assessment of patient dropins. In a large aspirin trial conducted in physicians (Peto et al., 1988) it was stated that dropins occurred at a rate of 2% of all patients each year. Some physicians took real aspirin in addition to (or instead of) their clinical trial medication because of their strong belief in aspirin's efficacy.

Patient Strategies to Drop Into a Prescription Medicine Trial

In the placebo-controlled zidovudine (Retrovir) trial, the medicine was unavailable commercially at the time of the initial trial. A number of patients were quite desperate to be in the active medicine group and resorted to a number of ploys to receive active medicine. These strategies included having their medicine analyzed by an underground laboratory and also sharing pills with other patients to increase their chances of receiving active medicine (Dr. D. King, personal communication).

Surgical Dropins

A number of surgical trials of coronary artery bypass grafts versus medical therapy for angina were conducted over the last two decades. Patients randomized to one treatment in some of these trials could opt to receive the other. This usually involved patients randomized to receive medical treatment who desired to receive (and did receive) surgical therapy. In addition, numerous patients assigned medical treatment eventually have surgical treatment. Because these crossovers are numerous, many surgical–medical trials do not actually compare two types of treatment, but rather immediate surgery with medical treatment, plus later surgery if indicated. When data are analyzed by intention-to-treat, numerous anachronisms arise (see Chapter 70 on Statistical Issues).

Determining the Occurrence of Dropins

If the phenomenon of patient dropins is suspected, efforts should be made to determine whether it is occurring. If so, then patients should be questioned carefully in a nonthreatening manner to identify the extent of this phenomenon. Another possibility is to sample the patient's blood or urine for the suspected medicine (Pitt and Costrini, 1979). The occurrence of dropins may be high enough to markedly affect the clinical trial's interpretation. If the decision is made to complete a clinical trial in which many dropins occurred, then the effect of patient dropins should be assessed by comparing results of the entire trial with those obtained in patient dropins.

REPORTING PATIENT NUMBERS IN CLINICAL TRIAL RESULTS

Data to Collect and Present on Patient Groups

Important measurements of patient refusers, nonqualifiers, dropouts, dropins, and discontinuers are (1) their numbers, (2) their characteristics (e.g., demographics, prognostic criteria, disease characteristics) (3) the reasons why they did not enter or why they left the clinical trial, and (4) how their data (if enrolled) compare with those of completed patients. These data enable the reader to determine how well the population that completed the trial represents the total population of patients exposed in one or another way to the trial's treatments or to patients who were considered for the trial but did not enroll. This information assists various professionals in extrapolating the trial's results to other patient populations, physicians, environments, and types of facilities. Simply totaling and presenting the specific numbers within each category of patient is not sufficient to understand the true significance of the data obtained in the trial. A number of authors (Lasagna, 1979; Calimlim and Weintraub, 1981) have presented data on some of these categories, but their presentations represent rare examples in the medical literature.

Extrapolations of Clinical Data

Extrapolations are made both by investigators who conduct clinical trials and by physicians who read reports of trials. Investigators may extrapolate their data to other types of patients, environments, or medical practices. These same extrapolations are also made by physicians who read the reports (usually as published papers). In particular, practicing physicians usually assess whether or not their patients are similar to those in the trial and whether the data presented are relevant. It is not essential that demographic and prognostic characteristics be similar in the group of patients studied and the group in the medical practice of the reader in order to extrapolate data reasonably well from one group to another.

It is certain that only a few clinical trials attempt to determine most of the information discussed above. However, of those few studies that gather even some of this information, little finds its way into the medical literature. Clinical trials that report these data usually restrict their presentations to the numbers of patients present at each stage of the trial, with a few comments about reasons for dropouts. Virtually no publication has presented a complete profile of these data. In fact, it is doubtful whether journal editors would accept a paper with all of these data because of space limitations, unless that topic was the main focus of the paper. It is hoped that additional demographic, prognostic, and disease data will be presented on each of these various groups (including patient completers) in future publications.

CHAPTER 32

Regulatory, Patent, and Legal Considerations

REGULATORY CONSIDERATIONS

Before protocols of investigational medicines may be initiated, a thorough evaluation of regulatory considerations must be conducted. This should be initiated as early in the protocol's development as possible, since there may be regulatory constraints that either preclude or have a significant impact on the initiation or conduct of the clinical trial. The vast number of potential regulatory problems and situations does not allow for more than a brief comment on this important area.

Sponsoring institutions of medicine trials usually have individuals or complete departments concerned with regulatory affairs and are able to address the various issues raised. Investigators who initiate an unsponsored clinical trial should seek a review at an early date of the regulatory aspects of their protocol from their institution, Ethics Committee/Institutional Review Board (IRB), the manufacturer of the medicine, or the appropriate government agencies. Investigators may obtain their own Investigational New Drug Application (IND) or other regulatory approval to study an investigational medicine. Even if no regulatory problems are anticipated, it would still be prudent for the investigator to confirm this impression with the appropriate individuals. Regulatory issues are presented in Chapters 126 to 128.

Academic or other investigators often conduct clinical trials that are not sponsored by pharmaceutical companies. Regulatory considerations for clinical trials of marketed medicines evaluated within their approved indications are primarily focused on informed consents and Ethics Committees/IRBs (see Chapter 27). If the investigator wishes to evaluate an unmar-keted medicine, or an unapproved use of a marketed medicine in the United States, he or she also needs to obtain an IND. Help could be solicited from the pharmaceutical company, if any, supplying the medicine, or the relevant group within the academic institution. Direct contact with a regulatory authority is also possible. Haakenson et al. (1987) described this process in detail, and their article may be used as a general guide.

PATENT CONSIDERATIONS

If the proposed clinical trial involves an investigational medicine, then there may be some patent issues to consider or discuss with relevant individuals. In sponsored trials, a clear understanding of the patent status of the investigational medicine should be obtained before any information is disclosed to outside individuals. By the time the protocol is being developed, these discussions should have been completed. It is important to realize that patent protection may be obtained for a novel use (indication) of a presently unpatented old medicine or chemical ("use" patent). Patent protection may also be obtained for novel pharmaceutical formulations or novel routes of synthesis of new or existing medicines in addition to "use" patents and a patent on the medicine per se. A patent on the medicine per se is the best type of patent to obtain.

Disclosure of a patentable invention before an appropriate patent application has been filed can have a profound impact on patent protection. In most countries, a nonconfidential disclosure (e.g., in discussion at a scientific meeting) becomes an immediate bar to patentability unless a patent application has been filed

242

prior to the disclosure. In the United States and Canada, however, one may file a patent application up to 1 year after such a disclosure.

The most critical evidence on which patent suits are often settled is in researchers' laboratory notebooks, particularly in the United States; the date of discovery rather than the date of filing (as in Europe) is of paramount importance in closely contested cases. Many patent cases depend on what is written as well as when it was written. A sponsor or potential inventor cannot let any original idea lie fallow for years without evidence that it is being pursued. The type and amount of work that constitutes pursuit of an idea is quite variable and open to interpretation.

In the United States an invention must meet three criteria to be patented. It must be new, useful, and not obvious. The method of synthesis for a compound must be the best method known. In the European system any synthetic method is acceptable, since 1 year is allowed to improve on the synthesis.

Investigators of unsponsored clinical trials should check with their institutional patent officers before publishing data on medicines used in a novel way. In order to clarify whether there are issues that must be considered and resolved in regard to patent protection, it is preferable for investigators of unsponsored trials to consult with their patent office prior to initiating a trial.

LEGAL CONSIDERATIONS

The following comments do not purport to provide legal advice relating to clinical trials but raise points that may be discussed further with your attorneys or other individuals who are familiar with the specific details in particular situations and the local laws governing them.

1. The informed consent cannot contain any exculpatory language that would waive or appear to waive any of the patient's legal rights or releases or appear to release the investigator, the sponsor, the institution, or its agents from liability for negligence.
2. Personal injury may result during treatment in the clinical trial; however, the occurrence of injury does not indicate that any liability attaches.
3. The investigator's legal obligations towards the patient include obtaining a voluntary informed consent from the patient or the patient's guardian, adhering to a proper and adequate clinical trial design and protocol that is approved by an Ethics Committee/IRB, and providing due care in conducting the trial.
4. Indemnification agreements may be entered into between sponsors and institutions, institutions and investigators, and sponsors and investigators.
5. Guidelines for compensation for medicine-induced injuries have been proposed in the United Kingdom by the Association of the British Pharmaceutical Industry (1983) with an accompanying commentary by Professors Diamond and Laurence (1983).

Liability Suits Resulting from Clinical Trials

A recall of a medical device has different meanings in various countries, including solely changing the device's label or changing a device in the field. Companies should develop a recall policy and program to use in case of need.

United States manufacturers are subject to three types of liability:

1. *Negligence*. If a company breaches a duty of care with its product and the risk was forseeable, then it is guilty of negligence. When companies are (or should be) aware of risks, they have the responsibility to warn users of their products.
2. *Warrantee*. If a company states something about its medicine or implies something that fails to occur or to be true, it then may be guilty of false claims or warrantees.
3. *Strict liability*. The manufacturer is liable if a defective condition renders the product unsafe to the user.

A plaintiff must prove three things to win a liability suit: (1) There was a defect in the product (i.e., medicine); (2) there was damage (i.e., problem) caused in the patient; and (3) there was a relationship between these two.

Attorneys in the United States can accept legal cases from a plaintiff based on obtaining a certain percent (contingency fee) of the final settlement if the case is either won or settled. This practice of contingency fees is unacceptable in many European countries. Other major differences are that the U.S. system allows for punitive damages and also damages based on pain and suffering, whereas many European countries do not.

Topics To be Included in a Contract Between a Clinical Investigator and Sponsor

If both the investigator and sponsor wish to sign a formal contract prior to a clinical trial (or if one party insists and the other agrees), the following aspects should be included in the contract. It is not suggested that a formal contract is required. A general letter of agreement including relevant details is usually sufficient for most investigators, institutions, and sponsors.

1. *Subject of the agreement.* The subject describes what the agreement covers (e.g., a clinical trial of medicine X in patients with disease Y, a preclinical study of compound A in test system B). The duration of the contract should be indicated.

2. *Obligations of the investigator.* This includes general statements relating to the ethical and regulatory standards of both the sponsor and the countries in which the trial will be conducted. Statements about adherence to the protocol and completion of data collection forms may be mentioned. Practical details such as the length of time that data must be retained should be identified.

3. *Obligations of the sponsor.* This includes the financial payments plus all relevant details as to the basis on which fees will be paid.

4. *Secrecy agreement.* The information to be kept confidential is specified as well as the duration of this agreement.

5. *Publications.* The review by the sponsor of manuscripts resulting from the study prior to publication is discussed, as well as any requirements to prepare such publications. The group that will prepare the publications should be identified.

6. *Cooperation between the groups.* The responsibilities and agreements are identified. Ownership of the data, medicine supplies, agreement for monitors to view source data, ability to conduct clinical audits, plus all other anticipated issues may and should be discussed.

7. *Patent rights arising from findings encountered during the clinical trial.* The topic is self-explanatory.

8. Any other legal statements required or desired.

9. Space for signatures, dates, and related items.

CHAPTER 33

Ethical Considerations and Issues

SELECTED AREAS OF ETHICAL CONCERN

Ethical and moral values often vary to a marked degree in different countries and often vary between different cultures within the same country. Although Ethics Committee/Institutional Review Board (IRB) and government regulatory bodies are "official" arbiters of ethical issues, every investigator should prepare the protocol with a cognizance of the ethical issues it raises. This sensitivity to ethical concerns is especially relevant when the protocol is intended for another country, social class, or group than that of the person who is developing the protocol. A number of ethical considerations raised in conducting clinical trials in developing countries were discussed by de Maar et al. (1983). These authors also discussed various other aspects of preparing protocols and conducting trials in less developed regions. Ethical considerations are definitely present in trials performed on infants, children, pregnant or lactating women, prisoners, mentally retarded or psychotic individuals, or other persons who are unable to protect their own rights fully.

Ethical questions concern not only which populations of patients are permissible to study and which clinical trial designs are ethical to conduct but also when it is no longer ethically acceptable to continue a trial to the scheduled completion (e.g., because of obvious changes in the medical outcomes from what was expected). The means used in terminating a trial may raise additional ethical concerns, which are discussed in Chapter 37. These and other ethical questions have been widely discussed in the last few years (Rouzioux, 1979; Levine and Lebacqz, 1979; Schafer, 1982).

This chapter focuses on ethical issues associated with a clinical trial (i.e., the micro-level), and does not discuss in any detail the large number of ethical issues that exist at a national or international level (i.e., the macro-level).

BASIC POINTS OF THIS CHAPTER

Three basic points will be made relating to ethical considerations in the design and conduct of clinical trials of medicine. The first point is that ethical questions involve all individuals and groups connected with a clinical trial, not just investigators and sponsors. The second point is that ethical questions are an important consideration in most aspects of a clinical trial, from the initial steps of developing the trial design through to the analysis, interpretation, and publication of results. Third, ethical questions are not merely present or absent, but range from the obvious to the strongly debated. Many ethical issues are not black or white and lie in a gray middle range.

OFFICIAL GROUPS CONCERNED WITH MEDICAL ETHICS

A collection of papers concerning medical research on the human fetus as well as the Declaration of Helsinki and The Nuremberg Code of Ethics in Medical Research are presented in the report by the National Commission for the Protection of Human Subjects of Biomedical and Behavioral Research (1976). The Declaration of Helsinki contains recommendations guiding

doctors in clinical research that have been adopted by the World Medical Association. The successor to the National Commission for the Protection of Human Subjects of Biomedical and Behavioral Research in the United States is the Presidents Commission for the Study of Ethical Problems in Medicine and Biomedical and Behavioral Research. Their first biennial report (Abram, 1981), provides information on policies followed by all individual U.S. government agencies that are involved in research on humans. This report also contains the numerous recommendations from this Commission.

UNIVERSAL STANDARDS

An early code for ethical behavior is the famous Hippocratic oath, which interestingly is not presented in many medical school programs and is only read at graduation at others. The Helsinki doctrine, which was approved by the World Medical Association, is an important example of a recent ethical code (see end of this chapter). These doctrines place responsibility for ethical conduct in medicine investigation directly on the physicians involved. Recent medical oaths and codes are summarized by Gillon (1985).

The term *ethics* is used in a broad context that includes and overlaps with legal responsibilities in some instances and with routine obligations of a medicine trial's sponsor in other cases. Some of the major ethical issues in medicine trials concern informed consent and Ethics Committees/IRBs at the institution where the clinical trial is to be performed. These issues have been widely discussed in the medical literature and will not be dealt with in detail in this chapter. Additional details relating to clinical trials were presented by the Committee for the Protection of Human Participants in Research (1982) and published by the American Psychological Association.

Balancing Individual Rights with Society's Rights

An important issue that is not discussed in any detail in this chapter is the balance between the rights of individuals and the rights of society. More specifically, to what degree can an investigator expose patients to an ethically questionable treatment for the potential benefit of many future (as well as present) patients? If serious harm results to many patients from potentially unnecessary or nonvalid surgery or medical practices, should these questionable treatments not be carefully evaluated in patients willing to sign an informed consent? The informed consent would describe risks as clearly and completely as possible. The issue is whether the apparent tradeoff of potentially compromising the welfare of a few for the benefit of many is ethical or not, given that all patients receive an appropriate informed consent.

The ethical basis for conducting clinical trials rests on the fact that doubt exists as to which of two (or more) treatments is better (or best) for a disease. If the preferred treatment is uncertain in the medical community, it is acceptable to conduct the trial, even though some investigators (possibly including the investigator conducting the clinical trial) have an opinion as to which treatment is better.

INDIVIDUALS INVOLVED WITH ETHICAL ISSUES

The first point to discuss relates to the conclusion that virtually all people and institutions involved in any aspect of a clinical trial must deal with at least some ethical questions. Examples of the types of ethical issues dealt with by nine different groups will be described. The ethical involvement of each group generally varies somewhat from trial to trial.

1. The Principal and Assistant or Co-Investigators

As physicians, investigators have a professional responsibility to maintain the highest ethical standards possible. These standards are enforced by State Medical Boards, peer review, and regulations of the hospitals and medical schools at which they practice. Specific ethical responsibilities of investigators toward their patients are to ensure (1) that the protocol adheres to appropriate and acceptable procedures, (2) that the protocol is approved by the relevant Ethics Committee/IRB, (3) that the patient gives a valid informed consent, and (4) that the protocol is followed according to appropriate and proper medical practice. The investigator has the ethical responsibility of notifying the patient of any relevant information that arises during the conduct of the clinical trial that might affect the patient's informed consent.

2. The Institution of the Investigator and Its Ethics Committee/IRB

There are specific regulations in the United States governing the makeup of IRBs (see 21 CFR 56). The IRB acts as the major ethical overseer of the clinical trial and usually requires the investigator to provide periodic reports describing progress of the trial, as well as information on any serious or unforeseen events. In some situations the investigator's clinical department must also approve the protocol. If the investigator uses facilities maintained by the institution to conduct the clinical trial, then the group that operates that facility

(e.g., a Clinical Research Unit) may also require the right to approve the protocol used. Roles and responsibilities of Ethics Committees vary to some degree from country to country and should be identified wherever clinical trials are to be conducted.

3. The Investigator's Staff

The major ethical issue involving the investigator's staff members is how they carry out the aspects of the protocol assigned to them, including contact with clinical trial patients when there would be significant consequences if their performance did not meet an acceptable standard. Protocol violations caused by the investigator's staff may range from minor incidents to issues of serious negligence.

4. The Staff of the Institution(s) Who Will Participate in the Clinical Trial

The staff at the institution who participate in the clinical trial (e.g., physicians who provide medical consults or evaluate electrocardiograms, staff who perform and interpret X-rays) must follow commonly accepted medical standards in meeting their responsibilities. This also applies to all personnel at sites other than those where the trial is taking place (e.g., at laboratories where biological samples are sent for analysis).

5. The Staff at the Sponsoring Institution

For those clinical trials that are sponsored by a different institution than the one where the trial is conducted, it is important that the sponsoring staff adhere to appropriate standards in each of their roles. These roles include those related to trial design, trial initiation, monitoring, trial termination, data analysis, data interpretation, publication, and all interactions between the various people and groups involved in the trial.

The sponsor chooses the investigator for a clinical trial. It is important to choose investigators who will maintain high standards. If this issue is not a concern of the sponsor, then the entire ethical conduct of the trial may be severely compromised. Monitors who follow the conduct of the trial must be cognizant of the standards that are followed by investigators, staff, and patients.

6. The Regulatory Agency

Protocols that are sent to a regulatory agency must be ethically sound, and it is the agency's responsibility to ensure that appropriate standards are maintained. In this manner, the regulatory agency acts as a safeguard to back up the formal and informal review processes that have already occurred at several points in the protocol's approval process. In a sense, various regulations promulgated by the agency govern the previous steps in protocol approval (e.g., having an Ethics Committee/IRB approve each protocol, use of good laboratory practices, use of good clinical practices), and thus the agency influences various ethical issues throughout the design and approval process.

Regulatory agencies in different countries adhere to different ethical standards. This may create a variety of difficult and often complex situations for companies that perform clinical trials in several countries and also submit regulatory dossiers in many countries. Many of the issues discussed in the rest of this chapter become more complex when standards and customs of different countries come into conflict.

7. The Patient (Plus the Patient's Parent(s) or Legal Guardian(s) When Relevant)

From an ethical perspective, the informed consent is one of the most significant issues relating to a clinical trial. In signing an informed consent, a patient accepts the responsibility of complying with the terms of the trial. Patients who are minors but above the approximate age of 7 years should be asked for their assent to participate in the trial, in addition to obtaining the legally required informed consent from their parent(s) or legal guardian(s).

There may be an ethical question as to whether patients who could otherwise afford to pay for and receive more expensive and perhaps medically "preferable" treatment should be enrolled in a clinical trial. Their enrollment would be acceptable if they are fully informed about alternative treatments.

8. The Press and Other Media

Important clinical trials are often reported by the press. The press has the responsibility to present data and conclusions honestly and not to distort or alter conclusions and interpretations of the trial. This may occur inadvertently when the medical language of the trial is changed to make it more easily understood by the public.

9. Clinical Research Contractors

Contract organizations that conduct clinical trials themselves would be considered in groups numbered 1 to 4 above. Contract organizations that place trials with investigators assume many of the ethical responsibilities of sponsors in choosing investigators (see number 5 above) and in monitoring the trial, as well as in conducting any other activities defined in their contract (e.g., data processing, statistical analyses).

ETHICAL CONSIDERATIONS RELATED TO THE CLINICAL TRIAL DESIGN

The second and third major points concerning ethical issues discussed in this chapter are related and will be discussed together. The second major point is that most aspects of a clinical trial involve ethical considerations. The third point is that ethical questions that arise in regard to clinical trials are not merely present or absent. Instead, they range from clear ethical issues to issues whose connection with ethics may be strongly debated. A wide range of issues to illustrate these points will be presented in the discussion that follows.

Almost all of the ethical considerations described are directly or indirectly under the control or influence of the investigator conducting the clinical trial and/or the sponsor(s) of the trial. If the sponsor believes that the ethical conduct of the investigators or patients is substandard then the sponsor has both the right and obligation to terminate the trial. Issues raised in analyzing and interpreting results of trials, as well as publishing data, will not be covered in detail. Many of the problems and issues in each category will be described, but possible solutions to most of these issues will not be presented.

Nine areas that relate to ethical issues raised in developing a clinical trial design will be described.

1. Is There a Need for the Clinical Trial?

The actual need for conducting a clinical trial should always be established first. Sometimes simple alternatives exist, such as conducting a literature search or discussing a topic with experts in the field. To conduct a clinical trial that is not truly necessary is contrary to commonly accepted standards, places patients at unnecessary risk, and may be considered unethical.

2. Is It Ethical to Include a Placebo Treatment Group?

The ethical acceptability of including a placebo treatment group in a clinical trial is often considered. The outcome of discussions and the guidelines used to assist a decision vary in some cases from country to country, even for the same trial medicine, conditions, and rest of the trial design. For example, the West Germans generally believe that a medicine must have the potential to offer patients benefit before it is acceptable to enroll them in a clinical trial, and also do not believe in using a placebo if an alternative treatment is available. This view is not as strictly held in the United States. Many aspects and considerations of this general issue are complex and will not be presented or discussed.

3. Choice of an Active Control

When a pharmaceutical corporation compares the activity of an investigational medicine with a marketed medicine the choice of the marketed medicine may raise important issues. For example, there may be a dilemma for the company if the medicine chosen for comparison with the trial medicine is also made by the same company. If unanticipated adverse reactions appear with the marketed medicine it could have a negative impact on the sales of that medicine. To avoid a potentially compromising situation some companies as a matter of practice do not compare an investigational medicine with one of their marketed or other investigational medicines.

4. Has the Clinical Trial Eliminated Obvious Bias and Deception?

Biases may be introduced into a clinical trial at any stage. It is the responsibility of both the sponsor and investigator to minimize bias. As major and minor biases manage to enter a clinical trial, the less value the trial generally has. At a certain point, biases of sufficient magnitude will have compromised a trial's value to the extent that it is unacceptable to continue.

In the past patients were sometimes given placebo medication without their knowledge. This deceit is generally unacceptable today and informed consents should indicate the probability that a patient will receive placebo. There are, however, circumstances under which certain types of deception may be condoned; such clinical trials should be approved by Ethics Committees/IRBs.

A few examples of deception are described below. One treatment group in a clinical trial to evaluate stress reduction by oxprenolol received a placebo but were led to believe they received an active medicine (Landauer and Pocock, 1984). In another study 80 patients were given a placebo liquid that was described to 40 patients as an "energizer" and to the other 40 as a "tranquilizer" (Dinnerstein and Halm, 1970). A third type of deception occurs when patients are given an active medicine, but they or others are told that a placebo has been given. An example occurred in a clinical trial with mentally retarded patients who were given active medicine, but the institution staff were told that the medication was a placebo (Breuning et al., 1980) (see Chapter 64).

5. Has Sufficient Attention Been Given to Sample Size?

In well-designed clinical trials that involve significant resources and numbers of patients, it is scientifically unacceptable to guess at the number of patients to enroll, even if this is done by experienced individuals. The number of patients required in a trial is often based, however, on assumptions that involve less than certain information (i.e., on educated guesses). A well-controlled clinical trial with too few patients will have minimal scientific value, and an important treatment difference may fail to be detected. Thus, it is not ethically acceptable to enroll patients in such a trial. Another problem that may occur if too few patients complete a clinical trial is that a false-positive or false-negative results may occur. Although such results may be found in all trials, the chances are higher in trials with too few patients.

When establishing the basis for determining sample size it is important to consult a statistician and to consider carefully: (1) Which variables are to be measured? (2) What size difference is important to detect? (3) What is the previous experience with the medicine?

6. Is the Statistical Power of a Trial Adequate to Show an Effect If It Is Present?

Power is defined as the probability of detecting the difference that is looked for, if it is present. It is the goal of any clinical trial to have a high power, i.e., a high probability of detecting a difference between treatments if one actually exists. A power of at least 80% (0.8) to detect clinically relevant differences is usually considered an adequate value for most controlled trials. If a trial with a low power is designed, there may be little chance of actually finding the difference sought, and it may be below commonly accepted standards (i.e., it is unethical) to enroll and treat patients in such a trial.

7. Are the Patient's Chances of Receiving an Active Medicine Acceptable?

Some statisticians advocate that all patients should have at least an equal (i.e., 50% in a two-arm trial, 75% in a four-arm trial) chance of receiving an active medicine rather than a placebo. Patients are usually more willing to enroll in a medicine trial in which their chance of receiving an active medicine is great. The relative importance of the patient's feelings in determining the ratio of group size in a clinical trial relates to a large degree to the particular disease studied and the severity of its symptomatology. A patient with severe chronic pain will be less willing to enter a trial when the chances of receiving placebo medication are 50% than when the chances are about 10%. When the chances of the patient receiving the active medicine are relatively low, it may be ethically unacceptable to enroll and treat the patients in a trial.

8. What Is the Safety of Patients Entered into Clinical Trials?

Normal Volunteers versus Patients

In Phase I clinical trials in which the initial safety of a medicine is to be tested, it is often possible to perform the trial with either normal volunteers or patients with the target disease. Phase I trials usually involve little risk to volunteers or patients despite the fact that these people are the first humans ever to receive the new medicine. Johnsson et al. (1984) stated that 157 studies were conducted using 1,325 normal volunteers between 1980 and 1982 at Hässle and there were no serious adverse reactions to medicines. Only one case of medicine-related sequela was reported in 29,162 normal prison volunteers tested over a 12-year period in 805 protocol clinical trials conducted in the United States (Zarafonetes et al., 1978). Cardon et al. (1976) surveyed 331 investigators who had conducted research on 133,000 human volunteers and patients over the preceding 3 years. Injuries were reported in 3.7% of the subjects. Of these injuries 80% were reported as trivial, 19% as temporarily disabling, and about 1% as fatal or permanently disabling. The total of 57 cases that were fatal or permanently disabling (out of 133,000 subjects) primarily occurred after cancer chemotherapy. This rate is less than risks of accidents in everyday life.

The death of a volunteer in a Phase I clinical trial was so noteworthy that it was written up in the *Lancet* (Darragh et al., 1985) and discussed in an editorial and several subsequent letters to the editors on February 9, 1985 (pages 343 and 344). An important point is that the volunteer had a psychiatric history and had received a depot neuroleptic the day prior to the trial. If this fact had been known, he would have been considered unsuitable for the trial, which points out the need for careful evaluation of all prospective participants in Phase I trials.

9. What Types of Patients Are To Be Entered into a Clinical Trial?

Volunteers versus Patients

Currently most Phase I clinical trials are performed with normal volunteers. There is, however, a growing belief that it may be appropriate to use patients in Phase I trials to test new medicines for safety. This may be especially true in epileptic patients who metabolize medicines differently than do normal volunteers. It is based primarily on practical considerations of learning more scientifically from epileptic patients, because it would not be ethical to treat volunteers with sufficient doses and durations of medicines to induce their hepatic microsomal enzymes. Another example of when patients may be used for Phase I trials relates to the use of medicines with expected toxicity, such as evaluating the safety of new anticancer or antiarrhythmic medicines that are potentially toxic. In this situation it is usually not acceptable to enroll normal volunteers in a Phase I trial.

Inpatients versus Outpatients

In various clinical trials either inpatients or outpatients may be enrolled. In reaching a decision on which group to use it is important to know if (1) the medicine has been well tested, (2) the pharmacological profile is well understood, and (3) it is safe enough to give to outpatients. Also, is it ethically acceptable to allow patients with the disease being studied to function as outpatients during the trial?

Types or Groups of Patients Who Require Special Consideration

Special ethical considerations are raised in clinical trials performed on infants, children, pregnant women, lactating mothers, prisoners, the mentally retarded, psychotic individuals, or other persons who are unable to protect their own rights fully. A major ethical problem encountered with these groups relates to the difficulty of obtaining a freely given informed consent (see Chapter 27).

ETHICAL CONSIDERATIONS IN PROTOCOL DEVELOPMENT

Fifteen separate categories relating to protocol development are discussed below.

1. Inclusion/Exclusion Criteria

A major area of any protocol involves inclusion/exclusion criteria. These criteria influence and control the types of patients enrolled. A number of specific types of inclusion/exclusion criteria are described that may raise ethical considerations on how these criteria are applied to patients who may enter a clinical trial.

Sex of the Patient

In studying most investigational (and many older) medicines, it is required to exclude all women of childbearing potential until appropriate reproductive and teratology studies have been performed in animals. In pediatric trials it is usually unacceptable to continue a female patient in the clinical trial after her first menses.

Age of the Patient

In both pediatric and adult clinical trials there are usually important ethical issues raised about which age to set as the lower limit for patient enrollment. There is also increasing concern about conducting clinical trials in the older population. Various constraints about the health status of older patients should be considered. Publications of ethics committees about their deliberations and decisions regarding inclusion of children and older patients in clinical trials would be valuable. Their conclusions would assist individuals developing protocols as well as other Ethics Committees/IRBs who must discuss and approve such protocols.

Pregnancy and Lactation

There is a general prohibition against evaluating medicines in pregnant or lactating women in clinical trials that are not specifically designed for this population. A pregnancy waiver is sometimes required from women of childbearing potential prior to enrollment in the trial. This waiver usually states that the patient is not currently pregnant and will either refrain from sexual relations or will utilize contraceptive methods approved by the investigator for the duration of the study. If an investigational medicine is being evaluated and a female participant in a clinical trial becomes pregnant the woman must be immediately discontinued. In addition, it is imperative to follow the course of her pregnancy closely and to evaluate the newborn infant.

Sensitivity to a Trial Medicine

It is not ethically acceptable in most situations to enroll patients in a clinical trial if they have a high risk of experiencing a hypersensitivity reaction to one of the medicines or tests used.

Concomitant Medicines

Although it is usually desired to study most medicines as monotherapy, it is not always ethically acceptable to do so. The basic reasons for studying a medicine as ''add-on'' medication are that (1) the efficacy and/or safety of a medicine have not been adequately tested or (2) other medicines are available that have been demonstrated to be efficacious and the patient should not be denied their use. As more information becomes known on a new medicine, it often becomes more acceptable to evaluate it as monotherapy.

Previous Medicine and Nonmedicine Treatment

There may be ethical reasons to exclude from a clinical trial patients who were previously treated with certain medicines or treatments. For example, if a mild analgesic is being evaluated, it would not be acceptable in most situations to include patients if they were previously given strong analgesics and failed to improve.

Washout Period of Nontrial Medicines

Whenever patients are being taken off one treatment and a different treatment is to be initiated, a period of time must elapse to eliminate or minimize the influence of the original medicine or treatment on the subsequent treatment. This interval is referred to as the washout or medicine-free period. Previous treatment effects often persist beyond the time of the medicine's known biological activity. The nature, intensity, and duration of possible carryover or residual effects of a medicine must be considered in determining the length of time that is necessary for an adequate washout period.

Many patients with numerous diseases cannot tolerate the medicine-free period required for an adequate washout. An ethical dilemma may be created when patients need constant medicine treatment and investigators cannot take patients off certain medicines for an adequate washout period. If the patient is not medicine free for an adequate period there may be a residual medicine effect that may alter the data obtained with the new medicine tested. One solution is to eliminate consideration of the first several weeks on the new medicine because of the possible carryover effect. This assumes of course that the previous treatment was discontinued when the new medicine was initiated.

History of Other Diseases

It is not generally ethically acceptable to include patients with certain diseases in a clinical trial, when those diseases would place them at a significantly higher risk than a patient who does not have those diseases. An exception is made when the anticipated benefits are believed to outweigh the risks. Individuals with many specific diseases are generally excluded from early trials of a new medicine until adequate data are obtained on how various types of patients are affected, and an initial profile of the medicine's safety is available.

Present Clinical Status

It is generally considered below currently acceptable standards to enroll patients with clinically *unstable* acute or chronic disease(s) unrelated to the trial disease. Even patients with *stable* chronic disease(s) unrelated to the trial disease are often excluded, especially from Phase II trials. Both the minimal and maximal severity of illness required to enter the trial are important to define, in order to enroll patients with an appropriate range of disease and disability.

Patients with clinically significant emotional problems or retardation are often excluded from clinical trials, unless the trial is designed specifically to include them.

Participation in Another Medicine Trial

Some patients engage in the unethical practice of enrolling in multiple medicine trials at the same time. Examples have been noted in which patients were enrolled simultaneously at two sites of a multicenter protocol, or in two separate clinical trials.

Some volunteers or patients enroll in clinical trials one right after the other. They usually do this for financial gain, to obtain temporary housing, or for other reasons. This is especially common in Phase I clinical trials. Carryover or residual effects from the preceding trial may occur that would confound the data obtained. Strict entry criteria about participation in other trials within X weeks are intended to minimize or prevent this problem.

Institutional or Environmental Status

Certain clinical trials are conducted with patients who reside in institutions or nursing homes, or who constitute a specific population (e.g., patients visited by a public health nurse). They may sometimes be coerced into entering or continuing with a trial, raising obvious issues regarding the validity of their informed consent.

Occupation

It may not be acceptable to include patients in an outpatient clinical trial if they are engaged in occupations involving the use of dangerous machinery. This may include patients who must drive a car. It is especially relevant when it is expected that there is a high probability of sedation, disorientation, or other effects on the central nervous system resulting from use of the trial medicine.

Litigation

Some diseases or problems such as cervical pain or back pain due to trauma are associated with a high incidence of litigation. When there may be secondary gain to the patient if he or she does *not* improve with treatment, the beneficial effects of a medicine may be compromised or completely unobserved if a patient with pending litigation is entered into a clinical trial. It is not a satisfactory ethical situation when patients have conflicting motives vis-a-vis improvement at the time of entering a trial.

Another aspect of litigation relates to patient compensation for medicine-induced injuries. This issue was addressed in the United Kingdom by the Association of the British Pharmaceutical Industry and a series of guidelines was issued (Association of the British Pharmaceutical Industry, 1983).

2. Choice of Efficacy Parameters

There are usually limits on the amount of resources available to conduct any clinical trial. In certain situations it might be medically desirable but financially impossible to utilize specific equipment. If, as a result, some or all important parameters cannot be measured, then it may not be ethically justifiable to conduct the trial.

3. Individuals Conducting the Tests

It is sometimes relevant to enumerate the individuals (by function) in the protocol who are permitted to perform certain tests. In addition, it may be relevant to specify the qualifications or credentials required of these individuals in terms of degrees, certification, or training. It is ethically unacceptable to have incompetent or poorly trained personnel (or investigators) conducting clinical medicine trials. This holds for all individuals in roles that may affect either the patient's care or the collection, analysis, and interpretation of data obtained.

4. Choice of Safety Parameters

Some of the ethical considerations and issues that relate to safety include the following: (1) proper tests must be chosen to ensure the patient's safety, (2) tests must be properly performed at appropriate time intervals, and (3) if problems occur the patient must be promptly and appropriately treated. If any toxicity is either anticipated or considered possible, then a specific attempt should be made to evaluate patients for their risk of having problems occur. Patients at high risk should be excluded unless there are strong reasons not to do so.

5. Modifying Dosing Schedules

When it becomes apparent during a clinical trial that a patient is experiencing difficulties with a trial medicine it may be necessary to modify either the dose of a medicine or the frequency of dosing. The most common safety reason requiring a dose modification is the occurrence of an adverse reaction. It is ethically desirable to determine the procedures, prior to initiating the clinical trial, that describe how this situation will be handled. If systematic plans for modifying doses have not been written into the protocol, then different patients who require dose adjustments may be treated differently. This situation might compromise the integrity and value of the data collected and of the trial itself. In trials using fixed doses of a medicine, dosage adjustments are usually unacceptable and patients who experience adverse reactions may have to be discontinued.

6. Compliance

Patients who fail to comply with the requirements of a clinical trial are not meeting the responsibility that they accepted when they agreed to participate. This occurs to varying degrees in most trials, and a great variety of tests have been developed to monitor patients for their extent of compliance. Many of these tests are straightforward (e.g., counting the number of pills remaining in medicine bottles that patients bring to clinic), but some other techniques raise ethical concerns about invasion of patient's privacy. These techniques must be discussed with a patient prior to the trial and preferably are included in their informed consent. For example, a member of the clinical team, such as the nurse, visits the patient's home at an unannounced time to collect a blood, urine, saliva, or other biological sample in which the amount of trial medicine will be measured.

Some of the reasons for poor patient compliance may be due to problems with the clinical trial that raise ethical considerations for those responsible for the trial design or implementation. For instance, the requirements of the trial may be too painful, stressful, or demanding on the patient (see Chapter 15).

7. Patients Lost to Follow-up

If adequate information is not obtained on how to locate patients enrolled in a clinical trial they may become lost to follow-up. This could pose ethical problems if patients had to be contacted during or after the trial about an issue that could affect their health. Methods of locating missing or lost patients are given in Chapter 30.

8. Patients Discontinued from a Clinical Trial

After a patient is discontinued from a clinical trial because of a medical problem it is the responsibility of the physician in charge of the trial not to discharge the patient from his or her care until the patient's condition has returned to its prior state or the patient is transferred to the care of another physician. Frequent causes of patient discontinuation include adverse reactions to the medicine and abnormal laboratory or test results.

Patients who are discontinued from a clinical trial because of adverse reactions may be rechallenged with the medicine at a later time under certain conditions. These conditions include: (1) the benefit outweighs the risk, (2) the abnormality was relatively mild, or (3) the information to be gained is considered substantial and the risk to the patient is relatively minor. If a patient is to be rechallenged, an additional informed consent should be obtained.

9. Early Trial Discontinuation

A clinical trial may be discontinued early for either positive or negative reasons. Negative reasons for discontinuing a trial include: (1) observation of serious adverse reactions, abnormalities in laboratory examinations or in vital signs that create an unacceptable risk for at least some of the patients to continue, (2) failure to enroll an adequate number of patients, (3) failure of the investigator or staff to maintain adequate clinical standards, (4) failure of the investigator or staff or patients to comply with the protocol, (5) termination of the trial medicine's development by the sponsor, (6) unacceptable changes in personnel or facilities at the investigator's site, and (7) determination that no statistically significant result can be obtained.

There are also a number of positive reasons for discontinuing a clinical trial early. The major reason is that beneficial effect of treatment is observed that raises ethical concerns for patients who are not receiving this treatment. If early termination for ethical reasons is considered possible at the outset of a clinical trial, then criteria should be established to define conditions under which the trial would be terminated early.

It is the investigator's responsibility to prepare patients for the trial's discontinuation once that course has been chosen. The investigator must inform patients in some manner about the results, arrange for continuation of their medical care, and collect the final data to be incorporated into the data collection forms.

10. Medical Emergencies

Patients may be given a wallet card indicating that they are in a clinical trial. The card should contain the name and telephone number of the investigator, coordinator, and other individuals who could be reached at any time. Another issue arises when a patient is in a double-blind trial and a medical emergency arises. It is imperative that a rapid means of breaking the trial blind be devised for all trials. Information on treating medicine overdose should be provided to all investigators by a sponsor prior to a trial. Information known to the sponsor for treating any serious adverse reactions should also be provided to all investigators, if that information might eventually be included in the medicine's labeling.

11. Amount of Data to Collect

Collecting either too little or too much data in a clinical trial may raise ethical issues. Too little data may lead to the situation in which data generated are inadequate for appropriate statistical analyses and clinical interpretation. In this situation the trial objectives are inadequately addressed. The opposite extreme occurs when the vast amount of data generated interferes with the conduct of the trial. In such cases the quantity of data collected may actually prevent the trial from being completed.

12. Instructions for Patients, Investigators, and Trial Personnel

During the initiation and conduct of any clinical trial, many different types of instructions must be provided to patients, investigators, and trial personnel. Although these do not need to be provided in a written form, it is essential that at least some communication is made. It would be unacceptable, for example, if patients went home, developed trial-related problems, and could not readily contact appropriate members of the trial team.

13. Continuation Protocols

An important ethical consideration in clinical trials of investigational medicines that have a specified duration is: will patients who have benefited from treatment be allowed to continue receiving the medicine after the trial is completed? If so, a continuation protocol is gen-

erally provided. Many questions relating to the necessary qualifications for patients to enter a continuation protocol have ethical implication. One dilemma relating to the design of a continuation protocol for patients completing a double-blind trial is whether patients who are receiving a placebo should be entered and remain on placebo in the continuation protocol. If these patients are either switched to active medicine in an open-label continuation trial or are not entered in the continuation trial because they had been on placebo, then the blind of the ongoing double-blind trial will be jeopardized and may be broken. If the continuation protocol is also double-blind there will be numerous ethical issues to consider (e.g., how long may a patient be treated with placebo).

If a continuation protocol emanates from a sponsor, then periodic review of data generated in the continuation protocol should be conducted by the sponsor. The sponsor should reserve the prerogative to cancel any continuation protocol if the medicine's development is discontinued, or for other reasons. Otherwise, the sponsor may be caught in the obligation of having to ''indefinitely'' supply a medicine to a small number of patients, even though the medicine is no longer being developed and will never be marketed. There is also a potential issue if the sponsor removes the only medicine that has benefited certain patients, and no suitable alternative therapy is available. Most sponsors would continue to provide the medicine under these circumstances.

14. Large Multicenter Trials

There are a few ethical issues involved in large-scale multicenter clinical trials that are not present in smaller trials. The larger scale of the trial requires more monitors and usually more monitoring groups concentrating on specific aspects. There may be a special group appointed with the responsibility of ensuring high standards at each site. This group will react to any ethical problems observed.

15. Confidentiality of the Data

There are several types of confidentiality associated with clinical trials. Confidentiality relates to information supplied by the sponsor to the investigator and to the Ethics Committee/IRB, in addition to information in the patient's medical record generated in the trial. This subject raises numerous ethical concerns in terms of deciding which, and from whom, information is confidential, as well as how the confidentiality will be maintained and under which conditions it may be breached. Discussions of confidentiality in protocols and informed consents must be consistent with government regulations and the policies of Ethics Committees/IRBs and sponsors.

Physicians involved in either a sponsored or unsponsored double-blind controlled clinical trial should not be made aware of results of interim analyses. If they are cognizant of one treatment being markedly better than another, it may be ethically difficult or impossible for them to continue treating seriously ill patients with a less effective medicine or placebo.

ETHICAL CONSIDERATIONS IN CONDUCTING A CLINICAL TRIAL

Five aspects of conducting a clinical trial that have ethical implications are briefly mentioned below.

1. Recruiting and Screening Patients for a Clinical Trial

There may be a temptation for investigators or sponsors in some Phase II and III trials to stimulate patient enrollment by offering overly generous inducements. It is unacceptable to offer a relatively large sum of money or other nonmedical inducements to patients so that their primary motivation to enroll in a trial is for financial gain. This view must be modified for Phase I clinical trials, plus selected other trials (e.g., pharmacokinetic trials) in which financial benefit is accepted as the primary motivating factor for many volunteers.

The opposite of paying patients to enter clinical trials is to charge them. In some clinical trials of medical devices, patients (or third-party payers) are charged for investigational devices. Patients in treatment-INDs or compassionate plea protocols may be charged (according to regulations) for the cost of a medicine, although this practice has rarely been followed.

During the screening phase of a clinical trial it is important for all data to be available on patients prior to enrolling and treating them. Otherwise, unanticipated abnormalities may be reported after the patient has been treated with a trial medicine that would have excluded the patient from the trial. The patient may be at high risk of a problem or may have developed adverse reactions that could have been avoided.

2. Providing Information to Referring Physicians

It is a responsibility of investigators to provide relevant clinical trial data and other information to colleagues who have referred patients for the trial. This usually takes the form of a letter or possibly a telephone call. This practice should be followed both as a matter of professional courtesy and as part of the responsibility

of temporarily caring for another physician's patient. If the trial has a significant effect on the patient's disease, then an account of all clinically relevant events and data should be communicated to the original physician.

3. Protocol Violations

Both investigators and sponsors must be sensitive to the issue of protocol violations. Although many minor deviations do not raise ethical issues, it is obvious that some deviations will raise significant dilemmas. These problems must be dealt with on a case-by-case basis in a prompt, sensitive, and effective manner.

4. Conducting a Clinical Trial in Developed Countries

During a trial many questions usually arise which were not anticipated during the development of the trial design and protocol. Many of these questions may raise ethical concerns.

5. Conducting Clinical Trials in Developing Countries

Some of the specific issues that should be considered in developing countries are:

a. Are the patients, investigators, or hospitals being exploited in any way?
b. Have all the practical and potential issues that would ensure patient safety been addressed?
c. Will the medicine, if successful, be marketed eventually in that country or are patients being exposed to a medicine that they can never obtain? This issue would be less serious for clinical trials evaluating patients with mild diseases or for diseases in which an adequate alternative therapy is available.
d. Are the medicines being tested ones that the population would not wish to use (even if marketed) because of local traditions or style of medical practice (e.g., testing oral contraceptives in countries where they would not be used)?

In conclusion, the numerous examples presented have demonstrated that a wide range of ethical issues may arise in any part of a clinical trial. Once an issue is accepted as an ethical concern, there are many complex questions about that issue which are subject to many interpretations and solutions. These matters affect all individuals involved in a clinical trial.

DECLARATION OF HELSINKI

Recommendations guiding medical doctors in biomedical research involving human subjects.

Adopted by the 18th World Medical Assembly, Helsinki, Finland, 1964, and as revised by the 29th World Medical Assembly, Tokyo, Japan, 1975, and by the 35th World Medical Assembly, Venice, Italy, 1983.

Introduction

It is the mission of the medical doctor to safeguard the health of the people. His or her knowledge and conscience are dedicated to the fulfillment of this mission.

The Declaration of Geneva of The World Medical Association binds the physician with the words, ''The health of my patient will be my first consideration,'' and the International Code of Medical Ethics declares that ''A physician shall act only in the patient's interest when providing medical care which might have the effect of weakening the physical and mental condition of the patient.''

The purpose of biomedical research involving human subjects must be to improve diagnostic, therapeutic and prophylactic procedures and the understanding of the etiology and pathogenesis of disease.

In current medical practice most diagnostic, therapeutic or prophylactic procedures involve hazards. This applies especially to biomedical research.

Medical progress is based on research which ultimately must rest in part on experimentation involving human subjects.

In the field of biomedical research a fundamental distinction must be recognized between medical research in which the aim is essentially diagnostic or therapeutic for a patient, and medical research, the essential object of which is purely scientific and without implying direct diagnostic or therapeutic value to the person subjected to the research.

Special caution must be exercised in the conduct of research which may affect the environment, and the welfare of animals used for research must be respected.

Because it is essential that the results of laboratory experiments be applied to human beings to further scientific knowledge and to help suffering humanity, The World Medical Association has prepared the following recommendations as a guide to every physician in biomedical research involving human subjects. They should be kept under review in the future. It must be stressed that the standards as drafted are only a guide to physicians all over the world. Physicians are not relieved from criminal, civil and ethical responsibilities under the laws of their own countries.

I. Basic principles

1. Biomedical research involving human subjects must conform to generally accepted scientific principles and should be based on adequately performed laboratory and animal experimentation and on a thorough knowledge of the scientific literature.
2. The design and performance of each experimental procedure involving human subjects should be clearly formulated in an experimental protocol which should be transmitted to a specially appointed independent committee for consideration, comment and guidance.
3. Biomedical research involving human subjects should be conducted only by scientifically qualified persons and under the supervision of a clinically competent medical person. The responsibility for the human subject must always rest with a medically qualified person and never rest on the subject of the research, even though the subject has given his or her consent.
4. Biomedical research involving human subjects cannot legitimately be carried out unless the importance of the objective is in proportion to the inherent risk to the subject.
5. Every biomedical research project involving human subjects should be preceded by careful assessment of predictable risks in comparison with foreseeable benefits to the subject or to others. Concern for the interests of the subject must always prevail over the interests of science and society.
6. The right of the research subject to safeguard his or her integrity must always be respected. Every precaution should be taken to respect the privacy of the subject and to minimize the impact of the study on the subject's physical and mental integrity and on the personality of the subject.
7. Physicians should abstain from engaging in research projects involving human subjects unless they are satisfied that the hazards involved are believed to be predictable. Physicians should cease any investigation if the hazards are found to outweigh the potential benefits.
8. In publication of the results of his or her research, the physician is obliged to preserve the accuracy of the results. Reports of experimentation not in accordance with the principles laid down in this Declaration should not be accepted for publication.
9. In any research on human beings, each potential subject must be adequately informed of the aims, methods, anticipated benefits and potential hazards of the study and the discomfort it may entail. He or she should be informed that he or she is at liberty to abstain from participation in the study and that he or she is free to withdraw his or her consent to participation at any time. The physician should then obtain the subject's freely given informed consent, preferably in writing.
10. When obtaining informed consent for the research project the physician should be particularly cautious if the subject is in a dependent relationship to him or her or may consent under duress. In that case the informed consent should be obtained by a physician who is not engaged in the investigation and who is completely independent of this official relationship.
11. In case of legal incompetence, informed consent should be obtained from the legal guardian in accordance with national legislation. Where physical or mental incapacity makes it impossible to obtain informed consent, or when the subject is a minor, permission from the responsible relative replaces that of the subject in accordance with national legislation. Whenever the minor child is in fact able to give a consent, the minor's consent must be obtained in addition to the consent of the minor's legal guardian.
12. The research protocol should always contain a statement of the ethical considerations involved

and should indicate that the principles enunciated in the present Declaration are complied with.

II. Medical research combined with professional care (clinical research)

1. In the treatment of the sick person, the physician must be free to use a new diagnostic and therapeutic measure, if in his or her judgment it offers hope of saving life, reestablishing health or alleviating suffering.
2. The potential benefits, hazards and discomfort of a new method should be weighed against the advantages of the best current diagnostic and therapeutic methods.
3. In any medical study, every patient—including those of a control group, if any—should be assured of the best proven diagnostic and therapeutic method.
4. The refusal of the patient to participate in a study must never interfere with the physician–patient relationship.
5. If the physician considers it essential not to obtain informed consent, the specific reasons for this proposal should be stated in the experimental protocol for transmission to the independent committee. (I.2)

6. The physician can combine medical research with professional care, the objective being the acquisition of new medical knowledge, only to the extent that medical research is justified by its potential diagnostic or therapeutic value for the patient.

III. Nontherapeutic biomedical research involving human subjects (Nonclinical biomedical research)

1. In the purely scientific application of medical research carried out on a human being, it is the duty of the physician to remain the protector of the life and health of that person on whom biomedical research is being carried out.
2. The subjects should be volunteers—either healthy persons or patients for whom the experimental design is not related to the patient's illness.
3. The investigator or the investigating team should discontinue the research if in his/her or their judgment it may, if continued, be harmful to the individual.
4. In research on man, the interest of science and society should never take precedence over considerations related to the well-being of the subject.

CHAPTER 34

Completing and Reviewing the Initial Draft

APPROACHES AND STYLES

Establishing clinical trial objectives and choosing a protocol design are usually the initial steps in developing a protocol. In writing a protocol, most of the steps described in Table 20.1 may be performed simultaneously or sequentially. If a sequential order is used, there is no "correct" order to follow for all protocols or for all individuals who could prepare the same protocol. One convenient method of preparing several sections simultaneously is to start rough drafts of each section on separate sheets of paper or by separate dictations. After all sections have been completed, the various parts may easily be brought together and interdigitated to form the first draft.

There are many individual styles used in writing protocols. Two different styles in writing that are discussed in this chapter are the slow and deliberate approach and the fast, "get-it-all-down-quickly" approach. Many individuals find it easier to adopt the latter approach and to improve their protocols through a series of revisions. Each individual who is involved in writing protocols develops his or her own approach.

The first draft of a protocol should be read and rewritten as often as necessary before copies are submitted to other individuals for review. In reviewing one's own draft, it is helpful to question whether (1) each section is placed in the appropriate order, (2) each paragraph within a section is placed in the appropriate order to carry ideas and statements forward smoothly and without gaps or sudden changes in direction or logic, and (3) each sentence has definite meaning and is required for inclusion in the protocol. Introductory phrases at the start of sentences that do not add meaning to the sentence should be deleted, as well as non-essential words such as "the" or "very" when not required. Check for colloquialisms or clichés that can be replaced by more appropriate terms. Ascertain that all statements are adequately qualified and that one has established the intended limits in latitude and scope that will be placed on the statements' interpretation. For example, it may not be appropriate to state "Include patients, who, in the opinion of the investigator, show little or no evidence of the symptoms of . . . ," since this statement does not adequately qualify the latitude allowed in the investigator's judgment. Finally, read each sentence by itself, for its connotations as well as denotations, before deciding whether it conveys the intended meaning and should remain in the protocol.

SHOULD ONE USE MULTIPLE TERMS WITH THE SAME DEFINITION?

Although the quality of fine literature is often enhanced by the use of a variety of expressions for the same concept, scientific writing is often made confusing when a number of different terms have the same or approximately the same definition. Thus, a concept such as adverse reactions should be written using the same single term throughout the protocol and not sometimes as adverse experiences, adverse events, medicine reactions, adverse medicine reactions, side effects, or untoward effects, unless different definitions are intended (e.g., adverse events and adverse reactions are defined differently in this book). Other examples of when a single word or term should be used throughout the protocol (unless differences are intended and are defined) include (1) medicine or drug, (2) volunteers, patients, or subjects, (3) clinical study or clinical trial, (4) disease, condition, problem, or risk factor, and (5) case report form or data collection form. Additionally, if two similar terms are to be used in a protocol with different meanings, then the specific meanings of each term should be made clear. For example, if the term "adverse reactions" is defined as the patient's signs, symptoms, and abnormal laboratory values but does not include other medical events, then another term, such as "adverse experiences," may also be used in a protocol. Each term used must be clearly defined.

WHAT IS THE APPROPRIATE AMOUNT OF REPETITION?

Some protocols are written with a substantial amount of repetition between various sections. Other protocols strive to avoid presenting any repetitive information. This aspect of protocol writing is highly individualized, and different authors have different opinions about the amount of repetition that it is appropriate to include in a protocol. If each section of a protocol is able to stand alone, and material may be repeated elsewhere, there is an advantage in generally being able to locate specific information quickly in the protocol. The major disadvantage of repeating information presented elsewhere is in increasing the length of the protocol. Each writer must determine the proper balance between avoiding any repetition and using extensive repetition. A number of the practical considerations described in this section, plus others not described, are listed in Table 34.1.

TABLE 34.1 *General considerations in writing and polishing a protocol[a]*

1. Avoid excessively long sentences
2. Use correct and consistent tenses
3. Limit the use of adjectives, adverbs, and other modifiers
4. Use concrete, graphic, and precise words
5. Eliminate unnecessary and hedge words (e.g., very, seemed, etc., presumably)
6. Eliminate clichés and trite phrases
7. Eliminate unnecessary sentences or paragraphs
8. Do not begin numerous sentences or paragraphs with the same word
9. Develop thoughts logically and in an orderly way
10. Describe each significant step in a complete thought or procedure
11. Define ambiguous or potentially ambiguous words or phrases

[a] There are exceptions to each of these points, especially when dictated by style.

CHAPTER 35

Improving the Quality of a Protocol

INTRODUCTION

The most obvious technique for improving the quality of a protocol is for the author to review it as critically as possible. It is often useful to conduct this exercise after laying the manuscript aside for several days. A fresh review after a lapse of time usually allows the author to view his or her own work more objectively.

IF–THEN EXERCISES

It is generally advantageous to check mentally every step required to complete all procedures or aspects of a clinical trial and to confirm that all steps have been both accurately and adequately described. All possible problems that can be envisioned should be considered, and a decision made as to which countermeasures to include in the protocol (e.g., if _____ situation occurs, then _____). Additionally, in reviewing one's own protocol, it is important to ensure that many common pitfalls have been avoided in the preparation of the clinical trial. A number of these common pitfalls are listed in Table 35.1.

"WHAT IF" SCENARIOS

A related approach to "if, then" statements is to speculate more on possible problems or issues by considering "what if" scenarios. Many of these will raise responses that could be described or listed in a protocol. Consider a patient calling or visiting the site and imagine every possible occurrence that could befall that patient, using the phrase "what if," as the hypothetical patient goes through the protocol having a series of mishaps and problems.

PEER REVIEW

Another established method for improving the quality of a protocol is to have other professionals and colleagues conduct a review and provide a critique for the author. If the investigator is not the same individual as the author, then the investigator's input is usually obtained, as is that of the statistician who will be analyzing the data. If a roundtable discussion among all investigators, monitors, coordinators, and the sponsor can be held, difficult points can be discussed and, one hopes, resolved. It is the author's assumption that the greater the attention paid to the planning phase, the greater is the likelihood that the clinical trial will be conducted as desired.

INSTITUTIONAL REVIEW

Protocols have to be approved by Ethics Committees/ Institutional Review Boards (IRBs), and if they are prepared by a sponsor, then the sponsor must also approve the protocol. The various steps followed in evaluating a protocol sometimes lead to useful suggestions for its improvement.

TRIAL ASSESSMENT PROCEDURE SCALE (TAPS)

A 15-page form titled *Trial Assessment Procedure Scale* (TAPS) has been prepared by the Pharmacologic and Somatic Treatments Research Branch of the National Institute of Mental Health to assist in the critique of protocols or completed studies. The TAPS procedure was designed to evaluate the quality of a clinical trial rather than the data obtained. One may use all or part of this form to evaluate one's own work, or request that a colleague use this form as the protocol is

TABLE 35.1 *Common pitfalls in preparing and writing protocols[a]*

A. Clinical trial objectives
  1. Expressed too generally to allow a specific trial design to be constituted
  2. Ambiguous or vague
  3. Not obtainable with the current clinical trial design. Trial may be too complex or include too many parts, or there may be inadequate resources to conduct the trial

B. Clinical trial design
  1. Not thoroughly discussed with a statistician, and the design will not adequately address trial objectives
  2. The design chosen is beyond current state of the art
  3. Efficacy tools chosen for the disease being studied have not been adequately validated
  4. There is inadequate statistical power for the particular clinical trial. The sample size chosen is too small to detect clinically meaningful results
  5. Inappropriate use of an active control in a pivotal clinical trial
  6. Lack of placebo or double blind in a clinical trial in which one or both should be incorporated
  7. Dose regimen too restrictive in terms of range of doses allowed, alterations of dosing for adverse reactions, or other factors
  8. Failure of the investigator or sponsor to consult with statistician before designing the clinical trial's randomization

C. Inclusion/exclusion criteria
  1. Too stringent to allow adequate numbers of patients to be enrolled
  2. Too loose to permit meaningful data to be obtained

D. Screen/baseline/treatment
  1. Periods of time for screen and/or baseline and/or treatment are used that are either too long or too short for optimal and appropriate conduct of the clinical trial
  2. Too few, too many, or an inadequate number of measurements are requested (i.e., the clinical trial generates too little or too much data)
  3. Patients may be inappropriately entered into the clinical trial and begin to receive medicine before all screening results are obtained and evaluated

  4. Excessive numbers of blood drawings are requested that may cause adverse reactions (headache or dizziness)
  5. An excessive period of fasting is required that causes adverse reactions (headache or dizziness). This is especially common in pharmacokinetic clinical trials

E. Medicine packaging/dispensing
  1. Medicine packaging that does not permit all options allowed by protocol to be followed

F. Clinical trial blind
  1. Clinical trial blind easily broken because of "obvious" characteristics (e.g., adverse reactions, changes in laboratory parameters, medicine odor) of one (or more) treatment groups (e.g., drowsiness caused by diazepam, colored urine because of phenolphthalein, garlic smell on breath caused by DMSO) that are difficult or impossible to mask adequately
  2. Study blind easily broken by observation of medicine interactions or other situations by the investigator (e.g., marked improvement in trial group or changes in blood levels of concomitant medicines)
  3. Clinical trial blind chosen for use is not appropriate or optimal for the trial

G. Data collection and analysis
  1. Poorly designed data collection forms
  2. Incorrect statistical methods used to analyze data

H. Overall
  1. Ambiguous language used in a protocol that may lead to different results or interpretations than desired
  2. Too many comparisons requested, which will probably lead to some significant results obtained by chance alone (5 of every 100 independent comparisons will be statistically significant by chance alone, if $\alpha = 0.05$ and there are no true differences between the comparison groups)
  3. Presence of conflicting parts of the protocol (i.e., internal consistency is absent)
  4. Discretionary judgments by the investigator are allowed, which may seriously affect the quality and/or quantity of data obtained

[a] Numerous pitfalls related to biases are presented in Chapter 5.

being developed. The eight general parts of the TAPS forms assess: (1) the research problem; (2) research management; (3) design characteristics; (4) treatment characteristics; (5) subject characteristics; (6) data collection; (7) data analysis; and (8) conclusions and interpretations. Each of these areas is divided into two to five sections, and each of the individual points is evaluated separately (Table 35.2). The full document and other systems for assessing reports of therapeutic trials are illustrated in Chapter 103.

TABLE 35.2 *Structure of Trial Assessment Procedure Scale (TAPS)[a]*

1. Research problem
   a. Background and rationale
   b. Objectives and/or hypothesis
2. Research management
   a. External review/monitoring
   b. Site selection
   c. Personnel
   d. Trial period
3. Design characteristics
   a. Independent variables
   b. Design configuration
   c. Subject assignment
   d. Control of treatment-related bias
   e. Control of extraneous variables
4. Treatment characteristics
   a. Description
   b. Dosage
   c. Duration

5. Subject characteristics
   a. Selection criteria
   b. Sample representatives
   c. Subject induction
   d. Subject compliance
6. Data collection
   a. Scope of assessment
   b. Assessment measures
   c. Assessment schedule
   d. Assessment performance
7. Data analysis
   a. Data preparation
   b. Data presentation
   c. Statistical analysis
   d. Data synthesis
8. Conclusions and interpretation
   a. Focus
   b. Logic
   c. Application

[a] Taken from DHHS, NIMH, Alcohol, Drug Abuse and Mental Health Administration.

CHAPTER 36

Preparing Data Collection Forms

GENERAL ORGANIZATION OF DATA COLLECTION FORMS

Three Basic Approaches

The forms for collecting information are also referred to as *case report forms* (or other terms) but will be called data collection forms in this monograph. One of the first decisions that must be addressed is whether or not to organize and group the forms on the basis of separate clinic visits or evaluations (e.g., day A, day B, day C), with all forms for day A separated from those for day B, etc. An alternative approach is to base the grouping on integration of similar or identical forms (e.g., forms for all physical examinations are placed together, followed by the forms for all laboratory tests, followed in turn by the forms for all efficacy measures, and so forth). In this approach, different copies of the same form (for any parameter) to be filled in on days A, B, and C are all placed together. A third approach is to combine both of the approaches described above and to have some forms arranged in a visit-by-visit grouping and other forms integrated by type of examination, test, or form.

Visit-by-Visit Format

The advantages of using a visit-by-visit format for data collection forms is that it is easier for investigators to complete them, especially if the original data collection forms are completed at the time of the patient's visit. One disadvantage of this method is that it is more difficult for either the investigator or a monitor to observe trends in the data. For example, a gradually changing laboratory parameter may be more easily missed, since the values obtained at each visit are in separate sections of the data collection form "book" and are not as easily compared as if all values were on the same or adjoining pages.

Combining Similar Forms

An advantage of combining all similar forms together in one section of the data collection form book is that data monitoring and trend detection are more easily accomplished. For example, if all the laboratory values obtained at one visit are placed in one column, and one page has several adjacent columns, then reading across the page allows one to scan quickly for any abnormalities or trends in the data. The major problem with this approach is that completing the forms is more difficult, since each form that must be completed at one visit is in a different section of the data collection form book and must be located.

Combination Approach

In certain circumstances it is advantageous to combine both the above formats. For example, it may be deemed important to observe specific parameters closely (e.g., laboratory results or seizure counts), but the investigator may prefer to use a visit-by-visit approach for the rest of the clinical trial forms. Also, selected data may be more easily kept together (i.e., integrated) in a trial of long duration (e.g., daily or weekly medicine doses in a trial in which the patients come at irregular intervals), and the remaining forms placed in a visit-by-visit section.

The needs of data processors and statisticians must also be considered in the design of data collection forms. Ideally, a group of individuals will discuss the optimal organization of these forms after the protocol has been written.

DESIGNING THE DATA COLLECTION FORMS

Standardized Information and Forms

Each page of the data collection form package may have a standardized section in which spaces are provided for the patient's initials, study number, and specific date relevant to the information on that page. Other standard information that may be printed on each page includes the title of the study, name of the sponsor (if any), page number, title of the information on that page [e.g., electrocardiogram (ECG), Medical History, Laboratory Examination], plus relevant information about the sponsor or medicine (e.g., regulatory submission, number, department organizing the clinical trial, code number of the medicine). To identify the general contents of any page at a glance when searching through a data collection form book, it is useful to print the title of the information contained on that page in much larger (and bolder) type than that used for the rest of the page. It may be relevant to specify on the data collection form whether the ECG as well as other tests [electroencephalogram (EEG) or X-rays] will be "read and interpreted" by nonexpert physicians or by physician specialists highly trained in their interpretation.

Investigators of unsponsored medicine trials may prefer to utilize some standardized preprinted data collection forms. A number of examples related to behavioral and performance tests as well as demograph-

ics, diagnosis, and adverse reactions are available from the Eastern Cooperative Drug Evaluation Unit (ECDEU) (see *ECDEU Assessment Manual for Psychopharmacology*, Guy, 1976).

Developing data collection forms requires the use of medical jargon and terminology that will be familiar and suitable for the physicians who will complete the forms. Precoded synonyms or codes for many of these terms will be useful for data entry and analysis. These terms or codes should be prepared prior to the clinical trial. Precoding of various responses in the data collection forms should be considered as a step to simplify data entry and analysis at the end of the trial. Discussing the forms with the relevant personnel who will process them after the data have been collected will provide important information on this point.

When multiple clinical trials are being conducted with one medicine, consideration should be given to designing generic data collection forms to improve the ease of combining data from different studies. Types of generic data collection forms are listed in Table 36.1. Various pitfalls to avoid are listed in Table 36.2.

Backward and Forward Approaches

In planning and designing data collection forms for multiple clinical trials a number of basic approaches may be followed. Both "backward" and "forward" approaches will be described. In the backward approach, one starts with an idea of what type of information and format one desires in the statistical reports or synopsis of data. This information is then tracked backward to the data collection form, which is designed to capture data in a manner that allows it to be easily converted or directly placed in the desired tables or figures.

The forward approach starts by considering the type and quantity of raw data that are to be collected and then designing the data collection forms to collect these data. The analyses of the data to be done determine the statistical tables and figures that may be generated. If the statistical tables (or figures) that may be generated are not considered optimal to use in integrating data from multiple clinical trials (or from a single trial) then the protocol and design of the data collection form should be modified to allow collection of more appropriate data.

One result of using either one or both of these approaches for designing data collection forms is that a group of generic forms is eventually established. These forms are presumably available in some type of "library" and may be modified as required for a particular study. The significant efforts that are generally expended in creating data collection forms for a specific study become lessened as more clinical trials are con-

TABLE 36.1 *Types of generic data collection forms that may be prepared*[a]

1. Patient demographics[b] (initials or name, address, birthdate, social security number, sex, marital status, race, education)
2. General medical history
3. Specific medical history focusing on the therapeutic problem being evaluated
4. Clinical chemistry
5. Blood sample: profile of time after medicine administration versus medicine or metabolite concentration
6. Hematology and urinalysis
7. Urinary, fecal, or other sample: profile of time after medicine administration versus medicine concentration
8. Urine screen for illegal drugs
9. Radiology reports
10. Electrocardiogram (specify lead II, 12-lead, Holter monitor)
11. Other laboratory examinations (e.g., pathology reports, biological samples, physiological examinations)
12. Physical examinations; forms for both complete and abbreviated examinations may be prepared
13. Vital signs, height, and weight
14. Neurological examination and/or other specialized physical examinations; forms for both complete and abbreviated examinations may be prepared
15. Disability tests
16. Psychological or psychiatric tests to be used
17. Quality of life measurements
18. Concomitant medications
19. Medicine dosing record for chronic trial—prescribed and actual daily, weekly, or monthly dose
20. Medicine dosing record for acute trial—precise amount and time of each dose given, plus amount prescribed
21. Medicine dispensing record
22. Compliance check—such as pill count
23. Adverse reactions—summary form for clinical trial
24. Adverse reactions—general form for times of onset and cessation plus number of occurrences
25. Adverse reactions—specific form for exact times of onset and cessation
26. Clinical global impression (to be completed by the investigator)
27. Clinical global impression (to be completed by the patient)
28. Premature discontinuation of patient
29. Efficacy measurements that are constant or similar between clinical trials
30. Termination record
31. Posttermination record for patient follow-up after the clinical trial would have normally stopped
32. Investigator's comment log

[a] Some of these topics may be combined on a single page of the data collection forms. For many of these categories several generic data collection forms may be prepared. These would include abbreviated and full reports. Different formats could be prepared for each form, which would allow for either one or multiple patient visits on a single sheet.
[b] Patient confidentiality must be maintained in sponsored clinical trials or if the data will be made public. Therefore, the patient's name should not appear on data collection forms that will be given to a sponsor or made public, nor on correspondence with the sponsor. Indicating the patient's birthdate is preferable to listing the patient's age.

TABLE 36.2 *Pitfalls to avoid in designing data collection forms or in determining the amount of data to collect at different time points*

A. Designing data collection forms
1. Requesting information without providing adequate instructions on the data collection forms (or elsewhere) regarding how to complete the forms
2. Using multiple pages for a single category of information that could easily fit on one page
3. Requesting an excessive amount of information to be put on a single page, which makes monitoring, editing, and data entry difficult
4. Using jargon unfamiliar to the person filling out the form. Some individuals advocate eliminating all jargon
5. Using a check-off system to obtain responses to a question, but not including all possibilities or an "other" category, in which different responses may be listed
6. Collecting all or almost all data in the form of write-ins, so that data obtained from multiple patients are difficult or impossible to combine rapidly and/or condense
7. Using codes on the form that are only relevant to data processors and make the forms difficult to complete by investigators or their staff
8. Not combining or attaching all of the pages of the data collection forms for each patient in a manner that is easy to use, store, and retrieve

B. Determining the amount of data to collect at different time points in one or multiple clinical trials
1. Not collecting sufficient data at baseline or posttreatment
2. Not collecting any data at the most relevant time points (e.g., taking an electrocardiogram before a medicine is given and after the effects have worn off, but not during the period of clinical activity while the medicine is in the plasma or the plasma levels are at or near their peak)
3. Not collecting adequate data at the relevant time points
4. Collecting unnecessary data

Closed versus Open Systems

Possible formats for data collection forms range from a "closed system" with almost 100% preprinted multiple-choice responses to questions to an "open system" with spaces or lines in which responses may be entered. In the former case, data entry and statistical analysis are immeasurably simplified, all investigators will respond in the same or similar manner, and the data obtained may be more easily combined with data from other clinical trials. There is the chance, however, that meaningful data may not be collected in a totally closed system, and some investigators will undoubtedly balk at this "regimented" approach. In the totally open system, different investigators will probably complete the forms differently, but some of the observations and comments collected on the data collection forms may provide valuable insights into the patients and their responses.

It is the author's opinion that a goal in designing data collection forms is to have a minimum number of write-in answers or responses. One essential write-in area is for "Investigator's Comments," located either in one central place or on several pages in the form. A list of

ducted. The potential danger in not considering this issue at the outset of a project is that similar data from separate trials collected on different forms may become difficult or even impossible to combine in an integrated manner.

alternative answers should be provided for questions on data collection forms with instructions to check, cross out, circle, or otherwise indicate the specific response. An additional space or spaces for "other" responses should always be considered. In recording the data from laboratory tests, some individuals prefer indicating the actual number of digits to be used in the answer (e.g., Hematocrit = __ __.__) rather than using a single line (Hematocrit = __), since this latter method may elicit a different number of digits in some written responses.

In multicenter clinical trials, the units of measurement used at each site must be compared for each test to ensure that all laboratories are utilizing the same system of units. This is especially relevant if trials are being run in two or more countries, since not all countries utilize standard international units, and several systems exist for expressing the results of certain laboratory parameters. It may be necessary to include conversion factors in the data collection forms or to use conversion factors on selected data after the data collection forms have been completed. A category of "NA" (not applicable) or another similar term should be used by investigators to avoid having certain boxes or lines left blank on the data collection forms. Blank spaces are undesirable, since they may indicate that (1) the patient did not respond, (2) the question was not assessed by the investigator, (3) the question was not found to be relevant at that site, (4) someone forgot to enter the response on the form, or any of several other possibilities.

Amount of Data to Collect

In determining how much data to collect in a clinical trial, two extreme positions may be taken. In the first scenario investigators collect too little data and collect it in a haphazard manner on various pieces of paper they have quickly assembled without conducting a thorough review of the forms required for recording data. Thus results of some tests may be adequately documented but relevant data generated in other tests are inadequate for appropriate statistical analysis. The "worst-case scenario" with this problem occurs when the trial objectives are inadequately addressed because of insufficient data collection.

The opposite extreme occurs when significantly more data are collected than are required to meet the clinical trial objectives. The vast amount of data generated may threaten the actual conduct of the trial as well as its analysis. The conduct of a clinical trial could be affected if trial personnel had to spend excessive time with patients to generate the data. The investigator, research coordinator, and other personnel may grumble at the redundant work, the patients may feel

hassled by excessive demands and testing, the individuals who monitor and enter the data into computers feel burdened, and the statisticians and clinicians who analyze and interpret the data may only utilize part of the data collected in an attempt to avoid being "swamped" by irrelevant information.

To avoid both of these extreme situations (which the author believes are rather common occurrences), the individual responsible for designing and assembling the data collection forms must analyze the overall approach to data collection as well as each data form used, adding important measurements and questions and culling extraneous ones. The touchstones for determining the amount of data to collect are (1) how necessary the data are to meet the objectives of the protocol, (2) how the data will fit with data collected from other clinical trials if they may be combined at some point into a regulatory submission, and (3) how the data will be treated in the reports that are generated.

Binders and Paper To Be Used

After the data collection forms have been prepared, evaluated, revised, and printed (or photocopied), they should be placed into loose-leaf or other binders or attached together by a different method. A method that allows for replacement forms to be used or for additional sheets to be inserted into the binder has obvious advantages over a rigidly bound set of forms. In addition, if a copy of an ECG, laboratory printout, or official interpretation of a test (or the original) is to be inserted into the record, it is preferable to have an easy means for accomplishing this.

An easy method of separating the different sections of the data collection forms is to place divider sheets with side tabs between relevant forms. The side tabs can be printed, or typed labels may be inserted into plastic side tabs attached to heavy stock paper sheets. If both integrated and visit-by-visit types of form organization are used, then the side tabs for each of the two parts may be printed in different colors for ease of identification. Side tabs can be labeled with the name or abbreviation of the test for integrated forms and with the day (week, month), visit number, or date for visit-by-visit forms. Numerous other approaches can be used in determining the titles to use on section tabs.

Some sponsors and investigators prefer to prepare data collection forms with noncarbon reproducing-type paper. Other individuals prefer single sheets of paper (usually white) that may later be photocopied to obtain additional copies. Noncarbon reproducing paper is often made in different colors. Instructions are often presented in the clinical trial that one color page of each form is retained by the investigator and two or more different colors of the same page are sent to the sponsor. If binders are chosen to hold the data collection forms together, then the outside color may be utilized either as a means to help identify the specific trial if multiple trials are being conducted by the same investigator (e.g., red binders for trial A, blue binders for trial B) or to identify different groups of patients within the same trial (e.g., green binders for group A and yellow binders for group B).

Specialized Data Collection Forms

It is often useful in designing data collection forms to include a separate checklist giving each procedure, test, or examination that will be performed or conducted at that visit. One of these forms may be prepared for each clinic visit or dosing period. It may also be relevant to prepare a checklist for all tests or procedures that are scheduled for a specific (or general) time period of a clinical trial. These checklists assure the investigator and/or others conducting the trial that they have not omitted any tests, procedures, or other details that should have been attended to at that particular time or visit. The checklist prepared for a clinical trial may indicate the page number of the data collection form for each item listed as well as include a space or a box next to each item to be marked after that item is completed. The overall time and events schedule (study flow chart) is a convenient reference for trial personnel and may be placed in the front of each patient's data collection form package as well as in other suitable locations. This schedule could be used as a checklist, especially in a long trial in which not all patients begin the trial at the same time.

Posttreatment Data

If patients cannot be discharged from the trial at their final posttreatment evaluation because of adverse reactions, abnormal laboratory measurements, or other factors, additional visits and possibly additional tests must be scheduled. To collect these data in an efficient manner, it must be determined how data will be entered into the patients' records. One means is to construct a separate form to be completed (see Chapter 125). Another is to have investigators utilize a form designated as the "Investigator's Comment Log," which is often included in data collection forms.

Recording the Time of Day

In noting the time of day at which specific events are scheduled and actually performed, a number of different systems may be used. Time measurements may be noted in terms of actual clock time (4:10 P.M.) or

TABLE 36.3 *Selected methods to measure and record time in data collection forms*

Tests performed at trial day (week) 4		Tuesday 7 2 80 Day of week Month Day Year	
Schedule time			
Hours post-medicine	Clock time (use a 24-hour clock)[a]	Actual time test was performed (use a 24-hour clock)[a]	Δ[c] (min)
0[b]	8:00	8:05	5
1	9:00	9:10	10
2	10:00	10:06	6
8	16:00	15:58	−2

[a] A 12-hour clock plus A.M. or P.M. may be used.
[b] Medicine is given at "0" time.
[c] Δ, difference between actual and scheduled times. This value may also be expressed in hours using decimals.

the elapsed time after a given point (2.50 hours after medicine administration) or both. Either a 24-hour "military" clock or a conventional 12-hour A.M. and P.M. clock may be used to specify the actual clock time. The 24-hour clock is usually preferable for data entry and analysis because it is more suitable for statistical treatment (subtracting or combining times), and it avoids potential problems created by any omission of the A.M. and P.M. notation. The time at which an event is scheduled to occur may be printed on the form used to collect the data. A brief summary of some possible notations relating to time is shown in Table 36.3.

MEASURING AND RECORDING PARAMETERS THAT ARE NOT EASILY QUANTITATED: USING RED BLOOD CELL MORPHOLOGY AS AN EXAMPLE

In examining safety or efficacy data after a clinical trial is complete, numerous options may be used in compiling, categorizing, and analyzing information. This book has stressed the principle that it is important to develop systems for collecting and processing data (insofar as possible) before the clinical trial begins.

Even data that may not appear to be easily quantitated should be dealt with in a systematic manner in data collection forms and analysis. The example that will be described relates to red blood cell morphology in a clinical trial in which this parameter is not being systematically investigated. If specific instructions or a data collection form are not provided for red blood cell morphology, then it is most likely that the data will be collected in the form of scattered comments in the data collection forms. To analyze these comments most effectively and to collect optimal data, it is initially useful to develop the categories that could be incorporated into the data collection forms to classify and quantitate the various comments. The four major categories of red blood cell morphology are: (1) poikilocytosis (abnormal shape); (2) anisocytosis (abnormal size); (3) color abnormalities (abnormal amount or distribution of hemoglobin); and (4) inclusion bodies (abnormalities inside the cell). These categories are not mutually exclusive; for example, a red blood cell may exhibit two or more abnormalities. After the categories are chosen, the terms that will be included under each category may be listed. Definitions of each term may be developed. The most common terms that would be included in the four categories above are listed in Table 36.4.

The next step is to designate a code or codes for grading the intensity of each abnormality. One sample code for categories 1, 2, and 3, shown below, is similar to the code used to grade various aspects of urinalysis.

```
  0 = None or negative
0.5 = Trace
  1 = Slight, mild, 1 +
  2 = Moderate, 2 +
  3 = Marked, 3 +
  4 = Severe, loaded, 4 +
```

The last of the four categories of red blood cell morphology (inclusion bodies) may be coded as "present" or "not present." If many abnormalities are noted in this category, however, then a more elaborate code may be developed.

Both the quality and quantity of data obtained in a clinical trial will undoubtedly affect how the categories and codes are used and reported. If there are few re-

TABLE 36.4 *List of terms included in four categories of abnormal red blood cell morphology*

1. Poikilocytosis

Common terms (old terminology)	New terminology
Burr cell, berry cell, crenated cell	Echinocyte
Acanthoid cell, spur cell	Acanthocyte
Mouth cell, cup form, mushroom cap, uniconcave disk	Stomatocyte
Spherocyte, microspherocyte	Spherocyte
Schistocyte, helmet cell, fragmented cell	Schizocyte
Ovalocyte, oval cells	Elliptocyte
Sickle cell	Drepanocyte
Target cell, bull's eye cell, Mexican hat cell	Leptocyte
Teardrop cell, tennis racket cell, poikilocyte	Dacryocyte

2. Anisocytosis
   Microcytosis
   Macrocytosis
3. Color abnormalities
   Hypochromic, pale color, thin cell, wafer cell
   Hyperchromic, dark color
   Heterochromasia, polychromasia (blue to orange coloration)
   Abnormal distribution of color
4. Inclusion bodies
   Basophilic stippling (noted in many clinical situations, the rest are seen in more specific clinical states)
   Howell–Jolly bodies
   Azuraphilic granulations
   Pappenheimer bodies
   Cabot rings
   Heinz bodies

ports of any abnormalities, then a summary sentence or even paragraph may suffice to treat the results. But if numerous abnormalities are reported, then a more sophisticated handling of the data will have to be developed.

SYSTEMS FOR CODING DATA

As data flows from the data collection forms to final medical reports (see Chapters 66 to 68) the flow is made easier when data are easier to handle. One means of accomplishing this is to code selected data either before or after the clinical trial.

Precoding Data

In some clinical trials all or almost all of the possible responses to questions or examinations are presented in the data collection forms. The investigator or research coordinator merely has to check off the box with the appropriate response (see Fig. 36.1, part A). In other trials, the investigator is asked to write the code of the correct answer (Fig. 36.1, part B). If each question is precoded, it becomes even easier to process and validate the data collected in a computer preprogrammed to associate question number X on page Y with the specific question posed.

If one assumes that the distribution of responses to the hypothetical question posed in Fig. 36.1 would elicit only a few "e's" in part B and little information is lost by not subdividing the "11 or more" category, then there would be little benefit to posing the question in the manner that used to be commonly asked on most data collection forms (Fig. 36.1, part C). In the particular example given, however, the responses to part C would be more amenable to determination of specific means, medians, and error measurements than would the data from parts A or B.

Assume a data collection form requests the patient or investigator to check off one of six categories: 1 to 10, 11 to 20, 21 to 30, 31 to 40, 41 to 50, and above 50. What would happen if the responses for all or even most patients were above 65? This could easily pose a statistical and interpretational problem. If the error was noticed early in a clinical trial, all data collection forms could be changed. If this problem was noted after the trial's completion, it could be a major problem, particularly if the parameter affected was essential to the demonstration of efficacy. Anyone caught in this predicament could only hope that the raw data would be retrievable.

Postcoding Data

In many clinical trials it is possible to go through the data collection forms after the trial is complete and to

A. During the last month, how many episodes has the patient experienced?

Check one:

0	☐
1	☐
2 to 5	☐
6 to 10	☐
11 or more	☐

B. During the last month, how many episodes has the patient experienced?

Place the code for the correct number inside the box. ☐

a	=	0
b	=	1
c	=	2 to 5
d	=	6 to 10
e	=	11 or more

C. During the last month, how many episodes has the patient experienced?

Write the appropriate number inside the box. ☐

FIG. 36.1 Options in designing data collection forms. Various means (A, B, C) of collecting data are shown in response to the question "During the last month, how many episodes has the patient experienced?" The box for the answer may also be labeled with the question number, to assist data entry.

assign codes as was done in the above precoded examples. There are several possible advantages to doing this coding after the trial is complete; one would be when confusion might arise if a long list of medical terms and associated codes were put on a data collection form and it was not clear which code or codes were to go in which places on the forms. Under these circumstances, placing a blank line next to each term with instructions to "check those answers or categories that are appropriate" would be clear to the investigator and a code (either printed or not printed) on the data collection form could be entered into a space or box at a later time. An example of this approach is illustrated in Fig. 36.2. Part A shows a simple response that will be extremely time consuming to enter in a computer and difficult to integrate with responses about other patients. Part B provides visual information, which is often useful as a supplement but is also difficult to integrate across patients. Part C is a postcoding example in which staff assign letter codes to

items checked by the investigator. A simpler version is shown in part D.

Data collection forms like the examples shown in Fig. 36.2 are not entirely satisfactory. If a patient experiences pain in one or two toes (or fingers), or only in his ears or eyes, it would be quite difficult to indicate this information accurately on a checklist. Using a drawing of the human figure would be a better method (Fig. 36.3), but the simple, open-ended example A (Fig. 36.4) would be best. Another approach is to divide the ten anatomical areas into many subdivisions.

Data obtained in the form of written comments, as in Fig. 4.4A, are very time consuming to enter into computers and take up significant space in a data base. Although the number and length of written comments may be minimized, it is usually impossible to eliminate them totally from data collection forms without losing potentially important data. It should be remembered, however, that data captured through comments are difficult to analyze statistically.

A. Location of Pain? _____

_____

_____

B. Location of Pain? Shade all affected areas on the drawings of the figure (front and back)

C. Location of Pain? Check All That are Appropriate:

Head	_____	
Neck	_____	
Chest	_____	
Back	_____	
Abdomen	_____	
Groin	_____ Right	_____ Left
Arm	_____ Right	_____ Left
Leg	_____ Right	_____ Left
Foot	_____ Right	_____ Left
Hand	_____ Right	_____ Left

**Do Not
Complete or
Mark**

a
b
c
d
e
f, g
h, i
j, k
l, m
n, o

D. Location of Pain? Check All That are Appropriate:

Head	_____	a
Neck	_____	b
Chest	_____	c
Back	_____	d
Abdomen	_____	e
Arm (s)	_____	f
Leg (s)	_____	g
Hand (s)	_____	h
Foot (Feet)	_____	i

FIG. 36.2 Options in designing data collection forms. Various means of collecting data are shown in response to the question "Location of pain?" The outline drawings of the front and back of a human for answering questions asked in part B would be attached to the form (see Fig. 36.3). Other variations are (1) to have "yes" or "no" boxes on the data collection forms alongside each body area or (2) to add a measure of intensity or duration. The former is acceptable, but the latter would add complexity and, probably, confusion.

McGill Pain Questionnaire

Patient's Name _____ Date _____ Time _____ am / pm

PRI: S _____ A _____ E _____ M _____ PRI(T) _____ PPI _____
     (1-10)   (11-15)   (16)   (17-20)   (1-20)

1 FLICKERING	11 TIRING
QUIVERING	EXHAUSTING
PULSING	
THROBBING	12 SICKENING
BEATING	SUFFOCATING
POUNDING	
	13 FEARFUL
2 JUMPING	FRIGHTFUL
FLASING	TERRIFYING
SHOOTING	
	14 PUNISHING
3 PRICKING	GRUELLING
BORING	CRUEL
DRILLING	VICIOUS
STABBING	KILLING
LANCINATING	
	15 WRETCHED
4 SHARP	BLINDING
CUTTING	
LACERATING	16 ANNOYING
	TROUBLESOME
5 PINCHING	MISERABLE
PRESSING	INTENSE
GNAWING	UNBEARABLE
CRAMPING	
CRUSING	17 SPREADING
	RADIATING
6 TUGGING	PENETRATING
PULLING	PIERCING
WRENCHING	
	18 TIGHT
7 HOT	NUMB
BURNING	DRAWING
SCALDING	SQUEEZING
SEARING	TEARING
8 TINGLING	19 COOL
ITCHY	COLD
SMARTING	FREEZING
STINGING	
	20 NAGGING
9 DULL	NAUSEATING
SORE	AGONIZING
HURTING	DREADFUL
ACHING	TORTURING
HEAVY	
	PPI
10 TENDER	0 NO PAIN
TAUT	1 MILD
RASPING	2 DISCOMFORTING
SPLITTING	3 DISTRESSING
	4 HORRIBLE
	5 EXCRUCIATING

BRIEF	RHYTHMIC	CONTINUOUS
MOMENTARY	PERIODIC	STEADY
TRANSIENT	INTERMITTENT	CONSTANT

E = EXTERNAL
I = INTERNAL

COMMENTS:

FIG. 36.3 McGill Pain Questionnaire (Melzack, 1975).

COMPLETING THE DATA COLLECTION FORMS

If the clinical trial is sponsored, the investigator(s) and research coordinators should both have an opportunity to evaluate the data collection forms before they are printed or photocopied. In unsponsored trials, a colleague should perform this task. The individuals who will be responsible for data entry and data analysis should also have an opportunity to evaluate these forms to ensure that the data collected are in the proper format for entry and analysis and may be integrated with data obtained from other studies.

When all of the various forms are brought together and put in order, it is useful to place individual forms in the order that the tests will be performed during the clinical trial. Similar types of forms should be grouped together (when possible), such as those relating to patient history, physical examinations, laboratory tests,

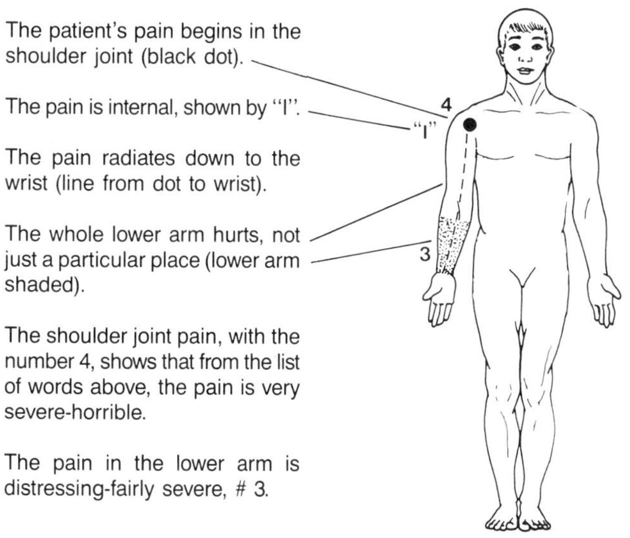

FIG. 36.4 Example of how the McGill Pain Questionnaire could be completed.

The patient's pain begins in the shoulder joint (black dot).

The pain is internal, shown by "I".

The pain radiates down to the wrist (line from dot to wrist).

The whole lower arm hurts, not just a particular place (lower arm shaded).

The shoulder joint pain, with the number 4, shows that from the list of words above, the pain is very severe-horrible.

The pain in the lower arm is distressing-fairly severe, # 3.

and specialized procedures or tests. This approach may be followed regardless of whether an integrated or visit-by-visit approach is used to organize the forms.

Several alternative methods are used to collect and enter data onto the data collection forms.

One Set of Data Collection Forms per Patient

All data are entered onto the data collection form directly or transcribed from laboratory or other forms. Forms may be bound or removable, as in a three-ring binder.

Two Sets of Data Collection Forms per Patient

One set is used as a rough copy to fill in during the patient's visit, and the other set is a clean copy that is filled out later. One set may be denoted as a "workbook," and this rough copy should be retained, at least until the monitor has edited the data, in case of any transcription errors. The clean set may contain "no-carbon-required" paper to provide additional copies. Using two sets of data collection forms may lead to

more errors than a single set and is not generally recommended.

Flow Charts Used with Data Collection Forms

A flow chart may be prepared and used to collect data as it is generated, at the bedside or under conditions in which it is not practical or convenient to use the complete set of data collection forms. The data written on the flow chart are later copied onto the forms.

The method chosen should be based on finding the most efficient approach to achieve the most accurate data in the most rapid period.

Partial Sets of Data Collection Forms for Different Functions or Individuals

The data collection forms for each patient may be divided into sections to provide one section to each individual, such as the physician, assistant, nurse, or coordinator who will complete that part. These separate parts are fitted together after they are completed.

It is usually preferable for one individual to enter all data onto the forms at one site. If this is not possible, then the smallest number of individuals possible should have this responsibility. In many studies, different individuals have responsibility for specific pages to complete (e.g., the investigator completes the physical examination, and the research coordinator completes the laboratory forms).

Signing the Data Collection Form

It is important for the investigator to sign each patient's data collection form. This can take the form of signing (and dating) each page or only the first and/or last page, of the form. Other options include having the investigator initial (and possibly date) each page and sign the last page or only sign the last page. Even computer-generated data collection forms should be signed.

Readers who desire to view an entire library of data collection forms or to find more details to help in form preparation are directed to *Data Collection Forms in Clinical Trials* (Spilker and Schoenfelder, 1991).

CHAPTER 37

Instructions for Patients, Investigators, and Study Personnel

After patients have been accepted for entry into a clinical trial, it is often helpful to prepare a summary of important information for them for easy reference during the trial. This may be achieved by preparing and giving patients an instruction sheet containing the

TABLE 37.1 *Types of information that may be supplied to patients*[a]

1. Discussion about the purpose of the clinical trial
2. Comments on the dosing schedule. A table of all medicines, dosages, and times of dosing may be appropriate
3. Comments on whether to take the medicine before, with, or after meals
4. Future clinic or laboratory visits—where, when, and other pertinent data. If all facilities are not located in the same building, a map may be useful
5. Information on possible adverse reactions of which patients should be cognizant
6. Information on whom to call with questions related to the clinical trial or if adverse reactions or medical problems occur (include telephone numbers for day and night calls)
7. Details on how to complete any self-rating scale, diary, or other patient-completed test included in the protocol
8. Instructions to bring all medicines and relevant records to all (or some) future clinic visits
9. Comment on types of permissible daily activities, including driving a car or operating potentially dangerous tools (machinery)
10. Instructions on when to take medicine doses prior to next (each) trial visit
11. Instructions on how to store the medicine
12. Comments on nonmedicine treatments that patients may also be receiving
13. Information on collecting biological samples (e.g., urine)
14. Comments on concomitant medications, food, alcohol, caffeine-containing drinks, or other beverages that may be relevant to the clinical trial
15. Patients may be given a wallet card that contains pertinent information[b]
16. A copy of the informed consent

  [a] The information to be given to patients may be preprinted and handed to patients or presented verbally (either formally by reading or less formally in a discussion).
  [b] Spilker, 1978.

names and day and night telephone numbers of the investigator and research coordinator plus salient points about dosing, appointments, self-rating scales (if applicable), contraindications, and any other related information (see Table 37.1).

An alternative to an instruction sheet is a text for the investigator to read to all patients prior to the start of a specific test or part of the clinical trial. This ensures that each patient has heard a standard set of instructions (information).

There are several additional types of instructions that may be prepared for use with a protocol. Many of these are listed in Table 37.2. The purpose of instructions is to standardize the conduct of the clinical trial and to help prevent problems in communication between the people involved. Instructions may be placed in an appendix to the protocol or in the data collection forms, or they may be prepared separately and not included in the protocol.

TABLE 37.2 *Types of instructions to be used in conjunction with a protocol*

1. Written instructions to be given to patients
2. Written instructions to be read to and discussed with patients by investigators; these instructions are not given to patients
3. Instructions prepared for investigators relating to the conduct of specific tests
4. Instructions prepared for investigators and research coordinators for filling in each page of data collection forms
5. Instructions for obtaining biological samples containing clinical trial medicines plus information on storage, handling, and shipping of these samples
6. Instructions prepared for pharmacists relating to their role in the trial
7. Instructions prepared for nurses or any of various specialists relating to their role in the trial
8. Other instructions pertaining to specific aspects of the clinical trial

Instructions may also be prepared to describe the accepted means of applying the inclusion criteria, arranging patient visits, completing the data collection forms, and dealing effectively with other aspects of the trial (see Table 37.2). These instructions and other information may be combined into a "manual of procedures," which is often extremely useful in achieving uniformity among different sites of a multicenter trial. When a multinational trial is relevant to conduct, a manual of procedures is even more important to create. Various suggestions for developing trial manuals are presented in Table 13-3 of Meinert (1986).

PART III

Planning Special Types of Clinical Trials

Extreme remedies are very appropriate for extreme diseases.

—Hippocrates

The modern minds in each generation are the critics who preserve us from a petrifying world, who will not leave us to walk undisturbed in the ways of our fathers.

—Edith Hamilton

CHAPTER 38

Single-Patient Clinical Trials

Clinical trials of medicines conducted in previous centuries usually consisted of an experimenter evaluating a single or a few patients. Patients were given one or more medicines and if they improved the materials were believed efficacious. This led to many cases of the *post hoc, ergo propter hoc* fallacy, i.e., if a patient improved, whatever substance was given shortly prior to the improvement was believed to have caused it.

For much of the last 100 years, many patients have been carefully evaluated in open-label case studies to discern a medicine's effects. While these studies are a major advance over the casual observation studies described above, they are still highly subject to many confounding factors and biases. When randomized, well-controlled clinical trials became prevalent in clinical medicine about 30 years ago, open-label trials were generally no longer regarded as providing the most valid results possible. Single-patient open-label studies still persist, however, in the form of case reports and case studies in the literature. These reports serve a valuable function by alerting the medical community to potentially important adverse reactions and previously unknown therapeutic benefits of a medicine. The characteristics of a single-patient clinical case study and trial are compared in Table 38.1.

Over the last 15 to 20 years a new type of clinical trial has been developed: a single patient is intensively evaluated in a double-blind, carefully controlled manner. These designs have raised the value of results from single-patient clinical trials to a higher level in carefully selected situations. Single-patient clinical trials de-

scribed in this chapter are all double-blind and prospective. Patients serve as their own control and often receive two or more treatments on multiple occasions, with each treatment presented in a randomized order.

PURPOSES OF A SINGLE-PATIENT CLINICAL TRIAL

Single-patient clinical trials may be conducted to treat a specific patient as well as to obtain information on a specific medicine. Reasons relating to the treatment of a specific patient include the following:

1. It is uncertain if the patient's current treatment is effective or is causing an adverse reaction.
2. It is uncertain if a new treatment would be beneficial for a specific patient.
3. It is uncertain if the patient's current dosage is correct.
4. It is uncertain if the patient reacts the same to a generic as to a brand name medicine.

Reasons relating to obtaining information on a medicine include:

1. Some rare diseases have extremely few patients available for clinical trials.
2. Patients with certain problems differ in important ways from others with similar conditions (e.g., physically disabled, mentally retarded), and it is not convenient to combine responses from multiple patients.

277

TABLE 38.1 *Characteristics of a single-patient clinical trial and a case study*

Characteristic	Single-patient clinical trial	Case study[a]
Orientation	Prospective	Usually retrospective
Protocol	Yes	No
Informed consent	Yes	Usually no
Real life situation	No	Yes
Use of blind	Usually yes	No
Controls[b]	Yes	No
May investigator modify approach during therapy?	No	Yes
Extrapolatability to other patients	Generally poor	Generally poor

[a] A case study is defined for this table as an in-depth investigation of a single patient. In other situations a single group or institution may be the subject of the case study.
[b] Usually a baseline or placebo is interposed between active treatment periods.

3. The treatment of certain intensely studied patients does not lend itself to multiple-patient trials.
4. When the protocol must be modified a number of times during the trial, along lines that cannot be fully delineated at the outset, it is difficult to treat many patients with the "same" protocol for a long period in these situations.

PROS AND CONS OF A SINGLE-PATIENT CLINICAL TRIAL

Single-patient trials usually differ from other prospective clinical trials only in the number of patients enrolled. All clinical trials require a protocol and data collection forms. All clinical trials involve data collection, analysis, and interpretation. Single-patient trials are always prospective, because a retrospective "trial" in a single patient would merely provide anecdotal information.

Advantages of utilizing a single-patient versus a multiple-patient clinical trial include (1) simpler patient enrollment, (2) less expense, (3) more rapid trial completion, (4) less involved data processing and statistical analysis, and (5) easier interpretation of results. Another advantage is greater flexibility in clinical trial design. For example, the most appropriate endpoint for a specific patient may be chosen, even though another endpoint might be more desirable for a different patient. The endpoint might be a specific behavior that is being modified or a specific speech disorder that is being treated.

The major disadvantage of single-patient clinical trials is greater difficulty extrapolating data to other patients. Although data may be compared with data from other clinical trials, no evidence of interpatient differences will be apparent unless a series of single-patient trials utilizing the same protocol is conducted.

Single-patient clinical trials are also unsuitable for new medicine development, except in a few situations described in the section on appropriate uses.

FLEXIBILITY OF SINGLE-PATIENT CLINICAL TRIAL DESIGNS

Single-patient clinical trials are more flexible than multiple-patient trials in three major ways. First, the design and protocol may be tailored to the specific patient studied. This is particularly relevant if a medicine's effect on a behavioral, psychological, or physical problem is being evaluated.

Second, a multiple-patient clinical trial should not, in general, have more than a single point during the trial at which a decision must be made about modifying the protocol in different directions (e.g., randomizing the patient to a treatment based on performance during the first part of a trial). This does not apply to dosage modifications made on the basis of safety. In a single patient it is possible to utilize multiple decision points within the same trial. This may be done to compare multiple medicine regimens chosen on the basis of the patient's response, or to evolve to the most appropriate medicine regimen and then to compare response(s) on that dosage with that of placebo or a standard medicine (i.e., active control).

Third, designs may be highly complex and sophisticated in a single-patient clinical trial, whereas it is often impractical to utilize complex designs in multiple-patient trials. For example, trial requirements may be physically or mentally demanding on patients or insufficient resources may be available.

TYPES OF SINGLE-PATIENT CLINICAL TRIAL DESIGNS

In the following discussion, "A" is used to denote a control treatment and "B" is used to denote an experimental treatment. Control treatments may represent an active medicine, a placebo, or no treatment. The periods of a clinical trial should only be changed from control to test treatment or vice versa (i.e., from A to B or from B to A) when the patient's data are stable.

Two-Treatment Designs

1. *Two periods.* This is the simplest design. A patient is crossed over on one occasion from treatment A to B, or from B to A (an AB or BA design).
2. *Three periods.* Patients are crossed back over to their original control (i.e., ABA design) or experimental treatment (i.e., BAB design) at the end of the second period. This design allows a stronger

interpretation of data to be made, because it tests the effects not only of introducing a new treatment in the second period, but also of taking it away.

3. *Multiple pairs of periods.* Each pair of treatments (i.e., AB) is presented two or more times in either an alternating (e.g., ABABAB) or randomized order (e.g., BAABABBA). In both situations there will be an equal number of A and B periods (see Fig. 38.1).

4. *Multiple periods.* Patients are assigned to treatment with an order determined by a statistically generated randomized pattern (e.g., ABBAAA-BABB).

5. *Multiple controls.* This design involves the use of control baseline periods of different durations. The same intervention is presented to a patient for different durations of baseline control to determine if the parameter measured changes only when the intervention is applied. Controls may relate to two or more different environmental settings when the same treatment is being evaluated in a single patient, or to two or more different behaviors in a single patient that are being influenced by a treatment in a sequential manner. Multiple controls are also used across patients to have a different initial control duration in various patients, each studied as a single patient. See Fig. 38.2 for an illustration. This technique is usually referred to as multiple baselines in the literature (Dattilo and Nelson, 1986; Kratochwill, 1978).

Three or More Treatment Designs

Three or more different treatments may be used for (1) test medicine, placebo, and active control medi-

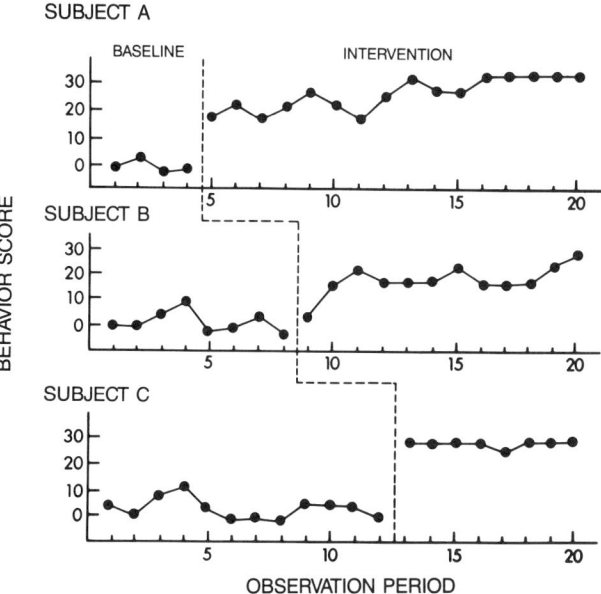

FIG. 38.2 Multiple controls (baselines) across three subjects. (Reprinted from Dattilo and Nelson, 1986, with permission of Human Sciences Press.)

cine, (2) two or more doses of a test medicine, plus placebo and/or active control, or (3) numerous variations of these patterns. Three or more treatments may use clinical trial designs described for two treatments. Care must be taken, however, to avoid introducing excessive complexity, which would compromise the interpretability of results.

Three or more arms of a clinical trial are especially relevant to use when separate components of a treatment are to be evaluated. Two basic types of ''component'' trials are conducted: those in which the *addition* of one (or more) component to a medical

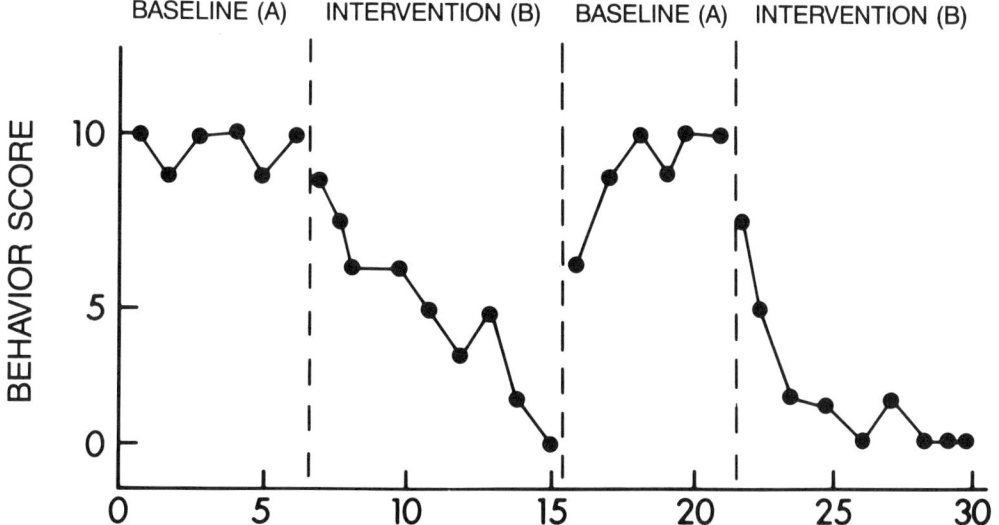

FIG. 38.1 Alternating periods between control (baseline) and intervention. The abscissa represents the number of days or sessions. (Reprinted from Dattilo and Nelson, 1986, with permission of Human Sciences Press.)

treatment is evaluated and those in which one (or more) component of a medical treatment is *deleted*. The objective in these clinical trials is to evaluate how separate components of a complex treatment or combination medicine contribute to its efficacy and/or safety.

In medicine trials, component designs may be used to study combination medicines using a factorial design (e.g., A, B, C, A + B, A + C, B + C, A + B + C). Innumerable variations of this design are possible utilizing concepts described above for the two treatment periods. Various component trial designs could also be used to evaluate add-on therapy to determine whether additional benefits are observed. An unstructured, informal evaluation of this type is often performed in patients with diseases usually treated with multiple medicines (e.g., epilepsy, hypertension). Medicine reduction trials may also be conducted using the component designs discussed. This is especially useful when it is desired to wean patients off one or more of their medicines. It may be done to simplify their therapy, reduce adverse reactions, or determine whether certain medicines may be used as monotherapy.

Other designs include the intensive design (multiple crossover) performed double-blind (Chassan, 1979) and various combinations of treatments and baselines (Barlow and Hersen, 1973).

WHEN MAY A SINGLE-PATIENT CLINICAL TRIAL DESIGN BE USED?

A number of circumstances should be present when considering single-patient clinical trial design. Those listed below are modified from McLeod et al. (1986).

1. The disease must be chronic.
2. The disease severity must be stable over the clinical trial duration.
3. The treatment's effect should be manifested within a reasonably short time.
4. The effect should be rapidly reversible once each treatment is stopped.
5. The efficacy parameters chosen should be the most appropriate ones available.
6. Both patient and investigator should be blind to treatment.
7. A period effect should not be present, but if expected then treatments may be randomly allocated.
9. Because most single-patient clinical trials resemble a crossover design, patients should return to preexisting baselines between treatment legs.

Single-patient clinical trial design issues are discussed in numerous articles (Barlow and Hersen, 1973;

Martin and Epstein, 1976; Kearns, 1986) and books (Kratochwill, 1978; Kazdin, 1982; Barlow and Hersen, 1984).

APPROPRIATE PATIENT POPULATIONS AND SITUATIONS IN WHICH TO USE SINGLE-PATIENT CLINICAL TRIALS

Medicines have been studied in single patients with numerous diseases (Guyatt et al., 1986; Kellner et al., 1979). The choice of the most appropriate clinical trial design depends on the considerations listed above as well as others (e.g., no carryover effect). The number of diseases that are appropriate for single-patient trials is limited, because the severity of many chronic diseases is unstable over the proposed trial duration and does not rapidly return to the original baseline each time a treatment is discontinued.

A single-patient clinical trial should be considered whenever a clinical trial is being conducted to determine the best means of treating a particular patient and results are not to be extrapolated to other patients. Several areas are particularly relevant for these trials, including mental retardation, psychological disorders (Kazdin, 1982), behavioral problems, patients undergoing occupational therapy (Ottenbacher, 1986), and hearing and speech disorders (Connell and Thompson, 1986).

Appropriate situations for single-patient clinical trials include: (1) to evaluate rare diseases when multicenter trials are impractical or inappropriate, (2) determine whether a particular patient's response to treatment is a placebo response, (3) when a small percent of patients respond to a specific treatment and it is relevant to determine a specific patient's response, (4) to evaluate a specific patient in detail to choose the best medicine therapy, and (5) to evaluate whether an adverse reaction in a specific patient is related to a specific medicine. Any rechallenge of a patient with medicine, following an adverse reaction in a multiple-patient trial, is actually a single-patient trial of type 5. Single-patient trials have also been used as pilot trials (McPherson and Le Gassicke, 1965; McPherson and Smythies, 1969).

INTERPRETATION OF DATA FROM SINGLE-PATIENT CLINICAL TRIALS

The interpretation of data obtained from a single patient depends on the trial design used. If multiple crossovers of treatment and baseline, or if two treatments were conducted (presented to the patient in a randomized pattern), there will be statistical tests that may be used to analyze the data. The interpretation will be conducted as for a larger trial, except that additional caution must be used in extrapolating the conclusions. If treatment was instituted at one time and the results are to be compared with baseline, the interpretation poses additional problems.

Data from single-patient clinical trials are often interpreted using methods that are inappropriate or rarely used in multiple-patient trials. The plots of two or more periods of treatment are often visually examined for changes in (1) magnitude of activity or response, (2) trend of response (e.g., upward, downward, level), (3) consistency of response (e.g., unstable, stable, widely varying), and (4) whether effects observed occur promptly after the new treatment is initiated or are delayed in onset (see Fig. 38.3). These characteristics must be examined, as well as determining whether conditions described earlier in this chapter are met. The visual method of Wolery and Harris (1982) allows both within- and between-treatment differences (or between treatment and baseline) to be observed. The interpretation of the visual analysis depends on the magnitude of the change, whether the

change in pattern coincided with the new treatment, and whether it recurred when conditions were changed in a repetitive way.

The visual analysis of these four characteristics considers both within- and between-treatment differences between treatment and baseline. Figure 38.3 illustrates the patterns of data that may be observed in two experimental conditions. Wolery and Harris (1982) described the role of statistics in single-patient trials. The interpretation of the visual analysis will depend on whether changes in the pattern coincided with a new treatment and whether the expected changes recurred when the conditions were modified in a repetitive way. If only one change was made (as in each example in Fig. 38.3), the strength or validity of the interpretation will be weak and will require confirmation in other patients and, if possible, subsequent replications in the same patient.

Wolfrum et al. (1984) evaluated three patients who received placebo, active medicine, or no medication in a randomized order for 21 days and a fourth patient who received placebo or active medicine for 27 days; medicines were changed in a randomized manner. All patients were treated for sleep disturbances in a double-blind manner. One of the major criticisms of these trials is their quasiexperimental nature. There is no doubt, however, that data from single patients may be convincing and have provided valuable insights in developing new treatments.

Figures 38.1 to 38.3 may be analyzed statistically in a variety of ways to confirm one's visual impressions. Parameters graphed should include those of clinical importance to both patient and investigator. A global impression of each treatment period may also be obtained from the patient. Each treatment may result in a graded response or in an all-or-none response. Either may be analyzed, although appropriate statistical tests differ for the two.

The manner of data presentation may greatly influence the interpretation reached. An excellent example of this (Gouvier et al., 1985) shows that results analyzed in four ways can be used to support three totally different interpretations (discussed in Chapter 101). Pitfalls in interpretation of data must be considered.

Another issue in interpretation concerns the ability of separate investigators to reach the same conclusions from a single patient's data. Ottenbacher (1986) described a study in which 46 therapists were asked to rate graphed data visually from a single-patient trial. He observed poor interrater reliability when compared with a statistical analysis of the data, but the raters only rated one pair of experiments (i.e., two treatments). If multiple pairs or periods were conducted it would probably have improved the agreement between raters and made the interpretation more clear.

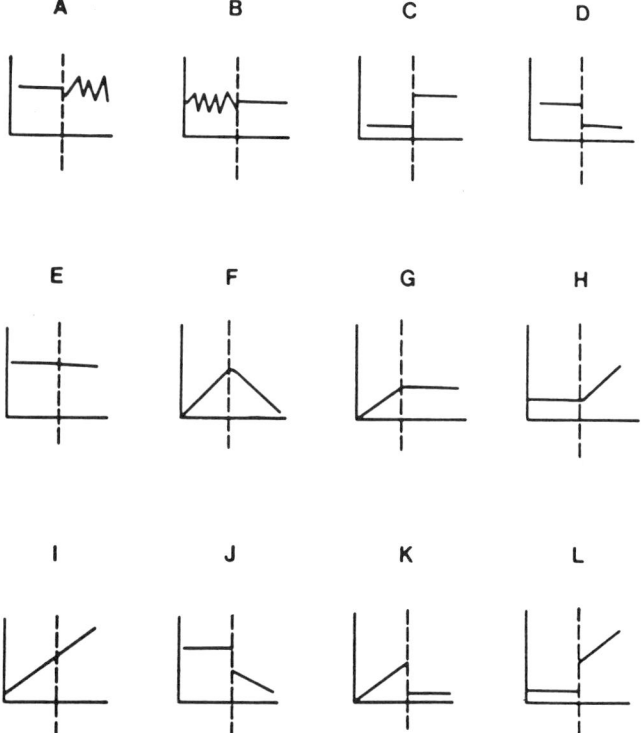

FIG. 38.3 Visual analysis technique of interpreting data from single-patient trials. Possible data patterns across two experimental conditions separated by a dotted line. The ordinate represents clinical activity, and the abscissa represents time. **A and B:** Changes in variability. **C and D:** Changes in level. **E and I:** No change in data. **F–H:** Changes in trend. **J–L:** Changes in level and trend. (Reprinted by permission of the American Physical Therapy Association from Wolery and Harris, 1982).

Interpretation of Individual Patient Data From Multiple-Patient Studies

One of the methods of reaching an interpretation with limited data is to make a separate graph (or table) of each individual's response and then to compare similar parameters for all individuals. Responses such as (1) increases or decreases from baseline, (2) length of time between exacerbations, or (3) other parameters may be sufficient to obtain a better understanding of the results. It may be useful to examine the data as well as individual data collection forms for patterns.

META-ANALYSIS OF SEVERAL OR MANY SINGLE-PATIENT CLINICAL TRIALS

It may be desirable to combine results of several or many single-patient clinical trials. This would be particularly relevant if results were not solely intended to optimize treatment of the patient studied, but were to be examined for relevance for treating other patients (i.e., the data were to be extrapolated). In such situations it *may* be possible to combine or pool data from multiple trials that utilize the same protocol. Traditional statistical tests could be used to analyze the combined data.

In many situations, it may not be appropriate to pool the data, and alternatives must be used. One approach, proposed by Chalmers et al. (1987), is to evaluate clinical trials using the same medicine treatment on the basis of how well or poorly the trial medicine compared with the control treatment, usually placebo. Each clinical trial is described by one mark along a continuum on Fig 38.4. The general interpretation is based on determining where the preponderance of marks lie on this scale. Although this is a visual interpretation of the marks, statistical analyses may be used if a sufficient number of clinical trials are being pooled. Although the outcomes of many single-patient clinical trials may be compared using this approach, caution should be used when different trial designs, endpoints, types of patients, and experimental conditions are present.

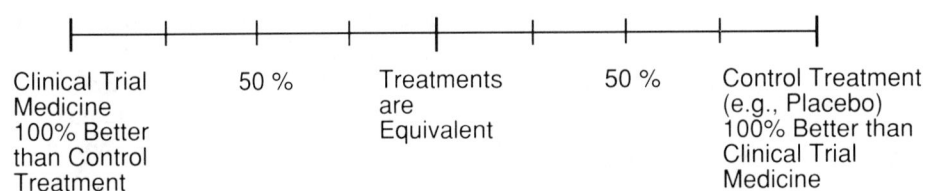

Clinical Trial Medicine 100% Better than Control Treatment   50%   Treatments are Equivalent   50%   Control Treatment (e.g., Placebo) 100% Better than Clinical Trial Medicine

FIG. 38.4 A continuum along which results of single-patient trials may be shown (e.g., by a mark).

CHAPTER 39

Multicenter Trials

ADVANTAGES AND DISADVANTAGES

By definition, a multicenter clinical trial utilizes one protocol at more than one site, although the protocol is usually implemented and conducted in a somewhat different manner and style at each site. Advantages and disadvantages are listed in Table 39.1.

TYPES OF SITES

In choosing the sites to include in a multicenter trial, one usually makes an attempt to include institutions (or investigators) that are either similar or different. The specific sites may be chosen on the basis of many factors, including geography, type of institution, or types of patients seen (other factors are listed in Chapter 59). A multicenter trial of a medicine used to treat chronic back pain could be limited to one type of medical practice (e.g., orthopedic clinics) or hospital (e.g., Veterans Administration Hospitals) or be expanded to include pain clinics, private (or hospital-based) practitioners in family medicine and/or internal medicine, rehabilitation centers, and other types of medical centers or facilities at which patients with back pain are treated.

GOLDEN RULES

The golden rules of multicenter trials are (1) that protocol designs be kept relatively simple and be the same

at all centers, (2) that careful planning of the initiation, conduct, and analysis of the trial be mandatory and that statisticians be involved in this process, and (3) that communication problems be minimized through all possible techniques. Both formal and informal systems of communications should be established to include consideration of all aspects and organizational levels of the trial.

CONDUCTING ADDITIONAL TESTS AT ONE SITE OF A MULTICENTER TRIAL

In numerous multicenter trials, one or more investigators often want to conduct an additional test(s) or evaluation(s) as part of the trial. These additional tests or evaluations are sometimes called add-on, tack-on, or side-arm studies. The major issue to consider before agreeing or refusing to allow any of these studies is whether they will affect the main clinical trial in terms of patient cooperation, enrollment, or compliance. Also, could these additional studies interact with other tests and, therefore, affect the interpretation of the data? Any studies in which these issues could arise should elicit a strong refusal to allow any add-on studies to be conducted, no matter how important they are to a particular investigator. The golden rule is that the primary clinical trial should not be jeopardized by allowing one or more investigators to conduct ancillary studies or tests that could affect the results.

The claim is usually made by the investigator that the rest of the trial will not be affected. The sponsor

TABLE 39.1 *Selected advantages and disadvantages of multicenter clinical trials*

A. Advantages
   1. More rapid patient recruitment
   2. More complex protocols may be able to be conducted because of additional resources utilized for certain large trials
   3. Less opportunity for one person's biases to influence the design or conduct of the clinical trial
   4. Greater likelihood for data processing and analysis to be conducted at a high standard
   5. Greater likelihood for a heterogeneous patient population to be enrolled

B. Disadvantages
   1. Administrative arrangements and management details are more complex
   2. Costs are usually greater for the clinical trial than if the same total number of patients were studied at a single site
   3. Statistical data analyses would be stronger from a single site
   4. Some Ethics Committees/IRBs may insist on changes to the protocol that create major delays or are unacceptable to the sponsor or other Ethics Committees/IRBs
   5. Individual investigators in large multicenter trials receive little recognition through the publication(s) of results

of the multicenter trial and the investigator's own Ethics Committee/Institutional Review Board (IRB) must approve this additional test. There may be strong reasons to either accept or reject this type of protocol amendment. If the proposed amendment to the protocol is accepted by the sponsor, its implementation may be limited to one site or made optional for the other sites as well.

STATISTICAL ISSUES

Should Data from Each Site Be Able to Stand Alone?

It is important to determine whether the expected number of patients to be enrolled at each site of a multicenter trial will be sufficient for the data to stand alone statistically, since data obtained from various sites may only be combined if they are determined to be compatible. Since the compatibility of data from different sites cannot be ensured in advance for multicenter trials, the possibility of enrolling adequate numbers of patients at each site should be considered. If this is done, then data from any site may be separated from the other sets of data. Each site may then be analyzed separately and still retain reasonable statistical power. On the other hand, one of the primary reasons for conducting a multicenter clinical trial relates to the inability of any single site to enroll an adequate number of patients. If there is a choice of conducting three separate "one-site" studies or one "three-site" multicenter study, the former choice is preferable.

May Multicenter Trials Be Divided into Multiple Single-Site Clinical Trials?

Many pharmaceutical companies conduct multicenter trials with two or three sites, enrolling a sufficient number of patients at each site with the intention of eventually separating them into two or three independent trials, if possible. Regulatory authorities often frown on this practice because they claim the sponsor should have initiated two or three independent clinical trials from the outset and not have the fallback position of combining the trials into a single multicenter trial if the separate sites cannot stand alone. Regulatory authorities often analyze the data separately from each site in a multicenter trial and pass judgments on any discrepancies found in the results. This issue is quite complex and no single approach will always be preferable, although the "sliced-meat" approach (i.e., making multiple trials out of one) is clearly desirable from the viewpoint of the pharmaceutical industry.

ADMINISTRATIVE CONSIDERATIONS

Central Reviewers

Quality assurance of data obtained in multicenter clinical trials may be conducted by establishing a group(s) to review various aspects of the trial. In order to ensure uniformity of standardization among centers on (1) criteria of patient eligibility, (2) diagnostic classification, (3) assessment of treatment outcome, or (4) other factors, it is often useful to have one individual or group not directly involved in the clinical trial review pertinent information on all patients. This individual or group would be assigned the function of reviewing any or all of the above points (e.g., diagnosis) according to a predetermined format and would thus function as an independent central reviewer. If questions arose on specific information reviewed, then it should be clarified whether the reviewer would contact the relevant investigator directly or contact the sponsor or monitor of the trial.

Individuals who are reading and interpreting medical data or tests [e.g., electrocardiograms (ECGs), X-rays, pathology samples] should be blind to patient treatment and should perform their tasks independently of clinical trial personnel if possible. If more than one individual will be involved in one activity, then inter-reviewer variability should be assessed.

Administrative Committees

In addition to clinical trial personnel plus clinicians and scientists at the sponsoring institution, a number of

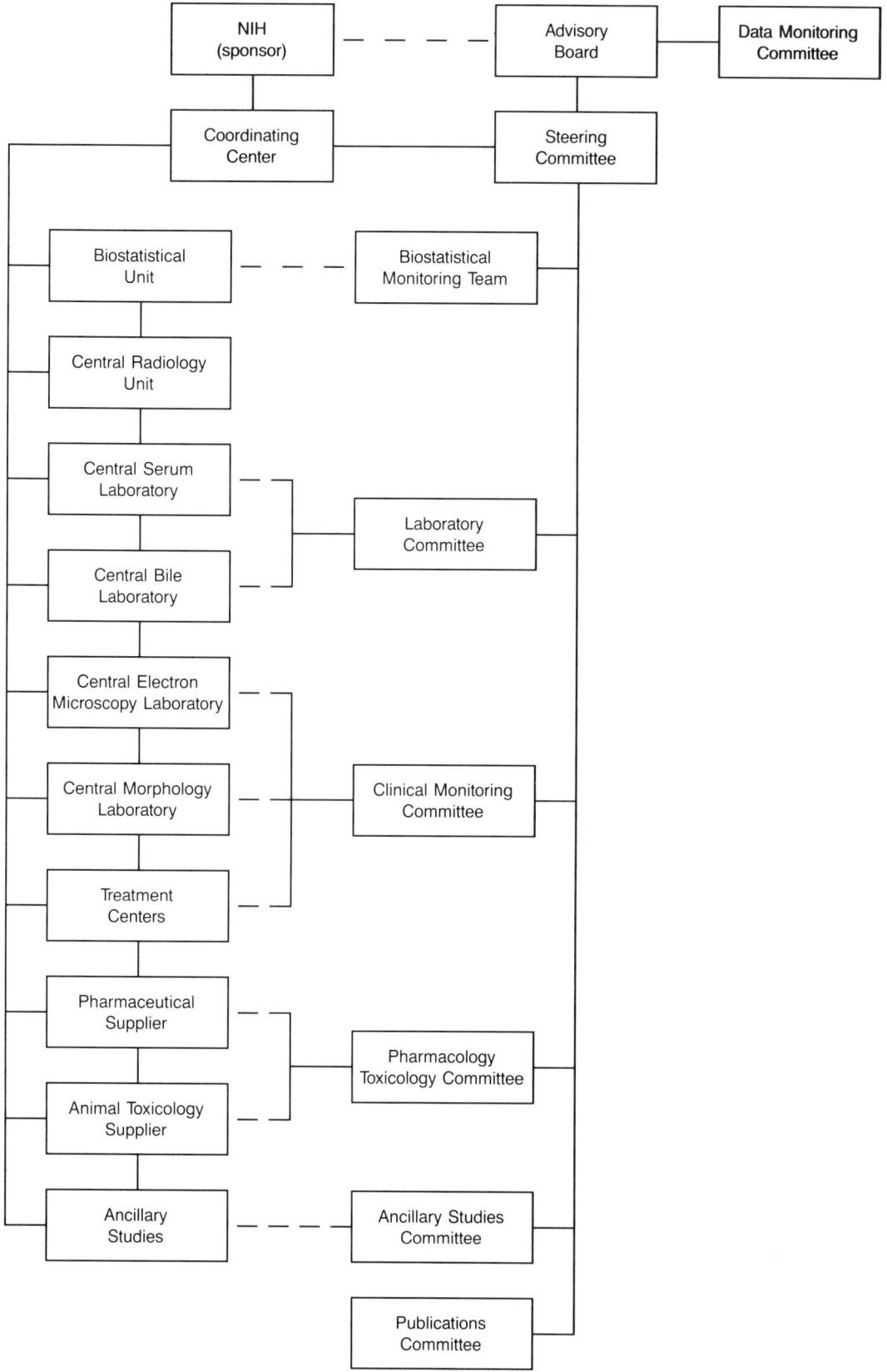

FIG. 39.1 Organizational structure of the National Cooperative Gallstone Study. (Reprinted by permission of Elsevier Science Publishing Co. from Lachin et al., 1981.)

administrative committees are sometimes established to help organize and run large multicenter studies. Many types of committees may be established, such as executive, data-monitoring, data analysis, publications, ethics, and outside advisory committees. A number of major clinical trials in recent years have utilized numerous committees, and their publications provide additional details on the procedures used (e.g., Anturane Reinfarction Trial Research Group, 1980; Winship et al., 1979; Lachin et al., 1981; β-Blocker Heart Attack Trial Research Group, 1981, 1982).

If the establishment of one or more monitoring and organizational groups to help run the medicine trial is contemplated, then it is essential to define clearly the role(s) of each group. A diagram of the organizational structure of one large multicenter trial is shown in Fig. 39.1. (There are numerous reports and papers on the conduct and logistics of multicenter clinical trials that may be consulted for additional details, including the following: Cancer Research Campaign Working Party, 1980; Chan et al., 1983; Friedman et al., 1981; Boissel and Klimt, 1979; Stanley et al., 1981.)

Cooperative Groups

A number of ongoing organizations are committed to conducting multicenter trials. Those "cooperative groups" focusing on cancer treatments began in the 1950s and now involve many groups, each with approximately 30 to 60 institutions, including many institutions from outside the United States. These groups may specialize in a disease (e.g., National Wilms' Tumor Study Group, National Surgical Adjuvant Breast and Bowel Group) or may be multidisease groups (e.g., Eastern Cooperative Oncology Group). Most institutions enrolled are tertiary care hospitals, but there is a movement to involve more community hospitals.

Ongoing cooperative groups have advantages over groups that start a clinical trial from scratch; these advantages are evident in recruitment efforts, statistical input, data processing, and internal monitoring and in having an administrative system in place.

Controversial Outcomes

Careful planning, conduct, and analysis of a large multicenter clinical trial do not ensure that the method-ologies used, data gathered, or analyses performed will be accepted by the medical community or by regulatory authorities. The last two decades have witnessed many of the largest (and most complex) multicenter clinical trials ever conducted, and yet the criticism of several of these trials has been strong, and the trials have been involved in controversy. For example, there has been criticism of the data gathered in the University Group Diabetes Program (UGDP) Trial (Seltzer, 1972; Kilo et al., 1980) and the analyses performed in the Anturane Reinfarction Study (Temple and Pledger, 1980). There is no simple solution to the dilemma of spending enormous sums of money, energy, time, patient involvement, and other resources on a large multicenter clinical trial and yet having the basic approaches or interpretation of the data strongly criticized. If the data are eventually going to be presented to the Food and Drug Administration (FDA) (or other government agency) in support of any claim, then the details of that large multicenter trial design should be discussed with the FDA (or other government agency) prior to its implementation. This approach is unfortunately not always possible with many other national regulatory authorities.

Periodic Meetings and Final Reports

It may be beneficial to the conduct of a large multicenter clinical trial to arrange for an annual or interim meeting of the investigators, monitors, and possibly other trial personnel. Meetings of the committees that are overseeing the trial may also be held on a periodic basis. If these types of committees are not established but situations arise in which outside input is required, then a group of consultants may be brought together to discuss relevant issues.

Finally, if the results of a multicenter clinical trial are published in a monograph, then one or more succinct articles in a widely read journal should also be considered in order to reach a wider audience. In addition to papers on the primary and secondary objectives, methodological papers should be considered. Methodological papers are quite valuable when they describe experiences in specific aspects of a clinical trial (e.g., recruitment, randomization, medicine storage, follow-up visits, dropouts), plus discuss the lessons learned.

CHAPTER 40

National versus Multinational Clinical Trials

BACKGROUND

A multinational clinical trial is a single trial conducted in two or more countries in which data are combined. All multinational trials are multicenter trials, but not all multicenter trials are multinational. The major reasons for conducting a multinational trial include (1) gaining more rapid patient enrollment, (2) expediting the development of a new medicine, (3) conducting a trial that otherwise might be impossible, and (4) gaining experience and being able to compare patients of different nationalities in the same trial.

The following discussion outlines some difficulties that may be encountered in conducting multinational trials. (Many are also encountered, to a lesser degree, in uninational trials.)

WHEN MAY MULTINATIONAL CLINICAL TRIALS BE CONDUCTED?

Multinational clinical trials are usually accepted if:

1. Patients with a rare disease are to be studied, and it is both impossible to enroll a sufficient number of patients in a single country and important to conduct a clinical trial (as opposed to collecting case studies).
2. Extensive resources can be devoted to the clinical trial; practical and other potential problems can be avoided with all necessary monitoring and steering committees.
3. A simply designed and brief data collection form and straightforward, simple clinical trial design are

used for similar patients enrolled from all countries.

In Which Therapeutic Areas?

Some therapeutic areas are more amenable to multinational trials than others. Those that are most amenable have a similar diagnosis, incidence, classification, and treatment in the countries considered for enrollment. The greater the difference in these and other factors, the less reasonable it is to conduct a multinational clinical trial. Many bacterial and viral infections lend themselves to multinational trials, whereas most central nervous system disorders do not. It is not possible to enumerate acceptable and unacceptable therapeutic areas because many factors affect the final determination.

In Which Phase of Development?

The phase of medicine development is a further consideration when determining whether or not a multinational approach is acceptable.

Phase I. Two or more countries should never participate in a single clinical trial.

Phase IIa. Two or more countries may conduct a pilot trial, though it is more desirable to conduct multiple pilot trials, each in a separate country.

Phase IIb. Unless the practice of medicine is almost the same in two countries and the patient populations are almost the same, a well-controlled trial should never be performed in two or more countries. Exceptions occur when extremely large amounts of resources are being applied or when the trial is extremely simple and few data must be collected.

Phase III. It is often acceptable to conduct multinational trials during Phase III, although this approach should not be viewed as a goal. Interpretation of data is facilitated by keeping similar patient groups together, even if each is quite heterogeneous in terms of concurrent medicines and diseases, age, severity of disease, and other factors.

Phase IV. It is sometimes desirable to combine patients from multiple countries in a safety surveillance study.

Safety versus Efficacy

Both safety and efficacy measures may be affected in multinational clinical trials. Efficacy evaluations should be conducted with validated scales or tests. When the tests are applied to patients from different cultures and a subjective component is involved, it may not be assumed that the test will yield equivalent results in each group of patients. Quality of life tests usually have a large degree of subjectivity and are particularly susceptible to this type of cross-cultural problem.

A method for developing tests or methods to conduct cross-cultural psychiatric research was proposed by Flaherty et al. (1988). They describe five dimensions necessary to establish cross-cultural equivalence.

Are Multinational Trials Necessary If a Disease Has a Low Incidence or Prevalence?

It is commonly stated that a compelling reason to do a multinational trial is when the prevalence or incidence of a specific disease is relatively low and few patients are available at a single site. This statement does not consider the following situations.

1. If the disease is extremely rare (e.g., less than 1,000 patients in the world), the entire clinical program may be completed based on case studies of individual patients without conducting any formal clinical trials.
2. If the disease has a low prevalence, many well-designed clinical trials may be designed with small numbers of patients and could be conducted within a single country. Countries would be chosen based on availability of sites and patients.
3. Single-patient clinical trials may be designed and conducted.

DIFFERENCES IN MEDICAL PRACTICE

Existence or Prevalence of Disease

Some countries are well known to have diseases not present in others (e.g., many tropical diseases). The reasons for this difference are usually well understood and accepted. On the other hand, many diseases exist (or at least are diagnosed) in one country but apparently do not occur in one or more nearby countries. Reasons for these differences often relate to the histories and traditions of medical practice in the countries. Diseases that appear to be different from country to country may result from true, spurious, or definitional differences. A few examples follow.

1. In Germany there is a disease often diagnosed in outpatients as low blood pressure (i.e., hypotension), although this finding is not diagnosed as a problem or disease in many other European countries. The disease is treated with medicines by physicians in Germany, but not by physicians in many other countries.

2. In Germany, irritable bowel disease does not exist as a disease, but it does exist in the United Kingdom and in the United States, where it is often treated with medicines.
3. In the United States and The Netherlands the prevalence of hyperkinetic children is said to be about 3%, but it is only about 1% in the United Kingdom. Why does this difference occur? Treatment of hyperkinetic children with medicine is common in the United States but not in The Netherlands. Many other examples of major differences in medical practice in different European countries are given in the book *Medicine and Culture* (Payer, 1988).

Classification of Disease

Different classification systems exist around the world for many diseases. For example, in the United States, depression is diagnosed according to DSM-III, whereas in Germany a different system is used. The diagnosis of a patient according to one system cannot readily be converted to the other system. Clinical trials that seek to enroll patients using two different classifications of disease are likely to encounter serious practical problems, as well as problems of extrapolation.

Genetic Background of Patients

Certain patient populations may have genetic differences that affect metabolism of various medicines (e.g., glucose-6-phosphate dehydrogenase deficiency, atypical pseudocholinesterase). In countries with a higher incidence of specific diseases, those diseases tend to be more readily recognized and diagnosed.

Therapy Used to Treat Patients

Concomitant medicines allowed in a multinational clinical trial may not be commonly used or even marketed in all countries participating in the trial. The difference could introduce a significant bias if concomitant medicines were stronger or worked better in some countries. Generic names of certain medicines differ among some countries (e.g., acetaminophen versus paracetamol).

Physician Styles of Practice

There are differences between countries in the vigor with which physicians adhere to clinical trial protocols, based on culture, training, peer pressure, and other factors, even among academic physicians. This factor is also relevant for multicenter uninational trials.

Regional Differences in Frequency of Medical Procedures

The frequency and type of certain medical procedures has been widely studied in surgery. See Chapter 85 for references and discussion. The overwhelming consensus is that great differences exist between countries and often between different areas or districts within a single country.

Differences in Medical Training and Practice Between Countries or Regions

1. Physicians are often trained differently in different countries or even in different regions within countries. In some regions, analytical skills are stressed and in others, more holistic care and skills are stressed. This may affect how investigators treat patients.
2. Sometimes physicians within certain regions or provinces of a country are said to prescribe more medicines per patient than their counterparts in other regions. This aspect may influence a trial's outcome in terms of how adverse events are treated.
3. Physicians may interpret a simple request like "obtain a family history" differently. It has been anecdotally reported that in one Canadian province physicians believed that this meant within the immediate family whereas others interpreted the phrase as including all uncles, aunts, and grandparents.

Cultural Heritage of Investigator

The general behavior of an investigator toward patients in a clinical trial may be strongly influenced by his or her culture of origin. For example, physicians from an Eastern culture who have not spent a long period in the West may find unexpected influences of their culture on their practice of medicine (Samra et al., 1988; Qureshi, 1989).

DIFFERENCES IN CULTURE

Cultural differences that may affect outcomes of multinational clinical trials include (1) language, (2) ethics, (3) diet, (4) customs, and (5) religion. Any of these cultural differences may influence patient compliance as well as the ease with which the trial is conducted and the ability to interpret and extrapolate the data obtained.

Language

It is important to note how the protocol and data collection forms are translated from the original language to the new one. What do each of the words mean and what are their connotations? If sufficient resources are available, a protocol can be translated and then re-translated (by someone else) back to the first language for comparison with the original protocol. This is a valuable method to ensure that a translation is correct. Some of the many medical terms that have different meanings in different countries include *cellulitis, chest pain,* and *chronic fatigue.*

Even when words are translated accurately, what do they mean in a different language? The connotations may be quite different and could lead to multiple difficulties. This is potentially the most critical factor in a trial. Again, this could be avoided in most cases by retranslating a protocol or data collection form back to the original language.

In oral contraceptive trials women were told to take the drug "every day." This instruction seems clear enough, but it was not. To some women it meant "every day I feel O.K.," to some it meant "every day I have sex," and to others it was interpreted as "every day my husband is in town."

When a simple phrase is interpreted in such different ways, it makes one wonder how investigators, as well as patients, interpret many statements made during a clinical trial, particularly one conducted in two or more countries. There are many bilingual or multilingual countries in which language may also be a major problem in uninational clinical trials (e.g., in Belgium, Canada, the United States, or India). Hunt (1986) describes some of the issues involved in translating a quality of life test (i.e., Nottingham Health Profile) from English into Arabic and Spanish.

Ethics

Different ethical views in each country may lead Ethics Committees to request or even to require different protocol modifications. These differences may be impossible to resolve and the trial may never be approved. A great deal of time may have been expended unnecessarily on protocol modifications that may not satisfy one or more Ethics Committees. Although this same situation may occur in a uninational clinical trial, its likelihood is greater in a multinational one.

Diet

While there is not a great deal of data on how diet affects multinational clinical trials, there are several folk myths and many anecdotes about patients on an Eastern diet reacting differently to medicines than Western patients. It is unlikely that these differences (to the degree that they exist) are solely the result of dietary causes. Other factors described in this and other sections are also likely to be involved.

Religion

Religious views may affect a patient's willingness to enroll in a clinical trial, and to adhere to its requirements. Differences in compliance between sites because of religious beliefs may lead to complications in interpreting data and could become a major issue.

DIFFERENCES IN REGULATIONS

Use of Placebo in Different Countries

The issue of placebo use really relates more to individual physicians, Ethics Committees, and regulatory policy than it does to medical practice. In some countries a placebo treatment group would be considered ethical, whereas it would raise strong objections in others.

Toxicology Data

The type and amount of toxicology data required to conduct a specific clinical trial vary among countries. This means that although one or more countries may be important to include in a planned clinical trial, it may be impossible to do so until additional or longer duration toxicology studies are conducted.

Ethics Committees/Institutional Review Boards

Ethics Committees/Institutional Review Boards (IRBs) may vary markedly among countries in their makeup and roles. A major difficulty that a sponsor will probably have to face is different types of Ethics Committees/IRBs reviewing (and having to approve) a single protocol. Because of differences in culture, medical practice, or for other reasons, Ethics Committees/IRBs may react differently to the protocol. An additional major issue is that a clinical trial must be acceptable to each national regulatory authority that will receive data from the trial in a regulatory submission. A clinical trial should be approved by an Ethics Committee/IRB in each country where the trial is conducted, even in those in which such approval is not normally required. If this is not done, serious questions could be raised at a later date by regulatory authorities in those countries where Ethics Committee/IRB approval is required.

Informed Consent

The same type of issues could arise with regard to informed consent as have just been cited for Ethics Committees/IRBs. The validity of a clinical trial could be quite easily challenged if patient populations were viewed as different from each other because each went through a different informed consent procedure. The issue of written versus oral informed consent is discussed in Chapter 27.

Import–Export Regulations

Import–export laws differ in each country and have many and varied effects on the ability to mount and conduct a multinational trial. For example, a monetary value must be declared for a finished medicine shipped between most countries for a clinical trial. The higher this value the higher are the taxes that must be paid. This might suggest that putting a lower value on the customs declaration is preferable. However, in some countries, the value put on this form strongly influences the price that may eventually be charged for the medicine.

Correct paperwork is not the only issue related to shipping and receiving medicines determined by these regulations. Some countries' procedures involve time-consuming delays to obtain approvals, and other countries have corrupt officials that must be paid to expedite the medicine's importation.

ECONOMIC DIFFERENCES

It would seem obvious that multinational trials should not include sites in both developed and underdeveloped countries, yet numerous examples of this practice occur that raise serious questions about pooling the data. Results obtained in the different countries will vary for many reasons, including economic ones, and not all of these reasons will be easily determined. For example, differences in storage of medicines may permit some supplies to deteriorate, and also poorer patients in some countries may not attend clinics as often as poorer patients in other countries.

PRACTICAL DIFFERENCES

There is no limit to the number of practical differences that invariably arise among the countries of a multinational clinical trial. While any conscientious group will attempt to prevent as many difficulties from arising as possible, the sense of urgency that is usually felt in starting a clinical trial, plus the lack of totally adequate resources in most cases makes this goal a difficult one to achieve. A few potential problems are mentioned, but most of the points raised in this chapter could also

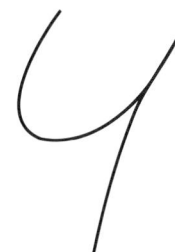

FIG. 40.1 A hypothetical number that could be any of several, depending on the national or regional characteristics of writing.

be considered "practical differences" between countries.

Writing Numbers and Dates

As mundane a subject as the different ways that people in different countries write numbers could lead to confusion and errors in data collection and processing. The number in Fig. 40.1 could be interpreted as 6, 4, 7, 1, or 9. The interpretation made would depend to some degree on the country. Additional samples could be given. The practice in United States of writing dates in the order: month, day, and year can be confusing to someone from another country who writes dates in the order: day, month, and year.

Using Central Laboratories

Many investigators who are willing to send samples or data (e.g., electrocardiograms) to a central facility for evaluation may balk if they are asked to send these to a site in a foreign country. This issue could lead to a lack of good will and potentially to less than adequate cooperation by an investigator in conducting the trial or in obtaining results.

DIFFERENCES IN PERSPECTIVE AND ATTITUDES

Prior to the initiation of a clinical trial to test an investigational medicine, the sponsor of the trial is the primary group involved with potential multinational issues. Later in the course of a new medicine's development, or even during the conduct of the clinical trial, regulatory authorities also become involved in these issues.

Attitudes of patients and investigators may differ in different countries. How patients accept their therapy often has a great bearing on how they respond.

Physicians may be asked to participate in clinical trials using methods with which they are uncomfortable. They may not share the same relationship with monitors as exists elsewhere, which may add stresses for both investigators and monitors. Physicians must accept the possibility of audits being conducted if they want to participate in a critically important clinical trial. Good intentions on the part of all investigators are important, but these are never as important as cooperation and diligence in adherence to the protocol and the spirit of the clinical trial.

A statement to the effect that a group understands the many requirements for conducting a multinational clinical trial is not proof that this is true. Direct experience with knowledgable people within each of the actual national environments is required.

Most European medical directors of large multinational companies who have a great deal of clinical experience believe they understand Food and Drug Administration (FDA) standards and requirements. Many who work (or have worked) in the United States have indicated that although they thought they understood FDA requirements, it was only after they moved to the United States that they truly understood what standards were actually needed to satisfy FDA regulations and reviewers.

PROBLEMS OF INTERPRETATION AND EXTRAPOLATION

Extrapolation of data from a multinational clinical trial is generally more difficult than from several individual single-country clinical trials. Data from a uninational trial are usually stronger and more convincing scientifically. Better quality data from one country can be extrapolated to other countries more reliably than weaker data can be extrapolated within the same country.

The quality of a multinational clinical trial's data, monitoring, and analyses must be evaluated before an interpretation may be developed. This ideally involves conducting a clinical audit of each site (see Chapter 63) to evaluate many points at each site, including: how much medicine was dispensed, how much data are missing, and how many errors occurred at each site? Large differences among the various countries in these or other values are more of a problem in multinational than in uninational trials with multiple sites. In the multinational trial the importance of national differences can almost never be ruled out. In a uninational trial the same types of differences are probably less significant for the interpretation of the results, and may often be ascribed to random variability.

Adverse Events

One of the major problems encountered in multinational trials relates to differences among countries in the diagnosis and treatment of adverse events. It is extremely difficult for monitors and sponsors to bring uniformity to the trial protocol when the participators differ so greatly in basic medical approach. For example, the basis on which a diagnosis of Stevens-John-son syndrome is made is extremely different in different countries. The implications of that diagnosis are also quite different in different countries in terms of the patient's prognosis and the sponsor's regulatory requirements.

Patients with a particular symptom or disease may be treated by a general physician in one country, a specialist of one type in another country, and a different specialist in a third country. Alternatively, the same patient could be treated by any one of many specialists within the same country. For example, patients with Stevens-Johnson syndrome are treated in the United States by infectious disease specialists, dermatologists, surgeons in burn units, and general physicians. In Sweden most cases of Stevens-Johnson syndrome are treated by infectious disease specialists, whereas in France and West Germany they are mostly treated by dermatologists. There are also some differences between countries in what signs and symptoms constitute the syndrome. A further difference is that the therapeutic approach by even a single group of specialists will differ from country to country. Another example of different diagnoses of a single condition is that the term *fixed drug eruption* has a fairly narrow definition in the United States, whereas in some countries (e.g., Finland) the term is used much more broadly to include conditions described as erythema multiforme in the United States. Adverse reactions reported as fixed drug eruptions in a multinational trial could not, therefore, simply be combined into a total number for the numerator of an incidence ratio.

Thus, even if a sponsor attempts to standardize the criteria required for diagnosis of a patient's primary disease and also standardizes the ways in which a protocol will be followed, it is still quite possible that results from multinational trials may lead to serious problems of interpretation when adverse events reported have vastly different meanings and regulatory implications in the different countries involved. If one investigator is taught to diagnose sepsis as a single event, and another as multiple events (e.g., infection, fever, headache), the resultant differences (i.e., in treatment) may be difficult to resolve satisfactorily without a great deal of effort.

Many of the issues involving adverse events are compounded when reports from multiple countries are involved. In this brief section there is only space for indicating some of the complexities:

1. Medicine is practiced differently around the world, and the type of physician or specialist who treats one kind of problem (e.g., skin problem) in one country may not be the type of physician or specialist who would treat patients with the same problem in another country. This means that the accuracy of diagnosis of the adverse event will vary depending on

both the nature of the disease being diagnosed and the physician's training. In addition, adverse events are often identified differently in different countries. Thus, the reported incidence of a single adverse event in a country may be greatly over- or underreported when compared with another country. The difference may represent an artifact based solely on diagnostic factors. Some diagnoses blend into or overlap others, and the lack of an objective method of identifying many adverse events means that resulting data may be skewed in different way. Achieving an accurate diagnosis is especially difficult for many syndromes (e.g., Stevens-Johnson syndrome).

2. The more precisely an adverse event is defined and diagnosed, the lower its reported incidence. However, different countries often use different methodologies in terms of processing and counting reports, in addition to differences in diagnosing reactions. All of these factors undoubtedly affect the incidence figures obtained.

3. Retrospective analyses of patient charts are fraught with problems in all countries, but when multiple countries are involved, the number of potential difficulties becomes substantially greater. One approach to this issue is to establish criteria for the diagnosis first. Second, design a data collection form and have medically knowledgable individuals who are unaware of the study's objectives review patient charts. Finally, the completed data collection forms may be reviewed by a panel of experts, who rate degree of improvement or another endpoint without knowing the treatment group of each patient. To evaluate the association of a medicine with an adverse event, charts from patients who had the adverse event but were not taking the suspected medicine should also be coded and examined. Any slides of biopsies, or any other documented evidence should also be reviewed in a blind manner.

4. Developing a unified interpretation of even a single adverse event from reports received from multiple countries is difficult, for various reasons, including the following: (1) allowable maximal doses may differ (it is necessary to know the dose that each patient received), (2) medical practice may differ (physicians may use the medicine differently), (3) concomitant medications may be unknown or unreported and the adverse event may actually represent an interaction between medicines, (4) excipients may differ for the "same" medicine and might explain the adverse event, and (5) the source of the report (e.g., physician, patient, public health service nurse) may vary and affect its accuracy.

OVERALL PRINCIPLES AND STANDARDS

The most important principle is that multinational clinical trials should not be conducted unless necessary.

The following procedures should be adhered to when such a trial is conducted:

1. Data should be examined for national differences.
2. One or two well-defined simple endpoints should be used. These should be the most well-validated measures.
3. High scientific and clinical standards should be used to obtain a clear signal above any noise present in the clinical trial.
4. Monitoring must be conducted at a high standard at all sites in all countries.
5. The clinical trial should be within a therapeutic area in which cross-national differences are not expected to affect diagnosis or treatment significantly.
6. The clinical trial should not be part of Phase 1, and ideally should not be part of Phase II medicine development.
7. The clinical trial should not be a quality of life trial because large cross-cultural differences will make interpretation of the data impossible.
8. It is important to hold a pretrial roundtable meeting, particularly if the clinical trial is conducted as part of Phase II. All aspects of the protocol and clinical trial should be discussed.
9. In most cases two or more uninational multicenter clinical trials provide stronger evidence of a medicine's efficacy than two or more equally well-conducted multinational clinical trials.
10. Careful attention to the data collection forms is essential to ensure that comparable data are collected. Translation, and retranslation to the original language, should be done. A no-carbon data collection form can be prepared so that one language is on the top sheet and another on the second sheet.

TABLE 40.1 *Specific pointers in designing, conducting, and interpreting multinational clinical trials*

1. Ensure that input is received from at least one physician consultant in each country participating in the clinical trial both prior to and during the protocol's preparation
2. Ensure that as many physicians as practical review the protocol prior to submitting it for Ethics Committee review
3. Only include sites in countries where clinical practice and culture are generally similar
4. Ensure that an appropriate audit of the data may be made by the sponsor or regulatory authority
5. Consider a limited feasibility trial both to show that the larger trial is feasible and to identify potential problem areas that will need to be addressed
6. Styles of interacting with investigators vary greatly among countries; if a single group of monitors visits all sites, they should be trained in appropriate manners and behavior
7. Countries that differ markedly in medical practice, culture, regulations, or practical aspects (e.g., Japan) should not be part of a multinational clinical trial

11. A feasibility trial (i.e., pilot trial) should be conducted, if possible.

When adequate resources are available to overcome many of the potential problems, it is possible to conduct trials that would otherwise be impossible (e.g., the 71-center, Extracranial/Intracranial Bypass Study, 1985). Some pointers for designing, conducting, and interpreting multinational trials are listed in Table 40.1.

Criteria for use in evaluating countries for inclusion in multinational trials and pointers for coordinating such trials are discussed in Chapters 121 and 124.

The final principle is that attitudes of sponsors should change *from* the prevailing view that multinational trials will be done unless a convincing case can be made to the contrary *to:* multinational trials will not be conducted unless someone is able to demonstrate convincingly that they should be done.

CHAPTER 41

Continuation and Compassionate Plea Trials

CONTINUATION PROTOCOLS

An important consideration in investigational medicine trials of specified duration is whether patients who have benefited will be allowed to receive the medicine after completion of the trial. If they will be, a continuation protocol is generally provided. Patients who enter continuation protocols may receive medicine under this protocol for a fixed, variable, or unspecified duration. The existence of a continuation protocol is often identified in the initial "feeder" protocol.

When Are Continuation Protocols Possible or Desirable?

It is possible to conduct continuation protocols during any phase of a medicine's development. Pros and cons of conducting continuation trials early in a medicine's development are listed in Table 41.1 and discussed below.

Phase I

A newly tested medicine that may be a breakthrough for severely ill patients is usually evaluated in patients rather than in volunteers, especially if the medicine is likely to be toxic. If those patients benefit it would sometimes be unethical to deny them the medicine at the end of a brief clinical trial. Provided that sufficient toxicology data are available, it would be advantageous in the situation described to obtain long-term data on both safety and efficacy parameters. Benefit-to-risk considerations for patients without alternative therapy would make an early continuation protocol desirable. The possibility of a continuation trial would also encourage patients to enroll in the initial clinical trial.

Phases II and III

Most continuation trials are conducted during this period of a medicine's development. If benefit-to-risk considerations indicate continuation even after a feasibility or pilot trial, it should generally be done.

The Case Against Continuation Protocols

Much of the material in this chapter assumes that a sponsor has unlimited supplies of a medicine and re-

TABLE 41.1 *Pros and cons of conducting continuation trials early in a medicine's development*

Pros
1. Such trials help patient recruitment in earlier clinical trials
2. They generate long-term data
3. They help with Ethics Committee/IRB approval of a concurrently run clinical trial of short duration
4. Dosage in the continuation trial may be flexible if the medicine's safety is acceptable
5. After treatment in the continuation clinical trial stops, the regression of patients' disease and symptoms may be evaluated[a]

Cons
1. If the medicine supply is limited the continuation trial may strain available, or even future, stock
2. Toxicology studies may be inadequate to justify a long-term clinical trial
3. Resources that could be reserved for other projects must be committed to the project at a relatively early stage when the chance for success is uncertain
4. Regulatory approval of the continuation trial may be a problem
5. The precise dose and dosing schedule may be unknown
6. Long-term data may be generated on a medicine that will never be developed

[a] This could also be evaluated after treatment in the feeder protocol.

sources to monitor clinical trials appropriately as well as staff to write protocols. The reality of most pharmaceutical development is that during the early years in the clinic the medicine is in short supply and resources to write additional protocols and monitor long-term clinical trials are limited. Often, a choice must be made between conducting additional short-exposure trials during Phase I and early Phase II, and initiating continuation trials. Supplies of medicines usually increase later in Phase II, when it is more certain that the medicine is effective. This is also the appropriate time to initiate continuation trials. During Phase III, continuation protocols are usually essential to a medicine's development.

PLANNING CONTINUATION PROTOCOLS

Many of the specific issues that arise when planning continuation protocols are discussed in the following sections, but a few broad concepts must be initially considered. These broad concepts are described by three initial spectra along which continuation protocols may be developed (Fig. 41.1).

Spectrum 1: Number

The number of clinical trials per continuation protocol may vary from 1:1 (i.e., each clinical trial has its own specific continuation protocol designed) to all:1 (i.e., all clinical trials utilize a single continuation protocol).

Spectrum 2: Complexity

The complexity of the continuation protocol(s) designed may vary along the spectrum shown in Fig. 41.1.

Spectrum 3: Artificiality

Artificiality is also illustrated in Fig. 41.1. Other factors (e.g., duration of the continuation trial) may vary along a similar spectrum.

ISSUES OF CONTINUATION PROTOCOLS

Designing Specific versus General Protocols

In developing a continuation protocol, it is important to determine whether it will be specifically tailored to follow one (and only one) protocol and thus exclude patients who have completed all other protocols with the same clinical trial medicine. An alternative approach is to design a generic continuation protocol that will accept patients from many protocols in which the same medicine was tested.

Essential Questions to Address

One must consider all the probable relationships of patients and clinical trial medicine that may be presented to the investigator and determine which patients will be entered and which patients will be excluded from the continuation protocol. For example, it should be determined whether patients who have completed their original protocol a number of weeks or months prior to the time of entry into the continuation trial will be allowed to enter. Similarly, will patients who have received only placebo treatment in the original protocol be allowed to enter the longer-term protocol? If patients have just completed the feeder protocol and are still receiving active medicine, it must be determined whether they must be taken off medicine prior to entry into the continuation protocol. Additionally, patients who were hospitalized with non-trial-medicine-related problems and then were dropped from the original protocol may wish to enter the continuation protocol. The manner in which any or all of these groups are permitted to enter the continuation protocol must be determined and specified in the admission criteria for the continuation protocol. Specific criteria for defining the minimal improvement on clinical trial medicine that qualifies a patient for entry into a continuation protocol also must be established. If the continuation protocol emanates from a sponsor, then pe-

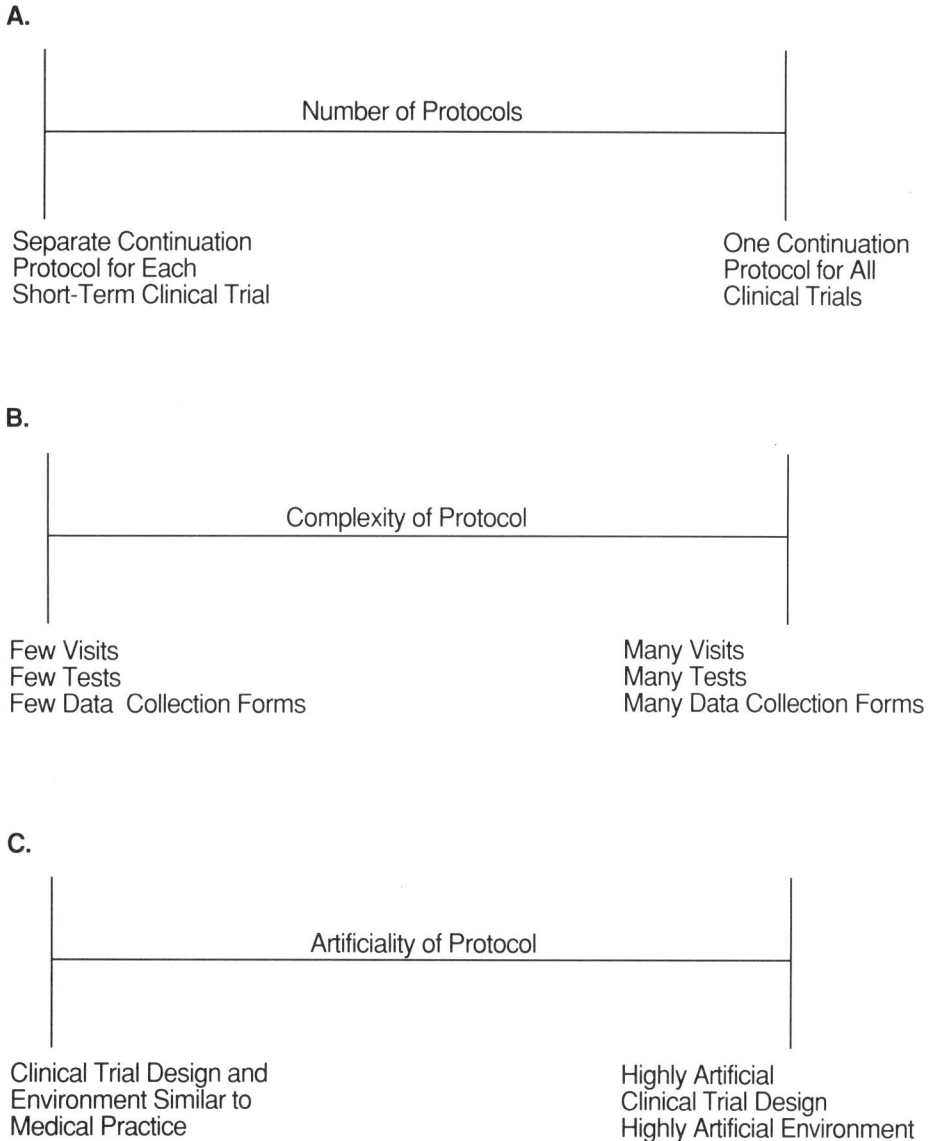

FIG. 41.1 Three spectra along which continuation protocols may be planned.

riodic review of the data generated in the continuation protocol should be conducted by the sponsor, who has the prerogative to cancel any continuation protocol if the medicine's development is discontinued, or for other defined (or undefined) reasons.

Semantic Issues and Combining Data

Many potential semantic problems may arise in describing the duration of patient treatment in continuation protocols. These can be illustrated by an example of two patients who enter a 1-year continuation protocol. The first question is whether "1 year" refers to a patient's total exposure to medicine or to 1 year of additional exposure to medicine beyond the time of original exposure. Assume that each patient had previously received medicine for 3 months but that patient 1 stopped receiving medicine 2 months prior to the beginning of the continuation protocol and patient 2 has not stopped medicine therapy but has entered the continuation protocol still receiving clinical trial medicine at a maintenance level. After 1 month of dose escalation, patient 1 is now at maintenance level. After the clinical trial is half complete, an interim analysis of the data is being prepared, and the question is raised of whether patients 1 and 2 have each received medicine for the same duration.

There are several different ways of combining data from these patients. The assumptions and details of the techniques used for data analysis should be established prior to the clinical trial. One issue is whether to define the duration of time that a patient has been on medicine as beginning at the time of the original exposure or from the time of entry into the continuation protocol. One solution is to group patients together who have been exposed to the medicine for different overall periods of time (e.g., 3–6 months and 6–9 months of exposure), but several other alternative methods of calculating exposure to medicine are possible. Data from patients 1 and 2 would be combined in some situations (e.g., total duration of exposure to medicine, since each would have been exposed to medicine for 9 months) but not in others (e.g., duration of exposure to medicine at a maintenance level in the continuation protocol, since patient 1 would have been receiving medicine for 5 months and patient 2 for 6 months).

Potential Dilemmas

The initiation of continuation protocols may be further complicated if the original patients entered in the clinical trial were previously evaluated in a double-blind trial and, at the time of their entry, there were at least some patients remaining in the original trial. At least three dilemmas may arise in this situation. First, if the clinical trial blind is broken for the original patients at the time or their entry into the continuation protocol, then the integrity of the original trial will be compromised. Second, if patients enter the continuation clinical trial in a double-blind manner, then some patients may be receiving placebo. This raises an ethical issue that must be considered. Third, when the double blind for the first clinical trial is eventually broken, there will be implications for the statistical treatment of the data in the continuation protocol if some patients' data were collected entirely in a double-blind manner, some in an open-label manner, and some under both conditions.

Admission of Patients Into Continuation Trials

Inclusion criteria may focus on demonstrating patient compliance with (1) attending the clinic according to schedule, (2) taking medicine(s) as prescribed, and (3) participating in the trial appropriately. The interest of patients considered for enrollment in continuation trials should be balanced against other factors, e.g., are there any severe adverse events that should preclude patient entry?

Escape Clause to Put Into Continuation Protocols

When a continuation protocol is written for an investigational medicine, it is important for the sponsor not to make an open-ended commitment to furnish the medicine permanently. An escape clause should be inserted in the protocol to indicate that the medicine will be provided as long as it is under active investigation, until an NDA is approved, or for only a fixed period. This clause enables the sponsor to gradually discontinue use of medicines that are no longer being investigated. Of course, the sponsor retains the prerogative of supplying the medicine to patients even after its active development is stopped, assuming that benefit-to-risk considerations are acceptable.

A related issue for extremely expensive medicines, or when few patients will ever use the medicine, is whether to charge for the medicine. Most sponsors supply investigational medicines without charge in continuation protocols, but numerous situations exist (e.g., a financially troubled sponsor) when charging may be desirable and appropriate.

COMPASSIONATE PLEA TRIALS

Other Terms Used for Compassionate Plea Trials

Numerous terms are used for describing investigational medicine protocols that are humanitarian in their purpose and intentionally have loose, or even virtually no entry (i.e., inclusion) criteria restrictions. The terms for such trials include *compassionate use, compassionate care, humanitarian, treatment-IND, dual-track, group C mechanism* (i.e., for some trials of the National Cancer Institute), and *parallel-track protocols.*

Justification for Compassionate Plea Trials

There are several reasons why investigators and patients want to receive medicines on a compassionate plea basis. The most basic reason is to receive medical benefit. This is justified on the basis of personal freedom of patients to have access to available treatments, even if those treatments are experimental. Nonapproved medicines are often part of reasonable medical care, because a great deal is usually known about the medicine prior to its approval. Sponsors usually like the additional usage and exposure to their medicines and benefit in a variety of ways when patients are helped. Issues raised by early access of patients to medicines are listed in Table 41.2.

When Are Compassionate Plea Trials Conducted?

At some stage of developing a new medicine the question may arise of whether to treat patients using a compassionate plea protocol. This type of protocol is for individual patients who are unable to enter formal clinical trials because they do not qualify or live too far from a trial site, or for other reasons. Sometimes it is

TABLE 41.2 *Issues raised by early access of patients to medicines outside of well controlled clinical trials*[a]

1. Potential risks to patients of serious adverse reactions that are presently unknown or for which the relationship to the medicine is uncertain
2. Lack of sufficient information about the medicine for patients to give an informed consent
3. The quantity and complexity of data collection requirements must not be too great for physicians to complete
4. Physicians who are unaccustomed to clinical trials must be provided succinct information (e.g., by audiocassette or videocassette) about how to use an investigational medicine
5. If a large compassionate plea program (e.g., treatment-IND) is initiated, it may become much more difficult to recruit patients for controlled clinical trials
6. The amount of professional staff and time required of the sponsor to administer a large compassionate plea program may be substantial
7. Physicians may use the medicine in inappropriate ways and raise issues for the sponsor to address. Moreover, these inappropriate uses may influence the medicine's image and its role in medicine more than the controlled clinical trials conducted
8. There may be public and various other pressures to approve a medicine before clinical trials are complete
9. An investigational medicine that is found to cause serious but unexpected adverse reactions may expose the sponsor to significant liability suits
10. The data collected may be incomplete and difficult to integrate or summarize

[a] Modified from a presentation by E. Andrews and P. Doi, with permission.

TABLE 41.3 *Considerations in determining the value of a compassionate plea program*[a]

A. Assess the appropriateness of a specific medicine for a compassionate plea program
   1. Are alternative therapies available?
   2. Are the efficacy and safety of alternative therapies adequate?
   3. Is the disease serious or life-threatening?
   4. What is the prognosis of patients who will not receive the investigational medicine?
   5. What is the relative safety and efficacy of the new medicine?
   6. How easy or difficult is it to use the new medicine correctly and appropriately?
   7. Does a clearly defined patient population exist?
   8. What is the likelihood that the new medicine will be misused?

B. Assess the impact of a compassionate plea program on the medicine's development program
   1. What are the views of the relevant regulatory authorities?
   2. What is the medicine's current stage of development?
   3. What is the likelihood that the program will delay rather than shorten the time to attain approval to market the medicine?
   4. What would be the impact on the development plans for the medicine (e.g., on Phase IV requirements, other clinical trials)?
   5. What are the implications for the labeling that will be obtained?

C. Assess the impact of a compassionate plea program on the sponsor's resources
   1. What will be the impact on developing other medicines?
   2. What is the sponsor's ability to monitor the sites of physicians who are supplied with the medicine?
   3. What are the anticipated expenses for the program's direct cost and administration?
   4. What are the requirements of various groups (e.g., information, public affairs, manufacturing) that might become heavily involved if the program is large?
   5. What is the commitment of senior staff at the sponsor's site to the program?
   6. Is the commitment by regulatory authorities appropriate?

[a] Modified from a presentation by E. Andrews and P. Doi, with permission.

advantageous to enter relatively large numbers of patients in compassionate plea protocols to gain additional safety data shortly before a medicine is to be marketed.

Some important considerations in deciding whether to utilize compassionate plea protocols are listed in Table 41.3. The clinical trial may include all or most of a physician's patients who are available and in need of treatment. It is not always necessary for patients to meet specific entry criteria to enter a compassionate plea trial. Physicians may be required to submit periodic data on all patients to ensure patient safety and to check on physician compliance with the protocol. A simple data collection form may be used for this purpose. Physicians who are noncompliant may be deleted from continued participation in the clinical trial.

Most compassionate plea clinical trials occur during Phase IIIa or IIIb, although many are started during Phase II. For investigational medicines that are medical breakthroughs, formal compassionate plea clinical trials may begin during Phase II after efficacy and safety have been initially demonstrated. When the medical need for the new therapy is less, fewer physicians will contact the pharmaceutical company to request supplies early in the medicine's development.

What Standards Are Used?

Humanitarian clinical trials should be designed and conducted to meet the highest standards of science

rather than current regulations or personal ideas of regulatory reviewers. Reviewers and even regulations will change, but aiming at high scientific and ethical standards are the best guidelines to use. Even though patients may be treated as individual cases and no actual protocol may exist, a form to collect relevant safety and efficacy data should be designed and sent to the physician along with the medicine. In some situations a formal protocol will be prepared to assist (and to some degree control) the treatment of individuals or groups of patients. Utilizing a written protocol for compassionate plea trials is the preferable approach.

TYPES OF COMPASSIONATE PLEA TRIALS

There are two major ways of categorizing the various types of compassionate plea clinical trials: on whether or not formal protocols are prepared and on when during a medicine's development the trial is conducted. With the exception of the currently experimental parallel-track program, all compassionate plea protocols are written after both safety and efficacy data are available.

Compassionate Plea Trials With or Without Formal Protocols

Type 1: Without Formal Protocols

Type 1 trials are individual patient trials in which no formal protocol exists and investigators evaluate the medicine according to their own assessment of the patient's response. Guidelines for the medicine's use are generally provided to physicians who are treating the patients, but there is usually no insistence that those guidelines be followed. Another way to describe this procedure is that medicine is supplied on a "named patient" basis. This means that the investigator supplies the name of the patient(s) to be treated and the sponsor supplies the medicine plus general information about the medicine. The sponsor may supply general instructions or a broad protocol and possibly data collection forms as well. These data collection forms are notoriously difficult for companies to retrieve, and when they do retrieve them, it is usually extremely difficult to combine the data received for different patients.

Type 2: With a Formal Protocol

In type 2 clinical trials a formal protocol exists. Investigators who contact the manufacturer or supplier of the medicine are sent the protocol and data collection forms along with the medicine. Investigators may be asked to sign a statement saying that they will adhere to the protocol and collect data as requested. Investigators are expected to return the data to the sponsor, and if data are not forthcoming, the sponsor usually initiates contact by telephone, letters, or visits to collect them. Data are combined to generate results that will, it is hoped, support a New Drug Application (NDA) or Product License Application (PLA) for the medicine. In some situations, (e.g., a very rare disease) valuable data may be obtained that may be the major evidence presented in a regulatory dossier.

Premarketing Surveillance

Long-term exposure to a medicine may be established in open-label humanitarian or compassionate protocols. These trials expose larger numbers of patients (than were previously exposed to the medicine) to a clinical trial medicine during Phase III, often at many different types of sites. Often, a single patient or a few patients are enrolled by each investigator. The protocols serve the function of decreasing the depth of the

clinical trial and increasing the breadth by including a broader population base. In essence, these clinical trials provide data that are useful for premarketing surveillance and serve as a methodological transition to the observational clinical trials often used in Phase IV postmarketing surveillance studies. Patients followed in this type of Phase III clinical trial could continue to be followed after the NDA has been approved and would form a pool of patients from whom postmarketing surveillance studies could be generated. Each of these possible scenarios, or others not described, must be worked out in advance.

Categorizing Compassionate Plea Trials Based on Their Time of Conduct

Compassionate plea protocols can be categorized by their time of conduct, that is, the phase of medicine development at which they are conducted. Most compassionate plea protocols of the types previously described are conducted during Phases III or II. Other types are described below.

Treatment-IND Protocols

Treatment-IND protocols are compassionate plea protocols for investigational medicines of major medical significance in the United States that are written after safety and at least initial efficacy tests are complete. The term is relatively new; there is a formal system for applying to the FDA to receive this designation. These protocols allow widespread use of the medicine

TABLE 41.4 *Administrative issues in organizing and running a large treatment-IND protocol[a]*

1. Determine the type and amount of data to collect
2. Define the adverse reactions that must be reported
3. Assess the expected level of protocol compliance
4. Define the frequency of data reporting by physicians
5. Determine the method of communicating information to investigators
6. Evaluate the methods to be used in monitoring clinical sites
7. Establish the process for holding physicians accountable for supplies of medicines
8. Determine if the costs of the medicine are to be recovered, and if so, choose the method(s) to be used
9. Assess whether a waiver of local Ethics Committees/IRBs should be sought in those countries where this is possible (e.g., using a national committee)
10. Establish patient access guidelines for special groups (e.g., prisoners, children in foster care) where informed consent issues exist)
11. Develop a plan and program to educate Ethics Committees/IRBs, military personnel, physicians, insurance companies and other third-party payers about the treatment-IND protocol
12. Establish a promotional program that defines the types and methods of advertising that are acceptable
13. Assess the impact on the ongoing and planned clinical trial program

[a] Modified from a presentation by E. Andrews and P. Doi, with permission.

until the NDA has been approved. Some of the controversies and issues that have arisen are described by Mattison (1988) and Barry (1990). There are few formal rules to follow and each situation and question must be judged on its own. A list of medicines that have received this designation is given by Shulman and Raiford (1990). Issues involving treatment-IND programs are listed in Table 41.4.

Parallel-Track Protocols

Parallel-track protocols are being widely discussed and debated as this book is being written, and their future makeup and use is uncertain. The major difference between parallel-track and treatment-IND protocols is that in parallel-track protocols only safety (i.e., not efficacy) has to be demonstrated before the community-based trial may be started.

ADMINISTRATIVE ISSUES

What Types of Medicines Are Candidates for Compassionate Plea Trials?

Literally any type of nonmarketed medicine may be considered for compassionate plea trials, but there are a few cases in which they are more common.

1. *Nonmarketed medicines not under active development*. This was the original type of medicine given out on a compassionate plea basis. Most research-based pharmaceutical companies currently have one or more medicines in this category. For one or more reasons, a company decision has been made not to develop the medicine further, but there are patients who still benefit from it. Depending on the philosophy of the sponsor, some or all of these patients are given the medicine. Medicine is usually given out on a named patient basis and generally without charge.

2. *Previously marketed medicines*. Some medicines withdrawn from the market continue to be provided as described above. Most manufacturers are quite responsive to requests from physicians, especially if the medicine is not easily replaced (Weintraub and Northington, 1986).

3. *Investigational medicines of great medical value*. Breakthrough medicines are usually provided with a protocol and data collection forms to standardize the use of the medicine and minimize the chance that it will be misused and create problems for the sponsor.

4. *Investigational medicines of minimal or moderate medical value*. Most new medicines are made available under certain conditions during Phase III. These trials may provide data that support a medicine's regulatory submission if handled appropriately (i.e., with a protocol and data collection forms, plus follow-up to collect the data.)

Common Errors in Designing and Conducting Compassionate Plea Trials

Some companies are apparently unaware of increasing regulatory requirements to collect data on medicines supplied on a compassionate basis. These companies create problems for themselves by making their medicines widely available without attempting to control their use. These companies apparently believe they are enhancing the reputation of their medicine and company, and that widespread dissemination of the medicine will eventually facilitate its approval, use, and sales. This is a naive belief for most investigational medicines in the 1990s, however. This approach merely accumulates a great deal of patient exposures that are unaccounted for and may create regulatory problems.

Another problem concerns physicians who obtain medicine from a sponsor but do not comply with requests to complete and return data collection forms. Physicians who request a medicine from a sponsor on a compassionate plea basis could be required to sign a legal document accepting liability for its correct use and agreeing to complete and return data collection forms.

Finally, some companies use compassionate plea clinical trials as a marketing technique to introduce physicians to a new medicine. Using a compassionate plea clinical trial as a type of seeding trial for marketing is not always a sound idea (see Chapter 51).

Obtaining Data

A sponsor usually has difficulty obtaining data from compassionate plea trials. Depending on the need for the data, there are several alternatives ranging from doing nothing to sending someone to each site to retrieve the data. Often, data can be obtained if the site requires additional medicine supplies. The medicine may be used as a quid pro quo to encourage the staff to complete a report about the patient or to return data collection forms.

One method for collecting data is to request a written report of unspecified length from the investigator describing his or her experiences with the treatment. An improvement on this approach is to request that specific topics be addressed in the report (e.g., degree of improvement, laboratory abnormalities, adverse reactions). A better solution is to have a few simple data collection forms prepared in advance that may be used to collect the most important information. The amount of data collected should be kept to a minimum. This last approach is virtually a necessity if the data from many patients treated individually are to be processed and used either in a publication or as supportive data for a regulatory submission.

CHAPTER 42

Pharmacoeconomic Trials

Pharmacoeconomic trials may be conducted separately from clinical trials designed to evaluate a medicine's safety and efficacy, or economic assessments may be incorporated in those trials. Pharmacoeconomic trials may be conducted at any point during Phases II, III, and IV, but are most appropriate during Phases III and IV. They are conducted for many purposes, including (1) pricing of a new medicine, (2) repricing of an already marketed medicine, (3) developing promotional material for advertisements or other marketing approaches, (4) convincing a formulary committee to place the medicine on their approved list, (5) helping to convince one or more regulatory authorities to approve a medicine, (6) addressing concerns of patients and patient groups, and (7) developing clinical strategies. Pharmacoeconomic trials may be conducted as a reaction to answer charges or questions raised by one or more groups or to influence various groups (Table 42.1), or they may be done proactively for one or more of the reasons mentioned above.

DEFINITIONS

The definitions below are slightly modified from those proposed by Bootman et al. (1989).

Cost-effectiveness analysis. Simultaneous measurement of costs and consequences of treatment (or diagnosis, or prevention). Costs are measured in terms of money, and effectiveness is measured in terms of obtaining a specified objective. A medical practice is considered cost effective if its benefits justify its costs.

TABLE 42.1 *Reasons for conducting economic analyses*

1. Influence policies of third-party payers
2. Influence formulary committees at hospitals, HMOs, government agencies, or other groups
3. Influence prescription behavior of physicians
4. Influence purchasing behavior of customers

TABLE 42.2 *Objectives of different types of economic evaluations*

Evaluation and objective
1. *Cost–benefit analysis:* To assess treatment X versus other treatments or no treatment
2. *Cost–utility analysis:* To choose the least expensive approach to achieve a set standard of gain, expressed in terms of artificial units (e.g., quality adjusted life years)
3. *Cost–effectiveness study:* To choose the least expensive approach to achieve a set standard of gain, expressed in terms of a meaningful medical unit (e.g., lives saved)
4. *Cost-of-illness study:* To measure the costs of untreated illness
5. *Cost–minimization analysis:* To identify the least expensive way to achieve the same therapeutic results
6. *Quality of life study:* To assess costs and economic benefits for individual patients and to assess their subjective evaluation of the importance of these costs

TABLE 42.3 *Selected types of financial costs relating to a treatment with medicines*

1. Costs of a medicine
2. Costs of medical devices or equipment used to administer the medicine (e.g., intravenous tubing)
3. Staff time in a hospital, clinic, or elsewhere
4. Laboratory tests to monitor patients
5. Physician visits to monitor patients
6. Transportation costs
7. Care for babies, elderly, or others during medical visits
8. Food and lodging costs
9. Wages lost if the patient must remain out of work as part of treatment
10. Wages lost if the patient must remain out of work because of adverse reactions experienced

Cost–utility analysis. Simultaneous measurements of costs and consequences of treatment. Measurements of quality of life consequences are usually made in terms of preference for one intervention over another.

Cost–benefit analysis. Simultaneous measurement of costs and consequences of treatment, where both are expressed in terms of money.

Cost-of-illness analysis. Identification and evaluation of direct and indirect costs of a particular disease.

Cost–minimization analysis. Analysis and comparison of costs for two (or more) interventions shown (or believed) to be equivalent in outcomes or consequences.

The objectives of these various analyses are described in Table 42.2.

Perspectives

The perspective of cost usually differs greatly among groups, primarily depending on whether they are receiving treatment or fees, or are paying. Major groups include patients, physicians, hospitals, insurance companies, and governments. Perspectives of each group also differ greatly between countries, depending on the nature of their health system and other factors. Some of these perspectives are discussed throughout this chapter.

COSTS OF A MEDICAL SERVICE

Costs of any single medical service (e.g., a clinical laboratory test, electrocardiogram) can be established according to many approaches. Selected types of costs are listed in Table 42.3. The official charge for the service listed by a hospital contains numerous assumptions and arbitrary decisions. For example, the cost of

an electrocardiogram is based on each of the following:

1. Supplies (e.g., equipment that is purchased or leased)
2. Disposable supplies (e.g., paper, ink)
3. Fixed costs of the group conducting the electrocardiogram (e.g., telephone, heart station computer, maintenance)
4. Personnel costs of the staff (i.e., salaries plus benefits)
5. Overhead costs of the clinic or hospital

If one electrocardiogram is not performed, the above costs are not affected, except for the negligible cost of the paper and ink. If many fewer electrocardiograms are not done, however, it may be possible for the hospital to have one fewer technician on its payroll. Thus, the major savings to a clinic or hospital is not a gradual savings (except for supplies), but is a stepwise savings.

Other means of saving money on a test are to increase the efficacy of the procedure, replace it with a less expensive one, or have interpretations made by a less expensive group of physicians.

Costs versus Charges

There is no agreed-on relationship between medical costs and charges, whether for a new medicine or a surgery. After a company establishes the works cost for manufacturing a medicine it must add a certain amount for research and development costs incurred in the medicine's development, and a further amount to pay for future research and development. Expecting research-and-development-based companies to price a medicine solely on the cost of the tablet produced is like expecting a surgeon to charge patients for an operation based on the value of the forgone earnings in office visits while they operate, with no allowance for investment in skill development; or expecting an accountant to charge his clients based on the cost of the pencils, pads, and calculator or computer time used. A company that is unable to pay for its past and future research will be unable to discover new medicines, leading to smaller profits and the possibility of bankruptcy.

GROUPS CONCERNED ABOUT PHARMACOECONOMIC STUDIES

Governments

Virtually all province, state, and local governments are concerned about costs of medical care. In some cases they pay the entire bill, but usually pay at least part of the costs. National governments have the perspective of being both the protectors of the nation's health and payers of at least some of their country's medical bills. This potential conflict of interest is rarely discussed in those countries where prices for new medicines are established by the same government that must also pay those prices.

Formulary Committees

Formulary committees control the medicine allowed for prescription by the hospital, health maintenance organization (HMO), government, or other organization they serve. They have the function of gatekeepers for medicines allowed into their institutions. Formulary committees must be convinced that a new medicine should be placed on a formulary, which primarily involves differentiating the medicine from its competitors, or from no-treatment in an important way (e.g., based on cost, efficacy, safety, quality of life, convenience).

It is not usually sufficient for a formulary committee to make decisions about including a new medicine on their formulary based solely on data that differentiate a new medicine from traditional older prototypes (in terms of safety or efficacy), if other newer medicines are also available and are already on the formulary. Clinical trials used to obtain regulatory approval of the medicine usually include the older prototype or standard medicines, even if they are less widely used in practice than newer agents.

In negotiating agreements with a formulary committee that has several choices of medicines, companies may offer to refund money spent by the institution on a treatment if the patient is not improved within a fixed number of months. Contracts between institutions (e.g., HMOs) and companies are often highly complex because they may include prices of several medicines, prices based on ordering certain volumes, contingencies based on new products being approved (e.g., a letter could be sent to physicians in the HMO saying that medicine X is the one of choice), and an understanding that prices agreed to must last for a defined period.

HMOs have a goal for a certain number of prescriptions per member per year, and also have a goal for a certain number of hospital days per 1,000 members per year. In the United States these numbers are currently about 5 and 400, respectively. A new medicine or other treatment that is able to influence either of these numbers would be looked at with great interest by the formulary committee.

TRADITIONAL VERSUS GATEKEEPER MODELS OF HOW COMPANIES INFLUENCE USE OF THEIR PRODUCTS

Traditional Model

The traditional model of how pharmaceutical companies indirectly influence the number of prescriptions written for their products has been operating for at least a half-century. In this model, the company reached physicians who prescribed their medicines by advertising their products, detailing their products through sales representatives, and promoting their products at professional meetings. The physician was therefore approached directly and was viewed as the primary customer of the pharmaceutical company for prescription medicines.

Gatekeeper Model

The traditional model has been declining in importance for several reasons, the most important of which is the critical role being played by many formulary committees. The formulary committee of an HMO, Preferred Provider Organization, hospital, government agency, or other group decides which medicines are allowed on an approved list for their physicians to prescribe. Unless they approve a new medicine, it simply cannot be prescribed in most cases. The formulary committee may be lenient or strict, have high or low standards, take a great deal of time to decide on each medicine or make rapid decisions. These formulary committees are thus gatekeepers in deciding which group of medicines may be given to their patients.

The gatekeeper model poses two challenges for pharmaceutical companies. First, companies cannot sell their new medicines in a growing number of markets until formulary committees approve the medicines for placement on the formulary. This means that regulatory agency approval of a new medicine no longer represents approval to market the medicine to almost all physicians, but to a more and more limited group of physicians. Second, companies must obtain data that convinces the formulary group to accept their new medicine.

The first medicine approved for treating a disease

has little need for new economic data beyond that required for regulatory approval in order to be placed on a formulary. One exception is if the medicine is extremely expensive. In that case, economic data demonstrating benefits versus no-treatment may be important or even essential to collect. For almost all other types of new medicines, it is important to demonstrate benefits of the medicine over existing treatments. Whereas benefits were traditionally viewed in terms of better efficacy and less toxicity, the benefits sought in an era of cost-containment in medicine are increasingly economic in nature. As a result, it is wise for companies to consider that all new medicines require economic data to support their inclusion on formularies.

The same data that are collected to convince formulary committees to include a new medicine may or may not be suitable for promotion to physicians using the traditional model. For example, a formulary committee of an HMO is prevention oriented, whereas most physicians in private medical practice are treatment oriented. This means that an HMO formulary committee wants to see data showing how the HMO can save money on the number of patient visits or costs of hospitalizations. These data will not be viewed in the same way by physicians who depend on the number of patient visits for their income. Those physicians may be more impressed by data demonstrating a better quality of life and better ability to treat patients' episodes as office visits. Hospital formulary committees may want to know whether their overall bill for medicines will be reduced without decreasing their annual revenues from patients with a certain disease. This discussion could continue, but the point has hopefully been made.

Physicians who prescribe medicines are usually interested in data on within-patient changes, whereas regulatory agencies and formulary committees usually focus on between-treatment comparisons.

COST–EFFECTIVENESS ANALYSES

Many, if not most, people use the terms cost–benefit and cost–effectiveness interchangably. In academic circles, however, cost–effectiveness analyses are often described differently from cost–benefit analyses. The former evaluate competing programs for which effects are measured in the same units, whereas the latter compare the costs and benefits of competing programs in which effects are measured in dollar terms (see definitions at start of Chapter and Table 42.2). The cost-effectiveness approach is designed to allow a choice between programs intended to achieve a specific set of targeted results. It often focuses on identifying the specific program that achieves set objec-

TABLE 42.4 *Difficulties in conducting cost–effectiveness analyses*

1. Straightforward assessments of costs in a study are difficult, particularly from a society's viewpoint
2. Benefits of a treatment also are difficult to measure, particularly if endpoints are soft
3. Costs for particular patients often vary widely depending on their complications, need for hospitalization, and need of follow-up care
4. Skills and charges of health care providers vary
5. Costs directed toward aspects of the clinical trial that would not occur in actual practice (e.g., compliance-enhancing techniques, monitoring, data entry into detailed data collection forms) as well as the additional time spent by investigators providing patient care bias economic calculations and should be considered

tives at the lowest possible costs. The targeted results or outcomes are often not expressed in financial terms. For example, one cost-to-effectiveness analysis focused on the question: Should donor blood be screened for elevated alanine aminotransferase to prevent non-A, non-B posttransfusion hepatitis (Silverstein et al., 1984)? Another focused on determining the cost per year of life saved (Edelson et al., 1990). A comparison of cost–benefit and cost–effectiveness analyses is given by McGhan et al. (1978). Various design issues in cost–effectiveness analyses are presented by Russell (1985).

Cost–effectiveness is described as an assessment of costs in economic terms (e.g., money, days in hospital, physician's time) and benefits in terms of cases detected (e.g., from health screening) or increased longevity for treatment methods. Quality of life is also used as a measure of effectiveness. Cost–effectiveness results are expressed as a ratio of costs to benefits (e.g., dollars per quality-adjusted life year saved, dollars per case of colon cancer detected). If multiple medicines are compared with the same parameters, then a hierarchy of medicine may be established as an outcome. Similar medicines are generally compared because benefits should be expressed in the same or similar terms.

A medicine that is cost effective for one type of patient, or for patients with a specified disease severity, may be cost ineffective for other groups of patients. Some difficulties encountered in conducting cost–effectiveness analyses are listed in Table 42.4. A five-step process for conducting a cost–effectiveness analysis is given by Beck (1990).

COST–BENEFIT ANALYSES

The cost–benefit analysis is primarily a tool to evaluate health programs and assist in the allocation of funds. This technique is used by legislators and administrators who want to determine how best to allocate resources to achieve the optimal medical health of their society. The analysis consists of identifying all of the costs of a given program and comparing this figure with the corresponding values for all of the expected benefits. The benefits are each converted to an appropriate monetary value. Some benefits are easy to convert to monetary terms, but others require subjective judgments. The actual process of computing the financial values of benefits includes discounting future benefits and costs at a determined rate to reflect their current value. This is done to make the comparison more fair, because all components are then measured in comparable dollars. The comparison of benefits and costs becomes straightforward at this point, because they both are expressed in similar monetary terms.

Willingness to pay is often measured in economic studies (Grabowski and Hansen, 1990) and is a variation of a cost–benefit analysis. Willingness to pay is an indirect measure: the higher the usefulness, and higher the willingness to pay (constrained by the ability to pay).

Difficulties in Measurements

Many benefits are difficult to measure adequately and/or translate into a monetary value. For example, some benefits are intangible, such as (1) improved patient well-being and (2) improved working conditions for physicians. Costs, too, are difficult to measure adequately and/or translate into a monetary value. Costs of a disease include direct costs (e.g., medical resources used to prevent, diagnose, and treat patients), indirect costs (e.g., loss of productivity), and intangible costs (e.g., pain, anxiety, depression). Each of these three types of costs is composed of various parts that may be individually influence by many factors. Intangible costs are clearly the most complex and difficult area to measure. Psychological and social costs are experienced by both the patient and the patient's family, friends, coworkers, and caregivers.

Problems found in this approach are similar to those of cost–utility analyses, including (1) difficulties in measuring utility, (2) difficulties in completely identifying all possible consequences, and (3) complexities associated with estimating probability. Another problem is that costs and benefits are often unequally divided among the population considered, so that some people may pay the costs while others receive the benefits. Because all programs compared are reduced to the same terms (i.e., money), it is relatively easy to compare different types of programs.

Diagnosis-Related Groups (DRGs)

The cost–benefit ratio ought to become more important in hospital and administrative management and in the sales of pharmaceuticals to institutions. The diagnosis-related groups (DRGs) are changing the way in which hospital medicine is being practiced in the United States. In the ideal system, DRGs compare the benefit–cost ratio of new versus old treatments and require that increased treatment costs of new medicines be justified by increased benefits if alternative cheaper treatment is available. Newly marketed medicines that are priced above alternative therapy without offering increased benefits will no longer achieve a major market share in hospital pharmacies. Decisions are often made, however, on the basis of costs alone and do not include all benefits to be accrued. This situation often arises when it is not easy to assign a cash value. For example, if a new medicine improves the quality of life for patients by allowing them an additional half hour of sleep every night, or reduces nausea by 15%, how much more can be allowed in the cost of a new medicine? If another medicine has an improved safety profile compared with standard medicines, but is slightly less efficacious, how would the new medicine's price be established and viewed by formulary committees?

Allocation of National Resources

Issues such as kidney transplants involve cost–benefit considerations for our society. There is a point at which the increased financial costs to society of the surgery, postsurgical care, and rehabilitation must be balanced against the benefits of increased patient productivity and patient life itself. Although this balance is markedly on the side of performing transplants for otherwise healthy and/or highly productive members of society, it becomes less clear whether society should bear the full costs for severely ill patients who have a limited life expectancy and/or limited potential for a productive life. In between these two extremes lies a gray area that up to now has not been well defined in the United States. The process of attempting to draw a distinction between those patients who will receive an organ (paid for through public taxes) and those who will not is fraught with difficulties. An important difficulty is that calculating benefits depends on the values of the individuals assessing benefits, and these may be limited to economic and not humanitarian values.

Cost–Benefit Assessments by and for Individual Patients

The cost–benefit ratio is often assessed by individual patients when they decide whether or not to (1) purchase a prescription that has been given to them, (2) revisit the clinic or hospital as requested, or (3) purchase an item suggested by their physician (e.g., firm mattress, filter for their air conditioning unit). Cost–benefit analyses of whether it is worth conducting large multicenter trials were reviewed by Hawkins (1984). These studies assessed the monetary benefit to society or to the patient of adhering to the regimen deemed superior in the study. Willingness to pay for specific benefits is a pecuniary measure and is a cost–benefit technique that is sometimes used.

Although cost–benefit analyses are usually applied to large health programs it is also possible to use this approach for a single individual. Benefits are summed in dollar terms and compared with costs. In addition, in decision analysis both positive and negative utilities are considered. Cost–benefit assessments differ from utility analyses. A utility is a measure of preference for nonpecuniary outcomes.

How to Conduct Cost–Benefit Analyses

Potential risks or adverse events associated with taking a medicine are itemized, along with the probability that each will occur. The costs associated with each are then listed and multiplied by the probability of each occurring. The sum of these individual numbers is the cost side of the equation for that particular medicine or treatment. The process is then repeated for benefits and the two numbers are compared with each other, and with pairs of numbers for other treatments.

No medicine has been as carefully examined from cost–benefit and cost–effectiveness perspectives as cimetidine. The interested reader is referred to a large case study (Fineberg and Pearlman, 1981) and proceedings of an international symposium (Bloom, 1982).

Cost–Utility Analyses

Utility measures include using tests that are referred to as feeling thermometers and standard gambles. Reliability and validity issues in utility assessments are discussed by Bursztajn and Hamm (1982). They point out some of the major issues involved with the use of this method. Quality adjusted life years, one of the important measures of cost–utility analyses, are discussed by La Puma and Lawlor (1990).

Cost-of-Illness Analyses

Four costs are measured. *Direct costs* are for the diagnosis and treatment of the disease or other problem. Ancillary treatments such as rehabilitation, long-term care, and medical devices are included as part of direct costs. *Indirect costs* result from morbidity or mortality from the disease, including a patient's lost wages, plus

TABLE 42.5 *Potential economic ratios*

1. First-year additional in-hospital costs per first-year death avoided
2. First-year additional in-hospital costs per additional normally functioning child at 1 year
3. Lifetime additional health care costs per life year gained
4. Lifetime additional health care costs per quality adjusted life year gained
5. Lifetime additional health care costs minus lifetime increased productivity
6. Lifetime additional health care costs minus lifetime increased productivity per life year gained
7. Lifetime additional health care costs minus lifetime increased productivity per quality adjusted life year gained

pain and suffering. Friends and family usually have indirect medical costs spent for transportation, food, babysitters, and so forth (for hospital visits, or to take the patient for medical appointments). *Social costs* include costs for marriage counselors to keep a family together. Counseling may also be required because of psychosocial problems and the inability to work. *Societal costs* include legal costs associated with suits brought for product liability, but are not usually included in economic evaluations, because they primarily represent transfers of money from one group to another.

Cost–Risk Analyses

A cost–risk ratio may be defined as the risk that patients encounter when they do not fill a prescription and/or do not take their medicine(s) as prescribed. It has been reported that between 3 and 20% of patients do not fill their prescriptions (Stuart, 1985). The cost to the patient is usually calculated as the cost of the medicine or nonmedicine item for the cost side of the ratio. Risks are physical, psychological, and emotional problems that may be incurred when the patient does not take the medicine as prescribed or follow the physician's directions. Obtaining data on these types of costs is not easy since they are difficult to measure.

Potential ratios that may be determined are listed in Table 42.5, and a comparison of the three basic types of analyses are shown in Table 42.6.

TABLE 42.6 *Comparison of the three basic types of economic analyses of medicines*

Types of analysis and comparison

1. *Cost–effectiveness.* Compares money value of resources used up to clinical effects produced
2. *Cost–utility.* Compares money value of resources used up to quality of life produced by clinical effects
3. *Cost–benefit.* Compares money value of resources used up to money value of resources saved or created

Other Types of Pharmacoeconomic Studies

Days-off-Work Study

To determine the number of days off work on different medicines a company could conduct a study at a large company with many thousands of workers (e.g., Ford, General Motors) where these data could be collected.

Broad-Brush (i.e., Quick-and-Dirty) Study

One of the most simple studies would be to take a retrospective look at the number of times a patient took a medicine and how long it was used, and then to calculate the cost. Ancillary costs for laboratory screening and other costs would be added.

SOURCE OF BIASES IN PHARMACOECONOMIC TRIALS

Apart from the many biases that may enter pharmacoeconomic trials in a similar way to other clinical trials (see Chapter 5), some biases are particularly relevant.

The major bias that may enter these trials is the choice of endpoints to measure, because of the arbitrariness of both methods and parameters chosen. There are so many possible ways of demonstrating that one treatment is economically superior to another (Table 42.7) that any results stating this conclusion must be initially viewed with skepticism. In fact, it is conceivable that cost–effectiveness could be shown for each me-too medicine of any therapeutic class by carefully choosing the tests to measure, as well as by carefully choosing the comparative treatments.

Another bias that may enter pharmacoeconomic trials is that by focusing on parameters measured at one level, costs may be shifted to other levels or groups that would make a treatment appear more (or less) cost effective. For example, if the hospital costs of one or more treatments were being assessed, patients could be discharged prematurely from the hospital to shift some costs that would usually occur in the hospital to the home. The practice of premature patient discharge may often be done in a way that is medically acceptable, even though the usual practice of early discharge may be uncommon or rare.

One approach to dealing with known biases in a pharmacoeconomic trial is to put them all in the same direction so that each of them lead to either an underestimate or overestimate of costs. This should be done after the biases are minimized or eliminated by methods that are consistent with the goals of the clinical trial.

In the evaluation of direct or indirect costs it is gen-

TABLE 42.7 *Selected parameters that may be measured in pharmacoeconomic trials*

A. Cost of medicine and treatment
  1. Medicine cost per day, per dose, or per tablet
  2. Cost per day or week for single-medicine treatment; this allows for an equitable comparison between a medicine taken twice a day and another taken four times a day
  3. Total medicine cost per episode (e.g., course of therapy)
  4. Cost per day for all medicine taken. Some medicines may require concomitant medicines (e.g., diuretics that require potassium supplements)
  5. Total medicine cost per year
  6. Ancillary costs (e.g., nursing care, dietary or other supplements)
  7. Medicine, clinical laboratory, and other monitoring costs per year
  8. Total hospitalization costs for the medical event or episode
  9. Additional physician fees required during hospitalization
  10. Number of office visits times the fee for each per month or other period
  11. Medical monitoring test costs per year
  12. Costs of treatment for any adverse reactions
  13. Total medicine and hospital costs per year
  14. Total costs per year for the disease
  15. Comparison of average total treatment costs of two groups of patients[a]
  16. Cost per year of life saved
  17. Present value of extra service costs per quality adjusted life year saved

B. Other costs to patient
  1. Total out-of-pocket costs for the patient per year
  2. Costs of transportation per year for medical emergencies

C. Times and numbers
  1. Length of stay of patients in hospital (e.g., days per year)
  2. Length of stay of patients in an intensive care unit (e.g., days per episode)
  3. Number of hospitalizations per year
  4. Number of episodes of disease per year
  5. Number of physician visits per year
  6. Time spent by physician with patient per year

D. Work
  1. Number of days of work lost per year
  2. Percent of patients able to work
  3. Percent of patients able to work full time
  4. Percent of patients able to work at their preepisode level

[a] This comparison should generally include costs of all patients who failed treatment and thus it would be a comparison of costs per successful treatment.

erally easy to bias the data by omitting an essential cost that is not obvious (e.g., many hours of patient care furnished by volunteers), or including costs for services performed by overqualified individuals (e.g., a registered nurse making beds, a dentist cleaning teeth). If professionals are overqualified for the task they are doing, the task should be valued as if the appropriate person was doing it.

CHOOSING AN ECONOMIC METHOD TO USE IN A CLINICAL TRIAL

The major question to address in choosing an approach, and also for choosing the specific parameters to evaluate, is: Who are you trying to influence with the results of the clinical trial? Possible answers (i.e., audiences) for this question include practicing physicians, government financiers, politicians, the public, patients, and formulary committees. Formulary committees may be located at HMOs, hospitals, or within government organizations. This wide group of audiences emphasizes the following truism: *No single pharmacoeconomic trial can provide appropriate data for all of these groups.* Rare exceptions only serve to stress how important this principle is.

There is often a temptation to obtain a partial picture of the pharmacoeconomics of a new medicine. A complete pharmacoeconomic profile considers the various audiences and the need for both macroeconomic as well as microeconomic evaluations. In addition, various severities of a disease, subtypes of a disease, and different patient groups (e.g., lower, middle, and upper class) all have different economic profiles. A single or a few pharmacoeconomic trials usually are insufficient to provide the full economic profile of a new medicine.

The major method to avoid biases in cost–effectiveness trials is to evaluate both the costs and consequences of a new medicine at three levels, the individual patient, the health care facility (i.e., institutional), and society (i.e., total patient population).

Validation of Economic Tests

Issues of validation in pharmacoeconomics are different from those in most clinical tests and measures. In pharmacoeconomics the major approach involves conducting a logic exercise about what parameters to include and measure, and which to exclude. One should ask if what was done (or is planned) is both logical and complete? One does not ask whether a specific test is validated. A checklist to rate the quality of published studies, as well as to plan new trials, was prepared by the Department of Clinical Epidemiology and Biostatistics of McMaster University (1984a).

It is important to ascertain that measurements were (or will be) made carefully, biases were (or will be) minimized, and confidence intervals are included to indicate the precision of the cost data obtained. If it is not possible to calculate confidence intervals, then it is important to present the ranges of values obtained in addition to means and standard deviations of the costs.

ARE ECONOMIC DATA OBTAINED IN CLINICAL TRIALS EXTRAPOLATABLE TO MEDICAL PRACTICE?

The answer to this important question is both yes and no. Part of the dilemma is that clinical trials represent an artificial environment. The degree of artificiality varies greatly and the more it differs from clinical practice the less the economic data from a trial may be extrapolated. A later section identifies some of the major factors to consider when this question is posed.

BASIC STEPS IN CONDUCTING A PHARMACOECONOMIC EVALUATION

Step One: Learn About the Issues. Discuss the situation with pharmacoeconomists and others who have relevant insight and knowledge. Read background information and ensure that the most relevant issues are clearly identified. Determine the group(s) for which the study is being conducted.

Step Two: Identify Alternative Approaches to Designing a Clinical Trial. The economic objectives may be evaluated in a separate pharmacoeconomic trial or as part of another (i.e., safety or efficacy) clinical trial. Advantages of each approach in terms of cost, time, quality of data, and suitability of methods must be considered.

Step Three: Determine the Level of Benefits and Costs to Evaluate. Are data to be collected on a micro- or macro-level? Are benefits and costs to be measured for a single patient or a group (i.e., micro-level), or for the health care of a large population of patients or even the entire society (i.e., macro-level)? The answer to this issue depends primarily on the target groups for which the data are being collected.

Step Four: Determine How to Value the Benefits. The method used to value the benefits has a major impact on the method(s) used for the study. The basic choices are in terms of natural units, money, or subjective terms.

Step Five: Evaluate the Possible Methods and Sites to Use. Choose One or More of Each. Given the general goals of the pharmacoeconomic trials and the specific objectives desired, determine which method is most suitable. Choose the type of site (e.g., tertiary care hospital, HMO), depending on the target group.

Step Six: Design the Pharmacoeconomic Trial. Determine all direct costs (e.g., medicines, nursing care, physician care, hospital charges) and indirect costs (e.g., equipment, transportation, loss of earnings, family assistance) that will be measured. The level (i.e., micro and macro) will match that of benefits. Identify all perspectives to be assessed (e.g., patient, institution, third-party payor, government). Consider ethical issues that might affect the trial. If the trial is to last for longer than a year then it will be desirable to use discounting. This process treats all costs and benefits as if they occurred during the same period and makes evaluations equitable. Other economic issues should be discussed with specialists in this area. If the trial lasts a long time then unrelated illnesses and their costs may affect the data.

Step Seven: Conduct the Pharmacoeconomic Trial. Monitoring is as important as for other clinical trials.

Step Eight: Analyze, Interpret, and Report Results. All assumptions and caveats about the trial and data should be assessed. Various analyses determined in advance should be conducted (e.g., break even, worst case, sensitivity analyses). Describe the degree of confidence in the trial outcomes.

COMPARING DATA FROM CLINICAL TRIALS AND MEDICAL PRACTICE

Are patients enrolled in the clinical trial similar to those who would be treated in the medical practice of interest? One problem is that a clinical trial is usually conducted in a single population of patients, but the medical practices of the physicians who will review the data and consider its extrapolation vary enormously (e.g., primary, secondary, tertiary care providers; medical practices catering to wealthy and poor patients). One must ensure that costs of the medicine or treatment were calculated, even though the patients in the clinical trial may have received their treatment without charge.

Another issue is whether the number of clinical safety and efficacy tests performed during the medical trial are also necessary to perform for patients in medical practice environments. Fewer tests are usually performed in a medical practice and this would decrease overall treatment costs, as would the fewer patient visits for medical practice versus an outpatient clinical trial. Clinical trials often include laboratory and efficacy tests that are seldom performed in medical practice. These tests are obviously appropriate for evaluating new medicines when insufficient information is available. Another factor in clinical trials that contributes to higher costs than in medical practice is the greater attention paid to assiduous follow-up of every complaint or potential adverse event with increased patient monitoring and consultations. These factors make the economics of a new medicine based on clinical trials appear more expensive than it is in the reality of medical practice.

One of the factors in a medical practice that may cause higher costs for at least some patients is related to the heterogeneity of the population treated. With the exception of some Phase III clinical trials, investigational studies are always conducted in more homogeneous groups of patients than are encountered in a medical practice.

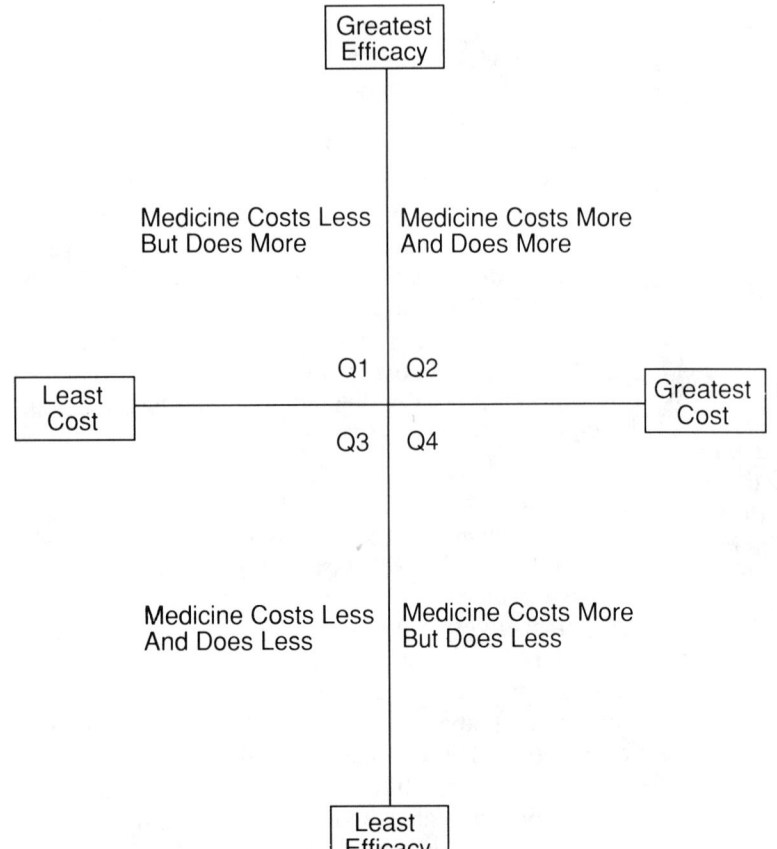

FIG. 42.1 Comparison of costs and efficacy for two or more medicines. The origin represents the status quo, and the axes measure change with respect to the status quo. Efficacy could be measured in terms of one parameter, a combination, or as quality of life.

Solutions

It should be clear from the above discussion that costs of treatment determined in a clinical trial usually differ markedly from those experienced in medical practice. When this issue is important to address, one approach is to include a usual care group in the clinical trial. Economic and clinical outcome data obtained in this group of patients would provide a better comparison than merely using historically controlled data or an active medicine control. To prevent physicians from treating both usual care and protocol patients similarly, a great deal of education about appropriate guidelines to use for each group may be necessary. Alternatively, physicians may be randomized to either usual care or formal treatment according to a protocol. However, relatively large numbers of physicians are needed to conduct this type of clinical trial successfully.

A frame of reference that may be used to compare costs and efficacy (or safety) for two or more medicines is shown in Fig. 42.1. This four-quadrant graph enables one to see both strengths and weaknesses of various medicines. Safety, patient convenience, or other parameters of a treatment may also be compared with costs.

In interpreting the results of quality of life and pharmacoeconomic tests, it is often possible to view data as predominantly in one of the four quadrants shown:
1. Higher cost and worse quality of life (or efficacy).
2. Higher cost and better quality of life (or efficacy).
3. Lower cost and worse quality of life (or efficacy).
4. Lower cost and better quality of life (or efficacy).

CASE STUDIES IN PHARMACOECONOMICS

This book does not have sufficient space to present detailed examples of the various pharmacoeconomic methods and to indicate how these methods can ac-

tually be applied. Tables 42.8 to 42.10 have brief examples. Readers are recommended to a few sources of multiple concise examples as well as to the pharmacoeconomic literature in general. Dao (1985) and Eisenberg et al. (1989) present numerous case studies using different approaches and methodologies. Feeny and Torrance (1989) present two examples of utility-based quality of life assessments. The Department of Clinical Epidemiology and Biostatistics of McMaster University Health Sciences Centre (1984a) present and discuss three economic case studies, and in a follow-up article (1984b) provide a detailed checklist for readers who wish to critique economic reports. Finally, a fairly complete source of examples is given in a monograph by Drummond et al. (1987). A series of tables used to present economic data is shown in *Presentation of Clinical Data* (Spilker and Schoenfelder, 1990).

TABLE 42.9A *Example of cost–benefit analysis*

Factor	Specifics
Treatment:	Taking cholesterol-lowering agent for 7 years, options: Cholestyramine resin; Colestipol; Oat bran
Costs:	Treatment, including medicines, physicians, dietician, and laboratory
Benefits:	Medical care costs of averted events (e.g., myocardial infarction, coronary artery bypass grafts, new angina) work time gained (earnings)

TABLE 42.9B *Cost–benefit per case (in dollars)*

	Cholestyramine	Colestipol	Oat bran
Cost	10,030	6,150	1,730
Benefit			
Averted events	240	240	240
Work gain	680	680	680
Total	920	920	920
Net economic benefit	−9,110	−5,230	−810
Effects per case[a]	0.08	0.08	0.08
Cost–effectiveness ratio (cost/life year gained)	117,400	70,900	17,800
Net economic cost/ life year gained	108,800	63,500	9,200

From Kinosian and Eisenberg (1988).
[a] In life years gained.

TABLE 42.8 *Example of cost–effectiveness analysis*

Factor	Finding
Treatment:	Beta blocker for 6 years after acute myocardial infarction
Costs:	Medicine, $208/year Assumed no savings in follow-up medical treatment costs Assumed no cost of side effects
Effects:	Gains in life expectancy (for age 55) Low risk, 0.10 years Medium risk, 0.34 years High risk, 0.47 years
	Cost–effectiveness ratio (for age 55) Low risk, $13,068/life-year gained Medium risk, $3,618/life-year gained High risk, $2,357/life-year gained

From Goldman et al. (1988).

TABLE 42.10 *Example of cost–utility analysis*

Treatment:	Neonatal intensive care of very-low-birth-weight infants
Costs:	Incremental (changes in) costs of: Neonatal period (hospital, physician) Follow-up (rehospitalizations, physicians, appliances, medicines, special services, special education) Future work time lost/gained (earnings)
Effects:	Incremental changes in quantity and quality of life measured in quality adjusted life years gained (QALYs)[a]
Cost–utility ratio	$1,000/QALY gained for 1,000–14,999 g, infants $17,500/QALY gained for 500–999 g, infants

From Boyle et al. (1983).
[a] QALYs are discussed at length by La Puma and Lawlor (1990).

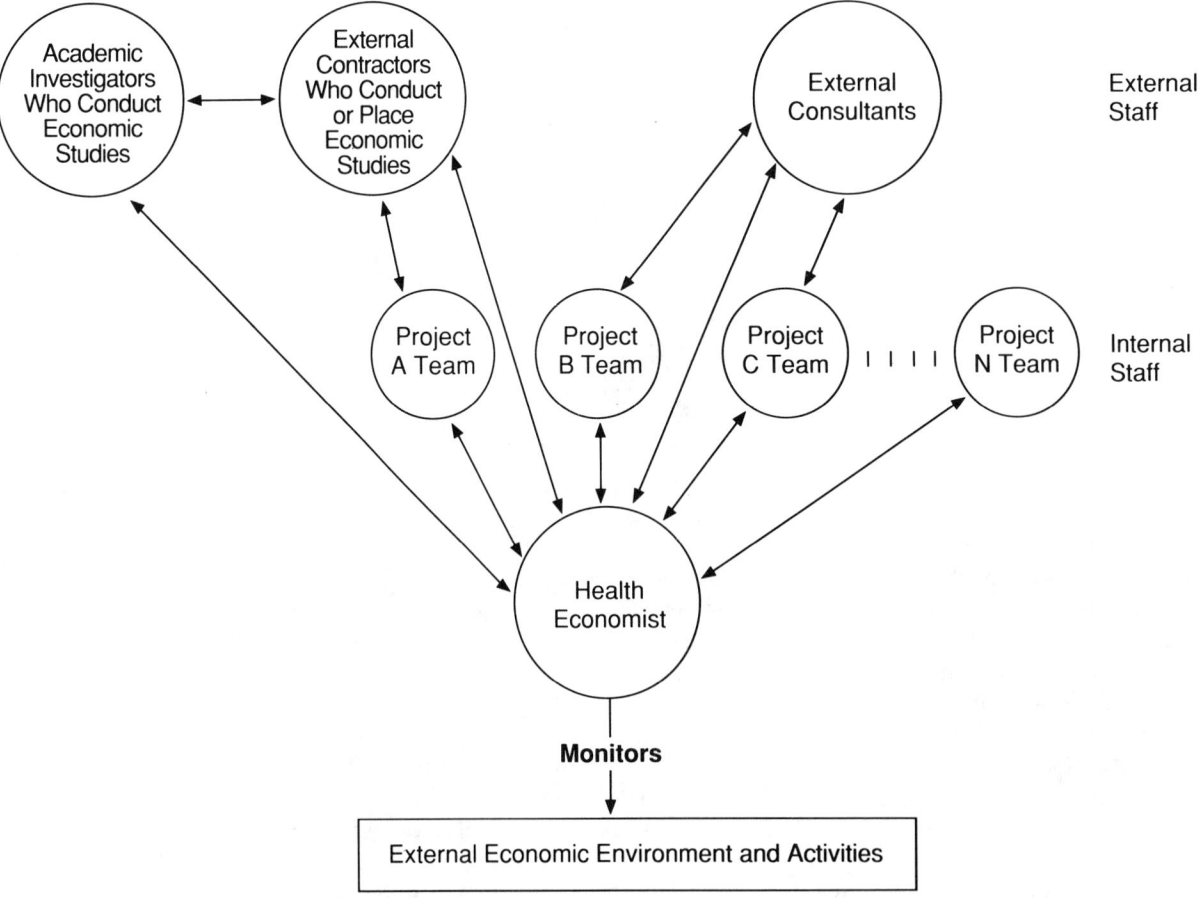

FIG. 42.2 Interactions and roles of a health economist within a pharmaceutical company, illustrating activities relating to the development and placement of pharmacoeconomic studies.

THE FUTURE

Two changes will hopefully occur in the field of pharmacoeconomics during this decade. First, the almost total freedom of investigators designing a pharmacoeconomics trial to focus on and evaluate any parameter and any approach arbitrarily will probably be decreased. This advance could arise because (1) a standard battery of parameters to be generally tested in all trials will be developed, or (2) the target audience for receiving the pharmacoeconomic data generated will inform the relevant group which tests to evaluate, prior to initiation of the trial.

The second change is that standards of pharmacoeconomic trials will increase dramatically, partly because of the first change, which will force standards higher. Consequent to both of these changes will be the development of pharmacoeconomics as a separate discipline within clinical medicine/pharmacology. More professionals with training in the methods describe in this chapter will be hired within academia, government, and industry to design and oversee these trials. Trials will be conducted (1) as part of clinical

trials, (2) as independent prospective pharmacoeconomic trials, and (3) as sound retrospective analyses of data gathered by others. The first two types of trials are at the two previously discussed micro-levels (i.e., individual patient, multiple patients) and the last is at the macro-level of society.

Pharmaceutical companies will coordinate their pharmacoeconomic activities with input from both medical and marketing groups. Trials at the micro-level will be planned and directed by medical groups, possibly by trained economists who solicit marketing input. Trials at the macro-level will generally be led by individuals (e.g., health policy planners) within the marketing function (Fig. 42.2). A coordination or even integration of these efforts is essential. These groups will plan specific pharmacoeconomic trials on a country-by-country basis, depending on where the medicine will be marketed. Cost data obtained in one country are generally inappropriate for another because of different cultures as well as health care systems. Within each country each type of customer or target group should be viewed separately.

CHAPTER 43

Validation of Clinical Tests and Measures

INTRODUCTION

Valid data are true and accurate. A validated clinical test is one that has been shown to yield true and accurate data. One of the major problems in clinical trials today is that many tests and scales used have not been adequately validated.

Need for Validation

Many preclinical scientists and research clinicians find it easy and fun to design new scales, questionnaires, and tests to evaluate relevant parameters in a particular or general area. When their method is used by others to generate data, those who developed the test have a feeling of accomplishment. However, some of these innovators do not fully understand that all scales, questionnaires, and tests must be *validated,* and that mere use by other investigators is not (usually) sufficient for validation, even if the original author's work

is confirmed. Data obtained with poorly validated tests may mislead people for many years. Moreover, the process of validation is generally a long, expensive, and painstaking process requiring several or many years or effort. Nonetheless, these steps are necessary to ensure that data obtained with a specific test are valid and are able to convince others. This chapter describes the process of validation.

Relative Validation

Validation is rarely an all-or-none process involving the demonstration that the results of a particular test are 100% true or 100% false. Rather, it is the demonstration of the degree of truthfulness of the results. This involves the establishment of the rates of false-positive and false-negative results obtained with the test. Unfortunately, this degree of validation has not yet been achieved with most tests and measures used in clinical trials.

313

Ideal Approach to Validating a Test

The major method of validating tests that yield objective data is to compare the results of the new test with results obtained using a gold standard. If a single gold standard exists (e.g., autopsy sample to prove a diagnosis) then the validation process may be a straightforward exercise achieved in one clinical trial and confirmed in a second. More frequently, however, no gold standard exists, and one is forced to use a "silver," "bronze," or even less reliable standard for comparison. It is therefore extremely difficult to validate tests that yield subjective data.

DEFINITION OF VALIDATION

Chisolm et al. (1985) state "To be valid a questionnaire needs to meet five criteria: (a) to be acceptable to the population under study; (b) to be easily completed; (c) to be consistent—that is, to elicit responses similar to those gained in a conventional doctor–patient interview; (d) to be reproducible when administered on two separate occasions; (e) to be of value or use when complete." The authors describe these five characteristics more simply as (1) acceptability, (2) feasibility, (3) reproducibility, (4) consistency, and (5) applicability. This is a clear, nonjargon definition that may be readily used when evaluating the validity of a new or old test, scale, or questionnaire. Nonetheless, this definition includes several concepts and is very broad. Numerous authors believe there are three separate concepts involved in validity (i.e., reproducibility, validity, and responsiveness) rather than a single unified one.

What Is Being Validated?

The process of validation is applied to:

1. Medical treatments currently used in practice. This includes specific treatments, dosages, and

TABLE 43.1 *Selected situations in which validation is performed*

1. A single piece of equipment used to measure or produce something
2. Multiple pieces of equipment used to measure or produce something
3. Overall process of producing something
4. A questionnaire or scale used in a clinical trial
5. Data from a study processed in a computer
6. Computer-generated results from a large, automated, multipurpose data base
7. Toxicology data after a study is completed

combinations of treatments. Other facets of current treatments may also be validated.
2. Tests, scales, and questionnaires used to measure clinical endpoints. These include safety as well as efficacy endpoints, and objective as well as subjective tests, scales, and questionnaires. Methods used with other types of clinical data and endpoints (e.g., pharmacokinetics, quality of life, cost–effectiveness) may also be validated.
3. Equipment used to measure clinical responses. The validation process should be completed before the equipment is introduced on the market and sold. It is the responsibility of the manufacturer or distributor to ensure that adequate validation of the products they sell has occurred. Validation is primarily important for class II and III medical devices.

Validation also occurs in numerous other processes that are only indirectly related to clinical trials (e.g., computers, manufacturing processes, animal models used to predict clinical effects). Table 43.1 summarizes situations in which validation is performed.

Gold, Silver, and Bronze Standards

The term *gold standard* is used in the literature with both a relative and an absolute definition. The relative definition defines the gold standard as whatever mea-

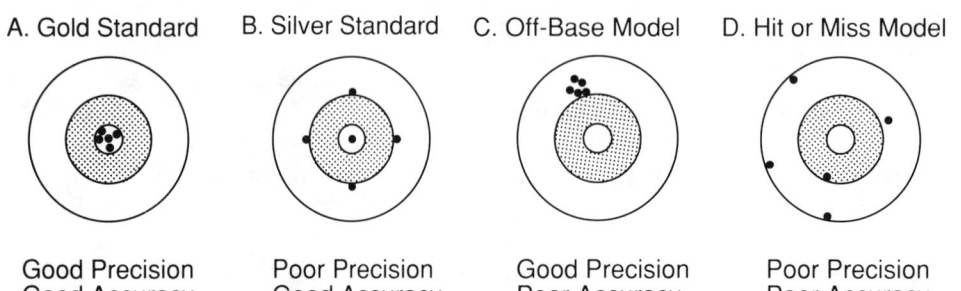

FIG. 43.1 The difference between precision and accuracy. The accuracy of a variable is defined as the degree to which it actually represents what it is intended to represent. The precision of results is the degree to which they are reproducible. (Modified from Hulley and Cummings, 1988, with permission of Williams and Wilkins.)

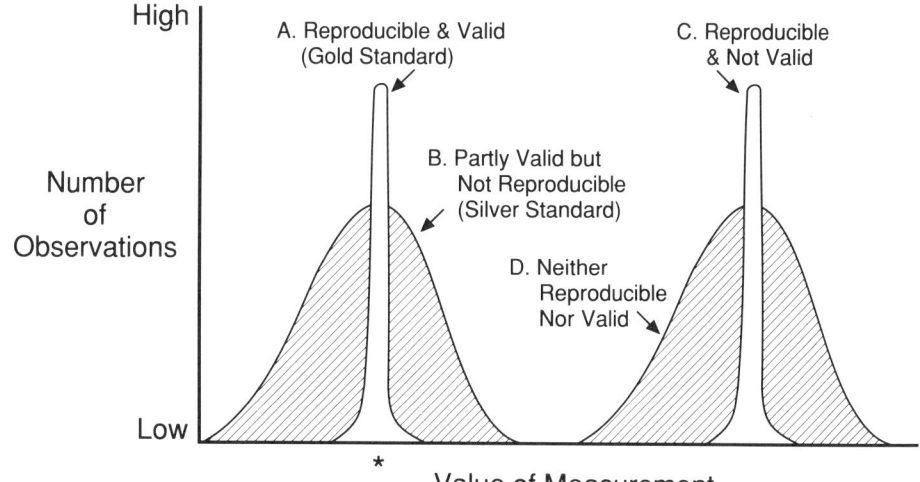

FIG. 43.2 Four hypothetical outcomes when conducting a test and evaluating the validity and reliability of the results. **A:** Valid and reliable. **B:** Valid but not reliable. **C:** Not valid but reliable. **D:** Neither valid nor reliable. *Asterisk* = true value. (Modified from Fletcher et al., 1988, with permission of Williams and Wilkins.)

sure is the best currently available means of diagnosing a disease. When a better measure is found, then the new measure becomes the new gold standard. In the absolute definition, no gold standard for diagnosing a disease exists until a method is found that is close to perfect. If a reasonable standard exists it could be referred to as a silver or bronze standard. This designation would indicate that it had value, but should not be considered a gold standard.

Two diagrammatic ways of viewing these standards are shown in Figs. 43.1 and 43.2. Both these figures are excellent examples of how precision and accuracy may be conceptualized and defined.

Reproducibility

Some authors describe reproducibility of a test (i.e., the measure of its consistency) as a prerequisite for validity, rather than as a part of validity. This distinction is primarily a semantic issue.

Responsiveness

For a test that yields reproducible results in a clinical trial to be valid, it must also be able to detect any differences resulting from the treatment. For example, a number of intelligence quotient tests are fairly reproducible and are generally considered valid, but these tests are not responsive to most treatments (e.g., medicines) that would be evaluated in clinical trials. Various psychological and behavioral tests that give reproducible and valid results may or may not be responsive to changes brought about in patients by medicines. This fact must be known before the tests can

be used in a clinical trial to measure clinically significant patient outcomes as a result of treatment with medicine.

Clinical tests cannot be adequately validated in a pilot trial or using retrospective data.

TYPES OF VALIDITY

The nomenclature for types of validity is far from standardized. Some authors discuss internal and external validity (Kazdin, 1982), whereas others discuss content, face, criterion, discriminant, and construct validity (Bombardier and Tugwell, 1982). Other terms describing types of validity are also found in the literature.

Kazdin (1982) describes internal validity as "the extent to which an experiment rules out alternative explanation of the results." He describes numerous factors that could affect results that are defined as threats to internal validity (e.g., selection biases, instrumentation, maturation of the patient). Internal validity therefore refers to factors within the clinical trial. External validity "refers to the extent to which the results of an experiment can be generalized or extended beyond the condition of the experiment." Kazdin also describes threats to external validity. This present book uses the term extrapolation or extrapolatability to describe external validity and dose not use the term internal validity. Instead, five types of validity are described. Definitions for the following five types of validity are adapted in part from Bombardier and Tugwell, 1982.

Criterion Validity. How well does the test, scale, or questionnaire obtain the same results as with other approaches measuring the same characteristic, particularly the gold standard? In a simple case, criterion validity is determined by the correlation coefficient that describes the relationship between the test and the gold standard. A test with criterion validity produces consistent results that reflect the true state of the patient. This type of validity is also called predictive validity. Some authors define criterion validity, however, as construct validity (described below).

Construct Validity. How well does the test, scale, or questionnaire measure what it is supposed to (or designed to) measure? This depends on the accumulation of scientific and medical evidence in support of a given construct's (i.e., description from someone's perspective used to explain one aspect of reality) being able to explain and predict a range of human behavior. The outcome of a test that has construct validity agrees with expected results.

Content Validity. Content validity is present when the choice and relative importance of each part of a test or questionnaire are appropriate for its purpose.

Face Validity. Face validity is the method of aggregating the individual components into an index or overall test that appear sensible, i.e., the measurements appear to be a reasonable approach to assessing the characteristic(s) of interest.

Discriminant Validity. Discriminant validity occurs when the test is able to detect the smallest change that would be considered as clinically significant both within and between patients.

Prospective, Simultaneous, or Retrospective Validation. Validation may be performed either before, during, or after a clinical trial or process is conducted. The terms prospective validation, simultaneous validation, and retrospective validation may be used to describe these three states. One (or more) of these types may be traditionally used as the process of validation in a particular situation.

Some clinicians approach the issue of validation by stating that merely conducting an extremely large-scale clinical trial will validate current treatment modalities (Remington, 1979). This is not generally true, and may lead to erroneous results. Moreover, the assumption that the test has been validated may lead to its widespread use for many years before its validity is challenged.

PROCESS OF VALIDATION

Some of the following steps are optional and others are not always possible to conduct.

1. Evaluate tests for reliability (i.e. reproducibility) by the same patient.
2. Evaluate tests for reliability by the same rater and also for different raters.

3. Compare data with the gold standard (e.g., autopsy results, biopsy results), or with definitive tests that yield unequivocal (or relatively unequivocal) results.
4. Compare data with other markers of the disease (i.e., a silver or bronze standard), especially when no gold standard exists.
5. Compare data from the scale being validated with data obtained using other validated scales.
6. Establish the rate of false positives and false negatives.
7. Convene a panel of experts to discuss the topic.
8. Have a professional society publish the results of their evaluation(s).

Protocols for Conducting a Validation Procedure or Test

It is desirable, if not mandatory, that the procedures used to validate a test or scale be written in detail. This enables the validation process to be evaluated.

The protocol for a validation procedure should address the following questions:

1. Is the process, equipment, or test measuring or producing what it purports to measure or produce?
2. Is it reliable (i.e., reproducible) both within patients and between patients? This is not considered a part of *validation*, although it is essential to establish before validation can be proved. Can two different people using the same test or equipment get the same results?
3. Is it accurate (i.e., correct)? This result makes data valid.
4. Is it as precise (i.e., detailed) as claimed?

CHOOSING TESTS FOR A CLINICAL TRIAL

Spectra to Consider When Choosing Tests

Validation is a relative concept; any objective test, subjective test, or scale varies along two spectrums that are of practical concern to people choosing tests to include in a clinical trial.

Spectrum 1 varies from perfectly valid to the other extreme of absolutely invalid.
Spectrum 2 varies from a statement that the test is completely evaluated as to its validity to the other extreme in which a test's validity has yet to be evaluated.

It is especially important to understand where a new test fits along both of these spectra before it is incorporated and used in a clinical trial. One pitfall that traps unwary clinicians designing a clinical trial is that a test

TABLE 43.2 *Desirable attributes of clinical tests*

1. Easy to administer
2. Easy to score
3. Measures clinically important changes
4. Easy to interpret the results
5. Sensitive to effects of medicines
6. Results are reproducible
7. Results are valid
8. Results may be extrapolated to other patients
9. Results may be extrapolated to other scales[a]

[a] A change of X units on one test correlates with a change of Y units on another test. Alternatively, a patient who is rated as severely ill with one test would also be ill if another specific test were used; or, a patient diagnosed as having disease A with one test would be similarly diagnosed with another diagnostic test.

or scale that appears to be reasonable to use and also appears to be clinically acceptable may actually yield misleading data and conclusions, either because it is insensitive to the intervention (e.g., medicine) studied or for other reasons. Desirable attributes of clinical tests are summarized in Table 43.2.

Tracing the Origins of a Test Back to Its Roots

Many clinical tests and scales are widely used and quoted, but have never been rigorously evaluated or validated. It is usually difficult, without a great effort, to trace a clinical test or scale back to its roots and discover the proof that it measures what it purports to measure. Subjective scales and tests used in medicine are particularly difficult to trace in this regard. The process of tracing the origins of tests to ensure that they are validated is rarely done.

Establishing the Validity of Objective Tests

Do objective tests have to be validated? The answer is definitely yes. There are also a variety of types of validation for measuring a laboratory analyte or parameter. One type of validation concerns the equipment used to measure the analyte (e.g., sodium in blood) or parameter (e.g., forced expiratory volume of air in 1 second). Every laboratory test procedure that uses biological samples (e.g., blood, cerebrospinal fluid, urine) to measure an analyte has its own sensitivity and specificity depending on experimental conditions. The value obtained must then be associated with a normal or abnormal clinical state. This abnormality is in turn often associated with a particular disease, syndrome, or condition. The degree to which abnormal values correlate with a specific disease is a second type of validation. Some laboratory tests are useful for identifying multiple diseases. This topic is discussed in Chapter 81.

CRITIQUING THE VALIDATION PROCESS FOR A CLINICAL TEST THAT IS PURPORTEDLY VALIDATED

Questions to ask about the validation of a method include:

1. What is the reliability when the test is used multiple times? How long a period was allowed to elapse between retests?
2. Who were the patients (volunteers) on whom the test was validated? How many patients were tested? What forms of disease did they have? What was the status of their disease? What were their demographic characteristics? What were their previous and current treatments (e.g., medicine, dose)? In what settings (e.g., inpatient, nursing home) were patients evaluated?
3. What was the interrater reliability and is it acceptable?
4. Was the validation conducted under generally similar conditions to the way the test is currently used? For example, it would be important to know if the test or scale was validated using a full 1-hour interview with each patient, although the scale is most often used during practice in a 5-minute interview. Also, the scale might have been validated in patients kept in a quiet setting, whereas the test may be generally used in clinical practice in a hectic group session.
5. How much experience and training for staff is required before the test may be appropriately used?
6. If the scale has many parts, has each separate part been validated? Are there differences in validity of the different parts?
7. Are the tests that were used to validate the method the best test available at the time?
8. Has the validation of the test been confirmed? Validation results, (just as results of well-controlled clinical trials) usually require replication before they are considered well established.

A validated scale or test that is used in a different setting or under different conditions from those under which it was validated may not be valid. Interpretations drawn from these results obviously may be incorrect. Many quality of life tests and scales have been shown not to be valid for different ethnic or national patient populations (Chapter 40).

ISSUES OF VALIDATION

Extrapolation Between Populations

Tests demonstrated to be valid in one population are usually assumed to be valid for other populations, although this is not always the case. It is unrealistic to have to validate each test in every population in which it could be used. Nonetheless, people may be misled by making this simple assumption. Generally, the closer the populations are to each other in major characteristics, the greater is the likelihood that a test is valid in both.

Static versus Dynamic Assessments

Tests that are valid for one purpose in a population (e.g., to characterize some aspect of behavior or disease) may be invalid for a different purpose (e.g., to assess how the same aspect of behavior or disease changes as a result of treatment). This is an example of comparing a test that captures a static measurement of a given state with one that captures a dynamic measurement as the state changes.

Ability to Measure Magnitude of Change

Some tests are not sensitive enough to capture small changes in a characteristic, even though the test may accurately assess the baseline state. The problem may relate to the test's inability to capture the magnitude of the change or the nature of the change resulting from the medical intervention.

Cultural Differences

A test that is validated in one culture may not be valid when used in a different cultural group. Five major dimensions of cross-cultural equivalence of tests were proposed by Flaherty et al. (1988).

1. *Content equivalence.* The content of each item of the instrument is relevant to the phenomena of each culture being studied.
2. *Semantic equivalence.* The meaning of each item is the same in each culture after translation into the language and idiom (written or oral) of each culture. This is often a major issue since the connotations of words and terms often differ markedly between cultures, even when the denotations of words are similar or identical.
3. *Technical equivalence.* The method of assessment (e.g., pencil and paper, interview) is comparable in each culture with respect to the data that it yields.
4. *Criterion equivalence.* The interpretation of the measurement of the variable remains the same when compared with the norm for each culture studied.
5. *Conceptual equivalence.* The instrument is mea-

suring the same theoretical construct in each culture.

Regulatory Standards Differ Between Countries

The quality and quantity of data required to establish the validity of a test or analytical procedure vary between countries. As an example, consider an assay to measure the contents of a capsule or tablet. Differences among regulatory standards exist when answering basic questions such as:

1. Can every impurity found during the preparation of the major chemical (i.e., active ingredient) of a medicine be identified both in quantity and chemical structure? How much of each impurity must be present before this must be done?
2. Can every impurity in each excipient (i.e., inactive ingredients) of a medicine be identified both in quantity and in chemical structure? How much of an impurity must be present before this must be done?
3. How much data must be collected on an analytical test or measure before it can be described as valid? How consistent must the data be?

Published Statements About Validation

Many authors are guilty of drawing sweeping conclusions about the validity of tests they propose, and the medical literature cannot be read uncritically. For example, a paper titled ''Validation of a self-administered questionnaire to elicit gastrointestinal symptoms'' (Chisholm et al., 1985) published in the prestigious *British Medical Journal* draws broad, sweeping conclusions on the questionnaire's validity, even though the questionnaire was tested in a relatively small patient sample that the authors themselves describe as a ''pilot study.''

Medical Histories

Most of the information in a patient's medical history comes from the patient. A little reflection (or experience) suggests that much of these data are unreliable or incorrect. Colditz et al. (1986) reported variable results when testing the accuracy of patient self-reports for different major diagnoses. For example, patient knowledge of the existence of their own cancers of the breast or thyroid were nearly 100% correct, but knowledge of primary cancers versus metastases were confused, and knowledge of a previous myocardial infarction was only 68% correct. Reports of family history, allergies to medicines, and past surgeries are often mistaken or poorly recalled by many patients. Validations of questionnaires in which patients are required to provide these types of data raise numerous problems. Nonetheless, a test that is validated based on the assumption of correct data cannot be expected to be valid when incorrect data are supplied.

Potential Problems of Using Patient-Completed Tests and Scales

When patients are asked to provide responses to a test, scale, or questionnaire using a validated instrument, poor quality or inaccurate data may result. Investigators who are inadequately trained in interpreting test results create another potential problem. Thus, a useful test, scale, or questionnaire based on patient responses requires much more than a previous demonstration of validation in order to be useful in many situations. Whether patient self-ratings are reliable depends on:

1. The subject being rated (e.g., intimate sexual questions versus the number of vaccinations received during the last year)
2. The psychological state of the individual doing the rating (e.g., normal patients versus mentally ill)

3. The emotional condition of the individual doing the rating (e.g., a high stress level versus a relaxed state)
4. The environmental conditions under which the rating is being made (e.g., crowded and noisy room versus a tranquil one)
5. The physical state of the individual doing the rating (e.g., presence of bothersome lesions)
6. Other factors (e.g., level of literacy or illiteracy)

STEPS IN DEVELOPING A NEW CLINICAL TEST OR MEASURE

The steps to develop a new instrument have been indicated and discussed by Guyatt and Jaescke (1990). This process is generally used in establishing a new test or scale, although it often requires many years to complete. The steps are as follows:

1. Selection of the item pool
2. Reducing the number of items
3. Choosing response options
4. Determining reproducibility
5. Determining validity
6. Determining responsiveness.

CHAPTER 44

Surgical Trials

INTRODUCTION

There has been a heated debate for many years as to the proper role of randomized and well-controlled trials in surgery. This chapter will not rehash each of the pros and cons of that debate, but will assume that it is both ethical and desirable to perform such surgical trials whenever possible. One argument supporting this view relates to the benefits for society. If a clinical trial involving 100 patients (50 in each of two treatment groups) can evaluate whether a questionable surgical procedure is of value, it is considered unethical to avoid this trial and subject large numbers of future patients to an operation that might be ineffective or even harmful. This assumes that all patients who enter the trial are fully informed and agree to participate. The other side to this debate claims that a number of patients may be unnecessarily subjected to sham surgery or a less than state-of-the-art surgery just to evaluate a point on which most surgeons may agree.

Surgical Operations that Disappeared after Controlled Surgical Trials

The history of surgery contains many examples of procedures that attained acceptance and were later shown to be without medical value. Many of those operations, which have been discarded in recent decades, were rejected on the basis of controlled clinical trials. Some of the stories about these events have been well documented and illustrate the great value that randomized trials may have in differentiating between useful and nonuseful surgeries. A classic example involved reputed benefits of the internal mammary artery ligation for improving the clinical status of patients with angina pectoris. This procedure became a national fad for a period during the 1950s. The true value of this particular surgery was not adequately assessed until two randomized controlled trials were performed, which included patients who underwent sham operations (Cobb et al., 1959; Dimond et al., 1960). This story is recounted well by Beecher (1961). One of the most salient points from the trial of Dimond et al. (1960) is that objective evidence of clinical improvement (improved T-wave changes in the electrocardiogram) was apparent in a patient who had received a sham operation. In addition, there were numerous reports of subjective improvement in the sham-operated groups. Other examples of accepted surgeries that were eventually rejected include: (1) prefrontal lobotomies for treating aggressive or schizophrenic patients, (2) laparotomy for tuberculous peritonitis or pelvic inflammatory disease, and (3) colectomies to cure epilepsy (Beecher, 1961). The extracranial/intracranial (EC/IC) bypass operation was also shown to have no advantage over medical treatment. This outcome caused a major furor in the surgical literature (Hawkins, 1987).

These few examples make one wonder if some surgical procedures used today are essentially no better than placebo, or may actually be detrimental to patients. By posing this question the author does not presuppose that any specific procedures are suspect. Nonetheless, surgeons with open critical minds should retain a healthy skepticism in their evaluation of currently used methods. The origins of some well-established surgical procedures may have been based originally on authoritative statements rather than on scientific evidence, even though many surgical procedures have been subsequently validated.

Case Series

Most surgeons previously believed that a retrospective analysis of a large series of patients who underwent a particular surgery would provide sufficient information to assess the value of that operation. Many surgical publications were of this type of retrospective review of a particular surgeon's (or group of surgeons') experience. The evidence has been overwhelming that even large series of sugical experiences often do not provide the correct interpretation of a particular operation's efficacy (Moses, 1984). There is a growing tendency away from this approach in surgery as a means of validating a particular operation.

DIFFERENCES BETWEEN SURGICAL AND MEDICAL TRIALS

Characteristics of Surgical versus Medical Treatment

In any particular comparison between a single surgical trial and a single medicine trial, the differences in protocol design and in patient outcome may be either minimal or substantial. There is no simple list of characteristics that may be used to evaluate or address all comparison studies. Nonetheless, many surgical trials

may be differentiated from most medicine trials by one or more characteristics. For instance, surgery usually consists of a one-time operation or procedure that is irreversible, although multiple surgeries are sometimes required as part of a single treatment or clinical trial. Medicines on the other hand, are usually taken multiple times to treat a problem.

Clinical Objectives of Surgery

Surgery itself has various objectives, which may be summarized in five categories:

1. To treat and cure an acute illness.
2. To treat and cure a chronic illness.
3. To treat a disease that is otherwise fatal and thus prolong life.
4. To palliate a slowly progressing disease.
5. To palliate a rapidly progressing disease.

Follow-Up

Some surgical trials measure parameters of improvement postsurgery prior to a patient's discharge and do not require follow-up visits. Nonetheless most major surgical trials include a follow-up period of evaluation after the patient has been discharged from the clinic or hospital. Obtaining adequate data during this period is often difficult and, depending on the length of follow-up, may be compromised by a patient's (1) lack of cooperation, (2) moving to a new location, (3) death, or (4) loss to follow-up for other reasons. Although the length of the follow-up period may be determined prior to the surgery, it is often unstated in the protocol (if a follow-up exists). The number of patient visits during this period is also usually left unstated in the protocol, as well as the specific parameters and tests to measure at each visit.

The majority of medicine trials have clearly defined endpoints that are measured, and most trials are completed at a certain point in time. After a trial is completed and medicine treatment is discontinued, patients are not continued in the same trial during a long-term follow-up period. In some surgical trials, however, patients are continued for an indefinite period (i.e., follow-up period) after the surgery has been completed. When patients are enrolled for a 1-year or even longer medicine trial, the number and schedule for all clinic visits (as well as the specific tests to be performed at each visit) are usually described in the protocol.

Endpoints

The term "endpoint" is often used differently in medical and surgical studies. In medical trials, an endpoint is usually a parameter that is measured to gauge the effect of the treatment or intervention. Endpoints are developed within certain categories of parameters (e.g., pharmacological, clinical, quality of life, physiological, biochemical) and a trial may include any number of endpoints. In surgical trials, an endpoint usually refers to either a certain time after the surgery or a certain clinical event that occurs (e.g., rehospitalization for the same problem, reoccurrence of the same problem, a new episode).

Risks

Many surgeries involve a greater risk than that associated with taking most medicines. Immediate risk is generally more apparent in surgical trials than in medicine trials. Risks include the potential for damage to nerves, muscles, and blood vessels during most surgeries (e.g., perforation, massive bleeding) as well as after the surgery is completed (e.g., bleeding, wound dehiscence). In addition, there are risks inherent in the use of both general and local anesthesia and risks of infection. Postsurgery, new diseases or problems may develop that are related or unrelated to the original problem that necessitated the surgery.

Technical Skill

Surgery also requires a greater degree of technical skill than is associated with providing most medicines to patients. Finally, surgical expertise for any specific operation requires special training, whereas special training is usually not necessary before a medicine trial is initiated. Surgical expertise varies greatly among surgeons and may be expected to influence the outcome of many surgical trials. Even for a single surgeon, his or her skills will be greater when performing certain operations. The technical skills of investigators in medicine trials are generally less critical to the outcome than are the technical skills of a surgeon. These distinctions are broad generalizations (see Table 44.1) and numerous exceptions exist.

TYPES OF SURGICAL TRIALS

Although it is logical to consider a surgical trial as a comparison of two surgical treatments, this chapter views surgical trials more broadly by identifying a number of comparisons that may be made under the general heading of surgical trials. It is certainly possible to limit consideration of surgical trials to one (or more) of the types of possible trials. These trials are listed in Table 44.2.

It is apparent from this list that the specific surgery conducted is paramount in some trials and not in others. Most of the considerations described in the following sections on surgical trial designs are concerned with those trials in which one type of surgery is being compared with another, or in which surgery is of major importance in the trial.

Randomized Controlled Surgical Trials

Types of surgical trials may also be described according to the trial designs used. The major controversy in this respect relates to the use of randomized controlled surgical trials. This topic has strong advocates and critics and the interested reader is referred to the literature, including the following articles by proponents of these trials: Spodick (1973), Gilbert et al. (1977a,b), Haines (1983), and Baum (1983); and by the opponents of this approach: Bonchek (1979), van der Linden (1980a,b), and Byer (1983). The article by Bonchek

---

TABLE 44.1 *Selected differences between development of new medicines, medical devices, and surgical operation*

Characteristics	Medicines	Medical devices	Surgical operations
Patient protection from risk[a]	Usually	Sometimes	Rarely
Source of innovation and development	Corporation	Corporation	Individual or group of professionals
Cost of development	Very high	Moderate	Low
Double-blind methods used to evaluate	Yes	Seldom	Almost never

[a] Often in the form of a detailed protocol reviewed by an Ethics Committee/IRB.

TABLE 44.2 *Types of trials involving surgical procedures*

1. Evaluation of medicines or anesthetic agents used during surgical procedures (e.g., neuromuscular blocking agents)
2. Evaluation of a disease treated either by surgery or medicines (e.g., angina, peptic ulcers)
3. Evaluation of a disease (e.g., cancer) treated either by surgery or nonmedicine modalities (e.g., hyperthermia, radiation)
4. Comparison of two (or more) surgical procedures (e.g., new versus old method, modified versus original method)
5. Evaluation of one surgical procedure (usually a novel technique) compared with historical controls
6. Comparison of a surgical procedure performed with and without medical (or other) adjunct therapy
7. Evaluation of equipment used in surgery (e.g., cauterizing machine, stereotaxic device) or medical devices (e.g., prosthetic heart valves), either used or implanted during surgical procedures
8. Evaluation of surgical materials (e.g., adhesives, suture materials, drapes, pins, staples) used during surgery

elicited a flurry of letters defending randomized surgical trials (Loh, 1979; Chalmers and Sacks, 1979; Fowler, 1979; Folland et al., 1979). Bonchek later expanded discussion of his position (Bonchek, 1982).

Gilbert et al. (1977a,b) reviewed the surgical literature and reported that about one-half of the surgical innovations evaluated with randomized trials demonstrated improvements, and that less well-controlled trials tend to yield more positive results than do well-controlled trials. Van der Linden (1980a,b) suggested that patients should be randomized to different surgeons who would perform the surgery they do best, rather than having the surgeon perform two different operations, one of which might be performed with less interest and possibly with less skill.

Use of Lasers in Surgery

The use of lasers in surgery has developed rapidly over the last 15 or so years. Lasers are commonly used in

ophthalmology, dermatology, plastic surgery, gastroenterology, gynecology, neurosurgery, otolaryngology, urology, and general surgery. A review by the Council on Scientific Affairs (1986) provides an overall introduction to this field.

DESIGNING SURGICAL TRIALS

This discussion primarily concentrates on those design aspects of surgical trials in which differences from medical trials are likely to exist. Various aspects of trial design particularly pertinent to surgical considerations are divided into a number of separate topics. These topics are listed below, and one is described in more detail (number 2):

1. Basic considerations (Table 44.3).
2. Identifying endpoints and parameters to measure (Table 44.4).
3. Preoperative considerations (Table 44.5).
4. Operative considerations (Table 44.6).
5. Postoperative considerations (Table 44.7).
6. Short-term outcomes (Table 44.8).
7. Long-term outcomes (Table 44.9).
8. Training and technique of personnel (Table 44.10).

TABLE 44.3 *Basic considerations in surgical trials*

1. Consider including a placebo or sham operation in the trial design
2. Determine the nature of the control group (e.g., historical control, placebo, standard surgery)
3. If a crossover design is contemplated (e.g., for a surgical procedure that is repeated, devices used in a repeated procedure, medical versus surgical trial in the same patient) evaluate whether patients will generally be willing to accept a second leg of treatment
4. Determine the magnitude of the difference between treatment groups needed to convince most surgeons to alter their clinical practice
5. Consider how tightly the protocol should be designed and how much flexibility is acceptable
6. Consider patient referral patterns and the treatment that referring physicians expect their patients to receive
7. Determine which parameters are to be used to establish the diagnosis and magnitude of the disease, condition, or problem
8. Consider whether multiple subsets of patients are to be included (e.g., cancer patients with different stages of one type of cancer)
9. Consider whether it is possible to have the patient evaluated independently, especially if the surgeon and patients will not be blinded to the trial treatment
10. Consider whether the patient's medical status may be monitored and controlled by a single internist at each trial site, who should remain blind to the patient's treatment
11. Monitor the surgeon's technique by a head surgeon or a quality control monitoring group
12. Incorporate a period of training into the trial as a "pilot trial"
13. If the objective of the trial is to evaluate a new method or type of surgery, determine whether the goal is to establish a high standard of performance which others may try to emulate, or to establish a standard that most surgeons can readily achieve and perform on a routine basis
14. Determine whether patients can be randomized to different surgeons who each perform the type of surgery they are most familiar with
15. Determine whether an algorithm may be useful in designing the trial[a]

[a] A comparison of surgical emergencies treated with and without an algorithm was published by Hopkins et al. (1980).

TABLE 44.4 *Suitable parameters used to evaluate surgical procedures*

A. During surgery
1. Technical ease or difficulty of surgery
2. Amount of practice required to "perfect" the surgical technique
3. Duration of surgery
4. Rate and nature of severe complications plus treatments given
5. Rate and nature of moderate and mild complications plus treatments given
6. Number and expertise of staff required to assist during surgery

B. After surgery
1. Morbidity and/or mortality rates
2. Improvement in physiological, pharmacological, biochemical, pathological, clinical, and/or other endpoints
3. Length of hospital stay
4. Total cost of hospitalization and total cost of the disease over an X-year (X-month) period
5. Quality of life at predetermined time points
6. Cosmetic appearance before and after surgery
7. Need for additional surgery or treatment
8. Amount of patient anxiety and stress prior to and after the surgery
9. Type and amount of medicines required to treat the patient's problem before and at specified times after surgery
10. Rate and nature of complications plus treatments required for these complications
11. Performance of patient on standardized tests (e.g., treadmill) before and after surgery
12. Clinical global impression rated by investigator
13. Clinical global impression rated by patient

TABLE 44.5 *Preoperative considerations in designing surgical trials*

1. Describe acceptable preoperative care (e.g., specific preoperative medicines, doses, time of administration relative to surgery)
2. Determine whether the procedures for obtaining informed consent should be standardized
3. Determine if a blind (single or double) is possible or necessary; if so, determine how it will be implemented and maintained
4. Determine whether contact between surgeons and patients should be limited or avoided in single-blind studies
5. Determine whether the surgeon's level of enthusiasm should be controlled or measured
6. Determine whether to measure each patient's anxiety and how this may be done
7. Determine whether to alter dosages of medicines patients may be taking
8. Determine type of bowel preparation (if relevant)
9. Specify patient's diet

Factors to Control

There is a great range in the definition of "standard surgical procedure" (DeCosse et al., 1980). Many of the details that make up the presurgical, surgical, and postsurgical procedures must be identified in a protocol to help ensure uniformity between surgical procedures and also to ensure uniformity of care given to different patients. An example of a presurgical issue that should be clarified in a protocol is bowel preparation. This may be done by mechanical means, elemental diet, antimicrobial agents, or any combination of these techniques. Another example relates to the number of lymph nodes biopsied during surgery. This number (or range) should be identified in the protocol and associated with the level or stage of the patient's disease. A typical postsurgery issue would involve identifying the technique of stimulating respiration (to prevent atelectasis) that is to be used, plus the frequency and other details of its use. Another issue involves whether prophylactic treatment to prevent deep vein venous thrombosis will be included as part of the trial, along with the details of this treatment.

TABLE 44.6 *Operative considerations in designing surgical trials*

1. Specify which anesthetic(s), neuromuscular blocking agent(s), and other medicines patients may receive during the operation
2. Specify types of dosing of neuromuscular blocking agents (e.g., by bolus or by constant infusion; specific doses or dose ranges may be identified
3. Specify instrumentation and equipment required to be present in the operating room; specific models and numbers required my be identified
4. Specify the calibration and use of the instrumentation and equipment
5. Specify relevant synthetic and biological materials to be used in the operation (e.g., suture materials)
6. Specify the pathological and/or X-ray or other examinations to be conducted during the operation

TABLE 44.7 *Postoperative considerations in designing protocols for surgical trials*

1. Describe both required and acceptable postoperative care and monitoring procedures in the recovery room
2. Describe both required and acceptable postoperative procedures and care after the patient leaves the recovery room (e.g., respiratory care, diet, activity)
3. For outpatient surgical procedures, indicate the time that patients must remain in the clinic or office prior to discharge
4. Provide instructions of how patients should behave at home and how they should handle and care for potential problems that may be anticipated; provide a telephone number for patients to use
5. Determine whether some or all patients will be placed in a special program postoperatively (e.g., occupational therapy)
6. Indicate how long a follow-up period is essential to include in the trial and how long a period is desirable

TABLE 44.8 *Potential factors to measure in assessing short-term outcomes after surgery[a]*

1. Amount of blood loss during surgery
2. Duration of surgery from the opening incision to closing the wound
3. Number of patient failures
4. Degree of improvement observed and measured
5. Rate of complications during and after surgery
6. Severity of complications during and after surgery
7. Rate of mortality and reasons for death
8. Number and severity of episodes of the medical problem requiring surgery
9. Improvement in laboratory parameters
10. Improvement in rehabilitation therapy (e.g., physical therapy, occupational therapy, other forms of therapy)

[a] The short term is defined as the period from initiation of surgery to the time of patient discharge from the hospital. Outcomes in high- and low-risk patients as well as in other groups of patients may be compared.

TABLE 44.9 *Potential factors to measure in assessing long-term outcomes after surgery[a]*

1. Length of follow-up
2. Number of patients lost to follow-up
3. Number of readmissions to hospital[b] and length of stay during subsequent admissions
4. Risk of mortality
5. Estimate of survival time
6. Covariates associated with long-term survival
7. Number and severity of episodes of the medical problem requiring surgery
8. Interval of time between episodes
9. Degree of improvement
10. Percent of patients improved by preset quantities or amounts
11. Improvement in laboratory parameters
12. Degree of functional disability
13. Improvement in rehabilitation therapy (e.g., physical therapy, occupational therapy, other forms of therapy)
14. Factors that place patients in either a high- or low-risk group
15. Total costs of health care for each treatment group

[a] The long term is defined as beginning at the time of patient discharge. The termination of this period will depend on the specific surgery. Each of the specific times at which measurements are to be made should be determined prior to the study (e.g., annual examinations).
[b] Only for reasons relating to the disease treated by the previous surgery.

TABLE 44.10 *Considerations of training and technique of personnel in designing surgical trials*

1. Specific qualifications may be indicated for surgeons who actually perform the surgery in a trial (e.g., residents, board-certified specialists)
2. Specify the required skills for the rest of the surgical team (e.g., anesthesiologists, pathologists, scrub team)
3. Specify the required training in the techniques to be evaluated (e.g., each surgeon to have conducted a minimum of X operations with an operative mortality of less than Y%, training for Z months, skills approved by the head surgical monitor)
4. Specify whether a single surgeon must perform all operations or whether a group of surgeons may operate and have their results combined
5. Determine whether a single anesthesiologist or group of anesthesiologists will assist during the operation
6. Determine whether to measure the skills of the surgeon for each type of surgery included in the trial
7. Determine whether the surgeon uses conventional dissection or "no-touch" dissection techniques
8. Determine whether a surgeon's preference for one of the test surgeries is a basis for assigning that type of surgery to the surgeon or for replacing him or her with another surgeon

Identifying Endpoints and Parameters to Measure

All surgical patients may be followed for a specified time (e.g., 10 weeks or 10 years) after surgery. When this duration is relatively long (e.g., 10 years), most published data include all patients who have been followed for at least a minimum period of time, although the durations for the individual patients will vary. If the follow-up period is relatively short (e.g., 10 weeks), then publications usually include patients who have all been evaluated for approximately the same period.

Another type of endpoint that is sometimes established in trials relates to (1) the occurrence or reoccurrence of certain adverse reactions, (2) rehospitalization, (3) exacerbation of problems related to the patient's disease, (4) death, or (5) other clinical occurrences. Any of these endpoints may be used to mark the termination of a patient's participation in a trial. If the surgery is primarily (or even secondarily) concerned with cosmetic appearance of the patient, then photographic depiction of the before and after appearance may be used to derive cosmetic endpoints. Photographs of control patients who were selected before their surgery was performed should be included for comparison purposes. Cosmetic endpoints such as 1+ to 4+ may be defined and independent surgeons kept blind to the patients' treatment should be used to rate all photographs.

In addition to these endpoints it is important to identify the parameters (e.g., mortality, postoperative sepsis) that are to be included in a trial to evaluate and compare treatments. A number of parameters that are more suitable for surgical, as opposed to medical, evaluation are included in Table 44.4.

Control Populations

The concept of a control population is alien to some surgeons who are used to evaluating new therapies without recourse to controls. It is clear, however, that more and more surgeons understand and accept the necessity of including control populations in surgical trials. There are also more surgeons who recognize the benefits that control populations offer in the field of surgery. This change in attitude is possibly related to recent changes in the training of surgeons. Training of surgeons is considered in Table 44.10.

Control populations may include a (1) no-treatment group (for open trials), (2) sham-operated group (see section below on placebos and sham operations), (3) standard accepted surgery, or (4) unmodified form of surgery. Murray (1986) has advocated the use of large banks of observational data to serve as a control population for comparing results of new surgical techniques. He describes a large international data bank that exists for severe head injury. This recommendation has value for some areas of surgery, but would not be suitable for all areas and can never provide data as strong as those from randomized controlled trials. Other forms of control are to identify two groups of patients in the trial whose results will be compared, although this type of comparison is usually weak in the degree of control it offers. This approach is similar to a subgroup analysis addressing questions such as: (1) Do men and women react similarly to the operation? (2) Is the operation equally effective in children as in adults? (3) Do patients with severe cardiovascular compromise tolerate the operation as well as patients with a normal cardiovascular system?

CHANGING STANDARDS IN SURGERY

Certain surgical techniques change over a period of time. For most newer techniques the rate of operative mortality and morbidity decreases because surgeons' experience with the technique increases. Thus, it is impossible to compare rates of operative mortality or morbidity for a new operation with rates obtained 10 years later. There is another factor that confounds the evaluation of a type of surgery at two or more time points. As operative mortality and morbidity decrease and as more surgeons become experienced in the methods, sicker patients are usually operated on and this tends to increase the overall rates of complications (i.e., mortality and morbidity).

PLACEBO EFFECTS AND SHAM OPERATIONS

There *is* a beneficial result from surgery that may be attributed to a placebo effect and to sham operations.

The evidence supporting this statement is strong, and some of it will be summarized below.

Use of Sham Operations Today

The ethics of conducting a sham operation have radically changed since the trials of Cobb et al. (1959) and Dimond et al. (1960) in the late 1950s. This is correct and patients are not given sham operations. Nonetheless, from society's viewpoint, would it not still be ethical to conduct sham operations if patients were fully informed of that possibility and gave their informed consent? They would serve to evaluate the value of a questionable surgery. If it was rejected, then mortality and morbidity would be decreased for many future patients who might otherwise have received the surgery. If the surgery was preferable to the alternative treatment, then more patients could be offered the better treatment. The author therefore strongly favors the use of sham surgeries to evaluate questionable surgeries, providing all patients receive a full informed consent, and also are tested for their comprehension of it. An additional ethical safeguard is the protocol review by the Ethics Committee/Institutional Review Board (IRB).

Dimond et al. (1960) and Cobb et al. (1959) used sham operations in double-blind trials and demonstrated that the sham procedures had positive subjective and objective effects on anginal symptoms. Ruffin et al. (1969) used a sham freeze in the double-blind evaluation of gastric freezing for treatment of duodenal ulcers. No difference in patient response to the sham and real freeze was observed. Other references are given in Chapter 85.

Placebo Effect in Surgery

In sham operations everything is done to the patient except perform the essential part of the operation. For example, in the internal mammary artery ligation trials of Dimond et al. (1960) and Cobb et al. (1959) the patient's chest was opened and a ligature placed around the artery, but it was not ligated as it was in the true operation.

A placebo effect has been widely attributed to surgical intervention and is partly responsible for both objective and subjective improvement observed after surgical treatment. Beecher (1961) estimated that the magnitude of the placebo response in surgery was the same (about 35%) as that observed in medical trials. The placebo effect was also enhanced by the enthusiasm of the surgeon. One way in which this occurs is when the surgeon alleviates or decreases the amount of anxiety a patient feels and encourages the patient to be optimistic about the outcome. This form of bias

may easily enter the trial and should be controlled and possibly evaluated (if a question of the bias arises) through patient interviews or questionnaires.

MANAGEMENT OF SURGICAL TRIALS

The management of well-designed surgical trials is similar to the management of well-designed medical trials. A few points of particular importance to surgical trials involve monitoring procedures. Monitoring may be performed by a designated surgeon who supervises, evaluates, or otherwise oversees surgical activities at one (or multiple) trial site(s), or by a team of surgeons or nonsurgeons who review and oversee the quality and consistency of the surgical trial.

It is extremely important for surgery to be conducted by surgeons who are patient oriented rather than surgically oriented. Surgeons chosen for trials should be well-trained physicians who are both experienced and interested in pre- and postoperative care. If the surgeons chosen, however, are less interested in pre- and postoperative care than performing the surgery it may be relevant to appoint a specialist in internal medicine to manage (or monitor) patient care. The potential advantages of this approach are several. First, it ensures a greater degree of consistency if a single nonsurgeon (or small number of nonsurgeons) takes care of all patients in a trial. Second, routine postoperative clinical care is usually allied with internal medicine. Third, this approach will tend to minimize or eliminate any influence of investigator enthusiasm on results, especially if the internal medicine physicians are blind to patient treatment. On the other hand, the internist's role should be limited because he or she usually lacks a great deal of detailed physiological understanding of the surgical procedure and the insight that accrues with having done the surgery.

Costs of a Surgical Trial

A special aspect of surgical trials that is indirectly associated with management are the costs of a trial. This is often an important factor in determining whether a particular surgical procedure becomes widely used, especially when alternative medical treatments are possible. Costs of a treatment include more than determining the total hospital bill for patients in two or more treatment groups. Costs do not merely refer to the cost or charge of performing the surgery, but to a determination and comparison of the overall costs of the comparison treatments. This often becomes an important factor that relates to how well new surgical techniques are accepted.

There are many types of costs associated with treatment and several are highly complex and subjective.

Costs relate to direct medical costs, indirect costs, and nontangible costs. These are discussed more fully in Chapters 42 and 130. Costs of treatment include the time in lost productivity resulting from the disease or condition and how this time is affected by each of the treatments evaluated. It is clear that a more expensive surgical treatment may be cost effective if patients are able to return to productive work sooner than patients who undergo a less expensive operation.

It is often impotant for costs of several types to be monitored in a trial, especially if the trial is evaluating a novel surgical technique. If costs are compared between two surgeries it should generally be on the basis of "per successful operation." This term must be carefully defined in terms of survival plus a specific quality of life for a specific period of time. Therefore, all patients who are operated on and die or who have an unsuccessful outcome in terms of established criteria are counted in with the costs of that surgery. This prevents an apparently inexpensive surgery with a poorer outcome from seeming to be much more cost effective.

METHODOLOGIES USED IN SURGICAL TRIALS

Control Groups

Some of the considerations for reporting surgical results are listed in Table 44.11. Except in some unusual situations, most surgical trials do not involve placebo control groups. An active control may be readily incorporated into most evaluations of new surgical techniques or procedures, but even this practice is not as widespread as it could be. The active control included in a trial is usually the standard surgical procedure, performed under conditions as identical as possible to the investigational surgical technique. Use of an active control has several advantages in an investigational trial, especially when patients are randomly assigned to receive either the new or standard technique.

Stepwise Development of New Surgeries

Many new surgical procedures do not develop *de novo*, but rather evolve slowly through a series of small steps

TABLE 44.11 *Reporting results of surgical trials[a]*

1. Report number of surgeries performed by each surgeon
2. If possible, describe the results obtained by each surgeon
3. Report the nature, number, and time of all specimens obtained during surgery and the pathologist's report
4. Describe monitoring systems used and the results of the monitoring

[a] Relevant factors listed in other tables in this chapter should be reported in a publication or report and will not be repeated in this table.

from established procedures. It is often neither practical nor necessary for a surgeon to approach an Ethics Committee/IRB for permission to perform a slight modification of a standard technique. In most situations the surgeon modifies an existing technique on his or her own initiative. Some surgical procedures are performed in many different ways. When a further modification is later considered and evaluated, the surgeon again might not approach the Ethics Committee/IRB. Eventually, a totally new procedure may have evolved and the surgeon will publish the results, using historical data from his or her prior experience as a control, or through reference to published literature for control data.

Ethics Committees/IRB Review

It is not firmly established which modifications of surgical procedures require Ethics Committee/IRB approval. A possible guideline is that any modification that places patients at an increased risk during or after surgery should be submitted to an Ethics Committee/IRB. At a certain point in developing minor modifications of a known method the surgeon should formally initiate a controlled trial that will not depend upon historical data to evaluate the surgery. It is understood that this suggestion is not always realistic or possible.

Types of Randomization and Blinding of Surgical Trials

One alternative to a completely randomized approach is to assign different surgeries to the surgeons who perform them best and to randomize patients to different groups and therefore different surgeons. Another alternative is to alternate patient assignment or to assign every third or fourth patient to the standard surgical procedure group. Surgery would be performed by surgeon(s) A. An independent surgeon (surgeon B) who is blind to patient randomization could be used to evaluate patients. If the two surgeries could not be blinded for an independent surgeon, then the independent surgeon (or surgeon A) could evaluate patients and code or describe surgery results on preprinted forms. These forms could then be evaluated by yet a different surgeon (surgeon C) who was blind to patient treatment.

Randomization of patients to one of two treatments (e.g., surgery or medicine) may not achieve the balanced groups desired (Fig. 44.1). This could occur if the population to be evaluated for a trial was composed predominantly of patients who could be treated with one modality, or if, because of inclusion criteria, patients from one group were selected out (Fig. 44.2). This situation could potentially lead to distortion in the

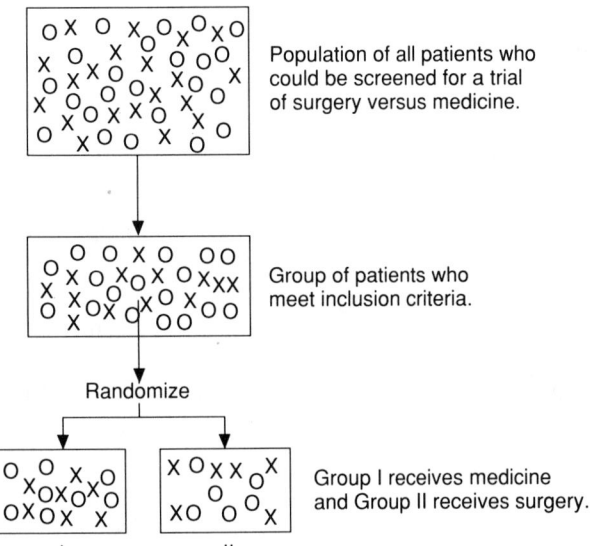

FIG. 44.1 Comparison of two groups of patients randomized to receive medicine or surgery in a comparative trial; equal randomization throughout the screening and randomization is illustrated. The two symbols represent patients who would otherwise receive surgery (X) or medicine (O), if they were not entered in the trial.

results and in the ability to extrapolate them to the larger population.

Use of Historical Controls

In some surgical procedures it is generally acceptable to compare new results with historical controls. For example, when there is a significant and consistent improvement in survival compared with well-documented historical controls or a significant and consistent decrease in surgical or disease complications, then one may use historical controls. Nonetheless, one must be wary of this approach because the rates of mortality and morbidity resulting from surgery, or even the natural history of a disease, often change over the years and apparently valid historical data will turn out to be invalid.

EVALUATION OF MEDICINES DURING SURGERY

A common type of medicine trial performed during surgery relates to prophylaxis against infection. Patients are treated with either a trial medicine, active control, or placebo at a defined time during the surgical procedure, and the occurrence of infection (defined by precise criteria) is measured and evaluated during a subsequent period. Patients may be randomly allocated to treatment groups, there may be double-blinding of the trial with a "double-placebo" technique, and the trial may be conducted at a standard as high as any double-blind medical evaluation.

Other medicines evaluated during surgery (e.g., anesthetic agents, neuromuscular blocking medicines, vasopressors) should also be evaluated in a rigorous and well-controlled manner. Methods for their study are described elsewhere in this book.

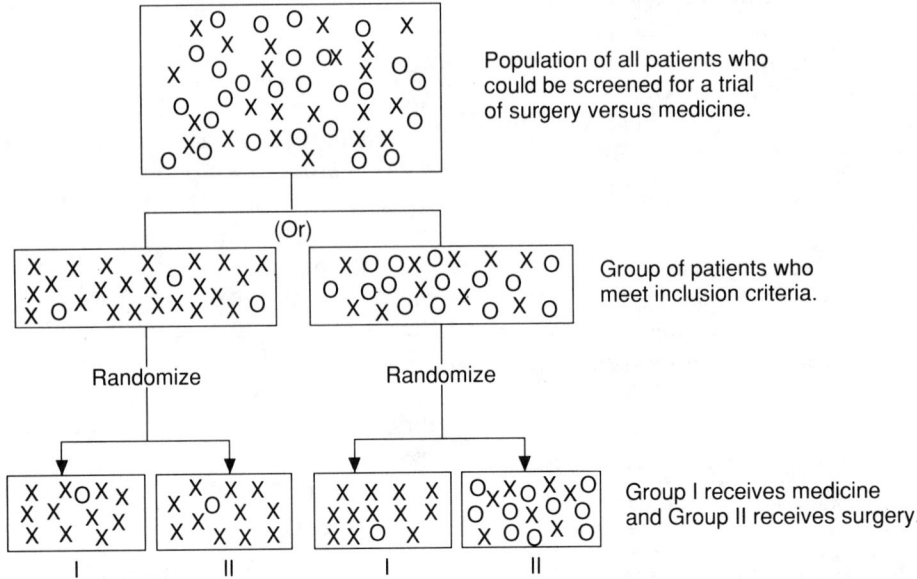

FIG. 44.2 Comparison of two groups of patients randomized to receive medicine or surgery in a comparative trial; a skewed distribution based on patients who meet inclusion criteria (left side of figure) or based on chance randomization (right side of figure) is illustrated. Inequality of patients could also emanate from an imbalance in the original population (not shown). For key to symbols, see Fig. 44.1 legend.

CHAPTER 45

Clinical Trials to Evaluate Medical Devices

With the passage of the Medical Device Amendments in the United States in 1976, the field of medical devices entered a new era. These amendments were incorporated in the Federal Food, Drug, and Cosmetic Act and require materials used in medical devices, as well as the devices themselves, to undergo comprehensive testing. The regulations were intended to raise the standards of introducing new medical devices on the market and to better ensure the safety of the American public. The statutes pertaining to medical devices are found mainly in Sections 501 to 521 of the Act.

TYPES OF DEVICES

Definitions and Examples of Classes I, II, and III Medical Devices

Medical devices have been divided into three classes, which are defined in section 860.3 of the Code of Federal Regulations.

Class I devices are the least hazardous and are subject to the "general controls" that had been used to regulate devices prior to the Medical Device Amendments. These controls include rules concerning good manufacturing practices, labeling, purity, banned devices, recalls, records kept, and reports. Devices are in Class I if they are not intended to support or sustain human life or prevent impairment to human health and do not present a potentially unreasonable risk of illness or injury. Class I devices make up about 29% of all types of devices and include elastic bandages, surgeon's gloves, manual surgical instruments, nasopharyngeal catheters, enriched culture media, and tongue depressors.

Class II devices are subject to specific performance standards, which the Food and Drug Administration (FDA) has developed or will develop. Many of these have not yet been written. General controls alone are deemed insufficient to provide reasonable assurance of their safety and effectiveness. Class II devices (63% of the total) have some risk associated with them. Examples include flexible laryngoscopes, surgical drills, stomach pH electrodes, arthroscopies, chin prostheses, and electrocardiogram machines.

Class III devices are subject to premarket approval. A device is in Class III if its safety and effectiveness cannot be ensured by performance standards. All devices that (1) are life supporting (or sustaining), (2) are for a use that is of substantial importance in preventing impairment of health, or (3) have a potential for causing risk of injury or illness are in Class III. New devices are automatically placed in Class III until the manufacturer or importer successfully petitions the FDA to reclassify them. Class III devices (8% of the total) require premarket approval from the FDA before they may be marketed. These devices include many orthopedic implants, artificial organs, intrauterine devices, tracheal prostheses, and herpes simplex serological reagents.

Classifications Based on Use

Although medical devices have been divided into three classes based on the degree of risk, there are also other means of classifying devices. A general four-category classification may be used relating to their use:

Type I—Internal devices. These devices are introduced into, or penetrate, the body for a month or less (e.g., cannulas, needles, i.v. catheters, drainage tubes); or for more than a month (e.g., heart valves, orthopedic prostheses, surgical clips).

Type II—Topical devices. These devices may be subdivided, depending on whether they come in direct contact with skin (e.g., surgical dressings, tapes, cast materials) or mucous membranes (e.g., catheters placed in the urethra, tubes placed into the trachea).

Type III—Indirect devices. These devices come in contact with drugs, fluids, or other substances that enter the body (e.g., oxygenators, hemodialysis machines, syringes, transfusion apparatus).

Type IV—Noncontact devices. These devices do not come in contact with the body or with substances that enter the body, but do come in contact with devices that contact the body (e.g., instrument trays, operating-room table covers), or materials from the body (e.g., dipsticks for testing urine).

Another classification of many medical devices could be made, depending on whether the device is intended for one-time use or limited number of uses, or is indefinitely reusable. Another aspect of this classification would be whether the device were intended for only a single patient's use, or for use in multiple patients.

Combination Products: Devices and Medicines

Although most medical devices are clearly devices and not medicines, there are some that have both characteristics and may be considered as a combination product. For example, a wound dressing or bandage that is placed on the skin is a medical device, but if it is impregnated with an antibacterial agent, growth factor, or other bioactive chemical, it could be considered as a combination product. This type of product is not necessarily difficult to study and evaluate, but identifying the regulations that apply to its approval could pose numerous complex issues that may not be easily resolved with a regulatory authority.

A sponsor developing this type of product should generally try to persuade regulatory authorities that the item should be considered a device. A recently marketed solution for organ preservation, Via Span (DuPont), was classified by the FDA as a device despite the fact that it contains several medicines or excipients, including allopurinol, adenosine, glutathione, and sodium hydroxide. Moreover, the recommended preparation of this product includes adding insulin, penicillin, and dexamethasone prior to its use.

A different type of combination occurs when a clearly identified medical device requires use of a concomitant medicine (e.g., kidney stone smasher plus dye).

DESIGNING PROTOCOLS

Types of Investigators and Trials

When designing protocols for studying a medical device it is usually relevant to consider who the intended user will be. If the device will be used by nurses and nonphysician therapists, it is important to include them in evaluations, as well as including relevant medical specialists. The investigator(s) must be provided with preclinical data as well as clear written instructions (and oftentimes training) in the device's use, in addition to warnings, hazards, and other information. Although clinical trials may be scientifically or marketing oriented, as with medicine trials, there is probably a higher percentage of medical device trials than medicine trials that are marketing oriented. This probably results from the fact that regulatory requirements are generally much less stringent for medical devices.

Stages of Testing

The two major stages of testing involve (1) an initial pilot stage in which the device's design and materials are being developed and tested and (2) a multicenter stage in which the safety and efficacy of the final product is evaluated. The former stage is analogous to early Phase II trials in evaluations of new medicines, and the latter stage is analogous to Phase III trials. Adequate testing must be conducted with the final medical device, regardless of the amount of testing with the pilot product. Most controlled studies use a parallel trial design. Crossover designs may be considered for a small number of medical devices (e.g., comparison of filters used in a dialysis machine).

Choosing Parameters: Number and Type

Although there is temptation to evaluate every parameter of interest and to obtain all or most of the answers to development questions in a single trial, this is not usually possible. When designing clinical trials it is important not to try to make any trial all-encompassing, which may hinder the process of development. An overly ambitious trial that tries to answer too many questions can create problems, which can only be resolved by further trials.

Control Groups

The literature on the clinical evaluation of medical devices is much smaller than that for most medicines. The quality of reported clinical trials varies enormously, and most trials suffer from lack of a control patient group that received a comparison medical device. Studies commonly describe a group of patients who received a device and who present before and after values for certain tests and parameters. There is usually no adequate control. One reason for this failure may be that the sponsor of most of these trials (i.e., device manufacturers) often do not wish to compare their device directly against a competitor's. In addition, it is rarely ethical to include a placebo or sham-operated group as a control. Placebo controls are often not necessary or possible in testing certain medical devices. Many situations in which Class II and III devices are used are not suitable for observation of a placebo effect (e.g., the patient may be unconscious, the interaction between patient and device may be minimal or nonexistent). There are several types of comparisons that may be used to evaluate medical devices (Table 45.1), and there are special considerations for designing protocols (Table 45.2) that illustrate differences between medical devices and medicines.

The need of many patients for a Class III medical device is often certain (e.g., heart valve replacement, hip replacement). In such cases it is generally unethical to consider including a placebo treatment group in a clinical trial. Therefore, clinical trials depend heavily on the patient's baseline values to evaluate the effects of the device. When open-label trials are conducted and no blinding is used, greater reliance should be placed on objective measures of change (e.g., ejection fraction) or semiobjective measures (e.g., distance the patient can walk without pain in a given period). Subjective parameters (e.g., quality of life measures) are usually more susceptible to influence by a placebo ef-

TABLE 45.1 *Types of comparisons that may be made in trials of medical devices*

1. Device A versus device B—usually performed single-blind
2. Device A versus medicine B—usually performed single-blind
3. Device A versus surgery B
4. Device A versus no treatment
5. Device A versus placebo device—preferably performed double-blind
6. Device A versus other treatment modality (e.g., radiation)

TABLE 45.2 *Special considerations in designing protocols for medical devices[a]*

1. In a double-blind trial it may be necessary to blind the identity of the device used; this may be done by disguising its outside appearance or by having the device inserted by one physician and having the patient evaluated by another physician
2. Describe all increased risks that patients may experience in the trial; indicate how these risks will be minimized
3. Label all devices appropriately, including the phrase "CAUTION: INVESTIGATIONAL DEVICE LIMITED BY FEDERAL LAW TO INVESTIGATIONAL USE"
4. Indicate appropriate methods of disposition of both used and unused devices
5. Describe all functional tests of range of motion, correction of deformity, relief of symptoms, and other criteria of improvement
6. Provide written instructions for use of the device, plus warnings, hazards, and contraindications[b]

[a] These points are in addition to relevant considerations for designing protocols for medicine trials.
[b] Evaluate the clarity of the instructions and their comprehension by potential users.

fect than are objective measures. Use of subjective measures should therefore be deemphasized whenever possible, unless they are validated parameters or there is no other choice. When one product is compared with another the parameters evaluated must be comparable.

Double-Blind Trials

There are a number of techniques whereby two or more medical devices may be effectively tested and compared in a double-blind manner. One process is to have two (or more) surgeons each implant or insert different devices and to have an independent surgeon (who is kept blind) review all patients. Each surgeon may implant only one type of device, or may be permitted to implant all of the devices being compared. In the latter situation, devices should be implanted in a random order. Since many surgeons will have preferences as to the devices they use and also will be more experienced in implanting certain devices, they will generally prefer being assigned to only one type of device. Since differences in surgical skill rather than the device implanted may influence patient outcome, it is preferable to have several (or many) different surgeons each implant one specific device and a different group of surgeons each implant the other device studied. Alternatively, all surgeons may be trained in the device's use so that they each achieve a minimum standard of technical competence. A third possibility is to measure and grade the skills of each surgeon and to consider this in the evaluation of the results.

If multiple hospitals are involved in a trial of a medical device, it is often necessary to control for differences in hospital care. This may be done by having at least one surgeon at each hospital assigned to insert device number 1 and a different surgeon or group of surgeons at each hospital chosen to insert device number 2. It is also important to ensure that all patients meet standard criteria to enter the trial, to eliminate the possibility that surgeons at one hospital select patients differently than surgeons at another hospital.

Other Tests

In addition to the clinical testing of the device in humans, it is necessary to conduct many other types of tests. These include clinical trials of shelf life (i.e., stability) and biocompatability. This latter term relates to the trials that demonstrate no untoward effects when the device remains in contact with skin, blood, mucous membranes, or other parts of the body for a prolonged period. Sterility tests must often be performed for medical devices. Various toxicity studies must be conducted on the separate materials (Northup, 1989).

Adverse Reactions

When commonly expected types of complications from a medical device are known, the data collection form may list these for the investigator to check off. Although this practice is not as common in clinical trials evaluating medicines, there are a number of advantages and justifications for its use in tallying "adverse reactions" due to medical devices. For example, the number of likely adverse reactions resulting from medical devices are usually fewer than for medicines and may be more precisely described.

Federal regulations in the United States require manufacturers and importers of medical devices to report device-related serious injuries and deaths to the FDA. Physicians and other health professionals are encouraged to report their experiences to the manufacturer, directly to the FDA Product Monitoring Branch, or indirectly to the FDA via the Problem Reporting Program administered by the United States Pharmacopeia. A newsletter of world medical device news (*Clinica*) is published by George Street Publications in Surrey, United Kingdom.

DIFFERENCES BETWEEN DEVELOPING DEVICES AND MEDICINES

Medical devices are a much more heterogeneous group of products than medicines in terms of their design, use, and purpose. Many devices never come in direct contact with patients, some have only brief direct contact, others attach to the skin or are inserted in the body for varying periods and then removed, and some become a permanent part of the patient. Each type of medical device has to be preclinically tested prior to

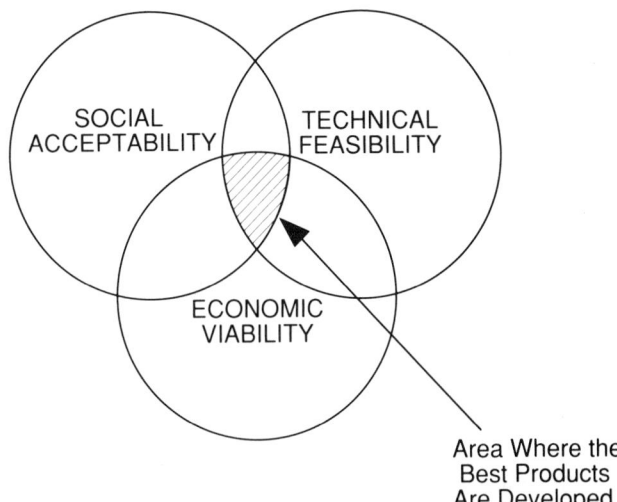

FIG. 45.1 Barriers to introduction of new medical devices. The greatest barriers exist in the areas outside the three circles.

its use. Implants, prostheses, and other devices must pass preclinical tests to confirm that they function electronically and mechanically in a reliable manner before they can be used in patients. Many of these devices must be sterilized after such tests are complete.

Some of the factors that must be considered in introducing new innovative medical devices are schematically shown in Fig. 45.1, and comparison of clinical trials, surgical trials, and device trials in Table 44.1.

Device Companies and Pharmaceutical Companies

The companies that develop and market most medical devices include a greater proportion of small companies than those that develop new medicines. Device companies generally have extremely small regulatory affairs departments and have relatively large marketing and research and development groups.

A major difference between medical device companies and medicine companies is that the goals of the device companies are more closely associated with specific needs of their customers. Device companies determine the specific needs of the users and often work closely with clients to develop prototypes of new products. Medicine companies are more dependent on inherent attributes of the medicines they discover or license to determine which specific indications to pursue.

EDUCATION OF INVESTIGATORS

Most investigators in trials testing new medical devices have to be educated about the correct use of the device. This is often a major issue and there is a period of learning necessary before the device can be used properly and efficiently. Therefore, it is necessary either to provide education and/or training prior to initiating the protocol or else to conduct the protocol in two stages. Data from the first part (pilot or training part of the protocol) would not be used to evaluate the device. Data from the second part of the trial would be of major importance. Objective criteria should be established to determine when the investigator is allowed to proceed from the first to the second part.

These considerations do not usually occur in medicine trials, especially when medicines are given orally. Investigators or their staff may have to be taught how to operate certain equipment used to measure parameters of safety or efficacy, how to assay for medicine levels in biological fluids, or how to perform other aspects of a trial unrelated to medicine administration. In unusual situations, technique may also be important in medicine delivery (e.g., placing radiocontrast dyes to perform myelograms, inserting depots of medicines, placing tubing from infusion pumps into intrathecal spaces, performing epidural or other types of anesthesia).

Modifying Devices and Developing a Final Product

Many device manufacturers do not create a final version of a medical device *de novo*, but proceed through a series of modifications. Many devices are continually being modified during their development and each clinical trial may actually test a somewhat different device. After a device is finalized it must be evaluated in a new and separate trial. It is not acceptable to state, in an application for marketing approval of a device, that each part was tested separately in different trials so that the entire device does not have to be studied in a new trial. It is possible that the whole may differ from the sum of its parts. This principle holds for Classes I and II medical devices, as well as for Class III devices.

When problems occur with devices, the company may involve many different groups to help resolve the issue, just as with medicine development (e.g., consultants, investigators). But device companies also involve design and other engineers to resolve many issues, whereas these people are rarely involved in a comparable role in developing a new medicine. Engineers are involved, however, in the manufacturing aspects of both medicines and devices.

Although medicines are provided without charge in almost all medicine studies, companies sometimes sell new devices to physician/investigators who will then use them (e.g., implanting them in their patients) in a clinical trial. This is one reason why investigators often want to make changes in the design or use of a device. This may or may not be desirable from the company's perspective, but many investigators are chosen because of their reputations as leaders and opinion setters in a specific field. The investigator may have his or her own way of testing the device and in such situations exerts greater control on the design and conduct of the trial than does the sponsor of the trial. This approach used to be more prevalent in the past in the pharmaceutical industry than it is at present. See Chapter 62 for a discussion of old-fashioned and modern approaches to monitoring, which describes an analogous situation.

CHAPTER 46

Evaluating Orphan Medicines for Treatment of Rare Diseases

There are estimated to be 4,000 rare diseases (or conditions), many of which are not presently treatable with effective medicines. Although the term *orphan medicine* is generally used to describe a medicine used to treat rare diseases, a close look at orphan medicines reveals a wider variety. To illustrate this point, three classifications of orphan medicines are described below. From the perspective of the pharmaceutical industry, orphan medicines represent a heterogeneous group of medicines that differ from each other in various ways: (1) patent status, (2) whether they are investigational medicines or are already marketed, (3) whether they are used only to treat rare diseases or both rare and common diseases, (4) degree of clinical usefulness, (5) availability to physicians, (6) cost to develop, and (7) commercial potential. It is therefore difficult to generalize about orphan medicines because each has its own set of characteristics and problems. Most orphan medicines also differ from nonorphan medicines in several ways (Table 46.1).

The decision to develop an orphan medicine is usu-

ally based on a combination of complex factors. Information about many or most of these factors is incomplete at the time the decision must be made to develop (or not to develop) an orphan medicine. More

TABLE 46.1 *Comparison between characteristics of orphan and nonorphan medicines*

Orphan medicine	Nonorphan medicine
1. Used in a limited patient population	1. Used in a large patient population
2. Often used only by a few specialists	2. Generally used by a wide variety or number of physicians
3. Often loses money for the manufacturer	3. Is more likely to make money for the manufacturer
4. May require fewer patient exposures to obtain approval for marketing	4. Usually requires a "standard"[a] quantity of data prior to approval

[a] The definition of the term "standard" depends on the identity and nature of the disease targeted, the nature of the medicine, the specific regulatory authority involved, and numerous other factors.

than 25 pharmaceutical companies in the United States are presently developing new orphan medicines. There are many incentives and disincentives for their development, and these are described later in this chapter.

CLASSIFICATIONS OF ORPHAN MEDICINES

Classification 1: Four Categories Based on Market Status

The first classification, consisting of four categories, is the easiest and most practical approach to use when describing orphan medicines.

1. Marketed medicines on or off patent used *only* to treat a rare disease.
2. Marketed medicines on or off patent used to treat *both* rare and common diseases.
3. Investigational medicines being actively evaluated in humans for treating a rare disease.
4. Investigational medicines that are available from a company for treatment of a rare disease, but that are not being actively developed for a New Drug Application (NDA) or a Product License Application (PLA).

Classification 2: Five Categories Based on Economic Status

A different classification of orphan medicines was proposed by Spilker (1990b), based on economic status (Table 46.2). This classification, as well as the one described below, is not meant as a refinement of the first, but as an alternative means of conceptualizing the various types of orphan medicines.

Classification 3: Eighteen Detailed Categories

A third, more detailed, classification of orphan medicines consists of eighteen separate categories (Spilker,

1985). It illustrates the heterogeneity of orphan medicines, and is based on market, economic, and patent status.

Complicating Factors

The above-mentioned classifications are complicated by many factors, a few of which are listed below:

1. There are various nonofficial definitions of an orphan medicine as well as definitions in federal laws and regulations; furthermore, the interpretations of these definitions may also change with time.
2. Most medicines and compounds that may be placed in a particular category will not always remain in the same category. Research ideas are often translated into investigational compounds, and eventually some investigational medicines are marketed while on patent and finally go off patent. Another example is when a medicine that was originally marketed for a rare disease is later found to be useful in the treatment of a more prevalent disease, or vice versa.
3. An investigational formulation of a medicine (e.g., intravenous) may be found to be useful for a rare disease, whereas the marketed formulation (e.g., topical or oral) may not be as useful or as effective for the rare disease.
4. The classification of orphan medicines described refers to prescription medicines. There may be a number of over-the-counter (i.e., nonprescription) medicines that are useful for some or all of the symptoms associated with certain rare diseases. A different set of considerations exists for these medicines, which are not discussed in this chapter.
5. A disease originally classified as rare may become more prevalent and no longer qualify as a rare disease [e.g., acquired immunodeficiency syndrome (AIDS)].
6. A variety of nontraditional orphan medicines and populations exist (Spilker, 1990b), including med-

TABLE 46.2 *Classification of orphan medicines by economic factors*

Type	Description	No. of patients in the US (prevalence)	Anticipated profits for a new medicine	Presence and adequacy of available treatment
I	Therapeutic orphans with little or no commercial potential	<200,000	Poor to marginal	None or highly inadequate
II	Therapeutic orphans with commercial potential	<200,000	Good to excellent	None or highly inadequate
III	Orphan medicine for a rare disease that can currently be treated	<200,000	Variable	Acceptable to excellent[a]
IV	Unprofitable medicine for a common disease	>200,000	Poor to marginal	None or highly inadequate
V	Orphan medicine used for both a rare and common disease	Both > and <200,000	Variable[b]	Variable

Modified from Spilker (1990b), with permission of Pergamon Press.
[a] In most patients.
[b] Each use of the medicine, as well as total profits, would be variable.

icines killed by publicity (e.g., Bendectin), "medicines that wouldn't die" [a term coined by Weintraub and Northington (1986) for unprofitable medicines removed from the market, but reintroduced as a result of pressure from professionals and orphan populations (e.g., children, pregnant women)], and vaccines.

INCENTIVES AND DISINCENTIVES FOR CORPORATIONS TO DEVELOP ORPHAN MEDICINES

There were incentives for pharmaceutical corporations to develop orphan medicines long before the Orphan Drug Act was signed into law in the United States in 1983. This act significantly improved some of those incentives and provided new ones as well. In addition to the incentives that will be described below, there are a number of disincentives, most of which were not addressed by the Orphan Drug Act. The major incentives and disincentives are described from the perspective of a pharmaceutical corporation in the United States. Congress is often exploring changes to the Orphan Drug Act, many of which would markedly change the incentives or disincentives described.

Incentives for Development of Orphan Medicines

1. In the United States, the term "rare disease or condition" includes but is not limited to, diseases or conditions affecting up to 200,000 patients (i.e., prevalence). This is an eminently fair and reasonable definition. Moreover, the definition allows one to consider medicine development for a subgroup of a more common disease, if a medicine is found to be only active in a subgroup of a total disease population.
2. Marketed medicines can qualify for orphan medicine status for new indications that are specific to rare diseases.
3. In the United States, medicines may qualify for orphan medicine designation if they are intended for populations larger than 200,000 patients, but the sponsor cannot recover sufficient revenues to cover costs of research, development, and distribution.
4. Companies may recover additional clinical research costs for medicines originally developed as a nonorphan medicine for major indications but where efficacy was limited to treatment of a rare disease. Tax credits are given for clinical studies on orphan medicines conducted between the time of designation of orphan medicine status and approval of the medicine's NDA.
5. Marketing exclusivity for 7 years post-NDA approval may be obtained on an unpatentable orphan medicine for a specific rare disease indication. This provides financial benefits to the sponsor and helps recoup costs.
6. Sometimes the regulatory authorities give clearer information on NDA requirements for an orphan medicine than they do for a nonorphan.
7. It is possible that an NDA application for an orphan medicine will obtain a more rapid regulatory review than if it did not have that designation.
8. If a company wishes to move into a new therapeutic area and has the potential to develop an orphan medicine at the outset, then it may be viewed as a means of enabling sales representatives to achieve easier access to offices of specialists in a new therapeutic field.
9. Publicity about new orphan medicines will enhance the image and prestige of the company in both the lay and professional community.
10. There is always the possibility that an orphan medicine may eventually be used to treat a common disease and some hope that an orphan medicine may become highly profitable.
11. Development of certain orphan medicines may expand a current product portfolio in a specific therapeutic area. This would allow a company to advertise and promote a more complete range of therapeutic, diagnostic, or prophylactic products within that area.
12. If the company has few medicines of major commercial potential under development, then orphan medicines may provide scientific stimulation and also utilize efforts of the staff while medicines for more common diseases are being sought.

Disincentives for Development of Orphan Medicines

1. The tax credits for developing an orphan medicine will usually have little impact on the total cost of a medicine's development. Major financial costs of developing a medicine often occur in areas where no reimbursement via tax credits are given under provisions of the Orphan Drug Act (e.g., toxicological studies, patent requirements, formulation studies, development of a practical route for chemical synthesis). Clinical trials would be expected to be less extensive in developing an orphan medicine and thus cost less than for most other medicines. Other development costs, however, may not be less. It is thus ironic that the tax credits are given in the one area (clinical trials) in which lower development costs are generally accepted for an orphan medicine.
2. A company may encounter difficulties in obtaining marketing exclusivity on an orphan medicine if a pending patent is rejected or awarded to another com-

pany. An approved orphan medicine may not be easily marketable if another company owns the patent. If the patent situation is not clear at the time of regulatory approval, then a company takes a great risk if it sells the medicine. If the patent is later awarded to another company, the first company may have to pay punitive damages that are greater than the amount of their sales.

3. A company that allocates its resources to developing an orphan medicine is not allocating them to developing medicines needed by larger patient populations. Since medicines for large populations are potentially more profitable than orphan medicines, there is generally a lost opportunity cost in developing orphan medicines.

4. When a marketed medicine (off patent) is being sold by generic companies and is found to be useful for a rare disease, it will probably be unprofitable for the primary manufacturer to conduct clinical trials to demonstrate the medicine's activity. This is because marketing exclusivity will be unenforcable if a generic manufacturer is already selling the same medicine for a more common indication. It may also be unnecessary for the company to study the medicine because physicians may legally use the medicine for the rare disease without formal NDA approval. In addition, it may be impossible to obtain NDA approval if the medicine is not sufficiently active in a high enough percentage of patients with the rare disease.

5. The time required to develop new medicines for some orphan indications is long, the problems encountered are usually tremendous, and the costs to develop them are among the highest of all classes of medicines. Given the enormous potential for difficulties, it is uncertain (when initiating the development of medicines for orphan indications) that success will be achieved.

6. The anticipated current and future competition and anticipated market share for a proposed orphan medicine must be evaluated. If there are medicines presently used to treat a rare disease, a new medicine must be compared with them in terms of both safety and efficacy. The need for the new orphan medicine should be assessed since there is a great difference between a medicine that will be the only treatment for a rare disease and a medicine that will offer limited benefits in treating a rare disease as an alternative therapy.

7. If the sponsor of the orphan medicine is not the original developer and current manufacturer, there may be great difficulties in obtaining the necessary development and toxicology data from the original developer. Such data must be submitted to the government to obtain marketing approval and the original NDA may only be referenced with the consent of the NDA holder.

8. Postmarketing studies may be required by the Food and Drug Administration (FDA) as part of the NDA approval of an orphan medicine. Since the tax credits for clinical trials on orphan medicines stop at the time that the NDA is approved, there is no reimbursement for any postmarketing studies. These studies may be extremely expensive, and the relatively small patient population treated with orphan medicines may make studies to monitor these patients even more costly than usual.

9. The possibility of liability exists for any new medicine. The magnitude of this risk will vary for each medicine, but there are no reasons to believe that liability of a manufacturer for an orphan medicine will be any less than for a more widely used medicine. Certainly there are no regulations stating that orphan medicines may be less safe than nonorphan medicines.

The Orphan Products Development group at the FDA is able to approve orphan status of new medicines rapidly, but is relatively ineffective in providing information to companies on requirements for approving an NDA, and helping other groups within the FDA to expedite the NDA review process.

Costs and Activities Associated with Orphan Medicine Development That Are Not Covered by the Orphan Drug Act

1. Preclinical studies conducted prior to initiation of clinical trials.
2. Nonclinical biological studies conducted after initiation of clinical trials.
3. Technical development costs.
4. All clinical trials conducted prior to the approval of the orphan medicine application, and subsequent to approval of the NDA, even if mandated by the FDA.
5. Administrative costs.
6. Patent costs.
7. Marketing costs.
8. Manufacturing costs.
9. Other support costs.

STIMULATING DEVELOPMENT OF NEW ORPHAN MEDICINES

It is generally inefficient and not cost effective for a pharmaceutical company to establish many highly specific animal models of rare diseases in their own laboratories to evaluate marketed medicines and promising chemical leads or to screen potentially interesting compounds. Sometimes, however, such testing can be useful. There is no single document available that provides information on most animal models suitable for evaluation of potential medicines for rare diseases.

Likewise, the names and addresses of leading experts involved in most rare diseases are not readily available.

Obtaining Information

To optimize the development of new orphan medicines within the pharmaceutical industry, it would be valuable to have a list of selected rare diseases and information about them. This document would provide additional opportunity and stimulus for collaboration between researchers in the pharmaceutical industry and academia. Information collected on individual rare diseases should include data on (1) animal models, (2) names and addresses of the most qualified researchers and leading experts, (3) names and addresses of relevant volunteer organizations, (4) medicines or chemicals presently used to treat the disease, and (5) any known chemical leads for treatment that are not patentable (either specific chemicals or classes of chemicals could be listed). Additional categories of information should be considered for inclusion.

This list would have to be updated regularly. The information obtained would *not* list priorities among diseases or medicines, nor would it include information of specific interest to patients or treating physicians. Although much of this information already exists, it is currently fragmented and not readily available. Such data would be sent to interested academicians, government agencies, volunteer organizations, individual pharmaceutical companies, and associations.

Potential uses for this information include:

1. Pharmaceutical companies with an interest in a specific disease or types of disease could privately pursue contacts with academicians or others. The companies could inquire about screening compounds for activity or about collaborating on a research project.
2. Academicians would readily see which orphan diseases did not have appropriate animal models or experts to serve as champions of that disease. The list might stimulate development of valuable new methodological techniques or encourage new champions. Little or no coordination of these activities would be required by the government.

Proposal

It is proposed that a government agency such as the National Institutes of Health or the Department of Health and Human Services prepare and disseminate this list, since the pharmaceutical industry is not generally considered to be in an appropriately neutral position, and most academicians would not have suffi-

cient time or resources. The National Organization for Rare Disorders (a volunteer group) in Fairfield, CT has been collecting many of these data and is playing an important role.

It would also be desirable if academicians could contact pharmaceutical companies to explore possible collaborations on projects of mutual interest. It is unlikely that most pharmaceutical companies have specifically explored their own research interest in all rare diseases or would be willing to have this information made public. On an individual basis, however, a frank discussion between an academician and company could occur after a statement of confidentiality was signed. The individual academician would have to explore company interests one company at a time and might find it difficult to identify the most suitable company with which to collaborate. Possible solutions to this dilemma should be sought since there are many academic scientists who seek to identify an industrial partner for collaborative research or medicine development.

ORPHAN MEDICINES UNDER DEVELOPMENT IN THE PHARMACEUTICAL INDUSTRY

How Are New Orphan Medicines Discovered and Developed?

There are usually no substantial differences between the specific processes used for developing medicines for rare diseases or common diseases. Orphan medicines (as all medicines) are discovered and developed through a variety of mechanisms. A company does not generally set up a program to discover medicines for a rare disease such as hairy cell leukemia. Instead, it sets up research programs to study biological activities in specific areas such as muscle metabolism, receptors, enzymes, or branches of medicine (e.g., immunology). The company may also establish therapeutic targets such as specific diseases or groups of diseases.

The company usually develops and creates animal models to screen compounds for interesting biological activity. If a compound with an interesting biochemical or pharmacological profile emerges, then a series of possible diseases will be considered against which the specific compound might be active. This list often includes both common and rare diseases. During the clinical testing program, it is common for companies to sponsor a pilot trial in a rare disease to evaluate the compound's activity, or to make their medicine available to an investigator who has reason to believe that the new medicine might have activity in a rare disease.

One can never know with certainty which diseases a medicine will eventually be used to treat. Many newly marketed medicines are given to patients with diseases or conditions other than the one for which they are approved, to evaluate the total spectrum of the medicine's activity. This often leads to serendipitous results, such as the discovery that the antiviral drug amantadine, originally approved to prevent and treat influenza, also had activity in patients with Parkinson's disease. This effect was unknown prior to marketing.

A different perspective on orphan medicines emerges by retrospectively examining medicines that have been marketed, rather than looking prospectively at medicines under development. Many medicines have been approved and marketed for multiple indications, and some of these indications would qualify as rare diseases. Yet, most medicines used to treat both rare and common diseases are virtually never thought of as orphan medicines. A few examples include the use of propranolol for idiopathic hypertrophic subaortic stenosis (IHSS) and cimetidine for the Zollinger-Ellison syndrome. Many of these indications were detected after the medicines were marketed for more common diseases. There are also examples of medicines marketed for a rare disease that were later found to have a more widespread market for another indication (e.g., carbamazepine, which was originally sold for tic douloureux, was later found to be active in treating patients with partial and other types of epileptic seizures).

Establishing Efficacy and Safety Data

Practical Issues. One of the greatest difficulties in developing an orphan medicine involves the conclusive demonstration of the medicine's efficacy. Patients with a rare disease are generally geographically dispersed, and unless they are brought to large referral centers, it is not possible to enroll a sufficient number of patients to conduct a well-controlled clinical trial. Evaluating a medicine in a few widely scattered patients may be possible if a clear and objectively measurable endpoint exists. If the prevalence of the disease is much less than 200,000, it will be necessary to conduct multicenter trials in Phase II. Phase I trials may be conducted in normal volunteers if the medicine is relatively nontoxic.

Efficacy. If clinical improvement is difficult to measure, then obtaining convincing efficacy data will pose major problems because of the low incidence and prevalence of the disease. It is especially difficult to evaluate dose levels, frequency of dosing, and other important clinical factors when few patients are available to enroll in a trial. A shortage of available patients also means that parallel double-blind placebo-controlled trials are usually impractical. Crossover trials require fewer patients than do parallel designed trials, but the

former design is often not suitable. Thus, innovative designs that seek to utilize all available patients optimally must be sought. Special considerations in designing protocols for clinical trials of medicines for rare diseases are indicated in Table 46.3.

In multicenter trials each center may call a central location when a patient is available to enter the trial. Depending on the number of centers and required speed necessary to start patients on therapy, the medicine may either be kept available at each center or flown to the site from a central location. Patients may be assigned to treatment in a double-blind trial by a central coordinator at the sponsor or at one of the trial sites. Each patient may be treated in a dose–response manner or, alternatively, patients may be initially placed in a cohort that receives the lowest dose of the test medicine or placebo. When the total number of patients enrolled reaches a predetermined number, a new cohort is begun, to receive the next highest dose or placebo. With both of these trial designs relatively few patients are needed to generate data that provide a dose–response relationship.

Evaluation of Safety. Significant problems may also exist in the evaluation of the safety of an orphan medicine. Patients with rare diseases desire medicines for treatment that are as safe as most other medicines. This raises an important issue when there are an inadequate number of patients with a rare disease to enroll in the clinical trials necessary to establish safety within a reasonable period of time.

TABLE 46.3 *Special considerations in designing protocols for medicine trials for rare diseases*

1. The number of available patients may be limited and their geographical location may require special procedures to ensure adequate enrollment
2. Inclusion criteria often must be more lenient than in other trials in order to include a greater proportion of available patients
3. Providing funds for transportation and meals or actual transportation may help minimize patient dropouts
4. Patients may be given reminders by cards at one clinic visit to inform them of their next appointment; telephone calls or mailed reminders may also be useful to minimize the number of missed appointments
5. Depending on the availability of useful alternative therapy, a financial inducement for patients may be required to obtain sufficient enrollment; the magnitude of this inducement must be determined for the trial after careful consideration of its projected effects on the patients and their family, but all patients must receive the same amount
6. The most knowledgable and experienced investigators in the field should be chosen to conduct the trial
7. A volunteer patient organization may provide valuable information that will help in designing the trial, identifying potential patients for the trial, and identifying potential investigators
8. Cooperation may be provided by a government agency (e.g., NIND[a] for certain epilepsy trials, National Cancer Institute for certain anticancer trials)

[a] NIND, National Institute of Neurological Disorders.

1. Is your company developing any orphan medicines for Rx use that are currently either investigational or marketed for other indications?

<u>28</u> Yes <u>22</u> No

2. If you answered "No", would you agree with those companies who do not feel that it is part of their mission to develop orphan medicines?

Agree that it is not part of our mission   8

The "No" reflects a different reason   14

3. What is the total number of orphan medicines that are:

	Total NCEs	No. of Cos.	Total Non-NCEs	No. of Cos.
A. Under development in preclinical stages?	2	2	0	—
B. Under development in clinical stages?	39	18	4	3
C. In the clinic that are already on the market for other indications?	9	7	4	3
D. In the clinic that are only being developed for orphan indications?	24	11	1	1

4. Regarding NCEs, was the Orphan Drug Act a minor or major influence in your decision to develop a medicine for orphan indications?

<u>20</u> Minor <u>8</u> Major

5. What types of incentives would encourage your company to develop more orphan medicines? How important are these factors?

On a scale from 0 (No Importance) to 10 (Marked Importance)

	Mean ± S.D.	Range	N
A. Reimbursement for preclinical studies	4.5 ± 3.0	0 — 10	22
B. Reimbursement for toxicological studies	6.1 ± 2.9	0 — 10	22
C. Reimbursement for technical development	5.4 ± 2.8	0 — 10	22
D. Reimbursement for retrospective expenditures	4.5 ± 2.9	0 — 10	22
E. Inclusion of tropical or other diseases that are common diseases in the "Third World" but not in the U.S.	2.5 ± 2.4	0 — 8	22
F. Reimbursement for clinical expenditures made outside the U.S.	5.7 ± 3.0	0 — 10	22

G. Others (written in): Expedited approval (9) (9) (8),

All clinical costs (8), Full reimbursement of clinical costs (10), Goodwill (6) and Tax credit (3).

( ) = Rating given by reviewer

6. Please check the range of your company's most recent annual sales of pharmaceuticals?

Under $50MM <u>9</u> $50 to 100MM <u>8</u>

$100 to 500MM <u>18</u> Above $500MM <u>15</u>

FIG. 46.1 Results of a questionnaire on development of orphan medicines in the pharmaceutical industry. NCEs, new chemical entities; Cos., companies.

The smaller number of patients used to establish the safety of orphan medicines is not necessarily a significant drawback, because the initial safety data on any medicine are usually the most important. Also, patients with the disease could be followed for a period after the medicine is marketed, to develop the safety profile further.

Benefit-to-Risk Ratio. The benefit-to-risk ratio must be considered in any discussion on the safety of new medicines. It is probable that an orphan medicine would be approved by a regulatory authority on the basis of data from fewer patients than the number required for most nonorphan medicines. Thus, the probability of observing rare but serious adverse reactions at the time of marketing is less for orphan than nonorphan medicines.

Current Status of Pharmaceutical Industry Activities and Perspectives on Orphan Medicine Development

To obtain an impression on current industry-wide development of orphan drugs, a questionnaire (Fig. 46.1) was mailed to the Head of Research and Development at each of 102 companies, chosen from the 121 members of the Pharmaceutical Manufacturer's Association (PMA). Nineteen of the subsidiary companies that belong to PMA were not contacted. Sixty-one responses were received. Of these, one company refused to participate, and ten replies indicated that their companies do not develop new medicines (e.g., medical device company). Fifty responders answered the questions and their responses are shown in Fig. 46.1. The survey was conducted in 1986, but numerous conversations suggest that the conclusions are still valid in 1990.

This questionnaire was not validated, and it may contain questions that were either unclear or misleading. It had a different purpose than the questionnaire used by Representative Waxman at the hearings on the Orphan Drug Act (Asbury, 1985). Although an in-depth analysis was not possible with the current questionnaire, a number of observations are pertinent.

1. The response rate (60%) was considered excellent. Some of the nonresponders are believed to be companies that do not develop new medicines.

2. Several of the negative replies to question 1 (Is your company developing orphan medicines?) were from companies that do not develop new pharmaceuticals (the exact number is unknown). This means that the percentage of companies that are developing orphan medicines, compared with the total possible number of companies, is somewhat greater than the current numbers indicate.

3. Of the 50 responding companies, 28 stated that they are developing at least one orphan medicine for prescription use.

4. Of these 28 companies, 8 (29%) stated that the Orphan Drug Act was a major influence in their decision to develop a medicine for orphan indications.

5. Potential incentives for stimulating additional efforts in developing orphan medicines were important to some companies and not important to others. There is a trend, however, suggesting that reimbursement for toxicological studies, technical development, and clinical expenses obtained from outside the United States would be the most important three incentives to the companies actually developing orphan medicines.

6. The 15 companies with the greatest yearly sales of pharmaceuticals (i.e., above $500 million) gave responses similar to those of the smaller companies. This indicates that orphan medicine development is not solely an activity of the larger pharmaceutical companies.

CONCLUSIONS

Orphan medicines are a heterogeneous group of medicines and offer valuable opportunities for pharmaceutical companies in carefully selected situations. Whereas legislators usually approach issues of orphan medicines as if they represent a single entity, pharmaceutical companies approach issues on the basis of the specific characteristics of each medicine. It is hoped that additional incentives for orphan medicine development will be enacted in all major countries where medicines are developed.

CHAPTER 47

Clinical Trials in Elderly Patients

This chapter describes some of the practical methodological considerations that are sometimes relevant in clinical trials conducted in the elderly. Chapters 16, 48, and 84 describe pharmacokinetic and other differences found in the elderly that are important to the interpretation of data. Many reviews and papers describe diseases that are more prevalent in the elderly, plus the therapeutic approaches and medicines that must be used with caution. These topics are not discussed here. Temple (1987) presents the Food and Drug Administration (FDA) perspective on this issue. Elderly patients are usually excluded from Phase I trials. Elderly patients often are enrolled in Phase IIb pivotal trials or Phase III clinical trials, and a subgroup analysis is all that is usually necessary to obtain adequate data on medicine behavior in this group.

SPECIAL PATIENT POPULATIONS

There are many operational definitions of "special patient populations"; this is because some are appropriate for only particular situations. The definitions depend to a large degree on the perspective and needs of the person (or group) defining the term. In this book, the term is loosely defined and includes groups of patients for whom medicines are not usually tested or for whom testing is usually not done until relatively late

in a medicine's development. Even this loose definition has several exceptions, since some special populations may be involved in a medicine's testing from the outset. Special populations that are often referred to include infants, pregnant women, lactating women, blacks, elderly patients, and patients with decreased renal or liver function. A more complete discussion of special patient populations is given in Chapter 87.

CONDUCTING STUDIES IN ELDERLY PATIENTS

It is important to note that age per se is not a good predictor of medicine response. The general public, as well as clinicians, have been sensitized to the fact that many individuals over 60, 70, or even 80 are both physically and mentally fit and have few or none of the attributes commonly associated with "old" people. Nonetheless, there are physical and physiological changes that occur with advancing age. Further, social and economic conditions often affect the aged. Because many elderly patients are not physically and psychologically well, it is important to understand how medicines behave in this group of patients.

Designing medicine trials for elderly patients or any other special patient population requires an understanding of the manner in which that population differs from other populations and also calls for an appreci-

TABLE 47.1 *Special considerations in designing protocols and conducting studies in elderly patients[a]*

1. Use reminder cards, mailings, and telephone calls prior to appointments
2. Arrange for transportation to and from the clinical trial site
3. Conduct periodic reviews to ensure patient understanding of protocol requirements
4. Conduct periodic checks on compliance
5. Include a sufficient number and frequency of tests of vital status and other safety parameters to ensure patient well-being
6. Avoid rigorous demands that might unduly strain some patients
7. Involve family members, nursing home staff, or other individuals to provide assistance and to observe the patient for relevant signs and symptoms
8. Consider previous data with the test therapy to determine whether elderly patients are at higher risk of adverse reactions than a younger adult population

[a] These methods are not endorsed for all clinical trials, but should be considered. They are often more important for elderly patients than for younger adults.

ation of specific factors that should be controlled or evaluated (Table 47.1). Knowledge of social, physical, psychological, physiological, and other characteristics of the group is essential. Many of these factors are listed in Table 47.2.

A greater percentage of elderly patients than younger adults have (1) pathological changes such as decreased renal and liver function, (2) decreased numbers of certain receptors, (3) altered homeostatic responses (e.g., altered blood pressure reflexes in response to stimuli, as a result of increased deposition of calcium and other substances in arterial walls), and (4) other physiological changes. Thus, it is important to collect data on how a given medicine affects the elderly, although it is usually not necessary to study

TABLE 47.2 *Selected physiological and physical changes in the older population*

1. Decreased lean body mass
2. Increased body fat
3. Menopause in women
4. Decreased flexibility of the lens, which is manifested as a decreased ability to accommodate to near vision
5. Increased opacity of the lens, which leads to cataract formation
6. Arteriosclerosis (i.e., hardening of the arterial walls) with accompanied increases in systolic blood pressure
7. Decreased pulmonary function (e.g., maximal breathing capacity, vital capacity)
8. Decreased renal function (e.g., glomerular filtration rate, renal plasma flow)
9. Decreased maximal heart rate achieved with exercise
10. Changes that mimic disease (e.g., decreased glucose tolerance, decreased plasma renin levels)
11. Decreased hepatic blood flow
12. Decreased immunological function[a]
13. Decreased cardiac output and cardiac index
14. Decreased gastrointestinal motility

[a] See King and Fenoglio (1983) for table of specific changes.

older patients in independent formal clinical trials prior to filing a New Drug Application (NDA) or Product License Application (PLA) on a new medicine. Elderly patients are at a higher risk of experiencing clinically important repercussions from adverse reactions to medicines than are younger patients because of their altered physiological and psychological state. Data from existing and planned clinical trials should be categorized by age so that any unusual or noteworthy effects in elderly patients may be perceived and subsequently explored to whatever degree necessary.

Practical Issues

The process of designing clinical trials for elderly patients is similar to that for trials to be conducted in a younger adult population. Nonetheless, there are some practical issues that require special consideration in the elderly, including patient recruitment, physiological status, physical status, parameters to measure, and social status.

Patients may be recruited from nursing homes, where a high incidence of debilitation often exists relative to the elderly patients who live in the general population. Recruitment in a poorer economic area will probably yield a patient group with substandard nutritional habits. Patients who live alone will probably have a higher incidence of loneliness and significant psychological problems than patients who have a strong support system or are in frequent contact with at least another person in close proximity to their living environment. Depending on the age and health status of the group, physical status may be important to evaluate. Important factors to assess in the group include increased incidence of debilitated physical condition, poor nutritional status, poor state of hydration, living alone with a decreased support system, living in substandard conditions, decreased compliance, and increased use of antacids, laxatives, and other medicines, which may lead to a variety of interactions. Some of these factors may be assessed with one or more questions, whereas others require use of a standard scale (e.g., to assess social interactions, physical status). Sources of recruitment are listed in Table 47.3,

TABLE 47.3 *Selected places and approaches to seek elderly patients in a community*

1. Health fairs
2. Senior cultural or social centers
3. Senior housing (e.g., nursing homes, retirement homes, retirement communities)
4. Pharmacies
5. Mailing lists provided by insurance companies or governments
6. Associations of older persons
7. List of retirees furnished by various organizations
8. Physicians specializing in gerontology

TABLE 47.4 *Selected types of medication problems reported for elderly patients*

1. Poor understanding of the purpose for taking one or more of their medicines
2. Poor understanding of the directions for taking one or more medicines
3. Use of expired medicines
4. Taking either excessive or insufficient doses
5. Using a medicine improperly (e.g., chewing a suppository)
6. Taking duplicate medicines with different brand names
7. Forgetting to take medicines
8. Simultaneously taking two or more medicines that should not be taken together

TABLE 47.6 *Characteristics of nursing homes that may influence their ability to participate in a clinical trial*

1. Location (e.g., urban versus rural, state or local)
2. Number of elderly
3. Percent of total occupancy over the preceding X months or years
4. Type of home (e.g., nonprofit, government, proprietary)
5. Range of severity of patients (e.g., in terms of disease or activities of daily living)
6. Distribution of patients by severity or type of pathology
7. Medical equipment available
8. Specialized nursing care available (e.g., ostomy care, wound care, skin care, respiratory care, medical appliance care)
9. Diagnostic categories of patients present
10. Range of patients present by age, type of insurance, and other factors
11. Staff available in terms of number, type, qualifications, and interest in the clinical trial
12. Ratio of number of staff to number of elderly

common medication problems in Table 47.4, and medical problems in Table 47.5. Characteristics of nursing homes that may influence their ability to participate in clinical trials are listed in Table 47.6.

An individual's physiological status changes with age (Table 47.2) and this factor must be considered when designing clinical trials in the elderly. If the population of patients studied excludes some who are debilitated, the physical requirements of the trial must be carefully considered. This includes evaluation of the time and effort needed to complete various tests and examinations. Interactions of function and physiological changes that occur in the elderly may be divided into many categories, including (1) cognition, (2) emotion, (3) mobility, (4) nutrition, and (5) elimination habits.

Why Study the Elderly in Separate Clinical Trials?

Major reasons for studying the elderly in separate clinical trials are (1) demographic (i.e., their number is rapidly increasing both in absolute terms and as a percentage of the total population), (2) commercial (e.g., they are the biggest users of prescription medicines), (3) regulatory (e.g., they are most at risk for adverse reactions because they have more complex and multiple diseases), and (4) medical (e.g., they take multiple medicines and have a high incidence of interactions

TABLE 47.5 *Common medical problems that frequently occur in the elderly and that should be monitored in clinical trials*

1. Psychiatric and neurological problems, including confusional states, loss of alertness, depression, dizziness, falls, syncope, gait problems, sleep apnea, sleep disturbances, tremor
2. Cardiovascular problems, including conduction defects, impaired blood pressure homeostasis, orthostasis, syncope
3. Gastrointestinal problems, including constipation and other forms of bowel dysfunction, hypochlorohydria and other gastric problems, impaired salivary function
4. Genitourinary problems, including urinary incontinence and other lower urinary tract dysfunctions, and impaired sexual function
5. Other problems, including impaired glucose control, anorexia, malnutrition

among medicines; their pharmacokinetic and pharmacodynamic responses to medicines also are sometimes different from those of younger adults), and (5) social–economic (e.g., their high incidence of loneliness, poor diet, poor hygiene, poor social support system, and debilitation often affect their compliance and responses to medicines). The elderly are a group who experience a progressive decline in their homeostatic mechanisms and homeostatic balance, particularly under stress.

Study Designs Suitable for Elderly Patients

Study designs of clinical trials used to evaluate medicines or other treatments in the elderly are no different from those described for other groups of patients.

PROBLEMS IN THE ELDERLY VERSUS PROBLEMS OF AGING

Numerous individuals have suggested that some of the recent increased medical attention to the elderly merely represents a fad. This view claims that most changes commonly observed in the elderly (e.g., debilitation, depression, dementia, incontinence, loneliness, poor nutrition, multiple diseases, multiple medicines) are not a result of age per se, but of other factors. If these other factors are addressed, many of the problems of the elderly will disappear. Even the most sacred cow of physiological changes reported in the elderly (i.e., an inevitable decrease in renal function with age) has been challenged by the Director of the National Institute on Aging (Williams, 1987). Williams also challenges the common notion that there is a natural decline in brain function with age, and stresses the distinction between aging and disease. Lindeman et al. (1985) reported that one-third of 254 normal elderly patients followed in a longitudinal study did not have any decrease in creatinine clearance over a period of 10 to 23 years.

The counter view states that pharmacokinetic and homeostatic factors differ in the elderly and that many, if not most, medicines must be prescribed differently. Elderly patients require additional care and attention to prevent or recognize and treat adverse events. Even the presentation of many diseases often differs in the elderly.

The author's opinion is that the increased attention paid to the elderly is extremely positive because many physicians overprescribe medicines to the elderly, who are also not observed as carefully as they should be for adverse reactions. Increased attention, particularly to the frail, will lead to improved medical care and more appropriate clinical trials. To learn about effects of medicines in the elderly, behaviors and reactions in patients above a certain age (e.g., 65, 70, 75, 80) should be sought that differ from those of younger adults. To do this in clinical trials it is necessary to control or evaluate problems commonly found in some groups of elderly patients (see list in following section). Evaluating these factors in patients of all ages will enable physicians to prescribe new medicines more accurately.

CULTURAL AND MEDICAL ASPECTS OF THE ELDERLY THAT MUST BE CONSIDERED IN CLINICAL TRIAL DESIGNS

Many of the problems associated with elderly patients described below are often more frequently observed in this group, but they are not related to age per se. These factors must be considered in terms of designing controls, choosing the clinical trial design, and determining methods of conducting the trial.

1. *Multiple medicines.* Polypharmacy is more commonly observed in the elderly than in other age populations. The number of irrational or unnecessary medicines is most likely excessive in the elderly.
2. *Multiple diseases.* The elderly are more likely than younger adults to have multiple diseases.
3. *Poor diet and eating habits.* Whether the elderly have a poorer diet and eating habits than other adults is uncertain, but many do not eat well because of insufficient funds, inability to prepare meals, lack of interest, or other reasons.
4. *Poor socialization and loneliness.* Many elderly live alone and have limited social contacts.
5. *Poor hygiene and sanitation.* This problem may be secondary to one or both of the following problems.
6. *General physical debilitation.* While not associated with age per se, it is more commonly found in elderly patients.
7. *General psychological debilitation.* This aspect too is not associated with age per se, but dementia is more commonly observed in elderly patients.
8. *Characteristics of presenting complaints.* The elderly are well known to present to physicians differently (i.e., have a different spectrum of complaints for a disease than do younger adults).
9. *Poor compliance with taking medicines.* This problem is often secondary to one or more of the others listed in this section. Table 47.7 presents selected methods to improve compliance in the elderly.

TABLE 47.7 *Mechanisms to improve clinical trial compliance in elderly patients[a]*

1. Utilize a service to deliver medicines daily or periodically to patients (e.g., "medicines on wheels," a pharmacist or study coordinator who makes house calls)
2. Have a small medication card placed in the patient's wallet or purse
3. Use patient package inserts
4. Provide a sheet of paper listing all medicines and the times they are to be taken. Tape one capsule or tablet of each type of medicine prescribed onto a sheet. This reinforces the medicine's name and its visual appearance
5. Provide a special medicine container with a week's (or month's) supply of each medicine laid out (e.g., oral contraceptive dial pack, large square medicine boxes with different sections labeled with days of the week and times of day)
6. Eliminate unnecessary medicines
7. Have the patient telephoned each time a medicine is to be taken (This may be done either automatically by computer or manually by staff)
8. Have a preset alarm ring at times when medicines are to be taken

[a] See also Chapter 15.

TYPES OF CLINICAL TRIALS ON INVESTIGATIONAL MEDICINES TO CONDUCT IN THE ELDERLY

Clinical Trials Specifically Conducted in Elderly Patients

The most important clinical trials conducted on an investigational medicine in the elderly are usually pharmacokinetic studies. These trials may be conducted either solely in the elderly, or in both elderly and younger adults. Omitting a young age control group is usually a mistake, because any unexpected effects observed might be unrelated to age, and this conclusion could not be made if one or more younger control groups were not included in the clinical trial. Another important type of trial is to evaluate cognitive function. To evaluate cognitive function many tests exist (e.g., card sorting, symbol digit substitution test, continuous performance). Practical issues may be evaluated by assessing the time to perform routine daily activities. Other types of clinical trials often conducted in elderly patients are dose–response efficacy and safety trials, and quality of life trials.

Subgroup Analyses

An alternative to evaluating effects of investigational medicines in the elderly is to analyze data from the subgroup of elderly enrolled in various clinical trials. Any unusual results found may then be pursued through separate clinical trials conducted in elderly patients. A failure to observe any different effects in the elderly through a subgroup analysis is interpreted as demonstrating no need to conduct specific trials in this group.

Pharmacokinetic Screen

A third approach is to conduct a general screen of pharmacokinetic parameters in various populations of elderly patients (e.g., patients with renal failure, patients over 70), where one or two trough plasma levels are measured. The presence of outliers indicates the need to conduct further trials to explore the relationship of dose, blood levels, and patient characteristics. Outliers are defined as patients with a tenfold or greater difference in plasma level than expected.

In most cases a screen should not consist of a single dose of a medicine. Multiple doses should be administered.

METHODOLOGICAL ISSUES

Longitudinal and Cross-Sectional Trials

There are two types of clinical trial designs that are typically used with elderly patients. In longitudinal trials, a group (cohort) is identified and is then followed for a period of time, with various parameters observed at fixed or variable intervals. Changes and trends in parameters measured are usually assessed.

One of the best ways of truly demonstrating age-related changes in responses to treatment is to conduct a longitudinal trial over time in a single population with a control group (Lindeman et al., 1985). Longitudinal trials are often administratively difficult to conduct and are usually quite expensive. Moreover, patients are subject to drifts in their methodological characteristics (e.g., they contract other diseases, are prescribed other medicines), which may affect results. Another approach is to conduct identical cross-sectional trials in two (or more) age strata, with each trial having sufficient power to stand on its own. Younger adults serve as a control group in this parallel design. Data obtained in each group are compared.

Choosing Patient Groups

It is essential to ascertain which groups to compare. Even if three different age groups of adults are used, the middle group of adults may not yield data that are in the middle. In addition, elderly patients may not show age-related differences at 65, 70, or even 75 years of age. The break point in the data should be found if it exists. Also, men may behave differently than women in groups of elderly patients; this factor should be considered when designing and analyzing a clinical trial.

Subgroup Analyses of Clinical Data to Evaluate Effects of Medicines in the Elderly

The data from a single large clinical trial or pooled data from multiple trials may be evaluated for differences in safety and in efficacy for younger versus elderly patients. One approach is to graph the percent of patients with a specific adverse reaction on the ordinate and the plasma level on the abscissa. If the plasma levels are unavailable, then other parameters (e.g., urine levels) may be used. Then data from two groups of patients (e.g., under 65 years and over 65 years) may be plotted to look for any differences. Each adverse reaction or efficacy parameter related to the medicine may be plotted separately. A cumulative graph of all adverse reactions or all adverse reactions of particular organ systems could also be graphed.

Plotting Treatment versus Age

Response to treatment versus the age of patients treated may be plotted. If the data have a significant correlation coefficient, they are usually interpreted as demonstrating an age-related effect. There are some logical problems, however, with this simple approach. For example, younger adults may differ from older patients in one or more important ways. If elderly patients have different (e.g., higher) baseline values of blood pressure, then decreases of these values with treatment would be expected to be greater for the elderly based on the phenomenon of regression to the mean. This has been discussed by Murray et al. (1988).

CHAPTER 48

Pharmacokinetic Trials

The field of pharmacokinetics (i.e., absorption, distribution, metabolism, and elimination) may be described as what the body does to a medicine (i.e., what tissues the medicine reaches and how long the medicine stays around in the human body); pharmacodynamics (i.e., biological and clinical effects) involves what a medicine does to the body. The coupling of these two processes in one sense occurs at the receptor level (Fig. 48.1) and in another sense relates to the therapeutic concentration range above the minimally effective dose. Basic principles and parameters of pharmacokinetics are described in Chapter 16. This chapter focuses on the various types of pharmacokinetic trials.

GOALS OF PHARMACOKINETIC TRIALS

The ideal goal of pharmacokinetic trials is to characterize the relationship between pharmacokinetic and clinical parameters. If this goal can be established, then one can predict the optimal dose to use, the optimal dosing schedule, and the therapeutic range over which patients can be treated. Furthermore, it becomes easier (1) to develop the medicine in Phases I, II, and III, (2) to review the regulatory submission, (3) to prescribe the medicine, and (4) to develop additional dosage forms more readily.

347

Pharmacokinetics Pharmacodynamics

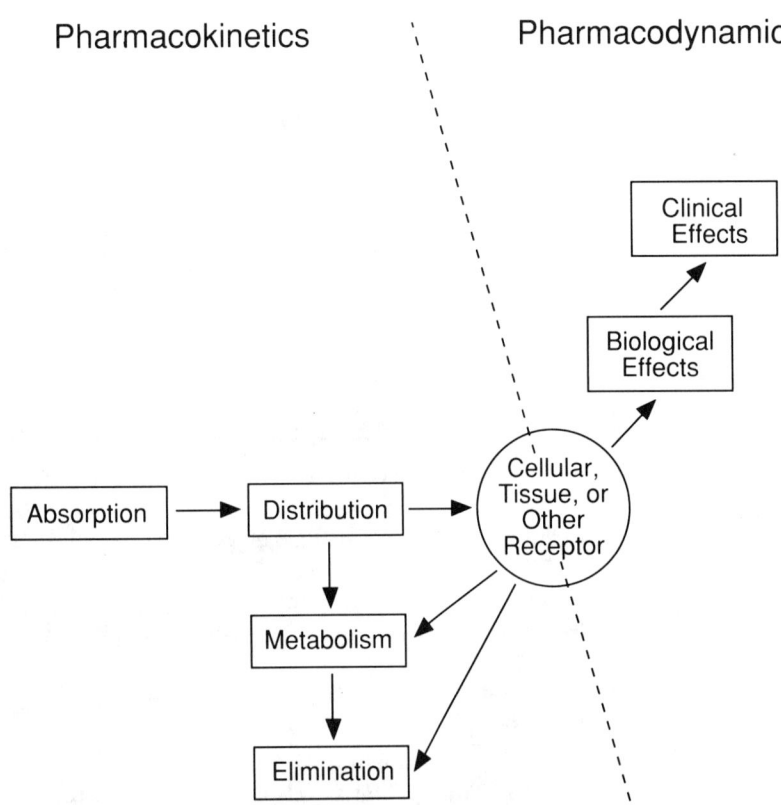

FIG. 48.1 Schematic illustration of the interface between pharmacokinetics and pharmacodynamics. In some cases a medicine leaves the receptor and is then metabolized. The receptor that leads to the metabolism of a medicine (primarily in the liver) is usually different from the receptor that leads to a biological and clinical effect at the site of action.

DEVELOPING A PHARMACOKINETIC PROFILE OF A MEDICINE

Comparison of Data Obtained in Animals and Humans

There is often a close relationship between results of pharmacokinetic and metabolic trials conducted in humans and those conducted in at least one animal species. When numerous animal species have been evaluated in preclinical studies, it is usually uncertain as to which specific species yielded data that will most closely resemble data to be obtained in humans. There is often little relationship between the position of the species on the evolutionary tree and the answer to this question, especially if only nonprimate species have been studied. When pharmacokinetic data obtained in animals are similar to those obtained in humans, there is a greater likelihood that toxicological data in animals will be predictive of the medicine's safety in humans.

Pharmacokinetic evaluations of a new medicine often begin during the initial clinical evaluation in humans and continue through all three phases of premarketing investigation. The major objectives and types of pharmacokinetic trials are listed in Table 48.1, and trials constituting a pharmacokinetic profile are listed in Table 48.2. It is usually unnecessary to conduct all of these trials on every medicine. The exact

trials required depend on the (1) biological, physical, and clinical characteristics of the medicine, (2) intended use of the medicine (e.g., acute or chronic treatment), (3) severity of the disease for which the medicine is intended, and (4) issues that arise during evaluation of the medicine. These latter issues include questions relating to clinical trials or parameters, toxicology, and technical development. The types of information obtained from pharmacokinetic trials are presented in Table 48.3, and the types of concepts evaluated are listed in Table 48.4.

Conducting Pharmacokinetic Trials

There are numerous reasons for conducting bioequivalence trials (Table 48.5). When data are obtained they are usually plotted as (1) concentration versus time and (2) concentration versus effect (i.e., pharmacological activity). Time, effect, and concentration are really three axes of the same relationship and may be plotted on a three-dimensional graph if desired. Criteria to relate concentration of a medicine to its effect are listed in Table 48.6, and reasons why a concentration–effect relationship may not be reproducible are given in Table 48.7.

Some individuals advocate a "shotgun approach" to pharmacokinetics by which a new medicine is evaluated in as many types of patients as possible and in

TABLE 48.1 *Examples of pharmacokinetic trial objectives*

To evaluate the:
1. Time course of blood and/or urine levels following a single dose (e.g., oral, i.v.) in a normal population and in patients
2. Time course of blood and/or urine levels during multiple doses, illustrating the ascension and achievement of steady state in a normal population and in patients
3. Routes and rate of elimination
4. Binding of medicine to plasma proteins to provide information on distribution and on potential medicine interactions
5. Distribution of the medicine to various tissues
6. Changes in medicine levels when enzymes have been induced with other medicines
7. Effects of a chronically administered medicine on the rate of its own metabolism (e.g., induction or inhibition of metabolism)
8. Effects of a medicine in patients with compromised renal, hepatic, cardiac, gastrointestinal, or other physiological function
9. Screening tests to establish a profile and identify potential problems in the elderly, children, and other special populations
10. Effects of food in general and of specific types (e.g., fats, proteins, carbohydrates) on the bioavailability of a medicine
11. Interactions of the trial medicine with other medicines and nonmedicines (e.g., walls or seal of the container, infusion sets)
12. Bioequivalence studies comparing two different dosage forms (e.g., solution and suspension, capsule and tablet), two different salts, or two (or more) different forms of the same medicine
13. Comparison of different patients to evaluate interpatient differences
14. Comparison of multiple samples from the same patient to evaluate intrapatient variations
15. Cumulative effects of the medicine under steady-state conditions
16. Mass balance study

TABLE 48.3 *Selected types of information obtained in pharmacokinetic trials*

1. Identification and characterization of special populations who are at risk of adverse reactions because of genetic or other factors (e.g., disease states)
2. Identification and characterization of special populations who may not demonstrate a benefit from a medicine because of genetic or other factors
3. Association of increased or decreased medicine absorption with special patient populations or special patient factors (e.g., age, sex)
4. Association of altered patterns or rates of medicine distribution or protein binding with specific factors
5. Identification of medicine metabolites
6. Identification of factors affecting medicine absorption, distribution, metabolism, or excretion
7. Identification of techniques to treat medicine overdosage

TABLE 48.4 *Selected concepts evaluated in pharmacokinetic trials*

1. Interpatient variability
2. Intrapatient variability
3. Steady-state kinetics of the medicine. This should detect the presence of medicine accumulation or altered metabolism
4. Relationship of therapeutic effect with medicine concentration in plasma or other fluids
5. Type of elimination mechanisms used to remove the medicine and the rate of removal
6. Relationship of medicine dose and blood level at various time points after medicine is given

TABLE 48.2 *Types of human studies involved in establishing a pharmacokinetic profile of an investigational medicine*

1. Bioavailability—compare the rate and extent of medicine availability in the systemic circulation after oral administration of a solid dosage form with that of an oral solution or an intravenous injection
2. Bioequivalence trials—Evaluate the comparability of two or more dosage forms, salts, or formulations of a medicine on the basis of rate and extent of absorption (area under the time–concentration curve)
3. Distribution studies—Obtain biological samples (e.g., biopsies) to detect presence and amount of medicine at various times in different tissues and compartments
4. Metabolism trials—Measure presence, quantity, and time course of formation and elimination of metabolites[b]
5. Elimination trials—Measure fecal and urine levels of parent medicine, metabolites, and conjugated products

[a] Any of the trials may theoretically be performed using radioactive labeled medicine. Labeled medicine trials are especially relevant if assays are not available to measure nonlabeled medicine or are not adequately sensitive to detect expected medicine levels.

[b] Clinical and biological activities of metabolites are measured in other studies. Numbers 4 and 5 are often combined in the same trial.

TABLE 48.5 *Selected reasons for conducting bioequivalence trials*

1. New formulation of a medicine is chosen to replace an older formulation (e.g., new excipients or new salt of the medicine are used)
2. New dosage form of a medicine replaces an older one (e.g., tablets replace capsules) or extends the product line
3. New physical characteristics of a medicine product exist (e.g., increased density of a tablet due to higher compression used in its manufacture)
4. An older supply of the medicine is to be compared with a newer one in order to determine the effect of age and "natural" changes in the overall composition
5. Two lots of an active medicine are compared in which differences are shown to exist[a]
6. A new manufacturing method is used to prepare the medicine, or a new manufacturing site is preparing the medicine and a question of bioavailability is raised
7. A new manufacturer[b] of a medicine desires to compare the new product with a standard

[a] *In vitro* and/or *in vivo* tests in animals may be sufficient to evaluate the possibility of differences [e.g., dissolution tests and other tests demonstrating that the medicine meets United States Pharmacopeia (USP) specifications].

[b] May be a generic manufacturer or a new supplier of a brand name product.

TABLE 48.6 *Criteria to relate concentration of a medicine to its effect*

1. Plasma samples are obtained at times, which are based on pharmacokinetic properties of the medicine
2. The analytical methods used to measure medicine concentration are sensitive, specific, quality controlled, and validated
3. There is no tolerance of the receptor sites
4. The medicine's action is reversible
5. If clinical effects are clear-cut and the endpoints may be objectively measured the relationship is easier to establish
6. Factors that modify the time course of medicine levels in plasma (e.g., metabolites) are considered
7. Total medicine concentration in plasma reflects the unbound concentration at receptor sites (i.e., binding must be relatively constant throughout the therapeutic range)
8. There is acceptable variability between the magnitude of individual clinical effects

TABLE 48.8 *Types of pharmacokinetic trials*[a]

1. Single-dose pharmacokinetics
2. Maximal tolerated dose pharmacokinetics
3. Intravenous versus oral pharmacokinetics to determine absolute bioavailability
4. Multiple-dose pharmacokinetics (e.g., at steady state)
5. Metabolism trial
6. Distribution trial
7. Elimination excretory trial
8. Dose–dependency pharmacokinetics
9. Absorption trials of multiple formulations
10. Bioequivalence of the final formulation
11. Steady-state kinetics of the final formulation
12. Pharmacokinetics in special populations (e.g., elderly, pediatric, smokers, renally impaired, hepatic impaired)
13. Influence of type and amount of food on absorption
14. Interactions with other medicines
15. Influence of disease severity[b]
16. Influence of concurrent diseases[b]

[a] Most of these clinical trials could be also conducted for sustained release formulations, different formulations, dosage forms, or routes of administration. The dosages used should be within recommeded ranges.
[b] See Koup (1989) for a discussion of appropriate methods.

as many ways as possible. This serves to screen the medicine for unexpected differences in its profile. Factors evaluated would generally include diet, cigarette smoking, gender, race, gastrointestinal disease, hepatic disease, renal disease, age, pregnancy, and others. Sheiner and Benet (1985) have advocated the use of premarketing pharmacokinetic screens of new medicines in populations of patients, not just in a few selected volunteers or patients.

TYPES OF PHARMACOKINETIC TRIALS

Most types of pharmacokinetic trials are listed in Table 48.8.

Various Patient Populations

Pharmacokinetic trials involve the assessment of one or more formulations of a medicine(s) in various types of patient populations:

- Volunteers versus patients
- Young adult patients versus elderly patients
- Patients with mild disease versus those with severe disease

TABLE 48.7 *Reasons for lack of a reproducible concentration–effect relationship*

1. The medicine is ineffective
2. Measurement methods of insufficient sensitivity are used
3. Effects of medicines are small or obscured because of difficulties in measuring effects
4. The medicine has an irreversible or long-lasting effect
5. Receptor tolerance occurs
6. Variable absorption, distribution, metabolism, and/or excretion
7. Genetic differences in the population
8. Age, sex, or other differences are present in patients studied and influence pharmacokinetics

- Young children versus older children or adults
- Renally impaired versus healthy patients
- Patients with and without induced hepatic microsomal enzymes
- Hepatic impaired versus healthy patients
- Males versus females
- Blacks versus whites
- Smokers versus nonsmokers
- Other subpopulations

Although many (and sometimes most) pharmacokinetic trials are conducted in healthy volunteers, pharmacokinetic trials are also conducted in patients to get a medicine approved for marketing. Eighteen to twenty-four subjects are usually enrolled. Medicines may be evaluated after a single dose or after a steady state is achieved.

Bioavailability Trials

Bioavailability is the rate and extent of a medicine administered that reaches the general circulation unchanged. It is measured by assessing the area under the curve for the graph of plasma concentration versus time. Relative bioavailability is the comparison of two oral forms and absolute bioavailability is the comparison of an oral or other non-i.v. form (e.g., intramuscular) with the i.v. form. Bioavailability trials using radiolabeled medicine evaluate the absorption of a medicine when biological sample (e.g., blood, plasma, urine) assays do not exist, or are not sufficiently sensitive, to measure unlabeled medicine concentrations in the plasma. The data to be obtained on bioavailability during Phases I and III are listed in Table 48.9.

TABLE 48.9 *Data on a medicine's absorption and bioavailability to be obtained during phases I to III[a]*

1. Absolute bioavailability
2. Relative bioavailability
3. Peak plasma concentration of medicine after different doses
4. Time to reach the peak plasma concentration
5. Factors that influence absorption (e.g., food)
6. Characteristics of absorption observed in various clinical trials

[a] These apply to a single route of administration. Each route of administration would require separate profiles as described.

Bioequivalence Trials

These trials are conducted to evaluate the rate and amount of absorption for:

1. Different formulations (e.g., brand versus generic, two formulations of the brand name medicine) or different dosage forms (e.g., capsule, tablet).
2. A medicine manufactured at two different sites (e.g., a medicine made by fermentation techniques).
3. A medicine manufactured by two different techniques (e.g., biotechnological methods and synthetic techniques). In most trials a pharmacokinetic endpoint (e.g., plasma concentration) is used.

Pharmacological endpoints may be used in some situations instead of blood levels (i.e., pharmacokinetic endpoints) of the medicine. For example, serum glucose levels versus time could be plotted for two (or more) formulations of a medicine that lowered serum glucose.

If neither pharmacokinetic nor pharmacological endpoints may be used, clinical endpoints may be employed to compare different medicine forms. These are the highest standards that can be applied to comparability trials. The trials must demonstrate not only that the medicine is absorbed and causes the biological effect desired, but that the clinical results of the two formulations are similar within a prespecified degree.

Dose-Proportionality Trials

A variation of the bioequivalence trial is a dose-proportionality trial. In this trial different dosage strengths are given to patients or volunteers to assess the area under the curve for the graph of concentration in plasma versus time. If three dosage strengths (e.g., 25, 50, and 100 mg) are assessed, the goal is to assess how closely the area under the curve (AUC) for the 50-mg dosage strength equals twice the area under the curve for the 25-mg dosage strength, and also how closely the area under the curve for the 100-mg dosage strength equals twice the area under the curve for the 50-mg

and four times the area under the curve for the 25-mg dosage strength.

If dose proportionality is not observed it could result from variability in single-dose pharmacokinetics or other factors leading to nonlinearity (e.g., Michaelis-Menton kinetics). If dose proportionality is not observed then one may evaluate patients at steady-state levels.

The importance of bioequivalence trials may be appreciated when one considers that there are over 180 brands of theophylline in the United States from 40 Food and Drug Administration (FDA)-approved manufacturing sources, and that numerous chemical configurations (e.g., anhydrous forms, different salts) and dosage forms (e.g., elixirs, suppositories) and more than 28 sustained release formulations exist. The real issue arises because the extent and the rate of absorption varies between "similar" forms.

To state that two or more test medicines are bioequivalent it is necessary to show that differences between them are no greater than 20% in terms of area under the curve. To ensure adequate statistical power in a bioavailability trial to attain this goal it is important to have input from a statistician to learn the necessary number of subjects to enroll.

Pharmacokinetic Screen Tests

Conducting a screen to evaluate effects of a new medicine in a variety of patient groups allows one to determine rapidly whether any subpopulations of patients are at greater risk of adverse reactions. If this is the case, then specific clinical trials may be conducted to evaluate that aspect in greater detail. One of the difficulties with this approach is that a screen with relatively few patients may reveal false negatives or positives. Reviewing the same subpopulations from multiple clinical trials should provide more reliable data.

Pharmacokinetics of Enantiomers

There is little doubt that the last decade has seen a dramatic increase in interest in the issue of differences in the pharmacokinetics of chiral medicines (i.e., optical isomers). A brief review of some of the differences observed is given by Jamali (1988). Methods of studying enantiomers are the same as for other medicines.

Isotope Trials

Radioactive labels are used for a number of pharmacokinetic trials, usually conducted in healthy men. These help determine distribution, metabolism, and elimination profiles of a medicine, plus its mass balance (i.e., percent recovery of administered dose). Radioactivity is measured in blood, urine, feces, and occasionally in expired air.

Medicine Distribution Trials

To observe where a medicine distributes in the body a radioactively labeled medicine may be injected or ingested. This type of trial is often conducted in animals that are sacrificed at different times after injection or infusion of the medicine, and autoradiographic techniques are used to identify where the medicine was distributed. The data on a medicine's distribution to be obtained during Phases I to III are listed in Table 48.10.

Metabolic Trials

To follow the disposition of a medicine as it is metabolized (i.e., biotransformed), blood samples are collected at various times and levels of all major metabolites identified are evaluated. Sophisticated analytical chemistry techniques are used to identify previously unknown metabolites. Each metabolite has its own spectrum of activity and toxicity and may interact with the parent medicine to antagonize or synergize with its effects. It is often necessary to synthesize or isolate metabolites (e.g., from urine) and then to test them for biological activity. Data on a medicine's metabolism to be obtained during Phases I to III are listed in Table 48.11.

Elimination Trials

To confirm that all of an administered dose is accounted for, it is common to use a radiolabeled medicine. The degree of recovery of the radioactivity can be assessed more accurately than that of the unlabeled medicine. Data on a medicine's elimination to be obtained during Phases I to III are listed in Table 48.12.

TABLE 48.10 *Data on a medicine's distribution to be obtained during phases I to III*

1. Volume of distribution
2. Degree of serum protein binding at different plasma concentrations
3. Characteristics of serum protein binding at different plasma concentrations and how this binding may be altered
4. Penetration of the medicine through capillary walls and cell membranes
5. Importance and nature of the blood–brain barrier
6. Importance and nature of breast milk excretion
7. Influence of other medicines on distribution
8. Influence of other diseases on distribution
9. Influence of other factors on distribution
10. Distribution to different tissues

TABLE 48.11 *Data on a medicine's metabolism to be obtained during phases I to III*

1. The nature of the first-pass phenomenon if it exists
2. The identity of metabolites produced and the pathway for their production
3. The amount of major metabolites produced
4. The manner in which other factors may influence the amount and type of metabolites produced
5. Production of any metabolites in humans not found in animal species used for toxicology tests
6. Biological activity of active metabolites in animals
7. Pharmacokinetics of active metabolites
8. Relevance and nature of hepatic microsomal enzyme induction
9. Importance of renal, hepatic, or other organ impairment in metabolism
10. Importance of various genetic conditions on metabolism
11. Existence of nonlinear or dose-dependent kinetics as a result of saturable metabolism

Food Trials

The most common reason to conduct a food trial is to assess the influence of food on a medicine's absorption. The pharmacokinetic parameters usually measured to assess the influence of food (e.g., in comparing a fed versus a fasted patient) are (1) maximum plasma concentration, (2) time to maximum plasma concentration, and (3) area under the curve.

It is useful to include a standard medicine in the clinical trial design if a standard exists. Any changes versus placebo or a different dose of the same medicine may be less important than how other medicines behave.

In addition to fed versus fasted states, the type of diet taken by patients may be of interest to evaluate. This could include giving patients high fat versus low fat, high protein versus low protein, high carbohydrate versus low carbohydrate, or any combination of these or other diets.

Many Phase I clinical trials are conducted on volunteers or patients who have fasted from 4 to 14 hours. Pharmacokinetic trials, in particular, utilize fasted patients or volunteers. During later Phase I or II clinical trials, when patients are not fasting, the presence of food may delay absorption of a medicine, though in some cases food speeds up absorption. Other potential

TABLE 48.12 *Data on a medicine's elimination to be obtained during phases I to III*

1. Major routes of elimination
2. Total body clearance
3. Plasma elimination half-life in patients with normal and impaired organs of elimination
4. Effect of age
5. Effect of disease severity or concurrent diseases
6. Ability to remove the medicine with dialysis
7. Effect on urinary pH on plasma half-life
8. Renal clearance
9. Urinary excretion half-life

effects of food include chelation or inactivation of a medicine. Any of these may affect the bioavailability of a medicine and, therefore, its efficacy or safety. It is for this reason that food interaction trials are conducted.

Food interaction trials should be considered early during a pharmaceutical's development if there is a low therapeutic ratio that could be affected by food. To evaluate the potential effect there are a few types of food trials to consider.

1. *Food spacing trial*. Use inpatients; the time between the meal and subsequent medicine administration can be controlled. The meal(s) evaluated may vary in content (i.e., percent of fats, carbohydrates, and protein), calories, and time prior to medicine dosage.
2. *Single-dose crossover food trials in fasted versus fed patients*. Various formulations and dosage forms may be compared in patients who are fed or fasted in a crossover design.
3. *Chronic dose food trials in fasted versus fed patients*. Food trials could be conducted for one or more weeks in patients using a parallel design. A crossover design could be considered. Food trials would evaluate spacing of food and dosage, different formulations with constant spacing, types of diets, or any of numerous other factors.

Metabolic Balance Trials

Metabolic balance trials usually use crossover designs in which patients (or volunteers) receive a placebo and medicine or a diet with and without a specific nutrient. To keep the diet controlled, patients are often kept within a special unit where the type, weight, caloric value, and chemical composition of their food may be controlled. In some of these trials it is crucial to know the precise amounts and composition of foods and liquids ingested. The extent of freedom allowed patients (i.e., to leave the unit) is a major issue, as is the extent of supervision of patients who leave the unit. Before these trials are initiated a baseline of sufficient length must be used so that all patients (or volunteers) are brought to a similar baseline. The time between the two parts of the crossover must also be of sufficient duration to prevent carryover effects from influencing the results.

CONSIDERATIONS IN DESIGNING AND CONDUCTING PHARMACOKINETIC TRIALS

Circadian Rhythms

Circadian variation in absorption occurs, so the blood levels achieved from an early morning dose may be different from those reached that evening or night.

Protein Binding

Protein binding of a medicine is important to measure because the unbound fraction of a medicine in plasma is available to elicit a biological and clinical effect. If all of a medicine is tightly bound to plasma proteins (primarily albumin or alpha-1 acid glycoprotein) then insufficient amounts may be available to cause an effect. Competition between medicines for binding sites on plasma proteins is common, and small changes in the total amount of a medicine bound may lead to relatively large increases of the unbound or free medicine. This may cause either greater efficacy or, more likely, greater toxicity (i.e., adverse reactions). Clinical effects are so dependent on free medicine concentration that pharmacodynamic effects are better expressed that way rather than in terms of total concentration of the medicine. Figure 48.2 illustrates the different curves obtained for concentration-dependent versus concentration-independent protein binding.

Analytical Method

A good analytical method must be available or developed to measure concentrations of the medicine, its metabolites and any other desired substances in the biological fluid or other tissues to be sampled. This is usually blood or urine, but could include feces, cerebrospinal fluid, tissue biopsies, saliva, or other biological substances.

Endpoints

It is also necessary to have an endpoint (i.e., parameter) that can be quantitatively measured. This parameter must be clinically relevant.

Should a Pharmacokinetic Trial Be Part of a Pharmacodynamic Trial?

Whether pharmacokinetics should be tested along with pharmacodynamics depends on the objective(s) of the clinical trial and the point during a medicine's development when this is being considered. Both types of clinical trials are usually combined in the first few safety trials conducted during Phase I and often during pilot trials in Phase IIa. Whether pharmacokinetic parameters continue to be measured depends on the specific situation. During Phase III when it is known that a regulatory application will be prepared and submitted, additional separate pharmacokinetic trials are designed and conducted to address outstanding questions and issues.

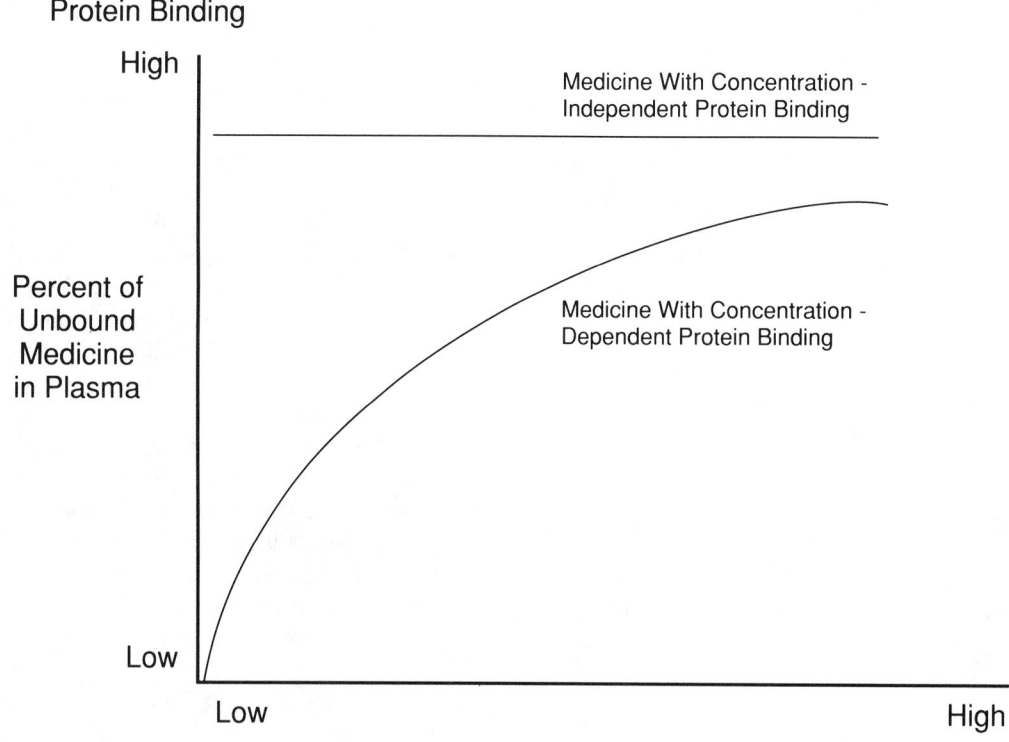

Protein Binding

High

Medicine With Concentration - Independent Protein Binding

Percent of Unbound Medicine in Plasma

Medicine With Concentration - Dependent Protein Binding

Low

Low

High

Total Medicine Concentration

FIG. 48.2 The influence of protein binding on total medicine concentration in plasma.

Variables to Control in Pharmacokinetic Trials

Pharmacokinetic trials are probably more rigorously controlled than any other single type of clinical trial. Some of the variables that are usually controlled include:

- Amount of food consumed
- Time since last meal
- Type of food consumed
- Age, sex, weight, and race of patients
- Drug history and alcohol history
- Amount of caffeine-containing beverages permissible

Collecting Biological Samples

The collection, fractionation, and storage of samples must be based on the stability of the material under various conditions. Preservatives may be required in the collection tubes. The time that a sample may remain in any state (e.g., unfrozen) should be determined and then specified in the protocol. Other conditions for obtaining, preparing, and storing the samples should also be evaluated and specified in advance.

Factors. The choice of an appropriate number of biological samples to collect and the optimal time points to collect them depends on four factors: (1) sta-

tistical considerations, (2) pharmacokinetic modeling requirements, (3) practical considerations, and (4) ethical considerations.

Statistical considerations are important in deciding how to cover best the time period of interest so that adequate samples are collected to achieve the goals set. For example, it is usually more relevant to collect several samples within the first hour of medicine administration and to then slowly start to space out additional collection of samples.

Developing pharmacokinetic models that fit the data is analogous to choosing clothes to fit a person. It is important to collect enough datum points at appropriate times to cover the medicine's profile. The more datum points one has at suitable times, the easier to select a model that will fit the medicine.

Initial Human Trials. If a medicine is being tested in humans for the first time, then it is not possible to make simulations of pharmacokinetic models using data from animal studies, because it is not known which species has a pharmacokinetic profile similar to humans. The first trials in humans basically looks at the pharmacokinetics without knowing what will be found. Later in the life of a medicine, data from human trials will be available on which to base simulations and models.

Approaches. Samples may be collected at the same fixed time points for all patients in a clinical trial (e.g.,

1, 2, and 5 hours after dosing), or a sequential strategy may be developed. In the latter approach, data from the first patient are used to derive optimal time points to collect samples from the second patient. Data from the first two patients are then used to choose the optimal time points for the third patient. This process may continue throughout the trial, or a fixed pattern may be established after a certain number of patients have been evaluated.

Practical Considerations. Practical considerations involve many different types of issues, including (1) total volume of blood that may be drawn on each patient in the clinical trial, (2) degree of inconvenience and bother to the patient (e.g., separate blood draws every 15 minutes may lead to emotional upset, especially if an indwelling catheter is not used), and (3) inconvenience and bother to staff (e.g., blood draws at 3 A.M. and 5 A.M. or on holidays will often lead to ire). There may be a limit to the number of separate blood draws permitted on each patient because of the quantity of blood necessary to perform duplicate assays. Up to 1 pint of blood may be taken every 8 weeks. It is sometimes necessary to balance the advantage of having duplicate assays performed on a patient versus the benefits of having samples taken at a greater number of time points.

Obtaining all of the appropriate blood samples in outpatient trials is usually more difficult than in inpatient trials because the patient (1) may be unavailable, (2) may not have taken the correct amount of medicine, or (3) may have taken the medicine too short or too long a period before the time when the sample is to be drawn. When patients collect their own samples (e.g., 24-hour urine) the number of additional factors that may complicate sample collection becomes even greater (e.g., patients may not collect the sample in the correct manner, or at the right time, or the patient may stop collecting samples too soon).

Usual times for blood sampling after an oral dose of a typical medicine would be at 0.5, 1, 2, 3, 4, 6, 9, 12, 24, 36, 48, 72, 96, and 120 hours. The actual times used are adjusted based on the expected half-life of the medicine in the body, and the purpose of the trial.

Some Problems Encountered in Pharmacokinetic Trials

Some of the characteristic types of problems often encountered in pharmacokinetic trials are listed below. These problems may affect the conduct of the trial or the interpretation of the results. Interested readers are referred to pharmacokinetic texts for additional information.

1. Ability of the assay methods to measure medicine levels in biological fluids accurately, precisely, and reproducibly.

2. Knowledge of the degree to which a medicine is bound by protein in plasma in various situations. In some cases the free fraction of medicine is markedly affected by certain pathological conditions or other medicines.
3. Differences in activity of optimal isomers.
4. Differences in activity of metabolites, whose concentration may be affected by many factors (see section on metabolites below).
5. Type and degree of binding to receptor may affect the clinical time course independent of the medicine's general concentration in plasma.
6. Nature of the medicine binding and interaction with receptors may be variable or unknown.
7. Variations in other aspects of medicine behavior (e.g., active transport, type of kinetics, tolerance, tachyphylaxis).

Determining the Importance of Medicine Metabolites

The presence of metabolites may be suspected in numerous situations, including when a medicine (1) has a highly different duration of effect in different species, (2) is an agonist in one species and a partial agonist or even antagonist in another, or (3) has a bioavailability profile that is markedly different in different species. Each of these reasons also may result from causes other than the presence of metabolites.

When a medicine metabolite is identified chemically it is essential to determine whether it has biological activity or clinical significance for the overall project. A preliminary biological profile of each metabolite should be established, but it may not be necessary to complete each profile before deciding that the metabolite has little or no clinical significance. Alternatively, it may be possible to determine that the metabolite's importance is so great (in a negative sense) that further medicine development of the parent medicine must be terminated. A profile of a metabolite may vary from a superficial characterization of its pharmacokinetic parameters, toxicology, and preclinical properties to a more detailed examination than that given the parent medicine. Representative types of biological and pharmacokinetic information that are often desired to profile a medicine's metabolite are listed in Table 48.13.

If the metabolite has a profile that is clinically preferable to the parent medicine in one or more important characteristics (e.g., less toxicity, longer duration of action), then serious consideration should be given to developing the metabolite as a medicine. If the parent medicine is already on the market (or close to the market) and the metabolite has significant advantages, then the metabolite may be developed independently and marketed as an improved version of the parent medicine. If the parent medicine has just started Phase I trials, then switching the development program to the

TABLE 48.13 *Selected aspects of establishing a profile of medicine metabolites[a]*

1. Chemical identify (i.e., structure)
2. Quantity produced based on amount found in blood and/or urine (e.g., percent of parent medicine converted to the metabolite)
3. Rate of production
4. Biological activities in animals
5. Clinical activity
6. Half-life
7. Evidence of cumulation
8. Toxicity (e.g., pathology, clinical chemistry, hematology[b]

[a] Each of these characteristics may be compared with the parent medicine and most are initially determined in animals.

[b] If a metabolite discovered in humans is not detected in the animal species used to evaluate the toxicology profile of the parent medicine, it may be necessary to (1) repeat the toxicology studies in a species that produces the metabolite and (2) evaluate the direct pharmacological effects of the metabolite in various animal test models.

metabolite may be relatively straightforward and highly desirable.

A metabolite that is to be tested in humans is viewed as a separate medicine from a regulatory viewpoint. In the United States it is necessary to obtain an Investigational New Drug Application (IND) based on a new set of data for the metabolite before it may be tested in humans. The disadvantage of pursuing development of a metabolite for the market is that it will probably cost almost as much as that spent on developing the parent medicine. Separate clinical trials, toxicological studies, and various types of technical development (including formulation development) must be conducted on any metabolite developed, even though it may be chemically (and biologically) similar to the parent medicine. Many examples illustrate that structurally similar chemicals have totally different biological, chemical, and/or toxicological activities.

Hierarchy for Adjusting Doses

The hierarchy for adjusting doses, either during a clinical trial or in medical practice, varies from the highly crude method based on overt clinical toxicity to the more finely tuned method based on tests of organ function. Between these poles are measures of clinical ineffectiveness and the method of using plasma levels.

Hepatic Impairment. No universal agreement exists as to the best hepatic parameter for titrating the dose of all medicines. The extraction ratio is usually considered best, although it is extremely difficult to obtain. Doses of some medicines metabolized in the liver should be decreased in patients with hepatic impairment. The degree of decrease is based on bilirubin levels in plasma for some medicines. Whatever guidelines are established for a medicine should be placed on its labeling. Serum albumin is probably the best single

parameter to adjust a medicine's dose as a result of liver abnormalities.

Renal Impairment. Creatinine clearance is usually the golden guide to use for titrating doses of medicines mostly excreted by the kidney in patients with renal impairment. A convenient table may be created for use in a package insert, with the first column listing creatinine clearances and an additional column listing weight ranges of patients. The body of the table lists the dose of medicine to use for each creatinine clearance and patient weight. Although plasma creatinine does not equal creatinine clearance, it is possible to go from one to another using a well-known formula.

MONITORING THERAPEUTIC LEVELS OF A MEDICINE DURING CLINICAL TRIALS

Criteria of When to Use Therapeutic Monitoring

Therapeutic medicine monitoring refers to the measurement of a medicine's plasma level and associating that level with either an acceptable clinical response, an underdose, or toxicity. The possibility of adopting therapeutic monitoring has been evaluated for many, if not most, medicines, but has only been found to be applicable for a small number. The reasons for this failure are numerous and generally relate to the criteria by which an ideal medicine and a therapeutic response are associated when performing medicine monitoring.

The necessary criteria for being able to use therapeutic medicine monitoring are:

1. Therapeutic effects of the medicine in patients must be able to be measured with accuracy.
2. Free medicine concentration in plasma (i.e., medicine that is not bound to proteins) should reflect free medicine concentrations at receptor sites.
3. The medicine should not be metabolized to active metabolites.
4. Tolerance should not develop.
5. Medicine effects should be reversible.
6. Plasma concentrations above a certain level should represent a medicine overdose or toxicity in almost all patients.
7. Medicine levels must be measured with accuracy.

When Is an Assay Developed?

An assay to measure blood, plasma or serum levels of a medicine during clinical trials is usually developed prior to initiating Phase I clinical trials. Considerations are given to measuring what are believed to be important metabolites and specific isomers if those issues are relevant.

Purposes of Therapeutic Monitoring

The major purposes of monitoring medicine levels during Phases I to III are identified in Table 48.14. Sample collection is usually done at the clinic for both in- and outpatient clinical trials. In certain clinical trials a traveling nurse collects a blood or urine sample from a patient at home to obtain a trough level. The patient then takes the medicine, and 1 hour later (or at another fixed time) the nurse collects a second sample to assess the medicine's peak effect.

Examples of Medicines Monitored via Plasma Levels

One medicine that meets the criteria listed above is phenytoin, but many other medicines measured routinely in laboratories fail one or more of these criteria. This is generally why data on their medicine levels are less useful clinically than the results of phenytoin measurements. Levels of digoxin, for example, do not accurately indicate whether a patient is under- or overdosed. The same is true for several anticonvulsants and many other medicines. In most cases it is not possible to establish a therapeutic plasma range in which a medicine's positive clinical responses occur. The medicines for which data of plasma concentrations are most useful include theophylline, lithium, aminoglycoside antibiotics, phenytoin, and possibly digoxin.

Value of Therapeutic Monitoring for Investigational Medicines

In developing new chronically administered medicines it is almost always worthwhile to evaluate whether a plasma concentration range of a medicine may be established that represents the therapeutic range for most patients. If so, and the other criteria listed above are met, then it will provide physicians with a valuable tool to titrate and control patient dosing of potentially toxic

TABLE 48.14 *Purposes of monitoring the concentrations of medicines within biological fluids during phase I to III clinical trials*

1. Characterization of the medicine's absorption, distribution, metabolism, and excretion
2. Characterization of the medicine's steady-state kinetic profile
3. Assessment of genetic influence on the pharmacokinetics of the medicine
4. Assessment of environmental influences (e.g., smoking, alcohol, diet) on the pharmacokinetics
5. Assessment of pharmacokinetics in special patient populations (e.g., risk factors, race, decreased renal function)
6. Assessment of concentration-dependent pharmacokinetics
7. Selection of the appropriate model of pharmacokinetics
8. Assessment of the degree of patient compliance
9. Assessment of interactions between medicines
10. Assessment of age-related changes in pharmacokinetics

medicines. Medicines with a large therapeutic index have little need of this approach, since there is a lesser chance of a therapeutic under- or overdosing and there is also a lesser likelihood of causing toxicity.

Dosing by blood concentration is expensive in terms of the costs to measure these levels, besides which it is often impractical for patients to schedule visits at certain times. Moreover, it is not the way that most physicians are trained, although epileptologists are a noteworthy exception. Both intra- and interpatient variability must be assessed to address this question. A clinical review of therapeutic monitoring of medicine levels that illustrates principles and problems is given by Friedman and Greenblatt (1986).

EXAMPLES IN WHICH A MEDICINE'S LEVELS IN PLASMA MAY NOT BE MEASURED OR DETECTED

Although it is usually desirable to measure levels of a medicine in blood, at least during its investigational period, this is not always possible. Four examples are given in which medicine levels may not be measured or detected in plasma. Approaches to evaluating pharmacokinetics in these situations are described below.

1. Medicines may be directly injected into the target organ (e.g., interferon may be injected directly into genital lesions). In animal studies it is possible to biopsy the tissues to evaluate pharmacokinetics. In humans this presents major difficulties except for skin and possibly muscle or liver. During surgery obtaining various biopsies is possible. Elimination may be assessed with traditional approaches.

2. The route of administration used may not involve significant systemic absorption, but only local effects (e.g., topically applied medicines, nasally inhaled medicines, antacids). Local kinetics may be evaluated with topical medicines when penetration into and through skin is evaluated with scrapings and biopsies. Other effects (e.g., blanching of skin) may be assessed, but the validity of these assessments must be demonstrated. Most traditional pharmacokinetic evaluations are impossible.

3. A medicine may enter the circulation, but may not be measurable as it breaks down or distributes rapidly (e.g., macrodantoin) or it may be a promedicine (e.g., an ester that is cleaved by esterases to the active medicine). Modeling experiments are used to evaluate pharmacokinetics of promedicines. For example zidovudine (Retrovir) is converted to a monophosphate, then to a diphosphate, and then to a triphosphate. The relationship between pool sizes of each intermediary may be studied and the pharmacokinetics may be modeled in vitro. Clinical data are used to confirm the model.

4. The medicine is administered in extremely small doses and the plasma levels are less than those detectable with existing assays (e.g., alpha interferon for hairy cell leukemia).

Tracer technologies may be used with either exogenous or endogenous labeled medicines. Alternatively, the sensitivity of the assay may be enhanced through other technologies (e.g., radioimmunoassays, chemical assays, bioassays, mass spectroscopy coupled with gas or liquid chromatography). Another approach is to develop an indirect assay and then assess if dose-proportionality may be demonstrated. Examples of indirect assays include the following: (1) biochemical measures (e.g., measure ammonia levels with lactulose), (2) physiological measures (e.g., blood pressure with tumor necrosis factor), or (3) clinical measures (e.g., *Pneumocystis carinii* pneumonia with aerosolized pentamadine).

When blood levels of an investigational medicine administered systemically cannot be measured, any other measures of pharmacokinetics must be validated. This usually means that more animal data must be collected prior to initiating Phase I trials than for other medicines.

WHEN SHOULD PHARMACOKINETIC TRIALS BE CONDUCTED DURING DEVELOPMENT OF A MEDICINE?

Advantages of Early Evaluation

Different companies and countries follow quite different strategies in addressing the question of evaluation time. Some companies attempt to collect fewer data and to conduct fewer pharmacokinetic trials (i.e., they use a lean plan) than others, who may use a fat plan. The comments in this section, however, focus on the timing of pharmacokinetic trials. Some companies stress conducting more extensive human pharmacokinetic trials early during a medicine's development so that they may identify the metabolites and determine their activity in animals, possibly consider their development as medicines, and ensure that no new major metabolites are produced in humans that are not found in animals. If this plan of early evaluation is followed, then toxicological tests may be more rapidly initiated and conducted on any important metabolites found in order to evaluate their safety.

Advantages of Delayed Evaluation

The counterview is that most medicines do not require an extensive pharmacokinetic evaluation until the medicine is in Phase III, apart from the basic pharmacokinetic trials incorporated into Phase I clinical trials. Proponents of this approach point out that numerous medicines are terminated during Phases I and II and that slowing critical efficacy and safety evaluations delays a medicine's progress. If a decision to terminate the medicine has to be made, it will be made earlier (in general) if efficacy and safety trials are not delayed. If this is not done, then resources expended on pharmacokinetic trials are generally considered to be "wasted."

Other advantages of delaying most of the important pharmacokinetic trials are that (1) the dosage forms to be marketed are more likely to have been developed, (2) the dosages to be tested are known with a far higher certainty, (3) the dosage strengths are more likely to be the same as those to be marketed, and (4) more information has been gathered about the medicine.

CHAPTER 49

Comparing Different Dosage Forms or Treatment Modalities

In some clinical situations it is important to compare two different modalities or dosage forms in the same clinical trial. For example, it may be relevant to ask whether radiation therapy or chemotherapy is a better treatment for patients with a certain type and stage of cancer. It may be important to compare medical and surgical treatment of unstable angina. In addition, there are many cases in which a tablet is compared with another dosage form (e.g., cream, suppository, implant).

CHOOSING AN APPROACH

A few simple approaches for choosing methods to compare different dosage forms or modalities are described. If the disease being evaluated is chronic and relatively stable, it may be suitable to use a crossover design. This design is often preferable to a parallel design because it requires fewer patients to demonstrate effects. There are various precautions, however, that must be considered before this design may be used, including the requirement that the patient's condition return to its original baseline between the two legs of the treatment (i.e., prior to the second treatment). Special care must be taken to prevent period or carryover effects from influencing data. An article by Dubey (1986) contains a description of some pertinent precautions (also, see Chapter 6).

DOSAGE FORMS

Comparing two (or more) dosage forms often requires a placebo medication of each form. This is often impossible when different modalities are compared. Be-

cause of the many biases that surround the usefulness of different dosage forms (or modalities) and the need for an objective evaluation, double-blind clinical trials must almost always be performed. Patients are usually instructed to take or use both medications (e.g., tablet and suppository, capsule and cream) simultaneously, knowing that one, or perhaps both, is a placebo. The usual design is to utilize a three-arm study of (1) dosage form A, (2) dosage form B, and (3) placebo. Patients in the two medicine groups receive one test medicine and a placebo of the other medicine. Patients in the placebo group receive two placebo medications. Either a parallel or crossover design may be used.

Trial Designs When Placebo Cannot Be Used. If a suitable placebo cannot be used for ethical or practical reasons then one can consider either (1) a three-arm study with two doses of the study medicine and an active medicine as control or (2) a dose–response relationship for only one of the dosage forms. In the former design each patient receives one study medicine and appropriate placebo(s) to keep the study double-blind, although no patient receives only placebo treatment (see also Chapter 6).

If a Suitable Placebo Is Only Available for One Treatment. If a suitable placebo can be made for dosage form A, but not dosage form B, it may still be possible to study both agents in a double-blind clinical trial. Conduct a dose–response trial in one or more groups for dosage form B. All of these patients should receive the placebo for dosage form A. A separate group should receive the single dose of dosage form A and the lowest dose possible of dosage form B. This dose of dosage form B will have been chosen to be homeopathic (i.e., equivalent to a placebo) and should be insufficient to interact with the other dosage form.

TREATMENT MODALITIES

Sham Procedures. Although some treatment modalities may not be easily blinded in clinical studies, it is often possible to conduct a sham procedure (e.g., sham radiation treatment, sham insertion of a medical device) that may serve as an excellent "placebo." Thus, it may be possible in either a crossover or parallel design to initiate a double-blind trial comparable to one of those proposed to evaluate two dosage forms.

Evaluating Two Modalities in Separate Trials. If both modalities cannot be compared in the same clinical trial it is important to evaluate each separately under double-blind conditions. In this situation of two separate trials it is preferable if each treatment modality is evaluated simultaneously at a single site by the same investigators. This will avoid the necessity of using historical data or data collected in a double-blind trial conducted under other experimental conditions. Controlling trials with historical data is usually the least desirable approach.

Current Standards. Current standards used in designing clinical trials vary for different modalities. Unfortunately, there are very different standards for introducing new medicines into medical practice and introducing other modalities, equipment, and techniques. Standards for new medicines are generally far higher than for other treatment modalities or for medical equipment. Challah and Mays (1986) describe this difference and illustrate that "Gastric freezing, high concentration oxygen for neonates, the use of hyperbaric oxygen in intensive care, and insulin coma for the treatment of schizophrenia are all examples of innovations introduced without evaluation and subsequently abandoned because they proved ineffective or unsafe." Clearly, it is in everyone's interest to utilize high standards before new nonmedicine modalities of treatment or diagnosis are accepted. Standards are influenced primarily by regulatory authorities and peer pressure.

CHAPTER 50

Combination Medicine Trials

INTRODUCTION

What Are Combination Medicines? Combination medicines consist of two or more separate active ingredients that are combined to improve the efficacy, safety, compliance, or another characteristic of the separate ingredients or medicines. In this discussion it will be assumed that the combination medicine is scientifically and medically rational and has a clearly defined clinical objective.

Types of Combination Medicines. The considerations in this chapter are for a single fixed-dose combination of two or more active medicines. There are also medicine "combinations": two or more medicines are given as a mixture or are given sequentially. The study designs and many of the considerations of developing a single combination described are also applicable in these other situations. The medicines combined may each be of the same therapeutic class (e.g., two analgesics) or differing therapeutic classes (e.g., an antihistamine and a sympathomimetic decongestant), or one agent may be almost therapeutically inactive on its own for the indication but in combination may potentiate the active medicine (e.g., probenecid plus penicillin). Combinations of these objectives may be present in the same product, especially if three or more medicines are combined. Readers interested in detailed discussions on combination medicines are referred to monographs edited by Lasagna (1975) and Mezey (1980).

FDA REGULATORY POLICY

The Food and Drug Administration (FDA) combination medicine policy states that each active ingredient in the combination must contribute to the overall safety and/or efficacy of the combination. The exact wording of the regulations in 21CFR 300.50 states: "Two or more medicines may be combined in a single dosage form when each component makes a contribution to the claimed effects and the dosage of each component (amount, frequency, duration) is such that the combination is safe and effective for a significant patient population requiring such concurrent therapy as defined in the labeling for the medicine." Note that no requirements for potentiation of effects is required, or even that effects be additive.

RELEVANT QUESTIONS TO ADDRESS IN DEVELOPING OR TESTING COMBINATION MEDICINES

1. Is there a patient population that needs or will significantly benefit from the combination?
2. If the combination medicine is significantly better than placebo, is it also necessary for each ingredient of the combination to be better than placebo? The answer is "sometimes," which means that this question must be applied separately to each combination. It may be more relevant to ask whether the combination must be better than pla-

cebo. It is not always necessary for this comparison to be made. The combination, however, must have advantages over each of its individual constituents given alone.

3. If it is impossible or impractical to demonstrate that a combination is better than either one or both of the individual ingredients in a proposed clinical trial is it possible to redesign the trial to:
   a. Study multiple doses of the combination?
   b. Measure two or more different objective endpoints (parameters)?
   c. Use multiple trial designs?
   d. Use multiple patient populations?
   e. Use less objective endpoints to measure relevant parameters (e.g., patient's clinical global impressions, quality of life measures)?

4. If it is not possible to demonstrate greater efficacy for the combination product over one (or both) of the single agents, but the safety profile is better and/or the medicine is better tolerated, can the combination medicine be developed and marketed?

5. What is the importance of patient convenience as a factor for deciding to develop a combination medicine?

TABLE 50.1 *Potential advantages of developing combination medicines*

1. Obtain an enhanced clinical effect by two (or more) medicines acting via different mechanisms (e.g., trimethoprim and a sulfonamide antibiotic for many infections, diuretic plus β-receptor antagonist in hypertension)
2. Improve the therapeutic ratio by utilizing a smaller dose of one or more medicines that avoids toxicity (i.e., decreases adverse reactions) (e.g., combination of L-DOPA and a DOPA decarboxylase inhibitor for treating patients with Parkinson's disease)
3. Multiple clinical effects are achieved in a disease or syndrome in which these activities are desired (e.g., various cough, cold, expectorant combinations)
4. Decrease the magnitude of peak-to-trough differences in physiological responses
5. Decrease the potential for medicine abuse (e.g., naloxone plus pentazocine)
6. Increase the duration of effective treatment by combining an immediate-release form of one medicine and a sustained-release form of another
7. Reduce the cost of medicine treatment
8. Increase the convenience for oral dosing
9. Obtain a lower Drug Enforcement Administration (DEA) scheduling than for a single agent
10. Enhance patient compliance because there are fewer tablets or capsules to take
11. Give a controlled ratio of two medicines to patients[a]
12. Enhance ease of administration (e.g., multiple vaccines are sometimes given in a single injection)
13. Decrease vulnerability to competition from generic medicines (e.g., one of the medicines may be protected by patent, the technology of medicine manufacture may be highly complex)
14. Allow for a more effective entry of a successful (or previously unsuccessful) medicine into new markets

[a] This may also be a disadvantage.

TABLE 50.2 *Potential disadvantages of developing combination medicines*

1. Physicians do not have adequate flexibility to adjust the dose of individual components
2. Cost of medicine may be more for the patient than if each medicine were prescribed separately
3. Combinations are sometimes prescribed by physicians as a "shotgun" approach to avoid careful diagnosis and/or therapy
4. Pharmacokinetics of the two medicines may be incompatible
5. Medicine combination may be used inappropriately by physicians or patients
6. Physicians may be unaware of the identity of the specific medicines in combinations
7. Certain irrational combinations may be prepared
8. Technical difficulties of developing certain combinations may be insurmountable

6. Which medicines should be combined and what is the scientific and medical basis for each medicine proposed?

7. How many different ratios of doses of the ingredients in a combination should be tested to evaluate the "ideal mix"?

Potential advantages and disadvantages of developing combination medicines are listed in Tables 50.1 and 50.2. Types of combination medicines are listed in Table 50.3; criteria to be met for most combination medicines are listed in Table 50.4.

TABLE 50.3 *Selected types of combination medicines[a]*

A. Both ingredients act on the same symptom, disease, or problem
   1. Two similar medicines of the same therapeutic class (e.g., two mild analgesics such as aspirin and acetaminophen; two diuretics with different, but complementary, mechanisms and sites of action, such as spironolactone and hydrochlorothiazide)
   2. Two medicines of the same therapeutic class, but of different potencies (e.g., aspirin and codeine)
B. Each ingredient acts on different symptoms, diseases, or problems
   1. Each contributes to the desired overall effect (e.g., triprolidine and pseudoephedrine)
C. Other type of combinations
   1. One active medicine plus one adjuvant[b]
      a. To enhance absorption (e.g., aspirin plus sodium bicarbonate)
      b. To delay excretion (e.g., penicillin plus probenecid)
   2. One active medicine plus a second medicine to decrease an adverse reaction or potential for one
   3. One active medicine plus a second medicine to decrease abuse potential (e.g., pentazocine plus naloxone)
   4. Mixtures of medicines [e.g., multiple vaccines such as diphtheria-pertussis–tetanus (DPT)]
   5. One medicine has an action that allows less of the other medicine to be used (e.g., DOPA decarboxylase inhibitor and L-DOPA)

[a] All examples are of two-ingredient combinations. Three-or-more-component combinations could also be described.
[b] An adjuvant is an inactive agent on the primary symptoms treated that increases the effect of the other medicine.

TABLE 50.4 *Criteria to be met for development of most combination medicines*[a]

1. Complete pharmaceutical compatibility (e.g., no interactions between the chemicals)
2. Dosage of only one component in the combination should be critical (e.g., if two or more components were critical then numerous ratios of the fixed combination would be needed to have a practical combination)
3. The combination provides an effect that is not possible to achieve from either medicine alone
4. Toxicity of the individual components is not synergistic or potentiated
5. Frequency of administration of the two medicines is the same
6. A population exists that can use (or needs) the combination

[a] These criteria are not intended to reflect a policy of any regulatory agency or sponsor.

DESIGNING CLINICAL STUDIES TO EVALUATE COMBINATION MEDICINES

Identifying the Optimal Doses of Each Ingredient

An initial step is to identify the optimal dose(s) of each medicine to use in the combination medicine. Holding the dose of one medicine constant and then varying the other will probably provide information on the dose of the second medicine to use. The clinical trial may be repeated, holding the dose of the opposite medicine constant. Nonetheless, this method will not definitely identify the ideal combination of doses to use with even two ingredients. This may occur because the two trials described were both designed to demonstrate the best dose of the variable medicine to use in relation to a fixed dose of the other medicine. However, if a smaller (or larger) fixed dose had been used, then different results might have been obtained. This is especially true if one medicine potentiates the effects of another. Because of the substantial knowledge that usually exists about at least one of the medicines when development of a combination product is considered, a small number of combination doses may usually be chosen on a rational basis. If the combination involves three (or more) medicines, then the number of possible dose combinations becomes extremely large and a definitive path to reaching the optimal combination is almost impossible to determine in advance of conducting studies. More "educated guesses" will generally have to be made in this situation.

Another approach to identifying doses to use in a combination is to utilize multiple dose ranges for each medicine. Patients in the first dosage group may receive from X to Y mg of medicine A and from V to W mg of medicine B (or placebo). A second group is given a larger dose and may receive from 2 to 4 times the dose given to the first group. A third group could receive an even larger dose. This study should provide data on which dose ranges were best (and least) tol-

erated and which ranges were most efficacious. Further studies could evaluate this issue in greater detail. Nonetheless, it is often only necessary to study one or two doses of one medicine in a combination. A summary of some methods to demonstrate clinical superiority of a combination product is given in Table 50.5.

Factorial Designs

The classic study design to evaluate a combination medicine uses a factorial design. The factorial design includes each active ingredient of the combination, the combination, and placebo. For a two-medicine combination (medicines A and B), there would be four treatment groups and in a parallel study each patient would receive two medications: (1) placebos of medicine A and medicine B, (2) medicine A plus placebo of medicine B, (3) medicine B plus placebo of A, or (4) medicine A plus medicine B. For a three-medicine combination, eight groups are possible (the full combination, three combinations of two medicines each, three single ingredients, and placebo). Several examples of study designs useful for evaluating combination medicines are illustrated in Fig. 50.1.

In most situations the effectiveness of one of the medicines in a combination is well established and it is then of interest to determine if its activity is enhanced with a second medicine. A semifactorial design could be considered in which the effective medicine is compared with the combination. In some ways this would be like testing a medicine versus placebo, since

TABLE 50.5 *Selected types of clinical results that demonstrate therapeutic superiority of a combination medicine over its individual constituents*[a]

| Scenario | Therapeutic value | | | |
	Medicine A	Medicine B	Combination of medicines A and B	Placebo[a]
1	+ +[c]	0	+ + +	0 to +
2	0	+ +	+ + +	0 to +
3	+	+	+ +	0 to +
4	+	0 to +	+ +	0 to +
5	−	0	+ +	0 to +
6	−	+	+ +	0 to +

[a] Clinical superiority of a combination product may also be based on an improved safety profile (e.g., decreased severity or incidence of adverse reactions), improved pharmacokinetic considerations, or decreased abuse potential, compared with each component. In such cases the efficacy of the combination may not be enhanced over the efficacy of the individual components.

[b] A placebo arm in the study design is not mandatory for evaluating the components of a combination, although it is usually desirable.

[c] +, a positive therapeutic effect; + +, a stronger positive therapeutic effect; + + +, an even stronger positive therapeutic effect; −, a negative therapeutic effect; 0, no clinical effect.

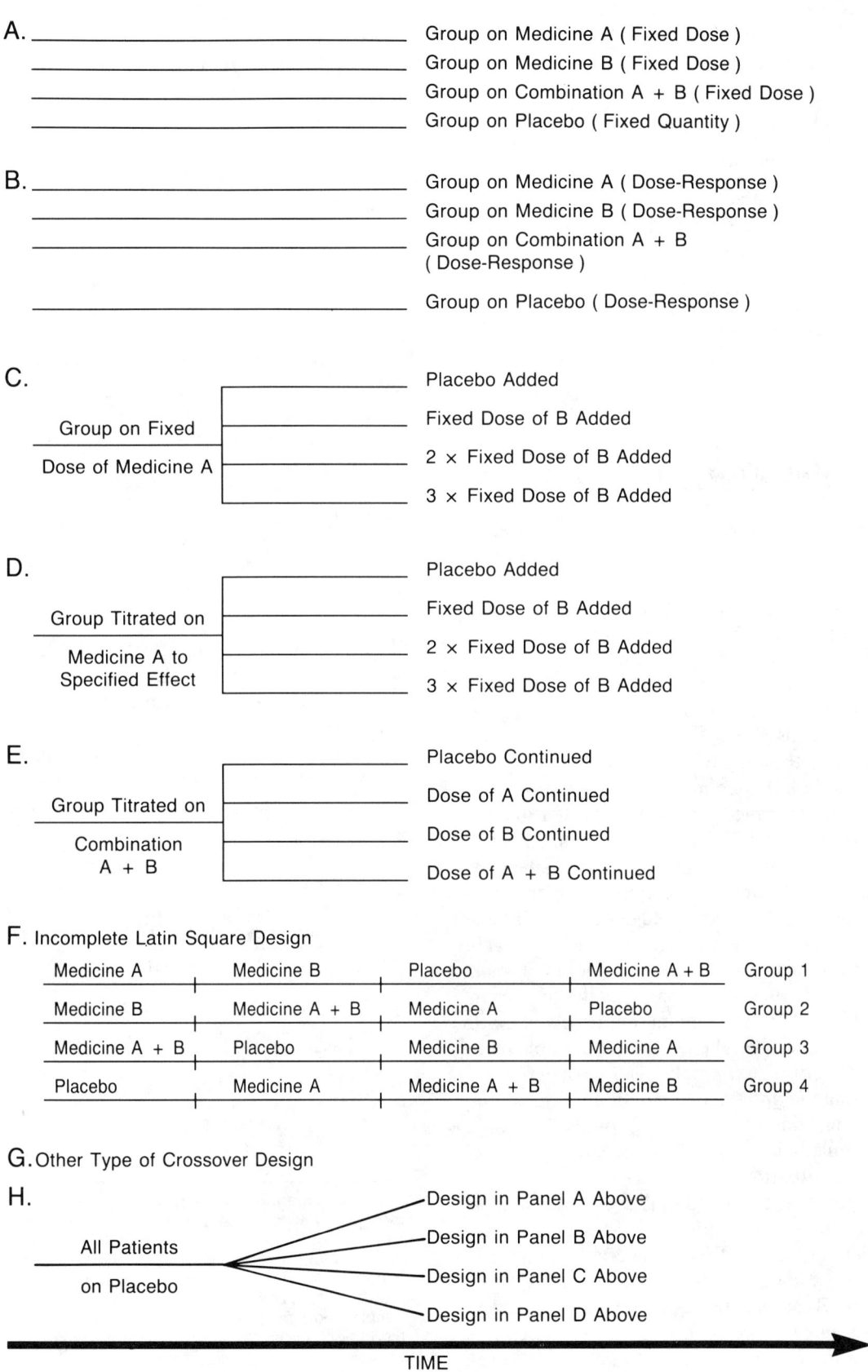

FIG. 50.1 Selected clinical trial designs to evaluate combination medicines. Many variations on these trial designs are possible.

the activity of the active medicine is equivalent to a baseline. This design may be used to study a medicine that potentiates another, but does not have any activity on its own (e.g., probenecid and penicillin). If potentiation is expected with an active medicine, then a lower than optimally effective dose may be studied in combination with various doses of the other medicine.

CREATING A SUITABLE FORMULATION

In developing a suitable tablet or capsule formulation of a combination medicine product numerous problems may be encountered. These are discussed under the headings of physical, chemical, and pharmacokinetic issues.

Physical Issues

Differences in bulk density, particle size, or particle shape between two medicines to be combined may cause problems during the mixing process from poor flow characteristics or particle segregation of the dry chemicals. Poor content uniformity of the medicines in the dosage form may result. Poor compressibility of one or both components may produce soft, friable tablets. Hygroscopicity or eutectic formation between the components may cause the formulation to stick to the tablet punch, resulting in an unacceptable appearance, or cause chemical degradation. These problems may be minimized by careful sizing (shifting or milling) of the particles to prevent segregation; inclusion of a granulating step to minimize differences in physical characteristics or overcome compressibility problems; careful selection of ingredients such as compression aids, binders, lubricants, dispersants, and antiadherents; by inclusion of adsorbents to remove excess moisture.

How will capsules be filled to ensure that each contains the precise amount of each ingredient? Capsules sold commercially are filled by machines and it is difficult to mix two large batches of powders sufficiently well in the correct ratio to ensure that every capsule is filled with, for example, 75 mg of medicine A and 25 mg of medicine B. If small beads of one (or both) medicines are prepared, then mixtures may be made and adequate samples of the capsules may be taken to ensure that they contain the correct weight of each compound. This same problem exists when tablets are compressed.

Numerous excipients must be added to almost all chemicals to make a medicine (see Chapter 18). Each excipient is carefully determined through many pharmaceutical tests. When two (or more) medicines are to be combined in a tablet then all these procedures must be conducted anew. There are many more difficulties in finding the ideal excipients for a combination than for a single medicine. If all appropriate excipients are found, then the physical form of the medicines may differ from each other and may not be adequately homogeneous for tabletting. For example, one medicine may be in the form of a light fluffy powder and the other in a hard granular form. In order to compress the dry powder and form a single tablet the two medicines must be brought closer together in physical characteristics.

Chemical Issues

Chemical interactions between medicines may adversely affect the long-term stability of the combination. These problems may be overcome by addition of stabilizing agents (i.e., antioxidants), use of a more stable salt of the medicine or a physical separation of the major components. For capsules, separation may be accomplished by inserting a tablet of one medicine in a capsule followed by a powder of the second medicine, or by filling pellets of each medicine separately into a capsule. Further separation of components may be accomplished by applying a barrier coating to the tablet or pellets to be filled into capsules. Separation of components in a tablet dosage form may also be accomplished using bilayered or trilayered tablets, or compression-coated tablets consisting of a core of one medicine coated with a granulation of the second medicine, or by microencapsulating one or both medicines prior to compression.

Because of all the potential physical and chemical problems described above, innovative technical solutions to these issues have been sought. Several approaches involve development of a slow-release form. Slow-release forms may be created in many ways, including (1) creating pellets of a medicine and coating them with a slowly dissolving polymer, or (2) coating an inert sugar granule with medicines and then coating this with a slowly dissolving polymer.

Pharmacokinetic Issues

In addition to the physical and chemical problems that have been described, there may also be a large variety of pharmacokinetic issues to address. A combination of two medicines that makes rational scientific and medical sense may involve medicines with vastly different half-lives and durations of biological effects. This may prevent a combination medicine from being developed if one ingredient had to be taken more frequently than the other and a suitable sustained-release form of that medicine could not be prepared. The pharmacokinetics of the two may differ greatly in terms of absorption, distribution, metabolism, and excretion.

An important point is that there should not be chemical or other interactions between the ingredients in a combination that affect pharmacokinetics in an unpredictable manner. The number of potentially important technical and clinical problems that may arise is almost limitless.

In conclusion, the successful development of combination products involves consideration of more variables and factors to be controlled than for a single medicine. This makes the entire process of developing a combination product more time consuming. There are often compromises that must be made (e.g., shorter product expiration dates). Production costs for combination medicines are usually greater than for single entity medicines, because of additional steps for granulating, microencapsulation, producing layered tablets, or other steps that must be incorporated into the manufacturing process.

Marketing-Oriented Clinical Studies

There is a widespread myth in some academic circles that marketing studies are the primary type of clinical study conducted by the pharmaceutical industry. Because some of these studies are poorly designed and conducted, even many well-respected academicians have an overall poor opinion of industry-sponsored clinical studies. The truth is that almost all Phases I and II clinical trials, and many Phases III and IV trials sponsored by the pharmaceutical industry are not marketing studies and are extremely well designed, conducted, and analyzed. Numerous marketing-oriented studies conducted during Phases III and IV have been relatively poorly designed and conducted in the past, but standards are beginning to improve.

GENERAL CONSIDERATIONS

A marketing group that intends to sponsor clinical studies to evaluate a new medicine, device, or therapy should carefully review its goals before designing or providing input. Their goals should dictate the type and quality of the study. The design of all clinical studies they sponsor should be determined in cooperation with medical personnel. Decisions about the study must be made based on (1) the medical specialty and reputation of investigators, (2) the type of safety, efficacy, economic, quality of life, or other endpoints to focus on, (3) the comparative medicines to include, (4) the ability of investigators to initiate and complete the study

within the desired time frame, and (5) the reputation of the facility. Various other factors described in earlier chapters may also be pertinent.

STUDY DESIGNS

Clinical studies conducted primarily for marketing groups may use any type of study design and may be conducted at any scientific level or standard. Because these studies are seldom submitted to regulatory authorities as a basis for the medicine's approval, the standards achieved are usually not as high as for most clinical trials (see Table 51.1). Some marketing studies in the past have used such poor designs that they would raise issues of questionable ethical standards if those studies were conducted today.

Choice of Endpoints

The most desirable endpoints to select for marketing studies are those that show advantages of the company's products over those of the competitors. If a study's results are to be targeted to formulary committees, then measuring financial endpoints to demonstrate economic benefits is desirable. To motivate practicing physicians to use the new medicine, improvements in efficacy or safety parameters are usually required. Other endpoints that are often useful to

TABLE 51.1 *Generally observed differences between clinical trials and marketing-oriented studies[a]*

Item	Phase I to III clinical trials	Phase III and IV marketing studies
Medical environment	Clinical laboratory, clinic, or hospital	Usual medical practice
Patient population	Restricted	Unrestricted
Number of patients	Few	Many
Investigator	Research-oriented	Practice-oriented
Protocol	Fixed	Flexible
Concomitant therapy	Uncommon in phases I and II, and more common in phase III	Common
Patient evaluation	As objective as possible	Less detailed, more subjective, and fewer objective tests are conducted
Design of trial	Formal structure	Informal or less formal approach
Blind of trial	Often double-blind	Usually open-label
Sponsor's goal in conducting the trial	Evaluation of safety and efficacy	Obtaining data for promotional purposes

[a] Numerous exceptions exist to each point.

assess in marketing studies include patient compliance, convenience, and quality of life.

Number of Patients

If an insufficient number of patients are enrolled and evaluated in a study, no effect of the medicine may be observed, or the effect may be opposite to what is expected. Even if a strongly positive (i.e., desired) effect is observed, there will be too few patients for the data to convince many (if not most) physicians. If the number of patients enrolled is too large some effects that are statistically significant may be trivial from a clinical perspective (e.g., heart rate may change by three beats per minute). Large numbers of patients furnishing anecdotal information provide little value. More attention is being focused on clinical significance of data, as well as on statistical significance.

SEEDING TRIALS

Seeding Trials That Are Published

In this type of Phase III or IV marketing-oriented seeding trial, data are collected from a relatively large number of physicians. Each physician is given sufficient medicine to treat X number of patients in a "real life" way. Physicians may be recruited by sales representatives, direct letters from the company, clinical monitors, or other methods. A simple data collection form is returned to the sponsor, data are analyzed, and the results are published. One of the problems with this approach is that medicines are not usually prescribed and used as intended (e.g., patients may be under- or overdosed). Also, no consistent endpoints are used to measure response. This type of study could potentially be advantageous to the sponsor, if the goal is to learn how the medicine will be initially used in the community or how the sponsor can better educate physicians to use the medicine appropriately. More important objections are that the clinical trials are open label

and are not sufficiently controlled to draw valid conclusions.

Seeding Studies Purportedly Conducted as Scientific Studies

Before 1980, numerous marketing studies were conducted in which pharmaceutical companies gave many physicians medicine samples to use. Physicians were asked to report their results and overall assessment of the medicine. The sponsor pretended that the collected data would be used for a publication. No publication was ever intended or resulted from the clinical "study." This practice is unethical and is not currently followed at most pharmaceutical companies today, but, seeding studies acquired a bad reputation with many physicians. A disadvantage of designing this type of study for the sponsor is that the data might include a large number of adverse events that must be reported to a regulatory authority and followed up with monitoring visits.

In some of these marketing studies, gadgets or money were given to physicians to "motivate them" to try a (usually) new medicine. These practices are usually questionable from an ethical perspective. It is similarly unethical to extract patient data from large data bases and apply them to studies of questionable

TABLE 51.2 *Selected problems with some marketing-oriented studies*

1. The number of patients enrolled and evaluated is too small to show the effect desired
2. Endpoints chosen were those known to show the effect desired rather than more appropriate ones
3. Study designs were usually open-label, even when a double-blind design was feasible
4. Studies were inadequately monitored
5. Seeding studies were thinly veiled attempts to get many physicians to use a medicine or new dosage form
6. Results were inadequately or poorly analyzed statistically
7. No control groups were included
8. Retrospective designs were used
9. Historical controls were used

value. Having an Ethics Committee/Investigational Review Board review all protocols should protect the public from such studies being used as "fishing expeditions" that might lead too inappropriate conclusions.

Seeding Trials That Lead to a Roundtable or Panel Discussion and Possible Publication

Another type of seeding study involves asking selected physicians to use a new medicine for a certain period of time and then bringing these professionals together to discuss their experiences. These physicians are often chosen because they are well-respected academicians. The transcript of the focus group they hold is edited and published in a "throw-away" (i.e., non-peer-reviewed) journal, house organ (i.e., newsletter or journal of a hospital), or brochure prepared by the company, or other sponsor. This latter publication is then widely disseminated as a promotional piece. Video and audiotapes of the clinical discussions may also be made and used. Some of the problems encountered in these and other marketing studies are listed in Table 51.2.

COMPARATIVE TRIALS

Focus of Comparative Trials

Marketing groups often compare new medicines with standard therapy during Phases III or IV. These comparative trials may focus on one or more aspects of clinical efficacy, safety, quality of life, cost–effectiveness, or any other area in which data are sought to demonstrate advantages for their product over those of their competitors.

Stacking the Deck (i.e., Biasing the Study) in One's Favor

Comparative marketing trials are frequently designed so that they have the greatest probability to show those advantages that are expected to be found. Ethical standards used in this approach may be questioned if the major parameters or endpoints evaluated are substandard, incomplete, or inappropriate, or are altered in such a way that the anticipated results are more likely to occur. Physicians who eventually read reports or publications about these trials are usually astute enough to determine whether the trial was inappropriately designed or poorly conducted.

Conducting open-label studies also stacks the deck in one's favor. The number of positive responses in open-label or active medicine controlled trials far exceeds those obtained in double-blind trials (see Chapter 4). Other means of stacking the deck in one's favor

TABLE 51.3 *Factors influencing the choice of a comparison medicine for marketing studies*

1. The market leader
2. The prototype
3. The expected future market leader
4. The major medicine in the same chemical class
5. The major medicine in the same therapeutic class
6. A similar type of combination medicine
7. Medicine on the market in a selected country

are to study too few patients or to study patients for too short a time period. A final method mentioned would be to look at subjective improvement assessed either by the physician or patient, without measuring the objective change from the patient's baseline status. Any other bias introduced (or not eliminated), or use of a poor study design, could also be described as stacking the deck in one's favor.

Choosing the Comparative Treatment(s)

The choice of a comparative medicine is based on a number of considerations (listed in Table 51.3). Any one of these may be paramount in the choice made for a particular trial.

Investigational medicines of a competitor usually are not chosen for comparison because (1) the other company is less likely to supply the medicine before it is on the market, (2) there may be excessive "red tape" if the medicine has not yet been imported into the country where the trial would be conducted, and (3) regulatory authorities may not accept the data obtained from such a trial, even as supportive evidence.

CHOOSING INVESTIGATORS FOR MARKETING STUDIES AND TRIALS

The criteria for choosing investigators for marketing-oriented studies may be very different from those used for clinical trials (see Chapter 59). While the criteria used in clinical trials may also be relevant (or even critical) for marketing studies, other factors may be relevant, such as (1) who are the best speakers, (2) who are the most influential in professional societies, (3) who are the most influential in political circles, or (4) who are willing to travel and speak about their clinical experiences with the new medicine. Speakers should be willing to answer questions about their presentation that are posed by the audience.

There is no reason why marketing studies cannot be designed, conducted, analyzed, and interpreted at the same level as clinical trials are done, to obtain regulatory approval. When lesser standards are used they should not only meet the highest ethical standards, but also meet those standards that the medical community finds acceptable.

CHAPTER 52

Quality of Life Trials

DEFINITIONS

It is ironic that despite the frequent use of the term quality of life, there are few formal definitions of the term in medical literature. Nonetheless, many authors discuss quality of life as if its meaning is generally understood. The term is used so loosely by so many that an extremely large number of usages, but not definitions, exist. This chapter discusses health-related quality of life, because total quality of life includes environmental issues (e.g., water and air quality), geographical issues (e.g., cultural opportunities), and other aspects.

A fairly complete, but rather general definition was proposed by Calman (1984). He wrote that "The quality of life can only be described in individual terms, and depends on present lifestyle, past experience, hopes for the future, dreams and ambition. Quality of life must include all areas of life and experience and take into account the impact of illness and treatment. A good quality of life can be said to be present when the hopes of an individual are matched and fulfilled by experience. The opposite is also true: a poor quality of life occurs when the hopes do not meet with the experience. Quality of life changes with time and . . . measures the difference, at a particular moment in time, between the hopes and expectations of the individual and that individual's present experiences." This is an excellent general definition at the level of an individual, but quality of life also exists for groups of patients, for an entire community, and also at the national level.

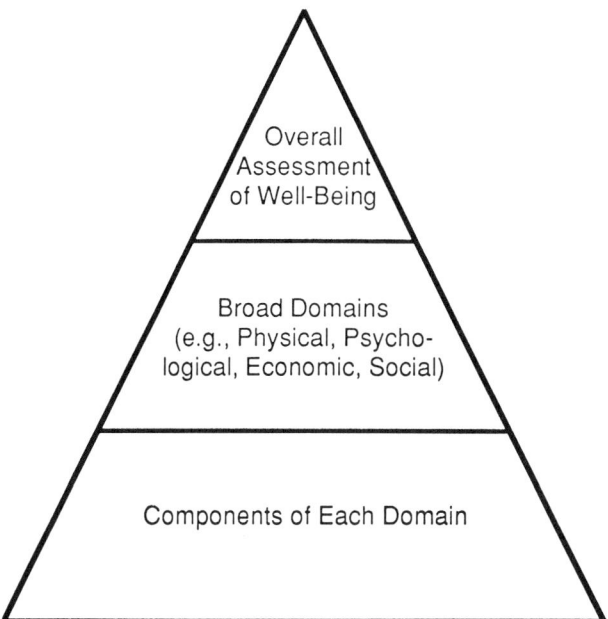

FIG. 52.1 Levels of quality of life. (Reprinted from Spilker, 1990a, with permission of Raven Press.)

Schipper et al. (1990) proposed the following definition: "Quality of life represents the functional effect of an illness and its consequent therapy upon a patient as perceived by the patient. Four broad domains contribute to the overall effect: physical and occupational function; psychologic state; social interaction; and somatic sensation."

A general frame of reference for viewing quality of life data for individual patients (or groups) was described by Spilker (1990a). This approach is illustrated with a pyramid (Fig. 52.1) to show the overall level, individual domains (e.g., physical abilities, social interactions, psychological well-being, economic status), and components of each domain.

PERSPECTIVES

Great differences are apparent in the perspectives of academicians, regulators, pharmaceutical companies, formulary committees, physicians, ethicists, and other groups who view quality of life trials, plus their need, appropriate designs, and interpretations. These and other perspectives are presented in detail in *Quality of Life Assessments in Clinical Trials* (Spilker, 1990a). Determining appropriate methods for quality of life trials depends primarily on the perspectives and goals of those who design the trial.

Cost–effectiveness trials are sometimes described as a subset of quality of life trials. Whether this is appropriate and correct is beyond the scope of this chap-

ter. Cost–effectiveness trials are discussed in Chapter 42.

Why Has Interest in Quality of Life Increased in Recent Years?

A number of factors, primarily economic and social, have combined to focus more attention on quality of life issues in recent years. There has been a rapid rise in the percent of gross national product spent on health care in several countries. In addition, patients are taking increased responsibility for their own care and are applying more rigorous standards when choosing medical care. Perspectives of some different audiences follow.

The concept of cost containment swept the United States during the late 1970s and 1980s. *Health administrators* are less willing to devote huge sums of money to health care, yet the costs of medical technology, which are currently high, are escalating rapidly. *Consumers* of medical care often feel that they are receiving many treatments, but not adequate care. To the consumer, it often seems that the physician focuses entirely on objective benefits of treatment, ignoring how patients feel. *Regulatory authorities* realize that in certain cases, quality of life endpoints represent viable surrogate parameters for measuring a treatment's efficacy. *Pharmaceutical companies* recognize that formulary committees are willing to use qualify of life data as a basis for accepting a new medicine onto a formulary.

CLASSIFICATION OF QUALITY OF LIFE TESTS

The simplest classification of quality of life tests divides them into indexes, profiles, and batteries.

Indexes. An index is a test that yields a single number at its conclusion. It usually evaluates multiple domains and often tests multiple components of each domain. The test may include measures of the quantity, as well as the quality, of life. The Quality of Well-Being Scale is an example of an index. Scores for subtests are not obtained.

Profiles. A profile is a test that covers multiple domains and components of these domains, but yields a number of separate scores. Each score is for a separate category of questions, and an overall score may also be obtained. Categories of the subtests scores may or may not be synonymous with domains. The Sickness Impact Profile Test is an example of a profile.

Battery. Multiple tests are used to measure several domains or several components of a single domain. These tests are chosen to cover a broad area of interest. Each test is interpreted independently, and results cannot be combined. Nonetheless, interpretations can be evaluated together.

METHODOLOGICAL PRINCIPLES

Validation of Tests

The validity of a test or scale should be documented and not assumed. Begin the search for the validation as far in advance of the quality of life trial as possible, because the process of determining the validity of a test may take a long time. This is discussed further in Chapter 43. Write to the scale's authors for information if a literature search is not productive. Given the critical importance of using validated tests, it is disappointing that authors of currently published articles in major journals are seldom using validated tests (Guyatt et al., 1989).

The applicability of a scale to the disease studied should be known. It is not generally necessary for a validated scale to have been validated in the specific patient population it is being tested in, but there should be a reasonable basis for its use in the group(s) evaluated.

Figure 52.1 illustrates three levels. It is unnecessary to validate the general question posed to assess the overall top level. For the other two levels it is best to validate tests within and across these three levels, particularly not by comparing with the top level. It is always important in attempting to validate tests to ask the question: Is it useful?

Sensitivity of Tests

The demonstration that a test or scale is sensitive to a patient's change during a clinical trial must be shown. The fact that a test or scale validity measures one or more domains (or components) does not mean that the test is able to measure the change brought about by a medicine.

Frequency of Test Administration

The correct frequency of administering the test or scale should be known. Baseline assessments should be obtained prior to initiating therapy. Whenever possible, baseline assessments should be obtained both prior to and subsequent to washout of any medicines the patient is using at the time of screening. Quality of life data are often presented as change from baseline. Follow-up mechanisms must retrieve sufficient data from each patient using a variety of methods (e.g., telephone, mail-in, home interviews). The recall period requested of patients in a questionnaire is usually any time up to 2 to 4 weeks.

Training Effect

The mere fact that a test is given on multiple occasions may enable patients to improve (or modify) their performance. This is referred to as a training effect. Whether a training effect occurs on repeat testing should be determined both for patients taking the test and for investigators or staff administering and interpreting the test.

Patient Stratification

The ability to stratify patients based on their baseline quality of life scores should be known or determined prior to the quality of life trial. This may be based on results from a single test or according to a complex weighting of multiple test results that are combined.

Maintaining a Blind

The staff member(s) rating a patient as well as the patient should be blind to the treatment group's identity and to responses of therapy. If patients are told that they are improving during the trial, or simply believe they are, then they may in turn feel better and report an improved quality of life. While patients may always believe whatever they choose, it is important to avoid feedback from the investigator or staff in a controlled trial that systematically influences patients. This is one of the major sources of bias in open-label clinical trials that leads to a high rate of positive results.

Statistical Analyses

The appropriate statistical methods to analyze scales should be determined. Close collaboration with a qualified statistician is essential to ensure that data are analyzed correctly.

The correlation of results with specific efficacy or safety endpoints studied should be determined after the quality of life trial is completed and the data are processed. This evaluation may be one of the primary or secondary objectives of the clinical trial.

It is impossible to merge results obtained from separate quality of life tests into a single overall outcome. This goal may sometimes be approached by rank ordering each patient's score on multiple tests and then combining these numbers. The issue of weighting of scales used in the quality of life assessment is important in this regard. The results of each individual test can also be presented in a manner that makes any clear trends become apparent (Fig. 97.1).

The question of how data from patients who are premature dropouts are to be handled should be discussed prior to conducting the quality of life trial. For ex-

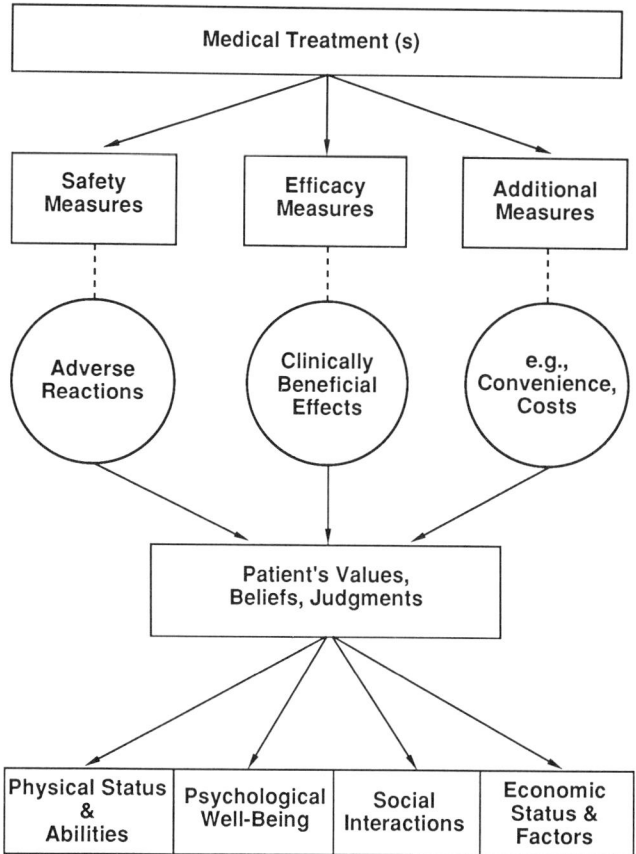

FIG. 52.2 Model of how clinical aspects of efficacy (i.e., benefits), safety (e.g., adverse reactions), or other factors filter through the patients' values and beliefs to influence his or her quality of life domains. (Reprinted from Spilker, 1990a, with permission of Raven Press.)

ample, an intent-to-treat analysis may or may not be appropriate.

Planning the Approach

The choice of a basic approach to quality of life trials can be summed up by the following question. Should one identify the categories of quality of life information one wants to know more about, and *then* identify the tests that can provide that information, *or* should one follow the opposite approach and choose tests of interest and then identify what information they will provide? Neither approach is correct for all cases, and differences of opinion exist on which approach is superior.

Standardizing the Methods Used for Interviews

Many quality of life tests utilize interview techniques to obtain patient responses. The tone and manner used to ask a question as well as the question itself should be specified in a protocol. Asking patients "How are

you truly feeling today" in a friendly manner may elicit different responses from the question "'You are feeling well today, aren't you?" The interviewer should be the same from visit to visit to avoid introducing confounding factors.

Watching video tapes of interviews can help investigators standardize their approach to diagnosis and categorizing adverse reactions.

Interrater reliability should be evaluated whenever two or more raters perform the same test. The nature of the tests chosen and objectives of the trial are necessary to consider before determining whether interrater reliability is essential to evaluate.

How Are Scales Administered?

Three basic approaches to completing scales are followed.

1. *Self-administered tests.* Patients complete the test entirely on their own, usually without a fixed time limit. The patient may or may not actually complete the test.
2. *Interviewer-administered tests.* Interviewer completes the test based on the patient's answers to specific test questions or the interviewer's assessment of the patient's responses.
3. *Interviewer-supervised self-administered tests.* This approach is a variation on the first method, whereby the interviewer confirms that the patient completely filled in each relevant question. The interviewer also should confirm that the patient understood each question.

The last method is particularly useful because it eliminates the implicit assumption in the first method—that all people interpret a test question the same way. The interviewer should know what each question means and be able to ensure that the answers obtained are realistic and appropriate. The last method also avoids the problem of patients who are semiliterate or actually illiterate. Picture charts are used in some tests to obtain reliable ratings from illiterate patients.

Must All Sites in a Multicenter Trial Measure Quality of Life?

If only some centers in a multicenter trial measure quality of life, various biases are likely to enter the overall clinical trial. If some sites agree to collect these data but do not, significant differences in patient treatment could result. Thus, all sites in a multicenter trial should utilize the same protocol vis-à-vis quality of life tests and evaluations.

Expressing Results of Batteries of Tests

Although each test may be separately interpreted and presented, it is often valuable to aggregate results. This could be done by stating that six of nine different tests showed X, four of nine tests showed Y, and so forth.

If no differences are observed in two or more quality of life scales, it may mean that no differences were present or merely that the tests were insensitive or improperly given. If differences observed on multiple tests are opposite to the clinical effects observed, various interpretations are possible (see Table 52.1). Finally, the same differences may be observed in both clinical parameters as well as quality of life tests.

What Types of Global Quality of Life Questions Exist?

Although physicians (or others) may provide an overall clinical judgment of patients' disease severity or degree of improvement, it is inappropriate for physicians to evaluate patients' quality of life. Quality of life information can *only* come from the patient. A single global question may be posed to the patient both at baseline and the trial's termination, or solely at termination. The types of overall quality of life assessments made by patients may relate to (1) patients' status at baseline, (2) patients' magnitude of change at a milestone point of the trial or at its termination, (3) the type of change that has occurred at any specified time point compared with baseline, or (4) the significance of the change obtained. Global quality of life questions do *not* need to be, and in fact cannot be, validated. Selected questions are: How would you evaluate your overall satisfaction with life? Overall, how would you rate your life as compared with the start of treatment? Overall, what is your assessment of the quality of your life? Answers may be given on a visual analog scale or using a Likert scale.

May Only Part of a Validated Test Be Used in a Clinical Trial?

Part of a validated test may only be used if the scale can be broken down and each part has been independently validated. Since this is rarely the case, it is generally necessary to conduct a new validation study. It is particularly important to validate a portion of a test if some questions are reworded or deleted, or if that section is changed in any way. Another criticism that could be raised if only part of a test is used stems from the suspicion that bias influenced the choice of selecting one (or more) parts. For example, there may have been a fear that the test treatment would not show up well in the sections deleted.

One strategy to validate the part of the test used is to give a subset of the total patient pool both the full and abbreviated test. Comparing results will help validate the practice of using only part of a test.

Can One Use a Validated General Test in a Disease Population in Which the Test Has Not Been Validated?

A validated general test not validated for the disease under study can be used if the test captures the domains of interest. However, a general scale may not capture all points of interest, particularly subtle ones. Thus, to capture at least some specific disease-related questions it is important to include a specific disease-oriented quality of life test, in addition to a general test. If such a test does not exist or has not been validated, then a few specific disease-oriented questions should be posed.

What Basic Questions Should Be Considered in a Quality of Life Evaluation?

The following questions are applicable whether the quality of life test(s) is included as part of a larger trial,

TABLE 52.1 *Comparison of quality of life and clinical effects of two medicines[a]*

Quality of life scale number 1	Quality of life scale number 2	Clinical effects measured	Interpretation of results
1. No differences observed between medicines A and B	No differences observed between medicines A and B	Medicine A better than medicine B	Quality of life tests may be insensitive to change or improperly given
2. Medicine A better than medicine B	Medicine A better than medicine B	Medicine B better than medicine A	Various interpretations possible
3. Medicine A better than medicine B	Medicine A better than medicine B	Medicine A better than medicine B	Results are supportive
4. Medicine A better than medicine B	Medicine A better than medicine B	No differences observed between medicines A and B	Medicine A is superior to medicine B
5. Medicine A better than medicine B	Medicine B better than medicine A	No differences observed between medicines A and B	Various interpretations possible

[a] Other scenarios and interpretations are possible.

or whether the test is the sole *raison d'être* of the entire trial.

1. How many domains must (should) be measured?
2. Which components of each domain should be measured?
3. How much time is available during the clinical trial to measure quality of life?
4. Are patients capable of adequately completing a self-administered questionnaire? For example, very old, debilitated, or illiterate patients are usually unable to complete these tests adequately without assistance.
5. Is it better to focus on the breadth (i.e., multiple domains and their components) or the depth (i.e., detailed examination of one or a few components of one domain) of the quality of life issue?
6. How much training is required before staff can satisfactorily administer and, if appropriate, interpret the test?
7. Are adequately trained staff available to administer the tests?

TEN STEPS FOR DESIGNING QUALITY OF LIFE TRIALS

1. Identify the purpose of the effort and nature of the problem. Decide whether data on quality of life are truly necessary to obtain. It is often unnecessary to measure how a new medicine affects a patient's quality of life. Henderson-James and Spilker (1990) summarize the desirability of measuring quality of life for a variety of medicines. Medicines that require cost–effectiveness scales are discussed in Chapter 42.
2. Decide whether an entire clinical trial must be conducted to evaluate quality of life, or whether one or more scales, or merely a number of carefully chosen questions, may be inserted into a planned clinical efficacy or safety trial. Assess resources available for this effort and keep choices within limitations of the resources.

TABLE 52.2 *Selected psychosocial conditions that may be measured in clinical trials*

1. Illicit drug abuse
2. Alcohol abuse
3. Physical aggression
4. Suicide attempts
5. Development problems
6. Memory impairment
7. Threatening behavior expressed verbally
8. Threatening behavior expressed physically
9. Number of social contacts
10. Quality of social interactions
11. Risk-seeking versus risk-averse behavior

3. Decide on which quality of life domains (and also which components of each domain) will be evaluated. If possible, measure all domains, even though data on only one or two may be of particular interest. The reasons for this statement are presented in the last section of this chapter. Table 52.2 lists several components of the social domain that could be assessed.
4. Determine what general scales and disease-specific scales exist for the population of interest? Which of these are well validated or at least reasonably well validated? Which are appropriate to consider for the clinical trial? Do not assume that disease-specific scales are either more or less preferable to general scales.
5. Decide on which specific validated scale(s) and tests to use in the quality of life trial to measure components of interest. Determine whether physician-completed or patient-completed tests will be used. For example, a patient-completed questionnaire might be inappropriate for psychotic patients, and only investigator-completed tests might be appropriate. Table 52.3 presents a method that could be used to compare various tests, and Table 52.4 presents the pros and cons of using telephone questionnaires.
6. As a general approach, attempt to choose a general scale(s), which can then be supplemented with a disease-specific scale or a series of unvalidated

TABLE 52.3 *A method to compare various types of quality of life tests*

Parameter	Test A, B, etc.	Patient-completed questionnaire	Personal interview	Telephone interview
		(fill in each column)		
Time to complete				
Number of items or assessments per test				
Personnel time to administer				
Personnel cost to administer				
Number of personnel necessary to train				
Time to train personnel				
Cost to train personnel				
Other costs per test				
Total cost per test				

TABLE 52.4 *Selected benefits and disadvantages of evaluating quality of life based on telephone interviews*[a]

A. Benefits
  1. Minimal personnel needs
  2. Minimal training of personnel
  3. Easy to standardize the interview technique
  4. Easy to coordinate activities and their management
  5. Patients do not need to travel or attend a clinic
  6. Interviewer does not elicit physician-pleasing behavior
  7. Data are available almost immediately
B. Disadvantages
  1. Limitations in types of questions and ratings that may be used (e.g., Likert scales may be used, but visual analog scales may not)
  2. Many questionnaires are insufficiently validated
  3. Potential loss of honesty and increase in evasiveness in answers
  4. Limited ability to assess deceptive, distorted, or dishonest answers

[a] This method refers to tests conducted entirely by telephone and not tests that are conducted by telephone when a patient misses a clinic visit.

questions related to the disease. Consider the seven dimensions described in the following section.

7. Decide who should conduct each test of quality of life and how each should be conducted and assessed.
8. Consider a pilot trial if a large, complex, long, or expensive clinical trial is planned primarily to evaluate quality of life.
9. Decide if a patient's family, friends, or others (e.g., healing physician) in addition to the patient should evaluate quality of life.
10. Consider each of the methodological issues described in the preceding section ("Methodological Principles") and conduct the trial.

CHOOSING THE MOST APPROPRIATE TESTS TO INCORPORATE IN A CLINICAL TRIAL: CONSIDERATION OF SEVEN DIMENSIONS

Tests of quality of life can vary along seven different dimensions. The choice of tests for any trial should be based on an overall assessment of each dimension.

Dimension 1—overall assessment of quality of life. If an overall assessment is desired, it may be obtained by asking an overall question, or by combining results of individual domains. This latter approach can only be used with a validated test that probed each domain and combined their separate results.
Dimension 2—domain(s) to be evaluated. Each domain and group of domains have specific associated tests.
Dimension 3—perspective to be used. These include marketing, pharmaceutical company, regulatory, ethical, and cultural perspectives.

Dimension 4—type of patient being evaluated. These include pediatric, geriatric, rehabilitation, and other types of patients.
Dimension 5—therapeutic area and specific disease. Specific quality of life tests have been developed to evaluate patients with various diseases.
Dimension 6—degree of validation of the individual tests.
Dimension 7—practical issues. Such issues include the length of time required to conduct each test, investigators' familiarity with the test, resources required, and cost of the test.

These dimensions are discussed in the book *Quality of Life Assessments in Clinical Trials* (Spilker, 1990a).

A Strategy for Choosing Quality of Life Tests

It is usually desirable to apply a general quality of life test in a clinical trial so that different patient populations can be compared. As discussed above, it is also desirable to include a disease-specific test or a few selected questions specific for that disease, which are choosen to address concerns of patients about their particular disease. Two problems often arise in trying to implement this strategy. First, for many diseases no disease-specific tests exist, especially validated tests. Second, numerous disease-specific instruments are broad in nature and substantially overlap with general tests or scales. In this situation either scale may be used, but it is preferable to use the one that is better validated.

When one is choosing between two or three similar quality of life tests, it may be desirable to have patients test them. Their comments can provide the basis for the investigator's choice.

A systematic means of comparing the attributes of multiple scales and tests is to create a matrix of relevant tests. This matrix would list the separate tests in one dimension, and would list relevant characteristics in the other. Relevant characteristics might include (1) domains covered, (2) time required to administer the test, (3) whether the test is investigator or patient administered, (4) amount of staff training needed, (5) validity of the test, and (6) cost of the test. These data would enable an investigator to choose the best test for a particular situation.

IDEAL QUALITY OF LIFE TEST

There is no ideal test at present to evaluate quality of life. A test that could become a gold standard would:

1. Be rapid to complete (i.e., up to approximately 15 minutes)
2. Be reproducible

3. Be valid either in a single patient population or across a large number of diseases
4. Be widely accepted
5. Not require excessive training of staff to administer
6. Be easy to interpret
7. Yield objective results.

The view of some researchers is that finding a test that meets all of these criteria is as difficult as finding the Holy Grail. It is an even greater challenge to devise a test that would be applicable to patients in different national cultures.

WHY PHYSICIANS SHOULD NOT EVALUATE A PATIENT'S QUALITY OF LIFE

A quality of life assessment is a value judgment. Only the patients have direct access to their inner thoughts and feelings, where the assessment of quality of life may be found. Patients may or may not choose to be open and honest with a physician or staff member about quality of life issues. Figure 52.2 illustrates this concept in part. (In some cases patients are unable to access their own personal assessment; certain patients do not know how to interpret their feelings and emotions.)

Patients outward actions should be examined to determine if they are behaving in a manner consistent with their stated views. Although there is rarely a complete correlation between anyone's stated views and their actions, it is usually apparent if a patient claims to be totally miserable, with an abysmal quality of life, but appears to lead a happy and carefree existence (or vice versa). A number of investigations have found that physicians are generally unable to assess changes in their patients' quality of life accurately (Jachuck et al., 1982).

Parents too should not complete forms, even for their young children. For example, a young asthmatic child may want to be very active even if it means visiting a hospital once a month. His parents may want to keep him inside and prevent any exertion. Frequent hospital visits will be interpreted quite differently by the child and the parents in terms of quality of life.

PREDICTIONS ABOUT THE FUTURE OF QUALITY OF LIFE TRIALS

Fad versus Significant Medical Advance

Quality of life trials are not a fad and will not disappear. They are an important subset of efficacy trials and may be viewed as an independent group or type of clinical trials. Useful methodologies are now available for most types of quality of life trials, and the quality and va-

lidity of methods should continue to improve over the next decade. Information on how specific medicines and treatments affect quality of life is desired, and in some cases demanded, by formulary committees, insurance agencies, patients, families, and other groups.

Arbitrariness of Scale, Parameter, or Domain Studied

At present, investigators and sponsors may arbitrarily choose *any* single (or multiple) parameter, test, or domain to measure as an index or indicator of quality of life. Their choice may be based entirely on identifying that parameter or scale that they believe, in advance of initiating the trial, will demonstrate advantages of one treatment over another. This is inherently a nonscientific approach because the most appropriate tests and parameters are not being used to evaluate one or more aspects of quality of life, but rather those tests and measures believed to yield the outcome desired. In some extreme cases this approach may be considered unethical: it is not a fair quality of life trial when the trial is actually conducted solely to prove the conclusion desired. The conclusion is then sometimes touted in advertisements or publications as a demonstration of improved quality of life for a particular treatment.

Standardization of Quality of Life Trials

Almost any type of clinical trial may be referred to as "quality of life," since the meaning of the term varies so greatly among investigators. It will undoubtedly become more clear to regulators, clinicians, and others during the 1990s. Quality of life trials will probably become more standardized, possibly through evaluation of all major domains and many of their components (e.g., Table 52.5); at the present time investigators or sponsors can select for evaluation only those domains or components that they expect will show spe-

TABLE 52.5 *Selected components of major domains in quality of life tests*

A. Psychological
  1. Neuropsychological functions (i.e., cognitive function)
  2. Emotional state (e.g., anxiety, anger, depression)
  3. Personal productivity
  4. Intimacy and sexual function
B. Economic
  1. Work status
  2. Amount of time worked
C. Physical
  1. Capabilities
  2. Dysfunction
D. Social interactive
  1. Number of contacts per week (month)
  2. Quality of social contacts at home, school, and job
  3. Quality and quantity of social contacts with friends
  4. Interactions at work
  5. Recreational activities

cific outcomes. In addition, the tests used are likely to be reduced to a small number that are well validated and accepted. Both general tests and disease-specific tests will be used, often in the same quality of life trial. When only general scales are available, a number of disease-specific questions may be incorporated to obtain additional information. [A relatively complete listing of tests for many specific diseases was recently published (Spilker et al., 1990)].

Data obtained in quality of life trials will be evaluated to determine how well they address the stated objectives. It is likely that many quality of life trials will generate a large amount of negative data on the effects of treatments on most domains and their components. That is an entirely acceptable outcome since it will assure readers that the results observed were not arbitrarily obtained by examining only selected domains and purposely ignoring others. A list of practical pointers is given in Table 52.6.

The problem of selecting certain domains to prove one's point only rarely arises in conventional efficacy trials, since the standard tests and parameters that should be included are generally well known and accepted. Any attempt to use unvalidated or questionable measures will be apparent to readers of the report or publication, and the clinical trial's results are more likely to be challenged.

TABLE 52.6 *Practical pointers on quality of life tests*

1. Certify certain staff to administer tests
2. Certify certain staff and monitors as teachers of staff
3. The test should be administered while the patient is in the waiting room (or other place), but before blood draws or physician interviews occur
4. Conduct a pilot trial of each major trial that will include the quality of life evaluations
5. The person administering the test should say every time "Fill in each question"
6. Clarify the time point that patients are to consider in answering questions (e.g., at this moment, usually, since the last visit, over the last week)
7. Obtain normative data to compare with data obtained in ill patients
8. Offer all patients who are to complete a self-administered test the option to have questions read to them; this gives illiterate or semiliterate patients a "no-fault" means of solving a potential problem and not admitting their illiteracy
9. The method described in point 6 above also applies to patients who are unable to write or too sick to complete the form(s); the data collection forms should be marked to indicate that the questions were read and the interviewer completed the test
10. Make a videotape to illustrate the correct approach for administering a test, particularly when multiple sites are involved
11. Patients should have privacy when completing tests; family members should usually not be allowed to interact with the patient during this period
12. Do not initiate a quality of life test after a trial has begun
13. Provide an extra set of tests for patients to keep at home in case they cannot attend a clinic and must complete the test via telephone

PART IV

Planning and Conducting a Single Clinical Trial

I never once made a discovery. . . . I speak without exaggeration when I say that I have constructed three thousand different theories in connection with the electric light. . . . Yet in only two cases did my experiments prove the truth of my theory.

—Thomas Alva Edison

The love of truth for truth's sake is the principal part of human perfection in this world, and the seed-plot of all other virtues.

—John Locke

- GOOD
- FAST
- CHEAP
  Choose any two

—Author unknown

CHAPTER 53

Introduction

Planning, initiating, conducting, and analyzing the results of a clinical trial require knowledge of and use of a large number of procedures. The specific steps followed usually differ among trials in terms of which steps are involved and how they are applied. The purpose of Section IV is to present a system that can be utilized to assist individuals in performing these steps in an efficient manner.

DIFFERENCES BETWEEN SPONSORED AND UNSPONSORED CLINICAL TRIALS

Important differences are usually present between unsponsored clinical trials initiated in academic institutions, clinics, or private practices and sponsored trials initiated by pharmaceutical corporations, government agencies, or other sponsors. These differences reflect the fact that in unsponsored trials the investigator usually assumes and modifies many of the responsibilities primarily carried out by the sponsor. For example, trial monitoring conducted by the sponsor is generally replaced by internal control mechanisms in unsponsored trials; medicine packaging by a pharmaceutical corporation in sponsored trials may be performed by a pharmacy for unsponsored trials. Most factors related to trial initiation, conduct, and data analysis are addressed by both academicians and sponsors, although the manner in which each addresses the same issue often differs.

The approach of Section IV focuses attention on the scientific method and is intended for use by pharmaceutical corporations (or other sponsors) and by clinical investigators involved in both unsponsored or sponsored clinical trials. Some modifications will be required by each group, depending on the perspective of the individual and nature of the clinical trial under consideration. The perspectives of academic investigators, physicians in private medical practice, and patients are presented in specific chapters. Perspectives of pharmaceutical companies are presented in several chapters, particularly those on choosing investigators and monitoring a clinical trial.

BASIC ASSUMPTIONS

The primary assumption underlying the procedures described is that the major goal of a clinical trial is to attain the objective(s) stated in the protocol. Obviously, this goal has a greater likelihood of success if the trial is planned, initiated, and conducted carefully and if the results are systematically evaluated. To achieve and maintain the highest standards of performance in carrying out these steps, quality assurance methods and an organized approach to the many facets of a trial should be incorporated into the overall trial, and the various components of the trial should be periodically assessed.

The strategy proposed to accomplish the above goals is discussed in terms of the nine categories listed in Table 53.1. A portion of this material was previously reported (Spilker, 1983). Other aspects that may be involved in a clinical trial (e.g., medical contractor groups, auditing a clinical trial) are also discussed in this chapter.

TABLE 53.1 *Conduct of clinical trials*

1. Interview and selection of investigators
2. Clinical trial initiation
   a. Internal documents and procedures
   b. Information for the investigator to send to the sponsor
   c. Information for the sponsor to send to the investigator
3. Pretrial roundtable meeting
4. Conduct of the clinical trial
5. Monitoring and troubleshooting a trial
6. Clinical trial termination or extension
7. Clinical trial data entry and analysis

CHAPTER 54

Training Professionals and Their Staff in Clinical Trial Methods

INTRODUCTION

Staff training should be an important and continuous activity at all pharmaceutical companies, regulatory agencies, and academic centers. It is an area that often has been neglected, and many professionals and their staff have been left on their own to learn their roles and how to play them effectively (colloquially referred to as *on-the-job training*). While self-taught and colleague-taught learning is an extremely important part of most people's education, it should not be relied on to provide adequate or complete training. Both formal and informal training programs must be developed and implemented by all organizations to address satisfactorily the steadily increasing complexity of conducting clinical research, analyzing and interpreting data, and discovering and developing new medicines.

Several for-profit groups have recognized the void that existed in training programs and have developed courses, video cassettes, workbooks, and other methods over the last decade. On a larger scale, a number of formal certificate or degree programs in medicine development or clinical medicine development have been initiated at several institutions in Europe and North America to help train people who wish to enter these fields.

Menu Approach. This chapter takes a broad general view of education by presenting many options currently available to train individuals in clinical trial methods and medicine development. A menu of possible approaches is provided. An organization should consider using any number of these for training any size group, from one or two junior staff to an entire division.

Informing Staff of Opportunities. It is desirable to inform all staff about educational opportunities that exist within the institution. Such opportunities could be classified by type and listed in a catalogue or on a simple sheet. Characteristics of each program should also be listed. This list should include the objectives, methods used, topics addressed, suitable audience, duration, format, type of homework, and instructors, plus any other pertinent information.

ONSITE TRAINING

The opportunities for on-site staff training primarily depend on the size and nature of the organization. Throughout this discussion, a large institution is generally assumed to be the type of organization planning an educational program. Most smaller groups are located near a large institution that could help in developing and conducting a training program. A site may consist of a single small clinic, a large university with teaching hospital, a pharmaceutical company, or another facility. Techniques commonly used for on-site training are described below.

On-the-Job Training

On-the-job training is one of the most important methods used in on-site training and usually involves experienced people who assist newly hired or transferred individuals to learn their roles. Some individuals are better teachers than others, and a number of people enjoy this role. Experienced people who are competent teachers should be identified by the organization and asked to help train some (or all) new employees for a set amount of time.

Usually people are trained by those for whom they work on a permanent basis. Training may be more effective and complete if those with an interest in teaching are assigned a new person to train for a fixed period. While the time required for training varies, clinical monitors could be assigned to a teacher for a 2- to 3-month period. Whether a separate teacher is assigned from the same clinical group in which the new employee works depends on the resources available.

During-the-Trial Training

Coinvestigators or other staff often join a study already in progress as a result of (1) staff turnover, (2) rotation of medical residents, (3) expansion of the study, or (4) other reasons. In all of these circumstances it is often important for an investigator or sponsor to review relevant information and techniques with the new investigator or staff. The sponsor usually has a clinical monitor serve this function, although it is possible for the project leader or others to coordinate and perform this role.

Personnel Assigned as Trainers and Training Coordinators

Some pharmaceutical companies and regulatory agencies assign the task of training new employees to specific personnel. These professionals may design an individual program for each new employee. The design of the program will depend on the employee's level of responsibility, previous experience, and educational needs. This program should be initially discussed with the employee and then reviewed on a periodic basis to assess the employee's progress and to revise the approach and goals. The tools used to create the training program are described throughout this chapter.

The person or group in charge of training may appoint a committee to advise on needs and suitability of proposed courses, and to provide other feedback. The committee should be composed of a few representatives from the groups receiving the training. If the groups are heterogeneous in their needs, then multiple committees could be formed. Each committee should meet on a periodic basis; otherwise its value will diminish.

In-House Courses or Workshops

Existing in-house training courses are usually an important resource. Courses designed for new employees should be offered frequently. All new employees meeting certain criteria may be automatically enrolled in one or more courses. Courses targeted for experienced people with a wide range of backgrounds must be evaluated periodically to ensure that they are effectively meeting people's needs. For example, courses organized by a medical department must be focused on and suited to that staff, whereas those organized by an entire company or university must have a broad appeal.

There is a tendency for most courses to be longer than needed to achieve their goals. The duration of each course must be evaluated from a time-expended-to-benefits-received perspective. Many courses, both within and outside organizations, present important material, but over too long a period for the courses to be totally worthwhile. This leads to boredom of students and wasted resources of the organization.

Small classes allow for more interaction among members. Such interaction, however, can be encouraged in other ways. For example, a large number of participants may be enrolled in a course and then divided into smaller teams to work on specific problems. Each smaller group could present their conclusions, consensus, or recommendations to the larger group.

Bringing Outside Courses Into an Organization

In-house courses or workshops are not always developed within the organization. Many are developed by outside groups and then brought in-house after internal staff have been trained as teachers. Alternatively, these courses may be conducted in-house by outside contractors. More and more individuals and groups are establishing themselves as independent consultants and contractors in this area. Their expertise must be carefully assessed through references and other standard techniques, including sending a few people to sit through outside courses to evaluate their content, format, and value critically for the group they represent.

Team-Building Exercises

Some courses are designed for groups of individuals who work together and may be intended as team-building exercises. A group of individuals does not automatically work together as a team when brought together. Planning, thought, and effort by appropriate managers are required to develop a cohesive team. The choice of a suitable leader is clearly important to the team's success. Once a team is developed, ongoing meetings, such as with the Quality Circles technique, may be a valuable method to maintain their spirit. In a Quality Circle, the group (usually 4 to 12) meets periodically to identify problems and after its analysis recommends solutions to line managers.

Mentors

The mentor approach may be pursued either formally or informally. A training coordinator could establish this system on a formal basis for new employees (e.g., person X may be appointed as mentor for new employees A, B, and C). The major requirements for a mentor are experience, accessibility, and compatibility. The trainee may meet the mentor on either an ad hoc or periodically scheduled basis.

This system often works best when people seek out a mentor on their own, or the relationship develops naturally. Nonetheless, a mentor may be assigned for a specific purpose (e.g., to accompany the person on one or more monitoring trips, to advise on protocol writing) or for general help in a broad area (e.g., to assist the individual in becoming an experienced project leader). Although a mentor could be an individual's immediate supervisor, it is generally advisable to have another individual serve this function.

Formal Seminars

Virtually all research and development departments sponsor seminars with both internal and external speakers. Seminar series of various types may be initiated apart from the traditional formal scientific or clinical presentations. For example, speakers from various departments can discuss their department's organization and function at a lunch seminar. Participants are invited to bring their lunch, or are given lunch by the sponsoring institution. Another type of series would be organized around issues of interest to those invited. The issues may be on a central theme and may involve only internal speakers. Having a panel of two to four discuss topics of current interest and answer questions is often an effective format to involve the audience.

Visual presentations (slides, overheads, or drawings on a blackboard or easel) are recommended teaching aids for all courses and seminars. These methods help the audience remember and retain important points. Some people believe that a realistic goal of an hour's talk on a scientific topic is to get the audience to retain a single point permanently.

Informal Meetings

Discussion sessions may be scheduled on an ad hoc basis. Selected topics, problems, or issues on medicine development may be discussed. These meetings may be led by a facilitator or a line management leader, or the leadership may rotate among individuals selected to focus on a particular topic. The subject matter may be scientific, practical, or specific to the institution's interests, or it may deal with other matters. Interactive sessions may be facilitated by posing questions, either verbally or on a screen, and writing down answers from the group on an overhead slide that everyone can read, or alternatively, on a blackboard or flip-chart.

Video Cassettes

Uses. Internally generated video cassettes on selected topics may be produced for use by medical personnel. These tapes may be made by either internal staff or external consultants, and should be based on scripts prepared or reviewed by internal staff. Seminars or a series of seminars of particular interest may be videotaped and added to the organization's library. Video cassettes could be played at small informal meetings at which the speaker would then answer questions "live" about the topics he or she discussed in the taped seminar. If the presenter was not available, then others could answer questions raised. A selection of suitable subjects for video cassettes is listed in Table 54.1.

Choosing a Group To Make Video Cassettes. In making video cassettes it is necessary to consider and identify precisely (1) who is the target audience, (2)

TABLE 54.1 *Selected topics for video or audio cassette presentations[a]*

1. Descriptions of the organizational structure of various departments, divisions, and groups within an organization
2. Descriptions and discussions of the functions and activities conducted by various groups within an organization
3. Description of an overall organization's history, functions, activities, or structure
4. One or more aspects of the pharmaceutical development process
5. One or more aspects of the clinical trial process
6. Standard operating procedures within an organization
7. Discussions of any issues pertinent to the overall organization or to one or more groups within the organization

[a] Any cassette may be accompanied by a workbook or other written material (e.g., a self-test to take after viewing or listening to the tape).

what is the major (and other) message to deliver, (3) how the information can be communicated most effectively, and (4) how the information will be received. It is essential to work with experienced groups to plan and create the video cassette. Before agreeing to hire any group, insist on viewing examples of its work in your field of interest. If the group's experience is entirely in a different subject area, its ability to produce the type of product you desire, as well as its creativity, must be carefully assessed. Ask for several references and contact each of them.

Determining the Content of a Video Cassette. Video cassette content may be as straightforward as taping a formal lecture accompanied by slides used at the lecture. These cassettes are often filmed during a live performance and are usually presented in a didactic format. Panel discussions present a more varied format, and the camera may show interactions with the audience. Neither approach has as much visual interest as a professionally produced video tape containing various bits of interviews, scenes, animation, or other approaches that enhance the visual appeal. Related scenes may be shown while the speaker delivers the text, or while the interview is being conducted. Professionally produced videotapes may be accompanied by a course leader's workbook to help the training coordinator use the cassette most effectively. If the cassette is to be viewed by individuals on their own, a workbook for their use may be prepared.

Case studies are often excellent subjects for a video format. Cases of actual patients help investigators define diagnostic terms and characterize and rate the severity of adverse events. Visual reinforcement is also a valuable method to teach personnel about particular medical problems. These cassette programs may be interactive: the viewer is asked to make decisions about specific situations. One or more relevant tapes would help ensure uniformity among different investigators in interpreting selected information (e.g., patients who present with different adverse reactions).

Book and Journal Clubs

Small groups of staff may be assigned readings in specific books or articles prior to meetings at which one or more topics are discussed. These meetings could have either a single leader, or the leadership could rotate among members of the group. The choice of leaders must be based on the people involved and the goals of the group. The formality of journal clubs varies widely.

SELF-DIRECTED TRAINING

The types of training previously discussed are primarily group activities focused within the relevant institution. The following discussion explores activities that may be conducted by individuals on their own, whether at an institution, at home, or elsewhere.

Books and Journals

A number of books have been written about clinical trials, clinical development of new medicines, and related issues. Articles have also appeared in journals, although it would take some effort for any group to identify the best ones. In terms of using the literature as a training tool, an important issue for training coordinators to address is whether to make formal reading assignments. Another issue is whether to expect individuals to locate their own literature sources, or simply to refer them to relevant literature. People in charge of training should prepare a list of major literature sources. These materials could also be collected and placed at a central site to be made available to relevant staff. An annotated bibliography could be prepared, which would enhance the value of the literature and facilitate choices of reading material. A representative list of books on development of medicines is provided in the appendix of *Multinational Drug Companies: Issues in Drug Discovery and Development* (Spilker, 1989a).

Self-Instructional Manuals, Guides, and Workbooks

Organizations can prepare their own manuals, guides, or workbooks. Typical subject matter for self-instructional material includes standard operating procedures or clinical areas of interest. These could be prepared by internal staff or contracted to outside individuals or companies. Materials could be based on published textbooks or on information found within the organization. A variation of this approach would be to prepare self-instructional guides that lead individuals through a prescribed course of instruction. These guides might in some cases be accompanied by video cassettes. Another type of self-instructional guide can be in the form of a computer-based tutorial complete with pre- and posttests.

Some companies spend an extremely large amount of resources to create education manuals for their staff. Such manuals should be placed in a loose-leaf binder so that new sections may be added or out-of-date pieces replaced. Titles and roles of key people (rather than names) should generally be used in organizational charts and descriptions of functions, since specific people tend to transfer, be promoted, or leave a group. On the other hand, an important group can be reorganized, rendering the chart obsolete. In this case, using a loose-leaf binder will facilitate the process of keeping the material current.

Standard Operating Procedures

Standard operating procedures are prepared by most organizations. These documents indicate how various activities are conducted within the organization. At some organizations the existence of these documents is little known and at others such documents are out of date. It is important to have a procedure to keep standard operating procedures up to date. Widespread distribution should be encouraged if these documents are easy to read and understand. See Chapter 125 for more information on this subject.

Audio Cassettes

Many professional societies and associations, private contractors, institutions, and other groups sell a wide variety of audio cassettes for educational purposes. One or more libraries of such tapes should be available within an institution or group for individuals to use or borrow. These tapes are particularly suited for listening to during periods of travel (e.g., during commuting). Tapes of individual sessions at various professional meetings are also becoming more widely available. These cassettes also should be deposited in a central repository for a department or larger size group to use, and information on their existence should be appropriately disseminated. These cassettes may also be circulated to interested staff, like journals are routed in many organizations. Table 54.1 contains a list of subjects suitable for audio cassettes.

Discussions Among Professionals

Although professionals in an organization generally discuss issues of interest without any prompting, this aspect of education could be slightly more structured

in a formalized educational program. It could be especially helpful for new employees, or those who are transferred to a different part of the organization. General discussions on a scheduled basis with relevant staff is one approach that could be used. The topic for each discussion may be specified in advance of the meeting. Alternatively, individuals could be encouraged to pursue discussions on an ad hoc basis.

Computer-Assisted Instruction

Interactive programs with computers that are designed to assist an employee's education may be created either within the organization or by outside vendors/contractors. Modules may be developed to focus on relevant topics and could include a pre- and posttest. This category differs from the self-instructional materials mentioned earlier in that those were based primarily on developing hard copy.

OFFSITE TRAINING

Almost all professionals in an organization receive part of their initial and ongoing training and education through activities conducted at places away from their organization. The major types of activities in this category are described below.

Courses

The number of available courses that provide information on clinical trials and development of medicines has increased markedly during the last decade. Courses are sponsored by professional societies, trade associations, academic institutions, nonprofit corporations, and for-profit corporations. The quality of these courses depends primarily on the staff leading the course and not on the affiliation of the group sponsoring the course. Therefore, a single group may offer courses of varying quality and it would be illogical to dismiss all of a group's courses because of someone's personal experience with a poor one.

Course Participants

One of the greatest problems faced by organizers of these courses is the great heterogeneity of people who attend. If a course is general in content, it will tend to attract a wide variety of people in terms of background, responsibilities, and experience. If a course is quite narrow and targeted to a specific group, however, the organizers often fear that it will fail to attract a sufficient number of attendees.

Halo Effect of Courses

There is often a "halo effect" after a recently completed course, particularly if the entertainment or social value was high. Participants usually are asked to review the course for the organizers, but on return to their institution they also should be asked to review the course by their own organization. Because a course can rarely be evaluated fairly or accurately shortly after the course is over, it should *also* be rated 2 to 4 months later. At that time most individuals can better assess whether the course has contributed to their education or professional performance. Most professionals have attended courses that were fun and appeared worthwhile at the time, but on hindsight were viewed quite differently.

Reviews of Courses

Single page check-off reviews of courses attended by professionals from an institution's department or division could be kept in a loose-leaf book for consultation by those considering a specific course. There are numerous arguments against this approach (e.g., changes in content and teachers, different people can rate the same course differently), and it is uncertain if the benefits of this approach would outweigh the disadvantages.

Professional Meetings, Conferences, Workshops, or Symposia

The value of these sessions varies. It is frequently stated that the greatest benefits come from informal discussions held in the hallways among participants, rather than at the formal meetings. It is for this reason (among others) that substantial time should be allotted for coffee breaks throughout meetings, and that a "quick 10-minute break" because time is short should not be substituted for a scheduled 30-minute break. Participants should not be penalized because one or more speakers went beyond their allotted time. Any topic can be presented in 1 minute, hour, day, or week. Therefore, any speaker who has prepared his comments carefully should remain within his allotted time. It is generally the more poorly prepared speakers who take more than their allotted time.

A particularly annoying policy of some organizations that sponsor these sessions is first to create all the titles of the talks and then seek the speakers. In theory, this approach is an excellent one and should create a unity and bring cohesiveness to the meeting that could not be attained if each speaker chose their own topic. What tends to occur, however, is that most

TABLE 54.2 *Selected objectives for retreats*

1. Developing plans and strategies to achieve short-term goals[a]
2. Developing plans and strategies to achieve long-terms goals[a]
3. Establishing priorities among activities competing for resources
4. Creating a mission, objectives, and goals for a particular level or function within the organization
5. Clarifying roles and relationships of various individuals or groups
6. Addressing concerns, issues, or problems of various individuals or groups
7. Identifying new opportunities or directions for the organization or one or more groups

[a] The goals may or may not be articulated and agreed on prior to the retreat.

speakers present their older rehearsed material on a related topic. Thus, listeners often find that the listed topics are not addressed and the presentations are generally unsatisfactory. This problem is particularly common when friends of the organizer, rather than respected experts in the field, are invited to give presentations.

Retreats

Retreats have gained in popularity over the last decade and are now *de rigueur* at many organizations. Retreats run from a half-day to a week, with the majority lasting from 1 to 3 days. They may be held close to the organization or at a distance. Spouses may or may not be invited. The decision to invite spouses should be based on the goals of the meetings. If the goals involve serious problem solving then spouses should not be invited. If the goals involve discussion of issues, plans, and strategies, or are mainly social, then spouses may be invited. A number of objectives for retreats are listed in Table 54.2. The place to hold the retreat (e.g., hotel, conference center, country club, resort, other facility) is based on availability, cost, level of participants within the organization, tradition, type of meeting anticipated, and personal wishes of the organizers.

ESTABLISHING A TRAINING PROGRAM FOR SPECIFIC GROUPS OF INDIVIDUALS

Organizing an Institution to Provide Training Programs

Figure 54.1 illustrates three basic approaches to organizing an institution's training program. No single approach would be preferable overall, and the most desirable approach for any group may change over time.

Model A - All Training is Centralized

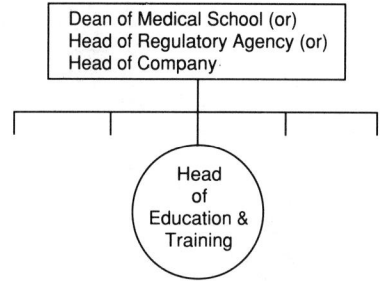

Model B - All Training is Decentralized

Model C - Hybrid Approach to Training

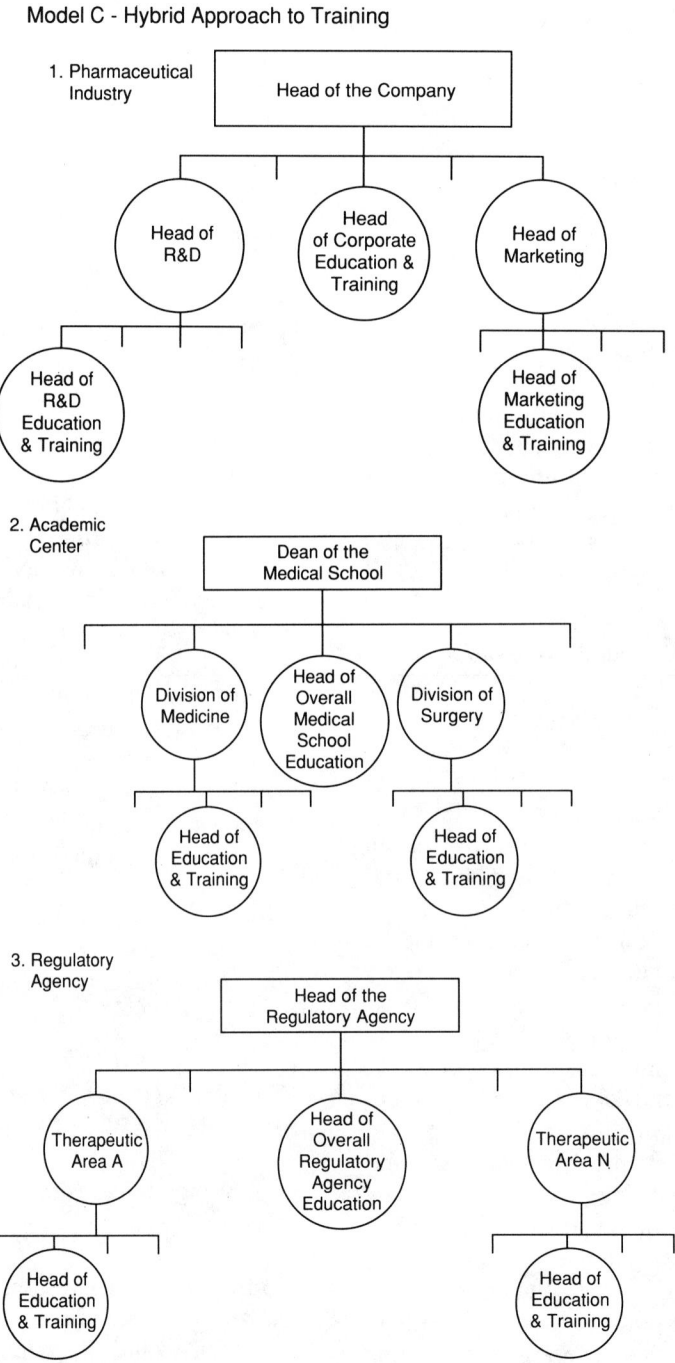

FIG. 54.1 Selected models for structuring the training function within an organization. In the decentralized model each department or unit has their own group to direct training, and no centralized function exists.

Training Programs for New Employees

A training program should be designed for all new employees who join a group, regardless of their level in the organization, previous background, or experience within the same organization. For some individuals (e.g., secretaries, clerks) this program will be minimal and may only involve a selected number of discussions and courses, plus activities that are part of the individual's responsibilities. For most professionals, a more extensive and formal program should be initiated. This may include having the person assigned to an individual to supervise his or her entire training for a fixed period. Mature individuals who are experienced at a company often volunteer their services to help educate others. All should view their own training as a continual and ongoing process. At a certain stage during this process, each person assumes more and more responsibility for establishing their own challenges and ongoing training program.

One advantage of creating individualized training programs is that the designer usually serves the additional role of helping the employee adjust and settle into his or her new environment. If problems develop for the new employee or questions arise, then the training coordinator is another person available to help.

Training Programs for Promoted or Transferred Employees

Individuals are always transferring or are assigned new responsibilities within an organization. The possibility of additional training should not be ignored at those moments, and a formal program should be established. A core program for new employees or new managers can also be developed, regardless of their level within the organization.

Sources of Additional Information

Education of clinical research personnel differs widely among companies. A few publications present approaches used at Upjohn (Metz et al., 1987), ICI (Sayers and Blake, 1989), and Glaxo (Cochetto, 1986). A source book that describes training methods was written by Laird (1985). Chapter 10 in that book describes many useful and unusual techniques (e.g., role-playing, reverse role-playing, doubling role-playing, rotation role-playing, simulations) that may be used to accomplish various training objectives.

Information on careers in various fields related to medicines (Spilker, 1989d) and career opportunities for physicians in the pharmaceutical industry has recently been presented (Spilker, 1989c). Courses in clinical research methods have been presented in greater detail in a recent article (Spilker, 1991).

CHAPTER 55

Interactions of Academic Investigators with Pharmaceutical Companies

NEW INVESTIGATORS

Many investigators who have initiated and conducted academically oriented clinical trials have never conducted sponsored trials for pharmaceutical companies or government agencies. These individuals often experience mild to strong surprise when they discover the large magnitude of data and the high degree of detail required in Phase I to III clinical trials. The industry-sponsored trial uses a 30- to 50-page protocol, on average, rather than the 2- to 8-page one commonly found in academic unsponsored trials. The 5- to 10-page data collection form of an academic trial contrasts sharply with that found in an industry-sponsored trial, which often ranges from 50 to 250 pages per patient. The steps to follow in the event that a patient experiences an unexpected situation may be dealt with in great detail, as may be other numerous courses of action.

New investigators are often provided staff to help complete these seemingly onerous forms to collect the data required by regulatory authorities before they can approve a new medicine. A clinical monitor from the sponsor's site will generally provide much help to the investigator and staff and will have the most contact with them. It is important for the investigator to develop a positive and professional relationship with this person (or persons).

COMMON MOTIVATIONS FOR CONDUCTING CLINICAL TRIALS

It is important for all investigators, whether new or experienced, to understand their own motives for undertaking a clinical trial. These motives often vary from trial to trial for a single investigator, and none of those listed below are considered inappropriate or unethical. It is common for two (or even more) of these factors to be relevant for a single physician.

1. Enhance one's career through association with an important clinical trial using a new medicine or treatment.
2. Participate in scientifically exciting clinical research.
3. Obtain medical benefits for one's patients, who may receive investigational new medicines or treatments.
4. Obtain new medical or scientific equipment either provided by sponsors as part of the trial or purchased later with money received for conducting the trial.
5. Obtain new staff, for a specified period, who will help with the clinical trial and may also help with other professional activities.
6. Obtain money that may be used for personal interests.

7. Obtain money that may be used to conduct unsponsored trials of professional interest.
8. Enhance one's standing in one's academic department because of bringing a grant into the department.
9. Publish scientifically and medically important articles.
10. Develop a relationship with a sponsor of particular interest.
11. Repay a favor.

PHYSICIANS WHO GENERALLY SHOULD NOT CONDUCT CLINICAL TRIALS

Not all academic physicians or physicians in private practice have the appropriate temperament or personality to conduct sponsored clinical trials. There are a few clues that should tell a physician to proceed with great caution. It may save both the investigator and sponsor anguish at a later date if the proposed investigator declines an invitation.

Clues that warn against becoming an investigator for a trial are:

1. A strong belief in individualizing treatment of all patients with the same disease.
2. Lack of the temperament for following a detailed protocol closely.
3. Insufficient staff to delegate large segments of the clinical trial that the physician would rather not do himself or herself (e.g., complete data collection forms).
4. Inadequate time to participate appropriately (i.e. at the level described) in a clinical trial.
5. Dislike of dealing with large amounts of clinical trial data and details.
6. Unwillingness to meet with the sponsor's representatives at periodic intervals.
7. Unreceptiveness to an audit of one's participation in the clinical trial. Audits could be conducted by the sponsor or the Food and Drug Administration (FDA). The probability of these events occurring could be estimated by the monitor.

Any questions about these or other issues should be discussed with colleagues who have conducted sponsored clinical trials, as well as with the sponsor's representatives.

QUESTIONS A POTENTIAL INVESTIGATOR SHOULD ASK A SPONSOR BEFORE AGREEING TO CONDUCT A CLINICAL TRIAL

Documents to Review Initially

The most important documents for an investigator to review before deciding whether to participate in a clinical trial are the protocol (if it has been written) and the investigators' brochure. The latter document describes previous experience with the medicine. This will consist primarily or entirely of animal data if the medicine is in Phase I, but primarily of clinical data if the medicine is in Phases II or III. A draft protocol is often, but not always, available when an investigator is initially contacted about a clinical trial. This document generally makes it clear to the potential investigator whether the clinical trial will be enjoyable or onerous. Every aspect of the protocol that is not clear should be discussed with the sponsor and clarified.

Specific Questions

Specific questions that a potential investigator may wish to ask a sponsor are:

1. *How did the sponsor get my name?* While there is no right or wrong answer, or even particular importance to this question, it may give the investigator useful information.
2. *Why should I conduct this clinical trial?* The answer to this question should be given by the sponsor before an investigator ever has a chance to ask this. In some situations (e.g., a major breakthrough medicine is to be initially tested in patients) the answer is so obvious that the question need not be asked. Nonetheless, if the question is not obvious or already answered it should be raised, even if it is only to learn what the sponsor is thinking.
3. *What are the sponsor's goals with the clinical trial and experience in the therapeutic area?* The quality of the sponsor's program should be assessed as well as their ethical reputation. Ask the sponsor for references to check, particularly of investigators who have worked with the same team.
4. *Who will analyze the data?* Although the answer to this question is almost always the sponsor for major trials, the investigator may wish (for special reasons) to analyze the data as well. Alternatively, an investigator participating in a multicenter trial may wish the sponsor to provide him or her with data and the results of statistical analyses from his or her individual clinical trial site. These results would usually be used to generate a publication that could include results of tests conducted only at that site. Small studies or marketing studies may be analyzed by the investigator.
5. *How will publications be handled?* In multicenter trials, the order of individual authors, or even the names of those who will be authors on publications, is often an issue. Does the investigator have the right to publish his or her results separately or to publish an add-on part to the study? What is the sponsor's policy about reviewing manuscripts prior to submission.

6. *How much of the investigator's personal time and effort is expected (by the sponsor) to be expended on the clinical trial?* For surgical trials the sponsor may not want the investigator to delegate the operations to others. In many medical trials the sponsor may be pleased to have the investigator as a figurehead and not mind delegation of the work to residents or other physicians on the principal investigator's staff.

7. *How often does the monitor intend to visit the investigator's site, and how much of the investigator's time does he or she anticipate requiring?* A busy investigator may be able to delegate these interactions with a monitor to a staff member or trial coordinator. Determine if this is acceptable to the sponsor.

8. *What help can the sponsor provide to recruit patients?* Is the sponsor willing to pay patients for transportation, parking, or meals? Is the sponsor willing to pay for newspaper or other advertisements? What types of advertisements and other recruitment techniques are acceptable?

9. *What is the sponsor's policy toward indemnification for the legal issues that arise?* This must be discussed with (or between) attorneys if it is or may be an issue. It could either be based on the likelihood of problems arising that would lead to suits or on institutional policy.

10. *Will the sponsor prepare a sample informed consent?* Many investigators appreciate receiving a sample informed consent from the sponsor that may then be modified for a particular trial. Not only does this practice save time, but it ensures inclusion of all essential elements that must be included.

11. *Is the clinical trial under discussion certain of being initiated or is it only a possibility?* Many sponsors expend a great deal of effort discussing potential trials that are never initiated. They do this because they want to know if the clinical trial is feasible and if they could identify the desired investigators. Representatives of a sponsor often contact investigators while they are still hoping to receive official approval to conduct the clinical trial. An investigator should know the precise status of any clinical trial discussed. Investigators who do not clarify this point may expend a significant amount of time that will never be compensated for and a feeling of resentment may result.

12. *On what basis will an investigator be chosen?* During an interview sponsors often give the impression that the potential investigator will definitely be involved in a clinical trial, whereas numerous investigators are actually being interviewed for one or a few openings. No ethical problem arises with this approach, as long as the potential investigator is clearly informed about the relevant facts. It is usually desirable to inform candidates about the basis on which the investigator(s) will be chosen. This information helps the potential investigator determine how much time and effort to spend on preparing for the clinical trial before the investigators are officially chosen.

13. *What is the starting date of the clinical trial?* This information is often important for scheduling purposes. An unrealistically short date that does not allow for Ethics Committee/Institutional Review Board (IRB) review and contractual negotiations should indicate to the investigator a lack of truthful information (or great naiveté) of the sponsor's representative(s). A surprisingly long period before the start of the clinical trial can indicate that the trial has not yet received the official "go-ahead."

14. *Discuss responsibilities.* All responsibilities of the investigator as stated in regulations and according to the sponsor's policies should be discussed. A number of these responsibilities are listed in Table 55.1.

15. *Is it possible to suggest modifications to the protocol?* It should be possible for the investigator to have input into the protocol in most cases.

16. *Does the investigator receive full or prorated*

TABLE 55.1 *Responsibilities of clinical investigators[a]*

A. Responsibilities to Ethics Committee or Institutional Review Board
   1. Submit protocol and informed consent forms
   2. Obtain their approval prior to initiating the clinical trial
   3. Submit for approval all modifications to the protocol that are not trivial
   4. Submit periodic (usually annual) progress reports on the clinical trial
   5. Submit a final report on the clinical trial
   6. Report any serious and unanticipated adverse events or unexpected events
   7. Report any significant events that affect the clinical trial (e.g., investigator leaves)
B. Responsibilities to sponsor
   1. Maintain records of receipt, storage, and disposition of medicines and other materials received
   2. Adhere to the written protocol
   3. Complete data collection forms
   4. Notify the sponsor if any serious and unexpected adverse events occur
   5. Meet periodically with representatives (monitors) and maintain a log of such visits
   6. Submit reports as agreed, including a final medical report
   7. Follow all jointly agreed-upon procedures
   8. Assist in data editing activities
C. Responsibilities to patients
   1. Obtain their informed consent
   2. Treat in a caring, ethical, and professional manner
   3. Discuss the trial in an honest and open manner
D. Responsibilities to regulatory agency
   1. Allow inspection by a regulatory authority of facilities and records
   2. Retain all records for 2 years after the medicine is approved by the regulatory authority or for 5 years after the regulatory submission is made by the sponsor, or according to other appropriate regulations and agreements

[a] These responsibilities are for a sponsored clinical trial. Other responsibilities may also be listed for relevant situations (e.g., for a committee overseeing use of the specific facilities used or of the academic departments involved).

payments for patients who drop out or are discontinued during the clinical trial? This question is listed to indicate that each aspect of the financial arrangements must be clearly described in the agreement. The relative importance of financial arrangements varies widely among investigators.

17. *Other questions.* Ask the sponsor about any aspects of the protocol that are unclear or appear to be unrealistic. Discuss the responsibilities of the investigator and the sponsor for each aspect of the protocol.

COMMON PROBLEMS ENCOUNTERED BY INVESTIGATORS DURING A CLINICAL TRIAL

Some of the problems that may arise during a clinical trial are listed below. These are followed by potential approaches to finding a solution.

Patient Enrollment. Patients are not being enrolled at the agreed-on rate. Numerous approaches to address this problem are discussed in Chapter 13, on recruitment. Both investigators and sponsors should track the trial's enrollment on a continual basis.

Staff Turnover. Important staff leave the investigator's employ. Call the sponsor to discuss alternatives. One possibility is to have staff from another site train the new staff. This may take place at either the trainer's or trainee's site. Another possibility is for a representative of the sponsor to act as trainer.

Cost Overruns. A clinical trial may cost more money to conduct than is included in the budget. Document all costs as well as possible and describe the reasons for their increase. Discuss this issue with the sponsor. Most sponsors react appropriately to legitimately incurred costs.

Protocol Changes. Modifications sometimes must be made to a protocol. Investigators should not make changes without contacting the sponsor to discuss the issue. All significant protocol changes must be approved by the Ethics Committee/IRB before they are initiated. "Significant" is defined in terms of risks to patients, generation of data that may affect the trial's outcome, or any change that could affect the integrity of the clinical trial.

Investigator's Responsibilities Change. The investigator's responsibilities or priorities change while the clinical trial is in progress and he or she cannot devote as much effort to the trial. If the basis for this change is legitimate (e.g., new responsibilities) the sponsor will usually be reasonable in reaching a mutually agreed-on solution.

Patient Death or Severe Adverse Reaction. A patient dies or has severe adverse reactions. Whether or not the investigator believes the problem is related to the medicine, the sponsor *must* be notified within 24 hours, even on weekends.

Personality Conflicts Develop. Personality conflicts occur with a monitor or other representative of the sponsor. Any difficulties that threaten the clinical trial's conduct or make the investigator unhappy should be discussed with the individual's supervisors.

Sponsor's Perspective Not Understood. The investigator has great difficulty understanding the sponsor's perspective on an issue. Any questions or issues should be brought up and discussed with colleagues or representatives of the sponsor.

ACADEMICIANS WHO APPROACH A SPONSOR WITH A PROPOSAL TO PARTICIPATE IN A CLINICAL TRIAL

A potential investigator may know (or believe) that a pharmaceutical company has a potentially exciting new medicine under development. Competition may arise among investigators who desire to participate in early-phase clinical trials. A few pointers are listed to help the academician who wants to convince a company to choose his or her site for a clinical trial. Relevant issues should be stressed during conversation or in writing. The potential investigator should consider which of the following are relevant and then:

1. Show enthusiasm for conducting the clinical trial.
2. Show a willingness to collaborate closely with the sponsor's monitors.
3. Show interest in the new medicine.
4. Demonstrate the presence of an appropriate patient population.
5. State that the local Ethics Committee/IRB is efficient and cooperative.
6. Describe the presence of adequate staff who can help conduct and coordinate the clinical trial.
7. Review his or her experience in conducting other sponsored clinical trials.
8. Show his or her knowledge of record-keeping requirements and claim the ability to do this correctly and efficiently based on past experience.
9. Describe his or her ability to obtain other services needed for the trial (e.g., laboratory studies, specialized tests, X-rays).
10. Be willing to provide references of other sponsors who can testify to his or her experience and quality of clinical trial conduct.

GAMES SPONSORS PLAY

Some sponsors use particular ploys to encourage an investigator to join a clinical trial but then fail to carry through on promises made. Anything that the investigator insists on should be put in writing prior to a clinical trial's initiation, if it is within the power of the sponsor to fulfill the statement. Many games that are played by sponsors' representatives (Table 55.2) are innocently perpetrated and many relate primarily to a lack of experience or knowledge on the part of the clinical monitors with whom the investigator interacts. Nonetheless, the investigator must constantly try to separate facts from beliefs, beliefs from desires, and actual commitments from sponsor's plans, intentions, and hopes. This approach will minimize or prevent surprise, disappointment, resentment, and other negative responses if it is later learned that the intended clinical trial will not be conducted, that the investigator was not chosen to participate, or that another undesired event occurred.

The category of games sponsors play is not meant to include examples of deceit, lying, or fraud, which are inexcusable and hopefully rare. Deception and misconduct are discussed in Chapter 64.

TABLE 55.2 *Selected games that sponsors may sometimes play with investigators*

1. Talk about starting a clinical trial at a certain date, but the date is unrealistic
2. Talk about a clinical trial they say is certain, but they are only evaluating whether it is feasible to conduct
3. Underestimate the amount of work involved in initiating or conducting a clinical trial
4. Underestimate the amount of work involved in completing the data collection forms
5. Underestimate the degree to which they will insist that the investigator adhere to every fine point of the protocol
6. Exaggerate how rapidly they can send medicines, supplies, and other materials to the clinical trial site
7. Claim that payments will be made promptly according to a schedule, but delay payment or pay investigators on a different basis
8. Claim that they will have a continuation protocol prepared at a later date, but do not furnish one, or furnish it too late to enroll all patients who complete the initial clinical trial
9. Claim that they would like the investigator to present his or her results at several important meetings, but do not follow through on this general statement
10. Claim that one or more publications will result from the clinical trial, but do not follow through
11. State that they will prepare a publication, but do not do so if the results turn out to be less positive than anticipated

CHAPTER 56

Roles of Private Practice Physicians in Clinical Trials

Most of the foregoing discussions centered on clinical trials that an academic or industrial group or individual scientist might choose to pursue. There are also trials that might be pursued by physicians in private practice. These require a number of special considerations that are described below.

The term *medicine trials* is used in broader context in this chapter than in the rest of this book. It includes participation in any type of medical research, including presenting posters at medical conventions and reporting cases in the medical literature, as well as participating in formal medicine trials using prepared protocols.

WHICH CLINICAL TRIALS TO CONDUCT

Possibly the simplest approach for many physicians who are interested in research is to analyze and write a report of an unusual case(s) that provides important lessons or information. Another approach is to contact the manufacturer of a medicine whose safety or efficacy profile is of particular interest. Many companies are willing to help private practitioners conduct small clinical trials on topics of mutual interest.

Physicians who have little training in conducting medicine trials would find it easier in most cases to begin with a Phase III or Phase IV trial. Such a clinical trial would generally be performed in outpatients and would not be as demanding for either patients or the investigator as Phase II trials. Phases III and IV trials usually have fewer demands in terms of patient visits

and tests that must be evaluated or performed at each visit; these trials may generally be integrated more easily into an outpatient clinic setting in a hospital or private clinic than Phase II trials.

SPONSORED TRIALS

There are numerous practical factors for a physician in private practice to consider in deciding whether to conduct sponsored clinical trials. These include the (1) number of staff members and time required to fill out and maintain the sponsor's data collection forms, which are often quite extensive, (2) amount of resources required to process and analyze data adequately (this step is usually performed by the sponsor or by a statistical collaborator), (3) liability insurance to protect oneself against unforeseen problems with a new medicine or treatment, (4) monitoring resources if several private practitioners are collaborating on a project, and (5) sufficient motivational drive and desire to withstand the demands of conducting a clinical trial throughout its duration. It is clearly better to conduct a simple trial and do it well than to attempt a more ambitious one and not succeed.

An investigator will want to ask a sponsor or its representatives many questions (see Chapter 55 for a list). Issues involve all aspects of the clinical trial, from initiation to data analysis to publication, and from protocol design to trial conduct to terms of financial payment.

INDEPENDENTLY CONDUCTED (NONSPONSORED) CLINICAL TRIALS

One of the major areas in which private practitioners may contribute to medical research, apart from conducting medicine trials, is to publish case reports of adverse experiences observed with new medicines. It is important when describing adverse reactions to indicate the number of patients with the problem and the number of patients with the same treatment who did *not* have the problem. It is only through such incidence data that a realistic perspective on the clinical significance of the reported event may be established. Details on severity, duration, outcome, rechallenge with medicine, and other factors are also important to include. These are more completely described in Chapter 80.

Overreporting of Adverse Reactions

Private practitioners may treat patients with a medicine and monitor prospectively for adverse reactions (Drury and Hull, 1981). One of the common traps of this type of approach is that it is easy to overreport and to speculate that an event is a result of a particular medicine the patient is receiving. It is usually a difficult, time-consuming, and sometimes expensive task to prove that this association is real and not a chance association or the result of a spurious relationship based on a bias of the patient or investigator. The consequences of false associations of medicines with adverse events may be far reaching and extensive. Significant medical resources and efforts may be unnecessarily spent by sponsors and by academicians evaluating nonexistent relationships. Patients may be unnecessarily deprived of a useful treatment that was withheld or withdrawn from the market. Patients may needlessly suffer psychologically or develop sequelae through stress, or they may experience physical complications during clinical trials conducted to evaluate the issue.

Underreporting of Adverse Reactions

The result of underreporting adverse reactions is equally undesirable. If physicians are either unfamiliar or uncomfortable with Food and Drug Administration (FDA) 1639 forms or the UK "Yellow Card" (see Chapter 126), then they will be less likely to use these systems for reporting potentially important adverse reactions. It was recently shown that an education program in Rhode Island greatly increased physician reporting (Scott et al., 1990). There are numerous other means for potentially important adverse reactions to be reported (e.g., through publications, directly to the manufacturer), but for this to occur the physician must (1) recognize the event as an adverse reaction, (2) recognize the potential value of reporting the adverse reaction, (3) have the knowledge of how to report it, and (4) have the interest and time to follow through on his or her good intentions.

Other Types of Clinical Trials

Nonsponsored trials that may be conducted by private practitioners include (1) those in which a small number of patients are required, (2) those with single straightforward objectives, and (3) various types of multicenter trials. If and when problems arise, the private practitioner may obtain advice or assistance from peers, nearby hospital staff, academic center staff, pharmaceutical companies, and individuals who have published related articles.

Golden Rule

The rules a potential investigator should follow are identical to those applicable to a group of experienced academicians who are conducting a large trial. Perhaps the single most important suggestion, or golden rule, is to enlist the aid of a statistician who is knowledgable about clinical trials, before getting too deeply involved in a project. Maintain this relationship throughout the trial.

Meaningful trials may be conducted in even a single patient under certain circumstances. Designs that may be used are mentioned in Chapter 38. See also Guyatt et al. (1986) and McLeod et al. (1986).

INVESTIGATOR'S INVESTIGATIONAL NEW DRUG APPLICATION

An investigator often approaches a sponsor with a request to study one of the sponsor's marketed (or nonmarketed) products for a new indication or in a new group of patients. Nonsponsored clinical trials may require the investigator to obtain regulatory approval. If so, it may be necessary to obtain an Investigational New Drug application (IND). Some companies prefer not to have investigators conduct this type of investigational trial under the company's IND. One reason might be that the company does not wish to dedicate the resources necessary to help design as well as monitor the trial. The company may be willing, however, to supply a medicine to an investigator who has obtained his own IND. An investigator who wishes to obtain his own IND to conduct clinical trials should communicate directly with the company that manufactures the medicine of interest and discuss the various possibilities for obtaining regulatory approval. If an investigator's IND is chosen as the most desirable approach, then the investigator must submit information listed in Figs. A1 to A3 (Appendix) of Spilker (1984) to the FDA. The company must provide a letter to the FDA allowing cross-reference of the investigator's IND to all previously submitted preclinical data.

CHAPTER 57

Patients' Perspectives About Clinical Trials

The term *patient* is generally used in this book to include normal volunteers, asymptomatic patients, and symptomatic patients who are entered into clinical trials. In this particular chapter the word volunteer(s) is used (when appropriate) in addition to the term patient. Volunteers are seldom used in Phases II and III clinical trials.

WHY VOLUNTEERS ENROLL IN CLINICAL TRIALS

The major reason that volunteers enroll in Phase I clinical trials is the money they receive. Payment to volunteers is ethically acceptable, as long as volunteers are not coerced to remain in a trial because the investigator or sponsor refuses to pay them if they do not complete it. The fairest way to pay volunteers is on a prorated basis depending on the extent of their participation (e.g., number of clinic visits, percent of total blood draws). It is ethically acceptable to encourage continued participation by offering volunteers a bonus if they participate in an entire clinical trial, but this should be stated in advance.

A small number of volunteers enter Phase I clinical trials to receive room and board, whereas others enter because of their desire to help society or the particular group conducting the trial. In some countries, volunteers may be employees of the pharmaceutical company that is conducting the trial. This raises issues beyond the ethical ones about coercion. The company must decide if it wants to allow employees to participate in clinical trials in lieu of spending their time at their job. The potential for lost production as well as productivity could be an important issue.

WHY PATIENTS ENROLL IN CLINICAL TRIALS

Patients enter most Phase II or III clinical trials to receive medical benefit from a new treatment, as well as the benefit of an increased level of medical care and monitoring. Personal reassurance from physicians and peace of mind are also important benefits. These benefits have been documented in two major cardiovascular trials (Mattson et al., 1985). Other benefits reported by patients in these trials included free medical and laboratory services, interaction with other patients, education about their problem, and physical improvement. A number of patients are motivated by a desire to help other patients with a similar disease, or by a desire to help the investigators. Other, less common reasons for enrolling in clinical trials are curiosity or a desire to pay back the medical system for help received in the past.

Unfortunately, some patients enter clinical trials because of fears and anxieties about how their physician(s) will treat them if they do not enter. This may apply more to patients with a severe chronic disease (e.g., cancer, renal failure) who require frequent care from physicians, although strong evidence that supports (or refutes) this view that patients who do not

398

enroll in clinical trials will receive inferior care appears to be unavailable. Counseling and support from nurses and others may be insufficient to allay this fear in some patients.

Additional information about patient enrollment based on patient interviews is found in articles by Cassileth et al. (1982), Kemp et al. (1984), Saurbrey et al. (1984), and Barofsky and Sugarbaker (1979). References on methods to use in interviewing patients are presented by Mattson et al. (1985).

DISCUSSING ENROLLMENT WITH PROSPECTIVE PATIENTS

Concepts

The physician, nurse, or other health professional who discusses a clinical trial with patients should describe the underlying conceptual difference, from the patient's perspective, between a clinical trial and usual medical care. The point should be made that in the latter, the physician guides the course of the patient's diagnosis and treatment whereas in the former (clinical trial), a protocol is written that directs the treatment the patient will receive. The patient should be assured that the physician can and will intervene whenever necessary to protect the patient's well-being.

Medical Information

Patients are often approached about enrolling in a clinical trial at a time when they are experiencing their maximum physical symptoms and psychological stress. It is precisely at those times that reaching a decision about enrolling in a clinical trial is usually most difficult. The professional staff should consider means of decreasing patients' fears, anxieties, and misconceptions about a proposed trial. Discussions must be tailored to the specific clinical trial and to the specific patient. A patient's willingness to join a clinical trial depends on factors listed in Table 57.1. A selected number of patient misconceptions are listed in Table 57.2.

Each patient likes to be treated with respect and many patients demand this right. While the amount of medical information desired by patients about a clinical trial varies greatly, in most countries where clinical trials are well designed and conducted, investigators are ethically required to provide patients with information about the trial and receive an informed consent. When relevant, a patient's informed consent may also be discussed with family members, close friends, or others. The participation of these other people is often vital to the enrollment of a patient, as well as keeping

TABLE 57.1 *Factors affecting patient willingness to enter a clinical trial*

1. Nature of their disease and type of disability it causes (e.g., are certain visible features of the disease embarrassing to the patient, is knowlege of their disability one they are ashamed about even though it is not visible to others)
2. Severity of the disease (i.e., very mild and very severe forms or stages of a disease generally make patients less likely to enter clinical trials)
3. Prognosis of various outcomes for the patient
4. Cultural and social background
5. Religious views and how these views relate to concepts of experimentation and helping others
6. Relationship with the physician conducting the clinical trial or whoever is referring them to the trial
7. Feelings about the medical establishment in general
8. Availability of time for participation and degree of inconvenience the trial entails
9. Personal safety issues that relate to traveling to the clinical trial site, including traveling within the site itself (e.g., parking lot, corridors)
10. Economic status and ability to pay for treatments, transportation, baby-sitting, and any other personal costs associated with the clinical trial
11. Distance required to travel to the clinical site and the ability to make these trips conveniently
12. Views of family and friends about the clinical trial
13. Frequency and length of clinic visits or duration of hospital stay
14. Quality of life and overall satisfaction with current therapy
15. Concerns about adverse reactions from the treatment
16. Personal values
17. Fears about needles and unpleasant tests

the patient in the clinical trial and ensuring the patient's compliance with the requirements of the protocol.

Counseling

Nurses, physicians, or others have an important role in counseling patients about entering and remaining in a clinical trial. This is particularly relevant for clinical trials involving serious diseases, major interventions, or long-term commitments. As Bujorian (1988) said, it is "helpful for some patients to explore their *feelings* rather than thoughts, about the opportunities to participate in a clinical trial."

TABLE 57.2 *Selected patient misconceptions about entering clinical trials*

Patients often believe that:
1. Physicians know in advance which treatment is preferable to receive
2. Physicians have some ability to modify the clinical trial design
3. Physicians have some control in assigning patients to specific treatment groups
4. Refusing to enter the clinical trial will endanger their own health[a]
5. Investigational treatments are definitely beneficial

[a] This belief may be associated with either vague or specific beliefs (e.g., the physician will no longer allow me to come to the clinic, or the physician will not take as good care of me in the future).

A nurse or other staff member may assist the patient in reaching a decision about whether to enter a clinical trial. Bujorian (1988) describes four main areas in which nurses play an important helping role by (1) evaluating the patient's retention and understanding of the information presented by the physician and given on the informed consent form, plus provide additional information or reinforcement; (2) assisting the patient in exploring personal and family issues; (3) guiding patients in evaluating priorities, benefits, risks, and other factors as a basis for decision making; and (4) supporting the patient's right to decide their own course of action.

Counseling ideally helps patients work their way through the process of reaching a decision. Counseling is *not* intended to be advice on whether or not the patient should enroll in a clinical trial. The choice of words and tone used are critical and influence whether or not patients are reassured and made comfortable about their decision. The terms investigation and investigational treatment are better to use when describing a clinical trial, rather than the terms experiment and experimental treatment. The term study may be an even more desirable term to use. A sympathetic and empathetic tone is important, as is taking an adequate period of time to discuss each of the patient's questions and concerns.

HOW EXPECTATIONS ABOUT RECEIVING ACTIVE MEDICINE AND IMPROVING THEIR CONDITION AFFECT PATIENT ENROLLMENT

Patient perceptions of how their quality of life will be affected by a clinical trial often influence their willingness to enroll, for example when a patient may receive a placebo and has a strong preference for receiving an active medication. The percent of patients in a clinical trial who will receive placebo is often an important factor that influences the patient's decision about enrollment. The lower the probability of receiving placebo, the greater is the likelihood of their entering the trial. Other examples of how perception of quality of life influences patients include almost all clinical trials in which the two (or more) treatment arms are perceived as having different impacts on a patient's lifestyle. These include trials in which comparisons are being made between medical versus surgical therapy (e.g., for treatment of angina), radiation versus amputation (e.g., for cancer of a limb), or major versus minor surgery (e.g., mastectomy versus lumpectomy as treatment for breast cancer). Two patients can have radically differing views about how any one treatment will affect their quality of life. This helps explain why it is more difficult to enroll patients in certain trials (Angell, 1984a, b). This situation is further complicated if the investigator has personal views as to which treatment is preferable for his or her patients who are candidates for the clinical trial.

Although the suggestion has been made (Weinstein, 1974) that patients be allowed to choose the treatment they prefer, this approach is improper in a clinical trial, because it is possible that patients who choose one treatment will differ in one or more important ways from those who choose the other treatment. On the other hand, patients who are *not* participating in a clinical trial should be involved whenever possible in the decision as to which medical treatment they will receive.

CLINIC VISITS BY PATIENTS PRIOR TO ENROLLMENT

It is sometimes useful for potential enrollees to visit the clinical trial site under relaxed circumstances, particularly when they are unfamiliar with either the setting or the nature of the trial and such unfamiliarity might adversely affect their willingness to participate. This visit, arranged for either individuals or groups, would enable potential enrollees to become familiar with details of the protocol, the equipment to be used, the staff, and the environment. Answers to questions about the protocol as well as discussions on specific details are likely to encourage patient enrollment and lead to cooperation and enhanced compliance. Audiovisual presentations describing both specific and general aspects of the clinical trial can also be utilized at this time.

Negative aspects of pretrial patient visits to a clinic site are possible and might include disruption of the investigator's and staff's workday, and intimidation and anxiety of patients in the medical environment. These potential difficulties may be prevented if the study site prepares a brief written agenda and description of what will take place during the visit and sends this to potential patients in advance. The agenda for patient visits should include (1) introduction of the staff, (2) tour of the facility, (3) discussion of the protocol, (4) discussion of patient's rights, (5) discussion of patient responsibilities, and (6) a question and answer period.

PATIENT CONCERNS ABOUT A CLINICAL TRIAL

General Concerns

A patient may become discouraged or disenchanted with a clinical trial, from failure to improve, or failure to improve at the anticipated rate. Other common reasons include adverse events, compromised quality of life, financial burdens, time commitments, and other problems.

The major concerns reported by patients enrolled in the two trials described by Mattson et al. (1985) were transportation to and from the clinic and the long time spent in the waiting room. Other difficulties included problems in scheduling visits, changes in clinic physicians, lack of adequate communication, feeling rushed at clinic visits, and blood draws. These (and other) concerns of patients should be monitored and addressed during the clinical trial as well as prior to the trial. In addition to maintaining patient enrollment, careful attention to these points will also enhance patient compliance as well.

Financial Concerns

Patients are sometimes concerned about the costs they will incur as a result of enrolling in a clinical trial or study. While the experimental treatment is almost always supplied without charge to patients, investigators may require patients to pay for professional services, laboratory tests, X-rays, and even administrative costs in academically sponsored trials. Not all patients have adequate health insurance to cover these costs, and even those patients who do may have significant out-of-pocket expenses. This issue rarely surfaces in pharmaceutical-company-sponsored trials, since the sponsor usually pays these costs. Patients usually have to pay for incidentals such as food and transportation, but sometimes even those costs are reimbursed.

The investigator should be astute enough to discern these feelings and discuss the situation frankly with the patient. An honest talk may serve to retain the patient in clinical trial. Alternatively, both the patient and physician may agree that the patient should be discontinued. Patients who do not have such discussions with investigators or staff often drop out of trials (see Chapter 31).

IMPROVING RELATIONSHIPS BETWEEN PATIENTS AND MEDICAL PROFESSIONALS

Views about a clinical trial often vary enormously among the enrolled patients. Physicians often are not aware of the reasons why a patient does or does not agree to a certain treatment (Churchill and Churchill, 1989). It is the staff's responsibility to assess patient views and to do whatever reasonable to answer questions, address needs, and anticipate relevant issues. Being interested in each patient and maintaining a sympathetic attitude will increase the probability that patients will share their concerns and feelings.

Relationships between patients and health professionals in a clinical trial may affect the trial's outcome more than any other single factor. When treatment options exist, shared decision making between patients and medical professionals should be an important goal. This helps create bonds that assist in maintaining patient compliance. If the physician or another professional attempts to impose his or her will on patients, it often backfires and promotes a lack of cooperation. The overall quality of the physician–patient relationship should be assessed during a trial by the monitor, particularly if the trial is experiencing problems. Methods to improve patient–physician relationships are discussed in Chapter 15.

WRITTEN AND ORAL INSTRUCTIONS FOR PATIENTS

Written Instructions

Written information should be given to all patients in a clinical trial at the time of their enrollment. This may occur after they sign the informed consent, at the first time they are given medicine, when the initially come to clinic, or at any other convenient time that is standardized for every patient in the trial. A checklist of pretrial or initial trial activities created either for or by the investigator should include the dispensing of these sheets. This practice ensures that all patients receive the same standard (i.e., minimum) amount of information.

Contents

The information sheets may include an opening paragraph that discusses the clinical trial's background and purpose, as well as reiterates some of the elements of the informed consent (e.g., you may leave the trial at any time). A copy of the informed consent should also be given to each patient enrolled, but that is not a replacement for the patient instruction sheet (or vice versa).

This instruction sheet may also describe how patients should (1) complete diaries or other data collection forms, (2) collect biological samples (e.g., urine), (3) comply with a diet, (4) conduct exercises, and (5) take precautions (e.g., not driving within 4 hours of taking their medicines, not standing up rapidly in the morning). The correct way to take medicine should be carefully described on this sheet. This information should also be presented verbally to patients, and their comprehension confirmed.

This sheet, as well as the informed consent, should contain the name and telephone number to call in case of problems or questions. The information sheet(s) must describe the first day in detail if it differs from the other days in the trial (i.e., patients often take fewer or additional doses). Patients should be told what to do if they miss one or more doses (e.g., take an extra one, do nothing) and whether to take the medicine with food, before meals, or after meals. If patients are allowed to adjust their dosage themselves, they must be informed about all appropriate details and caveats, preferably in writing as well as verbally.

Written instructions may use any format (e.g., terse bullets, prose, calendars) and any style deemed appropriate. Other items that are sometimes provided are listed in Table 57.3. A meta-analysis of 70 published evaluations of educational programs to inform chronically ill patients about their clinical trial has demonstrated the benefits of various interventions (Mullen et al., 1985).

Wallet Cards

It is also desirable to provide patients with wallet or purse cards containing information about the clinical trial (Spilker, 1978). These cards should list names and telephone numbers of contacts for the trial, and possibly some details (e.g., type of medicine). Patients should be informed that it is important to show these cards to other physicians, dentists, opticians, and other health care providers they visit during the trial.

Oral Instructions

When giving patients benefit and risk information about the treatments they may receive in a clinical trial it is important to inform them about the likelihood of each major benefit and risk. It is clearly difficult, if not impossible, for physicians to know precise probabilities for most potential occurrences of all adverse reactions and benefits. On the other hand, the general likelihood should be known. Likelihoods may be expressed in terms of either general categories (e.g., very likely, possible, highly unlikely, extremely unlikely) or as percent probabilities (e.g., over 90% likely, about 50%, less than 10%). It is also likely that patients will interpret the categories described differently than the physician or other professional intends. Chapter 72 discusses the fact that most general words used to describe probabilities (e.g., often, seldom, rarely, sometimes) are interpreted extremely differently by different people. This issue should be considered by the physician during interactions with each patient.

Some investigators may wish to present a more complete and balanced picture of the clinical trial to the patient and discuss whether or not a patient should enter. These investigators could describe reasons why a patient might choose not to enroll as well as reasons why a patient might choose to enroll. A frank, open, and honest discussion is the best policy to adapt and will lead to greater patient compliance. Video tapes may be prepared and shown to potential patients. These tapes could describe the treatment and trial in detail, or they could include interviews with patients who describe their experiences with (and reactions to) the treatment.

TABLE 57.3 *Items to include in written instructions provided to patients*

A. Information about other medicines
   1. Which other categories of medicines may be taken, or may not be taken with the trial medicine
   2. Conditions under which other medicines may be used
   3. Names of other specific medicines that may be used
   4. Names of other specific medicines that may not be used
   5. Should patients bring their medicine container to some or all clinic visits?
   6. If patients are being weaned off a medicine, the details of this should be described
B. Information about the clinical trial medicine and the patient's participation in the trial
   1. Methods that should be used to store the medicine (e.g., refrigeration)
   2. Instructions that patients should not take more or fewer pills than prescribed
   3. Whom to call (and when to call) if the patient believes their condition warrants a change of dose
   4. What to do if one, two, or more than two doses are missed
   5. How to complete a diary or data collection forms
   6. Instructions on how to collect biological samples (e.g., a 24-hour urine)
   7. A statement to inform other physicians seen for medical problems about this clinical trial
   8. Directions to show the wallet card at visits to other physicians and health professionals
   9. Discussion of adverse events and whom to telephone if they occur (telephone numbers must be included)
   10. Precautions to be used for driving motor vehicles, operating machinery, drinking alcohol, or doing difficult physical activities
   11. Suggestion to keep these instructions in a safe and easy to remember place
C. Information about clinic visits
   1. Amount of time to plan on spending at each clinic visit
   2. Instructions on how to reschedule any clinic visits that are difficult to keep
   3. What to bring to each clinic visit (e.g., diary, medicine container)
   4. How to prepare for each clinic visit (e.g., fast for X hours, do not take medicine the day of the clinic visit)
   5. Where to report first at the clinic
   6. When and how to inform clinical trial personnel if other physicians were visited and if other medicines were prescribed or given

CHAPTER 58

Roles of Medical Contract Organizations

At a meeting of the Pharmaceutical Manufacturers Association in 1988, a speaker was highly critical of the performance of medical research contract organizations. His sentiments were so widely echoed by company executives in the audience that the more than 100 medical and regulatory professionals appeared to be unanimous in their condemnation of such groups. Various people complained of exaggerated promises, poor quality of work, late deliveries, and excessive prices.

Are pharmaceutical company experiences uniformly poor? Of course not; if they were, most of the more than 300 contractors in the United States plus several hundred in Europe (Hughes, 1990) who depend on work from pharmaceutical companies would quickly go out of business. Subsequent discussions with many industry and contract company professionals have convinced me that these relationships can be improved. With a little foresight and planning by both parties, most of the problems encountered could be avoided. This chapter examines activities of contractors, reviews the types of relationships between contractors and clients, and suggests a number of methods to make those relationships more productive.

WHO ARE MEDICAL CONTRACTORS?

A wide spectrum of groups are referred to as contractors. Eleven types are described here, although many provide services in two or more areas. While most of the eleven types of groups defined are described as companies, some of these functions may be fulfilled by unincorporated individuals working as freelance contractors or as contractors working in academic centers.

Type 1: Independent companies that conduct clinical trials themselves. Contracted trials are usually Phase I safety or pharmacokinetic trials, but, in theory, almost any Phase I to III trial and some Phase IV trials could be conducted by these groups. Companies sometimes specialize in certain types of trials (e.g., quality of life, adverse reaction collection, sleep studies). Some of these companies are affiliated with academic centers or hospitals. Most of these contractors have a single clinic, although some have two or more clinics. Physicians may be employees of the contracting company or may rotate through the clinic on an as-needed basis.

Type 2: Academic departments or government agencies that conduct clinical trials. The former type may be administratively independent of the university. The department or group may specialize in a therapeutic area or it may be broadly based in clinical pharmacology.

Type 3: Medical practices that solicit sponsors for clinical trials to conduct. These trials may be either single-site or multicenter trials. In the latter case, the central practice may identify the other sites and may also provide monitors for the trial. They may have brokers to seek business from sponsors.

Type 4: Companies that place clinical trials primarily (or entirely) in a network of medical clinics that they have created. These clinics may be in hospitals, but they are more likely to be located in private group practices. A network of Health Maintenance Organizations (HMOs), nursing homes, or other types of medical practice may also be utilized or created.

Type 5: Contracting companies that place trials with investigators who are not part of a special network. This is perhaps the most common type of medical trial contracting group. Investigators are generally approached after a trial is identified that the contractor possibly or definitely will conduct.

Type 6: Regional monitors who act as independent contractors. These individuals may work independently for multiple contracting companies and/or sponsors.

Type 7: Contracting companies that focus their activities on performing statistical analyses of clinical data. A statistical report is usually their primary output. This role is often associated with the role described for type 8.

Type 8: Contracting companies that focus on data processing. Tapes of quality-assured, tabulated data are usually their primary output. See type 7.

Type 9: Contracting companies that focus on writing medical reports. These reports are prepared either from raw data or from a previously generated statistical report.

Type 10: Contracting companies that conduct retrospective medical studies and data analyses by reviewing primary patient medical records. Their usual output is a written medical and statistical report.

Type 11: Contracting companies able to have all clinical trials conducted that are necessary to proceed from the initial human trial to a regulatory submission. While the skills and even experience necessary to perform this role are easy to claim, few contractors are experienced in this capacity. This appears to be the goal of numerous contracting organizations. The ability to conduct most types of Phase IV trials may or may not be present in this type of group.

Some of these eleven types of groups focus their activities on specific therapeutic areas (e.g., cancer therapies), and some are able to write clinical protocols. Other types of contract organizations conduct toxicological studies, metabolic studies, screening evaluations, or nonclinical scientific studies. Contract

Ethics Committees/Institutional Review Boards (IRBs) are also available in Europe and in the United States.

Exemployees of a company who are not working for a competitor may serve some of these (or other) functions. For example, former employees could act as contractors to write final medical reports or serve as brokers to identify and possibly interview suitable investigators. The company would then pursue further contacts with the potential investigators. This service would be especially valuable for companies entering new therapeutic areas.

WHY SHOULD PHARMACEUTICAL COMPANIES USE CONTRACT GROUPS?

The major reason for a company to use a contract group is to conduct work that cannot easily or expeditiously be conducted internally. This could be a result of insufficient personnel or expertise. The contractor is essentially adding capabilities to the company without the company having to enlarge the staff on a permanent, or even on a temporary, basis. There are several advantages of this service for clients. The major advantage is that the client may rapidly achieve the total number of staff (including those of the contractor) necessary to meet temporarily greater work demands. This advantage is also felt at a later time when workloads decrease and no one must be dismissed. Another advantage relates to the ultimate savings in time required for a medicine's development. Companies have calculated that the increased costs for a contractor's services are often more than offset by future revenues of a medicine that is marketed earlier than it otherwise would be. In some cases the contractor's fee is more than offset by higher overhead of the client company, and, thus, use of a contractor may be cost effective.

In deciding whether to hire a contractor for a specific project, the client's resources and time required to complete the activities should be assessed. The amount of time and effort required to educate the contractor must be considered in determining the overall cost–effectiveness of using a contractor. For example, if a complex data processing project is being considered for contracting out, the sponsor will usually have to spend a great deal of time (e.g., 50% of the total time needed) just to educate and monitor the contractor. There is a strong probability in this situation that it is not worthwhile to contract out the project. On the other hand, if only 10% to 20% of the total staff time is required to educate and monitor the contractor (and an 80% to 90% savings in time is gained) then it makes much more sense to contract out the project. Sponsors must weigh direct and indirect costs plus the project's priority, commercial value, and importance to the company in reaching a decision on each particular project.

Some clients request proposals from multiple contractors before deciding whether to contract out a major activity. Under those circumstances, the client should inform the contractor that a firm decision has not yet been made to conduct the activity. The contractor may then judge better how much effort to put into the proposal it submits.

HOW SHOULD A CLIENT CHOOSE A GOOD CONTRACT GROUP?

One of the important rules in choosing contractors is to discuss the project with several independent contractors. The same information should be presented to each. Then, a client should obtain and compare proposals from two or more contractors for the same project. Meetings between contractors and clients that identify precisely what will and will not be done by each group are essential. Establishing a clear and open understanding between client and contractor is an important step to avoid misunderstandings and to ensure successful completion of a project.

The choice of contractors should never be based on cost alone. Contractors who propose lower costs than their competitors may be thinking of adding in cost overruns or of cutting corners on quality. If clients accept sloppy work, a poor relationship with the contractor will be ensured. Clients must interpret bids cautiously if the contractor has a history of cost overruns. This factor may be assessed by contacting several references. Differences in costs between contractors may also reflect differences in quality. A client that believes one specific contractor offers the highest quality service, but charges significantly more than others, may negotiate prices with this contractor.

Each of the following characteristics of contractors and their proposals should be evaluated, and these questions addressed.

Quality of the Proposal

Is the overall proposal logical and does it make sense? Is it complete or are important areas neglected? Does the proposal reflect an appropriate understanding of the problems involved? May the client make independent monitoring or comonitoring site visits during the clinical trial? What type of reports will contractors provide to the client and at what frequency?

Each of these issues must be discussed within the client's company, and any questions must be raised with the contractor. It is important for the client to know what it desires the contractor to propose for each

question or topic raised or to indicate to the contractor that the client's views are not fully determined. This enables the contractor to prepare meaningful proposals that may also be compared with those of others. Clients who do not provide clear information to contractors are placing them in an unfair position when proposals are created.

Reputation and Experience of the Contractor

Have they previously worked for you? If so, what were their strengths and weaknesses and how would each of these influence the current project? Obtain several references for each contractor and check them carefully. What weaknesses in the contractor's performance were observed by these referees, and how critical would the weaknesses be for the current project? Has the contractor previously conducted similar or identical types of work for other clients? If not, what is the likelihood that the contractor's work will be completed successfully? This question is essential to address, particularly if the client is unsure about using a contractor. If the contractors or studies they placed were audited by the Food and Drug Administration (FDA), what were the results?

Personnel at the Contractor's Group

How have the contractor's personnel been assessed? What is their experience and expertise and how closely do they relate to the current proposal? Are sufficient personnel available on the contractor's staff to be assigned to the client's project? What is the rate of personnel turnover at the contract group? This is particularly important for projects that are projected to last for longer than a few months. How strong are the relationships between the client and the contractor's staff who will manage the project? Judge the contractor's personnel at face-to-face meetings and not only by reading their qualifications on paper. Biographies and curriculum vitae may be written to make individuals appear far more qualified and experienced than they are.

Quality of the Clinics and Investigators That Are To Be Used

Clinic and investigator quality must meet a standard set by the client in terms of size, reputation, staff, and other factors. Practical considerations may also be a factor, including availability of the sites to conduct the clinical trial and the contractor's proximity to the client, to the investigators, and to adequate transportation facilities. A good airport with convenient, reliable regional carrier service is probably as good as a major airline service. Contractors may have either an easier, more difficult, or equivalent ability to enroll suitable investigators for a trial. This may be a relevant factor in deciding whether to use a contractor.

Costs of the Activity

Costs are often a difficult aspect of a proposal to compare among contractors. Each bidder may use different caveats and strategies in arriving at a total price estimate. Clarify each caveat used. If it appears that assumptions and caveats differ among the proposals, consider requesting new bids using standardized criteria. Contractors that are concerned about being underbid by competitors may choose to submit multiple bids, each with different assumptions. Alternatively, a range of bids could be given if the scope of the work is not precisely established.

Facilities of the Contractor

Is the contractor operating out of a one-room office or does it have impressive facilities? Does it have computers in-house or must it contract for outside computers? This would be particularly important for data-processing contracts. Can contractors perform various ancillary services efficiently, or do they subcontract some of these functions (e.g., statistical evaluations)? Are their standard operating procedures thorough, reasonable, and are they followed by staff? Relevant standard operating procedures of the contractor may be reviewed briefly or in great detail.

Marketing brochures of contractors often make substantial claims that must be evaluated carefully by prospective clients. Very little should be assumed by clients who are evaluating an unknown or little known contractor. For example, there are reports that some contractors who are awarded contracts actually subcontract the monitoring and data processing of some studies they undertake. While this may not compromise quality, the issue is whether the client is aware of this practice and whether adequate quality assurance procedures exist.

Time Required to Complete the Project

While no group can be strictly held to a tight schedule, speed is invariably important. Proposed timetables to achieve the project's milestones should be realistic. These milestones may be set by the client who insists that the contractor meet the deadlines or by the contractor who desires to impress the client with the speed at which a project proceeds.

There is a balance between proposing unrealistically short times and overly conservative times to complete project milestones. If the contractor has proposed the milestone dates, then the client may best judge them by calling numerous references about the contractor's performance, rather than comparing different proposals. Clients should also compare the time estimated to complete the project in-house with that estimated by the contractor. Contractors should follow comparable procedures if the time estimates are proposed by the client. Contractors should discuss milestone dates as openly as possible, to ensure that the client has not established unrealistic goals.

HOW CONTRACTORS MARKET THEIR SERVICES

Contractors are using more and more sophisticated techniques to market their services to the pharmaceutical industry. A few of these are listed.

1. Exhibits at conventions, symposia, and other types of professional meetings.
2. Hospitality suites at professional meetings.
3. Direct mailings of brochures, business cards, annual reports, announcements of new staff (or promotions), or marketing letters.
4. Direct mailings of professional publications of presumed interest to the client with a business card attached.
5. Advertisements in medical journals, newsletters, and medical magazines.
6. Telephone calls to selected industry staff. This is highly frowned on by many industry professionals and may be counterproductive if the potential client feels that he or she is being disturbed or harassed. Of course, if the contractor has knowledge of personnel who are planning clinical trials, then their telephone call may be welcome.
7. Luncheon meetings at sites outside the client's or contractor's facilities. Meetings designed to discuss a specific project often have a better chance of being productive than general discussions about the contractor's services, although this depends on the specific situation.
8. Invitations to key industry personnel to speak at the contractor's organization.
9. Seminars held at companies describing experiences and services of the contractor.
10. Meetings at a potential client's company to discuss the contractor's services. This approach is strongly discouraged unless the meeting is initiated or favored by the company.
11. Clients present data at major scientific meetings and give credit to the contracting organization.

COMMON REASONS FOR PROBLEMS BETWEEN CONTRACTORS AND CLIENTS

This list could include hundreds of different examples. A few basic types of problems, however, are mentioned. Careful attention to these issues and also to the final section on recommendations for clients will help make relationships between clients and contractors more productive.

Problems with Joint Causes

1. Inadequate understanding by both parties of exactly what the contractor has agreed to do. This is primarily an issue of communication: each assumes the other understands the project in the same way they do but neither confirms their understanding in writing or through active listening techniques. A clear understanding of each step of the process and agreement on each party's responsibilities is extremely important.
2. Either group haggles over details in the contract.
3. Communications start to lapse and one or both parties begins to feel ill at ease. Constant communication is a must, and enables contingency plans to be implemented, if necessary.

Problems Primarily Emanating from the Client

1. Inadequate understanding by the client of precisely what they want the contractor to do or exactly what they want the contractor to furnish as a final product.
2. The relationship is one-sided (i.e., the client does not view the relationship as one of joint collaborators working on a project). If this were unanticipated, then the contractor's staff may become rapidly displeased, and their cooperation and efforts on behalf of the client may diminish.
3. Clients ask contractor to do more than what was agreed to and refuses to pay for the additional work.
4. A competing situation is set up when sponsors have multiple contractors conduct the same clinical trial (using the same protocol) and compete for investigators, but do not tell them this fact in advance.
5. Clients insist that poorly designed protocols be used.
6. Clients add many protocol amendments after the clinical trial begins.
7. Clients are ill prepared to furnish supplies and clinical trial materials.
8. Clients do not allow the contractor to manage the clinical trial appropriately.

9. Clients may want to interact a great deal with the investigator because of inexperience or lack of trust with the contractor.
10. The client has set unrealistic deadlines for the contractor to meet, or the contractor has raised unrealistic expectations in the client because of foolish promises or deadlines.
11. The client is unaware of the true efforts or costs required to conduct the project. Clients may be unwilling to accept realistic information on patient availability.
12. The client's protocol contains flaws, is impractical, is incomplete, or has other serious problems. The contractor may be unaware of these problems, or may believe that to point them out would risk their losing the contract.

Problems Primarily Emanating from the Contractor

1. The contractor does not have the attitude that it will do whatever is necessary to ensure that each project it undertakes will be successful. This approach must be a hallmark of reputable contractors.
2. Project costs start to escalate beyond the original agreed-on amount, and the reasons for it are not fully justified in the client's opinion.
3. The quality of the contractor's work does not meet the standards expected by the client. Alternatively, the client's standards may be unrealistic.
4. The contractor does not understand the true reason(s) why the client decided to use a contractor.
5. The contractor should insist that the client indemnify it against product liability problems.
6. The periodic report submitted to the client is not adequately detailed from the client's perspective. For example, information may be lacking on (a) patient enrollment, (b) adverse reactions, (c) patient visits, (d) numbers and reasons for dropouts, (e) results of monitoring visits, (f) financial costs to date, and (g) any other areas in which information is expected to be reported. The amount of information to be provided must be established at the outset of each agreement.

WHAT TYPES OF PROJECTS MAY CLIENTS ESTABLISH WITH CONTRACTORS?

Types of projects are limited only by the imagination of the people involved. For example, a company may establish a relationship with two or more contractors for accomplishing a single project. One approach would be for contractor A to perform work X and then turn the project over to contractor B, who would perform work Y, who in turn would turn the project over to contractor C, who would perform work Z. In real terms, contractor A could conduct a clinical trial, contractor B could edit and process all the data, and contractor C could write the statistical and medical reports. The approach described would generally be quite risky to the client, because it must be concerned about the qualifications, performance, and cooperative nature of three serial groups. Any group that did not work well with the next group in the chain would lead to problems.

A contractor may subcontract parts of a project to other groups, but this should be agreeable to the client and discussed prior to signing any agreement. For example, laboratory assays of blood or interpretation of specialized examinations (e.g., electroencephalograms) from multiple study sites could be subcontracted to a central facility. This would generally lead to greater uniformity in measurements or data interpretation.

Reaching an Agreement

In detailing arrangements between sponsors and contractors who will not conduct trials themselves it is important to clarify all important areas, including the following:

1. How will investigators be chosen?
    a. The contractor may make the final decision.
    b. The contractor may choose the investigator, but the sponsor has the right of refusal.
    c. The sponsor must evaluate each proposed investigator and choose those who will conduct the trial.
2. Who will be responsible for monitoring the clinical trials?
    a. Only monitors from the sponsor.
    b. Monitors from the sponsor always accompanied by a monitor from the contractor.
    c. Monitors from the sponsor with or without a monitor from the contractor.

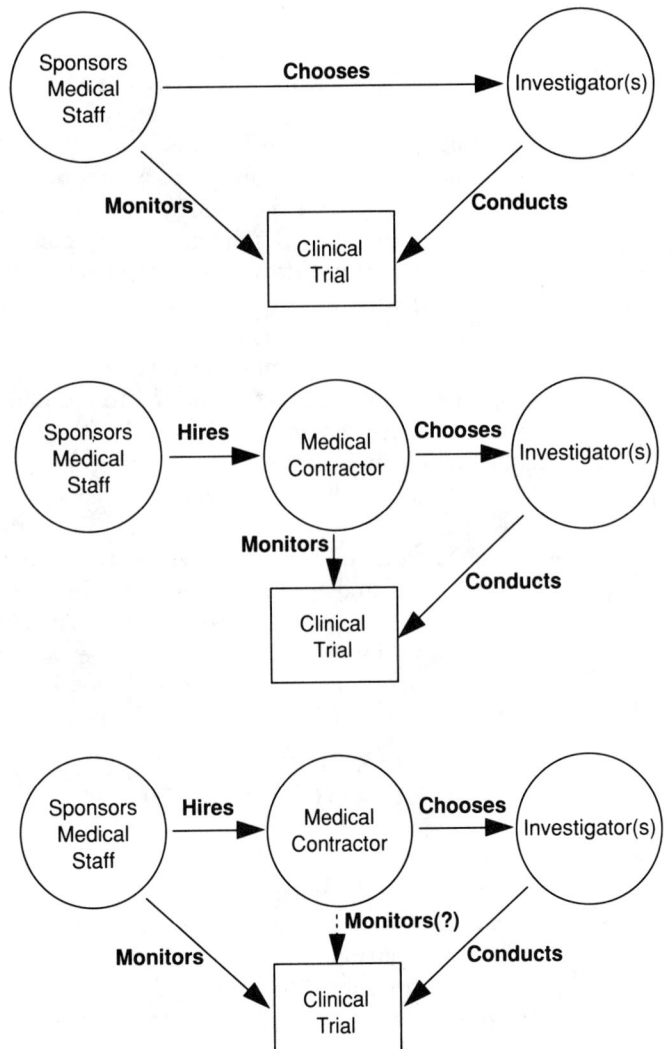

FIG. 58.1 Some of the relationships among investigators, monitors, and contractors that may be established.

d. Monitors from the contractor with or without a monitor from the sponsor.

e. Only monitors from the contractor.

3. How many monitoring visits will be made by the contractor?

a. Number to be determined solely by contractor.

b. Number to be determined solely by sponsor.

c. Number to be determined through joint discussions.

4. How will medicine supplies be handled and shipped to the clinical trial site? Various possibilities will be explored and agreement will be reached.

5. Who owns the data?

6. How will all payments be made?

Figure 58.1 illustrates some of the types of monitoring relationships that may be established.

RECOMMENDATIONS FOR CLIENTS

Develop an open and honest relationship with the contractor, since it will generally be able to help you better under those conditions. Explain why you are using a contract organization and what your major expectations are from the relationship. Monitor all clinical trials to the degree believed necessary for assurance that they are being conducted and monitored according to appropriate standards by the investigator and contractor, respectively. A primary contact person should be identified for both client and contractor.

Clients must always put the same overall effort into their interactions and relationships with contractors, even when they have previously had a positive experience with the same contractor. It is always wrong to assume that a clinical trial or other contract will be conducted well, because a previous one was. Decrements in performance may arise from many causes, such as staff changes, complacency, altered priorities, or an agreement that is unclear. Do not prolong a contract that is unsatisfactory—either correct it or agree to abandon it. Careful attention to all details of an agreement and interaction will help ensure that both parties are pleased at the end of the contract, which is the ultimate goal of the contractor–client relationship.

CHAPTER 59

Choosing Clinical Investigators

CHOOSING INVESTIGATORS TO VISIT

Many of the points discussed in this chapter are relevant for academic or other clinical investigators who are initiating clinical trials, in addition to sponsors. These factors concern trial planning and choice of collaborators, assistants, or research coordinators as well as interactions with pharmacists, laboratory personnel, and other individuals who assist.

Investigators are selected by sponsors on the basis of numerous factors, any one or combination of which may be decisive in reaching a decision for a particular clinical trial. A list of several factors that are involved in this process is given in Table 59.1.

The choice of a particular investigator for a single-site clinical trial or of several investigators for a multicenter trial may be made at any stage in the development of a protocol. Agreements may be reached before the trial design of a particular protocol is established or at any point prior to initiation of the trial. In addition, new sites may be added to multicenter trials that are already in progress.

In many clinical trials the choice of a specific investigator(s) is not made prior to the pretrial interview. This chapter is primarily focused on this situation and on the process by which an investigator(s) is chosen from among several who have been interviewed.

Identifying Investigators

The initial step in the process of choosing investigators for a clinical trial is to develop a list of potential candidates. This is often done by using the factors listed in Table 59.1 as a guide. Any one of these factors may be of major concern in a particular trial. If the sponsor prefers to have a contract organization locate and enroll investigators, then many of the processes described in this chapter would be performed by that organization.

Medical Contract Organizations

Contract groups are defined in this chapter as businesses or organizations whose primary activity is the conduct of clinical trials. Other activities are discussed in Chapter 58. They may function independently or be an integral part of an established medical school or hospital or associated with one or more schools or hospitals. There are a number of types of contract groups, but essentially they form two basic varieties: these groups either perform clinical trials themselves or serve as middlemen to place the clinical trials at other sites. In the former case, the location of the site used for the clinical trial may be at a medical school, hospital, private clinic, or building used primarily for the purpose of clinical trials. The contract groups may specialize in Phase I trials or offer to perform trials from Phase I to Phase IV. A few sites specialize in either Phase II, III, or IV trials. When the contract group initiates the trial at another site, the amount of planning, protocol writing, monitoring, data handling, and analysis by the contract group will vary widely, often based on the requirements of the sponsor. Trials may

TABLE 59.1 *Selected factors involved in investigator selection by a sponsor*

1. Reputation in the investigator's field of expertise, based on publications, references, and numerous other factors
2. Possession of equipment, techniques, or facilities essential or desirable for the clinical trial
3. Access to a patient population essential or desirable for the trial
4. Geographical location of the trial site in terms of ease of accessibility to the sponsor
5. Geographical location of the trial site in terms of conducting the trial in a desired location or region
6. Type of organization (e.g., VA hospital, nursing home)
7. Anticipated time required to initiate the trial
8. Anticipated time required to complete the trial
9. Relationship with individuals at the sponsoring institution
10. Budgetary factors (i.e., cost of the trial)
11. Previously made agreements
12. Desirability of utilizing a contract organization to locate and enroll investigators
13. Experience conducting other sponsored clinical trials
14. Presence of an experienced staff, including a clinical trial coordinator
15. Low turnover of the investigator's staff
16. Ability of the Ethics Committee/Institutional Review Board (IRB) to process protocols expeditiously and fairly

a Any one (or any combination) of these factors may be the predominant reason for selecting a particular investigator. These factors are not listed in any particular order.

be placed in private clinics, hospitals, or other sites depending on the specific contract organization that is contacted. Sponsors will usually be more aware of the quality and problems of a trial and the data that will be provided if they monitor the trial even though the contract group may also be monitoring it. Even if it is not possible to monitor each trial site periodically, the sponsor should visit the sites at which the actual trial will be performed on at least one occasion.

When Should Potential Investigators Be Visited?

There are several different times during the planning period of a clinical trial (or even during its conduct) when a potential investigator may be visited. The golden rule is that the sponsor should be honest with the potential investigator about the status of the clinical trial at the time of the visit. The status may be:

- A general concept only in the monitor's mind.
- A concept in which the company has expressed interest.
- A protocol is being written, but the sponsor is not yet committed.
- The protocol is complete, but the sponsor is not yet committed.
- The protocol is complete and the clinical trial will definitely be initiated.
- The clinical trial is under way and additional or replacement investigators are needed.

TOPICS AND INFORMATION TO DISCUSS

The sponsor of a clinical trial must evaluate a number of areas, such as those discussed below, at an initial meeting with the potential investigator, preferably at the site where the trial will be conducted. A list of the more important points to discuss may be prepared prior to the meeting, and a summary of the meeting is generally written after it has taken place. A synopsis of points to be covered is presented in Table 59.2. An important assumption underlying this chapter is that it is valuable to establish an open relationship with all personnel involved as well as a full understanding by each individual of his or her responsibilities in the medicine trial.

1. Determine the potential investigator's research experience in general and with new and marketed medicines in particular. Ascertain the major research interests of the potential investigator in clinical and nonclinical medicine.
2. Determine if the investigator has conducted similar medicine trials. This may be accomplished through computerized literature searches as well as by direct questioning. If the investigator has had previous experience, discuss the design, conduct, and entry rate of patients into previous trials plus other relevant aspects (e.g., overall quality and success of the trial). Obtain a copy of the published results if available.
3. Discuss the organization of the investigator's clinic, office, or laboratory, and whether a research coordinator, residents, assistants, laboratory personnel, nurses, or other individuals are to be included or will be available when necessary. If the site performs contract work for numerous sponsors, obtain a copy of the site's rules and regulations. Attempt to visit the site when a clinical trial is in progress and evaluate the atmosphere at the trial site.
4. Determine how often the investigator sees the specific type of patient to be included in the clinical trial, how many new or return patients the investigator sees each month or year, and how often the investigator obtains blood levels or performs other relevant tests on patients who are followed in the practice (i.e., how patients are treated and followed).
5. Determine how the investigator reacts to the actual or proposed protocol and how he or she feels about this type of clinical trial in terms of its design, efficacy measures, and other factors. Discuss why this trial is being conducted (i.e., what it expects to demonstrate or test and how it fits into the overall development of the medicine). Discuss specific areas in which additional information or input is

TABLE 59.2 *Selected topics to discuss with potential investigators*

A. Investigator
  1. Experience in conducting sponsored clinical trials (e.g., ask for names of companies or sponsor for use as references)
  2. Experience in conducting unsponsored clinical trials
  3. Problems or difficulties experienced in conducting clinical trials
  4. Research interests
  5. Availability of time to participate in the proposed clinical trial
  6. Interest in conducting the particular clinical trial
  7. Motivating factors for willingness to consider participation
  8. Priority he or she will assign the clinical trial in work load
  9. Responsibilities involved if another sponsor requests the investigator to initiate another clinical trial in the same therapeutic area
  10. Confirm that the investigator is not on any regulatory black list
B. Staff
  1. Number of staff present and their roles
  2. Experience of staff with aspects relating to the clinical trial
  3. Turnover of staff over the last year
  4. Special staff requirements relating to the proposed clinical trial
C. Site
  1. Clinic or office organization re: conducting the clinical trial
  2. Equipment required
  3. Ancillary facilities required (e.g., X-rays, laboratories, pulmonary function laboratories, pharmacy) and their ability to participate
  4. Hospital or clinic's policy about allowing monitors to view source documents in a patient's chart
D. Protocol
  1. Its current status and ability for input and modifications
  2. Policy on additional tests that may be performed by the investigator

  3. Review of general concepts and details (e.g., biological samples)
E. Patient availability
  1. Number of patients available in the investigator's practice who would pass inclusion criteria
  2. Investigator's anticipated rate of patient enrollment
  3. Basis for demonstrating patient availability to the sponsor (e.g., medical chart review by investigator or monitor)
  4. Characteristics of patients desired (e.g., disease severity)
F. Administrative issues
  1. Proposed (or firm) dates for conducting the clinical trial
  2. Budget (e.g., how it should be prepared, how the grant will be paid)
  3. Data handling and retention responsibilities
  4. Storage of medicines
  5. Dispensing of medicines (e.g., who, how)
  6. Publications (e.g., policies of the sponsor, order of authors, reasons for sponsor's review)
  7. Pretrial roundtable meeting (e.g., purposes, who will attend, where and when it will be held, input of investigators sought)
  8. Other responsibilities of the investigator (e.g, contents of regulations, policies of the sponsor)
  9. Other clinical trials under way or planned for the same medicine
G. Ethical issues
  1. Informed consent (e.g., who will write this, is a sample desired by the investigator)
  2. Ethics Committee/IRB (e.g., how often they meet, when documents must be submitted)
  3. Proposed relationship between sponsor and investigator (e.g., both are members of a team, investigators and staff will be available to monitors, everyone will be open and forthright)
  4. Basis on which an investigator(s) will be chosen to conduct the clinical trial (i.e., which factors in Table 59.1 are particularly important)

---

desired by the sponsor in order to develop a final protocol. It is the author's view that all potential or actual investigators in a sponsored trial should be given an opportunity to participate in the protocol's development if at all possible.

6. Determine the investigator's general motivation and enthusiasm for the proposed clinical trial. If it has been decided prior to the interview that additional tests can be incorporated by individual investigator(s) into the protocol, then discuss what types of tests are acceptable and determine the investigator's interest in conducting additional tests.

7. Discuss how the clinical trial would be conducted at the investigator's site in terms of the background of the personnel who would be conducting the actual trial, the amount of time and in what specific roles the investigator proposes to be involved, and the method(s) with which the investigator will review the work of assistants (or residents, nurses, and other personnel). Ascertain whether the investigator desires to have a colleague, partner, or other individual function as a co- or assistant investigator. The advantage of a

co- or assistant investigator is that he or she would be familiar with the trial and would be able to substitute for the principal investigator if that individual were unable to see patients. The investigator and co- or assistant investigator could each arrange to follow his or her own patients. The co- or assistant investigator(s) would also be empowered to sign data collection forms.

8. A discussion of the relationship between the sponsor and investigator(s) will include a review of the joint nature of the clinical trial to be conducted, since both the investigator and the sponsor will contribute to the overall project. Review the sponsor's contribution to the project, which is often in planning and implementing the trial plus monitoring and analyzing data. Discuss the role of the monitor, which is to help ensure a high degree of protocol adherence and attention to quality in the trial's conduct.

9. Discuss the basis on which a site or sites will be chosen to participate in the clinical trial and whether other sites are being considered. The standards of scientific quality and cooperation and financial arrangements must be discussed with the

investigator. Review the importance of the financial bid in site selection. The reputation of other potential investigators in this field may also be discussed. Indicate whether the investigator will have to sign a letter or statement of confidentiality.

10. Determine if the investigator has ever been audited by the Food and Drug Administration (FDA). If so, what were the conditions and results (i.e., was it a routine audit or was it "for cause")? Advise the investigator that he or she may be required to permit FDA inspectors to examine medical records with patients' names or previous medical histories.

SPECIFIC TOPICS TO DISCUSS

In addition to each of the areas discussed above, there are also a number of specific topics related to the proposed clinical trial that may be discussed with investigators. The specific topics listed in Table 59.2 are briefly presented. These subjects are intended to be representative of the types of areas that may be discussed in detail and are not intended to represent a comprehensive list.

Personnel. Define the number and roles of all individuals necessary to conduct the clinical trial. Review each of the specific people to be involved in terms of his or her training, experience, and other pertinent matters. Discuss how much time each individual will devote to the trial and in which specific roles he or she will be involved.

Determine if it will be necessary to hire additional staff. If new personnel are expected to join the investigator's staff, how certain is their arrival? Will all staff be present for the duration of the trial, or will residents and fellows, for example, rotate to other areas and be replaced by others who must be trained? This latter situation may pose serious problems for a trial in which the continuity of personnel dealing with patients is important or if it requires a long period to train the professional staff to conduct the clinical trial.

Laboratory and Pharmacy. Confirm that both the laboratory and pharmacy are accredited and have adequate facilities and personnel to perform all required functions. If applicable, confirm that they have previously performed similar functions and that successful conduct of all aspects of their role can be counted on with a reasonable degree of assurance. If the pharmacy will be involved in medicine packaging or dispensing, speak to the relevant pharmacist and review his or her role in detail.

Dispensing Medicines. Discuss the advantages and disadvantages of having medicines dispensed by a nurse, coordinator, pharmacist, or other individual. Discuss where medicines are kept and who has access

to a key. Inspect the facilities of medicine storage to confirm that they are adequate and meet reasonable standards for security.

Dates for Conducting the Clinical Trial. Discuss the proposed or firm dates for conducting the trial and, specifically, the expected starting date, the expected rate of enrollment, and the total duration of the trial.

Data Handling and Retention. Discuss how raw data will be collected, i.e., using a flow chart, data collection forms, or by other means. Determine who will complete the data collection forms. Indicate that clinical study files on investigational medicines must be retained for 2 years after the New Drug Application (NDA) is approved or for 2 years past the date the Investigational New Drug Application (IND) is cancelled. Discuss who will analyze the data and how it will be shared with all investigators.

Budget. Indicate how the investigator should prepare a budget, whether it will be itemized, and whether it will include the cost of the clinical trial on a per-patient basis (total cost divided by number of patients) or on the basis of a completed trial. Indicate how the sponsor will pay. Clarify whether costs for patients who fail to pass the screen or baseline are included in the budget. Clarify who will pay for patients who enter but do not complete the trial. The general basis for compensating patients may be discussed. Even patients who are not compensated may receive some funds for transportation or for other specific items (e.g., meals). See Chapter 130 for specific examples.

Ethics Committee/Institutional Review Board. Confirm that the investigator is familiar with the process of having a protocol reviewed and approved by the Ethics Committee/Institutional Review Board (IRB) and that obligations to them are understood. Review regulations (Food and Drug Administration, 1981a,b) and indicate that the sponsor of the clinical trial deals with the Ethics Committee/IRB (if at all) through the investigator and not directly. The Ethics Committee/IRB must be informed at periodic intervals about progress of the trial and advised immediately about any serious adverse reactions that may affect other patients in the trial; they must also be informed and approve any significant changes in the protocol. The sponsor should be sent a copy of relevant correspondence between the investigator and the Ethics Committee/IRB.

Informed Consent and Pregnancy Waiver. An informed consent and pregnancy waiver are to be written at each site by each investigator. Discuss the investigator's familiarity with these forms and the regulatory requirements that must be considered in preparing them. The elements that must be included in an informed consent, a sample informed consent, and pregnancy waiver are illustrated in Chapter 27.

Biological Samples Containing Clinical Trial Medicine. Blood, plasma, or other samples that contain the parent medicine or metabolites are often obtained in medicine studies. Usually these samples are sent to the sponsor or to another site for analysis. Instructions on how to obtain and treat these samples must be clearly delineated in the protocol, as must shipping instructions about how to send samples to the sponsor (or to another facility) for analysis (see Chapter 30).

Publications. Discuss any publications that are anticipated and how they will be organized and written. If the clinical trial is multicentered, discuss if it will result in a joint publication and at which point each investigator can write individual papers. Review the various criteria for establishing the order of authorship (e.g., seniority, number of patients enrolled, alphabetical order) and decide on one approach if possible. If the trial is sponsored, it may be relevant to discuss whether any individuals representing the sponsor will be coauthors.

Pretrial Roundtable Meeting. Indicate that a pretrial roundtable meeting will be conducted with relevant individuals to review and discuss all details and procedures to follow in a trial prior to its initiation. This is not generally carried out at the initial trial site visit, when the investigator is interviewed, but optimally is conducted within 1 month prior to trial initiation. Some of the above points may be discussed at the roundtable meeting rather than at the initial interview (see Chapter 60).

Other Responsibilities of the Principal Investigator. Other responsibilities of the principal investigator should be reviewed (see Table 59.2). A Final Study Report from the investigator is required by U.S. Federal regulations for the sponsor. This report will summarize the investigator's experiences with each patient in the clinical trial plus the investigator's general observations. The investigator may discuss the trial in terms of the overall safety and effectiveness of the medicine evaluated and compare it with known medicines used for the same clinical condition. An interim report may also be required by the sponsor (and possibly Ethics Committee/IRB), especially for trials of long duration. Investigators must send certain required information to the sponsor before a trial can begin (see Clinical Initiation Form II, Chapter 61). This list and the general information published by the Food and Drug Administration (1977b, 1978, 1981a,b) should be reviewed with each investigator.

EVALUATING PATIENT AVAILABILITY AND LASAGNA'S LAW

Discuss in detail the number of patients the investigator says can be entered in the clinical trial within the proposed time limits, how patients or volunteers are obtained, and how the investigator has derived these projections. Are patients to be recruited from a private practice, clinic, or other source? Discuss whether the investigator can get referrals of patients from other doctors or clinics for this trial or whether it would be advisable to advertise for patients. Review "Lasagna's law" (the incidence of patient availability sharply decreases when a clinical trial begins and returns to its original level as soon as a trial is completed; Gorringe, 1970), which is illustrated in Fig. 13.2, and discuss its implications for the current trial. Discuss the number of dropouts expected and how this estimate has been reached.

Reasons for the Existence of Lasagna's Law

The reasons for Lasagna's law must be well understood so that its influence in a clinical trial is minimized, if not eliminated. The major reason relates to inclusion criteria limiting those patients who may be enrolled in a clinical trial. There "always" seems to be one or more inclusion criteria that eliminates patients the investigator considered likely candidates. Those patients that pass all inclusion criteria and screening may live too far from the site, may not have available time to participate, may not be sufficiently motivated, or may decline for other reasons.

Lasagna's law can be invoked when an investigator is overly optimistic about the number of patients they will enroll. The investigator's optimism may reflect surreptitious behavior to obtain the clinical trial from a sponsor, or it may reflect inexperience and naiveté.

Methods to Avoid Lasagna's Law

A mechanism should be established whenever possible to ensure that adequate numbers of patients who meet inclusion and exclusion criteria are available to the investigator prior to commencement of the clinical trial. This may be accomplished for trials involving chronic diseases by review of patient charts selected by the investigator prior to the initial visit. It may be necessary to pay potential investigators to screen their records. If one has arranged for this procedure, then a preprinted form may be prepared to enter selected data pertaining to the inclusion and exclusion criteria. For trials in which the specific patients who could enter trial cannot be identified at this visit, other procedures must be used. These include (1) reviewing records of patients previously treated to obtain an indication of the nature and numbers of patients seen by the investigator, (2) assessing the performance of the investigator in previous medicine trials by contacting several references, and (3) contacting and assessing the proposed physicians or clinics who will be making patient referrals. The author believes that references from other sponsors should be obtained on all investigators in a sponsored trial. Ultimately, the potential of the investigators to enroll patients must be viewed as an educated guess based on all available information.

EVALUATING THE FACILITIES

Visit the facilities to be used in the proposed clinical trial. This includes the pharmacy, laboratories, and specialized testing areas as well as all rooms to be used. Evaluate the workload of these groups and determine whether they will be able to participate in the trial in a fully acceptable manner. Are the sizes of waiting rooms, offices, and laboratories adequate? Is all of the necessary equipment present and available? Determine that all laboratories to be used by the investigator have appropriate certification. Discuss calibrations, standards, and model numbers if relevant. It is important to meet and spend sufficient time with the personnel who will be involved in the trial, such as assistants, coordinators, nurses, administrators, pharmacists, laboratory personnel, or others.

INVESTIGATOR SELECTION FORM

Medicine: _____

Trial (Number and Name): _____

Completed By: _____

Date of Visit: _____

Name of Investigator & Title: _____

Other Staff Interviewed & Titles: _____

Address of Site: _____

Telephone: _____

Fax Number: _____

	Areas of Strength	Potential or Actual Problem Areas
Facilities and Equipment: Score ___		
Personnel: Score ___		
Experience of Investigator: Score ___		
Experience of Staff: Score ___		
Conflicts with Other Trials: Score ___		
Patient Population: Score ___		

FIG. 59.1 Investigator selection form.

	Areas of Strength	Potential or Actual Problem Areas
Attitude of Inv. & Staff: Score ____		
Budgetary Considerations: Score ____		
Time Considerations: Score ____		
Other Considerations: Score ____		

Documents given to site:

____ Regulations re: Obligations of Clinical Investigators

____ Regulations re: Informed Consent

____ Regulations re: Ethics Committee/IRBs

____ Protocol of Clinical Trial

____ Investigator's Brochure

____ Other (specify)

____ Other (specify)

Documents received from site (e.g., Investigator's resume, Assistant Investigator's resume, Reference laboratory values)

Overall Evaluation of Site:
Score ____

Comments:

Key to Score: 0 = Severe problems, enough to disqualify site
1 = Major problems
2 = Fair, may be considered
3 = Good, should be considered
4 = Excellent
5 = Outstanding, one of best encountered

FIG. 59.1 (*Continued*)

EVALUATING THE INVESTIGATOR

Assess how cooperative the investigator will be with the sponsor through his or her attitude, approach to the discussion, and willingness to discuss details and return telephone calls, plus any other available clues.

Testing the Investigator's Ability to Maintain Confidentiality of the Data

It may be desirable to test the potential investigator to determine how he or she will treat the information and details supplied by the sponsor. This may be done by asking questions that probe the investigator's previous experiences and observing how much information he or she keeps confidential. For example, a potential investigator should be willing to state whether he or she has conducted clinical trials for other sponsors. If the answer is positive, ask what kind of clinical trial and what specific medicine was studied, then request a copy of the protocol and/or data collection forms to view, and finally, if the potential investigator provides all of these, ask to view the data they obtained. The degree to which the potential investigator complies with these requests for information is a general indication of how much information he or she will be willing to give others about your clinical trial.

After the meeting has taken place, there may be a variety of materials to send to the investigator, plus items the investigator may have promised to send or has been asked to send. The completeness and quality of the material sent by the potential investigator and the time of its arrival may be an indication of the investigator's interest in the clinical trial and ability to handle relevant details and procedures. It is desirable to discuss the reputation of the potential investigator with other investigators or with other sponsors who have worked with him or her. When selection of investigators must be conducted, the above information plus knowledge of the sponsor's priorities, workload, and the factors listed in Table 59.1 will generally facilitate a decision. A form to use for selection is shown in Fig. 59.1.

The potential investigator(s) should be informed of both how and when an investigator(s) will be selected. If the person who visits the site will not be the clinical monitor, then that should also be stated. The types of investigators most often chosen are indicated in Table 59.3.

TABLE 59.3 *Types of clinical investigators most often chosen to conduct different types of clinical trials*

Type of clinical trial	Phase	Clinical investigators usually selected
Safety	I	Contract group with own facility
		Special Phase I facility at an academic center or hospital
		Pharmaceutical company with own facility
Pharmacokinetics	I	Same as above
		Experts in pharmacokinetics
Safety in patients	I, II	Experts at academic centers
		Others described above
Efficacy	IIa, b	Same as above
Safety and/or efficacy in a broad patient population	II	Same as above
		General practitioners
Safety and/or efficacy in a specialized population	III	Same as above
Marketing-oriented trials	III, IV	General practitioners
		Others
		Thought leaders

CHAPTER 60

Conducting a Pretrial Roundtable Meeting

PURPOSES AND GOALS

If a multicenter trial is being implemented, it is important to bring all investigators together prior to the starting of the trial to discuss various aspects of the trial and to agree on a uniform approach. Ideally, all research coordinators or assistant investigators will also be present at this meeting, or they will have a separate roundtable discussion. Since problems in communication are usually the source of most major difficulties encountered in multicenter trials, bringing all investigators together to review and discuss important points prior to the start of the trial will remove many sources of misunderstanding and help ensure a uniform approach. Table 60.1 lists various purposes of this meeting.

Even when a relatively uncomplicated clinical trial will be conducted by a single investigator with only a single monitor from the sponsoring organization, it is still important to hold this pretrial roundtable discussion. In an unsponsored trial the investigator may hold weekly or periodic meetings with his or her staff to plan and review the trial prior to its initiation as well as to assess progress.

LOCALE, STYLE, AND TIME

Where Is the Meeting Held?

There are almost no restrictions on where a roundtable meeting may be held. The number of people invited will have an obvious influence on the site chosen. If individuals will attend from geographically dispersed areas, then a central location is preferable. If time is limited, then a hotel near a major airport has more attraction, but if the participants will spend a full day or more discussing details, then a more interesting or even relaxing locale (e.g., a resort), may be chosen.

Meeting Style

It should be clarified prior to the meeting whether the roundtable is to be used as a working session to polish the protocol and data collection forms rather than a forum for discussion of a protocol (and data collection forms) that have been formally approved and fixed. It

TABLE 60.1 *Purposes of a pretrial roundtable meeting*

1. Achieve uniformity in approach by all investigators and staff
2. Review and discuss numerous activities described in the protocol
3. Answer as many questions as possible about the clinical trial
4. Generate enthusiasm for success
5. Get everyone to know each other and develop a sense of teamwork and trust
6. Review potential difficulties, issues, and problems
7. Have people practice important procedures or maneuvers that may not be straightforward
8. Indicate views on any subject (e.g., severity of patients who are definitely wanted and unwanted in the clinical trial) to those associated with the trial
9. Review administrative ground rules

is preferable to allow for input at this session, especially if there has not been a prior opportunity for input or if various issues remain unresolved. Any agreed-on modifications would be incorporated into the draft protocol prior to formal approval.

Time Required for the Meeting

It is important to schedule a sufficient amount of time for this meeting so that it is productive and may achieve optimal effectiveness. Although no firm guidelines may be given about how much time is required, it is the author's experience that a half day is necessary for most trials of average complexity and that multicentered trials often require a full day if numerous issues must be resolved. Major national trials with multimillion dollar budgets will probably require both more time and more than just a single meeting to accomplish all the tasks necessary to launch and maintain such a large-scale project successfully.

SAMPLE AGENDAS

The outlines of three sample agendas for a pretrial roundtable meeting are presented in Tables 60.2 to 60.4 and discussed below. They can be modified prior to the meeting to fit the particular nature of the trial under discussion. Although the agendas in Tables 60.2 to 60.4 are organized for a sponsored trial, most of the points covered must also be considered by clinical investigators of unsponsored trials.

CONDUCT OF THE MEETING

Background

After the introduction of all people present, the background of the project should be discussed in terms of the investigator's manual (also referred to as an investigator's brochure or by other terms) and either prior clinical experience (for investigational medicines) or published literature (for marketed medicines).

TABLE 60.2 *Sample agenda for pretrial roundtable meeting*

1. Introduction of all people present
2. Background of the medicine project
3. Protocol to be followed
   a. Introduction
   b. Materials and methods
   c. Conduct of the trial
   d. Data analysis and publication(s)
4. Administrative responsibilities of the principal investigator and other personnel involved in the trial
5. Financial matters
6. Additional topics

TABLE 60.3 *Sample agenda for pretrial roundtable meeting*

A. Introductions of all people present
B. Background of the clinical trial
   1. Standard research letter (request comments)
   2. Standard confidentiality letter (request comments)
   3. Standard letter of agreement (request comments)
   4. Investigator's manual (need specific information)
C. Protocol
   1. Where the clinical trial fits into the sponsor's global plans
   2. Materials and methods
      a. Details about packaging (instructions)
      b. Type and maintenance of blind (who will remain blind)
      c. Storage facilities and procedure to dispense medicines
      d. Drug disposition form and method of returning medicines
   3. Operational definitions of importance
   4. Conduct of the clinical trial
      a. Screening patients: review of each admission criterion
      b. Informed consent and pregnancy waiver
      c. Need for backup patients, assigning numbers, dispensing medicines
      d. Instructions for patients
      e. Dosing periods
      f. Modifying doses of medicine for adverse reactions
      g. Discuss timing of the clinical trial for each day and week plus for the overall trial
      h. Discuss basic policy for allowing patients to ascend to a higher dosing period (or to next step)
      i. Discuss timing and recording of adverse reactions
      j. Timing of vital signs (pre versus post blood-sampling)
      k. How to handle emergencies
      l. Follow-up visit(s)
      m. Policy for patient or clinical trial discontinuation
      n. Other instructions and any special forms to be completed by investigator
      o. Discuss data-processing requirements of the investigator and staff
      p. Turning data over to sponsor
   5. Administrative responsibilities of principal investigator
      a. Final investigator's report and interim report (if appropriate)
      b. Data collection forms (review each unique page)
         i. Data transcription onto data collection forms
         ii. Comment about legibility, and appropriate ink. How to correct, initial, and sign data collection forms
      c. Ethics Committee/IRB interactions, regulatory authority regulations
   6. Blood samples for measuring levels of trial medicine(s)
      a. Discuss obtaining and handling of samples
      b. Labels and tubes for samples
      c. Shipping samples to sponsor or core facility
   7. Procedures to follow for specialized tests (e.g., ophthalmological examination) and enrolling staff to conduct those examinations
D. Basic monitoring strategy
   1. Number of monitoring visits each month or year. Purpose of each visit (e.g., review of data collection forms from the previous period
   2. Telephone and other types of communications to be used in the clinical trial on an ad hoc or periodic basis
   3. Who will be allowed to interview patients
   4. Data and source documents that monitors may wish to check during or after the clinical trial
E. Financial issues
   1. Budgetary questions
   2. Methods to request payment of grants

TABLE 60.4 *Sample agenda for pretrial roundtable meeting*

A. Review of investigator's brochure and roundtable workbook
B. Obligations of clinical investigators and sponsors (use the roundtable workbook)
  1. Review the Ethics Committee/IRB submission documents and the laboratory certifications
  2. Discuss monitoring schedule and functions
  3. Review the system for dispensing and maintaining accountability of medicines
  4. Discuss record maintenance
C. Clinical protocol review
  1. Primary objective(s)
  2. Clinical trial design (e.g., double-blinded, stratified, randomized, one-week clinical trial)
  3. Dose(s) to be used and mechanism of dose changes, other than clinical trial discontinuation
  4. Medicine packaging and labeling
    a. How to decode patient's medicine in an emergency
    b. Accounting procedures for test materials
     i. Forms
     ii. Investigator dispensing
     iii. Patient usage—amount dispensed and returned
    c. Return of unused medication posttrial to sponsor or pharmacy
  5. Consent and clearance
    a. Ethics Committee/IRB approval
    b. Informed consent
  6. Experimental procedures
    a. Inclusion criteria
    b. Overall time and events schedule
  7. Adverse reactions
    a. Notification of sponsor or others
    b. Documentation required
    c. File report
    d. Follow-up of patient
    e. Rechallenge policy
  8. Protocol modifications and amendments
    a. Sponsor approval
    b. Ethics Committee/IRB approval
  9. Statistical analysis
    a. Interim
    b. Final
  10. Publications
    a. Policies
D. Data collection form review
  1. File original laboratory results, executing informed consent form and completing data collection forms
  2. Entry of each visit and telephone call must be made in the physician's office records for each patient; clinical-trial-related entries should be clearly apparent (e.g., possible use of colored ink)
  3. Edit records for legibility, completeness, and accuracy
  4. Review by investigator and signature
  5. Discuss method of corrections and how to deal with missing data
E. Communications
  1. Identify primary contacts at site and sponsor
  2. Establish system for clinical trial record keeping
  3. Discuss the establishment, maintenance, and completion of a site visit log
  4. Discuss method to ensure rapid and direct communications when needed

This should include a general comparison of the trial medicine with others in the same therapeutic or chemical class. Review the protocol's development (if relevant) and other background material. As an introduction to the present trial, review how it fits into the overall plans for the medicine's development and discuss the objectives of the present trial.

All investigators present should be asked if they have any concerns about entering patients into the clinical trial. Concerns or questions might relate to the (1) informed consent, (2) conflict between their physician and scientist responsibilities, (3) clinical trial design, (4) practical issues, or (5) physician–patient relationships. If these problems were not resolved prior to the meeting, they should be settled before proceeding.

Movement of Medicines

Indicate relevant details about packaging, labeling, storing, and dispensing of the trial medicine(s). Review all steps of medicine movement from shipping by the sponsor to receipt at the institution through dispensing to patients until the unused medicine is collected from patients, stored, logged in, and returned to the sponsor. Review the forms to be completed by the investigator to document receipt of medicines and return of unused medicines. Indicate whether all dosing bottles must be saved or whether the patients' returned medicines may be combined, and describe the method of returning unused medicines to the sponsor.

Foreign Sites

If a trial is being initiated in a foreign country, then discuss relevant questions as to import and export customs/regulations, language of the data collection forms, whether a different monitoring system will be used, regulatory requirements, patent considerations, legal concerns, and other related matters. Determine if there are potential problems relating to culture differences, availability of equipment, ability to perform necessary laboratory tests, and means of converting data from one system of units to another. Decide if the trial must meet Food and Drug Administration (FDA) or other regulatory standards. If so, then it must be designed, initiated, conducted, and analyzed accordingly. The various options for transmittal of data to the proper site must be considered (e.g., mail, telecommunications). See Chapter 40, "National versus Multinational Clinical Trials."

Degree of Blinding

If the trial is single- or double-blinded, describe the type of blind to be used and how it will be maintained. Discuss which of the monitors will remain blind and if any of the personnel at the site will be unblinded. Indicate how and when the blind will be for medical emergencies and at the end of a trial. If the trial involves a marketed medicine, discuss how the placebo has been prepared [i.e., is it identical to the medicine in taste, floating characteristics, and other factors (see Chapter 25) in addition to size, shape, and color?].

Various Details

Discuss any of the following points that are relevant for the conduct of the trial: admission criteria, operational definitions, informed consent and pregnancy waiver forms, assignment of patient numbers and medications, and enrollment of backup or alternate patients. Review any instruction (or other) forms to be handed out to each patient. Other points to consider for discussion are the randomization or stratification procedures to assign patients to different treatment groups, the criteria that will be used to determine whether to change doses or to move to another step in the protocol, and the frequency of monitoring visits plus availability of data to monitors. Also, question the investigators to determine if they anticipate any deviations from the protocol.

Time and Events Schedule

Discuss the time and events schedule for each day, week, and month. When will vital signs or other tests be performed, i.e., will certain tests be done before or after blood sampling, and how much leeway from the times indicated in the protocol will be permitted in performing each test?

Data Collection Forms

Review how data will be collected and kept until entered on the data collection forms and when such data will be available to the sponsor. If data are to be originally entered onto forms prepared by the investigators, such as "flow sheets," prior to being transcribed onto data collection forms, then the flow sheets should be reviewed and retained until all reports on the trial have been completed. In some situations, data may be initially recorded on one copy of data collection forms and rewritten on a second (final) copy.

During or after the clinical trial, the investigator must review each page of the data collection forms and sign or initial the forms in an agreed-on manner. At the roundtable, each unique page should be reviewed. Indicate how data, notes, and unscheduled tests and examinations are to be entered and how errors on the forms are to be corrected.

Adverse Reactions

Discuss the recording of adverse reactions on data collection forms. Discuss the adverse reaction dictionary to be used or establish and review a brief dictionary of the most common adverse events expected. This procedure will help ensure that similar symptoms will be described using the same term (e.g., fatigue, drowsiness, tired, sleepy, and sedated may all be described with one term by all investigators). This will prevent a list of many different terms for the same adverse event. Discuss the categories chosen for degree of association between adverse event and medicine (such as definite, probably, possible, none, unknown). Review the categories chosen to define the intensity of adverse events (mild, moderate, severe), their duration, and the steps taken by the investigator or sponsor to deal with them. Stress the importance of the investigator notifying the sponsor of all serious adverse events with 24 hours.

Patient Discontinuation

Review the policy for premature patient discontinuation and determine which tests or examinations must be performed at the time of discontinuation. The policy for replacing discontinued patients should be reviewed. Discuss the conditions under which patients will not formally be discharged from the trial in order to ensure that the patients' health had no adverse carryover effect from medicine treatment. Define a "completed" patient and under what conditions (if any) patients may enter a continuation trial protocol. Each of these points is discussed in other chapters in more detail.

Clinical Trial Discontinuation

In addition to individual patient discontinuation, a whole trial may be discontinued, for sponsor-, medicine-, or site-related reasons. The conditions under which the trial (or one site) will be discontinued for reasons relating to the investigator's performance or changes at the site should be discussed.

Medical Emergencies

Review how medical emergencies will be handled. Stress that the investigator must notify the sponsor and the Ethics Committee/Institutional Review Board (IRB) immediately of any serious and unexpected adverse events. The sponsor will contact the regulatory authorities according to regulations. If the investigator is conducting an unsponsored trial, he or she should be familiar with the adverse experience form (e.g., FDA 1639), which must be submitted to the relevant regulatory authorities for serious adverse events.

Technical Details

Discuss the source of syringes, needles, labels, tubes, and other items to be used for collecting and processing blood or other samples plus the procedures for obtaining, handling, and shipping of samples. Discuss the timing of biological sample collection relative to vital signs or other assessments scheduled at the "same" time. Review the availability of staff needed to conduct specialized tests such as ophthalmological examinations and indicate how patients will be taken to or arrive at the proper facilities for these examinations. Discuss whether special equipment will be required to perform any tests(s) at the site, and, if it is not present, how this equipment will be obtained and used.

Administrative Responsibilities

The principal investigator has some administrative responsibilities, which include writing a Final Trial Report (an interim report may also be required). Establish a time limit for this report to be received by the sponsor (and/or Ethics Committee/IRB). Discuss relevant Ethics Committee/IRB interactions and regulations, including what reports are required by each and whether the sponsor or investigator has primary responsibility. Discuss who will replace or fill in for the investigator if he or she becomes ill or goes on a trip.

Budget

Discuss with the principal investigator(s) which items are or are not included in the budget and how bills should be submitted to the sponsor. Review the number of fractional payments to be made and the time points in the trial at which each payment will be made. A commonly used arrangement is to pay investigators half of the agreed-upon budget at the start of the trial (often defined as the entry of the first patient) and the other half at the end of the trial, after the Final Trial Report has been received. Another common plan is to pay one-third at the onset, one-third when half of the patients are completed, and one-third at the conclusion of the trial. Various other alternatives are also used.

It is often acceptable to pay investigators an honorarium for attending the roundtable conference. Whether study coordinators or others who attend are also paid an honorarium depends on the sponsor, as does the amount paid. Full travel expenses and incidental costs are covered as a matter of course.

CHAPTER 61

Clinical Trial Initiation and Conduct

GENERAL FORMS TO USE AS CHECKLISTS

The steps to follow and consider in initiating a clinical trial after choosing the investigator(s) are presented in Figs. 61.1 to 61.3. These forms may be useful to both sponsors and investigators and can be modified as required for an individual trial. They are organized according to whether the documentation and procedures are performed within the sponsoring organization (Fig. 61.1), are sent by the investigator to the sponsor (Fig. 61.2), or are sent by the sponsor to the investigator (Fig. 61.3). Clinical scientists performing unsponsored trials can modify these forms to include only those steps and procedures that they must follow.

These forms are intended to serve as reminders of various steps or procedures that must be followed in organizing and initiating a clinical trial. In addition, they are designed to monitor the flow of paperwork as it is routed through various departments and individuals. In formulating the steps in Figs. 61.1 to 61.3, the assumption was made that government approval has been received to investigate the trial medicine. This approval is called an Investigational New Drug Application (IND) (in the United States) for new medicines or for marketed medicines being evaluated for nonapproved indications. If this step has not been performed, or if the investigator will be conducting the medicine trial under his or her own IND, then additional documentation must be prepared and submitted to the appropriate regulatory authorities.

RANDOMIZATION CODES

Figure 61.4 illustrates the process by which a randomization code is obtained and utilized. Each randomi-

zation code is checked by the individual who requested it unless that person will remain blind to patient randomization. In that situation, another individual will be assigned to check the code(s). Once it is confirmed that the code was generated according to instructions, it may be used to package the medicine. Medicine packaging may be performed either at the clinical trial site (e.g., at the pharmacy), at the sponsor's facilities, or at another location, possibly by an independent contractor. A copy of the randomization code may be sent to the investigator, pharmacist, research coordinator, independent monitoring group, or other person to keep during the clinical trial. If the trial is open label or single blind, then the code will usually not be sealed. If the trial is double blind, however, then the code must be sent sealed to the relevant individuals. This may be in the form of a group of individually sealed envelopes, each containing a patient number on the outside and the identity of the treatment inside. Another means by which information in the randomization code may be made available to the investigator in cases of medical emergency is for the third part of a tear-off label on the medication bottle dispensed to have the treatment's identity hidden within the label. This portion of the label would be placed either in the patient's data collection form or in another convenient place when the bottle is dispensed and only opened in case of a medical emergency.

Other more sophisticated systems to blind or unblind clinical trials have been developed (e.g., peeling back special printed labels, about 10 to 20 to a sheet, that cannot be reattached). These labels are relatively cumbersome to use and add unnecessary expense.

The randomization code is usually requested after

CLINICAL TRIAL INITIATION
Form I: Internal Documents and Procedures

Study Medicine: Investigator:
Protocol Number: Site:

Date and Check off each point when completed. NA = not applicable. Add Comments.

Complete

_____ **1. Protocol**
             Draft   With Author _____
                          With Typists _____
                          In Review _____
                          Section (group) _____
                          Statistics _____
                          Other Section(s) or Departments _____

             Final   With Typists _____
                          Department and/or Sponsor Review _____
                          Approved _____

_____ **2. Data Collection Forms**
             Draft   In Progress _____
                          In Review-Section _____
                          Statistics and/or Data Entry _____
                          At Art Department _____
             Proofs   In Review _____
                          At Printers _____
                          Completed _____
             Finals   Collated _____
                          Placed in Loose Leaf Binders _____

_____ **3. Randomization Code(s)**
                          Requested _____
                          Received _____

_____ **4. Medicine Supplies**
                          Bulk Medicine Availability _____
                          Specific Medicine(s) for Trial Requested _____
                          Specific Medicine(s) for Trial Prepared _____
                          Bottle and Carton Medicine Labels
                          Ordered _____
                          Bottle and Medicine Labels
                          Prepared _____
                          Forms Filled Out to Ship Medicine(s) _____

_____ **5. Regulatory Submittal Forms**
                          Packet of Forms Routed _____
                          Approved _____

_____ **6. Grant Request to Fund Trial**
                          Request Sent to Approve Grant _____
                          Grant Approved _____

_____ **7. Initial Grant Payment**
                          Forms Sent to Have Check Prepared _____
                          Check Received _____

_____ **8. Book or Forms Prepared to Monitor Trial** _____

_____ **9. Computer Base Set Up to Monitor Trial** _____

_____ **10. Other (ex: Medicine(s) needed from other Co.)** _____
                          _____

FIG. 61.1 Clinical trial initiation form I: list of procedures to be followed by the sponsor (sponsored trials) or by the investigator (unsponsored trials).

CLINICAL TRIAL INITIATION
Form II: Information For Investigator To Send To The Sponsor

Study Medicine: Investigator:
Protocol Number: Site:

Requested on _____ by letter, phone, visit.   Comments
Date and check off each item when received:

_____ 1. Curricula Vitae* _____

_____ 2. Signed FDA 1572/3 (or Other Regulatory) Form* _____

_____ 3. Signature(s) on Protocol Face Sheet* _____

_____ 4. Ethics Committee/IRB Approval Letter[1]** _____

_____ 5. Informed Consent (Sample)** _____

_____ 6. List of Reference Lab Values[2]** _____

_____ 7. Pregnancy Waiver Form (Sample)** _____

_____ 8. Budget for Trial _____

_____ 9. Names of Assistant-or
           Co-Investigators _____

_____ 10. Name of Coordinator _____
            (and/or other relevant individuals)

_____ 11. Details of How Checks are to be
            Drawn and Addressed _____

_____ 12. Other _____

_____   _____

_____   _____

* = Required for FDA
** = Required for Files
[1]Plus names and/or occupations of members
[2]The values for the specific population studied (ex: children, women) must be obtained. The name and address of the laboratory, as well as a copy of its certification must also be received.

FIG. 61.2 Clinical trial initiation form II: list of information that must be sent by the investigator to the sponsor (for sponsored trials) or considered by the investigator (for unsponsored trials).

the protocol design has been approved by medical and statistical personnel. It may not be requested until after the protocol itself is formally approved. Because the code may almost always be generated rapidly, the latter approach is usually acceptable. The size of the block used for the randomization is generally determined by the statistician.

INFORMED CONSENTS

Federal regulations covering informed consents (Food and Drug Administration, 1981a) should be reviewed with all investigators. Chapter 27 presents the elements of the informed consent that must be included in all

CLINICAL TRIAL INITIATION
Form III: Information For The Sponsor To Send To The Investigator(s)

Study Medicine: Investigator:
Protocol Number: Site:

Date and Check off each item when sent. NA = not applicable.

Comments

1. **Letter of Confidentiality**
   1. Sent _____
   2. Signed Copy Received _____

2. **Investigator's Manual (Brochure)** _____

3. **Protocol**
   1. Draft Sent for Comments _____
   2. Final Sent for Ethics Committee/IRB Approval
   _____

4. **Medicine and Medicine Disposition Forms**
   (Add Amount of Medicine Sent and Form Nos.) _____
   Additional Medicine Sent _____

5. **Data Collection Forms (Add No. Sent)** _____
   Additional Sets of Forms Sent _____

6. **Synopsis of Regulations on**
   Informed Consent _____

7. **Proposed FDA Regulations:**
   Obligations of Clinical Investigators _____

8. **Send on Request Only**
   1. References to Published Literature on the Clinical
      Trial Medicine _____
   2. FDA Regulations on Standards for IRBs
      _____
   3. Proposed FDA Regulations of Obligations Of
      Clinical Sponsors and Monitors _____
   4. List of Questions Prepared for and Used by FDA
      Inspectors _____
   5. Samples of Informed Consent or Pregnancy
      Waiver Forms _____

9. **Other Trial Material (If Applicable)**
   1. Prescription Blanks _____
   2. Pharmacist's Record Book _____
   3. Plasma Labels _____
   4. Plasma Tubes _____
   5. Forms for Mailing Plasma Samples
      (and Procedures to Follow) _____
   6. Boxes for Mailing Plasma Samples _____
   7. Patient Instruction Sheet _____
   8. Other (list): _____
      _____ _____
      _____ _____

10. **Letter to Authorize Trial** _____
11. **Initial Grant Payment Sent** _____

FIG. 61.3 Clinical trial initiation form III: list of information that may be sent from the sponsor to the investigator (for sponsored trials) or considered by the investigator (for unsponsored trials).

426

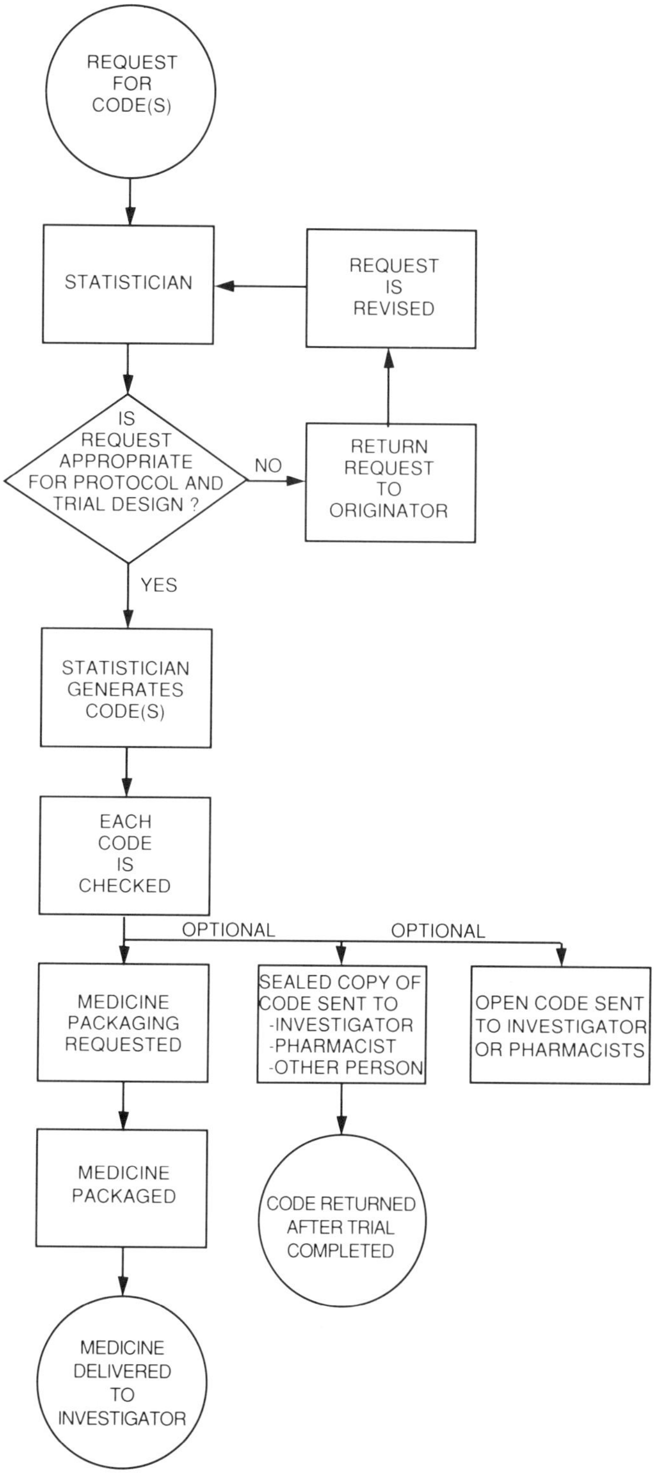

FIG. 61.4 Process for obtaining and utilizing randomization codes for packaging and dispensing of medicines and assigning patients to treatments. The code should not be used to package medicine until it is ascertained that the protocol has been finalized.

such forms according to Federal regulations (Food and Drug Administration, 1981a).

STRATEGIES FOR CONDUCTING CLINICAL TRIALS

At the time a clinical trial is being initiated, it is important to plan how its conduct can most effectively be handled. Some techniques are described that can be used to achieve the appropriate balance between "tight" and "loose" conduct as well as monitoring. A number of the more common aspects related to conduct of the trial are presented in Fig. 61.5.

PREPARING FOR UNANTICIPATED SITUATIONS

General Approach

Many unanticipated situations arise during the course of most clinical trials, and it is desirable to have a standard approach available for dealing effectively with the more common situations. This enables the trial to proceed (or to be discontinued) with the fewest problems. Some of the unanticipated situations that frequently arise during medicine trials include severe adverse events or death(s) after the medicine, changes in personnel, unapproved modifications introduced into the protocol ("unofficially"), or other protocol violations, and slower than anticipated patient enrollment. In order to minimize the impact of these and other problem situations on the overall conduct of the trial, it is advisable for sponsors to choose investigators carefully and to monitor the trial closely for early signs of what may later become significant problems.

"Dry Run"

It is advisable for investigators to conduct a "dry run" (prior to starting the actual clinical trial) with a fictional or trial patient. This patient is processed and taken through all steps of the protocol to work out procedures, time requirements, scheduling of tests and visits, and data handling. At the end of the "dry run," the investigator attempts to devise (or revise) a series of steps to conduct the trial efficiently, supply food to patients (if necessary), allow for recreation (if pertinent), and identify and solve potential or real problems that have arisen.

PATIENTS LOST TO FOLLOW-UP

In clinical trials of long duration, it is sometimes difficult or impossible to locate patients who do not attend scheduled clinics. In most cases, the location of these

CONDUCTING THE CLINICAL TRIAL

Study Medicine: Investigator:
Protocol Number: Site:

Check and Date. Add Number, if relevant, or comments.

1. **Initiation**
    All Forms Received from Investigator   _____
    All Forms Approved by Sponsor   _____
    All Forms Sent to Regulatory Authority   _____
    Investigator Told to Proceed   _____

2. **Monitoring**
    Identify Monitor(s) & Role   _____
    Plan Monitoring Strategy (see text)   _____
    Plan Frequency of Telephone and Personal Contact   _____

3. **Supplies Sent to Investigator(s)**
    Additional Trial Medicines   _____
    Additional Data Collection Forms   _____
    Other: _____   _____

4. **Plasma Samples, Data Collection Forms Received From Investigator(s)**
    Plasma or Other Biological Samples   _____
    Data Collection Forms   _____
    Adverse Reaction Report(s)   _____
    Other: _____   _____

5. **Financial**
    Additional Funds Requested by Investigator _____
    Forms Sent to Request Funds   _____
    Funds Sent to Investigator   _____

6. **Unanticipated Situations**
    Protocol Changes, Addenda or Extensions
        (Sponsor & Ethics Committee/IRB to Approve)   _____
    Severe Adverse Reactions or Deaths. Reports from
    (1) Invest. to Sponsor and Ethics Committee/IRB _____
    (2) Sponsor to Files, Regulatory Authority, and
         other Investigators
    Other: _____   _____
         _____   _____
         _____   _____

FIG. 61.5 List of procedures that may be utilized by the investigator or sponsor during the course of a clinical trial.

patients or their medical status is not especially important, but there are trials in which their vital status may be critical (e.g., if death is used as an endpoint). Methods for locating patients include contacting friends, relatives, and employers, as well as using social security numbers and national death registries (see Chapter 30).

If these steps might be envisioned as potentially necessary, then relevant information about the patient's outside contacts should be sought at the start of a clinical trial. It would also be relevant to indicate to the patients in the informed consent that a search might be conducted at a later date to determine their location, vital status, and medical condition.

Are Patients Who Can Be Followed Up After a Behavioral Change Program Similar to Those Who Cannot Be Readily Found?

Normal patients who can be easily found and readily followed up after a program to increase exercise differ in their main outcome variable from those who are more difficult to follow up (Lee and Owen, 1986). A greater current level of exercise was reported for those who were more easily contacted. Lee and Owen quote studies reporting that former alcoholics who are readily available for follow up have better long-term outcomes than those who are harder to locate. The conclusion is that as many patients as possible must be contacted to provide meaningful data if follow-up to a clinical trial is necessary.

CHAPTER 62

Monitoring a Clinical Trial

DEFINITIONS

Monitoring is a general term that is used in many different contexts in the pharmaceutical industry. The word monitor is used both as a verb and as a noun. As a verb it means "to watch, observe, or check," especially relating to a clinical trial. It also means "to keep track of, regulate, or control." As a noun, the word refers to individuals who are employed by a company and who monitor (oversee) the planning, initiation, conduct, and data processing of clinical studies.

These individuals also confirm that the execution of each step follows agreed-on plans. This chapter is primarily concerned with the latter type of monitoring. Many of the other uses of the term *monitoring* are listed in Table 62.1 and are discussed in other parts of this book.

FUNCTIONS

Clinical monitors have a wide variety of backgrounds both in their disciplines of training and in their expe-

TABLE 62.1 *Selected types of monitoring conducted in the pharmaceutical industry*

1. Monitor clinical trials (i.e., the primary subject of this chapter)
2. Monitor preclinical studies conducted at facilities outside the company (e.g., toxicological or specialized studies)
3. Monitor data processing or statistical analyses being conducted at facilities outside the company.
4. Monitor the status of, and progress on, projects at several levels within a company
5. Monitor potential and/or actual conflicts between projects in terms of priorities, problems that arise, or need for resources
6. Monitor the coordination between activities conducted at different sites and/or in different countries
7. Monitor the implementation of a divisional, departmental, sectional, or other strategy to conduct research and/or develop medicines
8. Monitor the quality of research being conducted
9. Monitor the quality of clinical data during the trial[a]
10. Monitor the quality of clinical data on the data collection forms after the trial is completed but prior to its statistical analysis
11. Monitor the quality of medicines produced (i.e., quality assurance)
12. Monitor the financial projections for new and upcoming medicines to reach a New Drug Application (NDA) status or other milestone
13. Monitor the costs of clinical trials

[a] A separate quality assurance group may perform this role.

TABLE 62.2 *Selected functions of a clinical trial monitor*

A. Related to protocol
1. Evaluate recruitment rate and number of patients entered into the clinical trial
2. Evaluate eligibility of patients enrolled
3. Evaluate randomization of patients to treatment groups
4. Evaluate conduct of the trial according to good clinical practices
5. Evaluate adequacy and accuracy of data obtained
6. Evaluate timely and accurate entry of data onto data collection forms
7. Evaluate transmittal of information on all important adverse reactions and other relevant matters to appropriate individuals at sponsoring institution or on monitoring committee
B. Administrative
1. Ensure adequacy of site with regard to good clinical practices
2. Ensure adequacy of professional treatment of patients
3. Transfer biological samples and data collection forms as directed
4. Arrange for payment of investigator
5. Arrange for the availability of adequate medicine(s), supplies, data collection forms, and other items
6. Confirm that proper contacts between the sponsor and Ethics Committee/Institutional Review Board (IRB) are maintained
7. Handle *ad hoc* problems and maintain communication with all relevant individuals
8. Encourage a positive interest and involvement in the trial by all trial personnel (i.e., attempt to keep morale high)
9. Assist in trial termination procedures
10. Assist in data handling, data analysis, and publications

rience with clinical medicine. Although many monitors perform similar functions they do so at highly different levels of expertise. Broad functions of general monitors include participation in most or all of the following activities: (1) planning clinical trials, (2) writing protocols, (3) initiating trials, (4) assessing the conduct of trials, (5) assisting in their termination, (6) assisting in data editing and analysis, and (7) assisting in data interpretation and extrapolation.

More specific functions of medical monitors during the conduct of a clinical trial may include (1) observing what is being done, (2) assessing or evaluating the quality of the trial's conduct, (3) comparing the quality to preset standards, (4) discussing results with the groups being monitored as well as with other monitors and supervisors, and (5) proposing improvements to be made in the trial or proposing solutions to problems. Other specific functions are listed in Table 62.2.

One of the rarely perceived functions of monitoring is to help maintain and improve the morale and enthusiasm of the staff. The means of achieving this goal vary among clinical trials and individual monitors, but some attention should be devoted to this consideration by all monitors. These and other functions are listed in Table 62.2. Investigators of unsponsored trials are also concerned with internal monitoring. Thus, the comments below are applicable to both sponsors and clinical investigators (of sponsored and unsponsored trials), even though various aspects will require modification.

STEREOTYPED STYLES OF MONITORING

The most important aspect relating to monitoring and choice of investigators is attitude or style. Two extreme attitudes may be characterized with stereotypes as either "old-fashioned" or "modern."

Old-Fashioned Style

In the old-fashioned style (Table 62.3) the investigator is usually seen as a highly respected individual (almost always in academia) who believes he is doing the sponsor a great favor by his willingness to conduct a clinical trial. "His" is used in the sense of "grand old man," and dates to a time before many women were permitted to enter the academic hierarchy. Even if the investigator was a virtually unknown clinician, the relationship with the sponsor was characterized as the investigator's "doing a favor" for the sponsor. Therefore, the monitor was never allowed to question seriously the investigator's decisions, comments, actions, or inactions. Little money was usually paid to the investigator to conduct the trial, and the investigator usually wrote the protocol without assistance from the sponsor. This protocol usually consisted of only a few pages, and these were often poorly written.

When the clinical trial was completed, the investi-

TABLE 62.3 *Old-fashioned stereotyped style of conducting and monitoring clinical trials*

Investigator: Male ("Herr Professor" or the "Grand Old Man")
Clinical trial site: Academic setting
Relationship with sponsor: Investigator appears to be doing the sponsor a favor by conducting the trial
Ability of the sponsor to influence the trial: Poor
Money paid for the trial's conduct: Usually little, but could be substantial
Preparation of the protocol: Usually by investigator
Quality of the protocol: Usually mediocre
Details in the protocol: Usually few
Statistical analyses: Conducted by the investigator and staff
Conduct of the trial: Delegated to staff
Quality of the trial's conduct and adherence to protocol: Usually fair to poor
Quality of the data: Usually fair to poor
Role of the monitor: Usually that of a menial
Adherence to time schedule: Usually fair to poor

TABLE 62.4 *Modern stereotyped style of conducting and monitoring clinical trials*

Investigator: Best qualified individual(s) are chosen
Clinical trial site: Wherever appropriate
Relationship with sponsor: Both are part of a team
Ability of the sponsor to influence the trial: Reasonable
Money paid for the trial's conduct: Fair market value
Preparation of the protocol: Usually by the sponsor with input of the investigator
Quality of the protocol: Very good to excellent
Details in the protocol: Substantial
Statistical analyses: Conducted by the sponsor or contractor
Conduct of the trial: By agreed-on personnel
Quality of the trial's conduct and adherence to protocol: Very good to excellent
Quality of the data: Very good to excellent
Role of the monitor: An important partner in the team
Adherence to time schedule: Reasonable to excellent

gator often performed the statistical analyses, interpreted the data, and then had the sponsor prepare the publication on which only the investigator's name appeared. As a result of this relationship, the sponsor had little or no leverage to exert on the investigator's activities. The sponsor could only hope that the trial would be conducted at a high standard, and was thankful if and when data were received. The data received rarely met the sponsor's expectations in either quality or quantity. If the investigator did not adhere to agreed-on patient entry rates or other commitments, the sponsor had little choice but to allow the trial to drag on, hoping that it would eventually be turned around and become productive. This miracle rarely occurred.

The monitor in the above scenario has a menial role and probably runs errands instead of acting in the role of a professional colleague. The extreme case occurs when development of an entire medicine program is turned over to an investigator. In this situation, the investigator is asked to evaluate the medicine in a number of clinical trials. After these trials are completed, the investigator is requested to inform the sponsor of his opinion about whether the medicine is worth developing further and whether a regulatory submission should be prepared. Protocols are generally prepared by the investigator and may be sent as a courtesy to the sponsor, who waits for a number of years while the investigator evaluates the new medicine. This stereotype is somewhat exaggerated to make a point, and hopefully does not occur any more to this degree. Nonetheless, elements of this style still persist in many countries.

Modern Style

In the modern stereotype (Table 62.4) the monitor interviews a number of potential investigators who each

have excellent reputations. The monitor's choice is based on the investigator's demonstration that he or she can conduct the clinical trial most efficiently and effectively. The protocol, often written by the monitor, has appropriate input from both the investigator(s) and sponsor. The investigator chosen is expected to adhere to the highest standards of clinical practice and maintain open communications and a sense of collaboration with the sponsor and monitor. The monitor is treated like an integral part of the clinical team by the investigator, and their relationship is based on mutual respect. The monitor's opinion on relevant issues is sought, carefully listened to, and evaluated. The investigator is paid a fair market value for conducting the trial. Through frank and open communications the monitor may exert pressure on investigators if their performance slackens or commitments are not achieved.

Although both of these patterns are idealized and represent extremes on a spectrum, the real world of the pharmaceutical industry has been gradually moving from the former pattern toward the more modern one. It is clear that companies in some countries tend to operate more closely to one style or the other. In addition, various idiosyncrasies tend to characterize the monitor–investigator relationship in certain countries, and certain rules of the game are generally followed.

MONITORING STRATEGY: WHAT, HOW, WHO, WHERE, WHEN?

Plan a basic monitoring strategy at the time of initiation of a clinical trial. This strategy will contain a number of different elements. Although the monitoring function may suggest that one is referring to a sponsored trial, in fact all unsponsored trials involve monitoring through periodic review and internal checks of performance and results.

In developing an overall monitoring strategy for a trial it is essential to determine the answers to several questions, including: (1) What will be monitored? (2) How will it be monitored? (3) Who will monitor it? (4) Where will it be monitored? (5) When will it be monitored? The answer to the question of *what* to monitor depends on the functions of the particular monitor(s). The most usual answer to this question includes four basic areas that must be periodically assessed. These involve confirmation that (1) the facilities remain adequate, (2) the trial is proceeding according to protocol, (3) the investigator and other trial personnel are fulfilling their various obligations, and (4) the data on the data collection forms are accurate and complete. The question of *how* to monitor is answered differently for each trial and for each monitor. Important principles are discussed throughout this chapter. The question of *who* will monitor is generally an obvious one. Monitors may be associated with the investigator, sponsor, or contract organization setting up the trial for a sponsor, or they may function independently and not be directly associated with either sponsor or investigator. This last method is sometimes used in large multicenter trials, for which an independent monitoring group is established. The numbers and functions of each monitor, and blinding of relevant monitors must be considered. The latter issue is discussed later in this section. Monitors include individuals with various backgrounds and experience, ranging from college graduates to PhDs, to MDs, and to medical specialists who monitor one aspect of a trial (e.g., pathologists, radiologists).

The question of *where* to monitor refers to the fact that monitoring must be conducted at each site where the clinical trial is being conducted, in addition to the monitor's own institution. It is usually more comfortable and convenient for monitors to rely on telephones, remote data entry, letters, electronic mail, and facsimiles rather than direct visits. This temptation must be avoided, or else monitors may be greatly misled about a trial's true status. The question of *when* to monitor refers to the timing of the visits to each site. Each clinical trial has its own appropriate times for visits (e.g., after the first two patients are entered, every 6 weeks, at 50% completion, during the entire clinical trial).

Standards of Performance

Monitors are members of the team that is developing a medicine (or device) whose primary responsibility is to work constructively with investigators and staff to ensure that each trial achieves the highest possible standards of conduct. An ideal standard of performance should not be used by monitors in judging a trial's conduct or in judging the staff, since that approach invariably leads to frustration and disappointment for the monitor. Nor should a lax or laissez-faire approach be adopted by the monitor. Learning the appropriate balance between these two extremes requires experience, knowledge, and tact. Questions that arise in this regard should be posed to more experienced monitors. The appropriate style and intensity of monitoring differ in different therapeutic fields of medicine. Moreover, the appropriate standards for one trial in a specific field will sometimes be totally inappropriate for another trial in the same field.

The feeling of a joint effort and common interests between the monitor and investigator plus staff should be developed and maintained. This can partially be achieved by the monitor's understanding the investigator's true motivation for participating in a trial. These factors are discussed later in this chapter.

Intensity of Monitoring

All trials have to be monitored with diligence and attention to detail. Certain clinical trials must be monitored more closely than most others to ensure that few problems/issues arise that could compromise the integrity and validity of the data obtained.

Monitoring Trials of Short Duration. A general principle is for medical monitors to remain at a site for the duration of a trial if it is only scheduled to last a few days. If a trial is of special importance to the sponsor then it is advisable for a monitor(s) to remain at the trial site for up to 2 (or even more) weeks.

Importance of the Clinical Trial to the Sponsor and Investigator. The intensity of monitoring should generally increase as the importance of a trial increases. The investigator's motivation, interests, and priorities may markedly differ from those of the sponsor, and even what the investigator views as the scientific objectives of the trial may differ. What may be a critical trial for the sponsor might be a minor fund-raising exercise for the investigator. In some occasions the opposite situation occurs, especially if an investigator contacts a sponsor for supplies of an investigational medicine to conduct a study of primary interest to the investigator. This type of trial is usually monitored less assiduously than a trial initiated by a sponsor. Other trials are of equal interest to the investigator and sponsor.

Phase III Trials. The intensity of monitoring some Phase III trials is usually relaxed as compared with Phase II trials. This is because the profile of a medicine's activity is better defined in Phase III, and many of the precautions and procedures necessary for the investigator to follow are better understood. Moreover, many Phase III trials are not as tightly designed and controlled as well-controlled Phase II trials.

Responding to Problems. Most clinical monitors should not consider themselves to be police officers who must crack a whip to correct problems. When problems arise a graded approach should generally be used by the monitor. Minimal actions should be initially tried because they may solve the problem. Progressively stronger actions may be taken, if necessary. The trial may be terminated if other approaches, including telephone calls, visits, or letters from senior management, are unsuccessful in improving a problem situation.

Monitors should be prepared to challenge any investigator whenever data seem strange, unexpected, too perfect, or unclear. If a significant problem occurs at a trial site, it may be relevant for the monitor to write a letter that is frank, but diplomatic. If the desired result is not achieved, a second letter may be more strongly worded. This is important to do, because inaction usually allows a poor situation to deteriorate and diminishes the possibility of exerting appropriate control over the trial if an important issue arises at a later date.

METHODS OF MONITORING

Telephone, Fax, Letters, Visits

Monitoring by telephone may initially appear to be a convenient and desirable technique. Nonetheless, excessive reliance on the telephone may lead to a false sense of security in regard to a trial's progress. A trip to the trial site may provide unexpected surprises. One possible exception to this principle would occur if data are being transmitted directly from the site to the sponsor and the telephone calls are made to discuss details of the data. The monitor may establish a regular as opposed to ad hoc system of placing telephone calls to the trial site, especially during the early phases of a clinical trial. If this is done then the site should be informed of this approach and a mutually agreed-upon time should be arranged.

Frequency of Monitoring Visits

The frequency of monitoring visits should be considered prior to initiating a clinical trial, but may easily be adjusted during the trial. In general, more frequent visits are made at the start of a long-term trial and fewer visits toward the end. The exact frequency should depend on (1) rate of patient entry, (2) time elapsed since last visit, (3) problems observed during the previous visit, and (4) problems reported since the last visit. Visits should therefore rarely be made on a fixed frequency (e.g., every 6 weeks) throughout a long-term trial. Monitors are often present at the initiation of a trial and often return after a few patients are enrolled to ensure that the trial is being conducted according to the protocol.

Confirm that the procedures to be followed for communication are explicit and discuss the purposes for telephone and direct visits. In planning the frequency of visits or internal assessments, consider the personality and reliability of the investigator and the staff plus the nature and relative importance of the medicine trial and also the resources of the sponsor. An independent consultant or group of consultants may be contacted at any stage of the trial to assist with the problems encountered, interpretation of data, or other matters. In addition, medical consultants at the investigator's site may be contacted prior to the start of the trial to evaluate patients if problems are anticipated that would require their expert help in diagnosis or treatment. Clarify that the sponsor will have access to all records generated in this trial to ensure accuracy of data transcription.

Maintaining the Triple Blind of Monitors

Inform investigators and the staff at all sites if monitors are blind to patient randomization. Monitors who interact with investigators should be blind. This may prevent misunderstandings that may arise if an investigator is interpreting the reactions and comments of the monitor, believing that the monitor is aware of the patient's treatment. If there are multiple monitors and only some are kept blind, it should be those who interact most closely with the investigator who remain blind. Types of monitoring methods are listed in Tables 62.5 to 62.7. Sample formats of tables to follow activities on multiple trials are shown in Table 62.8.

Monitoring is a continuous process. If problems de-

TABLE 62.5 *Types of monitoring methods utilized to oversee multiple projects*

1. Forms are completed by the investigator, research coordinator, or another individual at each trial site on a periodic basis; completed forms are sent to a single individual or group at the sponsoring or monitoring institution
2. Project leaders or managers prepare written reports on a periodic basis
3. Telephone calls, correspondence, and formal and informal meetings are used between the monitor and trial-site personnel; these may occur on an ad hoc or scheduled basis to review status of the clinical trial
4. Transmit data electronically from the trial site to the sponsor or to an intermediate contract group that has organized and is monitoring the trial for the sponsor; data are either sent online or transmitted at a later time
5. Monitoring groups are established that are independent of the sponsor and investigator
6. Each trial is periodically spot-checked, as opposed to monitoring all aspects of every trial
7. Every aspect of a trial is monitored as thoroughly as possible[a]

[a] Many specific aspects are listed in Table 62.6.

TABLE 62.6 *Aspects to monitor in a large group of clinical trials*

A. General data on each trial
   1. Protocol number and name
   2. Name, address, and telephone numbers of investigator and relevant staff members
   3. Total number of patients to be enrolled and number actually enrolled
   4. Number of data collection forms completed at the investigator's site
   5. Number of data collection forms received by sponsor
   6. Disposition and status of data collection forms
   7. Dates of initiation and completion of patient evaluation; dates of other milestones
B. Log of patients[a]
   1. Potential patients contacted about a trial
   2. Potential patients discontinued at screen
   3. Patients entered
   4. Patients prematurely discontinued during the trial
   5. Patients completing the trial
C. Log of monitoring site visits[b]
   1. Date of visit
   2. Names of monitors and staff members involved
   3. Important points covered and decisions reached
   4. Reference to a trip report (maintained at the sponsoring institution)
D. Status and projected dates of reports (e.g., generated, planned, or in progress)
   1. Statistical reports
   2. Medical reports (e.g., by investigators, by sponsors)
   3. Other reports
E. Outcomes of trials
   1. Brief synopsis of conclusions
F. Plans for overall program of trials
   1. List status of all trials (e.g., planned, ongoing, completed) and list actual or estimated dates of milestones
   2. Status of clinical protocols
G. Problem or "red flag" areas
   1. Follow details of safety or efficacy parameters in an open-label trial that are of particular interest or concern
H. Availability of materials for trials to monitor
   1. Bulk chemical available
   2. Needs of various departments for bulk chemical
   3. Bulk formulated medicine available
   4. Finished medicine available (e.g., number of tablets, capsules)
   5. Schedule for packaging of medicines
   6. Dates that medicine is needed by investigators

---

[a] See figures in Chapter 125.
[b] This log is maintained at the investigator's site until after the trial is complete, when it is sent to the sponsor for storage. A periodic site visit form is shown in Chapter 125.

TABLE 62.7 *Some potential problems to look for in monitoring clinical trials*

A. Concerning patient enrollment and randomization
   1. Ineligible patients allowed to enter trial
   2. Patients being enrolled more than once
   3. Patients assigned to treatment groups incorrectly
   4. Slow rate of patient enrollment
B. Concerning data collection forms
   1. Incomplete data collection forms (e.g., missing data or signatures)
   2. Errors in completing data collection forms (e.g., inconsistent data)
   3. Illegible data collection forms
   4. Vague or questionable entries
   5. Missing pages
   6. Excessive or unclear abbreviations used
   7. Blank spaces that should be filled in with "not done" or other terms
   8. Investigator's signature and date not appearing on pages as required by the protocol
   9. Previously observed errors not yet corrected with a line through the old data, correct data entered plus initials and date
   10. Patient number and clinical trial number not written or printed on every page as required
C. Concerning patient abnormalities
   1. Abnormalities in laboratory values, including unusual values recorded
   2. Trend toward abnormality in laboratory values
   3. Unreported severe adverse events
   4. Trends in the occurrence or nature of adverse events
   5. Any other abnormalities reported
D. Concerning clinical trial conduct
   1. Patients who are not compliant
   2. Lack of adequate efficacy noted when all patients are receiving active medicine[a]
   3. Efficacy noted in all patients on medicine, no efficacy noted for those on placebo, or other evidence that makes data appear too perfect
   4. Patients not examined by investigators, staff, or others who should have examined them
   5. Data or reports not being returned from outside groups as rapidly as desired and/or required (e.g., X-ray reports, pathology reports, pulmonary function studies)
   6. Scheduled tests not always conducted
   7. Tests incompletely conducted on some or all patients
   8. Unauthorized interim data analyses being conducted
   9. Errors in dispensing of medicine or in returning unused medicine
   10. Evidence that study blind has been broken
   11. Problems in storage of medicine (e.g., lack of refrigeration, lack of security)
   12. Study not conducted according to good clinical practices

---

[a] In studies where this is permissible (e.g., open-label clinical trials).

velop in this trial, such as if there are more dropouts than expected, the monitor must attempt to solve the problem. A number of possible interpretations are described in Table 62.9. After the correct one(s) is identified for the problem, a systematic approach to improving the situation must be developed.

WHAT AND HOW TO MONITOR

Site visits to conduct monitoring of records and facilities can be divided into previsit, onsite, and postvisit activities.

What to Do Prior to a Site Visit

Contact the investigator or trial coordinator prior to each visit so that he or she is aware of its purpose as well as an estimate of time requirements. This allows the investigator time to prepare for discussions that may focus on specific topics known in advance. Discuss the amounts of medicine and supplies that are at the site and whether additional medicine or supplies are needed. Reconfirm each trip approximately 1 to 3

TABLE 62.8 *Sample table formats used to monitor activities on multiple clinical trials conducted at various sites*

A[a]

Medicine or product	Indication or formulation	Trial doses, route, frequency	Trial sites	Principal investigator	Sponsor monitor(s)	Estimated start data (* = started)	Estimated end date (* = ended)	Current status and comments

B

Trial number	Principal investigator	Site location(s)	Trial objectives	Total no. of patients planned	No. of patients entered	Comments

[a] A, B are two separate examples of table formats.

days prior to its scheduled time to ensure that the meeting will be held as scheduled and that the monitoring trip is likely to be productive.

In an unsponsored trial, the principal investigator should establish procedures and guidelines for the conduct of periodic internal assessments of all aspects of the trial. This process of internal monitoring includes observations of physicians, other trial personnel, and patients, and assessment of data recording and entry. Discuss with trial staff how telephone and mail communications will be integrated into the monitoring strategy and how they will be implemented.

An informal agenda of activities prepared by the monitor will ensure that all major topics are covered and that the staff or investigator is available at desired times to review questions and findings. It may be desirable to provide this agenda to the site ahead of time. Experience at a site will enable one to judge the time necessary to allocate to various activities.

Monitoring Onsite

It is generally important that the monitor be seen as a colleague and a member of the team, rather than as a

TABLE 62.9 *Possible interpretations when "many" voluntary patient withdrawals occur at a single trial site*

1. Poor physician—patient relationship
2. Lack of incentives for investigator to try to keep patients in the trial[a]
3. Lack of incentives for patients to remain in the trial[a]
4. Incentives are present for investigator not to keep patients in the trial
5. Some attribute of the site or protocol is not conducive to a successful trial
6. Trial medicine is escalated too slowly, which yields an insufficient clinical response
7. Patients escalated too rapidly on medicine, which yields excessive toxicity
8. A specific factor is affecting the trial, which must be detected through careful monitoring
9. Trial medicine is not effective at the dose and/or conditions studied
10. Trial medicine is too toxic at the dose and/or conditions studied

[a] Includes both medical and nonmedical incentives.

policeman who arrives to inspect the troops or a nuisance who comes and gets in everyone's way. To avoid these and other images it is important to plan carefully to conduct monitoring meetings on a friendly but professional basis. Do not avoid discussing personal issues that do not go beyond types of conversations held with other business colleagues. Work around the staff and investigator's schedules to avoid interfering with their routine, insofar as possible, but do not allow them to "brush you aside" or refuse to cooperate.

The overall goal of monitoring is to ensure protocol and clinical trial compliance. Data collection forms must be reviewed for completeness and accuracy. There are literally hundreds of separate steps that may be taken to accomplish this. Those steps used depend on the specific clinical trial and the experience and knowledge of the monitor. A medically trained monitor with a medical degree should be able to conduct a greater in-depth evaluation of the records than someone without medical training. Each individual develops his or her own monitoring approaches and style over time and there is no single best approach for monitoring a clinical trial.

The types of activities to conduct on a monitoring trip are listed in Table 62.10 and the types of questions to pose about each activity monitored are listed in Table 62.11. A few of the specific items to monitor are listed in Table 62.12. Additional items are listed in Chapter 63, Auditing a Clinical Trial.

An important role of a clinical monitor is to review (edit) the data collection forms at each visit. It is usually more efficient for the monitor to review these rec-

TABLE 62.10 *Selected types of activities to conduct on a monitoring visit*

1. Talk to the staff and investigator about the status of the clinical trial, both before and after the data are reviewed
2. Inspect all relevant facilities involved in the clinical trial
3. Inspect all relevant administrative records being maintained
4. Inspect all relevant patient records
5. Document all errors and problems found
6. Confirm that all errors and problems found on the previous visit have been corrected or addressed
7. Complete the site's monitoring log

TABLE 62.11 *Selected questions to address about each of the activities monitored*

1. Are any problems being experienced by staff or investigator?
2. Are any problems observed by the monitor?
3. Are any procedural modifications desired by staff, investigator, or monitor?
4. What new questions does the monitor have?

ords prior to meeting with the investigator and research coordinator. The records should be reviewed for:

1. Problems of omission (e.g., missing or incomplete data, dates, or other information). Confirm that a properly signed and witnessed informed consent and pregnancy waiver (when appropriate) are in each patient's chart. The monitor should also confirm that the investigator's notes adequately explain missed visits or tests, patient dropouts, patients who are discontinued, and any relevant abnormalities that are noted by the monitor.
2. Problems of commission (e.g., errors that must be changed on the data collection forms by the investigator or coordinator).
3. Compliance with protocol requirements.
4. Legibility. If a monitor cannot read the form, other people probably cannot either.
5. Use of black ink, since blue ink does not usually microfilm well.
6. Corrections that have been properly entered according to established procedures.
7. Medical appropriateness and consistency within each patient. Are there areas to explain or clarify (e.g., abnormal or inconsistent data)?

TABLE 62.12 *Aspects to monitor in a single clinical trial at each site visit*

A. Clinic
 1. Are there any changes to the facilities?
 2. Are facilities still adequate?
 3. Are there any changes to the staff?
 4. Is the priority given the clinical trial adequate?
 5. Has the priority given the clinical trial changed?
 6. Are there training needs for either staff or investigators?
B. Clinical trial conduct
 1. Are there any changes or problems since the last visit?
 2. Are the previous issues raised being addressed?
C. Data management and administration
 1. Are medicines stored and dispensed appropriately?
 2. Are all samples being collected and sent as intended?
 3. Are data collection forms being completed on time, completely, and accurately?
 4. Are other administrative responsibilities (e.g., communication with Ethics Committee/IRB) being satisfactorily addressed?
D. Overall
 1. Are there other issues to address?

a For each of these questions, further questions, (e.g., who, what, where, when, why, how, and how much) should be asked.

One method to keep monitors from reediting a page on a subsequent site visit is to initial each page reviewed, either in a corner of the page or on a blank line titled "edited by" (if one was included on the data collection form). The procedure of initialing a page may be used only after the entire page is completed and has been signed or initialed by the investigator, if that is part of the protocol. Pages should not be altered after they are signed by the investigator without the monitor being informed.

Tools to Help Monitors

The progress of efficacy or safety parameters in some clinical trials is followed by collecting selected data on an ongoing basis in a "monitor's book." This book often consists of one or more forms per patient, kept in a loose-leaf or other similar binder. The monitor's book should be filled out at each visit or updated via telephone contacts. The information collected should concentrate on the most important efficacy and safety parameters. Computers may also be utilized to follow the conduct and results of medicine trials. This process will require careful organization and planning prior to trial initiation. In numerous trials, data are transmitted directly from the investigator's site to the sponsor by computer and telephone connections.

Examining and Interpreting Data

In addition to the editing function, a monitor should review the data and look for trends, problems, or relevant areas to discuss with the investigator or research coordinator. The monitor can perform this role most effectively in double-blind trials if he or she also remains blind to patient assignment. Some specific examples of reviewing data include an evaluation of whether the attribution of adverse events to the trial medicine (i.e., possible, definite, unknown, etc.) was the same at the patient's subsequent visits to the site. When terms such as "double vision," "dizziness," and other potentially ambiguous phrases are reported, the specific characteristics observed should be indicated.

The monitor should evaluate whether laboratory results are showing gradual changes or trends even if all values are still within the reference range. If a laboratory test is reported to be markedly abnormal in the data collection form, it may be worthwhile to compare the value with the original laboratory slip (report) to ensure that there was not a transcription error. Calling the laboratory to discuss the value may also be worthwhile. Determine whether a repeat laboratory test was performed. Consider having duplicate samples sent to two different laboratories. The monitor should confirm that the investigator is notifying the sponsor of all serious adverse events within 24 hours.

Checks for protocol adherence include evaluation of the number of missed visits and patient noncompliance as measured by pill counts, electronic monitors, plasma level fluctuations, or other methods. Some of the simpler mathematical calculations on the data collection forms should be checked to ensure that the numbers are being handled properly and that the numbers are added or subtracted correctly. The data collection forms should be corrected, if possible, during the same site visit. Otherwise, the questioned pages of the data collection forms should be reviewed at the following visit to confirm that necessary changes have been made.

Listing Questions and Issues to Discuss

The monitor can list specific questions or problems concerning data entry on the preprinted blank form for discussion at that visit with the coordinator or investigator. It is often convenient to use one of these forms per patient. In meeting with the investigator or coordinator, the monitor should review these forms as well as the specific topics mentioned on the telephone or in a letter that was sent to the investigator prior to the visit. Review questions and problems that concern the investigator and coordinator and discuss how these can be solved. Ascertain that the investigator is maintaining required contact with the Ethics Committee/Institutional Review Board (IRB).

Visiting the Pharmacy

The monitor should periodically visit the pharmacy (if relevant) and review dispensing records for the trial. A separate "pharmacist's book" can be prepared that will contain information on drug dispensing and returned medication if it will assist in the conduct of the trial (see Chapter 25 for an example). Ensure that returned medicine supplies are being properly documented and handled. Discuss questions and relevant procedures with the pharmacist. Examine the biological samples that are being collected. Confirm that the relevant samples have been collected and are properly labeled and stored. Labels may be preprinted with the trial number, patient number, sample number, and other relevant data. Adhesive may be required to affix labels to tubes or other containers, and waterproof pens may be sent to investigators if any writing is required on the label.

Monitoring During a Regulatory Audit

If a Food and Drug Administration (FDA) audit is being conducted when a monitor arrives at a site, or

an audit is initiated while the monitor is working at the site, a policy governing the monitor's behavior must be established by the sponsor. The monitor should obtain the results of any audits conducted at sites with which he or she is in contact.

Postvisit

A list of activities that require follow-up is generated at each site visit. In addition, it is usually important to notify the site in writing about any issues or problems found or discussed and the approaches to be taken on each. Other relevant information may be included (e.g., date of next visit), and the staff can be acknowledged and thanked for their efforts and time. Send investigators letters that document significant decisions or changes in the trial regardless of whether the decision was reached during a telephone conversation, at a site visit, or in a different manner.

Some organizations require that an official site visit form or prose report be written about each site visit. Drafts of these reports are often completed while traveling between visits to sites or on the way home.

MONITORING ACTIVITIES AT THE SPONSORING INSTITUTION

During the course of the trial, the monitor should confirm the arrival of all medicines, data collection forms, and supplies at each site. This process should include confirmation that the correct number of cartons was received in each shipment. A letter of transmittal should be sent separately for the items shipped to alert the investigator of the pending shipment. Complete any forms required by the sponsor after each visit and document all important decisions and changes related to the protocol or trial.

The monitor may assign unused medicines for backup patients at the trial site to patients if problems have occurred and additional medicine is required. This should be done with care and preferably after consultation with a statistician. Many unusual and "unique" situations seem to arise in almost all trials, which challenge the imagination and creativity of the monitor in arriving at a satisfactory solution.

Medical Emergencies

The monitor may be contacted if it becomes necessary to break the trial blind for a medical emergency and the randomization code for the patient is not readily available to the investigator. A copy of the randomization code should be accessible for such emergencies. Copies are often maintained both at the sponsor's office and at the home of one of the monitors. Provisions must be made for situations in which the monitor is out of town, "unavailable," or is blind to patient randomization. A standard series of procedures (e.g., obtaining blood and urine specimens and samples of medication for chemical analysis) may be developed for situations in which patients are discontinued for medical reasons.

Training of Monitors Who Are Untrained in Clinical Medicine

Many medical monitors at pharmaceutical companies are not trained in clinical medicine. Allowing interested monitors to go through the screening and possibly some testing procedures used in a trial personally will provide them with a better understanding of the trial. This practice will also help a monitor better appreciate various issues and problems from the investigator's perspective.

Monitors should be encouraged to attend relevant professional meetings, courses, and seminars to improve their medical knowledge and skills in interpreting data. Discussions with more senior monitors will provide important education and professional development. Some companies offer internal training courses for their monitors and provide appropriate educational materials (see Chapter 54).

Remote Data Entry

Workers at an investigator's site can enter clinical data into a computer and periodically (e.g., daily, weekly) transmit data to the sponsor's site. Variations on this flow of data are possible, such as having data initially sent to a central site or consultant's office prior to being sent to a sponsor (see Chapter 28).

The purpose of remote data entry is to increase the speed and efficiency with which data may be processed and analyzed. The computer assists the data entry operator by questioning inappropriate entries of data. Other advantages are that missing data may be easily flagged by the computer. The computer program may provide feedback if all entry criteria are not met, if visit dates are not entered in correct order, and if other preset criteria are not met. Simple calculations may be used both at the investigator's site and at the sponsor's site to maintain current information on total patient enrollment, trends in laboratory data, and other parameters of interest that do not affect the trial's blind. This topic is discussed in Chapter 125.

Geographical Location of Corporate Monitors

All monitors may be based at the sponsor's central location and may travel to and from the various clinical trial sites. Some sponsors utilize sales representatives and/or other individuals scattered throughout the country to monitor sites located in reasonable proximity to their homes. Various combinations of these approaches are also possible. When a clinical trial is sponsored by two different companies, a parent company and a foreign subsidiary, or by two subsidiaries of a single sponsor, monitoring is often performed by individuals from both groups.

In certain situations, a monitoring representative from a third country or group may be present. For example, when monitors of a subsidiary initiate a trial in a different country than that in which the main organization's headquarters are located, monitors may come from the parent, host, and subsidiary countries. There are also occasions when monitors of a contract organization accompany monitors from a sponsor (or vice versa) on a monitoring trip.

Travel

Monitors often travel a great deal to and from various clinical trial sites. It is usually necessary to balance taking fewer long trips versus more frequent shorter trips. Each situation differs, but most monitors attempt to cluster sites that are relatively nearby (or on a circle route) and that are to be visited in a single trip. Long trips rarely last for more than 10 days for most monitors. A few practical considerations for travelers are listed in Table 62.13.

Training of New Staff at the Trial Site

In most clinical trials of "long" duration there will be a need at different times to train new staff members who join the trial. Planning is required to develop appropriate means to do this efficiently. One useful method is to have the investigator, coordinator, or other staff member spend appropriate time (generally 1 day to a week) with a counterpart at another trial site. Another possibility is for the monitor and/or other individuals from the sponsor or another trial site (e.g., research coordinator) to spend time (at the trial site) directly training the new person and reviewing the trial with them. Whatever plan is adopted, it should not generally consist of merely allowing the person to gain their own "on-the-job training." A training manual may be considered as an adjunct in special cases, such as large multicenter trials. Flow charts should be included that illustrate how to change dosages when adverse reactions occur or the medicine is not sufficiently effective, plus how to perform various other modifications that may be necessary. However, this or other types of guides will never be sufficient to provide adequate training on their own. Ensure that only the final

TABLE 62.13 *Practical consideration for travelers*

A. Prior to a trip
 1. Copy the relevant airline, bus, ferry, or other schedule(s) that will allow for alternate arrangements to be made if changes are required en route or prior to return
 2. Consider an alternative plan if planes or other modes of transportation are delayed or canceled[a]
 3. Obtain maps of the area(s) to be visited
 4. Reserve all transportation and hotels as far in advance as possible
 5. Reserve hotel with guaranteed late arrival and become familiar with cancellation terms. Request an upper floor, lower floor, room with a specific view (if desired), or nonsmoking room
 6. Make arrangements for anticipated business and nonbusiness activities
 7. Reserve restaurants long in advance for important business meetings; it is often desirable to call the chef to discuss the menu, especially if everyone will be having the same meal
 8. Obtain currency for each country to be visited for international travel; consider obtaining traveler's checks issued in a foreign currency (or currencies)
 9. Set up as many business meetings as possible in advance and confirm each within 3 days of leaving
 10. Prepare a list of (1) activities and questions to cover at each appointment and (2) points to cover at each meeting
 11. Bring a copy of all relevant addresses, telephone numbers, and facsimile numbers
 12. Bring credit cards, including a telephone card
 13. Take sufficient traveler's checks in suitable denominations
 14. Evaluate the total cost and convenience of a car rental versus using taxis or other transportation; make arrangements that provide for the most efficient, cost-effective, and reasonable use of one's time
 15. Prepack a small suitcase with as many needed items as possible, to be ready to take on a trip, travel as lightly as possible
 16. Maintain a list of additional items needed for a warm and cold climate to add to the prepacked suitcase prior to leaving
 17. Check the weather forecast of the place(s) to be visited shortly prior to departure
 18. Put a change of underwear and socks (plus other essentials) in one's briefcase in case one's luggage is delayed or lost
 19. Consider membership in one or more airline lounges
B. En route
 1. Do not check luggage at an airport unless necessary
 2. Avoid scheduling airplane changes in cities where bad weather may cause delays (e.g., generally attempt to change airplanes in a southern city in the United States during the winter)
 3. Understand passengers' rights on public carriers (e.g., regarding smoking or nonsmoking sections)[b]
 4. Remove shoes on long airplane flights and carry lightweight slippers
 5. Bring a variety of work and reading material to suit one's mood at the time
 6. Allow ample time to reach each destination, thereby preventing most travel delays from affecting one's schedule
 7. Do not plan a tight schedule at airports or on the ground unless necessary. This is especially relevant for international travel
 8. If taxis are difficult to find at the airport terminal consider sharing one, renting a car, or taking a bus
 9. Use express services provided by many automobile rental companies
C. At the destination
 1. Request a hotel room with specific view or facing a specific direction if not done in advance; ensure that the room is not next to an elevator or in a particularly noisy location (e.g., immediately above a ballroom)
 2. Obtain directions to your meeting(s) or activities in advance, including information on where to park or how to obtain taxis for the return trip to the hotel
 3. Reserve seats for entertainment, restaurants, theater, or other activities as early in your stay as possible
 4. Allow extra time to get to appointments or an airport if the trip will be made during "rush hour" in a city; ask hotel or other personnel about the length of delay to expect and possible solutions
 5. Reserve a taxi in advance (if possible) whenever needed
 6. Consider express check-out from hotels
 7. Consider rapid return procedures for rented automobiles

[a] Delays of one air carrier to a destination because of weather problems does not necessarily mean that all other air carriers to the same destination are also delayed.
[b] Obtain *Fly Rights—A Guide to Air Travel in the U.S.* from the Civil Aeronautics Board, Washington, D.C. 20428.

version of the protocol is present at the site, plus any appendices if relevant.

Items to Monitor

Monitoring of a single clinical trial is primarily concerned with ensuring that the trial is well conducted and that all data are collected as efficiently and accurately as possible. Monitoring of multiple trials conducted on a single medicine is generally concerned with tracking progress, identifying causes of delays, allocating resources, and managing the project. Individuals who monitor single trials may or may not be the same people who monitor progress on a group of

trials. Monitoring is also performed at a more senior level in a corporation through formal and/or informal review and other mechanisms. Reports of each monitoring trip should be documented. This may be done with a note to the file plus completion of a log book or by completing a preprinted form (see Chapter 125 for an example), which is then distributed and stored. Many of the administrative functions of monitoring may be managed with a computer.

To identify all of the important points to monitor on multiple clinical trials or on multiple projects, it is necessary to determine the objectives of monitoring. There is certainly a balance between monitoring too little and too much. Once the objectives are listed the appropriate items to monitor should become more clear. These may be discussed with colleagues and supervisors to confirm that the list chosen is appropriate.

Monitors at the sponsor's site may better prepare for their site visit by concentrating on the known issues they wish to raise, rather than seeking issues to identify through a time-consuming review of the data collection forms at the site. It is also possible for the monitor and investigator to conduct some of these discussions by telephone.

Forms to Use in Monitoring

Each sponsor develops forms that are appropriately suited to the needs of the particular project and procedures in the sponsoring organization. Either of these factors may be the major one in determining the exact makeup of the forms used. A few sample forms are presented in Chapter 125 and Table 62.8 to assist in the design of forms for related purposes. Since the organizational makeup of sponsors as well as their "standard operating procedures" differ to such a great degree, it is not possible to describe in a generic way how these forms should flow between individuals, groups, or departments.

Individuals sometimes make up and use their own systems and forms to keep track of and monitor activities and status of clinical trials. Their forms may reflect those of their sponsor, or they may be highly individualistic. The forms may be handwritten on scratch paper, printed, or kept on a computer disk. These forms are usually the major means an individual uses to keep abreast of what he or she believes to be the most important items to monitor.

MONITORING LARGE MULTICENTER TRIALS

Monitoring large multicenter clinical trials presents special problems of ensuring intersite consistency. This is usually addressed by having many specialized monitoring groups, such as those illustrated in Fig. 39.1. Separate groups of monitors may be utilized to confirm diagnoses (e.g., through examination of pathology reports), observe treatment, and evaluate follow up. Groups may be established based on modality (e.g., radiation, surgery, clinical oncology, pathology in certain cancer trials), function, and therapeutic discipline (e.g., neurology or ophthalmological examinations) to monitor data collection or data analysis. It is clear that it may also be necessary to have one or more overall monitors whose function is to monitor the specialized monitors. Well-developed quality assurance programs have been used to monitor many large clinical trials (e.g., Glicksman et al., 1980).

When specialized monitoring groups are utilized they may be based at each clinical trial center and have responsibility only for that site. Alternatively, each specialized monitoring group may periodically visit each center. A third alternative is to use both approaches to monitoring and to have some specialized monitoring groups located at each site while other groups travel to the various sites of a large trial.

Sophisticated Monitoring

Monitors who are better trained (e.g., those with a medical degree) or more sophisticated will learn to look for subtle signs in clinical data. Countless examples relating to any safety or efficacy parameter could be given; a few examples of laboratory data are presented in Table 62.14. The point is that anyone may develop skills, but this development requires both knowledge and attention to detail.

How Often Should a Site Be Monitored?

No single answer applies to all sites; the answer usually ranges from every 2 weeks to every 6 months. Certain factors may be used to determine the correct response in a specific case, as listed below:

1. Priority of the clinical trial for the sponsor. The higher the priority, the more often a site should be monitored, if all other factors are constant.
2. Rate of patient entry into the clinical trial. The larger the number of patients entering the clinical trial, the more data are available for evaluation, and the greater the need to make frequent visits. A method should be chosen to learn when new patients enter a clinical trial (Fig. 62.1 and Table 62.15).
3. Staff members available for monitoring. If each person is forced to monitor many sites (usually over ten) the frequency of visits will tend to de-

TABLE 62.14 *Selected examples of sophisticated monitoring of laboratory values*[a]

1. Consistency of the type of disease (e.g., anemia) with specific values in the complete blood count and other blood tests (e.g., red blood cell fragility test)
2. Consistency of the severity of jaundice or hepatitis with liver function tests
3. Consistency of heart rate and respiration rate with body temperature and clinical findings
4. Consistency of the patient's diagnosis with required laboratory changes (e.g., in pernicious anemia, certain changes in the blood and bone marrow must be present)
5. Consistency of findings within laboratory reports (e.g., abnormal elevations of both lymphoid and myeloid cells in bone marrow may not be reported)
6. Hemolysis of blood affecting results
7. Over- or underdamped electrocardiogram (EKG) machine (e.g., make certain that a squarewave calibration is actually square)

[a] More specific relationships between patient diagnoses and laboratory parameters that must be present for anemias are presented by Rao et al. (1986).

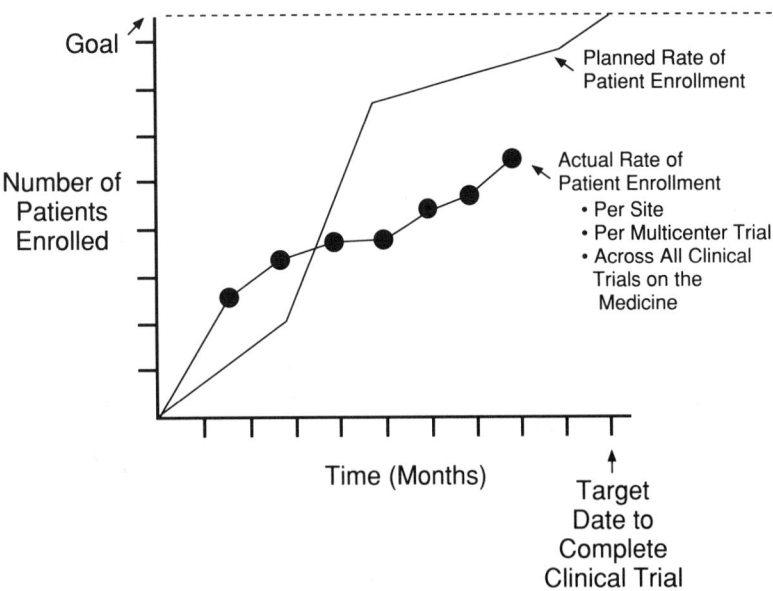

Goal

Number of Patients Enrolled

Planned Rate of Patient Enrollment

Actual Rate of Patient Enrollment
• Per Site
• Per Multicenter Trial, or
• Across All Clinical Trials on the Medicine

Time (Months)

Target Date to Complete Clinical Trial

FIG. 62.1 Tracking the status of actual patient enrollment, versus planned patient enrollment. The planned rate is often linear throughout the trial, rather than at different rates as shown.

crease significantly. Staff numbers may be temporarily enhanced by involving a contract organization.

4. Problems at the site. Special monitoring visits are made when problems arise. Therefore, a site that is performing at a high standard tends to require fewer site visits per year than a poorly run site or one with numerous problems.

5. The possibility for problems to arise is greater if the protocol is complex, if the medicine is relatively toxic, or if staff are new. Any factor leading or potentially leading to more problems encourages more frequent monitoring visits.

6. Location of the site. While the number of monitoring visits should be independent of this factor, the location of a site does affect the frequency of visits. Distant and more difficult-to-reach sites tend to be monitored less frequently. It is practical to visit several sites with major airline connections on a single trip.

TABLE 62.15 *Methods by which a sponsor learns about new patients enrolled in a clinical trial*

1. Telephone call placed by monitors at preselected times
2. Telephone call placed by the investigator or staff after every X number of patients or weeks
3. Facsimile sent by the investigator or staff
4. Remote data entry received by the sponsor on a periodic or ad hoc basis
5. A postcard is removed from the data collection form and mailed to the sponsor after each patient enters the clinical trial
6. Contacts may be received via a contract organization that serves as an intermediary between the sponsor and investigator
7. Monitor's observations made during a site visit
8. Data collection forms are received by the sponsor after every X number of patients complete the clinical trial

Different Standards of Monitoring

Everyone will agree that many standards of monitoring exist, but probably not everyone will agree on the value of having multiple standards. It is beneficial to have multiple standards available because all clinical trials should not be monitored to the same degree.

Standards are determined by (1) the experience of the monitor(s), (2) the frequency of monitoring visits, (3) the degree to which the monitor insists that the investigator and staff adhere to the protocol, (4) the completeness and accuracy of the data collection forms, (5) the investigator's communications with sponsor and the Ethics Committee/IRB, and (6) the relationship between investigator and monitor. Standards are established by the company, often through interactions with investigators and regulatory authorities. Selected standards are communicated to both monitors and investigators. The standards established depend on available resources, the medical value of the medicine, the commercial value of the medicine, its phase of development, its priority within the project system, and its overall importance to the company.

There is a minimal acceptable quality standard for each country that is appropriate for minor clinical trials. Higher standards also exist along a continuum. The highest standards are usually applied to a breakthrough medicine: data will be carefully scrutinized by various groups and, therefore, must be as scientifically and medically sound as possible. It is ironic, but it is in these very clinical trials that inexperienced or naive companies allow a lower standard of monitoring and investigator conduct. These companies (often biotechnology companies) believe that the medicine they are studying is so important and its value so obvious that both regulators and prescribing physicians will "have" to approve and prescribe it without critiquing the data as carefully as they do for routine medicines with "less obvious benefits" over existing therapy. It is astounding how this naive scenario seems to unfold with a promising new therapy every few years, markedly compromising the development of that therapy.

RELATIONSHIPS BETWEEN MONITORS AND INVESTIGATORS

It is always important to be considerate of the clinical trial investigators and all of their staff who assist and often have major roles. For example, it is wise to learn the names of the staff and something about their interests. It is also important to discuss relevant aspects of the trial and the medicine's development program with them. This often helps maintain cooperation, enthusiasm, and high trial standards. It is recommended to take the staff out for lunch and/or to provide other reasonable and appropriate benefits (e.g., snacks) at appropriate times.

Situations often arise during the career of a clinical monitor when the relationship with an investigator ceases to be solely concerned with, and limited to, business. This usually refers to development of a friendship (no other types of relationships will be considered). Furthermore, the motives for developing a friendship are assumed to be totally honorable and without any ulterior motives on the part of either individual.

In developing a relationship with an investigator (or possibly with a member of the investigator's staff) there are a number of questions for the monitor to consider. These include:

1. Can a satisfactory distinction be made between the professional and personal relationship to allow the professional relationship to continue in an appropriate manner?
2. Could the personal relationship potentially compromise the abilities of the monitor to act professionally with the investigator?
3. What is the potential for the personal friendship to compromise the conduct of the study and the professional career of the monitor?
4. What is the potential for the relationship to evolve beyond its present scope in a manner that is not presently desired?
5. Is it possible to define the limits of the relationship that the monitor considers acceptable?
6. Is it relevant to discuss the relationship with more experienced monitors or others at the sponsor's site?

Each situation will differ and there is clearly no single approach that is always appropriate. There are ways, however, of socializing as professionals that promote a cordial friendship while maintaining an appropriate and positive business relationship. No monitor should either encourage or participate in a greater friendship or social involvement than is considered appropriate and reasonable.

IMPROVING A POOR PERFORMER OR TRIAL

Step One: Identify the Problem

Monitors may perceive that the quality of an investigator's performance in a clinical trial has either diminished over a period of time, or else has never achieved an acceptable or agreed-on standard. In approaching this issue there are several stages to follow. The first is to identify the precise area or areas in which the investigator's performance is deficient. This may relate only to a single aspect of the trial (e.g., low patient enrollment). Alternatively, the problem may be more widespread and involve the investigator's overall motivation and morale, or overall performance of the trial. The seriousness of the problem must then be assessed.

A few common problems relating to the clinical trial and not the investigator are:

1. Incentives offered patients are inadequate to encourage or convince them to enroll in the trial.
2. The protocol is too demanding of a patient's time or efforts in performing tests.
3. The protocol is too demanding of an investigator's time or efforts.
4. Staff available at the investigator's site is inadequate in number, training, or other factors to handle the patient load effectively.
5. Patient visits are scheduled at inconvenient times of day or on weekends.
6. A schedule of patient activities is established that is too demanding (e.g., having patients go from one location to another for tests or examinations versus having professional staff visit patients at a central location).

Does the Problem Exist at One Site or Many?

Another aspect of problem situations at an investigator's site relates primarily to multicenter clinical trials. It must be ascertained whether the problem is isolated to one site or is a common problem at all or most sites. The situation is markedly different if nine of ten investigators in a single trial at different sites are performing well or if nine of these ten investigators are performing poorly. This balance may also indicate whether the primary problem is related to the specific investigator and location or to more general problems with the protocol or all sites. If each of the nine investigators are performing poorly for the same reason(s), this usually means that immediate attention is required to help the trial.

Step Two: Identify the Reasons

After the problem areas and degree of seriousness are identified, it is essential to discover the reasons for the problem. This may not be simple or straightforward, but usually should be attempted. The major reasons for the problem(s) may be unrelated to the clinical trial or to anything that a monitor may be able to affect (e.g., personal problems of the investigator, the trial site has moved to new quarters, students who are the major source of patient enrollment are on vacation). Many other reasons may directly relate to the problem and may be affected by the monitor, including those relating to the conduct of the trial (e.g., if the investigator overestimated the number of suitable patients available). The reason(s) per se usually does not provide the solution, but often allows an approach to be found that may be used to reach a solution.

Step Three: Finding a Solution

In seeking a solution to a protocol-related problem, consideration must be given to how the protocol may be modified while not compromising the value of data obtained. If the problem relates to conditions at the investigator's site, then possible alternatives should be considered and discussed. If the protocol is too complex to be easily followed, then steps must be taken to create flow charts, diagrams, and other aids to explain each step or factor in a sufficient and clear manner, or else certain parts of the protocol must be modified. If too many patients are dropping out because of adverse reactions then consideration must be given to steps such as eliminating the highest dose of the trial medicine. When the source of the problem lies outside the ability of the monitor or sponsor to affect or modify, then a decision of whether to terminate the trial must be considered.

Problems of Motivation

If the problem is believed to be primarily focused on the investigator's motivation as opposed to the protocol or other areas, then it is extremely important to understand the reasons why the investigator is conducting the trial. Reasons often vary widely among different investigators, even among those who are participating in an identical multicenter trial. Common motives involve (1) professional recognition resulting from being associated with an exciting new medicine

or special trial, (2) career enhancement, (3) scientific interest, (4) financial rewards as part of a professional medicine testing business, (5) financial rewards to obtain funds to support other research, (6) greater ability to treat one's patients, (7) obtaining medical or scientific equipment, and (8) doing a personal favor for, or returning a favor to, someone at the sponsor or another site. Numerous other motives exist that may be the investigator's primary reasons for conducting a trial.

Once the investigator's motivation is understood it is possible to determine ways to help solve the problem and also benefit the investigator. This could be in the form of a *quid pro quo*. The monitor should try to make the investigator share a stake in the clinical trial outcome and the problem's resolution. Enlist the help of others, if necessary, to solve the problem.

One of the most difficult roles for a monitor is to help maintain motivation at clinical trial sites during a long-term trial, or during a trial of short duration that is conducted over the long time period needed to enroll a sufficient number of patients. Knowledge of the positive attributes of a medicine, the potential value of the trial, the motivation of the investigator, and the potential problems that might arise will assist a monitor in both preventing and solving problem situations.

Varieties of Financial Incentives

When the investigator's primary motives relate to financial considerations it does not imply that the sponsor should merely increase the clinical trial budget to improve the investigator's motivation. This may only offer a short-lived stimulus to the investigator. A number of other approaches may be more effective. Providing assistance to the investigator by paying for a full-time (or part-time) research coordinator, nurse, or other individual to help with the trial may cause a dramatic improvement in the trial's conduct and the investigator's motivation. Paying for patient meals and transportation, or for previously unanticipated actual trial costs, is generally acceptable.

Paying a bonus to investigators to complete a trial by a certain deadline or to enroll a certain number of patients within a specified time is considered by some sponsors and investigators to be unethical. This practice places often strong monetary incentives on rapid enrollment. An investigator may thus be influenced to enroll a patient who would otherwise not be enrolled. Thus, the bonus may have the undesired effect of increasing patient risks and may have an adverse impact on the investigator's adherence to "good clinical practices."

An alternative to a bonus payment that is more acceptable, from an ethical perspective, is to pay investigators different per-patient sums for completed patients who meet a defined standard, as opposed to patients who do not meet the defined standard(s). These standards may be established in terms of duration of treatment (e.g., investigators get paid more for patients who remain in the clinical trial for a given number of weeks or months than for those who remain in the trial for a shorter period) or in terms of quality of data (e.g., investigators are paid a different rate for patients whose data collection forms are complete or meet certain criteria than for patients whose data collection forms have more than a preset minimum of missing or erroneous data).

GAMES INVESTIGATORS PLAY

Some of the common types of "games" or ploys are listed in Table 62.16. Many others could be included.

TABLE 62.16 *Games investigators play*

A. Prior to the clinical trial they may
  1. Overestimate the number of available patients who will enter; this is an example of "Lasagna's law"[a]
  2. Assure the monitor that they will conduct the trial themselves and then spend less time than agreed to or have assistants conduct the entire trial
  3. Indicate they are definitely able to conduct the trial, whereas they know their health is inadequate for the task
  4. Exaggerate their technical skills in trials in which their skills are important (e.g., surgery using medical devices, using sophisticated equipment)
  5. Place pressure on the sponsor to modify the protocol in a way that benefits the investigator
  6. Provide too optimistic a date for trial initiation or completion
  7. Indicate they have adequate staff to conduct the trial when they actually do not have staff available
  8. Complain about the budget and try to increase it
  9. Request a protocol to read, but not truly consider participating in the clinical trial
B. At the time of trial initiation they may
  1. Delay starting the trial
  2. Not obtain Ethics Committee/IRB[b] approval on the agreed schedule (e.g., delay submission)
  3. Include additional parts or tests in a trial because of personal interest, but that are not written in the protocol and are not approved by their Ethics Committee/IRB
  4. Share medicine supply with preclinical scientists
  5. Share the clinical trial's medicine with physicians who treat patients outside the protocol
C. Regarding patients entered in the clinical trial, they may
  1. Enter hard-core nonresponders despite requests not to do so
  2. Enter patients whose disease severity is too mild or too severe
  3. Enter patients (or volunteers) with a history of alcohol or drug abuse who are believed or known to be unreliable
  4. Enter patients and start treatment before the patients' screen or baseline laboratory values are returned; it is important to have these values in order to confirm that they are acceptable
  5. Enter the same patient two (or more) times in the same trial
  6. Enter the same patient in two (or more) different trials being conducted simultaneously by the investigator
  7. Enter patients after the date used for cutoff of new patient entry
  8. Enter patients who do not meet inclusion criteria
D. Regarding randomization they may
  1. Assign patients to treatment based on their own biases
  2. Take bottles of medicine from a box haphazardly, rather than randomizing patients according to the code provided
  3. Hide the fact that a patient did not qualify to enter the clinical trial
E. During the clinical trial they may
  1. Complete some or all tests on patients scheduled for one visit at a later date and fill in the data collection form under the original date
  2. Replace a departing staff member but not adequately train the new individual
  3. Change laboratories used to analyze samples without informing the sponsor
  4. Increase or decrease medicine doses inappropriately
  5. Fail to notify the sponsor about a serious adverse event or drug overdose
  6. Indicate additional costs that were not discussed prior to the trial, although they were known or could have been anticipated
  7. Initiate trials for other sponsors without any prior discussion with the original sponsor and the new trial slows or affects the original trial
  8. Not communicate with the sponsor as they agreed
  9. Hide the fact that a patient is violating the protocol, so that the investigator may keep the patient in the clinical trial
  10. Go on a long holiday and give patients more medicine than recommended
  11. Conduct some of the baseline examinations (e.g., chest X-ray, ophthalmological) after patients have already been enrolled in the clinical trial (and possibly are receiving treatment) because of scheduling conflicts
  12. Not adequately train their staff
  13. Change doses of one or more medicines inappropriately
  14. Use different equipment than agreed to when measuring one or more parameters
  15. Terminate some patients prematurely to complete the clinical trial as rapidly as possible
F. After the clinical trial they may
  1. Prepare and/or submit a publication without adhering to an agreed-on review and discussion procedure with the sponsor
  2. Analyze data independently of the sponsor in violation of an agreement
  3. Not complete reports by agreed-on dates
  4. Not prepare reports that adequately describe results for sponsor or for the Ethics Committee/IRB
  5. Not send reports to the Ethics Committee/IRB or sponsor on time

[a] Overestimating the number of available patients is usually inadvertent, but may be done purposely to obtain the sponsor's agreement to conduct the trial.
[b] IRB, Institutional Review Board.

The primary reason for listing these is to provide monitors with a sample list of undesirable situations that may be prevented or corrected. The major approach to solving most of these issues is to discuss them openly and frankly with the investigator. Reasons why these practices are undesirable or unacceptable must be given in a manner that does not criticize the investigator or staff. The monitor and investigator should aim to reach agreement on a course of action that is acceptable to both.

When monitors discuss or negotiate the contents of a protocol with an investigator, or discuss the conduct of a clinical trial, it is important to remember that each investigator has different needs and desires. Even assuming that an investigator does not have a "hidden agenda," there are numerous shortcuts, ploys, or actual protocol violations that investigators may introduce (or attempt to introduce) into the trial. It is the monitor's responsibility to keep the trial moving forward on as high a level as possible and to prevent undesirable or unacceptable variations. These deviations often arise from the investigator's lack of awareness of the importance and need to adhere strictly to a protocol. Deviations also arise from the investigator's busy schedule and desire to expedite patient treatment and care. Situations of actual deceit or fraud are not considered "games investigators play."

GOLDEN RULES FOR CLINICAL MONITORS

Clinical monitoring is an important cornerstone of clinical medicine development. Monitors conduct large number of functions, although some may not conduct all the functions discussed in this chapter. The major function of clinical monitors is to observe and assess the quality of a clinical trial's conduct.

Golden rules or standards of current monitoring practices are briefly described in four categories: (1) protocol preparation, (2) trial initiation and conduct, (3) conducting site visits, and (4) personnel interactions with investigators and their staff. Many additional principles could be added to these lists, and most principles have already been discussed in this chapter, but are given additional focus in this section.

Who the Monitors Are

Monitors include individuals at the study site itself, so-called "internal monitors" as well as "external monitors" from a sponsor, contractor organization, or government agency. They can also include clinical auditors, who often have a different function (see Chapter 63). Monitors may be professionals with an MD, PhD, or PharmD, in addition to professionals who do not have doctoral degrees.

Protocol Preparation

When a clinical protocol exhibits high quality, it results from deliberate decisions and efforts to utilize high scientific, ethical, and medical standards. The details of how high standards may be achieved are described in other chapters.

Every clinical protocol involving the medical treatment of patients requires a review by an appropriately trained physician prior to its initiation. PhDs, PharmDs and other nonphysicians do not have adequate training or experience to understand fully what aspects of a clinical trial may be too onerous, difficult, irritating, or inappropriate for patients and for the trial. PhDs are able, however, to create successful pharmacokinetic protocols or simple protocols mimicking others that were implemented successfully.

Monitors should actively seek input from the investigators who will conduct a trial to help in protocol development or review, except when this is impossible. This approach is often important in establishing a "bonding" or "buy-in" between the investigator and the clinical trial monitor. Without this commitment by the investigator to the success of the trial, it may proceed and be completed successfully, but the chances are somewhat less than if the investigator is more strongly committed. For example, the priority given by the investigator to the trial's conduct, the efforts expended to find patients, and the efforts to solve problems that arise all depend on the investigator's views. If he or she is handed a protocol and does not feel a sense of ownership, then efforts expended may be less. Even if all major aspects of a protocol are set in stone, the monitor should go through this exercise. Even minor adjustments to a protocol suggested by an investigator will usually achieve the same goals. A few of the situations in which this is not possible include: replacement or addition of an investigator during a clinical trial, multicenter trials that are ongoing, or when numerous Ethics Committees/IRBs have already approved the protocol.

Clinical Trial Initiation and Conduct

The roles of monitors in a clinical trial's initiation and conduct vary widely. Monitors who interact with investigators should remain blind to patient randomization in all double-blind clinical trials. Ensure that investigators are aware of this, or else they may make unwarranted interpretations of comments made about the trial or about specific patients (e.g., an investigator may interpret a physician monitor's calm manner upon hearing of adverse reactions as an indication that the patient is receiving placebo).

When a clinical trial is very important for the sponsor and several monitors are involved, hold weekly or twice-monthly meetings of all monitors to review its status and any issues that may have arisen. These sessions will serve to prevent issues being ignored that should be discussed.

It is important to look for patterns in data, both within patients and among groups of patients. Ask oneself if the data make sense. For example, in a treadmill exercise test there is an expected pattern of change in both heart rate and blood pressure. Is this pattern observed or not? If data appear bizarre, a little detective work may be needed (e.g., was the patient compliant, was the person who measured the parameter experienced, was the patient alert when the test was made).

Site Visits

Whether the monitor's visit is the first or tenth to a specific site, it is wise to confirm, *prior to departure*, that all essential and important preparations have been made that were previously requested. Many war stories are told of monitors stating that investigators were "supposed" to have had certain records or other things prepared, but when the monitor arrived at the site, they were greeted by an empty-handed investigator who had lame excuses. If the monitors had confirmed immediately (or shortly) before departure that the expected materials were prepared and ready, it could have saved them an unnecessary trip. A corollary of this principle is that monitors should be prepared *not* to go on a scheduled trip, if it is expected that it will not be productive. Even if the monitor planned the trip for 2 months, it is not only a waste of time and the company's resources, but it confirms in the investigator's mind that he or she may manipulate the monitor.

Prepare an agenda and list of people to see, things to do, places to visit, and questions to ask. Visit all relevant places at each site (e.g., clinical laboratory, microbiological laboratory, pharmacy), based on prior plans and intentions that arose during that visit. Allow sufficient time for the visit so that the monitor is not rushed and unable to conduct all the business planned. Titrate the frequency of visits according to the amount of work needed, the extent of any problems, and the importance of the trial to the sponsor. Do not rigidly adhere to an every X-week schedule of visits.

Personnel Interactions

Most standards in this category are rooted in common sense. Monitors learn to adopt a positive and nonconfrontational approach with investigators. Wise monitors also discuss changes they want the investigator to make in terms of why the change is in the investigator's interests. Understanding the investigator's motivation

in conducting the study is invaluable if it ever becomes important to modify their behavior.

Style

The style a monitor adopts in dealing with investigators at the outset usually persists throughout the relationship. It is therefore essential that monitors consider the style in advance of their initial meeting in order to establish the type of relationship they feel is correct and appropriate. Although individual styles vary enormously, the professionalism one projects is essential toward getting investigators' respect and their willingness to consider the monitor as a member of the team that will help move the trial from concept to completed report.

Monitors must be *polite*, *fair*, and *firm*. Use the broken record technique when appropriate: "Yes, I understand what you are saying, but I still want to see the X records." Attempt to settle all important issues during the site visit.

Respect

Without the investigator's respect for the monitor and a sense of teamwork it is possible that the investigator will treat the clinical trial with less respect. This may lead to critical concern by the sponsor for the clinical trial's success. For example, the liberties that investigators take with patient inclusion criteria may vary from none to 100%. Although adherence to these requirements and the overall trial quality depends on many factors unrelated to the monitor, there are many cases in which the investigator's feelings about a monitor have influenced behavior. For example, when the investigator considers entering a patient who clearly does not meet entry criteria into the clinical trial the investigator will usually consider the monitor's reactions. If the investigator believes that the monitor will not fuss, or may fuss a bit, but not do anything about it, or will exclude patients, but pay for them as if they were completed, the investigator is likely to enroll the patient in the trial. If the investigator believes, however, that the monitor will not only disallow the patient, but not pay the investigator at all for the patient, or only pay a minimal amount, then the investigator will tend not to enroll a patient that will probably cause unnecessary trouble and waste the investigator's time.

The opposite problems may also arise when an investigator has a great deal of respect for the monitor, but not for the clinical trial. This may result from the poor quality of the protocol or the investigator's lack of interest in the test medicine or treatment. In the former case, the sponsors should do whatever necessary to improve the protocol. In the latter case, the monitor may be able to inspire the investigator to perform well by (1) delegating some of the work, (2) providing special incentives, or (3) adding a test of particular interest to the investigator.

Dominance

Neither monitor nor investigator should be exerting undue pressure on the other. Unfortunately, both sides are sometimes jockeying for position where leverage may be exerted. Winning this tussle depends on the nature of the medicine, device, or treatment under study and the availability of other sites, and not on personalities. On the other hand, no matter how dominating the investigator, if there are many others available who want to conduct the clinical trial, even a weak-willed monitor will have more clout than an investigator.

CHAPTER 63

Auditing a Clinical Trial

THE GOLDEN RULE OF AUDITING

A major principle of any audit is that the auditor is independent of the auditee. Otherwise, a conflict of interest almost certainly will develop if problems are found by the auditor. This principle does not imply that one cannot audit one's own work, the work of one's boss, or the work of someone who at some point in the administrative hierarchy reports to one's boss (or one's boss' boss). It does mean that if the audit is to be credible to an outside group (e.g., the public, a regulatory agency), then a strong degree of independence of the two groups is required. Thus, quality assurance (QA) auditors of a company's manufacturing processors do not report to production personnel, and Good Laboratory Practices (GLP) auditors who audit toxicology data do not report to toxicology personnel.

PURPOSES OF AUDITING A CLINICAL TRIAL

The precise purposes of clinical auditors should be established prior to initiating this function within an organization. Specific purposes of auditing a clinical trial include helping to ensure that:

1. Clinical monitors are doing their job accurately
2. Investigators and staff are doing their job appropriately

3. Future regulatory inspections will be smooth and uneventful
4. The data will be suitable for a regulatory submission
5. The clinical development process is conducted as efficiently as possible

The outcome of an audit should be a clinical judgment that the trial is or is not acceptable. This judgment cannot be made by a junior level monitor, but requires a highly experienced physician or clinical scientist. A sponsor's audit is for internal use and therefore a copy is not usually given to the investigator audited.

Disseminating information about these purposes to relevant groups and individuals will enable the auditors to perform their role with greater cooperation of everyone involved. Cooperation will also be enhanced if the auditors report to a senior member of an organization. Individuals whose work is to be audited should be accurately informed as to the reasons for the audit, what is to be audited, and how they might benefit from the audit. Seeking the cooperation, or at least the understanding, of those being audited is important to achieve a workable, if not positive, relationship.

GOOD CLINICAL PRACTICES GUIDELINES

Good Clinical Practices (GCP) guidelines form a basis for determining what processes and activities should be audited. These guidelines have not officially been issued by the Food and Drug Administration (FDA) in final form, and the term GCP has no official definition in the FDA. The term is used in this book to include regulations covering the following five aspects of clinical research. The first three are covered by approved United States regulations, whereas currently proposed regulations cover the last two.

1. Investigational New Drug Application (IND). This is the regulatory submission necessary to initiate human trials in the United States.
2. Institutional Review Boards (IRBs). These committees are referred to as Ethics Committees in most countries.
3. Informed consents. Various types of informed consents are required around the world.
4. Obligations of sponsors and monitors.
5. Obligations of investigators.

Good Clinical Practices guidelines are being developed by several groups worldwide, and most appear to be generally similar in content and approach to each other. They also cover much of the material contained in the five approved or proposed regulations listed above. A much better, and more accurate, name for these guidelines is good clinical trial practices. It is hoped that more people will begin to use this name.

THE AUDIT TRAIL

The audit trail refers to the ability to track the flow of data retrospectively as it moved from the patient, via equipment or biological samples, to a laboratory, to a written report, to the sponsor, and through the steps of data processing and analysis to a final report. Steps involved in the flow of data include some or all of those shown in Fig. 63.1. Procedures of a group are necessary to put the system into operation, i.e., to turn on the process for moving data through the steps of the system. The audit trail consists of documentation (or the ability to document) what occurred at each step of the process, particularly if the data are transformed, corrected, or modified in any way. Records must be kept on all original and corrected values as well as reasons for the change and dates the changes were made.

The audit trail is important and useful for auditors or other individuals at the sponsor's site or at a regulatory agency who wish to follow the flow of the data. Even if the individual was not associated with the clinical trial he or she should be able to follow a specific datum in either a forward (i.e., starting with a source document with the patient's data) or backward (i.e., starting with a combined statistical–medical report) direction and to identify how it was combined, transformed, or otherwise handled at each stage. An audit

trail is usually followed to ascertain the accuracy of data as they moved from their original form to the final report. It is usually more difficult to accomplish this task if the data were recorded solely in electronic form (e.g., on disks) or in a computer, as opposed to having hard copy available to review all stages of the data's movement.

The audit trail may lead toward and potentially involve the follow-up of patients after the formal part of a clinical trial is completed. This type of patient follow-up may or may not be part of the formal trial protocol, but should be submitted to an Ethics Committee/IRB for approval. If a large number of patients are lost to follow-up during a clinical trial, then the investigator, staff, and sponsor should investigate the reasons for this event.

AUDITING CONDUCTED BY A SPONSOR

A sponsor may conduct one or two basic types of audits of a clinical trial: the activities of the sponsor itself may be audited, and the activities of the investigator or a contracting organization may be audited. A less commonly audited group is the data coordinating center of a large multicenter trial.

Auditing the Sponsor's Activities

No regulatory agency currently requires a sponsor to audit its own clinical trials. Therefore, any decision by a sponsor to initiate audits is to ensure that its monitors (and/or investigators) adhere to desired standards and to confirm that its clinical medicine development program is conducting its work efficiently.

When the sponsor's activities are audited, the audit may be conducted on (1) all (or most) clinical trials on all medicines, (2) all (or most) clinical trials of selected types (e.g., the most well-controlled trials), (3) all (or most) clinical trials on selected medicines, or (4) some clinical trials chosen as a spot-check whenever pertinent questions arise, or (5) some clinical trials chosen on a random basis. The choice of one of these approaches depends primarily on the reason(s) for undertaking a clinical audit. If a clinical department has previously experienced significant problems in the quality of its monitoring activities, or if most monitors are new and inexperienced, then it may be desirable initially to audit all clinical trials. As the monitors' performance improves or as they gain more experience, it may be appropriate to audit only selected types or randomly selected trials to ensure that appropriate standards are being maintained.

The choice of which sites to audit may be based on the importance of the trials (e.g., primary efficacy versus supportive trials), resources available for the audit,

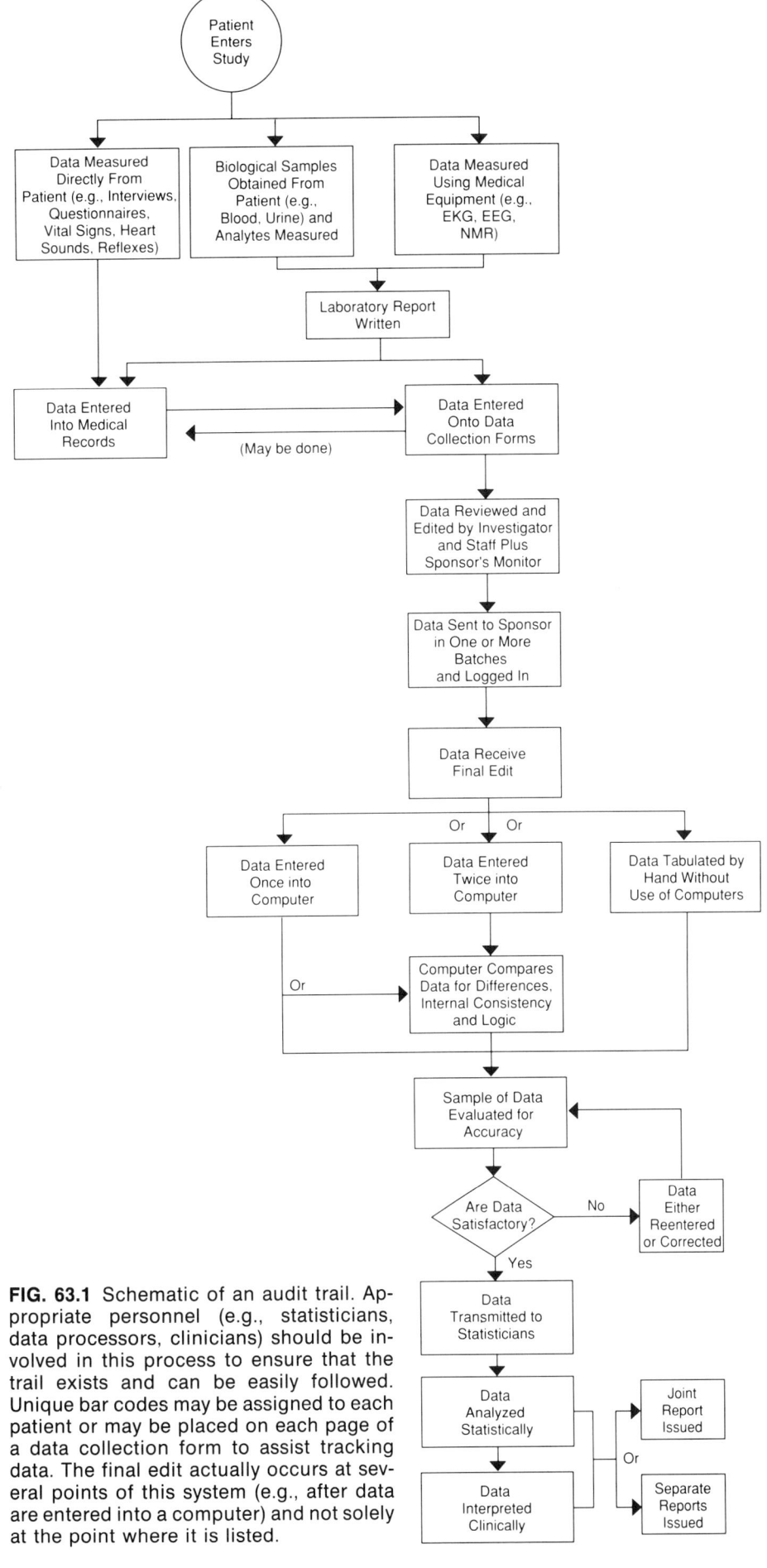

FIG. 63.1 Schematic of an audit trail. Appropriate personnel (e.g., statisticians, data processors, clinicians) should be involved in this process to ensure that the trail exists and can be easily followed. Unique bar codes may be assigned to each patient or may be placed on each page of a data collection form to assist tracking data. The final edit actually occurs at several points of this system (e.g., after data are entered into a computer) and not solely at the point where it is listed.

size of patient recruitment, sites where most problems were expected, or sites where the largest number of problems occurred during the trial.

It generally is more important for a sponsor to conduct some type of clinical audit when the sponsor's monitors are not based at the central headquarters in that country but are geographically dispersed. This is especially true if a large number of individuals (e.g., 50) are serving as clinical trial monitors. This may readily occur if a company utilizes part (or all) of its sales force for monitoring. These people may have had a training course in monitoring at the sponsor's central headquarters, but without frequent interaction with, and supervision by, medical personnel, some may not monitor trials in the manner desired by the sponsor. An audit conducted by the central headquarters is designed to provide both positive feedback to the monitors and assurances to the sponsor.

Auditing the Investigator's Activities

Any investigator who might be audited by a sponsor should be informed prior to initiating the clinical trial. The monitor and eventually the auditor should spend all the time necessary to discuss its importance and value with the investigator. Theoretically, this type of audit should not be necessary if clinical monitors are performing their roles ensuring that trial conduct meets appropriate standards. Nonetheless, sometimes a sponsor may question an investigator's performance and may desire reassurance from an "independent" auditor. For example, a sponsor may have received reports from a monitor that an investigator is not performing as expected. The monitor may not have sufficient authority to cause the investigator to modify his or her behavior. An independent auditor, or the monitor's supervisor acting as an auditor, may assess the situation at the investigator's site and then speak to the investigator in the appropriate manner.

An investigator's performance may also be audited after a clinical trial is completed, for example, when foreign trials are considered for submission to the FDA. To assess the quality of data and the investigator's performance, as well as the quality of the monitoring by a group from the sponsor's offices in the investigator's country, one or more individuals may be assigned to audit the investigator's site.

CONDUCTING AN AUDIT

Preparing an Auditing Protocol

Although it is not necessary to devise a protocol or specific forms to conduct an audit, if the following steps are followed prior to the audit, its credibility will be enhanced. This will minimize bias that could enter the evaluation and help to ensure that multiple audits are conducted in the same manner. The length of an auditing protocol may be only a few pages, depending on the depth of the audit.

At What Stage of a Clinical Trial Should an Audit Be Conducted?

An audit may be conducted by a sponsor, investigator, or Ethics Committee either while a trial is in progress or after it has been completed. The former procedure is particularly relevant if a monitor's performance is being evaluated or if it is believed there is a problem that should be addressed. Any of these individuals or groups may hire an independent contractor to conduct the audit. Audits conducted by regulatory agencies are conducted after a trial is completed.

The audit may take place after a certain *number of patients* are enrolled, after a certain *percent of patients* are enrolled, at a certain *time point* (e.g., 3 months after clinical trial initiation), or on a *random basis* because a problem is suspected. Problems uncovered while a clinical trial is still ongoing usually can be addressed and hopefully corrected, unlike those found after a trial's completion. The data's overall quality may be audited either during or after a trial. This audit could occur after the trial is completed, but prior to editing the data for processing and evaluation. The type of information sought in this kind of audit would relate to (1) acceptability of patients, (2) completeness of data, (3) accuracy of specific data, (4) requirement for significant editing, (5) adherence of the investigator to the protocol, and (6) any other specific requirements of the audit.

Who Conducts a Clinical Audit?

Ethics Committees/IRBs and clinical monitors each conduct quality assurance activities. Theoretically, there should not be any reason why a separate clinical audit is necessary. On the other hand, one or two individuals working for a sponsor could provide a valuable service to monitors or investigators by ensuring that files and records that would be subject to review during a regulatory inspection are accurate and complete.

A more thorough audit of monitors' activities could be conducted, but this raises the probability that the auditor would be viewed as a policeman and not as a helper. The appropriate degree for a company to audit its staff depends on its traditions and culture as well as the nature of any problems that exist.

Clinical auditors should not be the same individuals as those who conduct Good Manufacturing Practices

(GMP) or GLP audits of data, although some companies follow this practice. GMP and GLP auditors are mandated by regulations whereas clinical auditors are not. GMP and GLP auditors are generally perceived as adversaries, whereas clinical auditors are not. Companies that utilize clinical auditors have a wide variety of approaches to consider in establishing their function and reporting relationships, and this is a rapidly changing field. GMP or GLP auditors must not report to the same managers as the people in the groups being audited. This reporting relationship does not necessarily apply for clinical auditors. If a clinical auditing group is established by a company and the company desires the group to achieve the same degree of respect and autonomy as quality assurance and GLP auditors, then the clinical group, too, must report to nonmedical supervisors. On the other hand, the primary purposes of a clinical audit may be to train monitors and enhance the quality of their work, rather than to act as an enforcer of standards. In this situation, it may be acceptable to have the auditors based within the medical function and report to the same people whose workers are being audited.

Some companies believe that a staff ratio of one auditor for ten clinical research associates is appropriate, but most companies do not use so-called golden rules to decide on the appropriate number of staff.

HOW TO AUDIT A CLINICAL TRIAL

First determine if the audit is to focus on the policies, systems, and procedures used in the clinical trial or whether it will focus on validating the data obtained. In either case, the audit may be a global one or it may concentrate on one or more particular aspects of the trial.

Systems Evaluation

The goals of a systems evaluation are usually to assess how well one's systems are working, to identify those areas that require further effort, and to determine what changes may enhance the organization's procedures. The auditor should identify each of the systems and procedures to be audited and determine how clearly the policies and procedures that are to be audited were defined in advance of the clinical trial. Policies and procedures that are often audited include (1) frequency of monitoring visits, (2) documentation of monitoring visits, (3) conduct of pretrial roundtable meetings, (4) preparation and review of the protocol, (5) process for reporting adverse reactions to the sponsor, (6) process for reporting adverse reactions to regulatory authorities, (7) validation of computers used in the clinical trial, and (8) documents sent to the investigators.

Data Verification and Validation

Data validation is meant to provide the sponsor and regulatory authorities with greater assurance that the results are accurate and trustworthy. The major questions addressed in this type of audit are (1) what was done, (2) when was it done, (3) who did it, and (4) how was it documented? An auditor may go further, in selected instances, and ask (1) why was it done, and (2) what was the result or outcome?

Examples of quality assurance in clinical trials can involve literally hundreds of separate checks. General examples are listed in Table 63.1 and a few specific examples are listed in Tables 63.2 and 63.3. A few examples include (1) comparing unexpected laboratory results observed in data collection forms with actual laboratory slips, (2) comparing numbers in tables of reports with summary statements elsewhere in reports, and (3) determining whether patients were treated according to the protocol. Quality assurance evaluations are also made of data entered into computers to evaluate the accuracy of several steps in data processing (see Fig. 63.1).

If an auditor is not intending to conduct a global audit of a clinical trial, then he or she may focus on one or more specific areas. Selected areas that may be assessed include:

1. *Patient selection.* Evaluate demographics and medical histories of those enrolled. How do they compare with the natural history of the disease? How were patients recruited? Did this change during the trial?
2. *Patient enrollment.* Evaluate the screening process and the informed consent process. How many patients failed to progress through each step of the entry process?
3. *Patient response to treatment.* Evaluate how well patients kept appointments and the degree of patient compliance with their therapy. Were there problems that led to dropouts? Were laboratory

TABLE 63.1 *Selected examples of general areas to verify during a clinical audit*

1. All reported patients actually exist and were enrolled in the trial[a]
2. An appropriate number of monitoring visits were made and the monitoring reports were completed (if appropriate)
3. The number of patients who entered and the number that completed the trial
4. Data received at the sponsor's site agree with those at the investigator's site
5. Corrections in the data collection forms noted by the monitor were actually made
6. Grossly abnormal values are the same on original (i.e., source) documents
7. Data are transcribed accurately

[a] This may be confirmed by obtaining evidence that the patient's medical record is present and matches the data collection form.

TABLE 63.2 *Selected reports and items that may be audited in a clinical trial*

Reports generated periodically	Items to describe in each report
Patients discontinued[a]	Keypunch errors
Patient dropouts[a]	Missing forms
Patients lost to follow-up[a]	Missing data
Deaths[a]	Data inconsistencies
Adverse reactions[a]	Conflicting data
Summary list of records read by a reading center	Discrepancies between data bases
(e.g., electrocardiograms)	Duplication of forms
Plasma samples collected	Discrepancies between data bases and data collection forms
Patients receiving medicine and their dosages	

[a] The reasons for these events should be included as part of a report, insofar as the information is available.

results and adverse reactions reported of the type and frequency expected?

Any suspicions of serious misconduct or fraud must be handled with extreme caution. The auditor should discuss his or her feelings with the clinical trial monitor and relevant attorneys.

Specific Procedures Used to Audit a Clinical Trial

The procedures of a clinical trial audit are divided into four categories, which are described in more detail below:

(1) in-house evaluation of all clinical trial data, information, and documents; (2) onsite audits and interviews; (3) analysis of all information; and (4) reporting of results.

In some countries or clinics it is impossible to audit source documents, but it is permissible for someone to read data aloud from the source document for the auditor to check with the official data collection form. This procedure requires additional time but is acceptable.

TABLE 63.3. *Selected elements to evaluate the investigator's adherence to a clinical trial*

A. Administrative issues of the clinical trial audited
  1. Protocol name and number
  2. Sponsor(s)
  3. Names of investigators and staff
  4. Addresses and telephone numbers
  5. Name of monitor(s)
  6. Facilities used
  7. Name of contact person at the site
  8. Date of audit
B. Conduct of the clinical trial—technical points
  1. Regulatory documents acceptable for investigators
  2. Details of Ethics Committee/IRB approval
  3. Storage of data collection forms
  4. Storage of medicine before, during, and after use by patients
  5. Maintenance of randomization code
  6. Adequacy of equipment
  7. Adequacy of waiting rooms
  8. Adequacy of number of beds, rooms
  9. Adequacy of ancillary personnel
  10. Adequacy of appointment procedures
  11. Appropriateness of methods for obtaining informed consents
  12. Adequacy of the informed consent form
  13. Maintenance of a monitor's log
  14. Adequacy of laboratories (e.g., certification, reference ranges)
  15. Procedures for reporting adverse events
  16. Procedures for accounting for inventory and dispensing of the medicine
  17. Adequacy of randomization code
  18. Procedures for prescribing the medicine
  19. Procedure for the medicine getting from its storage to the patient
C. Conduct of the clinical trial—patients
  1. Adequacy of patients enrolled
  2. Register of patient refusers

  3. Register of patient dropouts and discontinued patients
  4. Number of patients enrolled to date and planned totals
  5. Number of patients enrolled who do not meet inclusion criteria, and a brief description of each such patient
  6. Number of patients lost to follow-up
  7. Number of deaths and severe adverse events, plus a brief description of each
  8. Reports on severe adverse reactions in accordance with regulatory requirements
  9. Quality of the interactions between patients and staff
D. Conduct of the clinical trial—data collection forms
  1. Completeness of the records
  2. Accuracy of the records
  3. Comparison with original medical records
  4. Patient informed consent present
  5. Concurrent illnesses
  6. Concomitant therapy
  7. Dosage adjustments
  8. Adverse event and reaction reports
  9. Names of the people who complete them
  10. Materials used as sources to complete these forms
E. Relationship between investigator and sponsor
  1. Frequency of visits by monitors and adequacy of reports
  2. Identity of names and affiliation of visitors to the clinical trial site
  3. Speed of transmission of data to core facility, laboratory, and sponsor
  4. Speed of correcting errors in data collection forms
  5. Speed and completeness of reporting serious adverse events and reactions to the sponsor
F. Other
  1. Reports of investigator sent to Ethics Committee/IRB
  2. Modifications of clinical trial sent to Ethics Committee/IRB for approval
  3. Systems used in the clinical trial and how well they are described in the final report

In-House Evaluation

This process is usually the most time-consuming of the four, particularly if the audit is conducted after the clinical trial is completed and all data have been received by the sponsor. In a step-wise fashion, the auditor proceeds chronologically through the history of the trial. The following points are usually ascertained.

1. Appropriate procedures were used to review and approve the protocol prior to initiating the trial.
2. Documents were filed with the regulatory authorities as required (e.g., protocol, consent form, amendments, investigator's curriculum vitae).
3. Approval was received from the Ethics Committee/IRB and any other peer committees at the site (if relevant).

The next stage would be to:

1. Evaluate monitoring reports to identify any outstanding problems and to evaluate how closely the clinical trial was monitored
2. Evaluate the protocol to identify the parameters that should be assessed most closely in the data collection forms evaluated at the site
3. Design forms to collect data and a data base to evaluate these parameters
4. Review medicine shipments as well as other shipments (e.g., samples, supplies)
5. Establish the audit trail that should be followed

The last stage would be to:

1. Review data collection forms and collect data desired on the newly designed forms
2. Review the data collected to determine what aspects should be checked more closely
3. Select specific cases to be audited more carefully onsite; choose both typical and atypical patients; select patients from all treatment groups and from all times over which the clinical trial was conducted; choose patients from subsets of particular interest. This approach means that cases to audit closely are not chosen at random.

Onsite Evaluation

This process usually involves one or two auditors visiting a site for 1 to 3 days. The visit should be scheduled through the monitor or clinical research associate, who may be invited to attend the audit. If the monitor does attend it is important that he or she is made to feel comfortable and is not interrogated. The staff should be interviewed to assess who was involved in each aspect of the clinical trial and how they were involved.

The audit should be a positive educational experience for the investigator, staff, and monitor (if present). This goal has a better chance of realization if the auditors make an agenda of their plans, rehearse relevant parts, and review their agenda with all people concerned. This should allay some fears about what the auditors are doing and planning to do.

The actual audit should evaluate the preselected data collection forms and other documents. Data collection forms should be compared to source records whenever possible. This poses problems in several countries, but an attempt should be made to conduct as thorough an audit as possible. The reliability of the source records themselves should be assessed if the data are unusual, highly abnormal, inconsistent, or suspicious.

Analysis of Auditing Data

It is often useful to create a timeline for a clinical trial in which major events are listed with their dates of occurrence. These events include protocol changes, Ethics Committee/IRB decisions, milestones of patient entry (e.g., first patient, 50% completion, last patient terminated), altered dosings, medicine shipments, and data collection form shipments.

The audit should identify questionable documents as well as any trends observed. Various groups should be assessed to determine if there are patterns to any errors or problems uncovered. The reasons for errors or problems should be determined and critiqued. Judgments about a clinical trial's quality must be tempered by consideration of acceptable rates of error in data management, test measurements, and personal behavior.

Report of Audit Results

The initial part of the overall audit report should contain a narrative of how the clinical trial was initiated and conducted. This should be followed by a narrative of how the audit was conducted, and conclusions about how well each aspect of the trial was conducted. Important deviations in documentation, patients' rights, monitoring, and other areas should be noted, as well as any follow-up steps suggested. The final section of the report should contain the detailed analysis and relevant documents (as an appendix). Because the sponsor's auditing report is available to regulatory authorities on request, it should not contain confidential analyses or comments on the sponsor's policies and systems used in the clinical trial. This information may be issued as a separate memorandum within the sponsor's organization.

Various reports on details of a clinical trial may be issued during or after a clinical trial is completed (Table 63.2). These reports may be assessed as part of the overall audit report.

Audit reports should be sent to the clinical expert writing the clinical expertise summary for those regulatory dossiers where it is needed.

PROS AND CONS OF AUDITING

Several medical directors believe that the auditing function tends to (1) keep people honest, (2) ensure that future unpleasant surprises will not occur because of data errors that should have been detected but were not, and (3) train clinical monitors. It is primarily for these reasons that the clinical auditing function has grown so rapidly over the last decade, but there is another perspective on the necessity of auditing.

Auditing is performed by companies that wish to enhance their performance and efficiency; it is not a requirement of regulatory authorities. Some critics of auditing point to the fact that it is often perceived as a policing force within an organization. Unfortunately, this perception can create a counterproductive atmosphere. The need for GCP audits should be periodically assessed. It is quite possible that this function will not be needed after certain standards are established and confirmed.

The goals of auditing can be achieved through a training function in a clinical department. One or more individuals who review data at an investigator's site and act in the role of trainer usually achieve a great deal more than those who serve as a policing force. The former approach will result in monitors and others who are informed of the ingredients that lead to quality clinical trials. High standards of design and conduct of clinical trials are the responsibility of investigators, their staff, and monitors, rather than auditors. Auditors often review trials after they are completed, when it is too late to influence standards or quality.

AUDITING POINTERS AND PITFALLS FOR SPONSORS

A few pointers and pitfalls are as follows:

1. Using regional or field auditors who are not well known to the monitors they audit is generally unwise. This practice often creates communication problems as well as fears in those audited.
2. Failure to obtain original source documents to confirm data put on data collection forms may lead to accepting invalid data as valid. Transcription errors occur commonly. In some countries it is difficult or impossible for auditors or monitors to have access to original patient records. This problem may often be overcome by deleting the patient's name from the photocopied records. Alternatively, the auditor should interview the investigator, study coordinator, other staff members, or a designated impartial physician to ascertain (insofar as possible) the validity of data.
3. The auditor should interview the investigator or patients in sufficient depth to explore the topic or question of interest adequately.
4. The auditor should strive to establish good rapport with all individuals. He or she should provide positive feedback, as well as negative, to help investigators improve the quality of their work and to feel good about their methodological strengths and abilities.
5. Quantify the percent of data collection forms that are useful for efficacy, the number of important items missing from these forms, and the time spent by the sponsor to correct errors in them.
6. Sponsors may have an internal and external auditing group. The internal group would audit good manufacturing and good laboratory practices. External groups would audit patients, investigators, Ethics Committees, and study sites as part of good clinical practices.
7. In the United Kingdom it is possible to see source data if consent is obtained from the patient, investigator, and owner of the medical records (i.e., Department of Health). Other countries may have other regulations. Suitable arrangements should be made in advance of the trial to ensure that source data may be examined.

AUDITING CONDUCTED BY INVESTIGATORS

Investigators sometimes have reasons to perform audits of clinical trials they are conducting or have previously conducted. The purpose of such an audit may be to uncover the reason for a known problem, or it may be to ensure the investigator that a staff member's questionable judgment, suspicious conduct, or misconduct has not had serious consequences. The focus may be on a particular aspect of the study or it may be global. The reason for initiating an audit may not reflect any problem; it could simply result from a desire to know that everything was conducted as intended and that the clinical trial contains no major surprises.

The methods used by an investigator, or person appointed by the investigator, to audit a trial are the same as those described in other sections of this chapter.

AUDITING CONDUCTED BY ETHICS COMMITTEES

Audits by Ethics Committees are rarely conducted today, but they may become more prevalent in the future. Investigators must currently submit all protocols for approval and usually provide annual updates on the trial's progress. It is conceivable that a proactive Ethics Committee/IRB could ask one or more people to conduct an audit of a trial the committee has approved. This could result from serious questions that have arisen about the trial's conduct or from direct accusations about the failure of the investigator to maintain patient's well-being.

The increasing importance of auditing general clinical practice has been recently documented (Shaw and Costain, 1989).

CHAPTER 64

Misconduct or Deception During a Clinical Trial

Research in science and medicine is built on trust. Data in publications are accepted at face value by reviewers and readers, although interpretations are often questioned or even challenged. Sometimes the data themselves are incorrect or false because of avoidable human error or misconduct. Misconduct or deception may result from inadvertent behavior or ignorance on the part of those involved in a clinical trial, or it may involve individuals who are purposely using unacceptable standards of behavior. There is an entire spectrum of misconduct that may occur during clinical trials ranging from poor scientific judgment all the way to fraud and other criminal offenses.

DEFINITIONS

Deception. Deception is defined as either providing incorrect information (i.e., lying) or failing to provide relevant information for the purpose of misleading another person or group. Both concealing information and providing misinformation are deception. Deception may be practiced by patients, investigators and their staff, sponsors, and anyone else connected with a clinical trial. Deception may occur at any time before, during, or after the trial.

Misconduct. Misconduct relates to behavior that is inappropriate; the more serious examples represent unethical behavior. Misconduct may be either purposeful or inadvertent, and may be practiced by anyone connected with a trial. When misconduct is purposeful and illegal it becomes a criminal offense.

Fraud. Fraud varies along a wide spectrum from purposely altering a single datum to fabricating entire clinical trials. It has been generally well described and discussed in the medical literature for the several cases exposed. Stricter guidelines of accountability for all coauthors and supervisors of clinical research have been widely disseminated and accepted as an important method of addressing this problem. Fraud, per se, is not discussed in this chapter, nor is the topic at the other end of the spectrum—poor scientific judgment. Deception and misconduct lie between these extremes and are the subjects of this chapter.

DECEPTION OF PATIENTS

It is the author's opinion that deceiving patients about a clinical trial is unethical. This view is not universally shared by physicians and in fact it may even be in the minority. Various types of deception are used with patients in clinical trials and many current publications report (without any apparent embarrassment) how patients were deceived. Most examples of deception occur in studies conducted in the social sciences, particularly in the field of clinical psychology. The use of deception is virtually taken for granted and is routinely justified as a necessity.

Deception in Medical Practice

Deception of patients about their treatment in everyday medical practice is widespread but difficult to quantify. For example, physicians often inform their patients that they will receive a mild medicine without side effects, when the physician knows that the medicine will cause adverse reactions. Other examples include patients who are given placebos and told that they are receiving an active medicine, while others are not told the truth about their diagnosis. Deceiving patients regarding their medical diagnosis, as well as treatment, is a common practice in Japan (Swinbanks, 1989).

Deception in Clinical Trials

A variety of deceptions are practiced in clinical trials and many are actually written into protocols. Examples of some types of deception practiced include:

1. *Giving patients wrong information.* Ross and Pihl (1989) told some patients that they received a negligible amount of alcohol, but in fact gave them enough to raise their blood alcohol level over the legal limit for driving. These patients were told that the test "alcohol tastes pretty strong because it's so highly distilled." Other subjects were told that they received a high dose, but were in fact given a low dose. They were told "the stuff's nearly tasteless, because the taste has been refined out of it." These patients were also "encouraged to sniff from the labeled jug to familiarize them with the smell."
2. *Giving patients placebo without their knowledge.* Landauer and Pocock (1984) gave one group of patients placebo, but these patients were led to believe that they received oxprenolol to reduce stress. In another clinical trial 80 patients were given placebo liquid that was described to 40 patients as an "energizer" and to the other 40 as a "tranquilizer" (Dinnerstein and Halm, 1970).
3. *Giving patients an active medicine, but informing them and others that they received a placebo.* Breuning et al. (1980) reported that mentally retarded patients were given an active medicine, but the institution and staff were told that the medication was a placebo.

Numerous Ethics Committees/Institutional Review Boards (IRBs) are willing to approve deception in clinical trials. Proponents of deception in clinical trials claim that the knowledge gained cannot be obtained without the use of deception. The absence of such deception would clearly make certain clinical trials ineffective. An important question to consider in this context is how much of a loss would the failure of conducting that particular trial be for society.

Minor forms of deception that are generally acceptable in a clinical trial include the following procedures conducted without the patient's knowledge: (1) washout of previous therapy, (2) placebo run-in period, and (3) dose taper of a medicine.

Drawing the Line Between Acceptable and Unacceptable Deception

It is worrisome when Ethics Committees/IRBs believe that a "certain amount" of deception is acceptable or may be tolerated in clinical trials. Where (and how) do they draw the line between acceptable and unacceptable deception? What about next year? Would the Ethics Committee/IRB accept a slightly greater degree of deception to conduct clinical trials that would otherwise be impossible? Once a new level of deception is widely accepted, the cycle can (and most likely will) begin again encouraging an even greater degree of deception. What about a protocol that contains just slightly more deception than previously allowed, which is submitted by the chairman of a department who is a personal friend or even a superior to at least one person on the Ethics Committee/IRB?

It seems that a clear line may be drawn only by allowing deception where proper safeguards are imposed and society would unequivocally be better off if it had the data from the clinical trial. If almost all trials practicing deception were never conducted, the field of medicine and society in general would be no worse off. Important clinical trials in which some degree of deception is necessary are rare exceptions; most of these are obvious, and rights of patients may be protected to a large degree.

UNDER WHAT CONDITIONS MAY DECEPTION BE TOLERATED?

Deception may be more acceptable to an Ethics Committee/IRB if:

1. The research objective is extremely important and there is no way to address the research objective appropriately without the use of deception.
2. All research subjects will be informed at the end of the clinical trial about the deception used.

3. Subjects on being told about the deception are expected to find the methods used reasonable and are not expected to be greatly upset.
4. Subjects may withdraw from the clinical trial at any time, and this is stated clearly in the informed consent. Although this principle is inviolate for clinical trials conducted in several countries, it is not widely practiced for psychological or social science research.
5. Investigators accept full responsibility for evaluating whether the deception used caused stress or otherwise upset the subjects. If such is the case, the investigator agrees to provide whatever treatment is required.

HOW WIDESPREAD IS DECEPTION IN HUMAN RESEARCH?

Deception is widely practiced in studies conducted by social and behavioral scientists; article surveys reported by Levine (1986) showed that 81% of conformity studies and 72% of cognitive dissonance and balance studies involved deception. Adair et al. (1985) reported that the percentage of studies using deception reported in the *Journal of Personality and Social Psychology* has increased for three decades, despite the promulgation of recent professional codes and regulations that attempt to decrease, or at least control, the use of deception.

DECEPTION USING PLACEBOS

Clinical Trials

Placebos are a form of deception if patients are not informed that they are receiving or have the possibility of receiving placebo in a clinical trial. In almost all clinical trials, however, the possibility of receiving a placebo is usually stated in the informed consent and is generally discussed with patients prior to their agreement to enter the trial. Therefore, the use of a placebo per se does not involve any deception of a patient. This is a separate issue from whether the use of a placebo in a clinical trial is ethical. That ethical question depends on the availability of suitable alternative treatment, the severity of the patient's disease, and other factors.

Medical Practice

In medical practice, most placebos used are given without the patients' knowledge, which is a clear example of deception. Some physicians in private practice maximize the deception of using a placebo by describing it as a medicine and emphasizing that the medicine (placebo) has therapeutic value for the particular patient and their problem. The physician's view is that by increasing the deception he or she is increasing the likelihood that the placebo will be effective. Other physicians in their private practice, however, discuss placebo use with patients in a positive and open manner. The physician describes the possibility of therapeutic gain, even though the patient is informed that the medication is literally a placebo. It is remarkable, but even when patients are informed that they will receive a placebo, it often still elicits a positive response. This benefit is usually attributed to the healing powers of the professional (essentially the "laying on of hands").

DOES THE MEASUREMENT OF COMPLIANCE INCLUDE DECEPTION?

Not all aspects of a clinical trial that are conducted without the patient's knowledge are considered deception. For example, to monitor patient compliance in taking their medicines, (1) pills are often counted outside the patient's sight, (2) a bottle cap's electronic circuitry is read privately to determine how often and at what times the bottle was opened, or (3) blood levels of a medicine are measured. In each of these (or other) methods of measuring compliance the patient's behavior is being monitored without their knowledge, but no misinformation was presented to any patient about these procedures, and no harm should result to patients. Nonetheless, information was withheld and it is possible that some patients would believe they were deceived. To prevent this, patients are sometimes informed that their cooperation will be assessed during the trial, but that they will be unaware of when this will take place, and that the assessment poses no risk or inconvenience. The methods to be used usually are not divulged prior to or during a trial. After the entire trial is completed, the methods used to assess compliance may be shared with patients, if both they and the investigator desire.

If attempts to enhance patient compliance are to be made *during* a clinical trial, then information on this topic should be provided to prospective enrollees prior to initiating the trial. This information may be stated in the context that monitoring of compliance will be conducted and patients will be (or will not be) informed about their results during the trial. Patients may be told that incompletely complying patients will be offered opportunities and methods to help them improve their compliance. The fact that poor compliers will not be considered "bad patients" by the professional staff should be communicated, to all patients. Furthermore, it should be emphasized that the quality of their medical care will not be affected by their compliance.

DECEPTION BY DIFFERENT GROUPS ASSOCIATED WITH A CLINICAL TRIAL

Deception by Patients. Patients who do not fully participate in a study and pretend that they are co-operating are being deceptive. This deception may take numerous forms, such as lying about their medical history, not exerting a full effort when asked to do so (e.g., in procedures to obtain various respiratory measures, such as forced expiratory volume in 1 second), not complying with the medication regimen (e.g., taking too few doses, taking doses at wrong times, taking wrong amounts at each time), or not complying with other protocol requirements (e.g., diet, exercise, completing their diary). While there are legitimate reasons why patients may not fully comply with any of the above, the patient should identify that fact. The reasons for patient behavior should be assessed so that their behavior can be modified.

Deception by Investigators. Investigators who conduct sponsored clinical trials may wittingly or unwittingly participate in many types of deception. A few of these are described in Table 64.1. Others are included in the list in Chapter 62 of "Games Investigators Play," although those games include many ploys and other behaviors that are not examples of deception. The critical assessment of clinical trials to determine the degree, if any, of misconduct is described in Chapter 63 ("Auditing a Clinical Trial"). Changing data in any way (e.g., discarding data, adding data that were not obtained) that is not described in full is an example of fraud and is not discussed in this chapter.

Deception by Sponsors. Sponsors may indulge in the same basic types of deception as investigators (Table 64.1). Differences usually are in the area of clinical trial conduct, since, with rare exceptions, sponsors do not conduct their own Phases II and III clinical trials. Additional types of deception by sponsors are included in Chapter 63 ("Auditing a Clinical Trial"),

and in Table 55.2 on games sponsors may play with investigators.

MEASURING SCIENTIFIC MISCONDUCT

Internal Audits

The major method for detecting scientific misconduct is to conduct an audit of a clinical trial, including all of its documentation. All organizations associated with clinical trials should have standard procedures in place to conduct audits of their own operations, whether the organization is a pharmaceutical company, academic institution, hospital, government facility, contractor, or some other group. It is conceivable that Ethics Committees/IRBs will conduct this function in the future for those clinical trials that they have approved. In some cases the investigators of a clinical trial have agreed to ethical guidelines prior to conducting the trial (Healy et al., 1989).

External Audits

This category primarily includes audits conducted by regulatory agency personnel. Another type of external audit would include those conducted by independent contract organizations hired by a sponsor or investigator. If the term external is narrowly defined as external to the group conducting the clinical trial (as opposed to external to all groups associated with the trial), then several of the groups listed under internal audits (e.g., Ethics Committee, sponsoring company) would be placed in the external category. The topic of external audits is discussed in more detail in Chapter 63. Rennie (1989) has suggested that authors certify to the journal editors that all primary data will be furnished upon request. This requirement could delay publication of some sponsored trials in which some of the data would be considered proprietary.

IMPACT OF DECEPTION, MISCONDUCT, AND FRAUD

Scientific errors (e.g., using incorrect hypotheses) or errors in logic have sometimes led to major advances in science and medicine. This happy result will always be a possible (though rare) outcome of poorly designed or even poorly conducted trials. The impact of adequately conducting poorly designed clinical trials or poorly conducting well-designed clinical trials varies along a negative spectrum, from mildly misleading people who read reports, to incorrectly influencing major health policy decisions. Results also may theoretically vary along a similar positive spectrum.

TABLE 64.1 *Selected types of deception conducted by investigators or sponsors*[a]

1. Choosing those parameters that are believed in advance to demonstrate a desired outcome, even though they are not the most relevant or scientifically appropriate parameters to measure
2. Deliberately including any bias in the clinical trial's design, protocol, conduct, analysis, or interpretation
3. Deliberately not eliminating known confounding factors that could readily be eliminated from any aspect of the clinical trial
4. Allowing carelessness to occur in the conduct of the clinical trial or its analysis
5. Incompletely reporting a trial's clinical data in a report or publication, e.g., omitting data that are or might be interpreted as contrary to the results or interpretation presented

[a] If these practices occur inadvertently, then they are examples of poor scientific judgment or incompetence and not deception.

A pharmaceutical company that is misled by false-positive results obtained as a result of misconduct in a clinical trial they have sponsored may initiate other trials to explore a medicine's profile of activity further. This approach is obviously a waste of large sums of money and years of ultimately fruitless activities by many individuals to bring a new medicine to the market. Unless the misconduct is identified, the truthful result that is eventually found will often not even be interpreted as an indication of misconduct per se, but as a combination of various hypotheses, conjectures, and data that led to a positive outcome. If gross misconduct or, more specifically, fraud is identified, the company has several options. In none of these cases will the data be of any real value to the company and can only cause problems.

MINIMIZING DECEPTION AND MISCONDUCT

One of the major causes of deception and misconduct, as well as fraud, in clinical trials is the pressure on investigators to publish papers. Data dredging, deception, and misconduct in the hopes of finding positive results that are worthy of publication are practices encouraged by this pressure. Pressure to publish also leads to the "sliced meat phenomenon"—dividing one trial's results into separate parts that are published separately. Another deceptive practice is to publish the same data multiple times.

One way to address this problem is for institutions to lower the number of publications considered or required for tenure. For example, assistant professors could be evaluated on their five best papers. Another approach is for journal to publish more negative clinical trials, and to consider asking for more information on questionable points in manuscripts submitted.

Guidelines for research promulgated by universities, hospitals, journals, professional societies, and other groups have made ethical standards clearer to all scientists and clinicians. These standards, plus the authors' increased awareness and responsibility for the entire contents of their papers, should help to decrease the incentives for purposeful misconduct in clinical trials. An example is given in the following section, quoted from the *Guidelines for Research at the University of North Carolina at Chapel Hill* with permission of the Dean of the Medical School (Dr. Stuart Bondurant).

Research Guidelines

There has been a good deal of concern in the U.S. Congress, among the Granting Agencies and among the general public about "fraud in research." The University of North Carolina at Chapel Hill has in place pertinent rules: "Policy and Procedures on Ethics in Research" as required by the granting agencies. All persons engaged in research should be familiar with these rules (copies available from the Office of Research Services, 919-966-5625).

Clearly it is important for the Institution as well as for the individual faculty member not just to know how to deal with fraud in research when it has occurred but—perhaps *a fortiori*— to prevent such fraud from occurring in the first place. In fact, we should comport ourselves in such a way that even the suspicion of fraud is unlikely to arise and, if it does arise unjustly, we have the records in hand to prove that the allegation was misplaced. Therefore the present guidelines, relating to Data Gathering, Storage and Retention, to Publication Practices and Authorship and to Supervision of Research Personnel were devised by the Faculty Committee on Research. Many are based on similar guidelines already extant at other institutions or in our School of Medicine. Although they do not have the force of law or regulation, they are strongly commended to your attention as desirable and prudent practices.

The most important ingredients in avoiding fraud are the integrity and high ethical standards of the research project leader. If one cuts corners and is more concerned with next week's publication or next month's research grant renewal than with a lifelong reputation and the integrity of the research, these guidelines are not likely to be of much help. They have been designed to assist those who are determined to maintain high standards in their research careers.

In making the following recommendations, the Faculty Committee on Research recognizes that there are wide variations from one field to another. Nevertheless we strongly urge adherence to these guidelines, if necessary with appropriate modifications to accommodate solidly established practices within a field.

General University Policies. Anyone engaged in research must abide by University, Divisional and Departmental policies and procedures concerning research.

Data Gathering, Storage, Retention. A common denominator in most cases of alleged scientific misconduct has been the absence of a complete set of verifiable data. The retention of accurately recorded and retrievable results is of utmost importance for the progress of scientific inquiry. A scientist must have access to his/her original results in order to respond to questions including, but not limited to, those that may arise without any implication of impropriety. Moreover, errors may be mistaken for misconduct when the primary experimental results are unavailable.

Recommendations:

1. Original research results should be promptly recorded, and should be kept in as organized and accessible a fashion as possible.
2. The research project leader should retain the raw research data pertinent to publication for a reasonable period of time (normally five years) after publication. In no instance should primary data be destroyed while questions may be raised which are answerable only by reference to such data.
3. Documentation of required approvals of Human Rights and Animal Use Committees should be retained in the research project leader's files for a period of five years.

Publication Practices: Authorship. A gradual diffusion of responsibility for multi-authored or collaborative studies has led in recent years to the publication of papers for which no single author was prepared to take full responsibility. Two critical safeguards in the publication of accurate scientific reports are the active participation of each coauthor in verifying that part of a manuscript that falls within his/her specialty area and the designation of one author who is responsible for the validity of the entire manuscript.

Recommendations:

1. An author submitting a paper should never include the name of a coauthor without that person's consent. Each coauthor should be furnished with a copy of the manuscript before it is submitted. Coauthorship should be offered to (and limited to) anyone who has clearly made a significant contribution to the work.
2. Anyone accepting coauthorship of a paper should realize that this action implies a responsibility as well as a privilege. If a potential coauthor has serious reservations concerning a publication the individual should decline coauthorship.
3. The senior author or authors of a paper, individually or in concert, should be prepared to identify the contributions of each coauthor.
4. Simultaneous submission of essentially identical manuscripts to different journals is improper.
5. As a general principle, research should be published in the scientific literature before reports of such research are released to the public press.

Supervision of Research Personnel. Careful supervision of all research personnel by their research project leaders is in the best interest of the trainee, the institution, and the scientific community. The complexity of scientific methods, the necessity for caution in interpreting possibly ambiguous data, and the need for advanced statistical analysis, all require an active role for the research project leader in the guidance of research personnel.

Recommendations:

1. All research personnel, such as technicians, graduate students, postdoctoral trainees, should be specifically supervised by a designated research project leader.
2. The ratio of research personnel to project leaders should be small enough that close interaction is possible for scientific interchange as well as oversight of the research at all stages.
3. The project leader should supervise the design of experiments and the process of acquiring, recording, examining, interpreting and storing data. (A project leader who limits his/her role to the editing of manuscripts does not provide adequate supervision.)
4. Collegial discussions among project leaders and research personnel constituting a research unit should be held regularly, both to contribute to the scientific efforts of the members of the group and to provide informal peer review of research results.
5. The project leader or supervisor should provide each investigator (whether student, postdoctoral fellow or other research personnel) with applicable governmental and institutional requirements for conduct of studies involving healthy volunteers or patients, animals, radioactive or other hazardous substances, and recombinant DNA.

CHAPTER 65

Clinical Trial Termination or Extension

PROCEDURES FOR TERMINATING A CLINICAL TRIAL

The process of terminating a single clinical trial may take less than a day or more than a year, depending on the complexity and nature of the trial as well as the efficiency with which it is dismantled. The major aspects to consider are indicated in Fig. 65.1. This figure is intended as a guide, for both sponsored and unsponsored trials, to many of the steps in complying with government regulations, Ethics Committee/Institutional Review Board (IRB) agreements, requirements of the sponsor, and good clinical practice (see Food and Drug Administration, 1977b, 1978, 1981b for details). Prior to following the steps in Fig. 65.1, the investigator must prepare the patients for the trial's discontinuation, inform them in some manner about the results, arrange for continuation of their medical care, and collect the final data to be incorporated into the data collection forms. The order and emphasis placed on each step will differ to some degree between clinical trials that are terminated normally and those that are prematurely discontinued. The investigator must also plan for the storage of trial documents and forms according to regulatory guidelines and regulations. These documents may have great value at a later date if questions arise on a patient's toxicity or on details of the trial; they may also serve as an aid in the development of a new trial. Another step is to ensure that the investigator's files are complete and can withstand a careful regulatory audit.

In double-blind trials, a decision must be made as to when the investigator will be provided with the randomization code. In general, this should occur only after the trial is completed and all data collection forms have been signed by the investigator and received by the sponsor. It should also occur after any end-of-trial questionnaire or interview has been completed. Fig. 65.2 is a form to track used and unused medicines.

EARLY TRIAL DISCONTINUATION (PREMATURE TERMINATION)

In a number of situations (because of ethics, accepted clinical practice, and statistics) discontinuation of all ongoing medicine trials must be considered. It may be appropriate to consider and indicate some of the major reasons in the text of a protocol. A trial may be stopped early for either positive or negative reasons. These topics are also discussed in Chapter 17. Termination of an entire project that involves multiple clinical trials is discussed in Chapter 131.

Termination for Negative Reasons

Negative reasons for discontinuing a clinical trial are listed in Table 65.1.

CLINICAL TRIAL TERMINATION

Study Medicine: Investigator:
Protocol Number: Site:

Date and Check when completed.   Comments

Data Collection Forms

_____ Returned to sponsor _____

_____ Copy retained at site _____

_____ Where store data _____

Biological Samples

_____ All samples sent (brought) to sponsor (or other facility) _____

Patients

_____ Obtain current address, telephone number, and name and address of nearest relative _____
_____

_____ End of trial questionnaire/interview _____

Pharmacy (or person who dispenses medicines)

_____ Records reviewed & copies sent to sponsor _____

_____ Forms completed, signed and returned to sponsor _____

_____ Unused medicine returned to sponsor _____

_____ Medicine samples retained in case questions arise _____

Principal Investigator

_____ Signed or initialed all Data Collection Forms _____

_____ Final Study Report received by sponsor _____

_____ Medicine forms signed _____

_____ End of trial questionnaire _____

_____ Final statement sent to Ethics Committee/IRB _____

Financial

_____ Determine number of completed and "partial" patients _____

_____ Final budget request received from investigator _____

_____ Memorandum to request funds[2] _____

_____ Money sent to investigator _____

Data

_____ Editing and processing of data _____

_____ Analyses of data[1] _____

_____ Publishing of data discussed _____

_____ Article(s) and/or abstract(s) prepared _____

_____ Article(s) and/or abstract(s) reviewed _____

Administration

_____ Discharge Data Review Committee _____

_____ Discharge all other committees _____

_____ Letters sent to referral physicians with trial results _____

FIG. 65.1 List of procedures to consider during the termination period of a clinical trial. Tracking finances, biological samples, and publications are usually conducted separately with more detailed forms.

TABLE 65.1. *Selected negative reasons for discontinuing a clinical trial*

1. Serious adverse reactions, including abnormalities in laboratory analytes or vital signs
2. Inability to recruit and enroll an adequate number of patients
3. Financial problems
4. The protocol is found to be impractical or unworkable
5. Investigator loses interest
6. A transportation (or other) strike prevents patients from attending the clinic
7. Problems arise in the medicine's stability or manufacture
8. New toxicological findings affect the benefit-to-risk ratio
9. Failure of the investigator and/or staff to maintain adequate clinical standards
10. Failure of the investigator, staff, or patients to comply with the protocol
11. Termination of the test medicine's development by the sponsor
12. Unacceptable changes in personnel or facilities at the investigator's site
13. Determination that no statistically significant result can be obtained

Termination for Positive Reasons

There are a number of positive reasons for discontinuing a clinical trial early. The major reason is the observation of a beneficial effect of treatment that raises unacceptable ethical concerns for patients who are not receiving this treatment. If early termination for ethical reasons is considered possible at the outset of a clinical trial, then criteria should be established to define conditions under which the trial would be discontinued. It may also be relevant to save valuable resources by terminating the trial early. If the trial is to be terminated early according to the criteria established, one must consider whether the data will be adequate to convince virtually all or at least the overwhelming majority of statisticians and clinicians of the conclusions. Criteria should be developed that will be impeccable from both a statistical and clinical viewpoint. If either is not fully achieved, then the value of the trial may be mitigated, and its potential to influence the treatment of future patients lost or at least compromised. In addition, discontinuing a trial for ethical reasons generally makes it difficult or impossible to conduct a similar trial in the future. If one is to err in choosing whether or not to stop a trial, then a decision to complete the trial is preferable. Another way of expressing this concept is that if there is doubt about terminating the trial, it should continue. Examples of trials that were discontinued early for appropriate and proper reasons are the collaborative β-blocker heart attack trial (β-Blocker Heart Attack Study Group, 1981) and the zidovudine (AZT) trial (Fischl et al., 1987).

When an investigator terminates a clinical trial, careful consideration must be given as to how to best phase patients back to their pretrial care and treatment. In many situations this will be a simple issue to address,

but when patients have benefited greatly from being in a trial, the transition from frequent contact with the investigator and staff, plus benefits of treatment, may present a challenge.

Early Termination Because a Positive Result Is Unlikely

Ware et al. (1985) observed that clinical trial protocols usually do not consider the possibility of premature termination arising from the situation that a positive result is found to be unlikely to occur. They proposed a new measure to deal with this problem, the "futility index." Such a measure would ensure that more trials would be ended early if appropriate.

Who Decides to Terminate a Clinical Trial Prematurely?

The decision to stop a clinical trial should not be made solely by those involved in its conduct. Impartial experts, such as a panel of outside consultants, may also be involved in the decision (see Chapter 17). When early termination is considered, there is a basic difference between those trials that are evaluating problems with severe clinical consequences (seeking to reduce mortality of a life-threatening disease) and those that seek to reduce relatively minor clinical problems (e.g., topical itching). Presumably, everyone would agree that the former type should explore early termination thoroughly prior to trial initiation, whereas the latter type can deemphasize the question (unless unusual medicine toxicity has been previously observed or is anticipated). The question of how much attention to give to early clinical trial discontinuation arises in the gray area between these two extremes.

Physicians involved in either a sponsored or unsponsored double-blind controlled trial do not generally participate in discussions on its early discontinuation. They must remain blind to patient randomization and should not be made aware of results of interim analyses. If they know that one treatment is markedly and significantly better than another, it may be ethically difficult for them to continue treating seriously ill patients with a less effective medicine (or placebo).

In conclusion, every clinical trial may be stopped early for negative reasons, but only some trials are liable to be stopped early for positive reasons. The latter should be identified in advance, and criteria established under which the trial will be terminated. Special considerations relating to the procedures for terminating a study are discussed in Chapter 65 and in a publication by Klimt and Canner (1979).

Special Considerations

For clinical trials that are discontinued prior to their scheduled ending point, there may be special considerations to evaluate. Should all patients be discontinued or only certain groups, and how should discontinued patients be treated? For trials in which only some patients are discontinued, all patients must be informed of the negative (or positive) data, and a new informed consent obtained. It may be useful to collect additional data not requested in the original protocol at the time of discontinuation. The decision on which specific data to collect will depend on the reasons for discontinuation and the circumstances related to the conduct of the trial (e.g., resources, time availability). The means by which patients will be discontinued must be established. If the scope of the trial or the implications of the reasons for discontinuing warrant public notification, then an announcement to the press must be considered.

Terminating One or More Sites of a Multicenter Trial

Terminating a single site of a multicenter trial is essentially identical to terminating a single-site trial. One of the few differences is that unused medicine and supplies may be sent (if appropriate) to those sites that are still enrolling or treating patients. Experiences of one group closing down a large clinical trial (Coronary Drug Project) are described by Krol (1983).

When Is a Clinical Trial Completed?

The answer to this question is obvious—or is it? A clinical trial may be said to be completed (1) when the final patient has completed his or her final evaluation, (2) when all analyses are completed, (3) when the final medical report is written, (4) when the publication comes out, or (5) when funding ceases. In this book, termination is considered to have occurred when the final patient has completed his or her final evaluation.

VALIDATING THE DEGREE TO WHICH THE TRIAL BLIND WAS MAINTAINED

It is often useful to incorporate an end-of-trial questionnaire into the clinical trial. This questionnaire may explore the adherence to and quality of the blind by asking patients to guess which treatment they believed they were receiving, how sure they were of their choice, and the reasons why they made that choice. Table 65.2 lists factors to consider in designing a posttrial questionnaire.

The degree to which the double blind was truly ef-

TABLE 65.2. *Factors to consider in designing a posttrial questionnaire*

1. Determine whether all patients or only a sample will be given the questionnaire
2. If a sample is chosen for this test, determine how they will be chosen
3. Determine if a telephone interview, direct interview, written questionnaire, or combination of approaches will be used
4. Appoint or choose the individual(s) who will conduct this phase of the clinical trial
5. Determine if a pilot project will be conducted with the questionnaire
6. Decide whether the data from the questionnaire will be analyzed to evaluate the trial blind
7. Design a standard series of questions to evaluate the trial blind, for example:
   a. Patients' guess as to their treatment
   b. Patients' "certainty" as to their guess
   c. Did patients' "test" their medication (e.g., taste, smell)?
   d. Other questions (e.g., about compliance)
8. Consider adding additional questions to evaluate different factors in the trial
9. If a similar questionnaire is to be given to each investigator, evaluate his or her guesses as to each patient's treatment and the reasons for these guesses (were the guesses based on adverse reactions, altered blood levels, clinical improvement, clinical deterioration, or other factors?)

fective should be evaluated by also asking the investigator to guess which treatment each patient received. The reasons(s) for the investigator's decision in categorizing each patient should also be recorded (was the decision based on adverse reactions, specific laboratory changes, improvement or deterioration in the underlying disease, or other factors?).

The data from the questionnaire will indicate how well the blind was maintained and whether investigators, patients, or both were able to break it and how (Brownell and Stunkard, 1982; Byington et al., 1985; Moscucci et al., 1987; The Parkinson Study Group, 1989; Swain et al., 1990). It is also important to collect data on how sure each group is of their choices (e.g., almost definite, fairly sure, fifty-fifty, unsure). This information could be used to defend a clinical trial and to quantify the validity of the blind in a publication. Patients' attitudes about the conduct of the trial and data on the trial's blind should be evaluated in more trials. This may allow better trial designs to be developed for use in future clinical trials. Examples of the data obtained with this type of questionnaire are presented in papers by Karlowski et al. (1975), Howard et al. (1982), and Rabkin et al. (1986). It has been clearly shown by Karlowski et al. (1975) that when patients break a clinical trial's blind, it may have a significant impact on the data obtained.

If questions relating to the trial blind are posed at the conclusion of a pilot trial, then the information obtained may permit a better trial design for future trials. For example, if certain clues, such as changes in blood levels of concomitant medicines or abnormal labora-

MEDICINE DISPOSITION FORM

After Completion of Form: Send
Copy 1 to Monitor
Copy 2 for Investigator
Copy 3 with Return Goods

I. Medicine Shipped to Investigator — Use One Sheet Per Dosage Form

Investigator: _____   Order Number _____

Monitor: _____   Formulation Code: _____

Protocol No.: _____   Batch Number: _____

Name of Trial: _____

Medicine Preparation No.: _____

Medicine Name: _____

Dosage Form: _____

Strength or Concentration: _____

No. of Containers: _____

Size of Containers: _____

II. Medicine Received — Initials and Date of Investigator _____

III. Medicine Returned to Sponsor (Use a Courier Service)

No. of Full Containers   _____   Size   _____

(Express Whole Cartons   _____   Size   _____
as Number of Full
Containers)   _____   Size   _____

No. of Partial Containers   _____   Size   _____

_____   Size   _____

_____   Size   _____

All Medicine Used   _____
(i.e., None Returned)

Is This the Final Shipment? Yes _____ No _____ (Explain) _____

Investigator's Signature and Date _____

IV. Medicine Received by Sponsor

Material Received as Described _____ Yes _____ No (Describe below)

Disposition: Destroyed _____   _____ Date

Method of Destruction _____

FIG. 65.2 Medical disposition form to track medicine disposal after a clinical trial is completed.

tory values, help an investigator break the trial blind, then this information may be kept from the investigator in a subsequent trial by utilizing a technique such as the ''two-physician method.''

Assessing Patient's Knowledge About Informed Consent

A different type of posttrial questionnaire was used by Hassar and Weintraub (1976). They evaluated whether patients in their trial understood the risks involved in the trial they had completed. The patients' memory of the informed consent that they had signed on entry into the trial was also tested. The authors found that patients committed three types of errors in memory. First, many patients did not recall one of the major risks inherent in the trial despite the fact that it was verbally reported to each patient on three occasions and each patient had read it twice. Second, patients made errors about the contents of certain discussions held with investigators, and, third, patients constructed entirely fallacious information. The authors suggested more careful means of obtaining an informed consent, which are presented in Chapter 27 of this book.

EXTENDING A CLINICAL TRIAL

Situations may also arise in which the duration of the trial should be extended. Depending on the nature of the trial, this may require an amendment to the protocol. The most common reason a trial is extended is that fewer patients enrolled than were expected. To extend a trial under these conditions, it is usually necessary only to increase the allowable recruitment time and not to modify the protocol: the original goal remains intact, i.e., to achieve the originally targeted sample size.

A second reason for extending a trial is that a larger placebo effect is observed than expected, and the original sample size is found to be too small to achieve the desired power. Increasing the duration of the trial to obtain a greater sample size than originally planned will be necessary to provide adequate power (i.e., the same power as originally intended). A third possibility is that fewer events being measured (to assess outcome) were observed than had been predicted (e.g., fewer deaths occurred in the population). In this situation, it might be necessary to modify the protocol and to follow patients for a longer period of time in order to observe the events that are being monitored

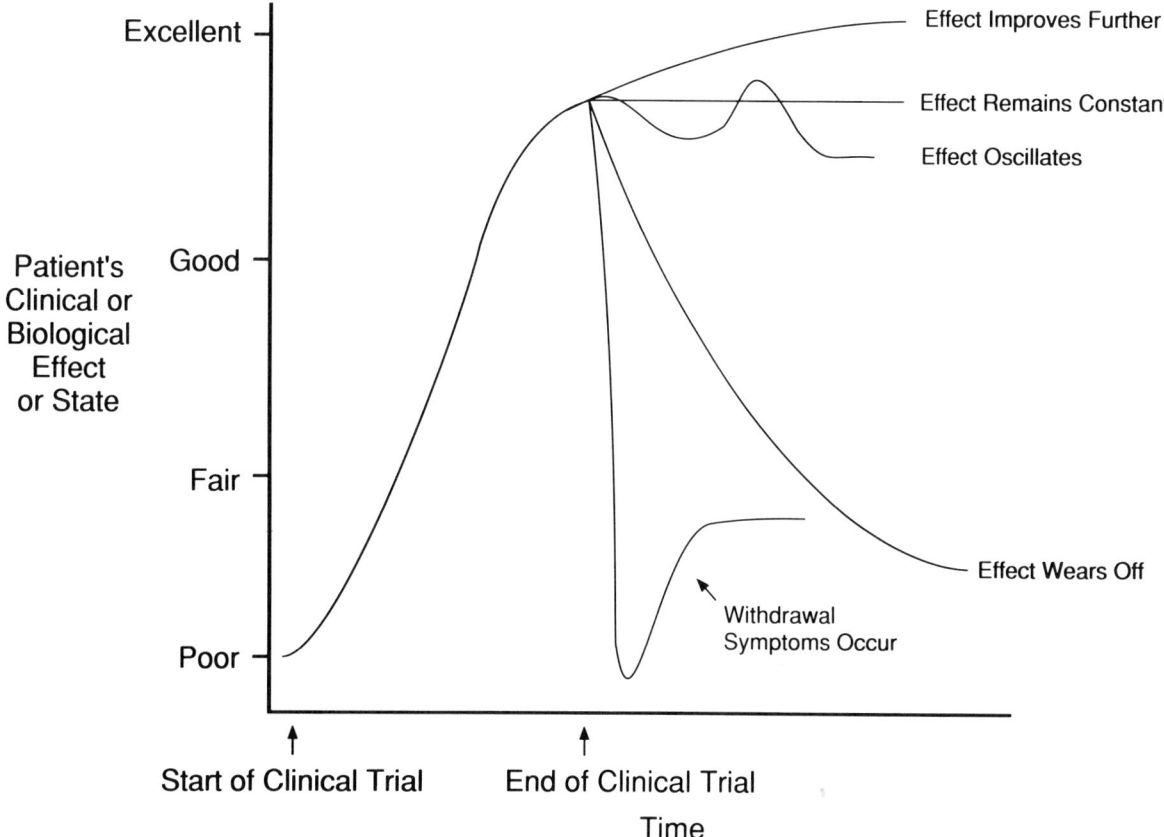

FIG. 65.3 Possible clinical outcomes after a clinical trial is completed and patients who improved during the trial are taken off treatment.

(e.g., death) or measured (e.g., a specific increase, decrease, or change in a physiological parameter). If patient deaths are being used as an endpoint, then prolonging the trial would be expected to increase the total number of events (deaths) observed.

It is often important to track the clinical course of patients after a trial is completed, since numerous patterns may result (Fig 65.3). These data help interpret and understand the medicine's effects.

Prior to incorporating a posttrial questionnaire into a trial, it should be reviewed and evaluated for clarity and content. In addition, both colleagues and patients should complete these questionnaires to determine that the instructions for their use are easy to understand and that the form is easy to fill out. It is possible to include an end-of-trial questionnaire in a trial even if it was not considered prior to initiating the clinical trial.

PART V

A Nonmathematical Approach to Statistics and Data Processing

After I had addressed myself to this very difficult and almost insoluble problem, the suggestion at length came to me how it could be solved with fewer and much simpler constructions than were formerly used if my assumptions (which are called axioms) were granted me.

—*Nicolaus Copernicus*

Human beings never welcome the news that something they have long cherished is untrue: they almost always reply to that news by reviling its promulgator.

—*Henry Louis Mencken*

A judicious man . . . looks at statistics, not to get knowledge, but to save himself from having ignorance foisted on him.

—*Thomas Carlyle*

Feinstein's Question: Do the data meet the traumatic interocular test? (Do they hit you between the eyes?)

—*Alvan Feinstein*, American biostatistician and clinical trial methodologist

CHAPTER 66

Developing an Overall Approach to Data Processing and Statistical Analysis

THREE-POINT APPROACH

One approach to the processing and analysis of data is to divide the entire procedure into three parts, as shown in Figure 66.1. This approach focuses on (1) handling of data collection forms by the monitor(s), (2) entering that data into a suitable computer by data processors, and (3) analyzing the data in conjunction with statisticians. These stages are essentially identical for both sponsored and unsponsored clinical trials, although modifications of the steps in Fig. 66.1 will be required for each trial. Clinical interpretation of data occurs after they are analyzed.

DATA EDITING AND PROCESSING

Data editing is part of the quality control system that is an important aspect of all clinical trials. The data-editing process refers to the procedures by which the coded and/or uncoded data on the data collection forms are reviewed for presence, completeness, legibility, accuracy, and consistency with prior and subsequent data. This is performed both during the trial by monitors and subsequent to the trial by monitors or specially trained data editors. Unusual or inappropriate values or codes in data entry should be brought to the attention of the data editor and evaluated at the proper stage of data evaluation. For many studies, data are entered twice into the computer, and a program is used to compare every datum in the two files to check for nonidentical information. Any discrepancies between the two files are printed by the computer, and an individual must determine which of the two values is correct. After all the data are correctly entered, a fur-

ther quality assurance process is utilized wherein a sample of the data entered is compared with the original data collection forms to determine an error rate.

PRESENTATION OF DATA

Prior to data analysis, the manner by which the data will be presented and evaluated should be determined. This involves the processes of setting up prototype tables and also determining the criteria and level of significance that will be utilized to define efficacy. The criterion setting should take place during the planning phase of the clinical trial and be completed by the time the protocol is approved. The prototype tables may be prepared during or subsequent to the trial. A series of prototype tables and figures to present safety data from a hypothetical multicentered double-blind evaluation of a trial medicine versus placebo is given in Appendix 2 of *Guide to Clinical Studies and Developing Protocols* (Spilker, 1984) and represents one of several approaches that could be used to present safety data. The major areas covered are study characteristics, physical examinations, electrocardiogram (ECG), laboratory examinations, and adverse reactions.

In addition to the tables referenced above it might be useful to include in an appendix to a Final Statistical Report (1) all raw data, (2) all data summarized by patient, and (3) all data summarized by center in those tables in which the data from all ten centers are combined (e.g., Tables A.8, A.10, A.11 in Spilker, 1984). Data on efficacy would require their own series of prototype tables and figures. Site-to-site differences in the data must be evaluated, and the data obtained at the different sites must be statistically comparable before

CLINICAL TRIAL DATA ENTRY AND ANALYSES

Study Medicine: Investigator:
Protocol Number: Site:

Date and check when completed.   Comments

Data Collection Forms (DCFs)

_____ Final Edit at Site or at Sponsoring Inst.   _____

_____   Completed   _____

_____ DCFs Received by Sponsor   _____

_____   Completed   _____

_____ DCFs Logged In   _____

_____ DCFs Sent to Investigator for Changes   _____

_____ DCFs Copied and Distributed   _____

_____ DCFs Sent to Computer Section   _____

_____ DCFs Received at Computer Entry   _____

Computer Entry

_____ Personnel Assigned   _____

_____ Data Entry Planned with Medical Input   _____

_____ Program Written to Enter Data   _____

_____ Data Edited   _____

_____ Data Entered (Single or Double Entry)   _____

_____ Data Quality Assured   _____

_____ Data Released for Statistical Analysis   _____

Statistical Analyses

_____ Personnel Assigned   _____

_____ Data Analysis Planned with Medical Input   _____

_____ Draft Report Prepared   _____

_____ Draft Report Received and Reviewed   _____

_____ Final Report Released   _____

FIG. 66.1 List of procedures to consider during the data entry and analysis period of a clinical trial.

the data may be combined. If data from different clinical trials are collected with the same data collection forms, analyzed in the same way, and presented in the same format, then the eventual combining of data from different trials will be expedited.

FINAL MEDICAL REPORT

After these procedures are completed and the data are analyzed, a Final Medical Report is usually written by the sponsor (see Chapter 125 for sample outlines). It differs from the Final Clinical Trial Report prepared

by the investigator participating in a sponsored trial. The latter is a brief synopsis of the investigator's experiences with the medicine and is often presented as a summary of experiences with each patient and a comparison of the trial medicine's overall safety and efficacy with known medicines of a similar class. The former report is generally prepared in a format suitable for submission to a governmental regulatory agency. The analogous report prepared by the investigator of an unsponsored trial is usually a paper intended for publication. In both sponsored and unsponsored trials, the investigator must adhere to and complete all re-

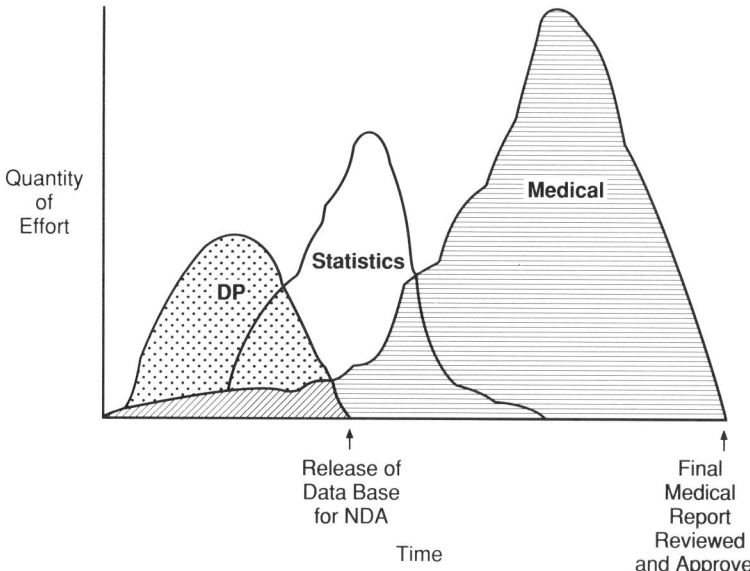

FIG. 66.2 Schematic illustrating the overlapping approach to data processing (DP), statistical analysis, and clinical interpretation and report preparation. Interactions occur among all three groups to prepare and review each other's reports. The relative amount and distribution of effort may vary enormously from trial to trial. NDA, New Drug Application.

quirements stipulated by the Institutional Review Board (IRB). Figures 66.2 and 66.3 illustrate how these reports overlap when they are created with the assistance of several groups. There is a current trend in some countries (e.g., United States) toward integrating the Final Statistical and Medical Reports.

ELIMINATING PATIENT DATA

Following good standards of protocol development and trial conduct optimizes the chances of achieving a meaningful clinical trial whose interpretations will be accepted. It is thus important not to allow the blind to

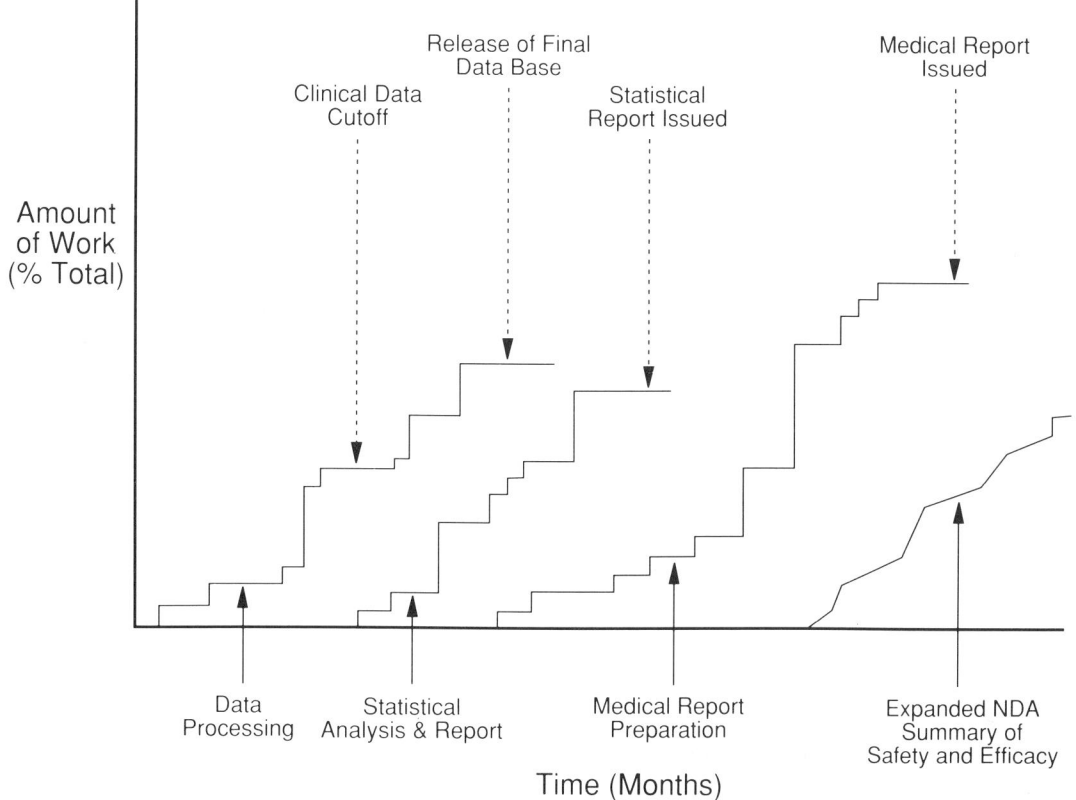

FIG. 66.3 Preparation of medical reports illustrating that effort often occurs in discrete boluses rather than as smooth continual efforts. A combined statistical and medical report may be issued instead of separate reports. NDA, New Drug Application.

be easily broken, introduce biases, peek at the data without proper allowances, or follow other procedures that would encourage the practice of eliminating some patients from the trial. Patients who are discontinued for any reason after randomization to treatment should be analyzed in the treatment group to prevent bias, since patient dropouts that are not related to medicine-induced adverse reactions may still be trial- or treatment-related. For example, patients may have dropped out of a trial if they improved on a medicine and no longer require treatment, did not improve on treatment and sought other medical help, or were unhappy with the requirements of the trial for some reason. Thus, patients should not be eliminated from consideration and analysis once they have been randomized to treatment, or, possibly, once they have begun to receive medicine treatment.

ANALYZING DATA

Finding a Statistician. Academicians who conduct clinical trials often become associated with a statistician whom they trust and find to be either knowledgable about their specific area of research or willing to collaborate in their activities. Statistical input is important (or essential) throughout the course of a trial but is almost always mandatory before initiation and after completion.

Blinding. There appears to be a growing trend to have statisticians kept blind to the identity of treatment groups and to analyze data from groups A, B, etc., rather than from groups labeled trial medicine or placebo. Some statisticians consider this approach preferable for interim rather than for final analyses and it may also be followed by committees who are deciding whether to stop a trial prematurely. An alternative approach is for statisticians to remain blind to treatments until after the tests to be used for data analysis are chosen. At that point the statisticians may be unblinded.

Choosing Statistical Tests To Use. Prior to the clinical trial it is important to identify the major statistical evaluations that will be conducted on the data. Data must be collected in a manner that will allow those methods to be used. During a trial unforeseen issues often arise, thus preventing the desired statistical tests from being used and requiring significant modifications of the statistical methods.

Each Patient Counts! A number of practical pitfalls in the statistical approach to clinical trial design and data analysis are discussed by Pocock (1985). He illustrates that even a single patient's outcome in a large trial may dramatically affect overall results and the interpretation reached.

Ensuring That Data Sets Are Complete. It is critical that the statistician not initiate and conduct analyses on data sets that are believed complete (i.e., have data from all patients to be analyzed) but are really incomplete (i.e., data of some or all patients are missing). This would lead to redundant work and the possibility of incorrect interpretations and decisions. Even the mildest of these problems would lead to frustration, inefficiencies, loss of valuable time, and possible deterioration of morale. A system of communications between the clinical monitor, data processor, statistician, and possibly others is important to prevent this problem. One element of this system should include a means of identifying which data are in which data set and how complete each data set is at all points in the data flow. Figure 66.4 illustrates a simple form of this type.

Subgroup Analyses. The question of whether to perform subgroup analyses not originally intended in the clinical trial is a controversial topic. After the data are examined, they may suggest comparisons or observations that were not expected or were not originally sought. The most appropriate use of these analyses is to design further clinical trials in which the new results found with this technique may be systematically examined.

Developing a Model Report. If several similar statistical reports are to be prepared on different (but related) clinical trials, then the initial statistical report may be used as a model. The approach used in this model may have input from the medical personnel who are involved with the trials, as well as the principal investigator in some cases. These medical personnel will help ensure that the trial analyses are presented in a format that can be clinically interpreted most effectively.

Complex Statistical Analyses. Sophisticated analyses that are not meaningful to the investigator will generally not be meaningful to most clinically oriented individuals who read the medical report or a clinical article prepared for publication. If statistical details are important to the audience of the report, then they should be included as a footnote or appendix to the clinical report or article. Statisticians should present data in a way that clinicians can readily comprehend the results, even if the clinicians are not statistically sophisticated. If multiple clinical trials are being conducted using a similar or related trial design, then each statistical report should be as similar as possible to the original model. Approaches used to analyze efficacy data are described in statistical texts. A few selected pitfalls to avoid in analyzing clinical data are listed in Table 66.1.

Eliminating Patients from Analyses. The specific patients who are eliminated from data analysis must be determined through nonbiased criteria, which should be enumerated before the clinical trial begins. This issue is extremely controversial because inclusion

Clinical Data Collection Form Reconciliation

Statistician to Complete Top Portion and Send to Clinical Monitor.

Medicine Number / Name _____

Protocol Number _____ Trial Number _____

Investigator _____ Investigator's Site _____

Name of Statistician _____ Date of Form Initiation _____

Clinical Monitor to Complete Rest of Form and Return to Statistician.

Name of Person Completing This Form _____

Number of Patients: **Total Number and Patient Numbers if Available:**

Scheduled (at this time) for Completion of Trial _____

Who Have Actually Completed the Trial _____

Complete DCFs Received From Site _____

Incomplete DCFs Received From Site _____

Complete DCFs Sent for Data Entry _____

Incomplete DCFs Sent for Data Entry _____

Data Entry Performed On _____

On Whom Data Should Have Been Received by Statistician _____

Comments, Qualifications, Modifications: _____

_____

_____

_____

_____

_____

_____

FIG. 66.4 Clinical data collection form reconciliation. Sample method to confirm that data entry and statistical analyses are being conducted on the correct number of patients.

of inappropriate patients in a trial analysis may bias data or create more "noise" in the results, which could mask true effects. On the other hand, if patients were treated with the trial medicine it is usually not considered acceptable to eliminate their data from analysis. An excellent example of this was reported by Sackett et al. (1985) in their Table 7-9 (see Table 70.1).

Analyzing Data From Patients Who Do Not Meet Entry Criteria or Do Not Complete the Trial. How does one deal with data from patients who did not meet entry criteria for a clinical trial? There are various situations in which it is uncertain at the time of enrollment if a patient will eventually be found to meet entry criteria, including trials in which all data are not available

TABLE 66.1 *Selected pitfalls to avoid in analyzing clinical data*

1. Analyzing data without a full consultation or association with a professional statistician
2. Using statistical techniques that fail to meet currently acceptable standards (unless there is a strong rationale for the choice of techniques used)
3. Analyzing incomplete data sets
4. Performing an unplanned interim analysis, which will compromise the analysis of the final data
5. Prematurely unblinding the clinical trial
6. Inadequately quality-assuring the data
7. Inadequately documenting the analyses conducted (e.g., the rationale for excluding specific data or patients from the analysis)

on entry. For example, when patients must be treated within a few hours of a myocardial infarction, patients with suspected myocardial infarctions may be enrolled but later found not to meet entry criteria. Another example is of patients with various types of infections who are of necessity treated with a trial medicine before microbiological culture results are available. These results are necessary to provide the evidence of whether their infections met entry criteria. Another complicating factor is that many patients are either mistaken or less than totally honest about their past medical history and are later found not to meet entry criteria.

Analyzing Data in Multiple Ways. There are numerous ways to deal with data from patients who either do not meet entry criteria or do not complete the clinical trial. The author agrees with those statisticians who advocate performing multiple analyses of the data. Multiple analyses have the advantage that all major views of the data are conducted and interpreted. Analyzing data from all patients treated in a trial is important since (1) the patients were treated in the trial, (2) in other situations similar patients will likely be treated, and (3) the ability to extrapolate data could be compromised if some treated patients were excluded from analysis. This analysis includes patients studied because of the investigator's "intention to treat."

Last Observation Carried Forward. In all analyses, it is possible to consider either those patients who completed the clinical trial or all patients who entered the trial regardless of whether they completed it. For those who entered the trial but did not complete it, it is possible to carry their last observed efficacy values forward to each of the times when no values were obtained or to simply ignore their missing values in the analysis from the time when they dropped out (of their volition) or were discontinued by the investigator. Patients who drop out and do not complete a trial because of adverse reactions are often considered as a separate

group. Their data are often treated differently than data from patients who drop out of their own volition for reasons unrelated to the trial.

Categories of Patients to Describe. There are different categories of patients who do not meet entry criteria including (1) patients entered legitimately who were later found to be in violation of criteria designed to preserve the integrity of the efficacy evaluation, (2) patients who did not meet entry criteria because of minor differences in age or another relatively inconsequential parameter, (3) patients who lied about their previous medical or nonmedical history, but met other criteria, and (4) patients who did not meet criteria designed to ensure patient safety.

These considerations indicate that various categories of patients should be reviewed when data are being assembled for analysis. These categories include

1. All patients entered in a clinical trial (e.g., those who signed an informed consent) regardless of whether they received any medicine treatment
2. Patients who received at least one dose of a medicine
3. Patients who completed at least a prespecified portion of the trial
4. Patients who completed the entire trial
5. Patients who dropped out of the trial on their own volition, because of lack of efficacy
6. Patients who dropped out of the trial on their own volition, because of clinical improvement
7. Patients who dropped out of the trial on their own volition, because of adverse reactions
8. Patients who dropped out of the trial on their own volition, because of reasons unrelated to the trial (e.g., moved, personal reasons)
9. Patients discontinued by the investigator because of safety considerations (e.g., adverse reactions, unacceptable benefit-to-risk ratio)
10. Patients discontinued by the investigator because of other reasons (e.g., lack of cooperation, poor compliance)

Some of these categories may overlap, may not be relevant for a clinical trial, or may have to be redefined (see Chapter 31). Once all relevant patient categories to be analyzed in a trial are chosen, it is essential to determine which type(s) of data analysis will be used. For example, will the "last observation carried forward" approach be used, will all data be presented, or will multiple analyses be conducted? After these choices are made the data may be analyzed with the tests and procedures considered most valid. Relevant within-treatment groups, between-treatment groups, subgroup analyses, and other comparisons are then conducted.

CHAPTER 67

Systems for Classifying Diseases and Adverse Reactions

There has been an increased use of dictionaries and systems in recent years to define diseases by code numbers, especially for patients entering hospitals. The spread of Diagnosis-Related Groups (DRGs) in hospitals will undoubtedly increase the use of these standardized categories. Some are created by professional societies (e.g., DSM-III in psychiatry was created by the American Psychiatric Society), and others (e.g., ICD-9) have resulted from international interest in this area. In some clinical trials the enrollment of patients with a standard diagnosis such as one listed in DSM-III is highly pertinent to obtaining the desired patient population. Nonetheless, in most clinical trials patient entry requirements are not tied to standardized diagnoses.

In certain therapeutic areas (e.g., epilepsy) most clinical researchers and many private practitioners adhere to a standard international classification for diagnosing patients. In other fields, however, there have been differences in the classifications used between countries. For instance, DSM-III is used in the United States to classify patients with various psychoses, but ICD-9, which is a morbidity and mortality coding system developed by the World Health Organization (WHO), is used (partially or completely) in many other countries for this purpose. In addition, numerous professional societies have prepared glossaries and/or classifications to assist in diagnosis of disease and treatment of patients.

A brief history of the classification of diseases is given by Côté and Robboy (1980). This article concentrates on Systematized Nomenclature of Medicine (SNOMED) and describes some of the problems with the International Classification of Disease (ICD) system. These authors propose that a merger of the two systems, using SNOMED as the starting point, would provide the most useful system of medical nomenclature. Various other coding systems and thesauri have been proposed for disease classification, including "Medical Subject Headings" of the National Library of Medicine in the United States.

In creating, using, and modifying codes a balance must be sought between excessive splitting and lumping of disease categories. It is particularly difficult to achieve the ideal balance because various groups have different needs and use these codes differently.

DICTIONARIES OF ADVERSE REACTIONS

Dictionaries of adverse reactions are created by individual companies, large professional societies, health agencies, and regulatory agencies. Those created by sponsors are developed for all clinical trials on a particular medicine or for all trials of the sponsor.

Purposes

One important reason for creating an adverse reaction dictionary is to allow different investigators (at different sites or at the same site) to identify the same adverse reaction with the same term and to identify different adverse reactions with different terms. Even one investigator may use different terms for the same reaction in different patients or for the same reaction in the same patient at different times. An investigator may label an adverse reaction as "drowsiness" at one visit and as "sleepiness" at a later visit if the patient is still complaining of the same problem. The investigator may not have the patient's data collection form from the previous visit readily available for reference and thus may write a different term in the medical record. This may be later transcribed as "sleepiness" on the data collection form, and without using a dictionary that describes these two adverse reactions as identical, a potential issue may be created.

Although the particular problem in this example is minor, the problem becomes much greater when magnified by 1,000 patients, by ten visits per patient, and by other synonyms that may be used by other investigators for the same symptom (e.g., fatigue, somnolence, tiredness). In addition, there are other terms that differ slightly in meaning but may actually represent the same symptoms (e.g., restlessness, irritability).

One counterargument to standardizing adverse reaction terminology prior to a clinical trial is that supplying even brief dictionaries to investigators or precoding data collection forms provides a stimulus that may increase the frequency of adverse reaction reports. Many clinical monitors prefer to assign the correct term to adverse reactions after all of the data have been collected.

Use of Adverse Reaction Dictionaries by Pharmaceutical Companies

A standard dictionary to be used in a clinical trial does not have to be many pages long, and it is generally easier for investigators and their staff to use if it is short. The most important and frequently observed adverse reactions observed with the same medicine in previous trials should be defined, synonyms should be presented, and a preferred term should be selected. If this practice is established, then when data are entered in a computer (or even written on a sheet) undesired terms may be removed and the appropriate synonym may be inserted. At a more sophisticated level, this process may be programmed into a computer.

When dictionaries of adverse reactions were first developed, each medicine under investigation or even each clinical trial had a home-grown list of preferred terms along with anticipated synonyms. In subsequent years some pharmaceutical companies (e.g., Eli Lilly, Merck) developed their own dictionaries or thesaurus of adverse reaction terms and synonyms (Gillum 1989). Some companies use the WHO Adverse Reaction Terminology (e.g., Schering-Plough: see Saltzman, 1985), or variations of the Coding Symbols for a Thesaurus of Adverse Reaction Terms (COSTART) system (e.g., McNeil: see Teal and Dimmig, 1985). These lists are

often divided by body system and certain terms carry an asterisk with the notation "Caution, other classification terms may be better suited." Other companies utilize standard systems such as COSTART.

The COSTART and WHO dictionaries have now been reconciled and the ability to move between these dictionaries represents a major step forward. It will obviate many problems that existed when one part of a multinational company used one of these systems and another part used the other.

COSTART System

COSTART provides a basis for vocabulary control of adverse reaction reports that emanate from a variety of sources. In that sense it is actually much more like a thesaurus than a dictionary. The orientation of COSTART is primarily anatomic. It has a hierarchical arrangement of terms, from the broadest (body-system categories) to narrowest (specific preferred terms or even special search categories). The COSTART dictionary is used and maintained by the Center for Drugs and Biologics at the Food and Drug Administration (FDA) for marketed medicine surveillance and has been endorsed by many senior managers in the various reviewing sections.

There are four indexes in COSTART:

Index A. Three lists of search categories: (1) body-system search categories, (2) special search categories (e.g., neoplasia, superinfection), and (3) special search categories for fetal–neonatal disorders.

Index B. An alphabetical listing of all the coding symbols, plus preferred terms and primary search categories (optional categories).

Index C. A listing of coding symbols by body-system categories.

Index D. An alphabetical list of terms commonly used by physicians to report adverse reactions to medicines, plus numerous related terms and the coding symbol to be used. This index is extensively cross-indexed.

WHO Adverse Reaction Terminology

The WHO terminology system of adverse reactions is relatively short, containing approximately 1,100 terms. A code number is assigned to each of these terms. This provides the advantage that the same code is retained when the term is translated into different languages, although between countries there are some differences in definitions of specific terms. The WHO system uses a hierarchy of "preferred terms" to describe adverse reactions. Other commonly used terms are called "included terms." These are listed with their preferred term.

FDA Adverse Reaction Drug Dictionary

The FDA and many pharmaceutical companies have gone through an evolution of systems in how they obtain, collect, process, and define adverse reactions. The medicine dictionary currently used by the FDA (*The Center for Drugs and Biologics Ingredient Dictionary*) is described by Forbes et al. (1986), and the processing of adverse reaction reports by the FDA is described by Turner et al. (1986).

Advantages and disadvantages of COSTART, ICD-9, Medical Subject Headings, SNOMED (2nd edition), and WHO Adverse Reaction Terminology are succinctly listed by Stephens (1985b).

Using an Adverse Reaction Dictionary

Dictionaries in use by pharmaceutical companies more and more use a single language, which is applied to adverse reactions collected by the company for both investigational and marketed medicines as well as those reported in the published literature.

Whichever dictionary and system are used, it is essential that an experienced individual be in charge and apply rules consistently in all cases. Any exceptions must be noted so that they may be identified if data are audited. It is essential that the system not be 100% automated since someone must check all questionable terms and obtain the clinical monitor's approval for any changes made (Nissman, 1987).

Potentially confusing terms that often must be defined to be clear include congestion (head or chest?), migraine (headache or true migraine?), and colloquialisms such as "patient feels bad" (malaise or something else?). Other colloquially used terms include shock and paralysis. Nissman (1987) reported that with COSTART, combined terms are divided by most users when it makes medical sense to do so. For example, if a patient has headache along with diarrhea, these are divided into two terms.

CHAPTER 68

Data Processing

This chapter describes in a general manner the various steps that data progress through after they are collected until a final medical report or publication is prepared. Because of rapid changes in the hardware and software used to process each step and the numerous options that exist, computers and technical details are not discussed. Integration of a data base management system with other data control uses also is not discussed. A recent book (Rotmensz, 1989) presents details of data management in oncology trials. Jargon used in this field is eschewed in favor of simpler terms.

TYPES OF DATA-HANDLING PROCESSES

After data have been collected and quality-assured there are three major processes that can be followed. The first is to *transfer data*, either by recopying or by electronic transfer from one computer to another. The second process is the *integration of data*, which are combined from different sources or from a single source over time. The third process is the creation of *data bases*. This chapter considers all three procedures but focuses on the integration of data and creation of

a data base used for the development of new medicines.

FLOW OF CLINICAL DATA

Clinical data obtained in a trial usually flow from investigator to monitors to data processors to statisticians to medical monitors and back to the investigator. Numerous variations in this pattern exist and depend on factors such as whether the trial is sponsored, whether data are entered directly in computers, and the nature of the sponsor's organization. The flow of clinical data after a trial is completed is shown in Figs. 68.1 and 68.2. Some means of improving data flow are listed in Table 68.1, and sample headings of tables used to monitor this flow are shown in Table 68.2. Three models of data collection, entry, and processing are shown in Fig. 68.3.

DATA PROCESSING IN 14 STEPS

Table 68.3 lists 14 steps used to process data from a clinical trial with a relatively short duration of patient

TABLE 68.1 *Means of improving the efficiency of clinical data flow*

1. Design standard operating procedures that make sense and are simple to use
2. Design standard data collection forms for use in multiple clinical trials on a project
3. Use data collection forms with responses that can be completed with a check mark or cross rather than requiring a fill-in
4. Design data collection forms to minimize write-in comments
5. Implement standard easy-to-use systems that take data step by step, from data editing to data entry to statistical analysis to clinical interpretation to report writing
6. Coordinate the procedures involved in data flow to allow integration of relevant systems and information with other divisions (e.g., marketing, production, technical development) and other countries
7. Explore automation of various steps (e.g., transfer of clinical laboratory data in machine readable form, use of optical scanners to "read" data collection forms, remote data entry)

TABLE 68.3 *Steps used to process data from a clinical trial with a short duration of patient treatment[a]*

1. Data retrieval
2. Programming computers for data entry
3. Editing data collection forms to prepare data for computer entry
4. Integrating data from samples sent by investigators to outside laboratories
5. Data entry
6. Editing of data after they have been entered into the computer
7. Obtaining responses to questions raised
8. Correcting data in the computer
9. Quality assurance and release of data base
10. Statistical analysis
11. Draft statistical report
12. Clinical interpretation
13. Final statistical report
14. Final medical report or final joint medical and statistical report

[a] "Short" usually means less than 3 months.

treatment (e.g., up to approximately 3 months). In the table each step appears to begin after the prior one is completed, but in reality a great deal of overlap usually occurs, which can shorten the entire process. Activities conducted during each of these 14 steps are briefly described. Some institutions have established general standards for the time allotted each one. While overall standards exist, individual clinical trial objectives must be established that explore what resources are needed and available to complete these activities. Charts of the proposed plan are often generated and used to schedule work.

The progress of clinical trial data as it passes through these 14 steps should be tracked and evaluated as a means of forecasting workloads and assessing whether there are bottlenecks or areas where new procedures are required. Such tracking should be repeated periodically (or even continuously) to document trends in these important time-requiring steps. Time saved here will enable Product License Applications (PLAs) and New Drug Applications (NDAs) to be submitted more rapidly and also (hopefully) approved more rapidly. Advantages of a centralized approach to data pro-

cessing are summarized in Table 68.4. The data-processing steps followed in a large clinical trial (the MRFIT) are presented by DuChene et al. (1986).

If the data from a few patients are not rapidly processed during the early stages of a clinical trial, then data entry problems may be continued by investigators and monitors. If such a problem is noticed at an early stage, however, it can be resolved, and "cleaner" data will be produced. The difficulty with entering data at an early stage, however, is that the clinical trial must have a sufficiently high priority in the group that writes the computer program to have the program written at an early enough stage. For extremely large clinical trials a variety of approaches should be considered for data processing. These are summarized in Table 68.5.

Step 1: Data Retrieval

Each clinical trial should have a strategy to retrieve data. Whether that involves collecting data on an ongoing basis, using a batch mode, or waiting until the clinical trial is completed before collecting the data will

TABLE 68.2 *Sample table heading formats used to monitor activities on multiple clinical trials during data processing, analysis, and report-writing periods*

A[a]

Category of trial	Trial number	Principal investigator	Number of completed patients	Projected[b] date of last DCF to sponsor (* = actual date)	Projected date of last DCF to data processor (* = actual date)	Projected date of draft statistical report (* = actual date)	Projected date of final statistical report (* = actual date)	Projected date of draft medical report (* = actual date)	Projected date of final medical report (* = actual date)

B

Trial number	Estimated[b] date of trial completion	Estimated date of last DCF to data processing	Estimated date of data-base release	Estimated date of statistical report completion	Author of statistical report	Estimated date of medical report completion	Author of medical report

[a] A and B are two separate examples of table headings.
[b] The term "Projected" or "Estimated" may be changed in the heading to "Actual" when all items in that column are completed. Alternatively, an asterisk or other symbol may be used to indicate that the task has been completed. DCF, data collection form.

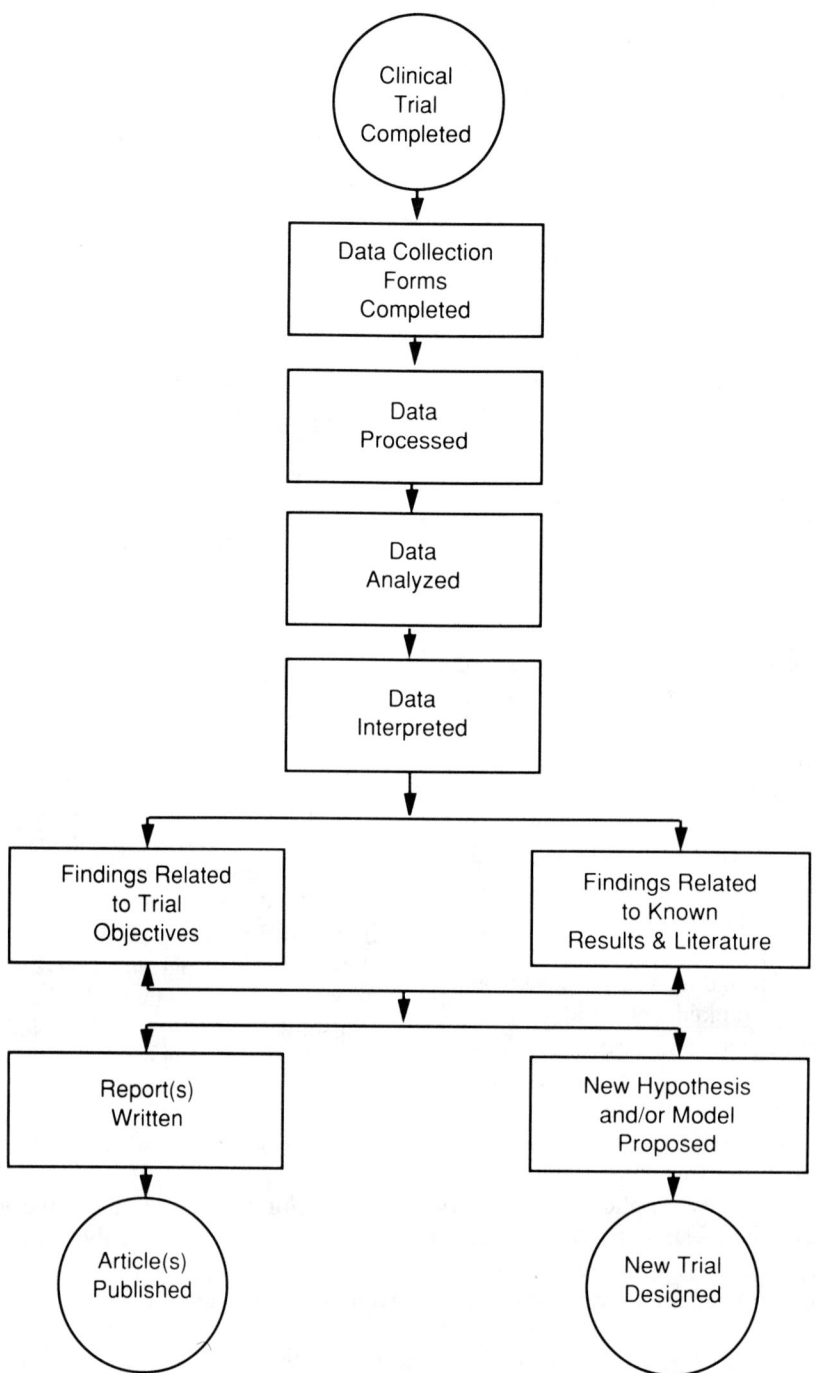

FIG. 68.1 Posttrial flow of clinical information and data. General flow of data after they are collected.

depend on numerous factors described in this chapter. The methods to be used in collecting data are also a part of the overall data-processing strategy developed.

Data are retrieved from sites by (1) monitors bringing data personally to the sponsor, (2) mail, (3) next-day courier services, (4) remote data transmitted via telephone lines, and (5) facsimiles. Telephone contacts are rarely used to transmit data, except possibly for reporting corrections or addressing questions.

It is often a goal of the sponsor to collect the complete data within a certain time period after the last patient has completed treatment at a site. This period must be established for each clinical trial and for each site within the trial. If the goal is to be realistic it cannot be set long in advance of the clinical trial's completion, because it will be impossible to know the priority of other activities (that may compete for resources) as well as the resources needed to achieve the goal.

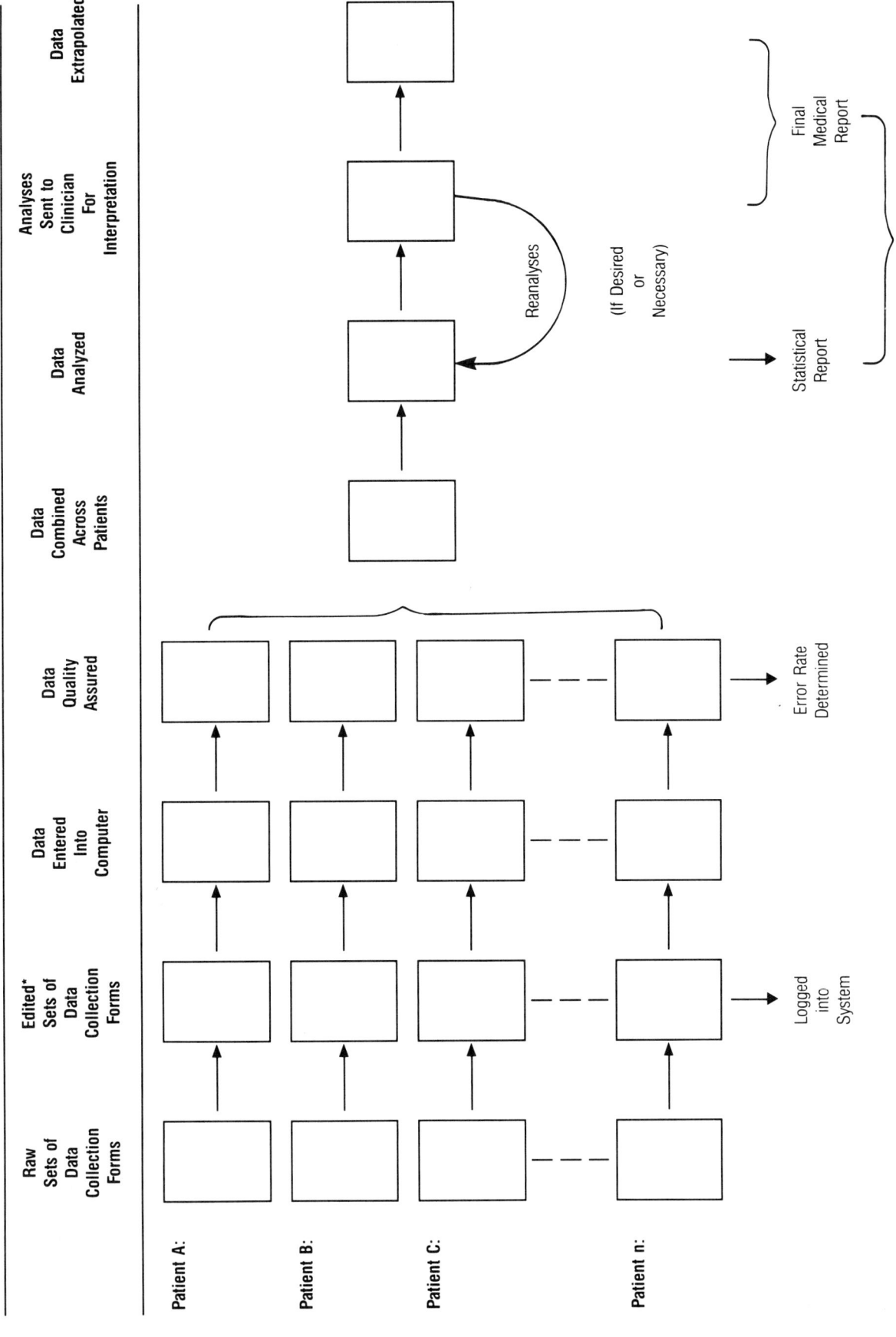

FIG. 68.2 Flow of data from data collection forms. General procedures conducted on data as they move from forms to a final medical report. *, edited at investigator's site and/or at sponsoring institution.

Model A: Conventional Approach

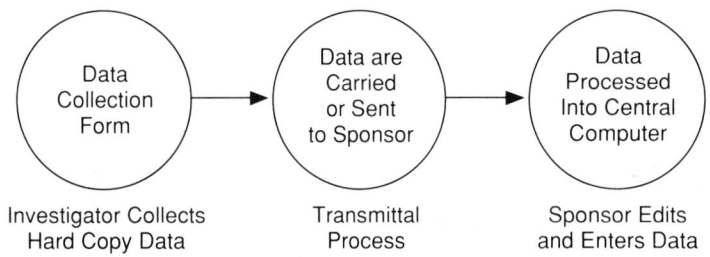

Model B: Remote Data Entry Approach

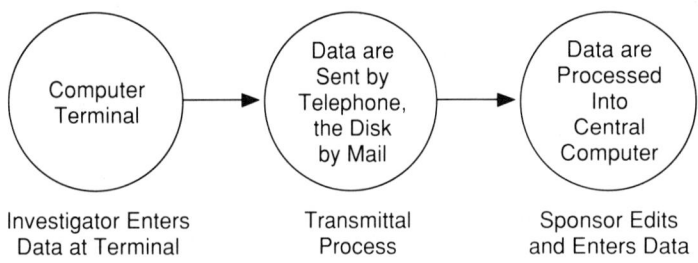

Model C: Direct Entry Approach

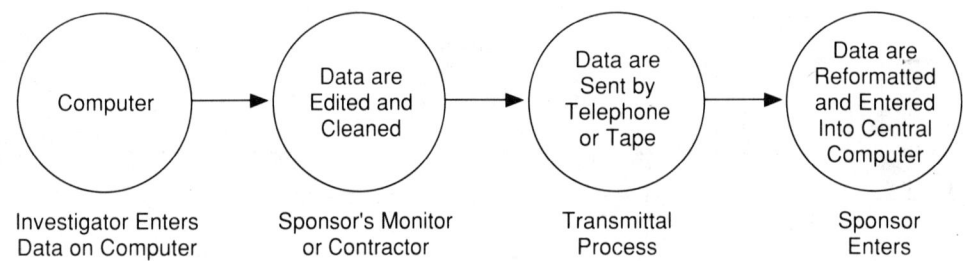

FIG. 68.3 Models of data collection, entry, and processing.

TABLE 68.4 *Advantages of a centralized approach to data processing for a large clinical trial[a]*

1. It is easier to initiate the clinical trial even if the entire system is not yet operational
2. Fewer training sessions are required for personnel
3. It is less expensive to have identical hardware and software at each site
4. It is less expensive for travel, installation, and development of detailed manuals
5. Greater security of data may be achieved
6. Changes to a protocol during a clinical trial or to data analysis are easier to implement
7. Various problems of communications may be avoided

[a] Most of these advantages also pertain to small and moderate-size clinical trials.

TABLE 68.5 *Approaches to dealing with a large amount of clinical data to process*

1. Use a contractor to process data, but not to analyze them statistically
2. Use a contractor to process data, analyze them statistically, and prepare a final report
3. Use a contractor to conduct a clinical trial and to do the other steps indicated in point 2 above
4. Decrease the number of clinical trials being conducted
5. Decrease the amount of data collected per clinical trial
6. Improve the quality of data arriving for data processing by increasing the monitoring and editing at each site
7. Use fewer variations of data collection forms
8. Use remote entry of data
9. Prioritize which clinical trials must have their data processed first
10. Eliminate services of data-processing groups that are not absolutely necessary
11. Use keyless data entry (e.g., with bar coded data, biological samples, or data collection forms)

Data retrieval strategies for long-term clinical trials (typically 6 months or longer) may be quite different from those for shorter trials. In long-term clinical trials, data may be retrieved after one or more selected milestones have been achieved by each patient. This allows more rapid completion of the final data base, or the creation of an interim data base.

Step 2: Programming Computers for Data Entry

The programmer uses the data collection forms as a basis for creating a suitable program. Entry screens must be designed for simplicity and to avoid eye strain. When building the data base, programmers must also consider the needs of the various groups who will use the data base (e.g., statisticians, adverse reaction personnel, biological sample analysis personnel).

Step 3: Editing to Prepare Data for Computer Entry

The purposes of the initial data edit by data-processing personnel differ from the edit conducted by the clinical trial monitor. Monitors are primarily concerned about verification of some or all data versus original source documents, ensuring completion of all forms, and looking for trends or abnormalities that might impact on the patient's treatment or the clinical trial's progress. Data-processing editors are primarily concerned that all entries are legible, all forms are complete, and entries are placed in the correct position (e.g., within a box, rather than between two boxes).

Some companies send data collection forms to these editors only after the monitor has completed an in-house edit, whereas other companies expect monitors to do this kind of editing at the investigators' sites. If the monitor does a poor job, this step may cause major delays in processing data. If the data are generally clean, this step may be conducted extremely rapidly. It is important to maintain high standards for monitoring edits, to allow for easy and onsite clarification and resolution of questions, rather than at a later time at the sponsor.

If investigators write many nonessential comments on a data collection form a great deal of time is wasted in transcribing them for entry into the computer.

Step 4: Integrating Data From Samples Sent by Investigators to Outside Laboratories

A number of clinical trials require investigators to send biological samples (e.g., plasma, urine) to outside laboratories or to the sponsor's laboratories for analysis. These samples often contain the investigational medicine and its metabolites that must be analyzed by the sponsor. Alternatively, samples may contain analytes (e.g., hormones) that cannot be analyzed at the facilities used by the investigator.

In such cases, a plan must be developed to ensure that each patient's laboratory data are entered on appropriate data collection forms and are integrated with the rest of their data. This may occur prior to computer entry of data, but often must be done at a later stage in the data-processing chain.

Step 5: Data Entry

Often there is a greater volume of trial data than can be entered into the computer (e.g., because of an inadequate number of trained personnel), and a backlog develops. Thus, it is essential to determine which clinic trials must enter data first. It is usually essential to enter data rapidly from clinical trials of an investigational medicine in Phase III approaching an NDA or PLA. Data from Phase I trials (in which it is uncertain if the medicine is effective) may usually be "analyzed by hand" to reserve resources for processing higher priority data. Typically, the priority of an investigational medicine increases as it progresses from Phase I through Phase III. Double-entry techniques are usually used (i.e., two separate operators each enter the data and a computer program compares each record). Future alternatives to key punch data entry are (1) bar code technology, (2) computer disk or tape, (3) optical character recognition, and (4) microcomputer-direct-to-large-computer transfer. These methods will undoubtedly become more widely used as data entry undergoes a transition, from (a) human to machine to (b) machine to machine.

In a large, high-priority trial, if data are entered in batches or only after the trial is completed, data processing may be delayed. This may be addressed by adopting a continual data-processing mode for selected trials.

Step 6: Editing of Data Entered Into Computers

The goal for computer data editing is to have it conducted by machines rather than by people. Differences are reported by computer and resolved. Machine edits include (1) range checks (e.g., are weights between 90 and 300 pounds, or is a 185-pound patient listed out of range as 815 pounds?), (2) value checks (e.g., Y or N), (3) logical edits (e.g., is a patient's weight listed as 200 pounds on one visit and 120 pounds the next time?), (4) numerical checks, and (5) some relational checks. Range checks are useful for most laboratory data, ages, and other factors bounded by reference, established, or normal upper and lower values.

Step 7: Obtaining Responses to Questions Raised

Obtaining responses is often frustrating for both the data processor and monitor, particularly if the clinical trial is not of sufficient priority to enable the monitor to give it full attention. This step requires the resolution of questions (even simple ones) that often require a relatively long time to address. The priority of the trial and the time of the investigator's staff are two factors that influence whether this activity is smooth or difficult.

Step 8: Making Corrections to Data Already Entered Into the Computer

Computer corrections are usually straightforward and rapid once one has the corrected data to be entered. Corrections in data collection forms should be annotated with dates and initials of the person doing the editing, according to established guidelines, and must leave an audit trail that can be followed, if desired, at a later date. It is important to ensure that all changes made to the data base also be posted to the data collection forms, and vice versa.

Step 9: Quality Assurance and Release of the Data Base

Quality assurance and data base release are also straightforward, and fast, in most cases. Release of a data base means that it is turned over to statisticians for analysis. Quality assurance estimates an error rate that indicates the accuracy of the procedures. An acceptable error rate is usually in the range of 1 to 10 errors per 10,000 fields, but may be higher.

Step 10: Statistical Analyses

Statistical analyses usually require interactions between statisticians and clinicians to ensure that all relevant subgroup analyses are conducted and that questions are addressed. The data are evaluated to affirm or deny the primary and secondary trial objectives. The protocol usually states which tests a statistician will use to address the primary objectives of the clinical trial. However, a large number of questions and issues may arise to challenge the use of planned tests, particularly if the data are not distributed and if the characteristics (e.g., amount of missing values) are not predicted in advance.

Step 11: Draft Statistical Report

The draft report is used as a basis for interaction between statisticians and clinicians, as well as for the initial clinical interpretation.

Step 12: Clinical Interpretation

Interpretation may be extremely straightforward or extremely complex, but it always begins with the clinical trial's objectives and statistical results. This process is described in detail elsewhere in this book.

Step 13: Final Statistical Report

Sometimes the medical and statistical reports are written as one. Even then, a final statistical report may be prepared as an appendix or separate part of the joint report.

Step 14: Final Medical Report

The final medical report is written by the relevant clinical staff member(s) associated with the clinical trial, another clinical staff member, or a professional medical writer. If the report is to follow a prototype report, it is easier for a professional writer to create the first draft, which is then reviewed by clinicians. Every report must be reviewed and approved by appropriately trained physicians. When multiple reports are being written, reviewed, and approved simultaneously, it is helpful to create a detailed schedule.

The final medical report must be reviewed by other major sites of the sponsor that will be expected to use the report in regulatory submissions. This will reduce problems when interpretations or other aspects differ significantly among professionals at the different sites.

CREATING A TEAM TO PLAN AND TRACK DATA PROCESSING

A loose or a highly formal system may be used to plan and track progress of the data as it goes through the 14 steps described. A small team composed of the data editor, programmer, monitor, statistician, and possibly data-processing supervisor or coordinator is created to plan and oversee progress of the data. At least one member of the group should be informed about actual and potential competition for resources from other clinical trials going through the same pipeline. This allows appeals for higher priority to be considered at an early stage, rather than after the competing trial has completed 50% of its path through the system. While

TABLE 68.6 *Some issues facing a data-processing coordination center for a large clinical trial*

1. How are data transferred to the center, and are multiple methods used to do this?
2. If data are transferred in electronic form, is a hard copy also received? Does the site maintain a hard copy?
3. Can a hard copy stage be omitted?
4. How does the center know that it has received all data sent or all data available at each site?
5. When are data sent in terms of time of day or night, and at what frequency?
6. Has a manual been developed after all problems and "bugs" have been resolved?
7. Are files transferred twice and results compared as a quality-assurance procedure?
8. Are hard copy printouts returned to each site for checking against the originals as a quality-assurance procedure?
9. Are all centers contacted if they do not transfer data within 24 hours of their scheduled time?
10. Are backup diskettes of data mailed to the center?
11. Are adequate local computer services available for each site?

competition may occur at any point during the system, it is most likely to be critical as the clinical trials are lined up in a queue waiting for their turn to enter the process.

Most of the very large clinical trials, whether sponsored by a government agency or pharmaceutical company, use a centralized system for data processing. Advantages of a centralized system are listed in Table 68.4, approaches to dealing with a large amount of data in Table 68.5, and issues facing a data-processing coordination center in Table 68.6.

Data processing is usually organized either as a batch flow (i.e., an entire trial's data or a significant part of the trial is processed together) or as a continuous process (i.e., data are processed as they arrive so that data from different trials are processed at the same time). The staff may be organized into teams to work together on individual clinical trials or medicines. A team is often headed by a data-processing coordinator and the members would include a (1) clinical monitor, (2) statistician, (3) medical writer, (4) database programmer, and (5) as many processors (e.g., editors, coders, reviewers) as appropriate.

DATA EDITS

The term *edit* describes the process whereby data are examined and corrected so all data make sense: forms are complete, correctly filled out, and legible; logic and range checks yield unambiguous results. Edits are conducted by investigators, their staff, and monitors prior to data processing. Edits are also conducted by data processors (step 3), data-entry operators (step 5), and after entry (step 6). Both steps 5 and 6 are done by the computer (i.e., machine edits).

AUDIT TRAIL OF CHANGES TO THE DATA BASE

Errors and Error Rates

When errors are detected at certain steps of the data review process, a record must be maintained of all changes made. This creates an audit trail, which the Food and Drug Administration (FDA) or other regulatory authority can evaluate if they wish. This audit trail of changes to the data base should not be confused with the clinical audit trail, which includes changes made to data during the conduct of the clinical trial. This point is discussed further in Chapter 63, "Auditing a Clinical Trial."

The later the stage of data processing at which errors on data collection forms are found, the greater is the work to reconcile all records. Errors found at the trial site during the trial's conduct only require changes to the original data collection forms, plus the appropriate signature and date. Errors detected by monitors during editing require changing the investigator's copy of the form as well as the original copy. A log of all such changes approved by the monitor and investigator must be maintained. Changes that occur during data processing require changing all data collection forms, plus maintaining a log and any other appropriate documentation desired.

Errors found in data entry or other data-processing steps that are *not* data collection form errors do not require this level of attention. In fact, most of those errors are simply corrected, except for quality-assurance steps, for which complete records are maintained.

The accuracy of most data collection forms is about 70 to 85%, online data entry keypunched into a computer is about 95% accurate, and double-entry data is about 99% accurate.

Once a data base is established and has been checked for errors, some companies may report the minor errors in the text of a report but do not correct the original data base. This is because a large amount of resources is required to modify the data base, particularly if it has also been transferred to other trial or sponsor sites. Rules of thumb for allowing minor errors to stand uncorrected may include (1) an acceptable error rate (e.g., up to 12 per 1,000 keystrokes), (2) an error that does not affect safety analyses, and (3) maintaining a list of uncorrected errors. A spelling error is rarely necessary to correct at this stage. Major errors of any type, however, must always be changed in the data base.

A heavily flawed data base with many major errors may have to be redone from the start (i.e., from an early stage) rather than corrected.

CHAPTER 69

Interim Analyses

TYPES OF INTERIM ANALYSES

The term *interim analysis* is broadly defined as either a formal or an informal analysis of data generated in a clinical trial prior to conducting a final analysis. Some authors define an interim analysis more narrowly, for example: A formal statistical analysis of response variables while the clinical trial is in progress for the purpose of decision making regarding continuation or termination of the trial. This definition is too narrow because an interim analysis does not have to be a formal analysis, it may occur after a clinical trial is completed, and several other purposes are possible. A comparison of formal and informal interim analyses is presented in Table 69.1. Informal interim reviews are also referred to as *administrative reviews*, or by other terms.

Spectrum 1: Time When the Interim Analysis Is Conducted

Any interim analysis exists at a specific point along each of four different spectra (Fig. 69.1). The first of these (A) represents the time when the analysis is conducted. Although a clinical trial is usually ongoing when the interim analysis is conducted, this is not a requirement. For example, an interim analysis may be conducted on the first X patients whose data are complete in an already completed clinical trial. In this situation, the analysis is only an interim one because the data base is not complete. Some people refer to this as a preliminary analysis, but that is a type of interim analysis.

Another aspect of time relates to the phase of medicine development. In Phases I and IIa most interim

TABLE 69.1 *Comparison of formal and informal interim analyses of data*

Issue or question	Formal interim analysis	Informal interim analysis[a]
How often does it occur?	Infrequent	Common
During what phase of development is the interim analysis done?	IIb/IIIa	IIa,b, IIIa,b
Is it generally stated in the protocol that it will be conducted?	Yes	No
What is the major purpose?	Should the clinical trial be modified or terminated based on safety or efficacy factors?	Should new trials be initiated?
Is an adjustment made to significance levels?	Yes	No

[a] This is also referred to as an *administrative review*.

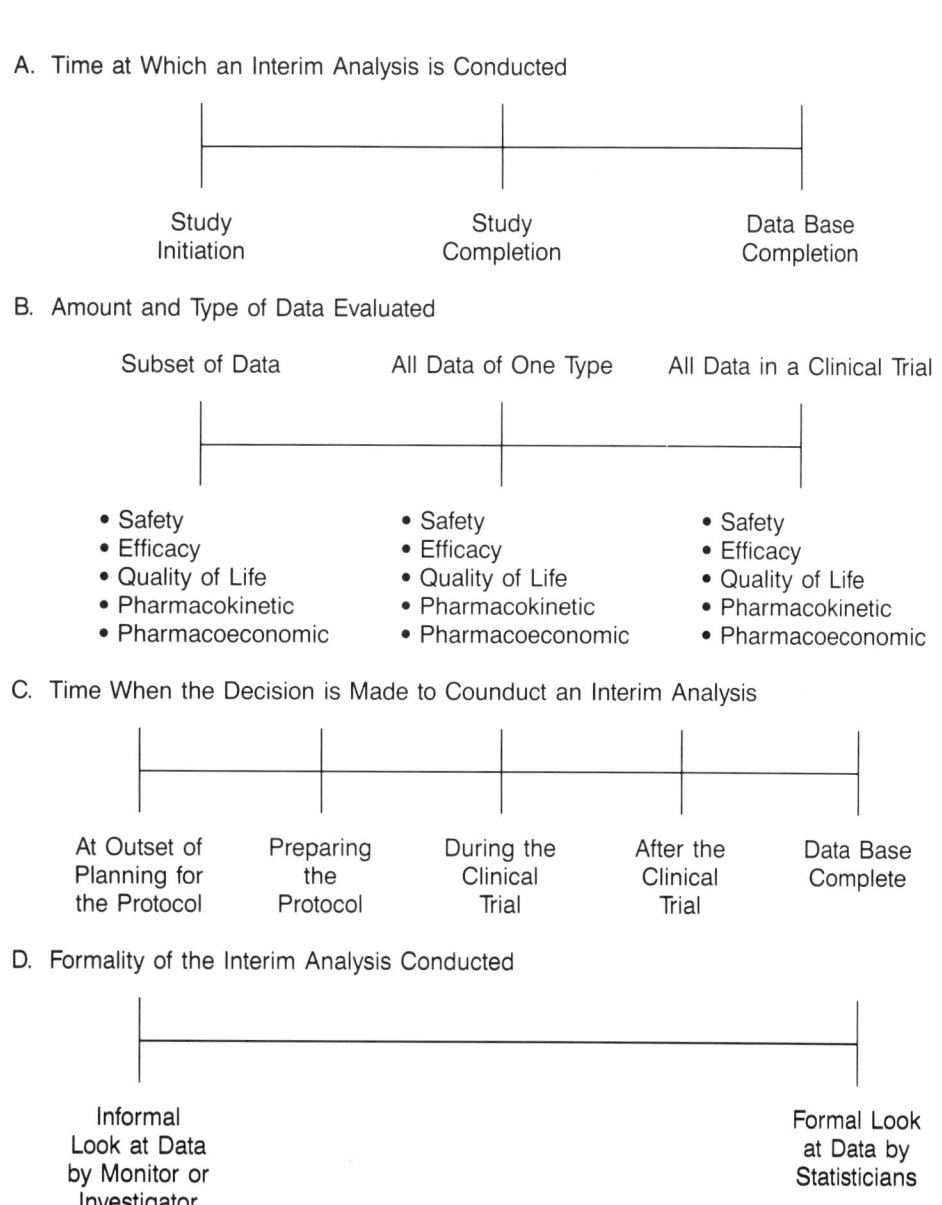

A. Time at Which an Interim Analysis is Conducted

Study Initiation   Study Completion   Data Base Completion

B. Amount and Type of Data Evaluated

Subset of Data   All Data of One Type   All Data in a Clinical Trial

- Safety
- Efficacy
- Quality of Life
- Pharmacokinetic
- Pharmacoeconomic

- Safety
- Efficacy
- Quality of Life
- Pharmacokinetic
- Pharmacoeconomic

- Safety
- Efficacy
- Quality of Life
- Pharmacokinetic
- Pharmacoeconomic

C. Time When the Decision is Made to Counduct an Interim Analysis

At Outset of Planning for the Protocol   Preparing the Protocol   During the Clinical Trial   After the Clinical Trial   Data Base Complete

D. Formality of the Interim Analysis Conducted

Informal Look at Data by Monitor or Investigator   Formal Look at Data by Statisticians

FIG. 69.1 Spectra along which interim analyses are conducted.

analyses are informal and are conducted to assist planning future trials. In Phases IIb and III interim analyses tend to be formal and are conducted for reasons discussed elsewhere.

Spectrum 2: Amount and Type of Data Evaluated

The second spectrum shown in Fig. 69.1 (B) represents the amount and type of data evaluated. An interim analysis may be conducted on all data obtained in a clinical trial. Nonetheless, most interim analyses focus only on efficacy or safety data. In fact, only a subset of either type of data may be studied in the interim analysis. Other types of data (e.g., quality of life, pharmacoeconomic, pharmacokinetic) may also be evaluated during an interim analysis.

Spectrum 3: Time When a Decision Is Made to Conduct an Interim Analysis

The various times during the conceptualization and conduct of a clinical trial when the decision is reached to conduct an interim analysis are shown in Fig. 69.1 (C). The earlier during this period the decision is reached, the more time is available for planning, and the more desirable is the interim analysis.

Spectrum 4: Formality of the Interim Analysis

The fourth spectrum shown in Fig. 69.1 (D) describes the level of formality of an interim analysis. If a formal data analysis is to be performed by statisticians, then it should be planned ahead of time, with appropriate statistical penalties (if required) incorporated into the study design (see section on interim analysis penalties for a further discussion of this point). If a decision is made to conduct an interim analysis after the clinical trial has begun, there will be more administrative difficulties in adjusting the necessary details if the number of patients and/or other factors (e.g., constituting a group to view the interim analysis) are changed.

Most interim analyses are clearly conducted *sub rosa*, i.e., few people are informed that it takes place,

no significant modifications (if any) are made to the clinical trial, and no statistical penalty is paid when the final statistical analyses are conducted. The final medical and statistical reports do not usually mention that an interim analysis was conducted. This approach may be strongly criticized. On the other hand, an administrative review could be accept if the outcome of the informal statistical analysis is limited to satisfying curiosity about the status of the clinical trial and possibly to helping plan future trials, and no modifications are made to the original trial. If the same type of *sub rosa* approach were followed, but the results were used to modify the clinical trial without mentioning the analysis and the resulting modification in appropriate reports, this practice would be unethical.

This informal interim analysis is beginning to be called an administrative review of data. It is uncertain whether an administrative review should be indicated in the protocol. Another issue is to determine who has access to the results of these informal analyses.

Group(s) That Receives the Results

Results of an interim analysis may be presented to many groups, from an independent Data Monitoring Committee to the investigator conducting the clinical trial (Fig. 69.2). In between would be a monitor or staff person who interacts directly with the investigator, those who do not, a sponsor's review committee, or another group apart from those who conducted the analysis. Various other groups could be described (e.g., staff of a contracting company). Possible outcomes of an interim analysis also range along a spectrum described later in this section. Except in an open-label clinical trial, it is inappropriate for interim analysis results to be given to the investigator conducting the trial. The results would clearly bias his or her approach to patients. Even in an open-label trial, this would be likely to occur.

PURPOSE(S) OF AN INTERIM ANALYSIS

The major reasons for conducting an interim analysis relate to ethics, science, finance, and practical con-

GROUPS THAT MAY RECEIVE THE INTERIM ANALYSIS

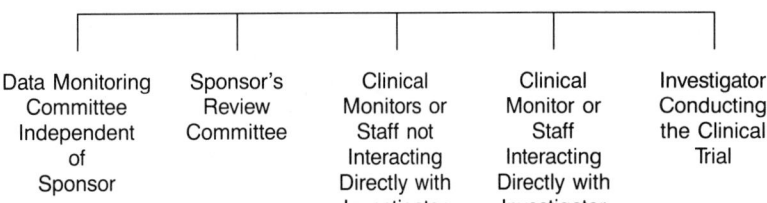

| Data Monitoring Committee Independent of Sponsor | Sponsor's Review Committee | Clinical Monitors or Staff not Interacting Directly with Investigator | Clinical Monitor or Staff Interacting Directly with Investigator | Investigator Conducting the Clinical Trial |

FIG. 69.2 Groups that may receive the interim analysis.

siderations. The precise purpose(s) of conducting an interim analysis must be clearly defined ahead of time. It is both reasonable and desirable to include this information in the protocol. The pros and cons of conducting the interim analysis should be debated and settled prior to initiating the clinical trial. Three examples of clinical trials in which interim analyses were conducted are the BHAT study (De Mets et al., 1984), AZT trial (Fischl et al., 1987), and the Enalapril Survival Study (CONSENSUS Trial Study Group, 1987).

Ethical and Scientific Reasons

Ethical reasons for conducting an interim analysis primarily relate to the importance of not withholding a better treatment from patients longer than necessary. If interim results of a clinical trial demonstrate an unequivocal positive result in treating seriously ill patients prior to the trial's completion, then the comparative trial should be stopped and all patients should be offered the opportunity to receive the better treatment. If a clinical trial clearly demonstrates that the test treatment is worse and patients are placed at greater risk of serious problems than with the comparative treatment (e.g., active medicine, placebo), then it also would be ethically unacceptable to continue the trial. A final ethical reason, but one that is not often looked for, is to show there is no possibility the test treatment will be found better than placebo (or ''no-treatment''). At that stage it is often unethical to continue the clinical trial, particularly if patients are placed at risk because of the treatment(s) they are receiving.

Additional ethical implications will occur if the results of an interim analysis are used to modify the ongoing clinical trial without indicating that the modification has occurred. If a clinical trial *is* modified based on an interim analysis, an evaluation must also occur to determine whether or not a statistical price must be paid for conducting the analysis.

Scientific reasons for conducting an interim analysis are related to those described above for ethics.

Financial Reasons

Financial reasons relate to the large costs of many clinical trials and the desire to stop expensive trials that cannot demonstrate desired differences. This conserves staff time, money, and other resources. However, financial reasons should never be the primary motivation for stopping a clinical trial.

Practical and Planning Reasons

A practical reason for conducting an interim analysis of a trial's data is to be assured that the clinical trial is progressing as planned. The analysis will also allow one to plan further trials (based on the interim results from a specific trial). These data enable one to assess the adequacy of the disease model used and the responsiveness of the efficacy variables chosen, and to determine whether any patient subpopulations of particular interest exist. Design assumptions such as baseline values, estimates of variance, and the magnitude of the placebo effect may also be assessed. Another practical outcome is help in deciding what types of patients should be sought for entry into the trial. At that point investigators may be encouraged to enroll patients of specific groups, based on demographics (e.g., racial, age, sex) or prognostic characteristics (e.g., disease severity), whose data warrant increased attention.

The protocol of any clinical trial analyzed may be modified in several important ways as a midcourse correction. This path must be taken only after extremely extensive discussions among clinicians and statisticians. Other groups (e.g., ethicists) may also be involved. If a protocol is modified during conduct of the clinical trial, it will always raise the possibility that the trial has become qualitatively different and that the data from the two parts should not be combined. Statisticians may assess the data to evaluate whether any differences occurred that would prevent pooling the two parts of the trial.

One of the ''dangers'' in performing interim analyses is that many statistical tests assume that the data are only being analyzed once, and multiple analyses of the data using these tests violate this assumption. This implies that if interim data analyses are planned, (1) they should be discussed with statisticians prior to the clinical trial, preferably while it is being designed, (2) the statisticians should perform the analyses under defined conditions, and (3) the potential ramifications of performing the interim analyses should be considered in advance.

OUTCOMES OF AN INTERIM ANALYSIS

A number of possible outcomes after an interim analysis is conducted and reviewed are shown in Table 69.2. Most informal interim data analyses are conducted to satisfy curiosity about the clinical trial's results, and no modifications are intended nor made to the trial. In other cases, however, these analyses help make decisions for other clinical trials. Should other trials be started? What designs, population groups, dosages, routes of administration, and dosage forms should be used? In such situations there is often no intention of modifying the clinical trial design or protocol of the trial under scrutiny. The analysis provides invaluable information, however, that helps a medicine's development program.

TABLE 69.2 *Selected outcomes of interim analyses*

1. No effect on the clinical trial
2. Minor modifications to the clinical trial that do not require Ethics Committee/IRB approval
3. Minor modifications to the clinical trial that require Ethics Committee/IRB approval
4. Major modifications to the clinical trial that require Ethics Committee/IRB approval
5. Modifications to other ongoing clinical trials
6. Termination of the clinical trial[a]
7. Termination of other clinical trials[a]
8. Modifications to plans for one or more clinical trials
9. Modifications to the development strategy for the medicine

[a] Termination of a clinical trial may occur for good (i.e., positive efficacy) or bad (i.e., adverse safety) reasons.

When it is difficult or impossible to gauge the correct number of patients to enroll prior to a clinical trial, the plan may be to use the results of the interim analysis to evaluate and possibly change the parameter. In other clinical trials, different parameters may be identified for possible modification (e.g., aspects of the inclusion criteria or testing procedures).

Clinical Trial Termination. The outcome that often receives most attention is termination of the clinical trial. The decision to terminate (or not) may have been specifically identified before the trial began for later consideration, or it may simply arise during the trial.

WHO CONDUCTS AN INTERIM ANALYSIS?

One of four different groups conducts most interim analyses, as described below.

Investigators Conducting the Clinical Trial

By definition, investigators may not conduct an interim analysis of a double-blind trial, but they may do so for a single-blind or open-label clinical trial. The major reason why investigators should not conduct *any* interim analysis of *any* clinical trial (i.e., introduction of bias) was previously stated.

Clinical Monitors and Staff of the Clinical Trial's Sponsor

Monitors who interact with investigators should neither conduct interim analyses of double-blind trials nor be informed of the results. This includes both the overall clinical trial results as well as specific results of particular patients. If monitors are aware of either detailed results or even overall trends, their communications with the investigator may be prejudiced and biased or may be misinterpreted if the investigator is aware of the monitor's knowledge. Clinical staff who do not interact with investigators often conduct highly informal interim analyses.

Statisticians Associated With the Investigator or Sponsor

Sponsor- or investigator-associated statisticians are usually asked to conduct *formal* interim analyses. As a matter of principle, they should be involved in the initial pretrial design discussions about whether or not to conduct an interim analysis. If protocol modifications must be made during a clinical trial (e.g., in the required number of patients) a determination must be made as to whether or not it is still desirable (or even reasonable) to conduct the planned interim analysis.

Statisticians Who Are Independent of the Investigator and Sponsor

In clinical trials with great potential impact on medical practice or public policy, when it is essential that no hint of impropriety be suggested, an independent group of statisticians may be asked to conduct the interim analysis. This group may be from academia or government, or may be part of an independent contracting organization.

WHICH CLINICAL TRIALS SHOULD HAVE AN INTERIM ANALYSIS?

Interim analyses are rarely relevant for Phase I clinical trials, which are usually short and involve few patients. Individual patient data are carefully followed to ensure patients' well-being. The same principles hold for pilot Phase IIa clinical trials. Careful monitoring of patients is essential in all of these trials. Interim analysis should be considered for all Phase IIb well-controlled trials and for all large Phase III clinical trials. Long-term mortality or significant morbidity studies could often benefit from interim analyses, particularly for those clinical trials with important national health policy implications and for those with the ethical requirement of a Data Review Committee (see Chapter 17).

STATISTICAL PENALTIES FOR CONDUCTING AN INTERIM ANALYSIS

This discussion presents the principle behind statistical penalties, but none of the mathematical details. Those details may be obtained from statisticians and the relevant literature. The concept of a statistical penalty is based on the fact that the more analyses conducted on a set of data, the greater the chance of finding a treatment effect, even if no effect exists. If data obtained in a clinical trial are examined periodically, it is likely that at least some analyses will yield statistically significant results. To compensate for this trend, the significance level at which the data are said to be statistically significant becomes progressively smaller the more times one looks at the data. It therefore becomes more and more difficult for the results to achieve higher statistical requirements (i.e., lower p value). For example, if a $p = 0.05$ was the level of statistical significance for only a single look, smaller p values would be necessary at each of the other looks. Whether these higher plateaus of statistical significance are considered acceptable to justify the clinical interim analysis must be carefully evaluated. Prior to initiating the clinical trial, one must decide exactly how many interim analyses are appropriate and justified.

The author believes that no penalty should be required if it is stated in advance that the interim analysis (to evaluate efficacy) will not affect the conduct of the clinical trial itself and in fact the trial is shown not to be affected. Thus, the clinical trial would not be stopped or modified because of a positive finding between two (or more) treatment groups. This type of statistical analysis would still be invaluable, if it was conducted for other reasons (e.g., to plan other studies). If there is even a small possibility that a clinical trial will be modified after interim analysis, the concept of a penalty is relevant.

The above comments do not apply to safety evaluations, since any clinical trial in which patients are exposed to unacceptable levels of risk must be stopped. This determination could be made by a Data Review Committee based on safety parameters measured in an interim analysis conducted for either safety or efficacy reasons.

REGULATORY CONSIDERATIONS OF INTERIM ANALYSES

Protocol Statements

The protocol should state the objectives of the interim analysis, which variables will be analyzed, the number of interim analyses to be conducted, and what types of decision options are to be considered. The existence (or not) of a Data Review Committee should be mentioned and its makeup described. The makeup may be described in terms of the types of people who will be on the committee and their affiliation with the sponsor and clinical trial staff. Termination rules must be described in full.

Regulatory Authority's Perspective

Regulatory authorities are concerned about how companies peek at their data and appropriately insist that any interim analysis be reported in a final medical report. The implications of the analysis(es) on the clinical trial's interpretation must also be dealt with in an appropriate and ethical manner. Regulatory authorities

recognize that many interim analyses are unreported in the published literature, but also are not used to modify the conduct of clinical trials. Each situation in which an interim analysis is conducted varies along the spectra shown in Fig. 69.1.

Sponsor's Perspective

It simplifies regulatory considerations for a sponsor if interim analyses are not performed, since questions may be raised at a later date that could place data from an important clinical trial in jeopardy. For example, if a clinical trial's data base is not yet completed, an interim analysis could be conducted for a more rapid evaluation. This would generally be unwise because the premise on which "no statistical penalty" would be based could be challenged by a regulatory authority at a later date.

Investigator's Perspective

Most nonsponsored clinical trials are never evaluated by formal interim analyses of the data. In those few that are, there are rarely any regulatory considerations.

HOW MANY INTERIM ANALYSES SHOULD BE CONDUCTED?

The appropriate number of interim analyses is both a statistical and practical question. The statistical aspects depend on which methods are chosen (e.g., repeat the significance tests and adjust alpha levels, use group sequential methods, use stochastic methods) and whether a statistical penalty must be paid. Practical aspects depend on the resources required and available to conduct the exercise.

The results of an interim analysis are usually prepared for the assessment and review of a specific person, group, or groups. Any decision to modify an ongoing clinical trial should be made with the full understanding of the ramifications it will have from regulatory, scientific, ethical, and other perspectives.

Continual Modifications to a Clinical Trial

It is unacceptable for an investigator to update a data base and modify any clinical trial on a continual basis. Even an open-label clinical trial would not be the same for one patient as for the next. When frequent interim analyses are desirable, it is possible to refer to the clinical trial as a pilot in which the optimal design is being developed. At a certain point in time, a new, more definitive clinical trial may be designed and initiated.

A similar situation often arises during the period when a medical device is being developed. Frequent engineering or materials modifications to the device itself, even with the same protocol, yield data that cannot (i.e., should not) be combined.

SELECTED ISSUES AND QUESTIONS

Informal Interim Analyses

Some interim statistical analyses are not considered "official" and are therefore not reported when the final analyses are conducted and the medical report prepared. To avoid conducting "official interim analyses," some investigators or sponsors will have analyses performed by nonstatisticians on informally gathered data that are not quality assured or rigorously reviewed. This may lead to a decision to modify a clinical trial that is not wise or correct, because it is based on incomplete, distorted, or incorrect data.

Should an Interim Analysis Maintain the Clinical Trial's Blind?

The blind in a clinical trial does not have to be broken when conducting an interim analysis. The blind may be maintained by referring to groups of patients by number or letter. Even after the analysis is complete and the data are reviewed by a Data Monitoring Committee that is considering clinical trial termination (or other possibilities), the groups could still be considered in terms of designated codes rather than by the actual treatments received.

If the data are to be used to modify a protocol or to plan additional clinical trials, the analysis should usually be conducted on unblinded data, or the code of the treatment groups should be broken after the interim analysis is complete. This issue should be considered and discussed prior to conducting the interim analysis because unblinding a clinical trial with interim analyses may introduce biases and compromise the trial's integrity.

Other Issues

1. Should a Data Review Committee be established to review the results of the interim analysis (see Chapter 17)?
2. How much data cleanup and quality assurance should be done during the processing of the data? The resources available for this effort and the time it will take must be considered, along with the importance of the interim analysis.
3. Who is authorized to conduct unplanned analyses of the data? How will these be controlled and results reviewed?
4. If termination of a clinical trial is being considered because of efficacy observed with a treatment, ensure that other variables do not allow a different interpretation. If so, then the clinical trial may fail to convince medical professionals and will lose most or all of its value.

CHAPTER 70

Statistical Issues

An extremely large number of statistical issues could be discussed without using formulas, equations, or detailed statistical reasoning. A selected number of issues were arbitrarily chosen for this chapter. The topic of interim analyses was felt to be so important that a separate chapter (Chapter 69) is devoted to this single issue. Also, a separate chapter explores Simpson's paradox (Chapter 75) because of its importance in questioning the premise that common sense reasoning is always appropriate. Statistical issues (e.g., data transformations expressing results as percents) are also discussed in numerous other chapters (see index for details). The following issues are somewhat interrelated, but the sections that follow are meant to be independent.

DEFINITIONS OF ERRORS AND TYPES OF STATISTICS

Type I and Type II Errors. Since types I and II errors are described and defined in virtually every book on statistics or clinical methods, definition by analogy is given here. If a weapons detector at an airport indicates that you are carrying a weapon, but you are not, that is a type I error (i.e., a false alarm). If the detector does not indicate you have a weapon (but you do), that is a type II error (i.e., a false negative). Another simple analogy is that a type I error occurs when the data suggest you have the disease, but you do not, and a type II error occurs when the data do not state you have the disease, but you do. It must be stressed that when the weapons detector or disease data are correct, then no error has occurred. This is the desired state from a statistician's, and also from a clinician's, perspective.

Types of Statistics. Statistics may be classified as descriptive, traditional analytic, or Bayesian analytic. Descriptive statistics use text and noncomparative techniques to analyze data and also may overlap the field of data interpretation. Analytical statistics use mathematical formulae, models, and tests to analyze data. Bayesian statistics also consider other events, data, and information from the past and incorporates that information when analyzing data. A comparison between classical and Bayesian approaches to statistics is presented by Gehan (1988).

497

SPECIFYING IN A CLINICAL PROTOCOL WHICH STATISTICAL ANALYSES WILL BE USED

The Argument in Favor

There are two general approaches toward specifying the type of analysis beforehand. One group of statisticians and clinical trial methodologists believes that a detailed presentation of the statistical methods and tests that will be used to analyze data from a clinical trial should be given in the protocol. This approach is designed to provide assurance that the statisticians did not use several approaches after the clinical trial was complete and simply chose the approach that made the data look best to prove the trial's hypothesis.

The Argument Against

The other group of professionals believes that only brief descriptions of the analyses to be used should be included in a protocol and that most details are unnecessary. This is because the data must be evaluated after the clinical trial is completed to ensure that their characteristics (i.e., distribution, number of missing data) justify use of the intended statistical tests and methods. Only after this step confirms that the planned methods are appropriate may they be used. If it is learned that the data from two or more sites differ in one or more characteristics, then alternative tests and methods must be found to use for data analyses. Therefore, the professionals who espouse this approach reason that it is not worthwhile going into detail in a protocol when the methods described may never be used, and the methods used may be unknown before the clinical trial is completed.

The Counterargument

The counterargument to this last view is that most statisticians assume that the data they receive after completion of a clinical trial do fit the characteristics anticipated, and they do not usually test the data to confirm this assumption. The lack of confirmation occurs because it is a time-consuming and expensive process to conduct, and no one is insisting that it must be done.

A Compromise

A reasonable solution to the dilemma described above is to indicate the proposed statistical methods with a moderate number of details in a protocol, but be willing to test the data if they appear different than expected in important characteristics (e.g., distribution). If it is anticipated that uncommonly used statistical tests will be necessary, it is essential to indicate those tests in the protocol. If this is not done, then regulatory agencies may question whether their use was based on an after the fact decision.

HOW LARGE SHOULD SAMPLE SIZES BE?

Sample size strongly influences the power of a clinical trial. The importance of utilizing sample sizes that provide sufficient power to detect an effect, if one truly exists, is discussed elsewhere in this book. *The point to stress is that it is necessary to have sample size determined by statisticians rather than relying solely on the investigator's clinical experiences or judgment.* While clinical experience or judgment is of inestimable value in diagnosing and treating patients, it can, at best only aid a statistician in determining the number of patients to enroll in a clinical trial. Clinical judgment is also valuable in estimating the magnitude of difference between the two treatment groups in the key end-point(s) of a trial, those that would encourage a physician to use the medicine in other patients.

The choice of sample size is based on the (1) desired power, (2) magnitude of difference desired to be detected, and (3) magnitude of the parameter in the control group. Choosing a sample size that is too large will tend to demonstrate statistically significant differences between groups that are not clinically significant.

INTENTION TO TREAT VERSUS OTHER TYPES OF ANALYSES

One of the most heated discussions in medical statistics today focuses on the situations in which it is necessary to conduct an intention-to-treat analysis. A related issue is whether a different analysis may be more valid than an intention-to-treat analysis. A strong case for intention-to-treat analysis is given by Armitage (1983).

Example of an Intention-To-Treat Analysis

Sackett et al. (1985) describe a case in which 16 patients in a study were "not available for follow-up" because of stroke or death during initial hospitalization. These patients were excluded from the analysis in Table 70.1. All but one were originally allocated to the surgery group in which ten patients suffered strokes and five others died *during* or *shortly after* surgery. When all 16 patients were reentered into the analysis, the data appeared totally different. This is a clear example of exclusion of patients from the analysis leading to a misleading interpretation of the results. The principle of including all patients in the analysis

TABLE 70.1 *Surgical versus medical therapy in bilateral carotid stenosis[a]*

	Rate of subsequent TIA[b], stroke, or death
A. Outcome among patients "available for follow-up"	
Medical therapy:	53/72 = 74%
Surgical therapy:	43/79 = 54%

$$\text{Risk reduction} = \frac{74\% - 54\%}{74\%} = 27\% \ (p = 0.02)$$

B. Outcome among all patients randomized[c]	
Medical therapy:	54/73 = 74%
Surgical therapy:	58/94 = 62%

$$\text{Risk reduction} = \frac{74\% - 62\%}{74\%} = 16\% \ (p = 0.09)$$

[a] Modified from table of Sackett et al. (1985) with permission.
[b] TIA, transient ischemic attack.
[c] The additional 16 patients had a stroke or died during their original hospitalization and were excluded from analysis. Fifteen of these 16 were in the surgery group. Moreover, five died and ten suffered strokes during or shortly after surgery. These data illustrate the importance of considering all patients who are randomized to treatment and not just those available for follow-up.

who are randomized to treatment, regardless of what occurs during the clinical trial, is referred to as intention to treat.

The Basis for Intention-To-Treat Analyses

Intention to treat means that all data from all patients are included in the analysis (in the group to which they were randomized), even if they never received the medicine. The concept of intention to treat has a great deal of validity in many clinical trials and is important in understanding results. A few years ago many patients were excluded from analyses of clinical trials for any one of many reasons. Examples include patients who (1) were later found not to have met entry criteria, (2) were found to be noncompliers, (3) did not attend all clinic visits, (4) moved, (5) had other illnesses, or (6) dropped out of the clinical trial before its completion. Excluding patients from efficacy analyses for any of these (or numerous other) reasons may initially seem reasonable but would often lead to excluding a large percent of enrolled patients. The analysis of a small subsection of patients who meet all criteria for inclusion is not reasonable from either a statistical or clinical perspective. The basis for this statement is presented below.

Excluding Patients Who Do Not Meet Entry Criteria

Patients who are found after a clinical trial is completed not to have met entry criteria include those whose birth date, laboratory value, duration of illness, or values of any of many other criteria lie just outside the inclusion criteria, or even well outside those limits. If the major difference between the inclusion criterion's limit and the patient's value could have a clinically significant impact on achieving the clinical trial's objectives, or the patient's safety, then the patient should have been excluded before the clinical trial began. One exception is for results that were reported after the patient was enrolled; this often occurs in clinical trials. For example, if a patient is suspected of having a myocardial infarction, but all of the laboratory results will not be available for a few days, the patient is often enrolled on the basis of a suspected myocardial infarction. The same situation occurs if a patient has a suspected type of bacterial infection, but laboratory culture results will not be ready for a day or two. Such patients are entered, treated, and later may be found to have been improperly included (i.e., they did not meet the inclusion criteria). The data from these patients are sometimes eliminated from the clinical trial's efficacy analyses, because the medicine could not have been expected to help these patients.

Is it acceptable to exclude such patients from an efficacy analysis? Definitely not! To exclude them opposes the purpose of the clinical trial: to evaluate how well the medicine acts in patients suspected of having the problem being treated. What would happen if all patients who were found not to have the problem were excluded from the data analysis and the medicine had a marked beneficial effect in those few entered who actually had the disease? The result would be relatively clean data and a great paper. Physicians in private practice and in academic hospitals would read the paper and many would treat their patients as described therein. However, the results these practicing physicians would see in their private practice would be quite different from the published results. In the real world, physicians treat patients *suspected* of having a myocardial infarction or special type of bacterial infection, not just the confirmed cases. Therefore, they would be misled by the paper's conclusions. For example, if 96% of the suspected cases enrolled in the clinical trial were later found to have the problem, the trial situation would generally reflect what physicians in practice confront, but if only 4% of suspected cases enrolled in the clinical trial actually had the problem, the publication would mislead readers to a major degree. This is because only 1 of 25 patients suspected of having the problem would be expected to respond to the therapy. The physicians might have expected nearly 100% of their patients to respond to therapy based on the published data. The assumption made by physicians is that patients treated in the original clinical trial would be the general types that would also be treated by other physicians.

Excluding Other Groups of Patients From Efficacy Analyses

The dilemmas over whether to exclude noncompliers, dropouts, and other groups of patients from efficacy analyses are generally similar. Cleaner data often result, but many of the types of patients who would be given the new treatment by other physicians in practice might be excluded from the data analysis. A distorted view of the treatment's efficacy could result. If a drug had a bitter taste and only 10% of the patients in a clinical trial were adequately complying with the protocol, this is extremely important to know. Solely stating that compliant patients had spectacular efficacy results is less important, even if the data are compared with those of poor compliers. Part of the appropriate approach is to do subgroup analyses after a clinical trial to illustrate how different strata of patients responded to treatment.

Can Intention-To-Treat Analyses Be Carried too Far?

It is believed that intention-to-treat analyses are sometimes pursued too far. Some propose that once a patient is randomized to a treatment group and drops out of a clinical trial, his or her data should be included as a medicine failure, even if the patient drops out *without ever having taken any medicine*. The author believes that a patient should only truly be considered as "in" the clinical trial itself when the first dose of medicine is taken or the first step of therapy is initiated. Other methodologists want to state that a patient enters the clinical trial (and by extension, his or her data must be included in an intent-to-treat analysis) at the signing of the informed consent, or at the initiation of baseline.

Some uses of intention-to-treat analyses make little clinical sense. For example, a patient with angina who is assigned to medical treatment but who crosses over to surgical treatment of his or her own volition is classified as a medical failure (and in some clinical trials as a "death" on the medical regimen). This truly muddies the data when one wishes to answer the question of which treatment is better—surgical or medical. Consequences of intention-to-treat analyses that result in this type of complex interpretation should be considered in advance of the clinical trial.

Importance of Background Noise

Background noise in a clinical trial from effects of the disease, concomitant illnesses, concomitant medicines, and so forth are a part of all trials. Trying to sanitize clinical trial results and eliminate noise by excluding specific patient groups does not help practicing physicians make the best decisions in the future when they treat all types of patients.

Conclusions

Intention-to-treat analyses should be prepared on data from most clinical trials, unless there is a sound reason not to do so. Other types of analyses may also be prepared. If the results of different analyses lead to different interpretations, then carefully check the comparability of the treatment groups in both data sets and seek the reasons for the difference(s) in results. There is no reason that both analyses cannot be described in a publication or presented in a regulatory submission. This helps readers better understand and interpret the data. The alternate analysis should not be viewed as an inferior one if a strong statistical case can be presented for its use.

IMPUTATION OF DATA

Definition

Often a patient is unable (or unwilling) to keep a scheduled clinic visit. The investigator may reschedule or cancel the visit. In the latter case, no data are available for that visit. Alternatively, a biological sample may be lost, destroyed, or may not yield valid results. When this patient's data are combined with those of others, there may or may not be an important consequence. One practice suggested by some authors is to adjust for missing data. Such adjustment can take the form of calculating the missing datum (i.e., *imputing* it) and using this value to fill the "hole" in the data set. For example, if laboratory values are not present at week 3, but are present at weeks 1, 2, 4, 5, and 6, values are calculated for the missing week. This practice leads to a complete data set for each patient to use when results from all patients are combined.

How Are Data Imputed?

The most usual method of imputing data is to average the values that occurred immediately prior to and after the missing value. The assumption is made that the missing value will lie between the two other values. Whether this is a reasonable assumption is often unknown. The validity of imputed data is particularly questionable if a long period of time has elapsed between the taking of the two values used to impute the missing number, or if the patient is clinically unstable.

Although the process of imputation described includes situations in which a patient missed an entire visit, imputation is more commonly used when only a limited number of values are missing. One laboratory test (or other test) may have been forgotten or omitted, or problems with laboratory equipment may have prevented the completion of all tests.

Guidelines for Imputation: Issues to Address

If a decision has been made to use imputation, then guidelines must be established to describe and limit its use. For example, if it is accepted to impute all values for a single patient visit, would it be acceptable to impute values for two successive missed clinic visits? What if the two visits were not consecutive? Which tests could be imputed and which not? Would both safety and efficacy parameters be fair game for imputation? The process of imputation definitely should not be considered until the statisticians and clinicians consider potential ramifications, including those at all regulatory agencies to whom the data will eventually be submitted. Any report of imputed data must describe what data were imputed and what method of imputation was used.

Other methods of imputing data, in addition to the use of averages, are available, but are not discussed here. Statistical procedures for imputing data and for analyzing results containing imputed data must be discussed with knowledgable statisticians. Any decision to use imputation should seriously consider comparing and publishing results of data analyses performed both with and without imputation. This practice will help convince readers that imputation has not qualitatively changed the trial's data and its interpretation. An example of imputation is presented by DeJonge (1983), who supports the concept. His example illustrates that imputation may have an enormous impact on a clinical trial's results. It is not clear, however, which set of results is more accurate and truthful.

A Counterargument

The practice of imputation of data is not supported by the author except in rare situations. The practice of *creating data* establishes a bad precedent that may be abused in a variety of ways. While the practice may make overall averages and data interpretations easier to derive, it does not make them more accurate. Moreover, an imputation may give a false impression if it obscures relevant facts (e.g., patients occasionally did not attend clinic because of problems related to the medicine).

CORRELATION COEFFICIENTS

Correlation coefficients test associations. Readers are supposed to be impressed when correlation coefficients are high and p values are significant. In numerous situations, however, correlation coefficients are low and nonsignificant, but the data may have great clinical importance. Some of these situations are listed in Table 70.2.

TABLE 70.2 *Reasons for a low correlation coefficient when data are clinically significant*

1. Relationship is not linear but curved
2. A few pairs of observations differ greatly from the rest
3. More than one pair of observations comes from one individual
4. A few of the groups that are mixed have quite different characteristics from the others

NUMBER OF STRATA USED TO ANALYZE DATA

In many clinical trials data are evaluated with subgroup analyses. Factors often evaluated in subgroup analyses are listed in Table 70.3. For many parameters tested (e.g., compliance, age, degree of improvement) it is possible to evaluate the data according to strata. For age, this could consist of two (e.g., above and under 65), three, or more strata. The more strata used, the fewer the number of patients there will be in each stratum. For large clinical trials, it is often possible to evaluate several or many strata to evaluate a parameter–response relationship. Thus, one could test the relationship for patients aged 0 to 20, 21 to 40, 41 to 60, and above 60 with any response of interest.

Avoiding Criticisms of the Choice of Strata

The number of strata used to evaluate data must be carefully assessed. For example, a recent study of over 4,000 patients used only two strata to test compliance. Serious questions can be raised about why only two strata were used and how the division between the two strata was chosen. Without supplying more information in a publication the suspicion will arise that multiple strata did not show the same relationship shown by using two strata, and also that the dividing line between the two strata was adjusted to show the greatest difference.

TABLE 70.3 *Selected factors to evaluate in subgroup analyses relating to either safety or efficacy endpoints[a]*

1. Age
2. Sex
3. Race
4. Concurrent illnesses
5. Concomitant treatments
6. Severity of disease at baseline
7. Response to previous therapy
8. Length of current illness or episode
9. Total length of disease
10. Dose of medicine
11. Each prognostic characteristic
12. Weight
13. Any other characteristic that appears relevant from a perusal of the data
14. Plasma level of medicine
15. Time to respond to therapy
16. Duration of therapy
17. Magnitude of clinical response
18. Decreased organ function
19. Investigational site
20. Season of the year

[a] Any of these could be the major objective of a clinical trial and thus would be part of a subgroup analysis. Also, almost any two of these could interact and be related to a safety or efficacy endpoint.

PART VI

Fundamental Principles, Considerations, and Techniques in the Interpretation of Clinical Data

The mind is an iceberg—it floats with only one-seventh of its bulk above water.

—*Sigmund Freud*

The foolish and the dead alone never change their opinions.

—*James Russell Lowell*

It is easier to fight for principles than to live up to them.

—*Alfred Adler*

Facts are not pure and unsullied bits of information; culture also influences what we see and how we see it. Theories, moreover, are not inexorable inductions from facts. The most creative theories are often imaginative visions imposed upon facts; the source of imagination is also strongly cultural.

—*Stephen Jay Gould*

CHAPTER 71

Summary of Principles and Procedures to Follow

INTRODUCTION

Interpretation denotes the process of discerning the clinical meaning or significance of or providing an explanation for data that are being evaluated. The term *data* usually refers to data collected from patients entered in a clinical trial. Numerous aspects of clinical data usually require an interpretation within the broad categories of safety or efficacy.

The major assumptions made in the descriptions given of data interpretation are that this process usually occurs after the clinical trial is completed and the data have been analyzed (usually statistically). The major procedures that are conducted prior to, and subsequent to, the clinical interpretation of data are illustrated in Fig. 71.1. Although each of the processes is shown as a separate event, there is often some overlap between two or more. Analyses of data are primarily

505

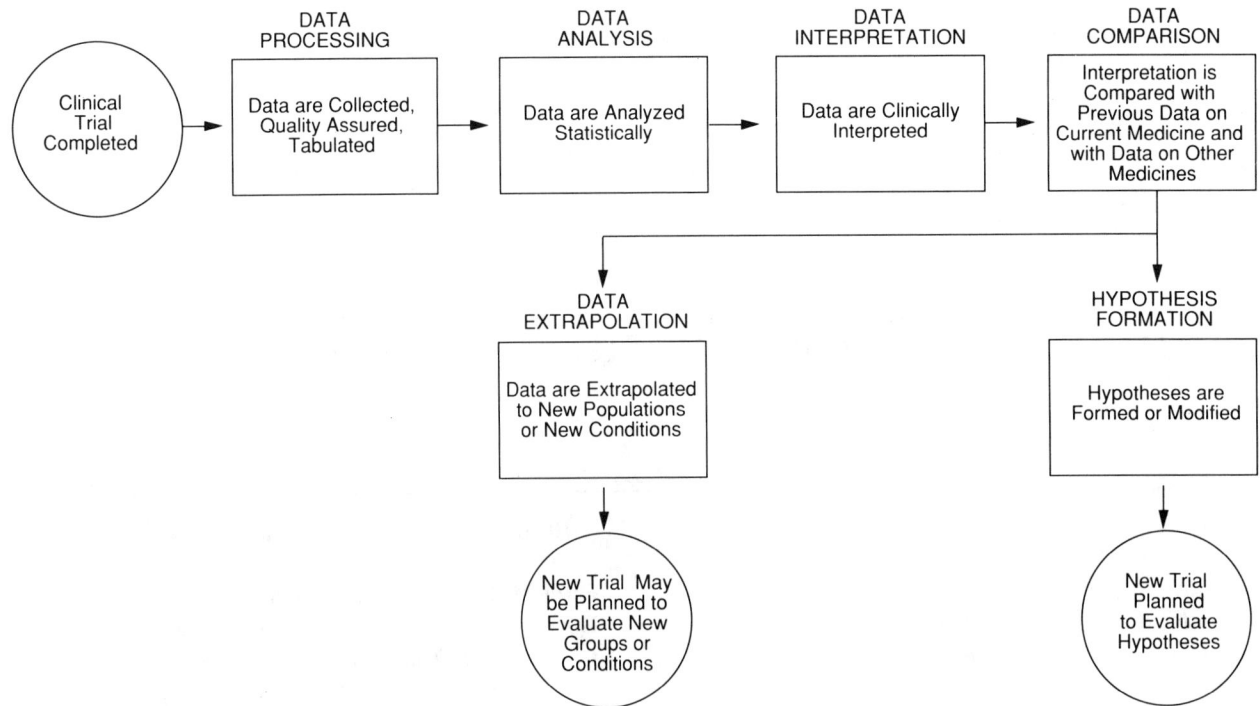

FIG. 71.1 Procedures to conduct after completion of a clinical trial.

statistical exercises, and the interpretation of data is primarily a clinical exercise. The same individual(s) may be associated with several (or all) of the steps shown. Also, the time between any two steps may be extremely short or prolonged.

A circular (or spiral-like) process is alluded to but not emphasized. This refers to the fact that interpretation of data from one clinical trial often leads to and contributes to the development of a follow-up trial, which generates data whose interpretation often leads to an additional trial, and so on (Fig. 71.1).

The Major Axiom of Clinical Interpretation

This entire book is based on the axiom that data analysis, data interpretation, and the extrapolation of data are three separate processes. The influences of one on the other and their interactions are described in many chapters.

Who Interprets Clinical Data?

Clinical interpretation of clinical data is performed by various individuals connected with a trial, including the investigator, the sponsor (for sponsored trials), and/or other individuals who evaluate the data. The sponsor of a medicine trial is primarily concerned with discerning the clinical significance of the data for its relevance in medicine development or evaluation; the academic clinical investigator is usually primarily con-

cerned with treatment of his patients, plus issues relating to publications, grants, and career opportunities. The primary care physician is mainly concerned with the significance of the data for its relevance in treating his or her patients.

Orientation of Interpretations

This book is primarily oriented toward the interpretation of clinical data insofar as it affects development of medicines. The topic of patient treatment, however, is considered throughout the text and is specifically addressed in several chapters, including that on clinical judgment.

Clinical investigators usually hope to attain an accurate understanding of the data, which may be extrapolated to other patients or situations. The process of extrapolation is dependent on many factors, the most important being an accurate interpretation of the data.

GOALS OF INTERPRETATION

Three major goals in clinically interpreting data are (1) to establish the most meaningful and relevant significance (i.e., importance) of the clinical trial overall, (2) to relate the results (i.e., data) to the original objectives of the trial, and (3) to compare data from the trial with data obtained in other trials. It is possible to consider additional goals after the data have been interpreted.

These include developing a hypothesis that may be evaluated in future trials and extrapolating the data to particular patients, environments, and types of treatment. Other goals are to assess the clinical significance the data have for the diagnosis, treatment, or prevention of disease in the patients studied or in other patient groups. Finally, the data may provide insight into interpretation of the nature of characteristics of the disease itself. The eventual goal of many trials is to attain an improvement in the practice of medicine.

PERSPECTIVES

Differentiating Between Data Analysis, Interpretation, and Extrapolation

It is important to differentiate between the processes of data analysis, data interpretation, and data extrapolation. The first involves primarily statistical procedures and evaluations, whereas the latter two are primarily clinical and do not necessarily require statistics. Interpretation and extrapolations of data require clinical judgment and often scientific logic. *It is the author's contention that data analysis, data interpretation, and data extrapolation are distinct processes.* Although two different individuals usually conduct these processes, they may be conducted by the same individual. Days or months may elapse between the two processes, or only a few milliseconds between analysis and interpretation or between interpretation and extrapolation.

Clinical interpretation primarily involves determining whether the results affirm the objectives or purposes of the clinical trial. This initially involves confirming that the treatment groups are comparable in terms of relevant demographic and other characteristics. Interpretation also involves a determination of clinical significance and relevance of data for patients treated in the trial.

Three Major Perspectives

The three major perspectives used to interpret data are discussed: (1) statistical significance, (2) clinical significance, and (3) relevance for medical practice. Interpretation begins when a clinical trial is completed; the data have been collected, edited, and entered in a computer; appropriate statistical tests have been used to analyze the data; and the statistical report has been written. At this stage the data must be interpreted.

Statistical Significance

Statistical significance on its own does not provide information on whether a data set is important for pa-

tients, and if so, how important. Clinical significance must be evaluated separately, although there is often a relationship between statistical significance and clinical significance.

Clinical Significance

The criteria used to evaluate clinical significance in terms of a medicine's efficacy are best established before a clinical trial begins. This is most often done by addressing the following question: How large a response in the most important parameter(s) measured would be necessary to convince physicians to use the clinical trial medicine or nonmedicine test therapy in treating their patients? This question may also be phrased in terms of a benefit-to-risk ratio. For example, what type and magnitude of patient response would be necessary for this medicine to have a greater benefit-to-risk ratio than that of other medicines (or nonmedicine treatments) used for the same indication? Other forms of the question may be raised that relate to safety, compliance, quality of life, or other characteristics. Each question involves comparisons with standard treatments, placebo, or the physicians' perceptions.

If the amount of change of an essential parameter necessary to achieve clinical significance is unknown, a group of physicians may be asked for their opinions. Although one might guess that their responses would be randomly distributed, experience has shown that such responses usually cluster in a given region. This is not surprising if one assumes that there is a value for a parameter's change that is clinically significant. If this exercise is conducted prior to a clinical trial it generally yields a response related to the specific disease being treated, and not to the specific medicine being tested. Hence, the amount of change of a critical parameter caused by any new medicine must equal or surpass the change caused by existing therapy. Exceptions might be for medicines with an important advantage not possessed by existing therapy, such as an improved quality of life or improved safety profile.

Relevance for Medical Practice

Relevance of data for medical practice means: What are the implications of the data for treating other patients? This is another way of stating that data from a clinical trial, from a group of trials, or even from a single patient must be extrapolated to new situations, new patients, and new conditions. Asking the question of how important or relevant the data are for other clinical situations may lead to a different interpretation from that based on the group of patients treated.

Extrapolation of Clinical Data

Extrapolation of data involves the determination of what the interpretation means in terms of treatment (or prevention) of disease, for different (1) patients, (2) physicians, (3) settings, (4) times, or (5) levels of interpretation. These points are discussed later in this chapter and in Chapter 90.

OVERALL OUTCOMES OF RESULTS OBTAINED IN CLINICAL TRIALS

At the most general level, the outcome of results obtained in a clinical trial may be viewed as either (1) positive, (2) negative, or (3) inconclusive. A few major types of each of these outcomes are described below.

Types of Positive (or Negative) Results

Positive (or negative) results obtained in clinical trials may be described in terms of three main types:

1. Well-designed, well-conducted, and well-analyzed clinical trials that demonstrate significant differences between treatments tested.
2. Poorly designed clinical trials that demonstrate significant (or nonsignificant) differences between treatments tested. The possibility that this outcome represents a false-positive (-negative) result cannot be excluded, even though the clinical trial may have been well conducted and well analyzed. For example, if too few patients were enrolled, the outcome might be a false positive (negative).
3. Well-designed but poorly conducted or poorly analyzed clinical trials that demonstrate significant (or nonsignificant) differences between treatments tested. The outcome might be a true-positive (-negative) or a false-positive (-negative) result.

Types of Inconclusive Outcomes

1. *Incomplete clinical trials.* These usually yield inconclusive results.
2. *Equivalence clinical trials.* These have an active control group and, rarely, a placebo or other control group. They are designed to show no difference between treatments. If this outcome occurs, then, to a small or large degree, the results are inconclusive. However, if the sample size is large enough and the efficacy of the active control is thoroughly established, then this result may be viewed as a positive result.
3. *Open-label clinical trials.* Negative results in an open-label clinical trial are usually more meaningful than positive results. Chapter 4 describes some

TABLE 71.1 *Classification of factors (sources of variability) that may bias data or affect their interpretation[a]*

1. Characteristics of the clinical trial design
2. Characteristics of patients
3. Characteristics of the disease or problem being evaluated
4. Characteristics of the clinical trial medicine(s)
5. Characteristics of the investigator and his staff
6. Characteristics of the environment
7. Conduct of the clinical trial
8. Characteristics of the tests and measures used
9. Statistical factors
10. Characteristics of data presentation and report
11. Errors of deceit committed accidentally or purposely before, during, or after the clinical trial
12. Other or unknown factors

[a] Each of these sources of variability represents a family or group of factors that are listed and described in Chapter 83.

of the reasons why positive outcomes in open-label trials must be interpreted with some skepticism.

4. *Case studies or poorly controlled clinical trials.* Clinical trials conducted using designs at the lower end of the "validity hierarchy" (Table 73.1) are more suspect in their results than better designed and controlled clinical trials.
5. When multiple endpoints of efficacy or safety are used and some yield positive results and others negative ones, the overall outcome of a clinical trial can be difficult to interpret, like the drawing in Fig. 71.2, which may be viewed as either a goblet or face. Situations like this should be avoided by carefully defining the criteria for success in advance. This problem may (and should) be prevented in most efficacy clinical trials by defining the specific criteria of a responder in advance.

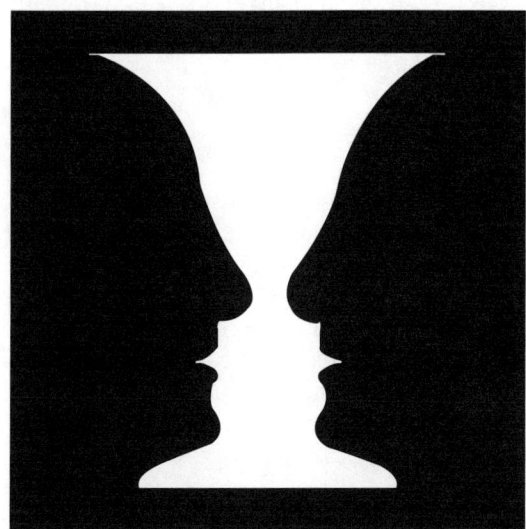

FIG. 71.2 A picture that can be interpreted in either of two ways.

Nonetheless, outcomes in a gray area may still occur.

6. The outcome may be statistically significant but the clinical significance may be uncertain.

COMPONENTS OF THE OVERALL CLINICAL RESPONSE

Although the clinical response of a specific patient is usually measured using single or multiple endpoints and/or parameters, an overall clinical response is observed by the investigator. A patient's overall clinical response is usually composed of two or more factors, such as those illustrated in Fig. 71.3. Each of these factors may lead to either improvement or deterioration, although some, such as the placebo effect, usually lead to an improvement. Not only is the patient's overall clinical response a summation of a number of these factors, but there may be a complex interaction between any two or more that makes it difficult if not impossible to separate out and accurately measure each individual factor. Utilizing separate treatment groups or specifically chosen trial designs is the most frequent means to obtain information on the importance and relevant role of the specific factors.

Sources of Clinical Variability

Well-designed clinical trials attempt to control the major sources of variation that could affect the data.

Well-designed trials are essential in certain stages of development to demonstrate efficacy. Well-designed trials also provide an opportunity to evaluate which sources of variation are important to measure and to understand better.

It is often useful to compile a list of relevant sources of variability that are believed to affect the data collected. This list could function as a guide both for interpreting data and for preparing an article for publication or for evaluating other articles on similar topics. There are many different categories of factors to be considered (see Table 71.1) and large numbers of potential factors within each category. A list of potential influences on the interpretation of data (see Chapter 83) provides the investigator with an overall guide to use when evaluating the clinical significance of the data.

Before a clinical trial is initiated, the originator(s) must consider many possible sources of variability. For instance, if the sex of the patient receiving treatment is thought to be an important variable (i.e., one that will affect the trial's outcome), then a decision might be made to randomize men and women separately to treatment groups. This procedure would equalize (or approximately equalize) the number of men (and women) in each group. Alternatively, a decision might have been made to analyze the data after the trial is completed for possible sex-related differences, in the hope that if any differences in response are observed, the numbers of men and women will be equally divided among treatment groups.

COMPONENTS OF OVERALL CLINICAL RESPONSE		CLINICAL EFFECT DURING TRIAL	
		Deterioration	Improvement
Natural Progression of Disease		and	/or
Nonmedicine Factors	+	and	/or
Concomitant Medicine(s)	+	?	
Nonmedicine Treatment(s)	+	?	
Placebo Response to Trial Medicine	+	?	
Biological Effects of Trial Medicine	+	?	

FIG. 71.3 Major components of the overall clinical response. The overall magnitude of the total clinical response varies during the clinical trial. There may be changes in the magnitude of any individual component during the trial, and there may be interactions between these components that will influence the observed clinical effect. The "?" symbol indicates that clinical deterioration usually does not result from that cause. The source of the deterioration (e.g., concomitant medicine, nonmedicine treatment) is usually removed after being identified. Observed clinical effect = "sum" of above components.

Outpatient versus Inpatient Trials

Data obtained in inpatient trials cannot always be interpreted (or extrapolated) to outpatients. An impeccably conducted trial of a new medicine compared with placebo in inpatients could unequivocally demonstrate that a medicine was clinically effective, but these data would not demonstrate that the same medicine would be effective if given to outpatients.

Some of the many sources of variability that are not usually present in inpatient trials and that will affect an outpatient trial include (1) diet, (2) exercise, (3) sleep, (4) environmental factors, (5) personal relationships, (6) stress, (7) concomitant medicines, and (8) compliance with the protocol. Unless these factors are controlled and/or evaluated in outpatient trials, a flawed trial may result, and it may not be possible to convince physicians to modify their therapeutic practices based on data obtained in inpatients.

Figure 71.3 illustrates the major possible components of a clinical effect observed in a trial. These include the natural history of the disease, placebo response of medicine, concomitant medications or therapy, personal factors, plus the response due to the medicine itself. It can be difficult to determine how much of a patient's response is due to the medicine, and how much to other factors. During a clinical trial that continues over a number of days or longer, any of these factors may vary in a simple or complex way. Simple or complex interactions between these factors may also occur, and may vary during the duration of the clinical trial. The "?" symbol in the figure indicates that clinical deterioration may, but does not usually, result from that cause.

Determining the Magnitude of the Placebo Response

Assume that one is interpreting the clinical response to a medicine in a double-blind clinical trial. When determining the magnitude of the effect due to a medicine, it is usual to subtract the magnitude of the effect observed in the placebo-treated group from that observed in the medicine-treated group. This is usually done on a group basis to obtain the "true" medicine response. The scientific evidence to support this practice is almost nonexistent, but few authors have questioned it. Little information is available about how the additional factors (shown in Fig. 71.3) actually interact. It is, therefore, naive to simply subtract the placebo response from the total response to obtain the medicine response. Unfortunately, no satisfactory solution to this issue has been proposed.

Including a No-Treatment Group

The patient's underlying disease is often assumed to remain constant throughout a clinical trial. This concept is sometimes tested, but in most trials it is not. Patients who have marked deterioration (or sometimes improvement) during a trial demonstrate that the status of their underlying problem has changed. In some situations a "no-treatment" group of patients who are merely observed would be an appropriate control group to study. This three-arm clinical trial (i.e., medicine, placebo, and no-treatment) would allow the extent of the disease's change to be evaluated and also the effect of placebo.

TYPES OF CLINICAL DATA

No single classification of clinical data is universally accepted. The simplest is to discuss data as related to safety or efficacy. While this differentiation is generally useful, it is also incomplete. Other categories of clinical data include pharmacokinetics, quality of life, compliance, and pharmacoeconomics. These categories may overlap and other categories of clinical data may also be defined.

CLINICAL SIGNIFICANCE OF DATA VERSUS THEIR STATISTICAL SIGNIFICANCE

In most clinical situations the statistical significance and clinical significance of the data are either both positive or they are not. If there is a clinically significant effect it is usually statistically significant and vice versa. Nonetheless, often one, but not both of these characteristics are positive. The four possible combinations are described below.

1. Statistical significance: Present (i.e., positive)
   Clinical significance: Present
2. Statistical significance: Present
   Clinical significance: Not present
3. Statistical significance: Not present
   Clinical significance: Present
4. Statistical significance: Not present
   Clinical significance: Not present

Variations could be described: clinical significance could be positive, equivocal, or negative (i.e., representing patient deterioration). These combinations could apply to data interpretation for a single patient, a single clinical trial, or a single medicine.

Both Statistical and Clinical Significance Are Positive

The first combination occurs when results of a clinical trial are both statistically and clinically significant. The most likely interpretation of this outcome is that the trial confirms the objectives. The data could also represent a false-positive effect.

Statistical Significance Is Positive but Clinical Significance Is Not

In the second combination statistical significance is positive, but clinical significance is not present. This is an extremely common occurrence that happens, for example, when (1) a vital sign changes by a small amount that is statistically significant because of the large number of measurements made, (2) the change in an efficacy parameter's amplitude is small, but statistically significant, often because of minimal variability, (3) the efficacy parameter changes at one or a few of many time points, but results are not consistent, (4) tolerance develops rapidly to a medicine, (5) the patient population studied was atypical, or (6) the parameters evaluated were not the most important ones indicative of activity.

A possible interpretation is that one of the results was false. The positive result might have occurred because too many measurements were made or the results occurred by chance (1 in 20 independent statistical tests will be positive because of chance alone). The failure to observe clinical significance might represent a false-negative result or be caused by confounding variables that may or may not be known.

Statistical Significance Is Absent but Clinical Significance Is Positive

A few examples of the third combination (no statistical significance, but clinical significance is positive) include (1) a positive treatment is found for a previously untreatable disease, (2) the number of observations are too small to achieve statistical significance, (3) the most appropriate parameter(s) was not measured, but an important clinical effect was observed, and (4) the most appropriate statistical tests or parameters were not used, but important clinical effects were observed.

Possible interpretations of this situation are that (1) there was an insufficient number of patients in the clinical trial, (2) an insufficient number of measurements were made, (3) inappropriate statistical tests were used, or (4) one or both results are false.

Both Statistical and Clinical Significance Are Negative

In the fourth combination, both statistical and clinical significance of data are negative. The most common interpretation is that no clinically important effect is present. Alternatively, one or both results could be a false negative. It is important to examine any unexpected negative results carefully and thoroughly to assure oneself that the data evaluated are not actually positive.

CLINICAL SIGNIFICANCE TO WHOM?

No single perspective may be used to evaluate clinical data and their clinical significance. The previous discussion described data primarily from the viewpoint of the investigator who collected the information, but there are other groups whose perspective may differ, including patients, treating physicians, pharmaceutical companies who sponsor clinical trials, and regulatory authorities.

Investigators and Treating Physicians. Investigators and treating physicians usually judge clinical significance by how well they are able to treat their patients. Other considerations for investigators relate to whether the data and publications will help their career and whether the money received will be sufficient to purchase new equipment, pay staff, or fund other clinical trials.

Patients. Patients usually judge clinical significance in terms of how a medicine affects their particular symptoms and quality of life. They want to know whether the medicine will help them feel better, help their disease, and prevent future problems. Some patients will appreciate benefits gained from reduction of risk factors. Judgment by a patient is usually based on their own personal experience.

Pharmaceutical Companies. Pharmaceutical companies judge clinical significance by whether the effect is of a sufficient magnitude and occurs in a sufficiently large population of patients to convince (1) national regulatory authorities to approve their medicine, (2) formulary committees to stock their medicine, and (3) physicians to prescribe their medicine. There is a heavy commercial slant to each of these judgments.

Regulatory Authorities. Regulatory authorities must interpret the clinical significance of a medicine in terms of how the medicine will affect their nation's health. The benefit-to-risk ratio, as well as the relative merits of alternative therapy, must be carefully considered. Medicines waiting to be approved are like high jumpers: the bar for each disease is set at a different height depending on the quality of available therapy. The bar becomes progressively higher for each new medicine, because other medicines and nonmedicine treatments that jumped before have improved on past performance of medical therapy and raised the standards. A specific standard height exists for safety and a different one for efficacy. A new medicine that raises one of the two bars by a large amount may not influence the other, or even cause it to be slightly lower under some conditions.

LEVELS OF EVALUATING CLINICAL SIGNIFICANCE

Although clinical importance has been described in terms of a medicine's effects in a single clinical trial or for a single patient, clinical significance may be evaluated on several levels. These levels include the following:

1. Single patient given a medicine.
2. Some or all patients in a single clinical trial given medicine.
3. Some or all patients currently receiving the medicine in all clinical trials as well as in clinical practice outside of formal trials.
4. Some or all patients who have received the medicine in the past.
5. Some or all patients with the target disease who are possible candidates to receive the medicine in the future.

CLINICAL SIGNIFICANCE OF TRIAL DATA VERSUS THEIR RELEVANCE FOR MEDICAL PRACTICE

Clinical trials have the greatest possibility of influencing medical practice if (1) the treatment is both medically and scientifically rational, (2) a dose–response relationship is observed for the most relevant parameters, (3) the response is clinically important in magnitude, (4) the effect is widespread in the patient population and not merely found in one or a few subgroups, and (5) the trial supports previous results.

Clinical trials generally have the least chance of influencing medical practice if (1) the major finding was an unexpected association found on subgroup analysis, (2) evidence of data dredging is present, (3) the results were not part of the trial's objectives, or (4) the results run counter to conventional medical practice.

Both clinical significance and medical practice relevance of data may be positive or only clinical significance may be positive. For example, assume that a clinical trial demonstrates a lowering of blood pressure in hypertensive patients by medicine X, and that the data are statistically significant. Further, assume that the data are clinically significant because all patients had falls in blood pressure greater than levels defined prior to the trial as clinically meaningful. The question to address is whether the data are relevant for medical practice. To answer this it is necessary to know some factors related to the relevance of medical practice.

Factors Affecting Relevance of Clinical Trial Data for Medical Practice

Relevance for medical practice depends on:

1. Availability of alternative therapy. If no treatment is available the medical practice relevance of a "poor" treatment may be high [e.g., the first investigational medicine reported in the media to treat patients with acquired immunodeficiency syndrome (AIDS), prior to Food and Drug Administration (FDA) approval of the medicine].
2. Suitability of alternative therapy. If the alternative therapy has serious deficiencies, then those characteristics will be important considerations in judging the medical practice relevance of a new medicine.
3. Capability of data to be extrapolated to a new situation. Some data lend themselves to the extrapolation process more easily than others.
4. Various other factors such as price, convenience, or adverse reactions of the medicine. Any of these factors could be an overriding factor in judging whether the data of a new medicine has relevance for medical practice.

Additionally, extrapolating data to other situations is not an all-or-none process. Most data may only be extrapolated to some situations, conditions, and patients. This may restrict the relevance of a clinical trial to a narrow spectrum of all possible aspects and types of medical practice.

Why Are Physicians Sometimes Unaffected by Clinical Trial Data That Are Relevant for Medical Practice?

Clinical trial data that are statistically significant, clinically significant, and relevant for medical practice are sometimes ignored by physicians and do not influence medical practice. It is important for pharmaceutical companies, professional medical societies, and others to consider why this is so. Companies desire to have their new medicines that possess medical advantages over existing treatment to be sold as widely as possible, and professional groups want their members to be using the most appropriate treatments.

Physicians may not be influenced by important clinical data and interpretations of a new medicine's effects for any of the following reasons.

1. They are unaware, or at least not fully aware of the significance and importance of the data. For example, are results of the clinical trial published, and if so, where? Also, are results of the trial widely discussed?
2. Results may be highly complex and unclear to the physician evaluating the report and data. This indicates the importance of presenting the results in a format that everyone can understand.
3. Results may not be consistent in all efficacy parameters or in all subgroups of patients studied.
4. The patients in the physician's practice may differ in one or more important ways from those entered in the clinical trials (e.g., outpatients versus inpatients, young versus old, mildly ill versus severely ill).

5. The clinical trials may have been conducted in other countries, in different types of patients, or by investigators from a different medical speciality. Physicians must believe that there is relevance for their present or future patients if they are to consider using the new therapy.

6. The physician's assessment of results may be counter to their own experiences and preferences. It is therefore important to know whether physicians accept the results as valid.

7. The treatment may be relatively new and not widely used. Many physicians are reluctant to use the "latest" treatment until their friends discuss their own experiences, colleagues or guests at local medical meetings discuss the medicine, or the company's sales representative describes the medicine.

8. The physician may be loath to change his established habits and methods of treating patients. The medicine may not address the particular aspects of the physician's current treatment that he considers a drawback.

9. There may be other drawbacks of the treatment (e.g., cost, adverse reactions, length of therapy).

Even if all of these points are considered and physicians believe in the new treatment, they represent only one-half of the total equation for using a new therapy. Patients must believe that they should visit a physician. Second, patients must follow through on their intentions and visit a physician. Third, they must fill the prescription given to them, and finally, they must comply with the advice of the physician and take the medicine as directed. This topic is discussed further in Chapter 132.

APPROACHES TO INTERPRETING DATA

After a clinical trial to evaluate a new medicine's efficacy is completed and the statistical analyses prepared, everyone wants to know "Did the medicine work?" They usually mean: "Is the response in the medicine-treated group of patients better than that observed in the placebo-treated group, or was the average response better on treatment than at baseline?"

Ten-Step Approach to Interpreting Clinical Data

A general ten-step approach to the interpretation of clinical data is given below. This approach is proposed for use after all data have been edited, processed, and analyzed statistically.

1. Compare the treatment groups in terms of demographic characteristics and prognostic factors. Statistically significant differences in demographics between the groups do not mean that the differences are clinically significant, but any differences mean that the parameter(s) should be carefully assessed. Differences in a critical prognostic factor can readily mean that the entire set of clinical trial data are worthless, or nearly so. Any demographic characteristic or prognostic disease factor that would be critical to the clinical trial should be used as a basis for randomization (e.g., mild and severe cases, or men and women, or low risk factor and high risk factor patients may be randomized separately). Alternatively, a different randomization system (e.g., minimization) should have been used. Other alternatives may be used to avoid having an important factor represented unequally in the treatment groups, which could invalidate the entire clinical trial.

2. Evaluate whether the data affirm or deny the primary objective(s) of the clinical trial. This is the real heart of the interpretation. It is important that the objectives be clearly indicated in the protocol before the clinical trial is initiated.

3. Evaluate whether the data affirm or deny the secondary objectives of the clinical trial.

4. Consider all the specific factors that may have influenced or biased the data and the interpretation reached.

5. Discuss the interpretation(s) with a statistician and other colleagues to determine whether any additional analyses or subgroup analyses should be conducted.

6. Adopt the "devil's advocate" perspective and strongly criticize one's own interpretation. Then evaluate each criticism and determine how it may be refuted or addressed. These evaluations or counterarguments will be helpful in the discussion section of a publication or report.

7. Compare the interpretations and data with those obtained using standard medicines or treatments. These may be obtained from data in the same clinical trial or from results in the published literature.

8. Discuss the interpretation with others and seek their input and reaction.

9. Extrapolate the interpretations to as many different patient populations, physicians, settings, levels of organization as may be justified and appropriate.

10. Develop hypotheses or plans to evaluate further new questions, issues, or models in future clinical trials.

Many of the subtleties and variations involved in each of these steps are discussed in other chapters. Step four of the general approach described above involves specific factors that may have affected the data or interpretation reached. These may be related to the

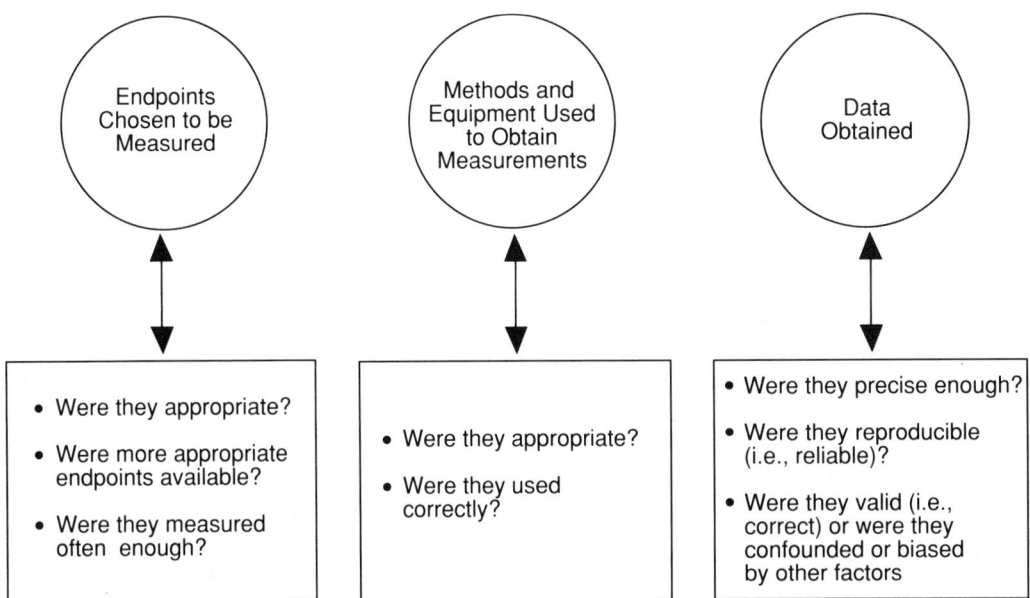

FIG. 71.4 General questions to pose about clinical trial data.

trial design, patients, medicine used, or several other categories (see Table 71.1). A detailed discussion of this topic, along with over 100 tables describing specific factors, is presented in Chapter 83. Figure 71.4 illustrates a variation on the approach described in this section.

DATA SETS OF DIFFERENT SIZES

Different types of data sets can be described along with possible approaches to deriving interpretations. The data sets described in this section are (1) a large quantity of heterogeneous or homogeneous data and (2) a small quantity of heterogeneous or homogeneous data.

Interpreting a Large Quantity of Data

Assume you have obtained 150 cartons of data on a new medicine you are licensing or will study. Difficulties may arise when an individual who is confronted with a vast amount of heterogeneous data does not know how to approach it to develop an interpretation. There are several ways that one may approach this situation. Even if the first approach appears to yield a meaningful interpretation, it is suggested that several of the other alternatives be followed (or at least considered) to determine whether an even "better" interpretation is possible. The same basic approaches may also be used for homogeneous data.

Before reviewing the data, it is important to determine which aspects of the data, or which data, are relevant. This decision is based primarily on the ob-

jectives of the clinical trials, which should be indicated in the protocols. If the objectives are not sufficiently delineated, it will generally be necessary to define more precisely exactly what objectives are to be addressed with the data.

Splitters. The first approach could be referred to as the "divide and conquer" or "splitter" method. In this system the data are divided (i.e., classified) into various well-defined categories, and each of the resulting smaller data sets is evaluated and interpreted separately. The first hurdle comes in choosing the categories that are to be considered. The categories may be obvious, but there is a reasonable probability that there will be more than one set of equally appropriate categories to consider. Under such circumstances a hierarchy should be created and followed so that each relevant category is tried, at least to the extent necessary to identify the best set of categories. Possible categories to use in approaching data might be based on (1) physiological function of patient, (2) length of exposure to the medicine, (3) age of patient, (4) concomitant treatments, or (5) any of many other possible sets of categories. In most situations, the possible categories to be used for classification will be suggested by the nature of the data.

Typologies versus Classifications. In some data sets it may be possible to discern certain common characteristics. Clusters of patients, events, or observations may stand out when the data are examined according to one or more of the "common" characteristics. This approach is referred to as a typological approach. The distinction between a typology and classification is that in the former, the categories are suggested by a combination of characteristic findings in the objects themselves, whereas a classification is based on well-defined categories that are chosen by the interpreter.

Lumpers. Another approach to consider is to seek a unifying theory, hypothesis, or model that will explain all or at least most of the data. The probability of achieving this unifying interpretation may be small but should be considered.

Comparison with the Literature. Data may also be compared with those in the literature. This assumes that the person who is interpreting the data is familiar with the literature. If this is not the case, then that individual should not attempt to interpret the data until (1) the relevant criteria to consider, (2) the types of data observed by others, and (3) the categories used to classify or present the data are known. Familiarizing oneself with the literature will also provide hints or indications of relevant qualities and attributes of the data that may be of particular importance in deriving an interpretation.

Bottom-Up versus Top-Down Approaches. Interpretations of data may proceed from a "bottom-up" or "top-down" approach. In the "bottom-up" approach, individual parts of an interpretation are fitted together in larger and larger patterns (i.e., more and more general patterns) eventually to create an overall interpretation. In the "top-down" approach, an overall approach is generally divided progressively to seek all of the possible ramifications of an interpretation. In the "top-down" approach, an algorithm may be used that could reveal unexpected or unanticipated conclusions or possibilities.

Flow Diagram Approach. The last approach described is to set up a logical order of events on paper and to attempt to use the data to support or modify the steps proposed. This approach is similar to that of using a flow diagram to explain a series of events that may or may not be directly linked. Depending on the nature of the data, one or more of these approaches may appear to be most likely to yield a valid interpretation of most or all of the data.

Contradictory Results and Loose Ends. It is clear that heterogeneous data cannot always be organized to create a single explanation. Moreover, data from even a single experiment are not always internally consistent, and contradictory results in different parts of an experiment or clinical trial may have been obtained. Some of these situations are described in Chapters 91 and 92.

It is important to realize that an experiment or clinical trial is not a failure if all parts are not utilized and fitted neatly into a single interpretation. Numerous findings that defy explanation are sometimes used in future years to explain a heretofore unexplained point, or the finding may stimulate a search for new information or explanations.

Interpreting a Small Quantity of Data

The approaches described above for large data sets may be utilized for some small data sets and should be attempted if there is a reasonable likelihood of interpreting the data. There are a number of other approaches, however, that may also be considered. These are discussed separately in other chapters for clinical trials with one or a few patients (i.e., Chapter 38), and for trials with multiple patients.

EXTRAPOLATING THE INTERPRETATION OF DATA

Whenever a patient is treated, the physician or other health care provider is extrapolating data from previous personal experiences, knowledge about clinical trial results, or experiences of others. In many instances the degree of probability is high that the medicine will do what the care-giver desires (e.g., an antibiotic used to treat a minor bacterial infection after culture and sensitivity tests have been performed). The magnitude of the extrapolation is relatively small in this example. In other clinical situations, the magnitude of the extrapolation is greater (e.g., treating a psychotic patient with an established medicine). Other extrapolations are even greater (e.g., treating a patient with a medicine not yet shown to be effective but with a scientific rationale to justify the treatment on an experimental basis). The dimension along which these extrapolations vary is related to the specific therapeutic area and disease considered.

Other dimensions exist along which an extrapolation varies. The body of medical knowledge and experiences used to generate the idea that a specific treatment is relevant for a specific patient's treatment may also involve an extrapolation. This extrapolation for treating a single patient might be necessary because of differences in the following:

1. Nature of the patient populations treated in clinical trials versus the current patient.
2. Characteristics of the physicians or other health care providers who conducted the clinical trials versus the current physician.
3. Characteristic of the environments in which the current patient lives or is being treated, versus those of patients and medical practice reported in the published clinical trials.
4. Period of time when the clinical trials and experiences were conducted (e.g., was the trial conducted 40 years ago when medical beliefs were different about treating the particular disease?) versus today.
5. Levels (or types) of interpretation.

Points 1 to 4 are discussed in Chapter 90, and point 5 is described below.

Levels of Interpretation

This chapter only mentions one of the levels of organization that can be used to interpret data. Levels of organization refer to the organization of matter whereby each successive level includes all of the preceding ones. These are shown in Fig. 71.5. Data are often obtained and interpreted at one level and are then extrapolated both up and down this chain to make projections about how a medicine acts at other levels. Clinical decisions (at an upper level) are often reached based on extrapolations of interpretations using results obtained at a lower level of organization.

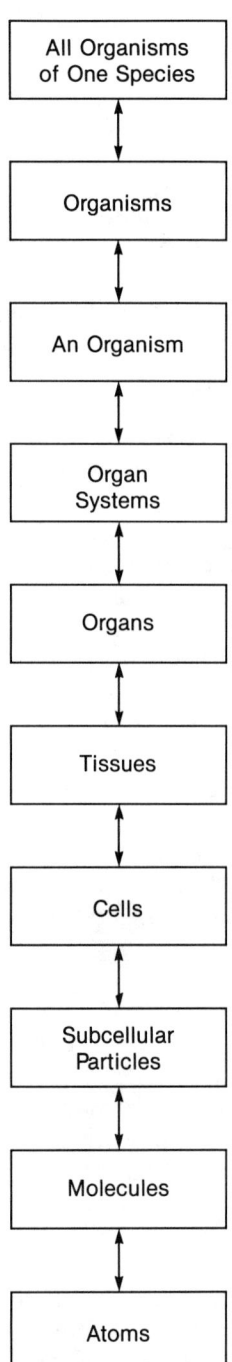

All Organisms
of One Species
↕
Organisms
↕
An Organism
↕
Organ
Systems
↕
Organs
↕
Tissues
↕
Cells
↕
Subcellular
Particles
↕
Molecules
↕
Atoms

FIG. 71.5 Successive levels of organization of matter from an entire population of one species to its constituent atoms.

PRESENTATION OF DATA TO SUPPORT AN INTERPRETATION

The specific tables, figures, and graphs used to present clinical data in a publication or report are usually chosen after the interpretations are reached. Reasons for this include the relevance of choosing those methods that most clearly present the interpretation and have the best chance of convincing readers. Moreover, when presenting data it is important to proceed in a stepwise manner that leads the reader (1) from more general to more specific points (or vice versa), (2) from past events to present events, or (3) from one set of conditions to another. To accomplish this most clearly it is generally necessary to complete the interpretation to determine the goal, and then to choose the best presentations to approach that goal. One goal of the presentation may be to extrapolate the data to a new situation or to develop a new hypothesis that can be tested or is currently being tested.

Before choosing the figures and tables to use, it is necessary to understand the pros and cons of each possible format. This knowledge would allow one to choose the best tables and figures to use when presenting the results. Unfortunately there are few (if any) people who have a complete understanding of these attributes. For the rest of us there are a few practical approaches that can be tried.

Practical methods for choosing figures and tables include (1) the trial and error approach of using those formats that occur to the individual or (2) using formats used by others in the literature or nonpublished reports. This issue should be discussed with statisticians, colleagues, consultants, regulatory authorities, or others. Additional information and a source of tables and figures to evaluate are shown in the book *Presentation of Clinical Data* (Spilker and Schoenfelder, 1990).

STRENGTH OR QUALITY OF AN INTERPRETATION

It is well accepted that the strength of an interpretation is related to the design of the clinical trial. There is a general hierarchy ranging from anecdotal case reports to double-blind, randomized, placebo, and active medicine controlled trials conducted to confirm a finding (see Table 73.1).

An important aspect of the hierarchical ordering concept of clinical trials and studies is that the chance of a false-positive response is decreased as one ascends the hierarchy. The reliability of the data and its interpretation is also increased as a more rigorous trial design is used. It is well known, for example, that open-label clinical trials are much more likely to demonstrate a positive outcome than are double-blind trials (see Chapter 4).

STYLES OF INTERPRETATION

Four styles of clinical interpretation of data are described briefly. These are (1) overinterpretation, (2) underinterpretation, (3) conservative interpretation, and (4) personal interpretation.

Overinterpretation and Underinterpretation

Overinterpretation is operationally defined as an interpretation that goes beyond the ability of the data to support the conclusions, whether or not the interpretation eventually proves to be correct. This is commonly observed when an interpretation of data is extrapolated to an entire population of patients with a disease when the clinical trial was conducted in a small subset of that population. Underinterpretation is operationally defined as an interpretation of data that is incomplete and does not fully describe the clinical importance of the results. When the "missing" part of the interpretation is obtained, it may render the new interpretation more positive or more negative, or may not affect the overall conclusions reached.

In general, data are either over- or underinterpreted either purposely or inadvertently. When someone purposely (i.e., deliberately) alters the interpretation, no discussion is required to describe how misinterpretation could have been avoided.

Why Are Erroneous or Distorted Interpretations Made? Inadvertent overinterpretation may result from (1) unbridled enthusiasm, (2) lack of experience in reaching a reasonable balance of how strongly the data may support an interpretation, (3) vested interests in supporting a personal hypothesis, point of view, or business venture, (4) desire to use data to support a given idea, (5) desire to achieve personal recognition, or (6) desire to achieve or continue grant support. Underinterpretation may result from (1) inexperience in knowing how data may be used to support an interpretation, (2) excessive caution on the part of investigators who require much more data than most clinicians before they are willing to reach a conclusion, (3) a mistaken belief that scientific credibility and reputation are enhanced by an overly conservative approach to data, or (4) vested interests in not interpreting data along certain lines that the interpreter specifically wishes to avoid. Vested interests could result in either inadvertently or purposely altered interpretations.

One of the most effective means of avoiding both over- and underinterpretation of data is to have one's colleagues and peers critique the results and conclusions of a clinical trial. Identifying and qualifying one's less firm conclusions as possibilities provides one type of modification of results that may otherwise be viewed as overinterpretations.

Conservative Interpretation

The third style of interpretation is the conservative style. This style is one in which minimal or no extrapolation of the data is made. The interpreter limits the interpretation strictly to those points that may be totally defended by the data generated in the clinical trial. This is a type of underinterpretation that is made purposely.

Personal Interpretation

The fourth style of interpretation is that of a personal approach to the data. Although most scientists follow generally similar approaches in developing interpretations and relating their conclusions to the pertinent medical literature, there are some scientists who take a highly individual approach to this process. These people often do not refer to previous models, hypotheses, and data. They often create a unique model of their own to explain their results and sometimes continue to develop their model for many years. This approach is sometimes used by scientists who appear to thrive on challenging traditional models or who wish to follow their own creative thought processes. It requires significant innovation and creativity to succeed at this approach and to convince the scientific "establishment" of the validity of one's views.

THE INSTITUTION OF THE INTERPRETER

Each individual who interprets clinical data draws from his or her own background, experience, and outlook. Thus, there are innumerable different perspectives. Additionally, these perspectives are influenced to some degree by the type of organization in which the interpreter is primarily employed or has been most strongly influenced. Academic, governmental, and industrial perspectives usually differ to a great degree in some areas (e.g., approval process of new medicines) and to a minor degree (if at all) in others (e.g., basic scientific data with limited or no commercial or regulatory implications). Consultants may be viewed in this schema as individuals whose perspective often changes to harmonize with that of their employer.

The ideal perspective to use in interpreting data should be the most objective one. However, no single perspective is considered to be ideal, and a group of scientists will usually be able to view the same data in several different ways. Objectivity in viewing data on a new medicine may differ for individuals in government who are charged with protecting the nation's health, for academic investigators who wish to have improved medicines available to treat their patients, and for individuals in the pharmaceutical industry who are attempting to develop new and profitable medicines.

It is an important and valuable talent to be able to understand another person's perspective. Nonetheless, stereotyping of an individual's perspective because of the source of his or her paycheck does a great disservice to both the ideas and the interpretations of many people. The clichéd view of academicians as "too theoretical," government employees as "too bureaucratic and rigid," and industrial employees as "too commercially oriented" does a great disservice to many people. The perspective of most clinicians is only partially influenced by their employers.

Many of the points summarized in this chapter are discussed in more detail in other chapters in Parts VI to IX of this book.

CHAPTER 72

Development and Use of Clinical Judgment

WHAT IS CLINICAL JUDGMENT?

Operational Definition

It is difficult to propose a single operational definition of clinical judgment since the term is used in numerous ways. In this chapter it is considered a combination of knowledge, skills, and abilities based on personal experience and reading about any area of medicine that applies to a clinical situation. The experience is usually acquired to a large degree from patient contact, although treating patients is not a mandatory requirement for developing clinical judgment. When the responsibility of patient care is not possible (such as for nonphysicians), then other techniques, including extensive readings in the medical literature and many hours of discussions with other more knowledgeable individuals, will assist in this process. Making judgments in clinical situations and then evaluating clinical outcomes to assess whether one was correct or not provides important feedback that is useful in improving one's skills. These experiences enable physicians to learn how to assign relative weights to evidence and to learn when less data are sufficient to reach a decision. A number of nonphysicians have been able to develop sound clinical judgment, at least in specific types of situations, through close association with physicians and through simulated exercises with real patients.

Uses of Clinical Judgment

Clinical judgment allows one to make correct diagnostic and therapeutic decisions based on information that is incomplete and uncertain. Clinical judgment is developed for both general therapeutic areas of medicine, including specific clinical situations, and specific patients. There are often occasions when applying standard clinical knowledge and practice is inappropriate. Clinical judgment is important in order to distinguish appropriate from inappropriate situations.

One important aspect of clinical judgment is that it represents an understanding of one's limits in various situations. Limits are based on consideration of technical expertise and intellectual understanding of a particular situation. Other aspects of clinical judgment include the ability to (1) choose relevant data from a larger set, (2) formulate an overall view of a clinical problem, (3) develop a plan to evaluate the clinical problem, (4) monitor and modify the plan as needed, and (5) determine what additional resources are needed (e.g., consultations, facilities, tests) to proceed effectively in dealing with the clinical situation in question.

Example of How Clinical Judgment Is Used

If a hypothetical patient is extremely ill and is in a hospital, usually many laboratory tests may be ordered to assist in diagnosis and treatment. It is only necessary to choose a small subset of this group to make the correct medical diagnosis in most patients. Of this subset of tests, certain parameters are generally identified and monitored on a periodic basis to observe the patient's progress and the effects of treatment. The specific parameters chosen to follow will depend on (1) the patient's major disease, (2) complicating medical factors, (3) which specific parameters were originally observed to be abnormal, (4) the nature of the medicine treatment given the patient, (5) fluids and other nonmedicine treatments given to the patient, plus other considerations. Reaching a decision about which parameters to measure and follow often requires a certain degree of clinical judgment in addition to clinical knowledge about the disease. It has often been stated that a clinical diagnosis may usually be made on the basis of a patient's medical history and physical examination without reference to laboratory tests.

It is clear that all laboratory abnormalities are not of equal importance in diagnosing or treating a patient nor are they essential to understand the current state of an individual's health. Some values are more important than others to use as guides to follow a patient's course. Knowledge of these parameters and how to evaluate their degree of abnormality is important in developing clinical judgment. Likewise, it is important to develop knowledge of other safety parameters that are important to follow and to be able to separate vital clues in a patient's history from nonessential medical details that will not assist in the decision-making processes.

Clinical Judgment versus Scientific Logic

The individual with a great deal of clinical judgment has usually mastered both the art and the science of medicine. This person is able to weigh and balance many disparate pieces of clinical information and to reach an informed decision within a short period. Sometimes, a decision must be made within a matter of seconds or minutes even though important information is missing, as in an emergency room or operating room. The clinician is trained through direct experience, discussions, disputes, and trial-and-error approaches so that his or her judgment can be applied in new clinical situations with a high probability of rapidly reaching an optimal decision. On the other hand, the training and logic of a scientist is quite different. A scientist is trained to collect systematically all necessary data on a question and to follow a structured and rigorous approach before reaching a decision. Scientists are rarely forced to make rapid decisions based on incomplete data, knowing that they have never faced the exact same situation and that their decision is often final. An interesting comparison of clinical and actuarial judgment was made by Dawes et al. (1989).

The tools of clinical judgment include both inductive and deductive logic. Scientific logic is predominantly analytical, uses both inductive and deductive logic, and also utilizes more formal methods to address issues. Clinical judgment is both analytical and nonanalytical, often reaches decisions on incomplete data, and uses less formal methodologies. On a practical level, it is the scientists that may withhold judgment, whereas the clinicians are often compelled to make a decision (e.g., when facing a patient who needs immediate treatment a physician cannot always elect to wait until the laboratory data come back).

Nonclinical scientists control most conditions of their experiments and try to study precisely defined situations. Clinicians usually deal with many variations and uncertainties, and cannot control most variables.

Medical School Education in the United States

Few medical schools attempt to educate students in a uniform way throughout their 4 years. Many, if not most, medical students go through an adjustment period between their second and third years. This period has usually been attributed to the transition from the classroom to the clinic, but another explanation is possible. Training during the first 2 years at most medical schools is disease oriented. Students are taught about diseases (i.e., the causes) and various signs and symptoms (i.e., the effects). Their training during the second 2 years, in the clinic, is patient oriented. Furthermore, they are asked to observe the effects (i.e., symptoms and signs) and to diagnose the cause. In the medical student's first 2 years, each cause leads to many effects, but in the last 2 years, each effect is seen to lead from many causes (i.e., the differential diagnosis).

DEDUCTIVE VERSUS INDUCTIVE LOGIC

Logic is the process of reasoning that is used to determine truth if the premises are correct. Logic differs from statistics in that statistics allows one to make assertions based on experimental or other types of evidence, whereas logic deals with the actual process of reasoning. There are two primary types of logic, deductive and inductive. Both types are used in clinical medicine, although inductive logic is used more widely.

Deductive Logic

In deductive logic, the conclusion is a necessary consequence of the premises. The usual form of deductive logic involves the syllogism, which is classically composed of two premises and a conclusion. The form is usually that if statement A implies statement B and if statement B implies statement C, then statement A will imply statement C. This type of logic was developed by Aristotle.

Scientists use deductive logic by beginning with known scientific principles or generalizations to deduce specific assertions or conclusions that are relevant for a particular situation. These assertions may be expressed as a hypothesis and may be evaluated through an experiment. Data obtained are then used to confirm, reject, or modify the original hypothesis. The greater the accuracy of the original principles, the greater will be the accuracy of the conclusions.

Syllogisms

A few clinical examples of hypotheses to be tested (in the form of syllogisms) are as follows:

1. Medicines excreted entirely by renal mechanisms are excreted more slowly in patients with diminished renal function (e.g., below 30% of normal). Medicine X is excreted entirely by renal mechanisms. Therefore, medicine X will be excreted more slowly in patients with decreased renal function.
2. Cells of a certain Y type are highly sensitive to radiation. Disease X has Y-type cells. Therefore, disease X cells of the Y type will be sensitive to radiation.
3. Medicines that are highly lipid soluble cross the blood–brain barrier. Medicine X is highly lipid soluble. Therefore, medicine X will cross the blood–brain barrier.

In each example given, the assertion (conclusion) may be tested through clinical studies. It is not suggested that all of these statements are true.

In addition to creating hypotheses to test, syllogisms may also be used to reach interpretations. For example: All medicines that lower the Hamilton Depression Scale are antidepressants. Medicine X lowers the Hamilton Depression Scale. Therefore, medicine X is an antidepressant. Another example is that medicines that lower diastolic blood pressure by 10 mmHg are clinically useful medicines. Medicine Z lowers blood pressure by 10 mmHg. Therefore, medicine Z is clinically useful.

Inductive Logic

In contrast, inductive logic is the basis of common sense and depends on experience. The process of using inductive logic begins with a particular experience and then reaches a conclusion (often a generalization) that is probably true based on the premises. The methods used to reach a conclusion may result from analogies, generalizations, or causal connections (i.e., cause and effect). This method does not achieve the logical certainty achieved with deductive logic.

Scientists utilize both types of logic in designing and interpreting clinical trials, although not necessarily in the same experiment. Inductive logic provides a use for clinical experience, and deductive logic provides a means of establishing relationships between facts. Repeated observations in a trial or experiment are made to establish valid data, from which a general conclusion may be drawn using inductive logic. Most clinical trials in which multiple observations are generalized to reach a conclusion (i.e., the data are interpreted) involve inductive logic.

Proof by Exclusion

One approach to using logic to interpret data is to prove something by exclusion rather than by demonstration. In this method the scientist demonstrates that all but one of the probable explanations are false and therefore the only remaining possibility must be true. This is not a good method to use in most areas of science, since it is preferable to show positive data rather than to reason by the process of exclusion. For example, if one believes that five possibilities exist and four are excluded, it is conceivable that there are other possibilities whose existence is presently unknown and that the remaining (fifth) possibility is also incorrect.

Critiquing Clinical Interpretations Based on Deductive Logic

The major questions to pose when reading clinical interpretations that use deductive logic are as follows:

1. Examine the general rule carefully. Is it known and accepted to be correct?
2. Does the general rule apply to the situation in which it is being used?
3. Are the examples relevant to the situation?
4. Are there a sufficient number of examples?
5. Are the examples presented in adequate detail?
6. Does the conclusion follow according to the rules of deductive logic?

Critiquing Clinical Interpretations Based on Inductive Logic

The major questions to pose in assessing clinical interpretations that use inductive logic are as follows:

1. Was an adequate number of examples used before the generalizations were made or conclusions were reached?
2. Were the parameters evaluated the most relevant ones to consider, or are there more relevant parameters that could have been used?
3. Were the parameters measured appropriately?
4. Were the examples chosen the most relevant ones to consider, or are there more relevant examples that could have been used?
5. Does the conclusion follow appropriately from the examples?

Analogy

The methodology of analogy is simpler than either induction or deduction. Arguments are based on a number of similarities or likenesses of two or more objects, cases, or situations to each other or to a third object, case, or situation. The assumption is usually made that one of the items compared is known, or at least accepted, to have certain attributes.

Many diagnoses of patients' diseases today are based on analogy. Similarities between a previous case treated by a physician (or merely read about as a typical case) and a patient currently in front of the physician are used as the basis of a (presumptive) diagnosis. This approach may be adequate to diagnose most cases of colds, hay fever, and insomnia, but for more serious diseases in which treatment has risks, and in which the consequences of a wrong diagnosis are greater, it is important to conduct corroborative tests. Overall, analogies help clarify, describe, and persuade, but they do not demonstrate or prove that two or more situations are identical.

Medical examples of analogies include situations in which historical accounts of symptoms experienced by one or many people who died are compared with present-day symptoms of a specific disease. The historical deaths are then assumed to be the result of the same disease, because their symptoms appear to be similar. Sometimes, the medical evidence is merely based on casual statements by a historian. Analogies may be based on physical descriptions of a patient's lesions, if they were recorded.

Critiquing Clinical Interpretations Based on Analogy

The major problem with the method of analogy is that two things may be alike in all characteristics except one. That characteristic may be important and may mean that the two (or more) objects, cases, or situations compared are, in fact, different and not the same.

Another problem with interpretations based on analogy is that each patient, object, situation, disease, or whatever is being compared has so many characteristics that a large number of characteristics may be found that are similar. But these characteristics may be either unimportant or may represent a highly incomplete sample.

A third problem is that even if all characteristics compared are the same for two objects, cases, or situations, the items being compared still could be different. Analogy is not a sufficiently strong method on its own to prove identity completely. Conclusions based on analogies must therefore be viewed as tentative and incomplete.

Assertions

When people make assertions in papers, reports, or presentations, the appropriate process of verification varies greatly. Some statements are confined to only an individual patient whereas others extend to an entire class or group of patients. Some assertions require a great deal of verification, while others require little or none. Some may be proved beyond doubt and others are impossible to prove at all.

Clear language must be used to identify whether statements made are fact, opinion, or preference. Signal phrases such as "in my judgment," "from one point of view," "it is certain" help the writer communicate the category of statement being made. Statements of medical facts usually are statements of beliefs, because most are subject to change over time.

Underlying assumptions are often of critical importance, both to understand assertions and to critique them. What one person takes for granted and does not feel obliged to state can create a misunderstanding in readers who do not share the same assumptions, do not understand the jargon being used in the same way, or are uncertain what the actual assumptions are. While it is not always critical to explain assumptions (e.g., when presenting results of laboratory tests), they may be initially important (i.e., when presenting results of psychotherapeutic interviews with patients). Assertions may be true even though the underlying assumptions are false or are unwarranted.

Relationship between Assertions. Many medical school examinations (at least in the United States) are based on relationships between assertions. Multiple choice questions present the choice of five possibilities in deciding about two statements: (1) statement A is true and statement B is false; (2) statement A is false and statement B is true; (3) statements A and B are are both true, and there is a causal relationship between them; (4) statements A and B are both true, but there is no causal relationship between them; or (5) both statements are false. Note that choices 3 and 4 examine the relationship between two statements.

The need to assess the relationship between assertions arises frequently in medicine, particularly when evaluating interpretations of data made in reports or publications. The author of a report usually states that medicine X had effect Y in a clinical trial and therefore it does (or does not) cause effect Z. For example, the statement that aspirin is an effective pain killer (i.e., is analgesic) because it inhibits cyclooxygenase is true. The statement that aspirin lowers body temperature (i.e., is antipyretic) is also true. These two statements, however, are not related as cause and effect. The example given is obvious, but much more subtle or complex illustrations could be given in which it is difficult to know whether the purported relationship is true.

Algorithms

Algorithms are sets of rules, usually in the form of a logical flow chart, that medical personnel use to make decisions about specific problems. They provide a decision path that enhances the probability of making correct decisions. Algorithms promote greater comprehension and retention of details than can usually be accomplished through traditional teaching methods. The typical basic form of an algorithm is: If A is found to be true, then do (or use) B. Thus, an algorithm may be viewed as a strategy or plan for solving a problem.

Although algorithms are usually presented as simple or complex flow charts, they may be shown as decision tables or computer programs. Algorithms differ from decision analyses in that they do not usually indicate the probabilities and utilities of choosing different paths.

Algorithms are widely used by physicians to diagnose a patient's disease and to plan and guide its treatment (Komaroff, 1982). They also allow nonphysicians to interact with patients more effectively and to communicate with physicians when necessary. Algorithms have been used to evaluate clinical performance and

help establish standards of care; they are also a valuable teaching aid. Algorithms are said to be most useful for common, nonserious clinical cases in which treatments may or may not work and patient care protocols have been worked out (Margolis, 1983). In these situations, if the medical treatment does not work, it is not a very serious issue. Decision analysis, on the other hand, is used for more serious cases when some actions may potentially harm the patient. Komaroff et al. (1978) show how both tools may be used together.

Algorithms are a useful device for integrating and condensing a large amount of information, organizing medical decisions, and facilitating choices, thereby optimizing the usefulness of known information and minimizing the roles of myth, ignorance, and misinformation. Thus, they enable more physicians to practice medicine at higher standards and to achieve desired outcomes more often. Algorithms are easily computerized and are being used more frequently in medicine. A few of the objections to their use are discussed by Margolis (1983).

Decision Analysis

Decision analysis is a logical method to reach decisions based on both probability theory and utility theory. One approach to decision analysis is presented as a four-step process.

1. Formulate the problem explicitly using a decision tree. This step specifies the problem and identifies alternative choices. The formulation is often presented in the form of a figure called a *decision tree*.
2. Quantitate the probabilities of each possibility occurring.
3. Quantitate the preferences or utilities of the various possibilities.
4. Determine the most appropriate decision based on choosing the path that yields the greatest utility.

An excellent example of how a type of decision analysis technique can be used to develop clinical strategies for treating disease is presented by Komaroff et al. (1978) for urinary and vaginal infections. Other examples are presented by Sackett et al. (1985).

Logical and Extralogical Proofs

Three major techniques are used to derive medical proofs: analogy, induction, and deduction. They have been briefly described as the basic methods of logical reasoning.

Science also employs other types of proofs, which are more commonly used in other areas of life. These methods include intuition, authority, and persistence. Although it would be fun to discuss these in some detail, they lie outside the main scope of this text, and are rarely accepted as the basis of reaching or establishing a valid interpretation in medicine.

DEVIL'S ADVOCATE APPROACH

A devil's advocate questions or proposes a different or opposite interpretation or possibility. The types of questions that a devil's advocate might ask initially are:

1. If it is observed that a medicine does "X," what does the medicine not do?
2. If it is observed that a medicine does "X," why did it not do "Y"?
3. If it is observed that a medicine causes a small effect, why did it not cause a large effect?
4. If it is observed that a medicine's effect is observed in volunteers, what would occur if the medicine were evaluated in patients?
5. If the trial evaluated a fixed dose of a medicine, what would occur if the trial were conducted with a variable dose?
6. If the trial's data do not prove theory "X," at least the data does not disprove theory "X."

In a follow-up discussion the devil's advocate will continue to adopt an opinion contrary to the other individual or group and will persist in challenging their assumptions and conclusions. This approach may be used constructively by individuals who wish to critique their own work and to determine alternate ways of viewing and presenting their data. It may therefore be used as a tool to develop statements or responses for reports, talks, or articles that both strengthen one's interpretation and also help to prepare a defense against possible criticisms.

Some of the traditional questions to pose when critiquing one's own data are listed in Table 72.1.

HOW TO DEVELOP CLINICAL JUDGMENT

The major techniques used to develop clinical judgment are (1) exposure to many patients with a wide variety of diseases, presentations, and courses in an area of medicine, (2) experience in treating patients and following their course, (3) reading the literature, (4) evaluating the validity of one's decisions in a sort of trial-and-error procedure, (5) attendance at lectures, seminars, and professional meetings, and (6) discussions with and feedback from peers and superiors.

Utilizing published exercises is one method of improving one's skills, and discussions with peers or more experienced clinicians are another. The degree to which an individual has acquired clinical judgment may be assessed through an evaluation of his or her performance in specific hypothetical or actual clinical situations.

Impediments to Clinical Judgment

Arkes (1981) discussed five impediments to accurate clinical judgment and suggested three strategies to minimize the impact of these impediments. The five impediments are:

1. Inability to assess covariation accurately. This is illustrated by an example of evaluating whether a specific symptom is associated with a specific outcome. The point is that many people overemphasize the percentage (or number) of cases in which both symptom and outcome are present. The cases in which the symptom is absent and the outcome is present are not accorded their full importance.
2. Preconceived notions or expectancies. Arkes describes the results of a classic study by Chapman and Chapman in which individuals were shown to associate certain personality traits with certain physical features. Most clinicians and scientists have many preconceived notions that undoubtedly influence their behavior in all areas of medicine and their interpretation of data.
3. Lack of awareness of factors that influence judgment. Every clinician has only a partial understanding of the identity and magnitude of the factors that influence his or her judgment.
4. Overconfidence by physicians about the accuracy of their judgment. There are numerous factors that support and tend to perpetuate this characteristic, including (1) placebo effect, (2) Hawthorne effect (the act of observing an event alters it), (3) gathering selective information that tends to support one's hypothesis, and (4) selectively disregarding evidence that contradicts one's present judgment.
5. Hindsight bias. Many data sets contain observations that may be used to support many different interpretations. If a physician is informed that a specific outcome occurred, then the data are observed and put together to support that outcome,

---

TABLE 72.1 *Selected questions to pose when critiquing one's own data*[a]

1. Do all components contribute equally?[b]
2. Are all results discussed?
3. What implications exist at other biological levels?[c]
4. Do data make sense clinically, physiologically, and theoretically?
5. May specific conclusions be extrapolated?

---

[a] Many other questions may be posed by using the checklists in the chapter on evaluating published papers.
[b] This may or may not be appropriate in the specific situation.
[c] See Fig. 71.4.

whereas if the physician is informed that a totally different outcome occurred, then the data are viewed in a different way.

Techniques proposed to avoid these potential problems are to (1) consider alternative explanations of the data, possibly including listing reasons for and against each possible explanation, (2) decrease one's reliance on memory because of the fallibility of recall, and (3) increase one's use of Bayesian statistics.

Psychological Aspects of Judgment

Additional information about judgment, and particularly about uncertainty, is available in two fine monographs, by Kahneman et al. (1982) and by Schwartz and Griffin (1986). These books explore the psychological aspects of judgment, a vast topic that is only briefly mentioned in this book.

BENEFITS OF CLINICAL JUDGMENT

Sound clinical judgment allows more accurate interpretation of data from clinical trials by focusing on the most meaningful data and deemphasizing abnormalities and other data that are not important to reaching conclusions. The greater one's clinical judgment, the greater is one's ability to reach accurate diagnoses and treat patients effectively. The ways that one specifically applies judgment in interpreting clinical data are described in other chapters.

An individual with well-developed clinical judgment about an area of medicine has developed a broad perspective about that subject. This skill enables him or her to interpret data better and to construct an overall clinical impression of a situation even when some important data are missing.

THE ROLE OF EXPERTISE IN INTERPRETING CLINICAL DATA

Chess experts and physicists have been widely studied in an attempt to learn how world class experts think and interpret data. The best experts are able to generate a limited number of highly likely hypotheses. Chess masters did not consider a larger number of moves than less expert chess players, nor did the masters follow the moves further into the game. They did think more about "good" moves, while less advanced players spent a larger portion of their time thinking about "bad" moves (de Groot, 1965). These mental abilities were developed by observing the impact of certain moves on a game's outcome.

The experts were able to focus more on optimal moves because of their ability to recall specific patterns of pieces, not because of a superior memory. Chase and Simon (1973a,b) concluded that chess masters have a large repertoire of chess patterns stored in their long-term memory, which may be compared with patterns on the board and then associated with good moves. This is why chess masters can play any number of simultaneous chess games and win almost all of them: in going from board to board they need only look at the pattern and recognize a familiar one to know which moves are best.

Expertise in medical diagnosis and treatment by highly experienced physicians is undoubtedly similar to this type of expertise, which is also found in those who can solve physics problems (Chi et al., 1981).

DEGREE OF INTERPHYSICIAN AGREEMENT ON DIAGNOSIS, TREATMENT, AND INTERPRETATION

Two or more medical experts of approximately equal stature and clinical judgment often reach opposite conclusions or decisions in specific situations. This may result from differences in their disciplines (e.g., a surgeon and an internist evaluating a patient with gastric bleeding), experiences, ethics, personal beliefs, and/or behavioral styles of practicing medicine (aggressive versus conservative). Each of these factors will influence how an individual physician utilizes his or her clinical judgment.

Numerous studies have evaluated interphysician reliability in terms of degree of agreement or disagreement. Such studies generally focus on physician ability to (1) elicit and measure physical signs, (2) interpret laboratory data, (3) establish a diagnosis, (4) recommend treatment(s), (5) evaluate the effects of treatment, (6) determine an overall assessment of patient care, or (7) communicate information accurately to peers or patients. Some studies use actual patients and clinical situations, whereas other studies rely on models or simulations (Table 72.2).

Several tentative conclusions were summarized in a review by Koran (1975). Most of these conclusions are rather obvious.

1. The greater the number of normal patients who are included in the study group, the higher is the rate of agreement, because agreement about normality is generally greater than agreement about abnormality.
2. Agreement about either/or types of judgments (e.g., present or absent, yes or no) is usually higher than for judgments about qualitative variables.
3. The larger the number of possible diagnostic categories to consider, the greater is the rate of disagreement.

TABLE 72.2 *Assessing agreement among physicians in medicine and language*

Area tested	Reference	Outcome
Peripheral pulses of 192 patients	Meade et al., 1968	Agreement 69% of time
Interpretation of chest X-rays	Herman and Hessel, 1975	
Electrocardiogram	Segall, 1960	Majority of 20 MDs agreed on 77% of EKGs
Electroencephalograms	Woody, 1968	Agreement on 53% of cases as normal/abnormal
Pathological diagnosis of tissues as benign or malignant	Coppelson et al., 1970	Disagreement 28% between same physician at two different times
Meaning of common terms expressing probability	Bryant and Norman, 1980	Poor agreement with a large range for most terms (e.g., "sometimes" meant anywhere from 5% to 75% chance)
	Nakao and Axelrod, 1983	Similar to above
	Toogood, 1980	Similar
	Robertson, 1983	Similar
	Kenney, 1981	Similar

4. The less severe the abnormality, the lower is the rate of agreement.

5. The degree of agreement among physicians diminishes as the number of physicians increases.

6. Pairs of physicians with more training relative to the decisions to be made will agree more than pairs of physicians with less training.

7. After physicians discuss terminology, criteria, and decision rules relative to the task, they tend to agree more often.

In general, the more objective the data, the better is the agreement between physicians, and the more subjective the data, the poorer is the agreement.

Fletcher et al. (1985) evaluated the ability of physicians from various specialties to detect lumps in manufactured human breast models. Detection rates varied widely, were far from perfect, and were described as "modest." The mean number of lumps detected by all groups of physicians was 44% of the actual number. Other studies on interobserver errors in detecting and measuring cancers or simulated cancers have also observed wide variation between observers (e.g., Moertel and Hanley, 1976; Warr et al., 1984). Warr et al. (1984) found that the error rate was influenced by simulation of tumor growth, multiple lesions, and sequential measurements. A bibliography of over 400 articles on interphysician variability was published by Feinstein (1985b).

Interphysician reliability also has been shown to be problematic when taking histories and conducting physical examinations as well as in the interpretation of X-rays, laboratory specimens, and other "objective" data (Koran, 1975; Department of Clinical Epidemiology and Biostatistics, McMaster University, 1980a). Verbal and written communications between physicians are also areas in which a significant amount of misunderstanding may occur, especially when terms such as "compatible with, probably, likely" are used (Bryant and Norman, 1980; Haynes et al., 1983). Factors influencing the presence and magnitude of inter-physician differences are listed in Table 72.3, and some methods to diminish these differences are listed in Table 72.4.

It is widely accepted that psychiatric diseases have a relatively high rate of interobserver differences (e.g., Fisch et al., 1981) as do angina (Rose, 1965), backache (Nelson et al., 1979; Waddell et al., 1982), abdominal pain (Gill et al., 1973), and breast cancer (Yorkshire Breast Cancer Group, 1977) under certain conditions.

Koch-Weser et al. (1977) evaluated interrater differences among three clinical pharmacology experts who assessed 500 identical reports of adverse reactions to medicines. The experts disagreed among themselves (1) in 36% of cases about which medicine was most likely to have caused the adverse reaction, (2) in 56% of cases about whether severe morbidity resulted from the adverse reaction, (3) in 57% of cases about whether the adverse reaction was responsible for the hospital admission, (4) in 67% of cases about whether the adverse reaction was responsible for prolonging hospital stay, and (5) in 71% of cases in which patients died,

TABLE 72.3 *Selected causes of interphysician differences*

A. Causes related to the physician
1. Technical variation in ability
2. Variation in experience
3. Inherent biases
4. Differences in training, attention to detail, and approach to a clinical situation
5. Differences in interest, alertness, and other subjective parameters

B. Causes related to the patient
1. Variation in clinical parameters measured over time
2. Inherent biases (e.g., recall bias)
3. Variation in cooperation and attitude

C. Other causes
1. Lack of precision of diagnostic tools
2. Lack of precision of tests used to measure efficacy and/or safety parameters
3. Lack of ideal environment for evaluating the patient (e.g., excessive noise)
4. Differences in methods used by physician to obtain data (e.g., different positions of patient)

TABLE 72.4 *Methods to diminish interphysician differences*

1. Increasing the number of categories that the physician may use (this may improve accuracy up to a point, but when distinctions between classifications become too fine, there will be a larger number of errors)
2. Having observers with more experience (generally diminishes disagreements up to a point)
3. Specifying clearer definitions and protocol instructions
4. Clarifying data collection forms and/or questions to address
5. Formulating more precise decision rules
6. Providing practice sessions for observers prior to the study
7. Monitoring such differences periodically tends to diminish them after they are recognized
8. Setting up discussions between physicians on reasons for differences observed and possible solutions

about the contribution of the adverse reaction the patient's death. Karch et al. (1976) and Blanc et al. (1979) also found marked disagreements among three clinical pharmacologists or "independent observers" in assessing adverse reactions. Even the use of algorithms to assist in characterizing adverse reactions did not improve the amount of agreement among three raters (Louik et al., 1985).

Ezdinli et al. (1976) observed disagreement in interpretation of the histological type and pattern of lymphoma in 40% of the cases evaluated by two groups of pathologists. They concluded that the method of classifying these lymphomas is not as objective as had been previously thought.

Minimizing Interphysician Differences

Six strategies to prevent or minimize clinical disagreement among physicians were presented by the Department of Clinical Epidemiology and Biostatistics, McMaster University (1980*b*). They recommend such techniques as "blinding" one's assessments of raw diagnostic test data, repeating key parts of the examination, seeking independent views of other physicians, and using appropriate technical aids.

Intraphysician versus Interphysician Differences

As a postscript to this section describing interphysician differences, it should be indicated that intraphysician agreement is usually greater than interphysician agree-

ment or consistency (Koran, 1975). Kirwan and Currey (1984) evaluated the stability of clinical assessments made for about 50 "paper" patients by seven rheumatologists about 1 year apart. The judgments of the rheumatologists at the end of the year correlated well with duplicates of their own judgments made at the start of the year. It is of interest that there were wide differences in judgments among the rheumatologists. Additional studies by this group (Chaput de Saintonge et al., 1988) showed little agreement over which patients improved and which had not.

ARTIFICIAL INTELLIGENCE

The use of knowledge-based expert systems, commonly known as artificial intelligence, became a new discipline in the 1980s. The thinking and evaluation processes of one or more experts on a particular topic is captured and transferred to a computer software program to enhance the application of that expertise. It is more developed in various engineering and nonmedical fields than in medicine, but experiments and uses for medical applications are growing.

Representative applications in medicine are listed in Table 72.5. Future uses and expansion of this field are expected.

TABLE 72.5 *Selected uses of artificial intelligence in medicine*

Use	Reference
Evaluation of human gait abnormalities	Dzierzanowski et al. (1984)
Online consultation and automatic screening for generating diagnostic hypotheses	Adlassnig et al. (1986)
Analysis of serial graded exercise electrocardiogram test data	Long et al. (1987)
Chemotherapy treatment advice	Kent et al. (1985), Hickam et al. (1985)
Assistance in cancer treatment plans	Musen et al. (1986)
Diagnostic assistance program	Todd (1987), Barnett et al. (1987)
Laboratory test monitoring	Clark et al. (1979)
Anesthesia and intensive care	Rennels and Miller (1988)
Clinical trial design	Malogolowkin et al. (1989)
Diagnosis of abdominal pain	Sutton (1989)
Decision making	Shortliffe (1987)

CHAPTER 73

Concept of Cause and Effect

INTRODUCTION

The determination of whether two events or phenomena have a cause-and-effect relationship is a basic objective in many clinical trials. Although this determination often appears to be straightforward and obvious, there are many pitfalls for the unwary. Feinstein (1985a, p. 39) wrote, "Perhaps the most difficult challenge in modern clinical epidemiology . . . is the evaluation of cause–effect relationships."

This chapter only briefly discusses some of the concepts involved in establishing cause-and-effect relationships. Many important statistical and epidemiological aspects are not described. Readers interested in additional details are referred to books oriented toward an academician's approach (Feinstein, 1985a), a practicing physician's approach (Sackett et al., 1985), a student's approach (Fletcher et al., 1988), or a general epidemiological approach (Susser, 1973).

In clinical trials it is not possible to establish a cause-and-effect relationship with 100% certainty. Cause and effect is a relative concept, and a degree of likelihood or probability is sought. Although probabilities may sometimes be expressed in mathematical terms, the clinical interpretation of a cause-and-effect relationship is most often expressed in more general terms (e.g., unlikely, probable, almost certain).

Levels of Cause and Effect

One approach to characterizing cause and effect is to view this relationship on multiple levels. Levels may be easily defined based on a series of questions. Two issues that may trigger these questions are (1) a medicine is *suspected* of causing an adverse reaction and (2) a medicine is *believed* to have had a beneficial effect. The specific questions to consider in evaluating the evidence on these issues at three levels are:

1. Could the medicine possibly do it in theory?
2. Does the medicine actually do it in practice?
3. Did the medicine do it in the particular situation of interest?

Only level 3 is actually concerned with the specific cause-and-effect relationship.

Influences to Rule Out

In evaluating whether a cause-and-effect relationship exists, it is important to rule out bias, chance, and confounding influences. Any of these three may give rise to apparent cause-and-effect relationships that may be shown to be nonexistent when the bias (or other influence) is carefully considered. Even when all known effects of these three influences (bias, chance, and confounding) are apparently eliminated, there is still a possibility that their presence is undetected. Future technical developments or evaluations may reveal that previously accepted associations were based on evidence later found to be faulty or incomplete. Fletcher et al. (1988) described the case in which neoarsphenamine had been considered to be a cause of jaundice because the medicine's use in syphilitic patients led in some cases to jaundice. It was later found that the jaundice (secondary to hepatitis) was a result of unclean syringes used to inject the medicine.

Of the three influences described that will affect the determination of the cause-and-effect relationship, the major factor is bias. Bias may affect the initial group of patients studied, the intervention that is being evaluated, the outcomes that are measured, and the interpretation of the data obtained. Bias may affect any part of a clinical trial and may also affect the determination of cause and effect. In addition, there are many types of bias that may affect each aspect of a trial. More detailed information on identifying specific biases is provided in Chapters 5, 83, and 87.

GENERAL APPROACHES

In evaluating the cause-and-effect relationship it is usually optimal to have two (or more) groups to compare. The groups should be as similar as possible except in one or a small number of differences, which are chosen for evaluation. The interventions imposed on the groups are usually identical or related according to a carefully planned clinical trial design. These interventions may relate to naturally occurring or imposed events. The objective of a trial often relates to a question of cause and effect. After the data have been collected and analyzed, they are interpreted to evaluate whether the objectives of the trial have been affirmed, denied, or neither.

Establishing Which Event Preceded the Other

Although it is essential for the cause to precede the effect, there are clinical situations in which it is not certain which event is the cause and which the effect. This may occur because the precise temporal relationship is unclear between two events. One example is in asthmatic patients with respiratory failure. Some of these patients have an exaggerated rhythm of bronchial constriction that maximally occurs at about 6 A.M., the most frequent time for respiratory arrests to occur. It is not certain whether the increased amplitude of airway resistance measurements contributes to (i.e., causes) or results from (i.e., is an effect of) asthma-related respiratory failure.

Association of Two Events in Time Does Not Prove a Cause-and-Effect Relationship

The hypothesis was advanced in the late 1960s that the increasing number of deaths from asthma was associated with use of bronchodilators, because sales had also risen and asthmatic patients had used the bronchodilators during their fatal attack. The history of this period is reviewed by Esdaile et al. (1987). Herxheimer (1972) and Conolly et al. (1971) hypothesized that tachyphylaxis was responsible in part for overuse and overdose of the bronchodilators. Thus, the temporal association of bronchodilator use with the fatal asthmatic attack was used as evidence in favor of a cause-and-effect relationship. Esdaile et al. (1987) and Lanes and Walker (1987) each independently evaluated available data and concluded that the true cause of death was related to the disease itself. Physicians had not considered asthma to have a high fatality rate during the 1960s, particularly because the patients' symptoms were dramatically relieved by the bronchodilators. This raises the interesting point that relief of a disease's symptoms does not mean that the underlying disease is not progressing. Similarly, control of a diabetic's blood sugar with insulin does not mean that underlying ophthalmological and renal complications are not progressing. The purported bronchodilator tachyphylaxis was challenged by Minatoya and Spilker (1975) and Spilker and Tyll (1976). These references summarize the results of numerous others who also failed to observe tachyphylaxis. The entire hypothesis associating the increase in asthmatic deaths with bronchodilators was challenged by Spilker (1973b), who suggested that the cause of the problem was deterioration of the underlying asthma.

CRITERIA FOR DETERMINING CAUSE AND EFFECT

Hierarchy of Clinical Research Designs

The strength of the research design and manner in which the clinical trial is conducted and the data are analyzed are important aspects in evaluating the probability of a cause-and-effect relationship. Table 73.1 lists the research designs in general order of their ability to provide clinical data that are accepted as being valid. The quality of the trial's conduct and data analyses may be determined with several formal or informal methods. Methods are described in Chapter 103.

Mill's Canons

Many clinical trials are conducted to investigate the cause of a problem or to establish whether a hypoth-

TABLE 73.1 *Relative strength of evidence (i.e., a validity hierarchy) in support of efficacy according to the general type of clinical trial used to obtain data[a]*

1. Anecdotal observations or comments of investigators or patients
2. Case reports
3. Uncontrolled series of patients
4. Cases obtained from computer data bases
5. A series of patients with literature controls
6. A series of patients with retrospective (i.e., historical) controls
7. Open-label trial
8. Randomized trial (single-blind)
9. Randomized active-medicine-controlled trial (double-blind)
10. Randomized placebo-controlled trial (double-blind)
11. Randomized active-medicine- and placebo-controlled trial (double-blind)
12. Confirmatory trial of a trial listed under 10 or 11

[a] These are listed in order from weakest to strongest.

esized cause is the true cause of a problem. The cause is sometimes referred to as the etiology or pathogenesis of a disease. A number of the criteria used to establish a cause-and-effect relationship are given in Table 73.2. This table includes the four types of tests referred to as Mill's canons, after John Stuart Mill who devised them.

Hierarchy of Cause-and-Effect Criteria

A hierarchy of criteria for establishing a cause-and-effect relationship was published (Table 73.3) by Sackett et al. (1985). These authors also described the relative importance of each of these nine factors in decid-

TABLE 73.2 *Criteria and methods that may be used to establish a cause-and-effect relationship*

1. The cause must precede the effect in time
2. The cause produces something that is defined as an effect, as opposed to the cause resulting from the effect[a]
3. Compare situations that are the same (or nearly so) in all but one variable[b]
4. Compare situations that only are the same in one condition. For example, many clinical trials are conducted on one topic, such as whether smoking causes lung cancer. Each trial differs from the others in trial design, but all demonstrate the same cause-and-effect association
5. Factors being studied vary in a systematic way with each other. When the "cause" changes, the "effect" also varies (e.g., dose–response relationship of a medicine or nonmedicine)
6. Factors that are established causes are eliminated from consideration, and the contribution of the remaining factors is measured (e.g., if smoking accounts for most cases of squamous cell lung cancer, then one may study causes of squamous cell lung cancer in nonsmokers)

[a] This relationship is not always easy to establish with 100% certainty. See text for example relating to asthma. Fletcher et al. (1988) provide an example relating to the use of estrogens and uterine bleeding.
[b] Points 3 to 6 are referred to as Mill's canons (Susser, 1973). These are named "method of difference" (3), "method of agreement" (4), "method of concomitant variation" (5), and "method of residues" (6).

TABLE 73.3 *Diagnostic tests for causation[a]*

1. Is there evidence from true experiments in humans?
2. Is the association strong?
3. Is the association consistent from trial to trial?
4. Is the temporal relationship correct?
5. Is there a dose–response gradient?
6. Does the association make epidemiologic sense?
7. Does the association make biologic sense?
8. Is the association specific?
9. Is the association analogous to a previously proven causal association?

[a] These diagnostic tests are listed in decreasing order of their importance.
Reprinted by permission of Little, Brown & Co. from Sackett et al. (1985).

ing whether a cause-and-effect relationship is established (Table 73.4). Finally, Table 73.5 describes a number of techniques that may be used to increase the probability of validating or disproving a cause-and-effect relationship.

Various Perspectives

Various scientific disciplines often view the "cause" of a particular disease from different perspectives. The clinician who observes a patient in a clinic and diagnoses a bacterial infection generally concludes that the bacteria caused the infection and views the clinical manifestations of the problem. A social worker, geneticist, surgeon, pathologist, or other scientist may view the cause as being quite different, depending on the conditions that predisposed the patient to be susceptible to the bacteria. The patient may also (1) have had a concurrent disease that diminished resistance to the bacteria, (2) have received a medicine that suppressed the body's ability to fight the bacteria, (3) have genetic factors that influenced susceptibility to infection, (4) live near someone who is chronically infected, (5) have malnutrition, and/or (6) live in crowded and unsanitary conditions. These or other reasons may have predisposed the patient to have acquired the infection. Other types of reasons include alterations in the patient's anatomy as a result of congenital problems (e.g., of heart valves) or previous surgery. Thus, the immediate cause of the infection (the bacteria) may be insufficient information to explain fully why a particular patient was infected with a particular bacterium at a particular anatomical location. Numerous additional factors that may have predisposed the patient to infection from the bacteria could also be proposed and investigated.

Direct and Predisposing Causes

The most effective treatment in many diseases is not one that solely acts at the final step in the process but is the treatment that is targeted to the predisposing

TABLE 73.4 *Importance of individual diagnostic tests in making the causal decision*

| | Effect of test result on causal decision[a] | | |
Diagnostic test[b]	When test result consistent with causation	When test result neutral or inconclusive	When test result opposes causation
Human experiments	+ + + +	− − −	− − − −
Strength of association			
From randomized trials	+ + + +	− − −	− − − −
From cohort study	+ + +	− −	− − −
From case-control study	+	0	−
Consistency	+ + +	− −	− − −
Temporality	+ +	− −	− − − −
Dose−response gradient	+ +	−	− −
Epidemiological sense	+ +	−	− −
Biological sense	+	0	−
Specificity of the association	+	0	−
Analogy with previous association	+	0	0

Reprinted by permission of Little, Brown & Co. from Sackett et al., 1985.

[a] Meaning of symbols: +, causation supported; −, causation rejected; 0, causal decision not affected. The numbers of +s and −s indicate the relative contribution of the diagnostic test to the causal decision.

[b] These tests refer to those criteria listed in Table 73.3.

cause(s) or risk factors that may have led to the problem or may even precipitate the problem on a recurring basis. A simplistic example of this is in asthmatic individuals whose attacks are precipitated by cold weather. Treating the symptoms is important, but if an individual were to move to a warmer climate it might break the overall cycle of asthmatic attacks triggered by low temperatures.

These points illustrate that diseases have both immediate and distant (predisposing) causes, some of which may be difficult to ascertain. Distant causes include both genetic and environmental factors.

Convincing, Strong, and Weak Evidence

Establishing the cause-and-effect relationship for a medicine (cause) and an adverse event (effect) was dis-

TABLE 73.5 *Methods to increase the probability of validating or disproving a cause-and-effect relationship*

1. Obtain measurements at multiple time points associated with the event (i.e., do not merely collect data at single before and after time points)
2. Change or modify the purported cause and observe how the effect is changed or influenced
3. Evaluate other clinical trials in which the same association was sought and/or detected
4. Extrapolate the association to different levels of biological activity and assess whether data exist to support this
5. Extrapolate the association to different populations or conditions and assess whether data exist to support this
6. Establish a dose−response relationship (if possible)
7. Remove the cause of the disease and evaluate whether the risk of disease is modified (e.g., people who give up smoking decrease their risk of getting lung cancer)
8. Determine if there are mutiple controlled trials that establish the same cause-and-effect relationship, which would strengthen its likelihood of being a real effect[a]

[a] The chance of an uncontrolled trial yielding a false-positive response is greater than that for controlled trials. See Chapter 4 for a discussion of this point.

cussed by Venning (1983a). He proposed five types of "convincing evidence" for establishing cause and effect: (1) rechallenge data, (2) dose−response data, (3) data from controlled studies, (4) experimental data on mechanisms of pathogenesis, and (5) close association in time and space (e.g., local reactions at the site of injection, acute anaphylaxis). He proposed three types of "strong evidence": (1) uniqueness of the adverse event, (2) extreme rarity of adverse event in absence of medicine usage, and (3) data that a medicine causes minor forms of an adverse event, which may indicate that it is responsible for a more severe adverse event. Finally, he proposed three types of "weak evidence": (1) association of a medicine with common or only moderately rare events relative to extent of medicine usage, (2) demonstration of pharmacological actions of a medicine not established as relevant to pathogenesis of adverse event, and (3) improvement after withdrawal without rechallenge.

Tests for Establishing Causation (i.e., the Relationship of Two Events as Cause and Effect)

The types of associations between events or factors in a clinical trial are listed in Table 73.6. The nine criteria

TABLE 73.6 *Types of associations that may be observed between events or factors in a clinical trial*

1. Causal, direct relationship (i.e., cause-and-effect)
2. Indirect relationship resulting from a confounding factor
3. Biased relationship resulting from an influence that should not be present[a]
4. A systematic artifact influences the relationship observed
5. No relationship (i.e., the factors function totally independently)
6. Chance relationship (i.e., no relationship exists, except one that was observed by chance)

[a] Error is introduced by biases, which introduce systematic variation into the trial and lead to a purported association.

mentioned in Table 73.3 as tests for establishing causation are described briefly.

1. *Is there evidence from true experiments in humans?* Data from well-controlled clinical trials providing strong evidence that two associated events have a cause–effect relationship should be combined with other criteria. For an adverse event, if the medicine is decreased or stopped (i.e., a dechallenge), does the adverse event disappear, and if the medicine is restarted (i.e., a rechallenge), does the adverse event reappear?

2. *Is the association strong?* When the relative risk of an adverse event occurring is two or greater, there is less likelihood that the association is a result of undetected confounding. The greater the magnitude of the response, or relative risk observed, the more likely it is that the association is a true one.

3. *Is the association consistent from study to study?* This is self-explanatory. An association observed by multiple people under a variety of circumstances at different times and places is more likely to indicate a real cause-and-effect relationship. A true association should be reproducible, and a single report must always be regarded cautiously.

4. *Is the temporal relationship correct?* Although the cause must always precede the effect, it is not always certain which event preceded the other in time. For example, it is not always immediately apparent whether the medicine a patient is taking caused the symptom or whether the symptom of the disease led to the patient taking the medicine.

5. *Is there a dose–response gradient?* Although it intuitively seems obvious that higher doses should lead to greater effects or greater risk, this is not always the case. For example, anaphylaxis does not exhibit a dose–response relationship. Moreover, the patient's response may be at the plateau phase of the dose–response, or homeostatic mechanisms may keep the clinical endpoints at a constant level, even though certain subcellular processes are more marked. An increase in the intensity of exposure of many people to a causative agent (e.g., toxic fumes) is associated with an increased risk of the resulting disease or adverse event.

6. *Does the association make epidemiological sense?* The association should be in general agreement with known facts about the natural history of the disease.

7. *Does the association make biological sense?* The association should generally make sense when other types of biological data are considered (e.g., animal data, pathological data, associations of related medicines, associations of related diseases). This criterion is not always met (e.g., scrotal cancer in chimney sweeps, birth defects in infants whose mothers had rubella during their first trimester).

8. *Is the association specific?* This criterion suggests that the association is stronger when the cause does not occur without the purported effect also occurring, and when the effect does not occur without the purported cause having previously occurred. Nonetheless, a high degree of specificity is rare in biology; one cause usually can lead to multiple effects and one effect can result from multiple causes. Thus, this criterion is rarely met.

9. *Is the association analogous to a previously proven causal association?* The probability of causality is enhanced if other related examples can be found in which causality was established.

MODELS OF CAUSE-AND-EFFECT RELATIONSHIPS

Models Focusing on Direct and Indirect Causes

Figure 73.1 illustrates four models that are used to help describe cause-and-effect relationships. Model 1 illustrates a simple and straightforward approach to describing this concept. A single direct (proximate) cause acts on a patient's baseline state and either immediately or through a series of processes leads to an outcome such as a disease. In many clinical situations there often appears to be a single direct cause of a disease, such as the tubercle bacillus causing tuberculosis.

The identity of a direct (proximate) or indirect (distant) cause is a relative matter. The identification of the variables that are being studied serves to determine which causes are labeled as direct and which are labeled as indirect. It is important that all direct causes operate at the same level of organization (e.g., cellular, organ, organism) as the effect that is being measured. Causes that are operating at a different level of organization are by definition indirect causes. Levels of organization are described in Chapter 71.

The second model illustrates several direct causes that act on the baseline to bring about an outcome. Some of these causes are more important than others (indicated by the thickness of the arrow), and only one (or more) may be needed to achieve the outcome. An example is noted in describing the cause of hypertension, which according to the mosaic theory suggests that several direct causes are often involved (e.g., consumption of salt, calcium, and other nutrients) in addition to numerous factors that affect the patient's baseline state (e.g., genetic predisposition, previous medical history).

Models 3 and 4 illustrate that direct causes and base-

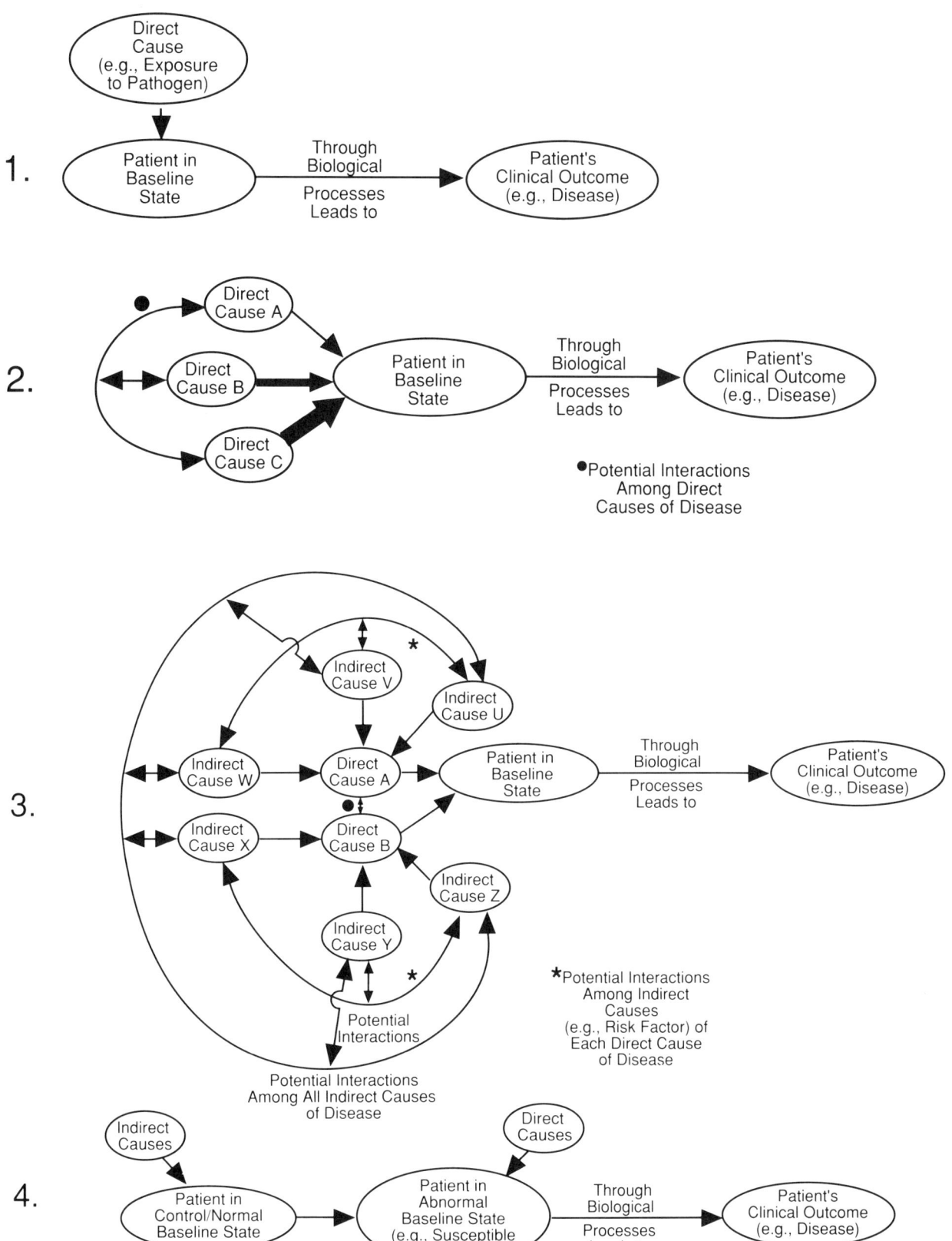

1.

2.

●Potential Interactions
Among Direct
Causes of Disease

3.

*Potential Interactions
Among Indirect
Causes
(e.g., Risk Factor) of
Each Direct Cause
of Disease

Potential Interactions
Among All Indirect Causes
of Disease

4.

FIG. 73-1. Models to illustrate factors involved in cause-and-effect relationships. Direct and indirect causes may be considered as proximate and distant causes of the outcome(s). "Processes" refer to biological steps whereby the baseline state is converted to a diseased state.

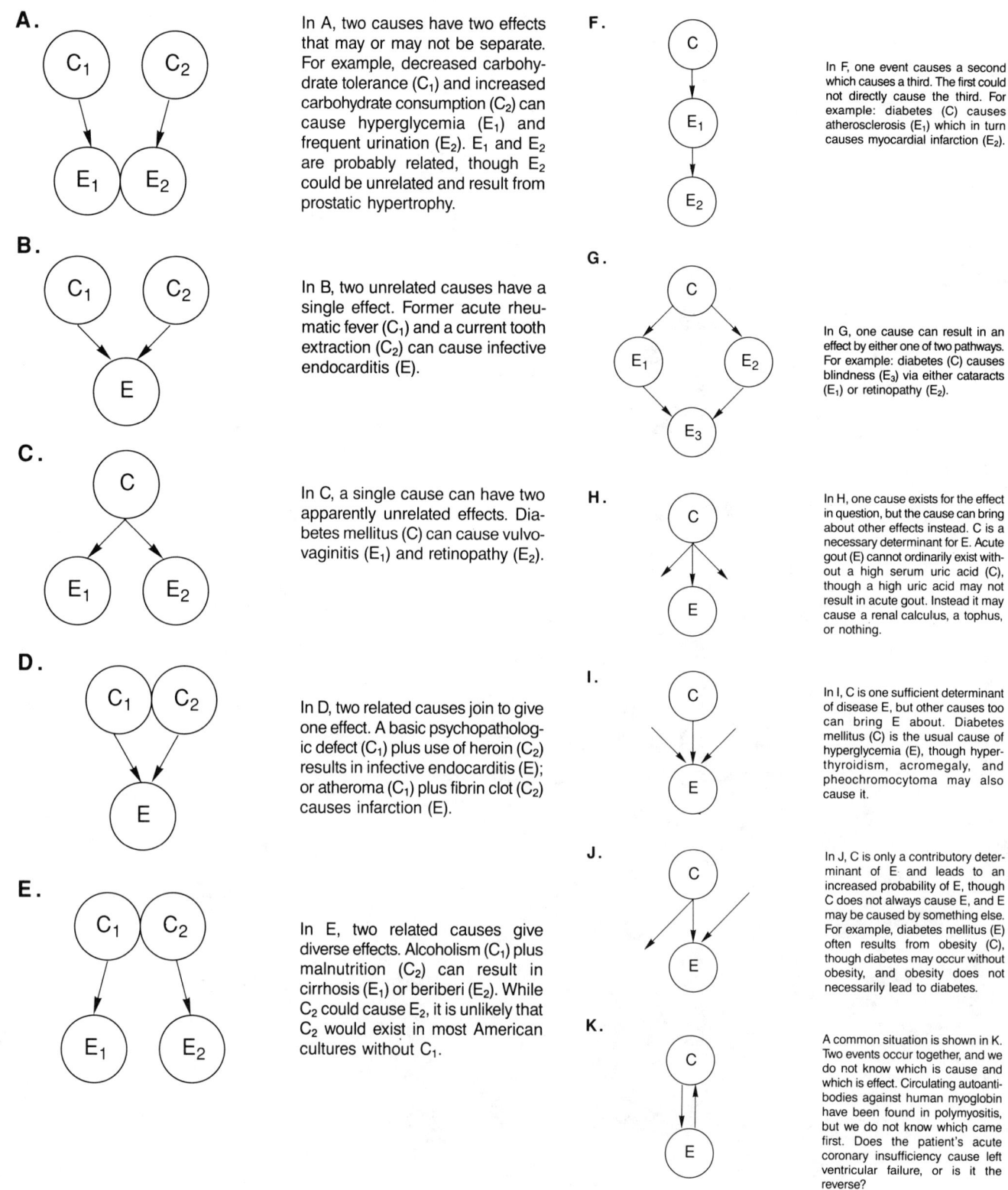

A. In A, two causes have two effects that may or may not be separate. For example, decreased carbohydrate tolerance (C_1) and increased carbohydrate consumption (C_2) can cause hyperglycemia (E_1) and frequent urination (E_2). E_1 and E_2 are probably related, though E_2 could be unrelated and result from prostatic hypertrophy.

B. In B, two unrelated causes have a single effect. Former acute rheumatic fever (C_1) and a current tooth extraction (C_2) can cause infective endocarditis (E).

C. In C, a single cause can have two apparently unrelated effects. Diabetes mellitus (C) can cause vulvovaginitis (E_1) and retinopathy (E_2).

D. In D, two related causes join to give one effect. A basic psychopathologic defect (C_1) plus use of heroin (C_2) results in infective endocarditis (E); or atheroma (C_1) plus fibrin clot (C_2) causes infarction (E).

E. In E, two related causes give diverse effects. Alcoholism (C_1) plus malnutrition (C_2) can result in cirrhosis (E_1) or beriberi (E_2). While C_2 could cause E_2, it is unlikely that C_2 would exist in most American cultures without C_1.

F. In F, one event causes a second which causes a third. The first could not directly cause the third. For example: diabetes (C) causes atherosclerosis (E_1) which in turn causes myocardial infarction (E_2).

G. In G, one cause can result in an effect by either one of two pathways. For example: diabetes (C) causes blindness (E_3) via either cataracts (E_1) or retinopathy (E_2).

H. In H, one cause exists for the effect in question, but the cause can bring about other effects instead. C is a necessary determinant for E. Acute gout (E) cannot ordinarily exist without a high serum uric acid (C), though a high uric acid may not result in acute gout. Instead it may cause a renal calculus, a tophus, or nothing.

I. In I, C is one sufficient determinant of disease E, but other causes too can bring E about. Diabetes mellitus (C) is the usual cause of hyperglycemia (E), though hyperthyroidism, acromegaly, and pheochromocytoma may also cause it.

J. In J, C is only a contributory determinant of E and leads to an increased probability of E, though C does not always cause E, and E may be caused by something else. For example, diabetes mellitus (E) often results from obesity (C), though diabetes may occur without obesity, and obesity does not necessarily lead to diabetes.

K. A common situation is shown in K. Two events occur together, and we do not know which is cause and which is effect. Circulating autoantibodies against human myoglobin have been found in polymyositis, but we do not know which came first. Does the patient's acute coronary insufficiency cause left ventricular failure, or is it the reverse?

FIG. 73.2 Types and examples of cause-and-effect relationships. (Modified from Cutler, 1985, with permission of Williams & Wilkins.)

line states may each have an indirect cause or causes. Multiple direct and indirect causes operate in almost all clinical situations in which cause and effect are considered. The practical ability to study effectively and interpret a particular phenomenon in a single clinical trial usually limits consideration to the major direct cause(s) and few (if any) indirect causes. In the case of tuberculosis, one may expand the frame of reference in model 1 to include some of the more indirect causes relating to the host organism and/or environment. These include factors that affect (1) the viability of the tubercle bacillus, (2) the patient's immune state, (3) tissue reactions, (4) exposure to the bacillus, (5) exposure to other patients with tuberculosis, and (6) quality of living standards in terms of air temperature, water supply, sanitation, health education, immunization, and nutrition.

Thus, a more complex pattern of proximate and distant causes (i.e., direct and indirect causes) usually operates in clinical situations in which the strength of the cause-and effect-relationship is being evaluated. In terms of multiple factors causing responses, there are usually many potential causes relating to patient characteristics, including both inherent and acquired characteristics.

Models of Related and Unrelated Causes and also of Effects

A series of models were described by Cutler (1985) to illustrate different examples of cause and effect. These were slightly modified and are shown in Fig. 73.2. Medical examples of each relationship are also presented in this figure.

CHAPTER 74

Clinical Significance versus Statistical Significance of Abnormal Data

ESTABLISHING CLINICAL SIGNIFICANCE

In order to evaluate the clinical significance of data, it is usually essential to know whether physicians would alter their practice of medicine based on the results from a specific clinical trial. To address this question, it is necessary to know how large a difference in the data would be judged clinically significant for the groups studied. This concept involves determination of the magnitude and overall quality of data that would be judged important enough clinically to encourage physicians to alter their therapeutic practices. The magnitude and type of data (e.g., reversal of coma, reverting arrhythmias to a sinus rhythm) required to influence physicians may be assessed by surveying or interviewing practicing and opinion-setting physicians, preferably prior to a clinical trial. The magnitude of effect and quality of data are then incorporated in the protocol as important goals for the trial to achieve. Other considerations of quality relate to how well the trial design, conduct, and analysis will stand up to close scrutiny. Considerations related to the target disease include whether (1) the disease represents an important clinical problem, (2) alternative treatments are available, and (3) alternative treatments are satisfactory.

Definition of Clinical Significance for Efficacy Measures

Clinical significance for efficacy measures may be defined as:

1. The amount of change in the parameter(s) of efficacy that defines a patient as a responder in a clinical trial.
2. The amount of change in the parameter(s) of efficacy that would encourage practicing physicians to use or at least try the new treatment in their patients.

These definitions are often the same.

Definition of Clinical Significance for Safety Measures

In a sense, safety is never proved, only disproved. A new medicine that has never been tested in humans could be considered 100% safe. Exposure of patients to this medicine will demonstrate the number, incidence, and clinical significance of observed adverse events. Each adverse event takes something away from the medicine's perfect safety profile. For some medicines, the risk of adverse events becomes so great that the benefits are not sufficient for physicians to use the medicine, and its development is either discontinued or suspended. If the medicine is marketed then it is either pulled off the market or it suffers a serious decline in sales.

The clinical significance of a medicine's safety profile may be considered from four viewpoints: (1) the individual patient receiving the medicine, (2) the patients in a clinical trial receiving the medicine, (3) all patients receiving the medicine, and (4) all patients who may potentially receive the medicine. The clinical significance of the first viewpoint is gauged entirely by the treating physician based on many factors, including severity, risk factors, type of treatment required, patient's views, degree of benefit obtained, and response to treatment. The second and third viewpoints are judged by the sponsor or proponent of the new treatment. This individual or group has more data to consider in evaluating the adverse event in comparison with other patients and in the context of other clinical trial results.

LEVELS OF CLINICAL SIGNIFICANCE

There are five levels of clinical significance for the impact and importance of clinical events:

Level 1: The individual patient. The event may be major or minor for that patient, but have no impact for other patients receiving the medicine.

Level 2: The group of patients in a clinical trial. The event may be protocol related or may result from conditions of a particular trial, but other patients are not affected.

Level 3: All patients currently receiving the treatment. An adverse event may have occurred that indicates a slower taper period is appropriate. This will impact all patients receiving the treatment.

Level 4: All patients who received the treatment in the past. There have been times when all patients who had received a treatment (e.g., radiation to their thymus gland, a medicine) are sought out to check for adverse sequelae (e.g., thyroid problems, liver enzyme elevations).

Level 5: All patients with the disease who may receive the medicine in future. Many adverse events have implications for patients who may receive a medicine in the future.

RELEVANCE OF THE TERM *CLINICAL SIGNIFICANCE* FOR CHARACTERIZING ABNORMALITIES IN A CLINICAL TRIAL

Because of various problems involved in the determination of whether an abnormality is clinically significant, it is useful to have an operational definition of *clinical significance.* The section on terminology in the beginning of the book presents a definition and considerations relating to this term in addition to those above. Use of a single definition improves the likelihood of intrarater, interrater, and intersite consistency in reporting abnormalities. Neither the sponsor nor the investigator, however, is obliged to include the term clinically significant in a trial protocol or report. The attribution of the abnormality to a medicine, plus therapeutic countermeasures used, should more than adequately describe whether an abnormality was in fact truly clinically significant. Prerequisite information needed by an individual who wishes to apply clinical judgment about an adverse reaction or abnormal laboratory result is presented in Table 74.1.

The term *clinically significant* to characterize an adverse reaction does not necessarily mean that treatment had to be instituted for the patient, since "increased observation" may have been a sufficient clinical response. Thus, the term *clinically significant*

TABLE 74.1 *Prerequisites to apply clinical judgment optimally as illustrated with two selected situations*

A. To treat a patient experiencing an adverse reaction
  1. Accurate diagnosis of the patient's disease
  2. Knowledge of available information on the pathology, physiology, and other characteristics of the disease
  3. Knowledge of the biochemistry, pharmacology, and pharmacokinetics of the medicines contemplated for use and those actually being given to the patient
  4. Knowledge of potential interactions and adverse reactions of alternative treatments
  5. Knowledge of optimal monitoring techniques to follow a patient's course
  6. Knowledge of the patient's medical history
B. To interpret clinical laboratory test results
  1. Experience in understanding when to order specific tests
  2. Knowledge of the test's sensitivity and specificity
  3. Knowledge of the relationship among test results, clinical diagnosis, and disease intensity in a broad population of patients and, if possible, in the particular patient(s) in whom the test was ordered
  4. Ability to discern the optimal interpretation(s) of the result
  5. Knowledge of the prevalence of the disease(s) for which the test was ordered
  6. Factors that may confound the results of the test (e.g., concurrent illnesses, concomitant medicines)

may not indicate that treatment was required but probably is an indicator that the investigator viewed the abnormality as worthy of special precaution (or treatment) and was alert to its actual or potential importance for the patient's health. If the designation of *clinically significant* for an abnormality provides the investigator with a useful guide to follow the course of an abnormality, then it probably does have value in a clinical trial. However, if this concept will not be used for following the course of a patient's abnormality, then the magnitude and severity of the abnormality and its association with treatment may be adequate information to collect. The potential value of this measure (clinical significance) must be determined separately for each trial.

The finding that an abnormality is clinically significant in 15 of 45 patients conveys less information than the statement that the abnormality had a severe intensity in 10 patients, a moderate intensity in 10 patients, and a mild intensity in 25 others.

INDIVIDUALS AND GROUPS WHO EVALUATE ABNORMALITIES

The patient and the investigator (usually a physician) are the central individuals in a clinical trial. Beyond this core group are many other people who may have some claim on the right to interpret the patient's abnormality in terms of its clinical significance. These other individuals include:

1. A coinvestigator or assistant investigator (who are often physicians) who has actually examined the patient and diagnosed, observed, or determined the abnormality.
2. Investigator's staff
   a. Nurses often interview patients and probe for adverse events.
   b. The Research Coordinator may have interviewed the patient and learned about the abnormality.
   c. Clinical assistants (e.g., fellows, residents, other medical faculty) often have examined the patient.
3. Study-related staff, usually at the trial site
   a. Specialists involved with testing or treating the patient in a specific part of the clinical trial.
   b. Consultants who are requested to evaluate a specific problem or condition.
4. Sponsor
   a. Physicians involved with the trial receive all data connected with it and have a thorough knowledge of the medicine and its clinical and preclinical characteristics.
   b. Nonphysicians involved with the clinical trial (e.g., monitors) usually have access to the patient's complete history and the entire pharmacology of the medicine.
   c. Statisticians or other staff at the sponsoring institution have possibly evaluated previous problems or other significant issues related to the medicine that are similar to the current problem.
5. Individuals connected with the patient
   a. Family members may have observed the present and possibly previous episodes (examples) of the adverse event.
   b. Friends may have observed the present and possibly previous episodes (examples) of the adverse event.
6. Others
   a. The Ethics Committee/Investigational Review Board (IRB) receives information from the investigator on all severe noteworthy adverse events plus periodic updates on others. This group may wish to define clinically significant events either using different criteria or applying the same criteria differently than the investigator.
   b. Regulatory agencies are in a somewhat similar situation as the Ethics Committee/IRB except that regulatory agencies usually receive information on abnormalities from the sponsor (for a sponsored clinical trial).

Almost all of these individuals, including the patient, may have input into the decision as to whether an abnormality is clinically significant, but the final decision is for the investigator to make. This decision is usually made according to one of the scales described below, although other scales or systems are possible. A scale that forces the investigator to weigh all relevant factors and to make a judgment about clinical significance (i.e., Yes, No, Unknown) is preferred.

Perspectives on Clinical Significance

1. *Regulatory authorities.* The regulatory authority's view of the clinical significance of data is based on a determination of how the nation's health will be affected—in a positive or negative way. This benefit-to-risk assessment concerns all patients with the disease, or the subset that would be affected by the decision. Regulatory authorities also focus on the clinical significance of one or more trials.

2. *Pharmaceutical companies.* When determining clinical significance, pharmaceutical companies focus on the probability that they will receive approval for marketing from regulatory authorities in a timely fashion for the dosage forms, indications, and other aspects of labeling they seek. The clinical significance of data is also associated with the forecast of sales. Small differences in a clinical profile can lead to much greater or smaller changes in forecasts and eventual sales.

3. *Clinical investigators.* To the investigators, the clinical significance of the trial is often related to their motivation for conducting the trial. Will the publications that result be viewed as important contributions? Will their careers be helped by the trial? Will they be able to treat patients better? Will the results be able to attract new trials from the same or other sponsor?

4. *Treating physicians.* Their major question is whether they will be able to treat their patients better. This answer depends on their seeing the data and believing the results.

5. *Patients.* Most patients would ask three questions relating to the clinical significance of a trial. Will the new treatment help me feel better now? Will the new treatment prevent future problems and help me feel better tomorrow? Will the new treatment help my underlying disease improve?

SCALES USED TO RATE CLINICAL SIGNIFICANCE

The question of whether a specific abnormality is clinically significant may be addressed through the use of a scale. Three scales are:

1. *Yes—No—Unknown*
2. *Always—Often—Sometimes—Hardly Ever—Never*
3. *Probable—Possible—Doubtful.* This scale is considered too vague and generally less useful than the preceding two scales.

Venulet et al. (1980) proposed that a physician working for the sponsor should make the final decision on the clinical significance of an abnormal event. This procedure has an advantage in that it avoids the problem that arises when more than one investigator or physician sees the patient at different times and they evaluate adverse events or other abnormalities differently. Another advantage relates to uniformity of approach to all patient abnormalities. Disadvantages include the following: (1) the physician making the decision about clinical significance is not the treating physician; (2) with rare exception, the physician at the sponsoring institution has not met or examined the patient; and (3) a charge of bias may be raised because of purported conflicts of interest at the sponsoring institution.

COLLECTING AND PROCESSING CLINICALLY SIGNIFICANT DATA ON ABNORMAL EVENTS

In designing clinical trials to detect clinically significant effects it is often necessary to bring experts together to assess which parameters to measure, in what hierarchy they should be ranked, and how large a change in each parameter constitutes a clinically significant change. Because all parameters are not of equal importance it is sometimes desirable to equalize them. This is most commonly done by assigning a numerical factor (i.e., a number) that is multiplied by the result to obtain a value indicative of its relative importance. This is called a *weight*. The larger the weight, the greater is the importance of the test. Weights attributed to efficacy parameters varied greatly according to rheumatologists (Chaput de Saintonge et al., 1988), but weights of parameters in disease areas with more standardized measures would presumably differ to a lesser degree.

The decision of whether an abnormal event (e.g., adverse reaction or laboratory value) has clinical importance may be indicated on the data collection forms. The most straightforward manner of doing this is to have a column or space printed on the data collection form next to each potential listing for indicating whether any abnormality observed is judged to be clinically significant. The column may (1) be blank to permit write-in responses, (2) contain separate boxes to be checked (e.g., Yes, No, Unknown), or (3) have printed words (e.g., Yes, No, Unknown) to be circled or otherwise marked.

If it is decided to collect data of clinical significance on the data collection form, this information must eventually be edited, entered in a computer (or tabulated), analyzed, and reported. If these events are relatively uncommon, then they may be reported with a simple listing and description in a report. The significance of these comments in the trial and for the test treatment should be evaluated and discussed. If there are relatively large numbers of a specific abnormality that is clinically significant, then these data may be organized according to various criteria (e.g., intensity of the problem, association with medicine, age, weight, sex, or race of patient). Incidence figures may be determined to indicate the scope of the problem.

A clinically significant abnormality will often be totally unrelated to the trial treatment and may be attributed to (1) concurrent illness, (2) chronic problem, (3) concomitant medicine, (4) trauma, or (5) other factors. It is important to consider each of these (and other) possibilities in deriving the most important association(s) and cause(s) of clinically significant abnormalities.

LIMITATIONS OF STATISTICS AND RELATIONSHIP OF STATISTICAL SIGNIFICANCE TO CLINICAL SIGNIFICANCE

The role of statistics in the planning of a medicine trial and in the analysis of data is critically important. Once data are analyzed appropriately, it is possible to interpret them. Choosing the optimal statistical tests and using them appropriately is neither simple nor straightforward. The choice of the most appropriate statistical tests to use lies in the purview of the statistician. Nonetheless, the clinician who will interpret the data should have an opportunity to discuss the anticipated types of interpretations to be made with the statistician prior to the choice of specific tests by the statistician. Ideally, there should be a joint collaboration between the statistician and clinician during both the analysis and interpretation phases of a clinical trial, although the former is primarily statistical and the latter is primarily clinical. The separation drawn in this book between the two processes is acknowledged to be somewhat artificial and arbitrary in some situations.

After all of the analyses are completed, their meaning in terms of the clinical trial objectives must be determined. Additionally, the implications of the interpretation for clinical care of patients must be determined. The overlap or integration between statistical and clinical significance will be separated and examined in some detail.

Strengths of Statistics

There are many strengths and weaknesses in statistics. Statistics can demonstrate the likelihood that the association of two events could have occurred by chance and assess whether the relationship is strong or weak. Statistics can provide essential information on the number of patients necessary to enroll in a clinical trial and the methods to use in testing a hypothesis. Statistics can also make many other important contributions to the overall successful initiation, completion, and analysis of the trial.

Weaknesses of Statistics

There are a number of statistical pitfalls that may trap the unwary interpreter, and this chapter describes a few of these. Some of the pitfalls that must be considered during the process of clinical interpretation of data are described more fully in Chapter 77.

What statistics cannot do is to make a clinical interpretation of the data. It cannot on its own provide a description of the meaningfulness or significance of data. Interpretation requires a consideration of the clinical situation that exists in individual patients in the clinical trial population and/or in a larger patient population. A p value of 0.0001 may relate to a trivial point with little or no clinical consequence, whereas a borderline p value of 0.055 may have enormous clinical relevance and significance. No p value on its own may establish a clinical fact or truth. A medicine-induced

change in heart rate of 4 bpm may be highly significant statistically but will rarely have even weak clinical significance. Feinstein (1977, p. 258) has stated that "Perhaps the most deleterious consequence of using conventional statistical theory in modern clinical science has been the widespread fantasy that a *statistically significant* difference is a *significant* difference."

Appropriateness of Statistical Tests Used

In order for there to be a strong relationship between statistical and clinical significance, the most relevant statistical tests for the situation must have been used. In most situations, some statistical tests that could be used to analyze the data are clearly applicable, others clearly are not, and yet others are of debatable acceptability. The appropriateness of the tests and measures used in a clinical trial (to generate the data) for the specific clinical situation or disease must have been established and preferably validated prior to the trial. Likewise, the appropriateness of the statistical tests chosen to analyze the data must be established and preferably validated prior to the trial. If this has not been done, then the most highly significant data in terms of statistical analyses may have absolutely no relevance for the clinical situation that it was intended to evaluate.

Biological Significance

It is possible to discuss biological significance as distinct from clinical and statistical significance. *Biological significance* refers to the value of a scientific interpretation of basic mechanisms and effects within the body. In the context of a clinical trial, the biological significance relates to the fundamental pharmacological, physiological, or other effects leading to the clinical effects that are felt, observed, or measured. Biological significance is considered as part of clinical significance in this book, and no distinction between the two is made from now on.

CLUSTERS OF EVENTS IN A COMMUNITY

What Are Clusters?

A *cluster* of events refers to a greater prevalence or incidence of a health-related event than would be expected within a specific time and in a specific place. Although one or more clusters never proves an association with a purported cause, it often establishes a hypothesis that may (or may not) be testable. Some clusters involve an event that may be tested in prospective studies. For those clusters a hypothesis is generated (e.g., exposure to a certain chemical causes cancer) and tested. Many clusters, however, are isolated events that will never recur, and prospective testing is impossible.

Why Investigate Clusters?

Clusters of events in a community must be seriously and thoroughly explored, because the mere perception of a problem in a community means that there is a problem. Nonetheless, most purported clusters involve only two to five cases and classical statistical methods cannot be used to test their significance. These events often represent a difficult public health issue, and coincidence can rarely be ruled out.

How to Investigate Clusters

One of the first steps in investigating clusters is to consider the biological plausibility of the trend they suggest and to develop alternative hypotheses (see Chapter 76). The susceptible population should be identified (if possible) and substantial efforts may have to be made to establish a reference rate. This process establishes the baseline incidence of the event, against which the new rate may be compared. A reference rate should not be based solely on a local area; a large geographical area is necessary for validation of a reference rate. When the investigation is complete, the results should be described in detail rather than in general. For example, one could say: "In a city the size of Akron, Ohio, two cases per year are expected and six occurred." An undesirable approach is to omit this sentence and merely say that the risk was three times the expected risk in Akron.

At a recent conference on clusters, many experts reported that almost all clusters are false alarms (Raymond, 1989). All purported clusters must be examined, however, even though only a very few turn out to be real. An event often occurs several times in a short period, without there being any change in the causative agent or its characteristics. For example, a hospital may not have any cases of disease X for 2 years and then three cases may be brought there in 1 week. This is shown most clearly by examining how random and even nonrandom events seem to clump together.

CLUMPING OF DATA

Random events tend to clump in various ways. Numerous examples illustrate this theory and also indicate that the data a clinician obtains in any clinical trial may lead to incorrect interpretations because of the clumping of results. For example, flipping a coin and counting the number of heads or tails is usually stated to yield 50% chance of either heads or tails occurring at each coin toss. In series in which a coin was flipped several thousand times, it was found that long "runs" occurred when only heads or tails turned up. Another example is that seven consecutive 3s occur in the value of pi. Data obtained by clinicians must include enough measurements to ensure that a clump of data has not overly influenced the results and yielded a false-negative or false-positive interpretation.

As the examples given above illustrate, there may be no correlation whatsoever between statistical and clinical significance, the relationship may be extremely tight and well established, or the relationship may fit anywhere between these extremes.

CRITIQUING STATISTICAL RESULTS

Huff (1954) proposed several questions to provide an impression of the value and validity of statistical information. These are questions that a skeptic might ask and are also appropriate to ask about clinical interpretations.

1. Who says so? This includes the necessity to look for biases, both conscious and unconscious.
2. How does he or she know? How complete is the survey, and is the sample large enough?
3. What is missing? This refers to data error values and other details.
4. Did someone change the subject?
5. Is there a *post hoc* cause-and-effect relationship?
6. Do the results make sense?

ALTERNATIVES TO STATISTICAL EVALUATIONS

Although most clinical investigators and professional staff are used to reaching decisions about clinical significance based on a statistical analysis of data, there are alternative means for arriving at a decision that can markedly affect clinical practice.

1. In cases of rare diseases or rare events, a few case studies can provide sufficient clinical evidence to influence clinical treatment of almost all patients with the disease, even though statistical analyses have not been performed.
2. If the response to treatment is so dramatic that controls are unnecessary, a few cases may greatly influence clinical treatment (e.g., use of Fab fragments to reverse otherwise fatal digoxin overdosage; Smith et al., 1976).
3. If the therapeutic value of two (or more) treatments is generally comparable and the costs are shown to be quite different, physician preference

may be swayed to favor the less expensive treatment.

4. A definition of clinically significant medicine activity may be established prior to a clinical trial. The numbers of patients who achieve (and who do not achieve) this standard may be determined in the trial. This type of simple computation, even without additional statistical analyses, may greatly influence therapy of other patients.

The Post Hoc Propter Hoc Issue

Using only a few patients to draw conclusions raises the possibility of making a major error of the *post hoc propter hoc* fallacy type. This occurs when an observation reached on a patient after treatment leads to a conclusion about the cause and is probably the main reason for the many thousands of worthless cures and remedies promulgated from ancient times through to the present. There are still discoveries being made about the relative worthlessness of commonly used medical practices. One relatively recent example is the purported barbiturate antagonist bemegride, which was highly promoted in the 1950s to be effective based on case reports. Subsequent evaluations have shown that bemegride actually decreases the chances of a patient's improvement. Experiences of some people with laetrile are probably of the same type, since controlled clinical trials have failed to demonstrate any beneficial effect with this highly publicized "medicine."

CHAPTER 75

Simpson's Paradox: A Case Against Common Sense

Although common sense is an extremely valuable skill to apply in most aspects of clinical trial design, conduct, and analyses (in conjunction with medical expertise), there are times when common sense may lead one astray. This brief chapter describes one such statistical case referred to in the literature as Simpson's paradox. It is clearly not the only example suggesting caution in applying common sense to clinical interpretation, although it is probably the most well known.

EXAMPLES OF SIMPSON'S PARADOX

Assume that two clinical trials were conducted. Clinical trial number 1 included 18 patients. Eleven patients received the active medicine and seven received placebo. At the end of the clinical trial it was found that five patients who received the medicine improved whereas six did not. Three patients who received placebo improved whereas four did not. Improvement in the active medicine group was 5 of 11, or 45%. Improvement in the placebo group was three of seven, or 43%. *Improvement was therefore slightly better in the active medicine group than in the placebo group.*

Clinical trial number 2 included 23 patients. Nine patients received the active medicine and 14 received placebo. At the end of the clinical trial it was found that 6 of 9 patients (67%) who received the medicine improved and 9 of 14 patients (64%) who received placebo improved. *Thus, a greater percent of patients in the active group showed improvement than in the placebo group.* This is the same result as in clinical trial 1 (see Table 75.1).

When the data from both clinical trials are combined, it is found that 11 of 20 patients in the active

medicine group (55%) showed improvement and 12 of 21 patients in the placebo group (57%) showed improvement. *Thus, the overall improvement in the combined clinical trials was better in the placebo group than in the active medicine group.* The combined results are thus opposite to the individual results.

Although the above example is hypothetical, a number of similar real examples have been presented in the literature. Hand (1979) discusses a paper in which the authors were exploring the changes in a mental institution over time. The probability of a patient being male in 1970 (343/739) was *greater* than in 1975 (238/515) suggesting that the overall proportion of males in mental institutions had declined from 1970 to 1975. To determine if this was primarily in the under-65 or over-65 age group, each group was evaluated separately. For the under-65-year age group the proportion of males in 1970 (255/429) was *less* than in 1975 (156/258), suggesting that the proportion of males under 65 had increased from 1970 to 1975. For the over-65-year age group the proportion of males in 1970 (88/310) was also *less* than in 1975 (82/257), again suggesting that the proportion of males had increased (Table 75.2).

Another quite well-known example involved the question of whether the graduate school of the University of California at Berkeley was discriminating against women. The probability of acceptance to grad-

TABLE 75.1 *Hypothetical data of two clinical trials*

Clinical trial	Improvement on	
	Medicine X	Placebo
1	5/11 = 45%	3/7 = 43%
2	6/9 = 67%	9/14 = 64%
Combined	11/20 = 55%	12/21 = 57%

TABLE 75.2 *Proportion of males in mental institutions*

Age Group	Year		
	1970	1975	
Combined	343/739 = 46.4%	238/515 = 46.2%	
Under = 65	255/429 = 59.4%	156/258 = 60.5%	
Over = 65	88/310 = 28.4%	82/257 = 31.9%	

uate school was much higher for men than for women, but if the acceptance rates of individual departments were examined, most of the 85 departments had equal probabilities of admission for women (Bickel et al., 1977). Bickel et al. noted that women tended to apply to departments in which the rates of rejection were highest. Thus, if women were admitted in the exact same proportion as men on a department-by-department basis, but mainly applied to the departments with the lowest percent admittance, fewer women than men would be admitted overall.

Another actual medical example is quoted by Hand (1979; electrical aversion therapy on alcoholics) and one concerning automobile accidents is described by Smith and O'Day (1982).

EXPLANATION OF SIMPSON'S PARADOX

This paradox arises because of the temptation we have to average rates. When data are combined from dif-ferent groups the aggregated data may have different characteristics than the individual sets of data. If the aggregate is opposite in outcome and interpretation, the effect is called Simpson's paradox.

The principle to remember is that an overall rate is not the sum or average of the component rates. Thus, the initial intuitive urge to ascribe an overall rate or probability that is the same as the components, or even to do the opposite, should be resisted. Most people are strongly tempted to average rates.

The Price of Wine

A straightforward explanation using the purchase of wine is paraphrased from Costain (1979). Assume that 1 year ago two cases of claret cost $50 a case and one case of Beaujolais Nouveau cost $20 a case. This wine together cost on average $40 a case. This year, with inflation at 20%, the same person can only purchase one case of claret at $60 and two cases of Beaujolais Nouveau at $24 a case. This year the wine cost an average of $36 a case. Thus, although the price (or rate) for each case has gone up, the changes in proportions purchased resulted in the overall price (or rate) going down.

Simpson's paradox dramatically illustrates that a subgroup analysis may be misleading when conducted after a clinical trial is completed.

The Art of Developing and Testing Hypotheses

Brilliant ideas come to some people as a revelation or in their dreams. While most people would like this process to occur on a frequent basis, it is difficult to train yourself for enhancing this method of developing hypotheses. It is possible, however, to improve one's ability to develop hypotheses utilizing more systematic methods. This chapter briefly describes some of these approaches.

Everyone seeking to develop hypotheses has a different amount of relevant knowledge and different goals. Therefore, some of the approaches and steps described will not apply to all individuals or all situations.

BACKGROUND STUDY OF A FIELD

Before it is practical to concern oneself with creating a hypothesis it is usually important to learn about the field of interest. This is achieved from reading, discussions, and experiences. Evaluate the various definitions used for key terms, and probe the underlying assumptions. Are each of these assumptions warranted and valid? Evaluate each of the accepted parameters used to study the field. Are each of them appropriate and what is their degree of validation? Meet with experts in the field and discuss issues and questions of particular interest that either may or definitely do relate to the area of the hypothesis.

During this background period it is important to gather and evaluate relevant data on the issue being addressed. Data gathered should be appropriate to the problem posed in both quality and quantity. Avoid gathering high-volume, low-value data.

DEVELOPING A HYPOTHESIS

Typically, an individual developing a hypothesis has an idea of either the starting point or the ending point in mind. People who are attempting to generate a hypothesis often know that they want to prove that something (the identity of which is currently unknown) will lead to or cause a known or identifiable effect.

Alternatively, people want to evaluate certain types of specific known activities to determine a currently unknown effect. Another possibility is that both the starting and ending points are known, but the connection between them is not. These three possibilities are described in somewhat more detail. A variety of approaches that may be used to develop an hypothesis are listed in Table 76.1.

TABLE 76.1 *Approaches to generating hypotheses*

1. Look for similar patterns in related pieces of information
2. Look for similar patterns in unrelated pieces of information
3. Look for trends in the information
4. Develop metaphors, analogies, or theories to assist one in thinking stepwise, either forward or backward, to develop a chain of causation
5. Mentally examine links in the chain of causation to test for plausibility
6. Assess which variables are most relevant to use in developing the hypothesis

Starting Point Is Known, but Final Effect Is Unknown

An assumption may constitute the starting point. An observation, fact, or idea may also serve this purpose. In this situation, only a forward method of creating a hypothesis may be used. To do this, one may list or describe each possible alternative that can be thought of as a result of going in different directions from the starting point. If more than one person is involved in this exercise, then joint as well as individual hypothesis-generating sessions should be held.

There are books on creativity that may help one use novel methods and approaches. "What if . . ." exercises are a well-known example. Either a realistic, far-fetched, or totally absurd statement is made that relates to the starting point and then as many answers are given as possible. Each of these alternatives is then evaluated and critiqued.

Starting Point Is Unknown, but Final Effect Is Known

The final effect that is known may be that a disease, symptom, or clinical sign must be modified in a specific way (e.g., improved, made worse, disappears). Alternatively, an enzyme may be inhibited or stimulated. Any biological effect may be considered as an endpoint. The means of eliciting the desired effect or change is what is sought. The methods to use in approaching this situation are the same as those mentioned above, except that backward thinking is used.

Both Starting and Ending Points Are Known but the Connection Is Not

If it is known that medicine A has a marked effect in disease B, the question may be: How does this occur? The answer to this common situation is to develop a hypothesis that can be tested using either a forward or backward approach.

Developing Intermediate Steps

In some cases it appears easy to say that A is hypothesized to cause B; therefore, it is necessary to measure

A and B so that this relationship may be tested. It is usually more fruitful to say that there may (or must) be one or many intermediate steps between A and B. It is extremely important to hypothesize as many of these intermediate steps as possible, and then determine how one (or more) of those steps may be tested. Many types of intermediates may be observed in Chapter 73, on cause and effect.

TESTING THE HYPOTHESIS

Making the Hypothesis as Detailed as Possible

The hypothesis should be as detailed and as realistic as possible, so that each of the individual points in the chain that can be tested with known and available technology is identified. A series of methods that could be used to detail hypotheses are listed in Table 76.2. Once these points are known it is then necessary to determine which parameters can (or could) be used at each step to assess the connection (i.e., association) between subsequent steps in the hypothesis.

Evaluating Known Data

Before designing clinical trials to test one part of a hypothesis, it is important to determine if data are available that address any of the individual steps in the causal chain that has been created. Are the data reliable? What do the data suggest? If data are unavailable, which individual steps that are amenable to study are most important to the hypothesis? What is the most appropriate order of study for intermediate steps? Once these questions are answered, a series of clinical trials may be planned and ordered, and the objectives of each established.

Possible Outcomes of a Clinical Trial to Test a Hypothesis

The clinical data hopefully will affirm or deny all or part of the hypothesis being tested. At that point it may be necessary to modify the hypothesis and retest that modified hypothesis. Another possibility is to test another step in the causal link created as part of the hypothesis. A third possibility is to test the same link in

TABLE 76.2 *Selected techniques to use in developing and testing hypotheses*

1. Decision trees	7. Pattern recognition
2. Algorithms	8. Developing cases
3. Flow charts	9. Intuition or guesses
4. Euler diagrams	10. Exclusion of all incorrect possibilities
5. Venn charts	11. Boolean algebra
6. Bayes' theorem	12. Hard or soft evidence

greater detail or in another manner. Finally, one may completely reject the hypothesis.

What to Do After a Hypothesis Is Rejected

If a hypothesis is rejected several steps may be taken. A few possibilities are to (1) look for and test alternative hypotheses following procedures discussed earlier, (2) conduct subgroup analyses of the data collected looking for ideas or possible research leads, (3) analyze retrospective data looking for possible research leads, (4) discuss the issue with colleagues and others, (5) use techniques to enhance one's creativity (e.g., lateral thinking).

WHAT MAY BE DONE IF REASONABLE HYPOTHESES CANNOT BE GENERATED

The problem may be with the environment in which the hypothesis generator is operating. Something may be bothering the person and inhibiting his or her thinking. Whatever factors are negatively affecting thinking and the free association process should be removed (if possible) to create an environment in which the person can focus more appropriately on the topic. This may include going offsite, having a different leader, bringing in a facilitator, holding the session at a different time of day or night, providing more or different food, and so forth.

Written Methods

If it is difficult to formulate one's ideas and create the hypothesis, a few approaches might help bring the hypothesis to life.

1. Use a flow diagram to show how events are connected. Do this in pencil to erase easily. Can new associations be established or tested? Are other associations possible? Ask "what if" questions.
2. Outline one's thoughts and determine which parts are missing or where they belong. Use a classification that makes sense. Also use a classification suggested by the items with which you are working.
3. Write down everything you know about a central point. If that would be too much material, limit the scope of the exercise. Include all possible information on the theme, and use a stream of consciousness approach. Now attempt to organize the materials as described above, evaluate them, and determine if an appropriate hypothesis can be developed.

Conceptual Methods

1. Search for relevant clues in the material that may assist in developing a hypothesis. How do the clues fit together? Do clues have something in common? Develop alternative models to explain them. Look for the absence of an expected item or clue.
2. Search for patterns in the material present. Think first about the various types of possible patterns or trends and then attempt to find them.
3. Attempt to build a case to support a given perspective or view and then determine how one may test the case developed.
4. Starting with a rudimentary hypothesis, develop it further either in depth by focusing on additional levels in important areas, or in breadth by exploring related areas looking for another approach.

CHAPTER 77

Specific Techniques and Issues in Interpreting Clinical Data

GENERAL CONSIDERATIONS

Major Steps in the Movement and Interpretation of Clinical Data

A general approach or orientation toward interpreting data is usually developed before a specific approach is created. An experienced investigator or interpreter of clinical data usually follows a similar approach in all clinical trials unless the nature of the data requires that a modified or totally new approach be used. Most experienced scientists interpret data without consciously considering each of the individual steps involved. These scientists often use a trial-and-error method whereby a tentative hypothesis is established, challenged, and then modified, accepted, or rejected. After a general approach has been chosen to be used in the interpretation of data, it is appropriate to consider specific approaches. The types of specific techniques useful to apply to interpret data vary from situation to situation.

The major steps in collecting, processing, analyzing, and interpreting data are as follows:

1. Data are usually entered on data collection forms.
2. Data are verified for completeness and accuracy.
3. Missing data are recovered (if possible).
4. Data are appropriately copied, shipped, stored, edited, and then (usually) entered into a computer or otherwise tabulated.
5. Quality-assurance procedures are conducted on the data to ensure their accuracy.
6. Data are analyzed by statisticians, and a report is prepared with appropriate clinical input.
7. Data are interpreted clinically.
8. Data may then be extrapolated to a larger or different population of patients.
9. Specific hypotheses or models may be developed for future clinical trials.
10. Further trials may be considered and planned to extend or evaluate the interpretations and/or hypotheses.

548

Personnel and Personal Issues

Prior to or during a clinical trial, it is often helpful to assemble a team of individuals who will assist in the steps described above. Confirm that they are available to participate in the data handling and that they have the requisite abilities and skills. Their training and experience will usually overlap to some degree, which generally facilitates communication. At that point in the process, it is necessary to make workload assignments. Whenever possible, multiple tasks should be conducted simultaneously, but this cannot always be done (e.g., data analysis cannot usually proceed at the same time as data entry).

In addition to assembling a team of individuals to assist in the editing, processing, and analysis of data, it is necessary to have one or more people coordinate these activities. The coordinator may prepare a schedule, keep track of activities, assist in "troubleshooting" when problems arise, and also periodically revise the schedule. This individual may or may not be the person primarily responsible for interpreting the data. He or she could be the clinical monitor, the planner of project activities, or the data processor.

To achieve a nonbiased clinical interpretation, it is highly desirable for the interpreter not to have a vested interest in the outcome of the clinical trial. This is, however, not always practical or possible. If the interpreter can honestly state that he or she does not care how the trial turns out, then a relative degree of objectivity is more likely to be present. The more strongly the investigator, coordinator, or other individual is concerned about how the interpretation turns out, the more pressures he or she will exert to view the data in ways that could be biased. Some techniques to minimize this influence are to (1) request colleagues to view the data and develop their own interpretation, (2) interpret the data jointly with a colleague or statistician, or (3) remain blind to the randomization throughout the period when the major clinical interpretations are developed.

PROCEDURES TO FOLLOW IN DEVELOPING THE INTERPRETATION

Consider Physical Environment

The physical environment in which the interpretation is considered and developed is important. Each person has individual preferences in terms of room, time of day, amount of noise tolerable, and other related factors. This aspect should be considered, at least briefly, prior to interpreting the data.

Stepwise Approach

Some people prefer to read a statistical report completely before attempting to interpret the data, whereas others proceed stepwise (i.e., interpreting the data as one reads the analyses). The stepwise approach is acceptable if the statistician has been requested to place his or her analyses in a specific order in the report, which allows the stepwise procedure to be followed. Otherwise, there is a possibility of reaching one or more tentative conclusions that must be revised or discarded after considering statistical analyses that are presented later in the report. Chapter 71 presented a ten-step approach toward interpreting data from a clinical trial.

Obtaining an Impression of the Statistical Report

A general impression and understanding of the statistical analyses should be obtained. In some cases this impression will be developed during the initial reading of the statistical report. In other cases the investigator (or clinical representative of the sponsor) will have participated in the draft version of the report and will have confirmed through discussions with the statistician that the statistical methods used for the analyses were appropriately chosen to address the objectives of the trial.

Comparison of Demographic and Prognostic Factors

In an ideal clinical trial, the groups being compared should be comparable in their demographic and prognostic factors. In practice it is not always necessary for the treatment groups to be totally comparable (i.e., without statistically significant differences) in all characteristics. Any factors considered essential to the outcome should generally be stratified prior to the trial, if, for example, men are expected to react differently than women or whites to react differently than blacks. Factors may also be evaluated after a trial is completed, but a random distribution may not have yielded balanced groups, and this could present major problems in one's ability to interpret the data.

Interpreting the Data Regarding the Major Objective

At this point in the process, it is appropriate to interpret the data pertaining to the major objectives. Interpretation of data pertaining to secondary objectives and other facets of the clinical trial should usually be considered at a later time. Determine how strong and well supported the interpretation is that was reached.

It should be as clear, simple, and straightforward as possible. List all of the pros and cons that relate to the interpretation. Describe alternate interpretations that could be proposed to explain the data. Develop any corollaries of the interpretation that have significant (or even minor) implications for the nature or mechanisms of the disease or problem studied or for future clinical trials. Consider additional analyses that can be conducted to provide new data to confirm the interpretation. Conduct subgroup analyses to help plan future clinical activities, even if the numbers are small.

Hypothesis-Forming versus Hypothesis-Testing in Clinical Trials

In interpreting data, it is preferable initially to use the data to address the objectives of the clinical trial rather than to develop an interpretation to explain the data. This latter approach is "hypothesis forming," whereas the former is "hypothesis testing." The hypothesis-forming stage looks forward to the next clinical trial and usually occurs only after the hypothesis-testing phase of the current trial is completed.

PITFALLS IN INTERPRETING DATA

The total number of possible pitfalls to avoid in almost any part of a clinical trial's plan, conduct, analysis, or interpretation is extremely large. It is impossible to focus on how to avoid each possible problem in a short space. There are almost no clinical trials that could not be criticized, if desired. An investigator should have an awareness of the most common and important pitfalls to avoid and should concentrate on positive steps to improve the standards with which data are analyzed and interpreted. Improving the quality of these standards will also serve to guard against most pitfalls without overemphasizing them.

Regression to the Mean

A common trap of inexperienced investigators occurs when a patient improves after taking a medicine or using a new therapeutic modality. Many medicines and other modalities have been credited with causing a beneficial effect when the true reason for the patient's benefit was related to the natural history of disease (e.g., nature, time, human healing, faith) and regression of disease severity to the mean. Patients seek clinical help and enter clinical trials when their medical problems tend to be at their worst. Most problems improve to some degree over time, regardless of the intervention. Likewise, patients whose medical problems are better than usual will tend to worsen over

time. Another way of viewing regression to the mean is that if all the flies in a room are on the ceiling at one time when their position is measured, then when a second measurement is made more flies will tend to be at a lower point in the room. Likewise, if all the flies are on the floor at the first measurement, more would tend to be at a higher point at the next measurement. This means that a graph of the general changes observed in a group of patients over time would show the most ill ones improving toward the mean of the group and the most healthy ones deteriorating, also toward the group's mean. This occurs independently of treatment and has been demonstrated in a number of diseases (e.g., epilepsy, Spilker and Segreti, 1984).

Humorous Examples: Of Frogs and Worms

A number of humorous stories aptly illustrate some of the pitfalls that may trap unwary scientists who interpret data. The first is a fictitious story of a young researcher who was measuring the distance that a certain species of frogs can jump. After carefully placing a frog on a line the investigator shouted "jump" and the frog jumped 24 inches, which was carefully measured and entered onto a data collection form. The investigator then cut off one of the frog's legs and repeated his command. This time the frog could only jump 20 inches. This was duly entered on the data collection form. After the investigator cut a second leg off, the frog could only jump 10 inches. Another cut and the frog was hobbling around, barely able to move. The investigator shouted "jump" and the frog could only muster 5 inches. Finally, the investigator cut off the fourth leg and shouted "jump." The frog didn't move. The investigator shouted again, but there was no movement. The data were entered on the data forms and the data were then analyzed. The investigator then interpreted the data and concluded that when you cut off all four legs in this species, the frogs become deaf.

The other tale concerns a third-grade class in which the teacher was trying to impress on her class the evils of drinking alcohol. She pondered on how to get this message across and then hit on what she considered to be a splendid idea. She brought two extremely large jars to school and filled one with water and the other with alcohol. Then she put a worm in the jar containing water, and the worm swam about, doing various strokes and dives. The teacher then took the worm out and put it in the jar containing alcohol. The worm swam well for a while, then swam more and more slowly, until it stopped and sank to the bottom of the tank—dead. The teacher turned in triumph to her class, and, just to emphasize the point, she asked who could tell her what that episode meant. A young boy in the back raised his hand, and when the teacher called on him, he said, "It shows me, teacher, that if you drink enough alcohol you won't get worms."

These tales illustrate two of the pitfalls that may arise when interpreting data. In the frog story, data were used inappropriately to support the interpretation, and the interpretation had nothing to do with the data and did not make sense. In the worm story, an alternative far-fetched interpretation was proposed. In conducting the processes involved in the interpretation of data, there are many pitfalls to avoid. A few of the common pitfalls that may arise in interpreting efficacy data are listed in Table 77.1.

Searching for Causes of a Disease

An important pitfall occurs when a specific disease is shown to be highly correlated with different factors or "causes." The pitfall to avoid is ascribing a cause-and-effect relationship to a single factor and a disease merely because a statistically significant correlation between the two is observed. Strong correlations do not provide evidence that other factors or events are not also correlated with the disease. Knowledge of the

TABLE 77.1 *Common pitfalls in interpreting efficacy data*

A. Problems that may occur prior to clinical trial
1. Failure to contact a statistician until after a trial is completed to correct mistakes introduced into the trial that affect data collected
2. Collecting inappropriate data to address objectives and support interpretation(s)
3. Collecting insufficient data to address objectives and support interpretations
4. Failure to control an important variable
5. Failure to randomize patients appropriately, yielding unequal groups according to an important variable
6. Introduction of bias(es)[a]
B. Problems that may occur after a clinical trial is completed
1. Failure to consider one or more critical factors in reaching a conclusion
2. Using inappropriate data to support interpretation(s)
3. Using inappropriate statistical methods to analyze data
4. Interpretations extrapolated too broadly to inappropriate populations or to quite different experimental conditions
5. Qualifications and limitations of the data are not adequately described
6. Introduction of bias(es)[a]
7. Failure to include (or at least consider including) appropriate data from patients who were discontinued during the trial
8. Failure to consider the possibility that the data yielded a false-positive or a false-negative result[b]
9. Failure to consider the effect that methodological errors may have introduced into the trial[c]
10. Failure to consider that patients usually enter trials when doing poorly and tend to improve even without treatment (i.e., the phenomenon of regression to the mean)
11. Failure to consider that investigators often enroll their most nonresponsive patients in a new medicine trial[c]

[a] See catalog of biases listed in Chapter 5 plus tables in Chapter 83.
[b] See Chapter 96.
[c] This factor is also relevant to include under group A.

specific disease being studied and knowledge of data from other clinical trials are essential prerequisites if one hopes to derive meaningful interpretations of the data and to avoid pitfalls that trap inexperienced or unknowledgeable interpreters.

An example of this may be described in essential hypertension. Strong correlations have been shown between elevations of blood pressure in hypertensive patients and (1) the quantity of salt consumed, (2) calcium levels in food, (3) lead levels in blood, (4) amount of a patient's weight, (5) genetic history, and (6) a number of other factors. The "mosaic theory" has been developed to explain the etiology of hypertension. In this theory, numerous factors combine in an as yet undetermined manner to cause essential hypertension in patients predisposed to developing this disease. The strong correlation of different factors with hypertension that occurs in different trials is therefore reasonable. If a new clinical trial stated that a single factor was solely responsible for hypertension, it would initially (at least) be met with a great deal of skepticism.

In a disease process or syndrome such as sudden infant death syndrome (SIDS), there have been numerous reports of associations or possible leads between SIDS and a single approach or factor, which was then intensively studied to determine if it was in fact the major factor responsible for SIDS. Each of these potential or actual associations has created a flurry of research activity and investigation (e.g., looking for markers at postmortem examinations, evaluating the possibility of delayed development, altered sleep physiology, preexisting markers, apnea monitors, search for infections and immunological disorders). A search for positive risk factors has identified several. Another approach also followed in SIDS research is to look for subgroups of patients that fit specific data or theories.

These studies demonstrate that a strong correlation of a factor and disease is usually insufficient on its own to understand the cause of a disease. In the absence of knowledge about established risk factors associated with a disease or problem (as does exist for myocardial infarctions), a strong correlation may not represent a cause-and-effect relationship. See Chapter 73 on cause–effect relationships.

CRITIQUING ONE'S OWN INTERPRETATION

A number of questions should be asked of one's own work in order to identify potential weaknesses in interpretation. A few of these follow.

1. Some parameters (e.g., ejection fraction, cardiovascular resistance) are actually the result of various components that are measured separately and are combined using a defined formula. It is important to evaluate whether all components of

each observed effect contribute equally, or whether some play a more substantial role. Are there some minor components that actually yielded the opposite result than that caused by the majority or the most important components? Perhaps when these minor components were summed or combined with the more prominent components, an overall effect was observed that was opposite to that observed with the minor component. If this situation occurred, then describe how it affected the overall interpretation and what interpretation(s) or conclusions may be drawn about the individual components?

For example, two medicines may be compared for their effects on cardiac ejection fraction. Ejection fraction is determined by dividing stroke volume by end-diastolic volume. Resistance is calculated from mean arterial blood pressure and cardiac output. Assume two medicines have equal effects on resistance. Does one medicine have a greater effect on one component and the other medicine on the other? Also, how are the medicines influencing resistance? Is an overall increase due to an increase in one parameter or to a decrease in the other?

2. May specific conclusions be extrapolated to other groups of patients, to specific patients, or to different clinical situations, settings, or conditions?

3. May general conclusions be better supported by specific data?

4. Does the interpretation have implications for other biological levels, either toward smaller or larger units of organization (e.g., receptors, molecular level, subcellular level, cellular, tissue, organ, organ system, organism, population)?

5. If results appear to be nonspecific (e.g., a general depression of physiological function), could they become more specific and selective if different doses, conditions, or populations were studied?

6. Are all patient responses discussed? For example if medicine A is claimed to be superior to medicine B because medicine A causes a 65% cure rate and medicine B causes a 25% cure rate, and the response is either a cure or not a cure, then one should discuss possible reasons why 35% of patients treated with medicine A do not benefit.

7. Have the following variables been determined and compared where possible: (1) interpatient versus intrapatient responses, (2) interrater versus intrarater measurements, and (3) intersite versus intrasite results?

8. Does the interpretation make sense from practical, theoretical, physiological, clinical, and other relevant perspectives?

9. Cross check data collected by different means or techniques to confirm that data that should balance actually do.

10. Is it possible that what is being interpreted as the cause is really the effect and vice versa? For example, it is uncertain whether the increased amplitude of airway resistance contributes to or results from asthma-related respiratory failure. Also see discussion under "Devil's Advocate Approach" in Chapter 72.

CHAPTER 78

Relevance of Clinical Trials for Medical Practice

BACKGROUND AND APPROACHES

Dr. Thomas Chalmers is one of the first individuals to have carefully evaluated the impact of clinical trials on medical practice (Chalmers, 1974, 1982). He has described examples of clinical trials that should have influenced medical practice but did not, and also trials that should not have influenced medical practice, but did. Three medical treatments that were continued for "many" years past the time they should have been discarded are (1) use of diethylstilbestrol for preventing spontaneous abortion, (2) bed rest for viral hepatitis, and (3) use of the "Sippy" milk diet for acute peptic ulcers. Various treatments have been abandoned after well-controlled clinical trials were con-

ducted. Several are discussed later in this chapter and Guyatt and Newhouse (1987) mention others. A general review of this topic is presented by Hawkins (1984).

Medical practice could and should certainly move a great deal closer toward the ideal by which clinical trial results influence medical practice in proportion to their true importance. Two central questions should be addressed.

1. What are the actual factors that influence which clinical trials affect medical practice?
2. How may these factors be modified so that important clinical trials have a greater influence on medical practice?

553

One approach to evaluate this area is to start with important clinical trials and then work forward to assess their impact on medical practice. Another approach is to assess current medical practice and then proceed in a backward manner to determine whether current medical practice is consistent with important clinical trials.

FACTORS THAT INFLUENCE WHICH CLINICAL TRIALS AFFECT MEDICAL PRACTICE

Should Clinical Trials Mimic Medical Practice?

The precise factors that influence which clinical trials affect medical practice vary from case to case, but certain characteristics are commonly observed. Some people believe that controlled clinical trials should be more like the actual practice of medicine and that if this occurred, medical practice could be more efficiently influenced. The author disagrees, because the purposes of Phases I, IIa, and IIb clinical trials, as well as many Phase III and Phase IV trials, are not to evaluate a medicine under actual medical practice conditions, but under selected and often artificial conditions to answer best the trial's objectives. Moreover, controlled clinical trials, even in Phases III and IV, cannot by definition mimic actual medical practice conditions.

Medical Importance of the Question Posed

The ability of the clinical trial to address an important medical question is an important prerequisite to the outcome affecting medical practice. Some medical issues are so important that a major clinical trial will have an immediate impact on medical practice (i.e., the demonstration that Retrovir was effective in treating patients with AIDS). Other medical issues have little direct importance to the overall medical community, although a clinical trial may address an issue of great importance to a small number of physicians.

Clinical Significance of the Results

The clinical significance of the results may be the most important factor influencing medical practice, although it overlaps with the factor described above. Even if several of the factors described below are absent, a major clinical breakthrough should lead to a relatively rapid change in medical practice.

Place of Publication

Publication in a highly prestigious journal is usually an important requirement, partly because it ties in to some of the other factors mentioned below (e.g., medical reporters read specific journals each week and report on important papers).

Presentation of the Data

Data that are not clearly and accurately presented may be confusing or otherwise not well understood by readers. Inappropriate or confusing tables or graphs will contribute to this dilemma and compromise the value of the data.

Extent of Media Publicity

For the media to learn about a clinical trial and to publicize it, it either has to be published in one of the prestigious journals they cover, or it has to be presented to them by an individual or group [e.g., sponsor, academic scientist(s), professional association]. Any of these groups may call a press conference, and if the medical story they report has merit it will probably be disseminated. The term media includes both medically oriented and lay media.

Reputation and Influence of the Authors

Reputation and influence of the authors are really two separate factors, but these often overlap in a variety of ways. The importance of these two factors on influencing medical practice varies enormously.

Types of Medical Practice of the Authors

Publications by academic clinicians who treat a different group of patients (e.g., with more refractory disease) than general community practitioners, or who treat patients differently, are sometimes viewed skeptically or even totally ignored. This depends on the specific disease and type of patient being treated by the reader of the publication.

Amount of Promotion for the Clinical Trial

Sponsors of some clinical trials go to great expense and trouble to promote their results. They may do this through advertisements in newspapers and magazines, reprints distributed widely, discussions by sales representatives, speaking tours by distinguished academicians, symposia, printed supplements in prestigious journals, and various other methods.

Statements by Thought Leaders

In most fields there are particular individuals who are very well respected and whose opinions are usually sufficient to influence treatment practices of some or many individual practitioners. These opinions may be stated in editorials, at professional meetings, or in other forums. In some therapeutic areas and in some countries the "thought leaders" wield enormous influence over medical standards and practices.

Organizational Endorsement and Support

Which organizations are promoting the clinical trial's results? If prestigious organizations promote a clinical trial's results through editorials, sessions at annual meetings, presidential addresses, and other means, an important "seal of approval" on the validity and relevance of the clinical trial's results is provided.

Designs and Standards of the Clinical Trial

A clinical trial designed and conducted by state-of-the-art standards has a much better chance to affect medical practice than a poorly designed and conducted one. Numerous exceptions to this principle exist, however. Clinical parameters and endpoints measured should also be the most well accepted ones.

Political, Social, and Economic Implications

Are there particular political, social, or economic implications of a clinical trial's results? Those with important implications have a better chance of influencing medical practice. If a clinical trial demonstrates a means of important cost savings, it will be carefully evaluated by many experts.

Are Results Comforting or Disquieting?

Are the results of a clinical trial what people expected or desired? If either of these conditions are met, it is more likely that the clinical trial's results will be widely believed and its recommendations followed. Whenever clinical trials demonstrate an unexpected and/or an undesired result, there is always a backlash attempting to discredit the clinical trial's design, conduct, analysis, or interpretation. If there are strong economic implications [e.g., the extracranial intracranial bypass surgery trial suggested that this major surgery was not as good as medical therapy (EC/IC Bypass Study Group, 1987)], then the vehemence of the affected group may be expected to be extremely strong. Hawkins (1987) summarizes the strong debates that followed publication of this surgical trial.

Is Supportive Evidence Available?

Whenever there is supportive evidence to confirm the results, a clinical trial is viewed as being more definitive.

Extrapolatability of the Data Obtained

Although there are no formal rules on how broadly one may extrapolate from a set of data, the more far-reaching an extrapolation is, the greater is the probability that it will be inaccurate and will be challenged. If investigators desire to convince practicing physicians to alter their therapeutic practices based on data in a particular trial, the practicing physicians must (1) be aware of the trial, (2) appreciate the quality of the trial, and (3) understand how the data may be extrapolated to their own patients. Phases III and IV trials conducted in a general population are especially important in providing information on how many specific types of patients will react to a new medicine. These trials usually have minimal or even no controls on the types of patients with a particular disease who may be treated. A good perspective on how a broad range of patients will respond to therapy can thus be obtained. In Phase II pivotal trials conducted in smaller and relatively homogeneous groups of patients, it is impossible to determine responses in many special types of patients who are purposely excluded (e.g., infants, renal compromised).

The better validated the clinical models and chosen endpoints, the more likely it is that a well-conceived and well-conducted trial's interpretation will be accepted by the medical community. The converse is also true, which emphasizes the importance of choosing the most appropriate and well-validated clinical model(s) and endpoints.

HOW MAY THESE FACTORS BE MODIFIED?

Consensus Conferences

Professional associations are often in an excellent position to influence their members and other practitioners through newsletters, publications, the media, meetings, and other vehicles. If the association believes that a particular clinical trial's interpretation is being promoted incorrectly, then they may take steps to counter those impressions. These associations may also hold a consensus conference to determine what most people in the field believe to be correct. The results of a consensus conference are sometimes viewed like a trump card that asserts itself as the force that should influence medical practice (Lomas et al., 1988).

Guidelines for the Classification and Diagnosis of Diseases

Some professional organizations publish guidelines for the classification of diseases within their discipline, for the diagnosis of those diseases, and in some cases for the treatment of diseases (i.e., amenable to treatment). Periodic updates are based on views of the contributors and editors, which in turn are influenced by clinical trials.

Reviews and Meta-Analyses

Meta-analyses conducted by individual scientists and clinicians often influence medical practice. Even a narrative review may summarize data or conclusions of clinical trials in a way that says something new, and then influences medical practice.

Direct Appeal to the Public

The public may be used as a target by groups that wish to affect medical practice indirectly. If results of a clinical trial are presented to the public, then people may be stimulated to approach their physicians to request a certain treatment. This approach has been successful in the United States, at least to some degree, for a male hair growth stimulator, for a nonsedating antihistamine, and for a medicine to help patients stop smoking. The influx of patients requesting certain treatments in physicians' offices throughout the United States undoubtedly affected the prescribing habits of physicians and the ways in which they treated their patients.

INFLUENCE OF IMPORTANT CLINICAL TRIALS ON MEDICAL PRACTICE

Numerous instances show that current medical practice (which was based on nonrandomized studies) was changed drastically after randomized controlled studies were conducted. A few examples include the abandonment of (1) gastric freezing treatment of patients with peptic ulcer, (2) clofibrate in patients with elevated serum cholesterol, (3) internal mammary artery ligation as a treatment for angina, (4) laetrile for cancer, and (5) use of pure oxygen for treating premature infants (because of the problem of blindness from retrolental fibroplasia). Results of some controlled trials have been rapidly incorporated into medical practice (e.g., in the second to fifth examples above, which criticized a current practice). Other controlled studies (e.g., those on diethylstilbestrol in pregnant women) have sometimes taken many years to influence a change in medical practice. The above evaluations of the literature support "Muench's second law" as quoted by Ederer (1975): "Results can always be improved by omitting controls."

ENHANCING THE IMPACT OF CLINICAL TRIALS ON MEDICAL PRACTICE

Attention to all of the factors described earlier in this chapter is an important means of potentially enhancing the impact of clinical trials on medical practice. A few factors are described in greater detail.

Appropriate Presentation of Clinical Data

The presentation of a clinical trial's data may greatly enhance or obfuscate the message it is trying to deliver. Expressing results in terms of how many patient years of treatment are required to add 1 year of life or to prevent one stroke is often an effective means of capturing the reader's attention. Choice of optimal formats for data (e.g., tables, graphs, figures) as well as choice of the data themselves for presentation have a major impact on how the results of a clinical trial are perceived. Of course, the interpretation and implications of the data are of paramount importance. This topic is discussed in *Presentation of Clinical Data* (Spilker and Schoenfelder, 1990).

Measures of Expressing Clinical Benefit

The way(s) in which clinical benefit is expressed can make results easier or more difficult to understand and can make it more or less likely that results will be influential on medical practice. Laupacis et al. (1988) present and discuss three ways in which data are often presented and propose a fourth method as preferable in their view. The first three methods are relative risk reduction, absolute risk reduction, and odds ratio. The method they propose is the number of patients needed to be treated to prevent one adverse event.

Relative risk reduction is the difference in rates for an adverse event between control and treated groups, divided by the rate in the control group. Absolute risk reduction is simply the numerator of the above category (i.e., the difference in rates between the control and treated groups). Odds ratios are similar to relative risk reduction and are determined from a ratio of the odds of the adverse event in each group rather than the probabilities. The number who must be treated to prevent one adverse event equals the reciprocal of the absolute risk reduction, and has the advantage that the number can be more readily and completely understood by medical practitioners (e.g., how many patients must receive surgery X to save one life after Y years of follow-up, how many people must be vaccinated to prevent one case, how many women must be examined to prevent one death from breast cancer).

The same four methods may be used to express the

concept of measures of harm, or bad outcomes of medical treatment.

RELEVANCE OF SMALL CHANGES OF AN IMPORTANT PARAMETER MEASURED IN A LARGE POPULATION

Expressing Results in Terms of Percent

Many large clinical trials detect statistically significant mortality differences between a treatment group and placebo or between two treatment groups. Some of the arguments given for or against treating patients with new medicines depends on how results are presented. An overall mortality that decreases in a group from 1.0% to 0.75% represents an absolute reduction of $\frac{1}{4}$% (0.25%). However, these data may also be expressed as a 25% relative reduction in mortality:

$$\frac{1.0 - 0.75 \times 100}{1.0}$$

The fact that both the absolute reduction and proportional reduction have the same numbers (though 100 times different values) is pure coincidence, as can be seen by describing a decrease from 1.5% to 1.0%, which is an absolute reduction of 0.5% and a relative or proportional reduction of 33.3%.

The interpretation is often made that physicians should therefore start to prescribe the "better" treatment for their patients. Assume that the data are correct and that the most relevant parameter was measured. What should one's response be to the data?

There are a few major issues to consider in this example.

1. Was the noted magnitude of difference clinically significant as well as being statistically significant?
2. What would the difference be for a single patient's risk of mortality expressed in readily understood terms?
3. What are the risks of the medicine(s) and what impact would it be expected to have on a patient's quality of life?
4. What factors (if any) might challenge the interpretation?

Judging a 25% Decrease in Mortality

Proponents of change to a new therapy, whether clinicians or reporters, usually present the larger numbers to describe the relative decrease in mortality. These data may not be properly interpreted by the readers and make no sense if the actual data are not also presented. For example, a 25% relative decrease

in mortality may represent an actual decrease in mortality from 100% (i.e., a totally fatal disease) to 75%, from 8% to 6% (i.e., a serious disease), or from 0.008% to 0.006% (i.e., a less severe disease). Clearly, the first example represents a dramatic increase in patient survival, in which all physicians should prescribe the new medicine, and the last example would require consideration of many other factors than mortality to determine whether the new treatment should be prescribed. The middle example was chosen to lie in a gray or intermediate zone. Assuming that the difference is statistically significant, the question is whether the difference is also clinically significant. A difference of 2% in mortality will generally be viewed differently by various physicians. This will depend on questions such as "did the medicine that caused the effect have a similar effect in most patient groups?" and "what adverse reactions were observed?"

An actual example of this occurred in the Hypertension Detection and Follow-up Program. Proponents of treatment stressed the 20% reduction in mortality whereas others viewed the raw data differently. Mortality was reduced from 7.7% in the untreated group of hypertensives to 6.4% in the treated group, i.e., only an average of 1.3 treated patients for every 100 patients treated with medicine experienced a decreased mortality.

Reasons Why Data Should Usually Not Be Expressed as Percent Change from Baseline

It is often unwise to express results as percent change from baseline. For example,

1. Increases in percent are unlimited in how high they can go. A baseline of 5 units that increases to 25 units on treatment is expressed as a 500% (i.e., five-fold) or 400% (25 minus 5 divided by 5) increase depending on how percent change is defined and calculated. Decreases can only go down by 100% (e.g., 5 to 1 is an 80% decrease) unless negative values are possible to attain. It is thus difficult to compare percent increases with percent decreases in a clinical trial when a specific parameter (e.g., number of seizures) may either increase or decrease. Moreover, the ease with which a number (e.g., 5 units) can increase *or* decrease is often different. A simple percent change tends to obscure this fact.

2. Changes may seem large in terms of percent changes, but small in absolute terms. A baseline of 3 that decreases to 2 is a 33.3% decrease. If most patients have a baseline of 12, they would also have to have a 4-unit fall to have a 33.3% decrease.

3. Authors of clinical reports do not always present all raw data; thus readers cannot determine the actual

baseline values. This makes interpretation difficult and sometimes impossible.

4. A medicine may improve survival from 90 to 92% by decreasing mortality from 10 to 8%. The medicine may be said to cause a 25% reduction in mortality but only a 2% increase in survival. Groups that have their own agendas to promote may stress either the large reduction in mortality or the relatively modest increase in survival.

These points illustrate again the adage that p values of 0.05 do not separate fact from fiction.

Clinically Significant Responses

The magnitude of a clinically significant response should be established prior to the study. Nonetheless, that does not mean that all physicians would agree with the magnitude chosen; stating that a difference of 2% in mortality prior to the study is clinically significant might have led to the same difference in opinion between physicians. Another factor relates to which physicians are establishing the magnitude of response that is clinically significant. If it is those who are organizing and conducting the study at large tertiary care hospitals, their opinions may be challenged by primary care physicians or those who treat a different group of patients.

Influence of Treatment Cost on Assessment of Clinical Significance by Third-Party Payers

Costs influence the assessment of clinical significance by third-party payers. No health insurance company or third-party payer would refuse payment for an expensive new medicine that decreased mortality from 100 to 75%. Nor would any third-party payer approve an expensive treatment that reduced mortality from 0.008% to 0.006%, particularly if other treatments were available. In the middle situation (i.e., decrease from 8% to 6%) the costs of treatment would be expected to influence the determination of the clinical significance of the treatment.

Validity of Data

It is important to consider the validity of clinical data. A single clinical trial, no matter how large, may contain a number of flaws in design, conduct, analysis, or interpretation. These may be major flaws that invalidate the results; more commonly, however, the flaws are minor, but raise questions about the clinical trial's validity. Repeating very large clinical trials to confirm

the results is usually impractical, and when it is done, the trial design is invariably different and there are differences in conduct; therefore the results are not totally comparable. Thus, some question of the validity of a clinical trial's data usually remains.

PHYSICIANS' REACTIONS TO CLINICAL TRIAL RESULTS

Different groups of physicians have vastly different perspectives in viewing the influence that clinical trial results have for medical practice. Their perspectives often relate to their activities and research focus, in addition to their basic personalities. For example, epidemiologists study large patient populations and often seek and observe small effects or trends in the data on which they base their interpretations. Private practitioners treat individual patients and must extrapolate data from large groups to the specific case. As a result, each physician may arrive at different interpretations of a single set of data.

Any previously untreatable disease or medical problem that may be treated with a new therapy with a positive benefit-to-risk ratio will generally be rapidly used in medicine. When the advantages over previously used therapy are not dramatic, physicians must be convinced to use new treatments.

A simple table (Table 78.1) illustrates which groups of patients will generally be treated with new medicines by most physicians.

Physicians should be better trained to weigh and judge clinical evidence regarding new therapies and claims. This training could be developed through education about clinical trial designs and practice in critically evaluating clinical research reports. This subject could and should be taught more extensively in medical school, and would lead to physicians making better judgments in assessing the value of new and old treatments.

TABLE 78.1 *Patients who will generally be treated with new medicines*[a]

		Did the patients have adverse reactions to previous or currently used medicine?	
		Yes	No
Is patient's disease well controlled by current (or previous) medicine?	Yes	+	−
	No	+ +	+

[a] −, patient is highly unlikely to receive the new medicine.
 +, patient may receive the new medicine.
 + +, patient is highly likely to receive the new medicine.

PART VII

Interpretation of Safety and Efficacy Data

If we would be guided by the light of reason, we must let our minds be bold.

—Louis D. Brandeis

A man must not swallow more beliefs than he can digest.

—Havelock Ellis

Our firmest convictions are apt to be the most suspect, they mark our limitations and our bounds. Life is a petty thing unless it is moved by the indomitable urge to extend its boundaries.

—José Ortega y Gasset

CHAPTER 79

Patient Demographics and Accountability

DEMOGRAPHICS

After data have been processed and tabulated, clinical researchers who are anxious to interpret the data are tempted to evaluate the major parameters relating to the clinical trial's objective. While this may, in fact, be the first step followed, it should occur after the demographics and patient accountability tables are created and the groups compared.

Demographics are often presented in a table that includes relevant prognostic factors. Prognostic factors or characteristics of patients are those that influence the outcome of a clinical trial or disease. While even statistically significant demographic differences between groups are often unimportant, significant differences between groups in prognostic characteristics are always important. It is so essential that prognostic characteristics between groups be similar that they are often the major basis for randomization and stratification of groups. For example, if older patients react differently than younger patients, it is unwise to trust to chance that both older and younger adults will be evenly distributed to different treatment groups. The wise, and probably mandatory, approach is to stratify patients by age into two groups and to randomize each group separately.

A table is usually prepared of all relevant demographic criteria. If few patients are entered in a clinical trial, their data may be individually presented (Table 79.1). If many patients are entered, group averages are usually presented. Other characteristics may also be listed (Table 79.2). Prognostic criteria are listed either separately or in the same table. There is a large category of demographic data that may be collected, but that usually have little bearing on a clinical trial. These factors include marital status, employment, number of children, economic status, and social status. A list of demographic data for presentation in a publication or final trial report is given in Chapter 4 and many formats of both demographics and patient accountability data

TABLE 79.1 *Demographic characteristics of individual patients in a clinical trial or trials*

Patient number	Treat-ment	Age (years)	Sex (M, F)[b]	Race (W, B, O, *)[c]	Height (cm)	Weight (kg)
Group 1[a]						
101						
102						
103						
104						
etc.						
Group 2						
201						
202						
203						
204						
etc.						

[a] Each group could represent patients from different centers in the same trial or from patients enrolled in different clinical trials.
[b] M, male; F, female.
[c] W, white; B, black; O, oriental; and *, other. If other, specify.

TABLE 79.2 *Selected characteristics of the clinical trial population[a]*

	Treatment group		
	A	B	C
1. Marital status			
Married			
Single			
Divorced			
Widowed			
2. Living arrangements			
Apartment			
Home			
3. Admission service at hospital			
Surgery			
Medicine			
Psychiatry			
4. Duration of hospitalization (days)			
5. Functional status			
Independent			
Semidependent			
Dependent			
6. Mental status			
Test one or more aspects			
7. Number of prior episodes			
8. Treatment for prior episodes			

[a] Values may be presented as means with standard deviations and ranges.

561

TABLE 79.3 *Potential categories to indicate the number of patients present at different stages of a clinical trial*

Total number of patients in a practice, clinic, population, or other category who:
1. Are potentially available to enter a trial
2. Are contacted by the investigator or staff
3. Contact the investigator
4. Pass a preliminary interview
5. Are screened
6. Pass the screening examinations and procedures
7. Consent to enter the trial
8. Actually enter the trial
9. Complete the baseline period
10. Enter the treatment period of the trial but do not complete the entire trial
    a. Patients who drop out of their own volition
    b. Patients who are discontinued by the investigator
    c. Patients who drop out or are discontinued who cannot be defined as completing the trial
    d. Patients who drop out or are discontinued who are defined as completing the trial
11. Complete each part of the trial (for multipart trials)
12. Complete the entire trial including drug taper and withdrawal periods
13. Complete the entire trial including the full follow-up period

a The number who do not complete each part of the trial (for categories 4–12) should also be determined, since there is a patient dropout and investigator discontinuation rate at each phase. The most important discontinued and dropout patients to account for are those who enter but do not complete the treatment period of the trial (category 10).

TABLE 79.4 *Possible definitions of the term "number of patients in a clinical trial"*[a]

1. Those who verbally agree to enter the trial
2. Those who sign the informed consent
3. Those who start or complete the screening period
4. Those who start the baseline period
5. Those who start the treatment period
6–10. Any of the former groups minus patients who were discontinued or dropped out during that period for reasons judged to be unrelated to the trial
11–15. Any of the former groups minus patients who did not complete the period because of reasons defined in the protocol

a The author prefers definition 4 or 5, depending on the particular trial and its design. An explanation should be provided as to why each patient who did not complete the trial dropped out or was discontinued.

LOGSHEET OF POTENTIAL PATIENTS CONTACTED ABOUT A CLINICAL TRIAL

Protocol Number _____ Title _____

Month: _____ 19 _____

Date In Month	Number of Patients Contacted re: Clinical Trial	Number of Patients Contacted But Not Screened	Number of Patients Screened
1	2	1	1
2	3	0	3
3	0	—	—
4	4	4	0
5	2	1	1
6	1	0	1
7	6	3	3
8	2	1	1
•••	•••	•••	•••
31	7	7	0
TOTAL =	N	X	Y

FIG. 79.1. Logsheet of potential patients contacted about a clinical trial and screened.

562

LOGSHEET OF POTENTIAL PATIENTS DISQUALIFIED AT SCREEN

Protocol Number _____ Title _____ Month & Year _____

Date In Month	Number of Patients Screened	Number of Patients Disqualified at Screen	Reasons for Disqualification of Patients at Screen[a]												
			1	2	3	4	5	6	7	8	9	10	11	12	Other:
1	2	1		✓											
2	4	0													
3	4	4					✓			✓		✓			✓ Pain resolved spontaneously
4	2	1													✓ Primarily due to anxiety
5	0	0													
6	3	3				✓✓					✓				
7	6	1		✓											
8	1	0													
•	•	•													
•	•	•													
•	•	•													
31	11	7		✓		✓					✓		✓✓	✓✓ Pain in wrong location
TOTAL =	Y	Z	A	B	C	D	E	F	G	H	I	J	K	L	M

[a] 1 = Patients age or weight outside of inclusion criteria
2 = Previous medical history unacceptable
3 = Alcohol or drug abuse
4 = Recent surgery
5 = Insufficient severity of symptom

6 = Insufficient duration of symptom
7 = Presence of concomitant medicine
8 = Previous participation in clinical trial
9 = Medicine allergies
10 to 12 = Other defined reasons

FIG.79.2. Logsheet of potential patients disqualified during screen and the reasons for their disqualification. A footnote may be used to describe patients disqualified for multiple reasons.

LOGSHEET OF POTENTIAL PATIENTS ENTERED IN A CLINICAL TRIAL

Protocol Number _____

Title: _____

Week	Dates	Number of Patients Screened	Number of Patients Passing Screen	Number of Patients Enrolled In Trial	Reasons for Nonenrollment by Successfully Screened Patients					
					No Interest	Insufficient Inducements	Informed Consent Not Signed	Inadequate Time	Lives Too Far	Other (List)
1	Jan 14-20	17	12	10			1	1		
2	Jan 21-27	24	20	14	1	2	2			
3	Jan 28-Feb 3	14	14	13		1				
4										
5										
6										
7										

FIG 79.3. Logsheet of patients entered in a clinical trial and reasons for nonenrollment by successfully screened patients.

are given in *Presentation of Clinical Data* (Spilker and Schoenfelder, 1990).

PATIENT ACCOUNTABILITY

There are a large number of potential listings and comparisons that may be considered as part of patient accountability. In essence, patient accountability is the indication of each patient's status who entered the clinical trial. Patient status may be presented in few or many details. Moreover, the category of accountability is being expanded steadily over time. It now often includes those patients who did not enter the clinical trial, but who were screened and failed, or who passed the screen but refused to sign the informal consent. Calimlim and Weintraub (1981) present an excellent discussion on this subject. The characteristics and possibly even the outcome of patients who did not enter the clinical trial should be understood to allow for more meaningful extrapolation of data from the clinical trial.

The nature of the patients who entered and completed the trial should be compared whenever possible with those who either did not enter or did not complete the clinical trial.

Table 79.3 shows potential categories to indicate the number of patients present at different stages of a clinical trial. Possible definitions of the term "number of patients in a clinical trial" are shown in Table 79.4.

To generate tables of demographic and patient accountability data on patients who do not enter a clinical trial, it is necessary to collect these data from the outset of a clinical trial. A suitable approach is to create and use either hardcopy or computer forms such as in Figs. 79.1 to 79.3. It is particularly important to document the major reason(s) why patients did not meet the inclusion criteria or did not enter the trial, and to assess their prognostic characteristics. This process will indicate if one or more inclusion criterion are especially stringent, resulting in the disqualification of many potential patients. It may be desirable to modify the protocol to enhance patient recruitment.

CHAPTER 80

Interpretation of Adverse Reactions

In interpreting safety data, the first question to address depends on the interpreter's particular perspective in assessing safety data. For a practicing clinician, it may relate to the information that is relevant to the particular patient(s) and situation. For an epidemiologist, the basic issue is to understand the data at a population level to evaluate its importance in the context of broad social needs. For other individuals there will be other orientations.

Although certain tests or parameters may be viewed as providing either safety or efficacy data (e.g., electroencephalogram), the identification of most tests that are used in a study to obtain safety data is quite straightforward. These tests are listed in Table 23.1 and include physical examinations (including ophthalmological, neurological, and other examinations) plus various laboratory tests, electrocardiograms, and the questioning of patients about adverse reactions.

This chapter discusses interpretation of adverse reactions. Adverse reactions are usually the most complex issue relating to safety and are the issue that has the least uniformity in approach. This chapter describes the clinical presentation of adverse reactions as distinct from laboratory aspects. The next chapter discusses interpretation of data obtained from laboratory tests and other safety examinations.

TYPES OF ADVERSE REACTIONS

Adverse reactions are usually viewed as an indication of a medicine's toxicity. Nonetheless, they may have a number of beneficial aspects: (1) adverse reactions are sometimes welcomed as an indication that a medicine is absorbed in adequate amounts, (2) dosages are sometimes titrated against the presence or magnitude of adverse reactions, and (3) an adverse reaction observed in patients using a medicine for one indication may reveal a novel indication that may be used for other patients. A well-known example of this latter principle relates to the sedative effect observed with most traditional antihistamines of the histamine-1 receptor type. This effect is considered an adverse reaction when antihistamines are used to treat allergies but serves as the basis of the newer indication for certain antihistamines as sleep-promoting agents. A number of other adverse reactions have become therapeutic effects (e.g., minoxidil for hair growth).

Some adverse reactions are predictable and almost always occur when a medicine is used, either dependent or independent of the dose administered (e.g., constipation with opiates). The occurrence of other adverse reactions is impossible to predict (e.g., most rashes, anaphylactic reactions). Many medicines cause both types of adverse reactions. In other words, adverse reactions range from those caused by intrinsic toxicity of the medicine at a target organ (e.g., direct hepatic toxicity) to idiosyncratic reactions that are sporadic and nonreproducible. Idiosyncratic reactions include (1) hypersensitivity reactions to medicines, (2) metabolic idiosyncratic reactions (e.g., a toxic metabolite formed by certain individuals), and (3) reactions based on autoimmune mechanisms.

In reviewing the adverse reactions observed in a clinical trial, there sometimes is value in categorizing (or describing) them on a scale ranging from idiosyncratic reactions to those resulting from intrinsic toxicity. Some adverse reactions have both types of characteristics. For new investigational medicines it is often impossible to make a distinction until additional information becomes available. Phase I clinical trials essentially only measure a medicine's intrinsic toxicity because of the relatively few patients enrolled. Phase II trials measure both types of toxicity, and Phase III trials primarily uncover idiosyncratic toxicity, since most or all of a medicine's intrinsic toxicity will have been discovered by that time. Phase IV trials are almost entirely devoted to discovering and/or evaluating idiosyncratic toxicity. Some individuals believe that the distinction between intrinsic and idiosyncratic reactions is artificial and that all adverse reactions may be classified on the basis of their frequency. This issue is not settled.

ISSUES INVOLVING ADVERSE REACTIONS IN CLINICAL TRIALS

There are many issues in clinical trials that involve adverse reactions. Each of these issues has facets that may affect the interpretation of data, although not all are necessarily present in every trial and some overlap with others. Thirty-three of these issues are presented below. Some of them should primarily be considered prior to the initiation of the trial; others are usually dealt with during or after the trial.

Levels of Adverse Reactions

One factor that makes consideration of these issues more complicated is the question of whether one is discussing a single patient, a single clinical trial, or multiple trials of a single medicine.

1. Single patient. This level involves consideration of one or more adverse reactions that occur in a single patient. Each type of adverse reaction may occur on more than one occasion.
2. Single clinical trial. This level involves consideration of one or more adverse reactions that occur in a single trial. Consideration of each type of adverse reaction may be limited to those experienced

by a single patient, multiple patients, or by all patients enrolled.

3. Multiple trials of a single medicine. This level involves consideration of one or more adverse reactions experienced in multiple trials (possibly in all trials conducted with the medicine). All patients exposed to a medicine in the relevant studies are usually included in the data considered whether or not they have experienced the adverse reaction.

Categories of Adverse Reactions

Adverse reactions may be categorized as measured in numerical and objective terms or in subjective and descriptive terms (see Table 80.1). Although this distinction is arbitrary and oversimplified because of significant overlap, it points out a reason why many of the problems associated with collecting data and interpreting the importance of adverse reactions occur. These problems include several of the issues discussed in this chapter (e.g., association of the adverse reaction with a medicine).

Operational Definitions and Classifications of Individual Adverse Reactions (Issue 1)

Definitions of an adverse reaction may vary, and this will have a large impact on how they are counted, interpreted, and dealt with by sponsors, regulatory agencies, and practicing physicians. Definitions may be narrow or broad and may or may not include reference to the cause. Three representative definitions of adverse reactions are given to illustrate how differences in interpretation of data may arise. An adverse reaction may be defined as:

1. An undesired and unintended event or phenomenon that initially occurred after medicine treatment was initiated, or, if present at baseline, became more intense or severe after medicine treatment was initiated.
2. Any undesired event or phenomenon that occurred while a patient was receiving a medicine.

A definition used by Koch-Weser et al. (1977) is: "Any noxious change in a patient's condition which a physician believes to be due to a drug, which occurs at dosages normally used in man, and which (1) requires treatment, (2) indicates decrease or cessation of therapy with the drug, or (3) suggests that future therapy with the drug carries an unusual risk in this patient."

The last definition does not include trivial and expected adverse reactions that do not require any change in treatment or events that result from deliberate or accidental overdosage. It is also difficult to know when a change becomes noxious, particularly for laboratory changes that occur without symptoms. These definitions do not deal completely with the question of attribution (i.e., association with the medicine).

Serious Adverse Reactions

Three definitions of a serious adverse reaction are:

1. Adverse reaction of sufficient clinical concern to warrant discontinuing the patient from the clinical trial
2. Adverse reaction that produces a significant impairment of functioning or incapacitation, is a definite hazard to the patient's health, and warrants counteractive treatment, or alteration of therapy
3. Adverse reaction that is rated by the investigator as clinically significant and severe

This last definition is the most general, since the classification of an adverse reaction as "severe" is often left to the investigator's discretion and does not require that the patient be discontinued from the clinical trial or that the patient's functioning be significantly impaired. Nonetheless, a list of criteria may be used with this or any of the other definitions that would be used to define the adverse reactions as severe.

The definitions and classifications of adverse reactions must be determined prior to a clinical trial since they may have great impact on the clinical interpretation of data. If adequate definitions and appropriate

TABLE 80.1 *Sample categories of adverse reactions*[a]

A. Adverse reactions that are measured primarily in numerical or objective terms[b]
1. Clinical laboratory abnormalities detected in blood, urine, cerebrospinal fluid, or other biological samples
2. Clinical laboratory abnormalities detected in the patient (e.g., electrocardiogram, pulmonary function tests)
3. Abnormalities detected on physical examination (e.g., vital signs, nystagmus, depressed deep tendon reflexes, abnormal heart sounds)
4. Scores on written tests to evaluate behavior, performance, social, psychological, or other parameters
B. Adverse reactions that are described in subjective and/or descriptive terms
1. Spontaneously reported symptoms
2. Symptoms reported as a result of a probe
3. Psychological, social, and/or behavior abnormalities determined through various tests and interviews

[a] This list does not include categories of adverse reactions that are not considered to be directly related to the trial medicine or treatment (e.g., trauma, concomitant illness, accidents). These events are included with adverse reactions under the broader term "adverse experiences" or "adverse events."

[b] Many of these tests are subject to (1) patient influence (e.g., voluntary effort in pulmonary function testing, cooperation and honesty in written examinations), (2) physician or rater expertise (e.g., determination of heart sounds, interpretation of much of the data obtained), and (3) errors that may arise for innumerable reasons (see Table 81.2) for examples of errors associated with clinical laboratory tests).

classifications are not completed prior to initiation of the trial, then the interpretation of adverse reactions will be complicated, and the final results may be seriously obfuscated.

In addition to the classification of adverse reactions in Table 80.1, adverse reactions may be classified as dose-related or non-dose-related (e.g., pharmacological reactions, immunological reactions). Another classification is of short-term, long-term, or delayed effects. A final classification based on the incidence of the adverse reaction is shown in Table 80.2.

Terms Used to Describe Adverse Reactions

The specific terms used to describe individual adverse reactions may be decided prior to initiation of a clinical trial, or coding systems may be used to deal with this issue after a trial is completed, although the former practice is preferable. It is important to determine which terms will be avoided and which will be viewed as synonyms. For example, if sleepy, drowsy, fatigued, tired, and somnolent are all defined as being identical in a trial, the preferred term to use should be chosen, defined operationally, and made known to all individuals who are responsible for determining and describing adverse reactions. If distinctions are to be drawn between apparently similar terms, then clear operational definitions of each should be created. This is discussed further in Chapter 67.

When a medicine has been associated with an extremely serious and rare adverse reaction (e.g., Stevens-Johnson syndrome, toxic epidermal necrolysis) it is important to specify the diagnostic criteria of each and to indicate these in the protocol and data collection forms. Recommended methods of treatment for adverse reactions may also be indicated, although each physician will want to reserve the right to treat every seriously ill patient in the most appropriate manner and not be committed to following a prespecified plan.

Types of Toxicity (Issue 2)

Adverse reactions imply some degree of causal relation with a medicine or treatment and are therefore a subset of all adverse events (adverse experiences). This is shown in Fig. 80.1.

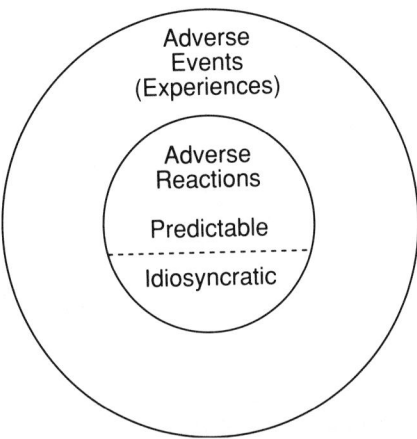

FIG. 80.1 Schematic of adverse events, illustrating that adverse reactions are a subset, and also showing two categories of adverse reactions (i.e., predictable and idiosyncratic).

Toxicity resulting from a medicine may be divided into four types:

Type 1 toxicity results from an excess of a desired beneficial pharmacological effect. This is the effect for which the medicine is used (e.g., a barbiturate used as a sleeping aid that has a long duration of action and causes fatigue the next morning).

Type 2 toxicity results from an excess of an undesired pharmacological effect. This effect is one that could be turned into a beneficial effect in some situations (e.g., hair growth occurring with the antihypertensive minoxidil, sedation occurring with older type 1 antihistamines).

Type 3 toxicity results from effects not observed at therapeutic doses. These pharmacological effects are generally predictable and are observed in patients taking an overdose of a medicine. Although overdoses are usually purposeful, some are inadvertent (e.g., low weight of patient, genetic difference of patient). Another instance of type 3 toxicity relates to those adverse reactions that occur from abusing the drug, i.e., not using it in the manner specified, although not necessarily overdosing.

Type 4 toxicity is unexpected. Such idiosyncratic effects occur at extremely low rates and rarely can be predicted in advance. Risk factors may be known that place certain patients at greater risk than others.

TABLE 80.2 *Ability to detect medicine-induced adverse reactions[a]*

Incidence of medicine-induced adverse reactions	Background incidence of an adverse reaction in population		
	Rare	Moderate	Common
Rare (<1 in 10,000)	Difficult (1)	Extremely difficult (2)	Extremely difficult (3)
Moderate (between 1 in 100 and 1 in 10,000)	Relatively easy (4)	Requires a study (5)	Difficult (6)
Common (>1 in 100)	Easiest (7)	Relatively easy (8)	Requires a study (9)

[a] Examples of the nine possible cases are given in Table 80.3 and correspond with numbers in parentheses.

TABLE 80.3 *Examples of adverse reactions for the nine categories of Table 80.2*

1. Phenylbutazone-induced aplastic anemia
2. Halothane-induced liver toxicity
3. Formation of cataracts induced by photosensitization (e.g., ultraviolet light)
4. Phenformin-induced lactic acidosis
5. Estrogen-induced endometrial carcinoma
6. Small increase in sedation by certain medicines
7. Thalidamide-induced phocomelia in offspring of pregnant women
8. Thiazide-induced potassium deficiency
9. Chlorpheniramine-induced sedation

Adverse reactions include undesirable effects, as defined above, that occur as (1) psychological symptoms, (2) physical symptoms, (3) physical signs, (4) laboratory values obtained using biological samples, (5) laboratory values on data obtained directly from patients (e.g., electroencephalogram, electrocardiogram, pulmonary function tests), and (6) other factors relating to quality of life (e.g., social interactions).

Therapeutic Index (Issue 3)

The therapeutic index (also known as the safety index, therapeutic ratio, or safety ratio) is defined as the ratio between the minimum toxic dose (numerator) and the maximum effective dose (denominator). It is possible that the denominator's dose may be defined somewhat differently (e.g., mean effective dose). This index or ratio represents the safety factor of the medicine; the larger the therapeutic ratio the greater is the safety.

Risk factors often influence the size of the therapeutic index for a particular patient or group of patients. Medicines usually have multiple therapeutic indices because they are used in patients from multiple patient populations, each with their own risk factors.

Collecting and Monitoring Data on Adverse Reactions (Issue 4)

Careful monitoring is necessary to identify adverse reactions, especially those that are imprecise and require clarification. For example, problems may arise in interpretation of adverse reactions if they are imprecisely listed on data collection forms as "gastrointestinal problems," "feels bad," or "double vision." The actual event must be defined if a term such as "double vision" is written, since true "double vision" is a potentially serious adverse reaction. Often, the patient may have casually described his "blurred vision" as "double vision," and an inexperienced investigator may not have probed further or may not have appreciated the distinction and implications for the trial medicine. Terms such as "gastrointestinal problems" and "feels bad" are too general and too vague. Whenever possible, the precise meaning of each potentially vague term must be better elucidated. Even the term "malaise" connotes a general feeling that is better understood than the vague term "feels bad," which may refer to a specific part of the body or organ system, whereas "malaise" generally relates to the entire patient.

Probability of Observing an Adverse Reaction (Issue 5)

Table 80.4 illustrates that the probability of observing an adverse reaction (with 95% certainty) depends on both the background incidence of the adverse reactions in the population and the number of patients in the clinical trial. If one wants to be able to observe relatively uncommon adverse reactions, it is necessary to have a large number of patients in the trial. These probabilities may also be expressed on the basis of the rela-

TABLE 80.4 *Likelihood of observing an adverse reaction (95% likelihood)*

Number of patients in adverse reaction trial	Background incidence of an adverse reaction					
	1/100	1/500[a]	1/1,000[b]	1/5,000[c]	1/10,000[d]	1/50,000[e]
100	0.63	0.18	0.10	0.02	0.01	0.002
200	0.86	0.33	0.18	0.04	0.02	0.004
500	0.99	0.63	0.39	0.10	0.05	0.01
1,000	0.99	0.86	0.63	0.18	0.10	0.02
2,000	0.99	0.98	0.86	0.33	0.18	0.04
5,000	0.99	0.99	0.99	0.63	0.39	0.10
10,000	0.99	0.99	0.99	0.86	0.63	0.18
Number of patients required to be 95% likely to observe an adverse reaction	300	1,500	3,000	15,000	30,000	150,000

Reprinted by permission of J. B. Lippincott Co. from Sackett et al. (1980).
[a] For example, lymphoma from azothioprine.
[b] For example, eye damage from practolol.
[c] For example, heart attack in older women from oral contraceptives.
[d] For example, anaphylaxis from penicillin.
[e] For example, aplastic anemia from chloramphenicol.

tive difficulty of observing an adverse reaction (Table 80.2). Examples of the nine categories are listed in Table 80.3.

The examples given demonstrate the types of adverse reactions referred to by each of the nine categories. They also point out the relative ease with which common medicine-induced adverse reactions may be observed and attributed to the medicine if the adverse event is rare in the general population (i.e., category 7).

The consistency of events reported for any patient at each examination or interview should be confirmed through monitoring and data editing. Any problems in data collection will make the eventual interpretation of adverse reactions more complex and may make a meaningful interpretation impossible. Some of the major issues relating to the collection of data involve the question of (1) whether to probe for adverse reactions or to collect only unsolicited comments, (2) how to define the precise method of probing for adverse reactions, (3) how to record and monitor the adverse reactions elicited, and (4) how large a clinical trial is required to be able to detect adverse reactions. Points 1 and 2 are described in Chapter 26. The easiest system for both recording and analyzing data is a "closed" system in which all responses are entered as check marks, circles around the correct answer, or another similar procedure. A totally "open" system allows any relevant comment to be placed on a blank line. This open approach may or may not convey more information on adverse reactions observed but is certainly more difficult to enter into a computer and to analyze.

It is interesting that in a study designed to evaluate whether patients were more or less conservative than experts in attributing adverse reactions to a medicine, patients were more conservative (Mitchell et al., 1988).

Measuring the Intensity of Adverse Reactions and Determining their Clinical Significance (Issue 6)

A classification system for measuring adverse reaction intensity is generally established for each individual clinical trial but usually is similar or identical across most studies conducted on a single medicine. The most commonly used system is to classify adverse reactions as "mild," "moderate," or "severe." These terms must be defined clearly prior to the trial, and it should be clarified whether individuals other than the investigator will rate the intensity of adverse reactions.

The rating of each individual patient's adverse reactions should be done by a single physician whenever possible. This technique will present variations arising from having different raters (physicians) evaluate the intensity of a single patient's adverse reactions at dif-

ferent clinic visits or at different times. If different physicians evaluate a single patient at each time point, each physician may identify different adverse reactions based on his or her interpretation of the patient's history and physical examination. In addition, two or more physicians will sometimes hear the same complaint but will probe it differently and identify it as two different adverse reactions. It is also desirable in any clinical trial that the intensity of all patient's adverse reactions be rated by a single physician to prevent interpatient variation arising from differences between raters.

The question is often raised of whether a specific adverse reaction is clinically significant (also referred to by some authors as clinically important). The individual who is most qualified to rate adverse reactions or abnormalities as either clinically significant or not clinically significant for the patient is the treating physician who observes and measures the adverse reaction. This individual may require additional information from other staff or from the sponsor (e.g., metabolic data, pharmacological activities) before arriving at a decision. It is inappropriate for the decision of clinical importance of the event for the patient to be made by the investigator's nonphysician staff or by the sponsor. In the former case, clinical judgment must be brought into the decision, which cannot be assumed in nonphysicians, and in the latter case there could be issues of conflict of interest, besides which the sponsor's medical personnel have not treated and usually have not observed the patient.

The company or sponsor rates the clinical significance of the adverse reaction for the medicine or for the clinical trial. Venulet et al. (1980) describe what occurs in the Medical Department at Ciba-Geigy in Switzerland. In their company, the "evaluator" is a physician at the company rather than the investigator who treated the patient. The sophisticated checklist and assessment form used at Ciba-Geigy plus a key to how answers are weighted are provided in their article.

Association of an Adverse Reaction with a Particular Medicine or Treatment (Issue 7)

Why Attempt to Establish Causality?

At the patient-care level, understanding causality enables the treating physician to decide whether to alter a patient's treatment. From a regulatory perspective, information about certain types of adverse reactions (e.g., serious and unexpected) allows physicians to protect other patients better who are receiving the medicine or who might receive it in the future. From a sponsor's perspective, such information helps determine protocols for future clinical trials (e.g., to include or exclude certain patient populations, dosages, titration schedules, tests). It also helps sponsors determine whether to withdraw a medicine from the market.

Three basic approaches have been used to assess the association of an adverse reaction with a particular medicine. These are global introspection, algorithms, and formal logic. These methods lie along a spectrum relating to the application of formal logic. At one end of the spectrum are uninformed guesses. Next is informed opinion, followed by group discussion among informed individuals or experts, simple algorithms, complex algorithms, use of algorithms plus discussion among experts, and, finally, Bayesian logic. This spectrum does *not* relate to the accuracy of these methods and no gold standard exists.

Global Introspection

Global introspection was the first major method developed. Experts and others would consider all of the relevant data in a specific case, including data obtained at their request (e.g., concomitant laboratory data, effects of dechallenge and rechallenge), and reach an opinion on the cause–effect relationship. The factors to consider are listed in Table 80.5. The overall judgment is based on knowledge of the case and the experience and intuition of the experts. In many cases of adverse reactions occurring today, it is impossible to achieve a more informed or accurate assessment of causality. On the other hand, several studies of experts have shown that there is often poor agreement between raters (see issue 9). Kramer (1986) discusses problems associated with global introspection. For a period in the early and mid-1980s this method was out of favor (see recommendations below about its current status).

Algorithms

During the decade from approximately 1975 to 1985 about 20 different algorithms were proposed to help determine the association of an adverse event with a particular medicine. These algorithms varied from simple (only a few questions asked) to highly complex. It soon became clear that more complex algorithms did not necessarily yield more accurate assessments of causality, often because many of the questions posed in complex algorithms could not be answered completely for specific cases. Complex assessment was particularly difficult for a new medicine because sufficient data had not been collected. Moreover, it was difficult to know which factors were relevant in specific cases. A growing sense of frustration about lack of reproducibility and validity led a group of interested clinicians and scientists to explore methods using formal logic to assess causality.

TABLE 80.5 *Factors to consider in utilizing global introspection to associate a medicine and adverse event*

A. Previous experience with the medicine
   1. How many years has the medicine been available for use?
   2. How many patients have been treated with the medicine?
   3. How often have patients experienced the particular adverse reaction?
   4. What is the background incidence of the particular adverse reaction in the absence of treatment with the medication?
   5. What data exist in animal studies (either pharmacological or toxicological) relating to the adverse reaction?
   6. What data exist for structurally or therapeutically similar medicines relating to the adverse reaction?
B. Patient's medical history
   1. Previous exposures of the patient to the medicine
   2. Previous episodes of the adverse reaction
   3. Association of previous episodes with the medicine
   4. Association of previous episodes with other medicines or other factors
   5. Genetic, racial, social, or other factors that are risk factors for experiencing the adverse event
C. Characteristics of the adverse event
   1. Timing of its onset in comparison to the expected occurrence (i.e., use of the medicine must precede the event)
   2. Timing of its onset in relation to the purported mechanism of action if the medicine is believed responsible for the event
   3. Levels of the medicine in plasma at the time of the event
   4. Possibility of overdosage
   5. Laboratory test results
   6. Duration of the event
D. Effects of dechallenge, rechallenge, and treatment
   1. Events after the dose was decreased or the medicine was discontinued
   2. Evidence of tolerance
   3. Time that treatment was initiated
   4. Effects of treatment
   5. Effects of rechallenge
E. Alternative explanations for the adverse reaction
   1. Other therapies
   2. Underlying disease
   3. Other concomitant illnesses
   4. Diagnostic tests and procedures
   5. Spontaneous events

Formal Logic

The Bayesian approach to statistics or formal logic considers past experiences as a guide to help reach a decision of causality. If an adequate volume of suitable data are available, it is possible to address the question, "Does medicine X cause adverse reaction Y"? It is not possible, however, to ask, "Did medicine X cause adverse reactions Y in patient Z at a specific time?" It is also not possible to answer the first (legitimate) question for medicines in Phases I or II because an inadequate amount of data are usually available at those early stages of a medicine's development.

This method takes a significant amount of time to use. It is best suited for those few cases in which it is important to apply the highest standards possible because the answer has important implications and it is appropriate to apply the large amount of resources required. Naranjo et al. (1990a,b) show how this method may be applied using the example of Guillain-Barré syndrome and zimeldine, and to neutropenia associated with antiarrhythmic agents.

Recommendations for Clinical Trials

In almost all Phase I and II clinical trials, global introspection techniques *or* a simple algorithm is appropriate for mild and moderate adverse reactions. For severe adverse reactions that are previously unknown, both global introspection *and* a simple or somewhat more complex algorithm should be used. If the results of the two approaches do not agree, the global introspection assessment should be used as the final arbiter. For severe adverse reactions that have previously been associated with a medicine, an intermediate method, or the method for moderate and known adverse reactions could be used.

More data on adverse reactions should be published in reports of clinical trials. Venulet (1985) reported that only 21% of 1,379 publications contained an adequate amount of information to determine causality, and moreover did not include sufficient information to interpret the clinical significance of adverse reactions.

Classifying the Association between Adverse Reactions and Trial Medicine or Nonmedicine Events (Issue 8)

This concept may be addressed at all three levels of interpretation (i.e., patient, single trial, and multiple trials on one medicine), although this section concentrates on the first two. The protocol should include a description of both the classification and definitions of the associations to be used for both the individual patient and trial. The common systems used in medicine trials usually include from three to nine categories. A widely used approach includes five terms: Definitely related, Probably related, Possibly related, Not related, and Unknown. See Chapter 26 for additional details.

Operational definitions may be created to meet the needs of a specific clinical trial, or the definitions may be relatively standardized across multiple trials. Although specific definitions may be devised for each term, it is often difficult and sometimes impossible to distinguish clearly between "possibly" and "probably" medicine related when evaluating the association with an adverse reaction. Moreover, certain investigators believe that certain terms, such as "definitely related" or "not related," should almost never be used, since complete assurance is almost never achieved. Thus, some investigators essentially eliminate these terms from consideration, whereas other investigators use them somewhat loosely.

Operational definitions may include a scale of probabilities (e.g., "possibly related" is sometimes defined as less than a 50% chance of the adverse reaction resulting from the medicine), but it is difficult in many cases to know whether the probability of an adverse reaction being associated with a medicine is greater or less than a given percentage. Thus, although a "precise" system of three to nine categories may be established and clearly defined, there is usually a large subjective factor and often great variation in how these categories are applied to a specific adverse reaction by different investigators. Some investigators use simple or elaborate algorithms, and some rely on clinical judgment to derive a decision as to whether the relationship is possibly or probably associated with a particular medicine.

It is doubtful that the use of one of the more formal systems (i.e., algorithms) yields a more definitive conclusion on the association of a medicine with an adverse reaction than the more subjective system. The case against using algorithms is based on many points, several of which are described by Girard (1984). Nonetheless, the optimal system to use in a medicine trial is considered to be one that (1) uses specific categories, defined as clearly as possible, (2) is utilized by one or as few investigators as possible at each site, and (3) is monitored assiduously and periodically to ensure that it is consistently applied to all patients and by all investigators. The types of evidence that associate a medicine with a particular adverse reaction were reviewed by Venning (1983a). Techniques of formal logic may be useful in analyzing specific cases of attribution, but will probably not be widely used.

Improving Interrater and Intrarater Reliability in Assessing Adverse Reactions (Issue 9)

If a large multicenter trial is being undertaken, it is usually important for the sponsor to instruct the investigators who will identify and rate the severity, determine the association, and choose the clinical treatment or response for each adverse reaction. This process may be performed with various types of teaching sessions and will help ensure that both interrater and intrarater consistency will be high and remain relatively constant throughout the trial.

Some techniques that are useful to improve interrater reliability are (1) to prepare video or audio presentations illustrating each important or controversial adverse reaction, (2) to prepare a list of synonyms or definitions, (3) to have practice sessions with actual patients, (4) to prepare instructions, and (5) to conduct workshops or roundtable discussions to increase the probability that a common approach will be applied to each aspect of dealing with adverse reactions. Another type of approach is to obtain movies of interviews or patients and to have all patients reviewed by a single independent evaluator.

Influences of nonmedicine factors should be evaluated by the same individual who evaluates the possible association of the adverse reaction to a trial medicine. There are many medicine- and non-medicine-related events that may be wholly or partially responsible for eliciting adverse reactions. Some of these factors are listed in Table 80.6.

Determining the association between nonmedicine events and an adverse reaction depends in part on common sense, experience, and clinical judgment.

How Adverse Reactions May Be Related to Clinical Trial Design or Conduct (Issue 10)

A few examples of how adverse reactions may be primarily related to clinical trial design rather than trial medicine are described below:

1. If patients are required to fast for a relatively long period before receiving a trial medicine, it may increase the frequency of headache, abdominal discomfort, or pain plus possibly cause or contribute to other adverse reactions.
2. If the dosages are given too frequently relative to medicine excretion, blood levels may reach a toxic range resulting from accumulation of medicine. Adverse reactions will markedly increase under these circumstances.
3. A trial in which patients are required to remain awake or alert or are frequently tested during an

excessively long period (e.g., for 18 hours instead of 6 or 8 hours) will lead to additional adverse reactions.
4. If patients are questioned about adverse reactions every few minutes for a prolonged period, they may become irritable and even "create" responses.
5. Long periods of relatively little activity in quiet dark rooms will generally increase reports of sleepiness and fatigue.

The occurrence, frequency, and nature of adverse reactions may also be related to the conduct of the clinical trial in terms of staff behavior or uncontrollable factors. A few examples are given:

1. Frenetic activity on the part of the investigator or staff may create adverse reactions. For example, rushing patients through tests and in general increasing their level of anxiety and stress will tend to increase various subjective complaints as well as gastric or other types of distress. This approach would have a marked effect in an acute trial but could also seriously affect a long-term trial.
2. An intense heat wave that occurs during a trial may cause a variety of additional adverse reactions.
3. Assassination of a beloved national leader may lead to reactions of grief and even depression that may affect patients in a trial.

An unusual case in which one medicine (penicillin) was mistakenly dispensed as another (ascorbic acid) was described by Golbert and Patterson (1968). Recurrent anaphylaxis occurred that was particularly difficult to diagnose because the patient refused to admit use of the medicine.

How to Treat Adverse Reactions (Issue 11)

The manner of treating patients with adverse reactions is rarely specified in a protocol, since there are many more possibilities than can be anticipated or addressed in a simple or generic manner. Prompt and appropriate medical treatment adhering to current standards is ethically required of physicians. The types of commonly used medical treatment are often categorized into a small number of general classes. These classes include (1) continued treatment without modification, (2) increased surveillance of the patient, (3) using a counteractive medication or treatment, (4) changing the medicine's dose or frequency of administration, (5) temporarily discontinuing the medicine, (6) permanently stopping the medicine and discontinuing the trial, (7) rechallenging the patient after the medicine has been stopped, (8) combining two or more of these techniques, and (9) other procedures.

Whether a physician chooses a proper clinical re-

TABLE 80.6 *Adverse reactions obtained in a specific clinical trial may be related to any one or more of the following factors*

A. Characteristics of the patient population treated[a]
B. Characteristics of the medicine and its administration
  1. Rate of dose escalation
  2. Rate of infusion
  3. Specific doses used
  4. Blood levels achieved
  5. Specific dose regimens used (e.g., alternate-day doses, medicine holidays)
  6. Quantity of capsules or tablets ingested or fluid administered
  7. Dosage forms of medicine
  8. Duration of exposure to medicine (e.g., acute, chronic)
  9. Number of doses administered in a given time (i.e., degree of cumulation)
  10. Interactions with other medicines
C. Characteristics of the trial, home, and/or other environments
D. Techniques of eliciting and interpreting adverse reactions including the personalities, approaches, and behavior of individuals eliciting and interpreting them
E. Characteristics of the trial design (e.g., periods of fasting, demands of the tests)

[a] See Table 83.25 for a listing of numerous specific factors that may influence adverse reactions.

sponse to treat an adverse reaction depends on the accuracy of his clinical assessment of the nature and severity of the problem and his or her clinical judgment about how best to resolve it. Inappropriate or inconsistent methods for treating adverse reactions may lead to an incorrect or biased interpretation of the clinical significance of specific adverse reactions.

Influence of Baseline and Concomitant Medicines on Adverse Reactions (Issue 12)

Some adverse reactions observed in a clinical trial of an investigational or marketed medicine are not induced by the trial medicine. Before starting to analyze adverse reaction data to consider benefit-to-risk ratios and clinical importance of the adverse reactions, it is necessary to eliminate from consideration those adverse reactions that were related to nontrial factors. Thus, it is usually worthwhile to eliminate adverse reactions present at baseline that were also observed during the trial. There are two caveats, however, to this approach. The first is that if adverse reactions present at baseline worsened during the trial, they are generally considered to be related in some manner to the trial medicine. Second, adverse reactions in patients receiving concomitant medicines may be caused by a medicine interaction and not result solely from the trial medicine. This is an example of how the use of concomitant medicines in a study makes interpretation of data more complicated (i.e., confounds the data). In early phases of medicine development it is usually not desirable for patients to be maintained on other medicines. On the other hand, avoiding use of concomitant medicines may render clinical interpretation more difficult, since the trial may not reflect the nature of actual clinical practice. Moreover, it is sometimes ethically and medically necessary to use concomitant medicines (e.g., in most epilepsy trials).

Impact of a Trial's Adverse Reactions on Other Trials Performed with the Same Medicine (Issue 13)

There are numerous possible actions that can be followed to modify the conduct of an ongoing clinical trial as a result of adverse reactions. In addition to requiring possible modifications of an ongoing trial, the adverse reactions observed or reported may be of such a nature or intensity that other trials using the same medicine may also need to be modified. The procedures that are usually followed to modify other medicine trials depend primarily on the importance placed on the adverse reaction and the risk assigned to current patients in continuing in the trial. Thus, the question of who

assesses the clinical significance of the adverse reaction and how it is assessed is of major importance to the trial.

There is a wide spectrum of possible interpretations and modifications of a clinical trial resulting from the determination that a severe adverse reaction has occurred that requires further action. A useful means of obtaining a balanced perspective in reaching a reasonable decision as to how to modify clinical trials is to involve several or even many individuals in the decision-making process. Consultants, colleagues, peers, and others may be brought together or consulted individually to reach a consensus of which action(s) appears to be the most reasonable response to the adverse reaction. This course ensures that the views of one individual do not arbitrarily direct a trial or group of trials in a given direction. The decision-making group (whether formally or informally constituted) should include both the principal investigator or a designee and representatives of the sponsor for sponsored trials. Each group or individual may wish to evaluate his or her position independently, both prior and subsequent to joint discussions. All decisions to modify significantly the trial or group of trials must be made with approval of the Ethics Committees/Institutional Review Boards (IRBs) involved. Because of the significance ascribed to these meetings vis-á-vis patient safety and the entire medicine development program, even a decision not to modify a medicine study should generally be presented to the relevant Ethics Committee/IRB for information or ratification.

Obtaining Additional Data on Adverse Reactions During a Clinical Trial (Issue 14)

Additional data on adverse reactions may be obtained during a clinical trial by increasing the frequency of monitoring of patients both with and without the specific adverse reaction. Increased monitoring activities will help uncover early signs of the problem, determine its natural history, and allow medical treatment to be instituted as soon as indicated in those patients in whom it is required.

Other sources of additional data on adverse reactions involve evaluating supplemental data requested from a laboratory. This approach may be used on patients with the adverse reaction and, if the adverse reaction is serious enough, with all patients. A third approach is to obtain the services of a consultant. This is especially important in complex situations in which the identification or treatment of the adverse reaction is not established or other questions need to be addressed. The requisition and accumulation of additional data will allow more appropriate and complete interpretations to be made.

What Are the Implications If Few or No Adverse Reactions Are Reported in a Clinical Trial? (Issue 15)

This result is not a real issue if few adverse reactions are expected (e.g., a pharmacokinetic trial comparing two doses of a medicine and placebo or two formulations in which no adverse reactions should arise). Actual situations have arisen when more adverse reactions are anticipated than are reported. This includes a population of Veterans Administration Hospital patients who wanted a place to stay and believed that reporting adverse reactions would lead to their being discontinued from the clinical trial. Another example is a clinical trial conducted in West Germany in which patients were implicitly told (or at least understood) that they were not to experience adverse reactions. Although the power of positive thinking is a valuable method when used appropriately in clinical practice, its use in the example given is clearly inappropriate.

What Are the Implications If an Excessive Number of All Adverse Reactions or Only Severe Adverse Reactions Are Reported in a Clinical Trial? (Issue 16)

Too many adverse reactions could be reported because of cultural differences in the patient populations compared, or because of differences in physician training or practice. This issue is discussed further in Chapter 40, "National versus Multinational Clinical Trials."

Another possibility is secondary gain. For example, a physician who receives a fixed amount of money for all patients regardless of how much of the clinical trial they complete may be tempted to exaggerate the severity of complaints and to discontinue a patient prematurely.

Adverse Reactions on Brand versus Generic Medicines (Issue 17)

All reports to companies and regulatory agencies should include information on whether the adverse reaction occurred in a patient given the brand name medicine or a generic equivalent. In some cases adverse reactions are known to result from an excipient in the formulation, and there are almost always at least some differences in excipients present. Cases of this nature have been well documented with use of tartrazine.

Reporting of Adverse Reactions by Sales Representatives (Issue 18)

During visits of sales representatives with physicians, the physicians may mention one or more adverse reactions observed with the company's products. The representative may leave an official regulatory agency form for the physician to complete and mail to the regulatory agency. In most situations, the sales representative may be asked or may volunteer to complete the form for the "busy" physician. The representative should also inform the company directly about each adverse reaction.

This situation leads to the ironic conclusion that the larger the sales force and the greater the number of contacts between physicians and representatives, the greater will be the number of adverse reaction reports obtained. Another result is that a company that asks their sales representatives to file the regulatory (or company) forms themselves will uncover more adverse reactions than if the representative leaves the form for the physician and his staff to complete.

How Should Adverse Events Be Characterized that Are Part of a Medical or Surgical Procedure? (Issue 19)

If a patient develops pain during an endoscopy procedure conducted as part of a clinical trial, the pain is definitely trial related, but it is probably not medicine related. It is an adverse event but not a treatment-related adverse reaction. The same conclusion may be drawn if a patient experiences dizziness after several blood draws or headaches after a long fast that is part of a clinical trial.

On the other hand, the clinical trial medicine may make the patient more susceptible to these or other adverse events and may not be a totally independent factor. The correct approach is to assess whether the incidence of adverse events of a particular type is greater in a clinical trial than anticipated and is greater in one treatment group than another. If so, then the cause(s) of this finding should be explored.

Time of Occurrence of Adverse Reactions Relative to Medicine Administration (Issue 20)

There are two separate issues relating to the association in time of medicine administration and occurrence of the adverse reaction. The first issue is how soon after the dose is ingested or administered the adverse reaction is observed or occurs. This is an important consideration in establishing the association of the medicine with the particular adverse reaction in question. In general, the longer it takes for an adverse reaction to be manifested (after a specific time period during which it is expected), the less likely it is that the adverse reaction is associated with the medicine in question, and the more likely it is that there is another cause for the adverse reaction. With increased time between purported cause and effect, there are some associations that become almost impossible to establish firmly, even though they may be biologically plausible (e.g., long-term outcomes of single exposures to ionizing radiation). The same principle applies to a beneficial clinical effect. There are some noteworthy exceptions to this principle (e.g., carcinomas and other effects in offspring of mothers given diethylstilbestrol during pregnancy, acute myocardial infarctions and use of oral contraceptives).

The second issue is to determine when the adverse reaction occurred during the course of treatment. Adverse reactions may occur during (1) the initiation of therapy, (2) the dose ascension phase, or (3) the maintenance period. Development of tolerance to the adverse reaction often occurs.

Adverse reactions may also occur during taper and on discontinuation of a medicine. Three different types of signs and symptoms are observed after medicine discontinuation. Symptoms that gradually recur as the patient relapses to his former state are generally assumed to be related to the disease. Symptoms that suddenly recur with a greater intensity than at baseline are referred to as a rebound phenomenon and are related, at least in part, to the medicine. A third type of symptoms are those of medicine withdrawal, which had not previously occurred and are generally believed to be caused by the medicine, although withdrawal symptoms are sometimes also noted after a placebo is stopped. A mixture of these three types of responses may be observed.

Adverse reactions may also periodically recur for a long or short time after a medicine has been stopped. Sometimes an adverse reaction will occur for the first time after the medicine has been stopped. Many of these adverse reactions are referred to as "flashback" symptoms. Numerous other patterns of adverse reactions over time may occur, especially during a period of chronic treatment.

Interpretation of the clinical significance of adverse reactions requires careful consideration of these concepts. These concepts may affect numerous aspects of interpretation conducted during the clinical trial (e.g., establishing the association with a medicine) as well as after the trial is complete (e.g., establishing the significance of the time and number of doses required for certain adverse reactions to occur after medicine dosing is initiated).

Statistical Evaluation of Adverse Reactions (Issue 21)

This topic is not addressed in the present discussion. The interested reader is recommended to refer to standard statistical works by Feinstein (1977), Gore and Altman (1982), Bailar and Mosteller (1986), and Ingelfinger et al. (1987).

Processes to Determine Clinical Significance of Adverse Reactions (Issue 22)

Various aspects relating to interpretation of data obtained from a single patient and from a single clinical trial have been discussed above. This section focuses on the types of assessments that are considered in relation to the overall development or marketing of a medicine.

The interpretation of adverse reactions is important primarily for how the data affect the index patient(s) and, secondly, for the risk of other patients who are presently receiving the medicine or who may receive the medicine in the future. This issue includes consideration of (1) the remaining part of the index trial, (2) concurrently run trials with the same medicine, and (3) trials to be initiated in the future with the same medicine.

Five processes are considered in determining the clinical significance of a medicine's adverse reactions. These evaluations are (1) overall incidence of the adverse reaction, (2) clinical consequences for those with the adverse reaction, (3) risk for different groups to experience the adverse reaction, (4) identification of specific factors that make the adverse reaction more serious and, (5) determining how patients with the adverse reaction may be treated.

Incidence

The first process is to assess the chance that individual patients will experience the specific adverse reaction (i.e., to evaluate the overall incidence in the population exposed to the medicine). The incidence figure is often expressed as a fraction or as a percentage. To obtain this information, it is necessary to know both the total number of patients who had (or have) the specific adverse reaction (numerator of the fraction) and the total number of patients exposed to the medicine who potentially could have experienced the adverse reaction (denominator of the fraction). Patients included in the numerator are also included in the denominator. Denominators often include a factor relating to time (e.g., period of exposure, duration of exposure, period of risk).

Clinical Risk

The second process is to assess the clinical risk for a particular patient who experiences the adverse reaction. Clinical risks may be measured through a combination of methods.

1. Determine the percentage distribution of patients whose problem is mild, moderate, severe, or life-threatening.

2. Assess whether it is likely that the problem will worsen over time.
3. Evaluate how long the adverse reaction generally persists after the medicine is discontinued and whether it will recur on rechallenge with the medicine.
4. Calculate whether patients develop tolerance to the adverse reaction.
5. Assess if the adverse reaction occurs after the medicine is discontinued, either during the acute withdrawal phase or possibly a long period later.

Third, assess whether all groups of patients have an equal likelihood of acquiring the adverse reaction or whether there are certain risk factors that increase the likelihood of experiencing the adverse reaction. Determine whether the adverse reaction occurs with equal severity in each group of patients treated with the medicine (e.g., high- versus low-dose group, geriatric patients versus adults, children versus adults, patients with decreased liver or renal function versus patients with normal function).

The fourth process is to assess whether there are medicine interactions, concurrent illnesses, concomitant medicines, or other risk factors (e.g., smoking, lifestyle) that make the adverse reaction occur more frequently or make it worse when it does occur. The fifth and last process is to assess how patients should be treated and whether all patient groups with the problem react similarly to treatment.

The answers to these questions will help establish which if any particular patient groups are at high risk of experiencing this problem. If it is possible to identify such groups, then precautions, warnings, and contraindications for using the medicine should be developed. If there are groups of individuals who may be identified as high-risk patients based on laboratory tests prior to exposure to the medicine, then the use of such tests should be recommended. This assumes that the benefit-to-risk ratio and the benefit-to-cost ratio suggest that use of those tests would be worthwhile.

Risk versus Benefit

The risk of an adverse reaction must always be balanced against potential or actual benefits. The presence of an adverse reaction (even a serious one) does not mean that the medicine should be discontinued. There are many circumstances when continued treatment is medically and ethically acceptable. This topic is discussed in Chapters 41 and 99.

Outcome

If a portion of the potential patient population is excluded from using the medicine (because of their ele-

vated risk), then it should be assessed whether the remaining patient population has sufficient medical need of the medicine to pursue its development or to continue its marketing. The revised market size and projected sales for the medicine must also be assessed to ensure that continued development is commercially feasible. Even when a negative marketing assessment is made, there may be other (e.g., humanitarian) reasons to pursue the medicine's development.

Clinical Significance of Adverse Reactions (Issue 23)

The question of assessing clinical significance involves clinical judgment and can be addressed in several ways. One approach is to define all adverse reactions that are rated as moderate or severe (or only severe) as clinically significant. Another approach is to develop an operational definition of the term clinically significant that can be applied by the rater to each adverse reaction (or other abnormality of a safety parameter). Without any definition to use as a guide, the association of the term clinically significant to a particular adverse reaction will vary from rater to rater and possibly within each rater from time to time for any one patient.

Problems of interpretation may arise if different physicians reach different decisions as to the clinical significance of an adverse reaction at one point in time. A clear operational definition will minimize the possibility of this situation occurring. If two physicians reach different decisions about the clinical significance of an adverse reaction that has occurred or continued at two different times in a trial, then it is necessary to resolve this difference. The resolution could be that both were correct and the condition of the patient changed between their separate observations, or that one physician's rating should be modified. When differences in assessment of the clinical significance of an adverse reaction are observed in the data, the case records should be examined further and discussed. The clinical monitor should attempt to settle this discrepancy through review of the data (e.g., was the intensity of the adverse reaction rated differently by the two physicians?) and discussions with all physicians involved, preferably together if two or more were involved.

When a single physician rates an adverse reaction as clinically significant for a patient on one occasion but not at another, careful monitoring of the data and discussions between the monitor and staff will ensure that such differences were intended and were not accidental. To minimize the chance for discrepancies, the data collection forms should be designed to have a place for rating each adverse reaction as "clinically significant" (or "clinically important"). A check-off system (Yes, No, Unknown) can be used alongside the place where each adverse reaction is written.

When three "experts" in clinical pharmacology were each given identical information on adverse reactions, there was nonetheless a great degree of difference in several important questions posed, including the attribution of medicine to adverse reaction (Koch-Weser et al., 1977). These authors stress the need for standardization of definitions of adverse reactions and their attribution to medicines.

Discovery of Novel Indications for Medicines Based on Adverse Reactions (Issue 24)

Many current uses of medicines are based on adverse reactions. Some of the most well-known examples include (1) hair growth with topical minoxidil (originally marketed as a systemic medicine to lower blood pressure), (2) antihypertensive effect of clonidine (originally developed as a decongestant), (3) diuretic activity of sulfonamides (originally developed as antibacterials), and (4) sleep-promoting activity of antihistamines (originally developed for allergic rhinitis). The stories of some of these and others are described by Blumenthal (1989).

Presentation of Sufficient Data on Adverse Reactions (Issue 25)

In a presentation of data from a single clinical trial, the interpretation of adverse reactions is enhanced when the reader is provided specific information on (1) specific nature of the adverse reaction, (2) number of patients and number of reports, (3) indication for which the medicine was used, (4) doses of the medicine associated with the adverse reactions, (5) identity, doses, routes, and timing of concomitant medicines used, (6) attribution or degree of association of the medicine with each adverse reaction, (7) concurrent illnesses, (8) to what degree the adverse reaction was reversible, (9) the time that was required for the patient to return to "normal" or baseline, (10) whether patients were rechallenged with medicine, and if so, what occurred, and (11) what the basic demographics were such as age, sex, race, and weight of the patients who were affected and, in some situations, those who were unaffected. A comparison of these data with results of similar medicines is generally useful.

Iceberg Effect

To obtain a realistic understanding and perspective of a medicine's adverse reaction profile, it is important to describe nonserious as well as serious adverse reactions. If there are two reports of a serious adverse reaction in the presentation of data on adverse reactions, it would be important to know if there were 100 nonserious reports (i.e., mild or moderate intensity) of the same adverse reaction as well, or whether there were just two or three nonserious reports. If there were 100 nonserious reports, were they from one or two patients only, or were they observed in a much larger number? The clinical significance of an adverse reaction can best be assessed by consideration of all cases in the data base. Evaluation of the total data allows one to assess whether a few serious cases are isolated or represent part of a much larger problem, analogous to the tip of an iceberg. Knowledge of even apparently trivial cases of an adverse reaction provides a more complete perspective, which allows a better interpretation of the clinical significance of the adverse reaction to be achieved.

Presentations of data on adverse reactions in reports or publications vary from extensive lists of a trial's "raw data" to brief "summary data" of a trial, from full case reports replete with background data and description of outcomes to detailed FDA 1639 forms to one-line descriptions of each patient's adverse reactions, or to summary descriptions of a medicine's entire clinical history, as in the *Physicians' Desk Reference*.

A variety of formats used to present adverse reactions was given in *Presentation of Clinical Data* (Spilker and Schoenfelder, 1990). Those tables and figures illustrate a number of formats that may be used to combine all data on one adverse reaction into a single or several tables, although other formats have also been used. The completeness of information on adverse reactions presented in published articles has been evaluated (Venulet, 1985). It was found that most articles presented insufficient information for the reader to be able to evaluate the adverse reactions. This report proposes guidelines for presenting information on adverse reactions from the Morges Conference on adverse reactions. Three categories of publication reports on adverse reactions are described: preliminary reports, single cases, and multiple cases.

It is important to describe how the adverse reaction reports were obtained, i.e., by (1) reading a checklist to the patient, (2) collecting only spontaneously reported adverse reactions, (3) using a general verbal probe, (4) having the patient read a checklist, or (5) by other techniques. Other details relating to the systems used to measure (and define) intensity and attribute the reaction to the medicine, and to the clinical treatment provided to the patient with the adverse reaction are all important factors to describe prior to presenting the actual data.

It is also important to describe whether tabulations of adverse reactions are based on the number of patients experiencing the event, the number of events reported, or both. If one uses a narrow operational definition, then a lower incidence figure will result. If one includes multiple reports from individual patients as adverse reactions, then an exaggerated incidence value may result. Incidence figures may also reflect chronic medicine use and will be inappropriate to apply to patients who receive acute or short courses of the medicine.

Many published reports of clinical data do not

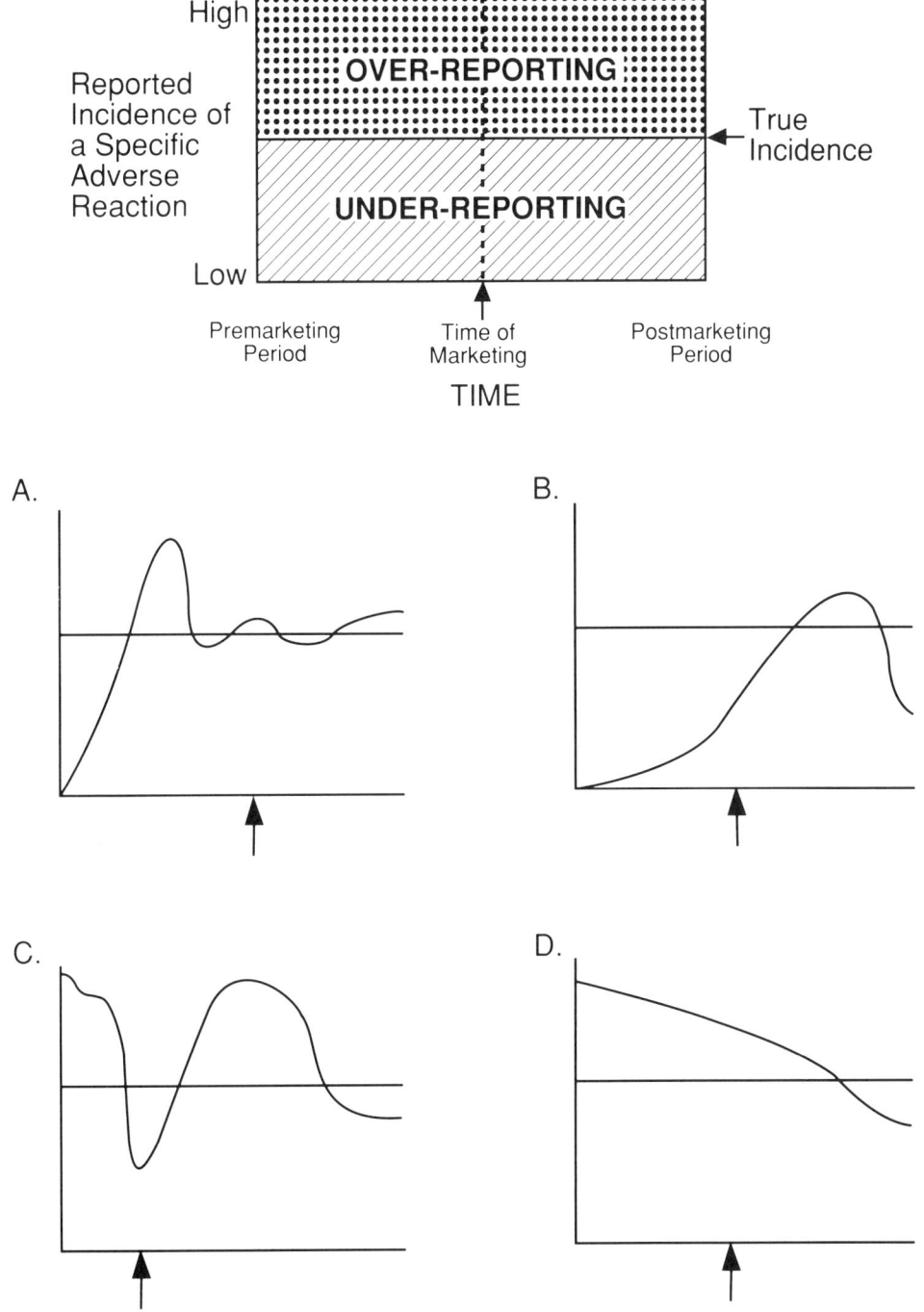

FIG. 80.2 Four hypothetical types of reporting patterns of adverse reactions over time. Innumerable variations of these and other patterns are possible. The assumption that the true incidence of an adverse reaction is constant over time is probably incorrect in many cases. The arrow indicates the time of initial marketing. (Reprinted from Spilker, 1989a, with permission of Raven Press.)

present sufficient details about adverse reactions to allow readers to obtain a complete perspective of their clinical significance. This lack of information affects and limits the assessment of the interpretation that may be reached by readers of the report. A glowing report or publication about a new medicine may not contain an adequate balance of the risks to patients in terms of potential adverse reactions. Inclusion of adequate information about adverse reactions allows the reader to achieve a more balanced interpretation and understanding of a patient's true risks.

Changes in Adverse Reaction Incidence Over Time (Issue 26)

Insufficient attention is paid to how adverse reactions change over time (Figs. 80.2 to 80.4). Figure 80.2 refers to reporting patterns for all patients receiving a medicine, and Figs. 80.3 and 80.4 refer to patterns observed for individual patients over time. A number of major factors responsible for changing patterns are mentioned below.

Factor I—Time of Onset. The pattern of occurrence varies among adverse reactions for a single medicine, as well as among medicines. Some adverse reactions usually occur shortly after a medicine is ingested (e.g., anaphylaxis), whereas others only arise after several weeks or months of therapy.

Factor II—Duration. Various patterns of adverse reaction duration are illustrated in Figs. 80.3 and 80.4. Numerous variations are possible.

Factor III—Intensity. If tolerance develops rapidly to an adverse reaction, patients may continue their treatment, otherwise they often discontinue treatment. Some adverse reactions persist unabated, although the intensity of most improves or worsens.

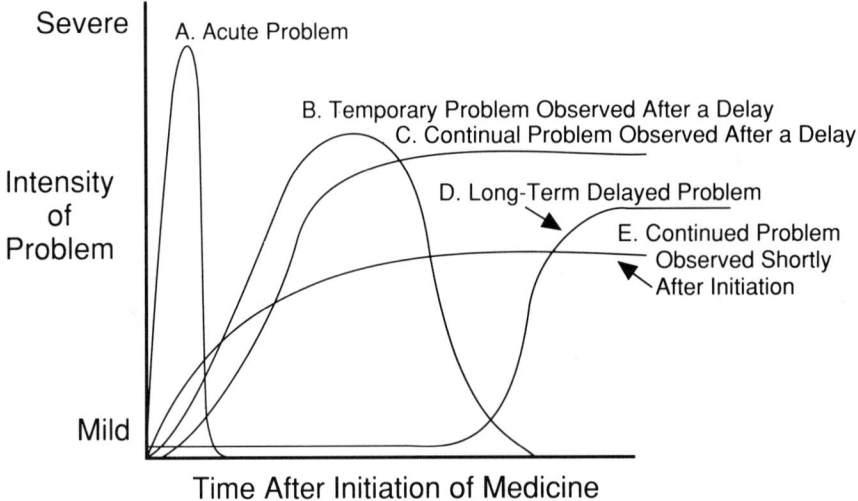

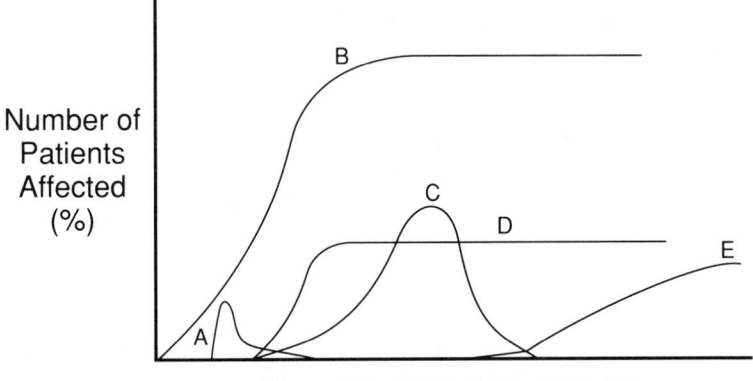

FIG. 80.3 Temporal patterns of adverse reactions, showing a few hypothetical patterns relating to the intensity of the problem (*upper graphs*). Examples in the lower graph could be anaphylaxis (*graph A*), cancer (*graph E*).

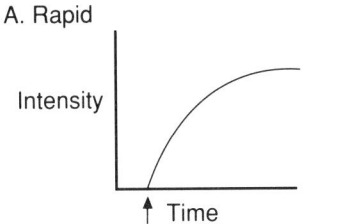

A. Rapid

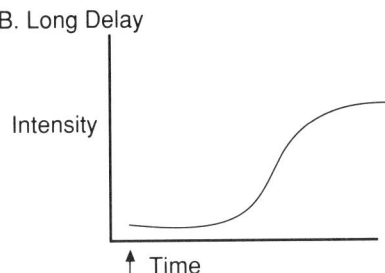

B. Long Delay

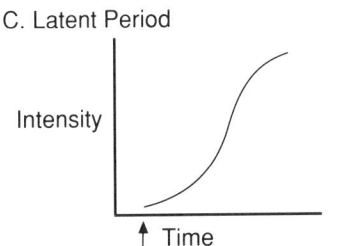

C. Latent Period

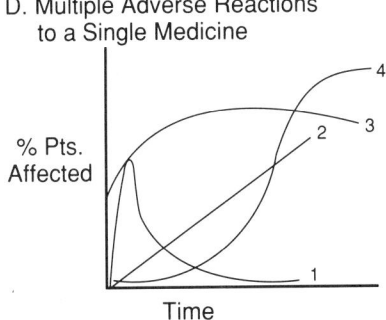

D. Multiple Adverse Reactions to a Single Medicine

FIG. 80.4 Various patterns of adverse reaction onset. The arrow is the time when the medicine is started.

Factor IV—Dose. The various patterns of dose-response relationships are shown in Fig. 80.5. If physicians start to prescribe gradually higher (or lower) doses of a medicine, it will probably influence the dose–response relationship and incidence of adverse reactions reported.

Formation of Hypotheses about Adverse Reactions (Issue 27)

In developing a medicine's adverse reaction profile, it is important to determine all important factors to which the adverse reactions are related. Many of the major factors are listed in Table 80.6. Adverse reactions resulting from a medicine have clinical significance in terms of (1) medical problems that are caused, (2) duration of effect, (3) reversibility of effect, and (4) interaction with other medicines.

There may be a number of adverse reactions that appear to occur in a cluster or constellation. These may be worth investigating to gain additional knowledge about the medicine and diagnostic clues for physicians to look for in patients receiving the medicine, and possibly as an aid in treating adverse reactions effectively.

There are special clusters of adverse reactions to certain medicines that are defined as syndromes. An example is the syndrome of systemic lupus erythematosus (SLE), which occurs as an adverse reaction in some patients given procainamide or other medicines. In this situation, a number of apparently unrelated symptoms (adverse reactions) may be associated and should be recognized as such. Many such syndromes resulting from medicines (e.g., Parkinson's disease-like syndrome) are listed in the *Physicians' Desk Reference* and may be identified by experienced clinicians. In some syndromes certain symptoms or adverse reactions always occur, whereas in others such as SLE there are numerous symptoms that may or may not be present.

With newly marketed and investigational medicines there are usually insufficient data available to know whether various adverse reactions constitute syndromes that may be caused by a medicine or, if syndromes are identified, whether they are related to a medicine. It is during investigational and early postmarketing periods that it is important to generate and test hypotheses about the association of multiple adverse reactions as constituting a known (or previously unknown) syndrome. It may take a short or long period of time to test the validity of each hypothesis. Similarly, an association of certain congenital abnormalities may be hypothesized to be associated with a medicine [e.g., VACTERL syndrome (vertebral, anal, cardiac, tracheoesophageal, renal, and limb), which is associated with progestational agents given during pregnancy]. These hypotheses are then evaluated through subsequent clinical experience and also through animal experimentation.

Postmarketing Surveillance of Adverse Reactions (Issue 28)

Studies conducted during Phase IV may be classified in broad groups discussed in Chapter 7. These include epidemiological data collected in a passive manner, in which data are generated under normal use conditions. This type of study has been referred to as epidemiological intelligence. The second type of study is an active one in which a cohort or other group is established

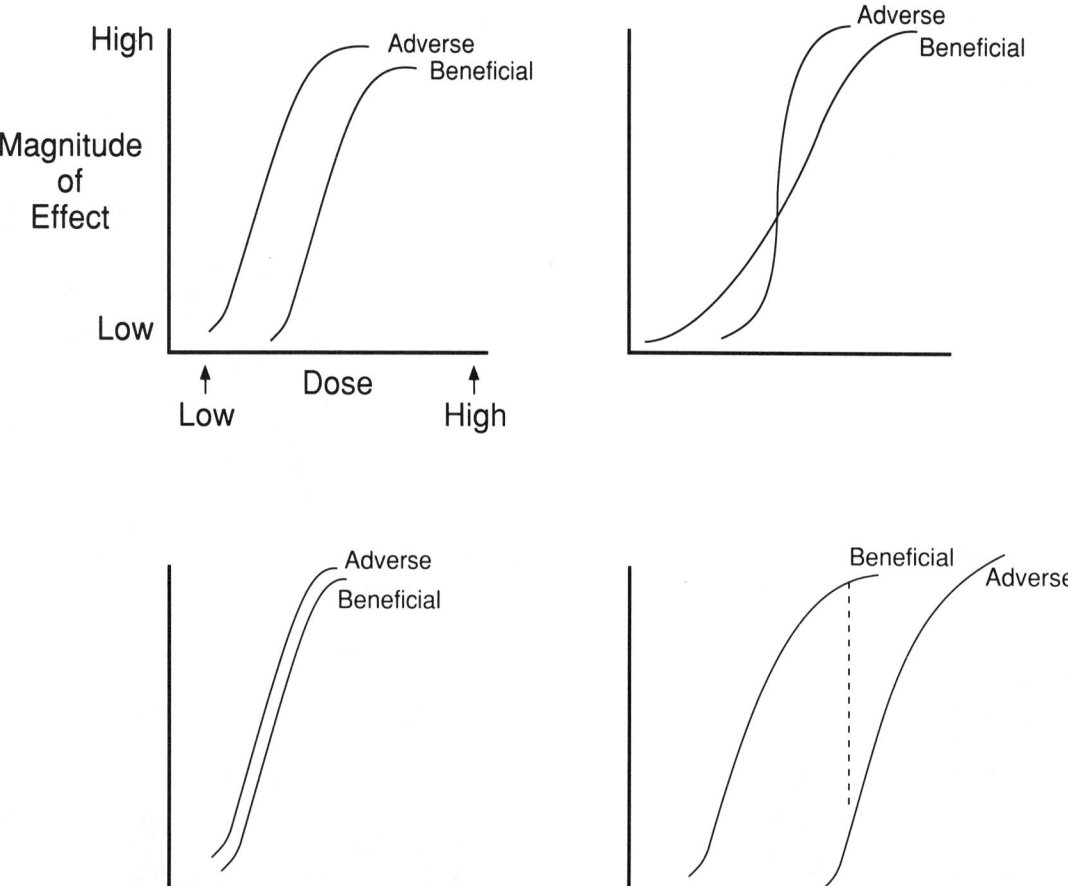

FIG. 80.5 Dose–response relationship of beneficial versus adverse effects of hypothetical medicines. The most desired pattern is in the *lower right panel*. The other panels illustrate that adverse reactions may (1) occur prior to the beneficial effect such as with many oncology medicines (*upper left panel*), (2) occur at the same dose as the beneficial medicine such as the sedation that occurs with many older antihistamines (*lower left panel*), or (3) predominate at higher doses of a medicine and often prevent those doses from being used (*upper right panel*). Other adverse reactions occur in an all-or-none manner, and no dose–response is present.

and followed in time or assessed retrospectively. The third type of study is a Phase IV randomized control trial or one using a different trial design.

Postmarketing data may be obtained by direct patient contact via telephone interviews, questionnaires, or diaries with appropriate follow-up. Data may also be obtained by medical record screening for occurrence of key terms. This latter process is becoming more widespread as more medical data are being entered on computers. These data can be used to help assess the incidence and clinical significance of adverse reactions for the population of patients that is exposed to the medicine. The actual incidence of serious adverse reactions in the population and risk for patients to acquire the adverse reaction can better be defined with those additional data. Thus, postmarketing surveillance data may be obtained either with or without patient contact, consent, and involvement.

Reputation of a Medicine

One value of high-quality postmarketing surveillance data is that it can help prevent unsubstantiated data, poorly analyzed reports, or even slander from giving a medicine an undeserved bad reputation. It is unfortunately true that a medicine's reputation built through many years of careful work and enormous efforts may sometimes be destroyed by a brief press conference focusing on questionable or incorrect accusations. Accusations that may never be proved or substantiated often require years of effort to counteract effectively. In some cases the stigma of an unproven accusation will persist despite well-designed trials that demonstrate the accusation to be false.

Potential new benefits, possibly leading to new indications, may also be uncovered through postmarketing studies. This byproduct of postmarketing studies is primarily a theoretical consideration, since potential new indications have rarely been uncovered through this type of clinical study. Nonetheless, it should be remembered that postmarketing surveillance is a relatively new discipline, especially in the pharmaceutical industry. The second type of postmarketing study using a cohort or other design to collect data should provide more concise data on adverse reactions than using epidemiological intelligence.

Well-designed clinical trials conducted during Phase IV (e.g., randomized controlled trials) are another means of obtaining safety data. In this situation more clearly defined patient populations are usually studied rather than the entire range of all patients given the medicine. This latter group (i.e., all patients given the medicine at specific sites) is the usual population used for passive postmarketing surveillance studies. Careful techniques in Phase IV controlled trials may compare adverse reactions obtained in the group of patients exposed to a new medicine with another group exposed to placebo, no treatment, or an active control. Thus, more tightly designed Phase IV trials provide data that primarily assist in the overall understanding of a medicine's safety and enable a more accurate interpretation and clinical assessment to be reached.

Tracking the Pattern of an Adverse Reaction's Incidence Throughout the Life of a Medicine (Issue 29)

Two common types of patterns occur in the study of adverse reactions over time (Fig. 80.2):

No. 1. Illustrates the time to onset, peak, and total duration of adverse reactions associated with a particular medicine. Both the pattern of intensity, time to onset, and number of patients may be graphed.
No. 2. Reporting patterns of adverse reactions change over time, particularly after a medicine is marketed. Both under- and overreporting occurs and the proportions of these also change over time. Data on the "true" incidence of adverse reaction are difficult to collect. Few studies have ever been conducted to examine this aspect of overreporting or underreporting of adverse reactions. The extent of adverse reaction reporting appears to be related to type of medicine (e.g., illicit and abused medicines are more frequently reported), time after approval (adverse reactions to newer medicines are reported more often than those to older medicines), and type of adverse reaction (e.g., deaths and unusual or rare adverse reactions are reported more often than are less severe and common adverse reactions).

Tracking adverse reaction reports accurately requires a large volume of data, an understanding of the magnitude of the background incidence (i.e., "noise")

of each adverse reaction, and knowledge of the indication for which the medicine is being used.

Most commonly noted adverse drug reactions are observed to have a different incidence in investigational trials than in postmarketing studies. Rossi et al. (1984) reported incidence rates for individual adverse reactions to various medicines to be 6 to 200 times greater in premarketing clinical trials than in postmarketing Phase IV studies. There was an 18-fold greater incidence for the cumulative incidence rates of ten expected adverse reactions in investigational studies.

Methods to Decrease the Incidence or Minimize the Severity of Adverse Reactions (Issue 30)

There are often medicine-related adverse reactions that may be reduced in incidence or severity. It is essential to obtain information as to how this may be accomplished with new medicines so that a balanced impression of the medicine's adverse reaction profile may be obtained. This effort is also important to protect patients from experiencing medicine-induced adverse reactions and will increase the benefit-to-risk ratio, at least for some patients.

An example of this approach is to administer a concomitant medicine that speeds up or slows down certain physiological events, such as renal elimination or hepatic metabolism of a medicine. Specific cases include the use of probenecid with penicillin or of antiemetics with chemotherapeutic agents. Other methods to decrease medicine-induced adverse reactions exist and are widely used. A list of selected techniques is presented in Table 80.7.

Reaching an Overall Impression of the Clinical Significance of Adverse Reactions (Issue 31)

A definitive clinical impression of a medicine's adverse reactions is rarely, if ever, achieved because of (1) additional data that are constantly being generated, (2) frequent reassessments of data, and (3) difficulties in arriving at a uniform consensus. One notable exception is for medicines that have been removed from the world-wide market, since no additional data are being generated and a consensus opinion is less likely to change over time.

Overreporting of adverse reactions in clinical trials may occur because (1) the detailed methods used for eliciting adverse reactions, (2) the tremendous attention focused on each patient, and (3) the desire, insistence, or regulatory requirement to enumerate each adverse reaction observed or reported. On the other hand, Phase IV studies may underestimate the true incidence of adverse reactions because of (1) deficien-

TABLE 80.7 *Techniques that may decrease the incidence or severity of adverse reactions*

A. Techniques related to patients
 1. Do not give the medicine to patients at high risk of having a serious adverse reaction (e.g., those with a genetic factor that predisposes them to having an adverse reaction)
 2. Monitor all patients frequently and carefully for early signs or symptoms
 3. Identify patients who are at high risk of experiencing adverse reactions and monitor them intensively
 4. Inform patients of signs or symptoms to check for and steps to follow to minimize or prevent adverse reactions
 5. Contact patients periodically by telephone to detect any adverse reactions that are minor and nonserious before they have a chance to become serious
 6. Select patients to receive medicine on the basis of predetermined criteria
B. Techniques related to medicine administration
 1. Use lowest possible effective doses
 2. Decrease amount of medicine given per administration by dividing the dose into two or more separate doses
 3. Instruct the patient to take the medicine with food or after meals to delay absorption and avoid high peak plasma concentrations
 4. Evaluate the optimal route of administration for minimizing adverse reactions of enteral medicines (sublingual, buccal, rectal, oral)
 5. Give parenteral medicines by routes that lead to a slower rate of absorption (e.g., depot injections)
 6. Give intravenous medicines by constant infusion or by slow or intermittent injection rather than by a bolus
 7. Develop enteric coated or other formulations that retard the rate of absorption and reduce peak plasma concentrations
 8. Explore other dosage regimens for maintenance therapy of chronic diseases (e.g., alternate-day dosing, medicine holidays)
 9. Give the dose with a concomitant medicine that may enhance renal elimination (e.g., probenecid is used to slow the elimination of penicillin)
 10. Administer the entire dose or largest dose at bedtime so that the patient sleeps during the period when adverse reactions are expected to occur
 11. Administer concomitant medicines that antagonize expected adverse reactions (e.g., antiemetics are given concomitantly with some chemotherapeutic agents)
 12. Administer concomitant medicines that modify the absorption, distribution, metabolism, or excretion of the medicine
 13. Administer concomitant medicines that affect biological receptors and lead to a decreased incidence or severity of adverse reactions
 14. Utilize a slower rate of dose escalation and/or dose taper[a]
 15. Stagger the time of administration of two (or more) medicines that might otherwise interact

[a] Dose escalation or taper may be modified in various other ways that may decrease adverse reactions.

cies in the methodologies used, (2) lack of recognition of adverse reactions by patients or investigators, and (3) lack of reporting of observed adverse reactions by patients or physicians.

It is facile to conclude that the true incidence of adverse reactions lies between these two values, but there is little or no evidence to support this common sense view. It is possible to conclude that the true incidence either lies closest to those data that were most

appropriately and accurately collected, or else both sets of widely differing data may be correct but for differing clinical conditions. A summary of reasons why a clinical trial may have an overreported or underreported incidence of adverse reactions is presented in Tables 80.8 and 80.9.

It was indicated that Phase IV studies may underestimate the true incidence of adverse reactions. The incidence and type of adverse reactions reported to three countries (United Kingdom, Sweden, and The Netherlands) were also found to vary substantially even though the three countries are similar in ethnic, dietary, and economic factors (Penn and Griffin, 1982). It is often difficult or even impossible to combine data on the same adverse reaction from different clinical trials. This may occur for many reasons including different types of definitions used for the adverse reactions or because the denominators differ (e.g., patients, patient years, patients plus duration, no denominator).

Excessive numbers of adverse reactions may be reported by overzealous investigators who are anxious to publish case reports, establish their reputation, or otherwise advance their careers. These individuals often elicit adverse reactions in their patients by asking

TABLE 80.8 *Selected reasons why a clinical trial may have an overreported incidence of adverse reactions[a]*

A. Reasons related to investigator or protocol design
 1. Overzealous investigator is overinterpreting patient reports and comments, possibly as a result of inexperience or various incentives
 2. An excessive number of adverse reactions are attributed by the investigator to the medicine
 3. Investigator's assessments of adverse reactions are exaggerated because of naiveté, ignorance, incompetence, or for other reasons
 4. An excessive number of medicine doses are given to patients because of protocol requirements or a desire to "push the dose," which elicit more adverse reactions than under normal use conditions
B. Reasons related to patients
 1. Patients have compromised physiological function (e.g., decreased liver or renal function) that leads to elevated blood levels of the trial medicine and thus to an elevated frequency of adverse reactions
 2. Patients are fasted for a relatively prolonged period prior to receiving the medicine
 3. Some patients have a genetic or medical history that differs from the control group or other patients in the clinical trial
 4. Patients weigh less than the average of those previously treated with the medicine and therefore receive a relatively excessive dose of the medicine on a milligram-per-kilogram basis
 5. The patients' disease process is worsening during the trial which leads to an increased number or severity of symptoms that are attributed to the medicine
 6. Intensity of adverse reactions is reported by the patient at a higher level than it should be (i.e., the patient exaggerates the magnitude of the adverse reaction)

[a] These reasons may relate to all adverse reactions in a clinical trial or to a subset of the adverse reactions that occurred.

TABLE 80.9 *Selected reasons why a clinical trial may have an underreported incidence of adverse reactions*[a]

1. No attempt is made by the investigator to discover either any adverse reactions or a subset in specific medical areas (e.g., sexual dysfunctions)
2. Adverse reactions that occur are not recognized by patients and/or investigators
3. Adverse reactions that occur are recognized but not reported by patients and/or investigators
4. Adverse reactions are reported by patients as less intense than they actually were
5. Adverse reactions are attributed by investigators to causes other than the trial medicine
6. Patients do not admit to experiencing adverse reactions because of "loyalty" to investigator, embarrassment, vague fears, or for other reasons
7. Patients' disease improved spontaneously (and unexpectedly) along with their symptoms. The incidence of medicine-related adverse ractions does not reflect what it would have been if the patients' disease did not improve
8. Physicians may not report certain adverse reactions if they fear lawsuits

[a] These reasons may relate either to all adverse reactions in a trial or to a subset of the adverse reactions that occurred.

leading questions. They may unconsciously bias their interpretation towards a stronger association between an adverse reaction and a medicine and conclude that a specific medicine is more toxic than it actually is. This group of individuals may adversely affect general medical use of a particular medicine by creating a stigma around it. There are, unfortunately, examples of investigators publishing the same group of adverse reactions in numerous publications. This inaccurately inflates perceived incidence rates and creates an unfounded belief that the medicine is more toxic than it truly is.

Careful and attentive physicians usually detect more adverse reactions than casual physicians. It must be concluded that the true incidence and overall impression of medicine-induced adverse reactions require substantial time and patient exposure after marketing to eliminate many sources of bias and to achieve a balanced view of a medicine's toxicity. Unfortunately, a 20-year reputation of medicine safety can easily be destroyed by some biased or unfounded results presented by someone with ulterior motives. A misinterpretation of real data based on an overreaction may have the same outcome.

The general impressions and reputation of a medicine's adverse reaction profile in the medical profession and literature often relate to the number of patients taking the medicine rather than to the true incidence of the problem. This is a situation in which the perceptions of prevalence and incidence figures become mixed. For example, adverse reactions resulting from interactions of a new (or marketed) medicine with either alcohol or diazepam may occur less frequently than interactions of the same medicine with

other medicines. If the severity and clinical importance of all adverse reactions caused by the above interactions are all approximately equal, there will often be an impression in the medical community that the interactions with alcohol or diazepam are more common. This perception arises since the number of patients taking alcohol or diazepam is much greater than the number of patients taking most other medicines. Thus, physicians may acquire an incorrect impression of the incidence of a problem (rate at which the interactions occur) based on prevalence data (total number of patients experiencing the adverse reactions). The longer that medicines are available on the market, the more likely it is that there will have been severe and unpleasant cases that may affect the medicine's reputation, even though the incidence may be extremely low.

In assessing a medicine's overall profile of adverse reactions, it is important to understand the pattern of how adverse reactions change in an individual patient over the course of therapy. Are they likely to increase, decrease, remain constant, or exhibit a bimodal or other pattern? A high incidence of some specific adverse reactions is noted to occur after the first dose of a number of medicines (e.g., prazocin) and then markedly to decrease. Another characteristic sometimes observed in clinical practice is for more severe adverse reactions to occur when a medicine is initiated after a lapse of time (e.g., zomepirac).

Various types of scales or formulas may be derived to help judge or interpret the clinical importance of a medicine's overall profile of adverse reactions. The scales or formulas will consider characteristics such as severity, number of days an adverse reaction persists, and various other factors. No single scale or group of scales have yet been widely accepted and used as an indicator of a medicine's adverse reaction profile.

Profile of a Medicine's Adverse Reactions during its Initial Investigational Period versus during its Marketing (Issue 32)

Although many reasons could be given for differences in a medicine's adverse reaction profile during clinical trials and during marketing, few studies have been published on this topic. The most extensive survey the author is aware of was published by Johnsson et al. (1984) on metoprolol (Table 80.10). Communication with the authors (Wallander and Johnsson, personal communication) has brought out several pieces of information relating to Table 80.10.

1. The indications evaluated during clinical trials for metoprolol were both hypertension and angina pectoris. The medicine was launched for those indications, and data in Table 80.10 are primarily for

TABLE 80.10 *The percentage distribution of adverse reactions to metoprolol for different system–organ classes, reported in clinical trials and in clinical practice (1975–1981)*

System–organ class	Percentage of adverse reaction reports	
	Clinical trials	Clinical practice[a] 1975–1981
Skin and appendage system	2.4	25.3
Musculoskeletal system	0	2.1
Collagenous system	0	1.4
Central and peripheral nervous system	22.0	8.9
Autonomic nervous system	19.0	11.8
Vision	2.4	11.2
Hearing and vestibular system	0	1.2
Special senses, other	0	0.4
Psychiatric	10.4	15.3
Gastrointestinal system	19.6	3.7
Liver and biliary system	0	2.3
Metabolic and nutritional system	0	1.7
Cardiovascular system	0.1	1.1
Myo-endo-pericardial and valve	0.1	0.4
Heart rate and rhythm	0	0.4
Vascular (extracardiac)	0.6	2.1
Respiratory system	7.0	6.0
Platelet, bleeding and clotting	0	0
Urinary system	0	0
Reproductive system	0	0.2
General disorders	16.4	4.3

Reprinted by permission of Almqvist and Wiksell from Johnsson et al. (1984).

[a] The total number of reported adverse reactions to metoprolol was 658, and the use of the medicine was 4 million patient years during this period.

those indications, although the proportion of each disease treated differed during the period of clinical trials and marketing.

The authors of the Johnsson et al. (1984) report have stated (personal communication) that the major investigational use of the medicine was in patients with angina, whereas the major marketed use was in patients with hypertension. This difference, however, does not account for some of the major discrepancies noted in Table 80.10.

2. Data for the marketing period were primarily obtained through spontaneous adverse reaction reports to the company or regulatory authorities.

3. Most adverse reactions during clinical trials were mild or moderate, whereas many more during marketing were severe. This is readily understandable, based on the fact that all adverse reactions in clinical trials were solicited, whereas information on important serious adverse reactions is usually reported after the medicine is marketed.

4. The duration of treatment was much greater in patients treated during the marketing of the medicine. The relatively short duration of clinical trials is the main reason for the lower percentage of skin problems.

5. The relatively high percentage of central nervous system disorders during clinical trials resulted from nonspecific complaints of headache and dizziness. These were also reported to a large extent in patients on placebo.

6. Autonomic nervous system adverse reactions included bradycardia, palpitations, vasopasm, diarrhea, and constipation.

7. Rates of adverse reactions for patients over 60 years of age versus the rate for those under 60 did not show differences.

Coles et al. (1983) examined the profile of adverse reactions for six nonsteroidal antiinflammatory medicines, as reported in the *Physicians' Desk Reference*. These profiles were compared with numerous studies on each medicine conducted in clinical settings, with computer-based records of private practice experience, and with data from patients who had been evaluated in clinical trials or in a clinical practice. Coles et al. found wide ranges of incidence of particular adverse reactions, depending on population characteristics, methods of calculation, and other factors. Medical records of patients in private medical practice showed a lower rate of adverse reactions compared with formal clinical trials, resulting from the lack of consistent reporting. Patient reports obtained via a mailed questionnaire yielded a rate of adverse reactions greater than those reported in clinical trials, particularly severe reactions.

TABLE 80.11 *Sources of data on adverse reactions[a]*

1. Premarketing clinical trials (Phases I, II, III)
2. Postmarketing studies (Phase IV) in a large population
3. Epidemiological studies
4. Spontaneous reports to regulatory authorities (e.g., yellow card system in the United Kingdom and FDA 1639 forms in the United States)
5. Data collected in a large Health Maintenance Organization (HMO) or large collaboration of hospitals (e.g., Kaiser Permanente HMO, Boston Collaborative Drug Surveillance Program)
6. Case reports published in the literature
7. Clinical trials and reviews published in the literature
8. Data bases available on subscription (e.g., Medlars, Excerpta Medical, Toxline)
9. Anecdotal reports published in the public media (e.g., newspaper, television, or magazine stories)
10. Publications by government or international agencies such as the Food and Drug Administration[b] and World Health Organization
11. Disease-oriented registers
12. Data bases established by governments (e.g., Medicare, Saskatchewan Health Care System)
13. Evaluations of old medical records in hospitals (e.g., Mayo Clinic), private practice, or in other locations

[a] These relate to prospective or retrospective trials or to spontaneous observations.

[b] For information on the Adverse Reaction Data Base, contact the Freedom of Information Staff at the FDA. Started in 1970, the data base contains over 100,000 records of all prescription medicine adverse reactions reported to the FDA.

The major difference in percentage of reports relating to the gastrointestinal system may relate to the attention focused on this system during clinical trials. Patients are often asked if they are able to take or tolerate a medicine or whether it makes them feel sick. Patients too often focus on how the "experimental" medicine makes them feel, and an important aspect of this relates to gastrointestinal symptoms. Most marketed medicines, however, are believed to be well tolerated by most patients.

The two most noteworthy differences in Table 80.10 (i.e., the tenfold difference for skin and appendage system, and almost fivefold difference in vision) are surprising. It would be particularly interesting to compare these results with those observed for other medicines. Pharmaceutical companies have a great deal of data of this type in their files, and it would be valuable if more of it were analyzed in this manner and published.

Planning Future Clinical Trials to Evaluate Adverse Reactions (Issue 33)

Numerous approaches are possible to obtain additional information on adverse reactions. The major source for obtaining scientific data relates to modifying existing or planned clinical trials to explore questions relating to adverse reactions. Another approach is to initiate premarketing surveillance studies, usually during Phase III, in which larger numbers of patients may be screened and followed to obtain information on the incidence, severity, predisposition, and other factors relating to an adverse reaction. Other sources of additional data on adverse reactions are shown in Table 80.11. The roles played by various sources of adverse reactions in establishing the cause-and-effect relationship of important adverse reactions to 18 new medicines were presented by Venning (1983b).

CHAPTER 81

Interpretation of Laboratory and Other Safety Data

USES OF LABORATORY DATA

Laboratory data are used for numerous purposes, including (1) routine screening, (2) diagnostic evaluation of a patient, (3) identification of risk factors, (4) monitoring progress of a disease or treatment, (5) detection of medicine-induced adverse reactions, (6) determination of appropriate medicine dosage (e.g., in patients with compromised renal or hepatic function), (7) to ensure therapeutic levels of a medicine, and (8) to confirm an unexpected result. A laboratory test result is of no value until it is interpreted. This is best done when results are interpreted in the context of information from the patient's history, physical examination, and underlying pathophysiology. A few examples in which laboratory data are diagnostic are listed in Table 81.1. Figure 81.1 shows how laboratory analytes are used to help reach a diagnosis.

For laboratory data the most important points to consider prior to evaluating a particular patient's value(s) are (1) reference limits of the test (previously referred to as *range of normal values*), (2) precision

TABLE 81.1 *Selected examples in which laboratory results are diagnostic[a]*

1. Hyperkalemia	5. Acidosis
2. Hypercalcemia	6. Alkalosis
3. Hyperglycemia	7. Hypercapnia
4. Hyperbilirubinemia	8. Ketosis

[a] In this simple model the disease is always present or absent based on the laboratory value. In other cases a disease may only have elevated levels in its advanced stage, or patients without disease may have false positives resulting from confounding factors.

and accuracy of the test, (3) degree of overlap with values indicative of disease or biological variation related to age, sex, diet, physical activity, medicines, or other factors, and (4) the predictive value of the test,

which depends on its specificity and sensitivity (i.e., magnitude of false-positive and false-negative data obtained). This information must be kept in mind as one evaluates specific data for a single patient or for a group of patients and assesses the clinical implications of any abnormality observed.

REFERENCE VALUES

Concept and Application

The *reference values* (range) of a test usually refers to the mean value and two standard deviations on each side of the mean. The term *normal values* is being re-

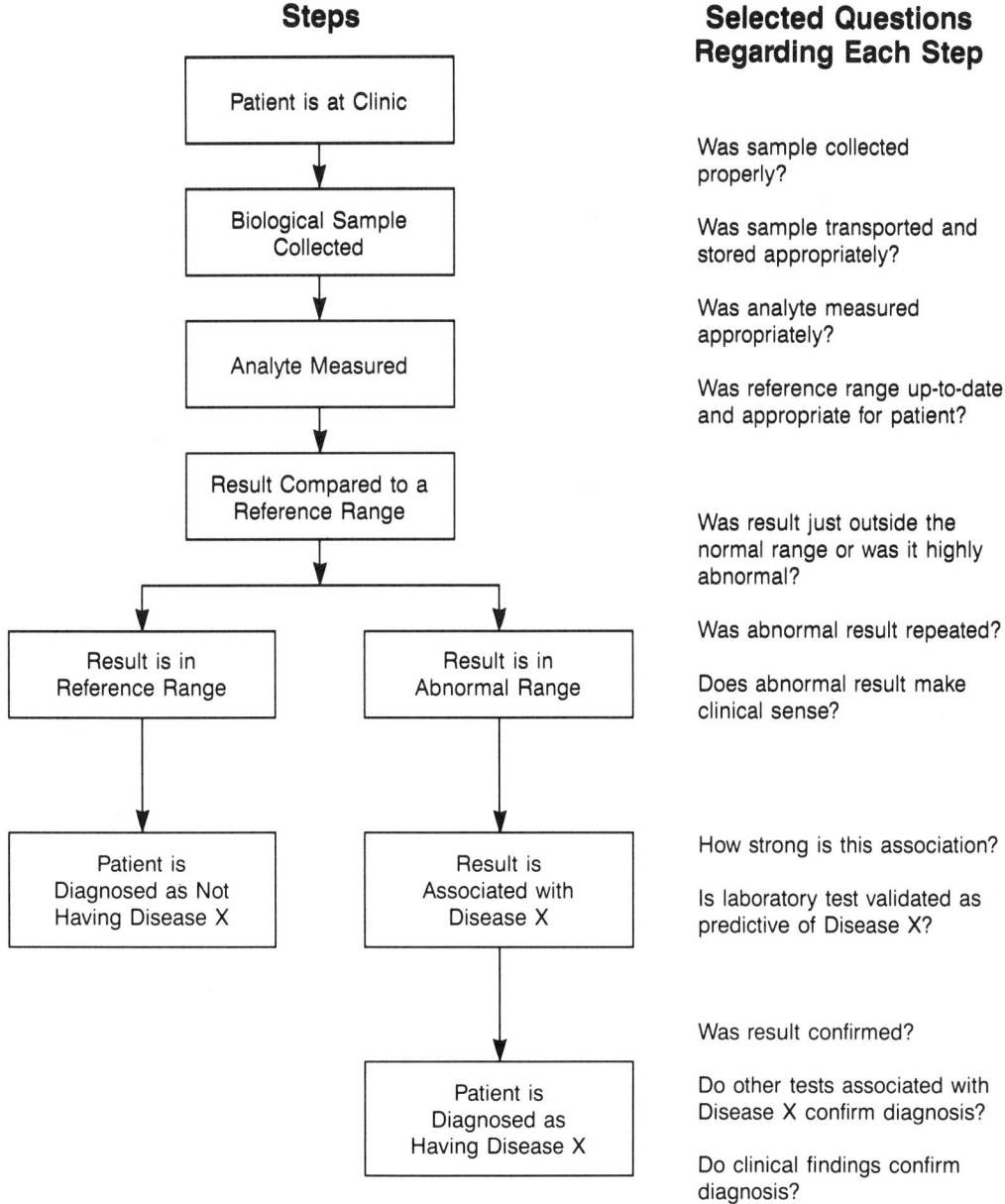

FIG. 81.1 Schematic illustration of the diagnostic process when a laboratory analyte is used as the basis of the diagnosis.

placed and should not be used (Sunderman, 1975). This range is a guide that illustrates values found in 95% of a sample population who are free of disease. This means that 2.5% of normals will be expected to have values below the lower limit defined as normal and 2.5% will be expected to have values above the upper limit defined as normal. The values are transformed (if necessary) so that a normal bell-shaped (i.e., Gaussian) distribution is achieved. Many laboratory tests of analytes have to be transformed since they do not have a normal (Gaussian) distribution (Elveback et al., 1970). Instead, the majority of tests have skewed, peaked, or flattened distributions.

Most laboratories periodically update their ranges of reference values to reflect the population(s) they serve. These updates are made because of changes in their analytical methods or subtle alterations in the population used to derive the ranges (e.g., changes in the demographic or genetic makeup of the people whose samples are used). The population used to determine the reference range is subject to strong debate between advocates of using objectively healthy people and advocates of using hospitalized or ill patients. The best choice would seem to depend on the population of people for whom the range will be used. On the other hand, that approach might suggest that multiple reference ranges be created at each laboratory, which is impractical. A combination cohort of both normals and patients may be used to create a reference range, and often is a reasonable compromise.

Problems of a Reference Range

There are a number of problems associated with a reference range, some of which are correctable and some of which are not. The issues of new analytical methodologies and shifts in the characteristics of patients served by the laboratory are correctable by updating the reference range of values. Problems with skewed results are usually handled through data transformation. Problems that are not as easily solved relate to (1) diseased patients who are included in the reference population and tend to create ranges that are too broad, (2) outliers who constitute about 5% of the group studied and are rated as abnormal but are nondiseased, (3) the laboratory not having adjusted the reference range for patients who were atypical of the population at the time the sample was drawn (e.g., diet, age, posture, physical activity), and (4) the test being used for various purposes so that one reference range is not usually suitable to confirm disease, exclude disease, and determine when it is necessary to initiate treatment. Many of the specific factors to consider in developing a reference sample are described by Sunderman (1975).

False Positives and Negatives

Figure 81.2 illustrates three hypothetical situations. In panel 1 there is a small overlap of the two populations (patients with a disease and those who are disease-free), such that 97.5% of each population does not overlap the other. There is a 2.5% rate of false-positive and 2.5% rate of false-negative responses. In panel 2 there is a much greater degree of overlap in results obtained, and in panel 3 the reference range and even outliers have no overlap at all. Since multiple diseases are usually evaluated with any particular laboratory test, the actual situation encountered in diagnosing a disease usually involves a combination of these patterns, at both the upper and lower limits of the normal range. This is illustrated in Fig. 81.3 for both calcium and albumin.

Depending on the degree of overlap between the reference range and that of a particular disease, both false positives (i.e., normals with abnormal data) and false negatives (i.e., abnormal patients with normal data) will result. Since a reference range of values for patients with a disease will be based on 95% of the data from abnormal patients, 2.5% will have lower and 2.5% will have upper values outside the range established. This also means that the probability of at least one abnormal result based solely on chance (i.e., a false positive) for a normal patient who has a battery of tests is reasonably high. The more tests that are run, the greater is the chance of a false positive.

The sensitivity and specificity of tests are described in Chapter 96 on false-positive and false-negative data. Briefly, the sensitivity of a test is a measure of its ability to detect a disease when it is present and the specificity is a measure of its ability to indicate the absence of a disease when it is absent.

Size of the Reference Range

The width of a reference range may be of diagnostic value since it is related to interindividual variation in the test values of the sample population. For certain tests, intraindividual variation is much narrower than the range of values defined by the reference range. Examples include serum immunoglobulins, transferrin, triglycerides, hemoglobin, and platelet count. The importance of this observation is that changes in a patient's test values that do not go beyond the limits of the reference range may still be clinically important.

Individual Reference Ranges

The previous discussion was based on a reference range created in a population of normals and/or patients. Alternatively, an individual patient's reference

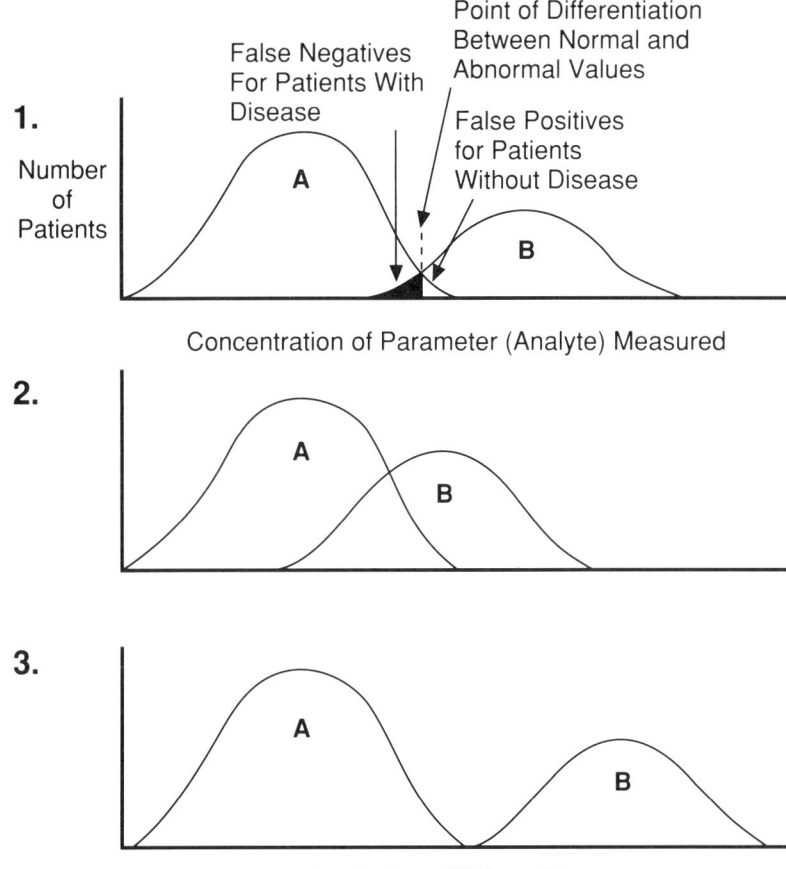

FIG. 81.2 Models of frequency distribution of laboratory values in populations of normal and diseased patients in a single test.

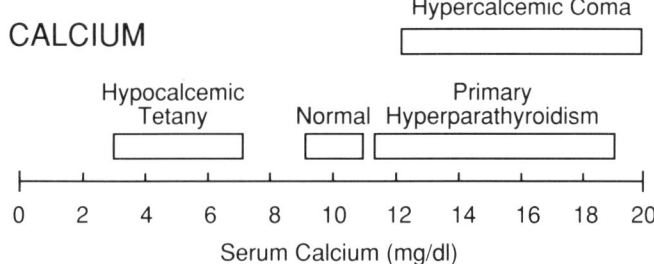

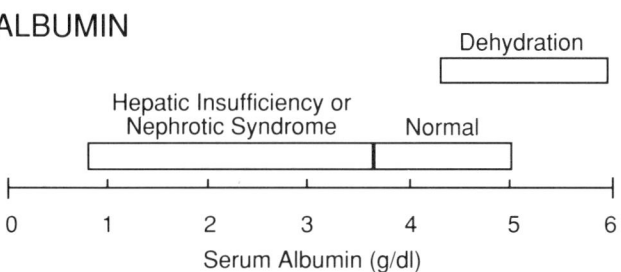

FIG. 81.3 Selected examples of ranges of serum values for calcium and albumin for various diseases. This illustrates a number of patterns that may be obtained.

range may be created, particularly if it is narrower than that of the entire population. This approach would be utilized for specific reasons (e.g., serial tests of serum ceruloplasmin to detect impending relapse in patients with leukemias and lymphomas).

Expanded Reference Ranges

An expanded reference range may be used as a triggering device to inform one when a patient's value has reached or passed a point at which some action is deemed necessary. The range represents the limits beyond which clinically significant effects are stated to have occurred. This range may be determined through a consensus of expert physicians or by other methods. A single analyte would be expected to have multiple ranges for different groups of patients, which would depend on their risk factors. In fact, the range created for some analytes would probably be less than the total reference range. These values also enable one to create summaries of patients who exceeded this value and required treatment or special observation.

INTERPRETATION OF CLINICAL DATA

Looking for Patterns

When a variety of laboratory values are abnormal and these abnormalities fit a previously described pattern, then reaching (or confirming) a diagnosis may be quite straightforward. It is ironic that it is often most difficult to interpret an abnormal laboratory result when it is an isolated finding and the other values are found to be normal. This often necessitates repeating the test and employing other confirmatory procedures such as measuring additional analytes that also measure the same or a related function (e.g., using both urea nitrogen and creatinine as indicators of renal function).

LABORATORY DATA ERRORS

To interpret laboratory data correctly, it is necessary to discern whether the data are valid. This requires some knowledge of the potential errors that may have affected the results. A list of possible errors is given in Table 81.2. When requesting laboratory tests, it is usually important to provide information to the clinical laboratory that will assist in preventing unreliable data from being reported back to the physician. The most relevant information usually consists of the patient's diagnosis and list of concomitant medicines. Once these potential errors are considered and the data are believed to be valid, the process of interpretation is initiated.

TABLE 81.2 *Selected sources of error in laboratory measurements*

A. Patient-related
  1. Inadequate or excessive physical activity (e.g., creatinine phosphokinase increases with activity)
  2. Emotional stress (e.g., stress increases hematocrit, glucose, and catecholamine release)
  3. Medicines that interfere within the patient with the biochemical parameter(s)[a] measured (e.g., phenobarbital affects triiodothyronine levels)
  4. Nonmedicine treatments that interfere within the patient with the biochemical parameter(s) measured (e.g., a sauna causes dehydration)
  5. Inappropriate posture of patient (e.g., renin and cerebrospinal fluid are important to measure with the patient in a specific posture)
  6. Samples taken at an improper time based on circadian, circaseptan, or other biological rhythms (e.g., menses, steroid levels)
  7. Patient has ingested food, caffeine, or alcohol, and the sample is taken too soon (e.g., triglycerides measured after an inadequate fast)
B. Sample collection and transport-related
  1. Incorrect container used to collect sample (e.g., without necessary preservative, incorrect preservative present)
  2. Sample taken improperly (e.g., tourniquet applied incorrectly, blood hemolyzed, air bubble present in blood gas determination, heparin lock not flushed, unsterile urine collected, poor sputum sample obtained)
  3. Sample taken from wrong patient
  4. Sample incorrectly labeled
  5. Sample stored incorrectly (e.g., not refrigerated, not taken promptly to laboratory)
  6. Sample contaminated with intravenous fluid resulting from using inappropriate arm or site on arm to obtain sample
  7. Sample taken from venous return side of dialysis machine
  8. Sample allowed to evaporate (e.g., moist bacteriological specimen)
  9. Commingling samples inappropriately from two or more anatomical locations
  10. Sample lost
  11. Reports completed illegibly
C. Analytical technique related
  1. Machines not accurately calibrated (e.g., wrong standard used, excessive length of time since last calibration)
  2. Standards not used to check machine
  3. Technical problems with the equipment, reagents, or other aspects of the procedure(s)
  4. Aliquots inappropriately taken (e.g., wrong amounts were used)
  5. Variability in conducting the assay (e.g., regular technician was absent)
  6. Delays in performing test resulting in deterioration of the analyte (e.g., sample thawed too rapidly with applied heat or was allowed to remain at room temperature too long)
  7. Inappropriate reference range reported by laboratory (e.g., range reported for different methodology, out-of-date range reported, range for newborns reported)
  8. Medicine taken that interacts with the analytical assay
  9. Use of overaged reagents
D. Postmeasurement related[b]
  1. Worker-related errors in measuring the value or writing it on the report (e.g., 0.075 written as 0.75)
  2. Incorrect report sent to investigator
  3. Report incorrectly written in the patient's chart
  4. Failure to report results
  5. Failure to act on results
  6. Report written in wrong patient's chart

[a] The term *parameter* is used to denote an analyte measured.
[b] Although not strictly an error, reports are sometimes lost.

Sources of Error

The processes of interpretation involve consideration of (1) errors that occur prior or subsequent to test analysis, (2) analytical errors at the time of test analysis, (3) biological variability, and (4) pathophysiology. Many of the various types of errors and influences on test results are listed in Table 81.2. Specific examples of laboratory errors that had severe consequences are listed by Belsey et al. (1986). The individual interpreting the data should be reasonably confident that the abnormality is not a reflection of one of these situations. The simplest means of gaining reasonable assurance is to repeat the test. If the second test reveals a similar result, then the chance of the value being correct is enhanced. In general, the more surprising the abnormality is, the greater the effort should be made to eliminate the possibility that it resulted from an error, problem, or factor that was not adequately considered.

Analytical Variability

Analytical variability refers to the range of values that would be reported for a particular plasma or other sample that is tested on different occasions. For some clinical chemistry tests, repeated determinations on the same plasma sample are highly reproducible, in the range of 1 to 3% (e.g., sodium, potassium, chloride, calcium). For others there is a range of imprecision between 5 and 10% (e.g., amylase, bilirubin, creatinine). When a single value is observed, there is really a "plus or minus" value that is not reported.

This analytical variability may be important if a patient's progress is being monitored to evaluate the course or the effect of treatment. As the values change, it is desirable to know whether the change represents an improvement, deterioration, or only random variation in the test results. For example, sodium has a variability of ±3 mM such that a test value of 137 really means that there is a 95% chance of the real value being in the range of 134 to 140. Thus, values of subsequent samples that lie within this range may not indicate a true change in the patient's status. Even values that lie outside the normal range may not represent a physiological abnormality (see Table 81.3).

Clinical interpretation of laboratory abnormalities should consider the factors described in this chapter to determine the relative importance of the abnormality and subsequently to identify the options to deal with the abnormality. For some parameters (e.g., potassium), there is a narrow range of biological variation possible, whereas for others (e.g., triglycerides), there may be a large range, and it may vary greatly between patients.

TABLE 81.3 *Selected reasons why a laboratory value outside the normal range may not represent a physiological abnormality*

1. The normal range may be inappropriate to compare the patient's results with because it was obtained using individuals who were different in terms of:
   a. race (e.g., differences in acetylation)
   b. sex (e.g., females have lower hematocrits)
   c. age (e.g., cardiac outputs differ in the elderly)
   d. body build or weight
   e. biological rhythm (e.g., circadian, menstrual, menopause)
   f. diet (e.g., vegetarians may differ from others)
   g. physical activity
2. The patient may be normal, but the value lies outside the reference range, usually 95% of the range of values encountered in a healthy reference population
3. The normal range was obtained using different analytical techniques to measure the parameter (e.g., different temperatures to assay an enzyme, different reagents, equipment, pH of the assay mixture)
4. The patient may have eaten a meal, engaged in strenuous exercise, or done something else that affects the values (e.g., most reference ranges are based on fasting samples)

FACTORS AFFECTING INTERPRETATION OF LABORATORY DATA

A number of factors may affect the interpretation of laboratory data, as described below:

Current Values

The patient's value for the test in question is considered, as well as other concurrent test values: It is usually preferable to interpret a particular laboratory result in the context of all the other results obtained at the same time. Other values may provide clues to unexpected "abnormalities," which might be related to variables such as sex, diet, physical activity, drugs, pregnancy, and clinical status.

Previous Values

Looking at the patient's previous test values since treatment was initiated allows one to discern whether treatment is having its desired effect and whether that effect's magnitude is adequate.

Baseline

Baseline data allows one to compare the before and after values and also provide a perspective for interpreting the value. For instance, if the baseline value was abnormally low (or high) and the value on treatment is also abnormally low (or high) to the same degree, it would be interpreted differently than if the baseline value were normal.

Trends

The presence of a trend is extremely important in interpreting laboratory data. This is so important that charts are often used to document all of the values obtained on one or more laboratory tests. Putting serial values on a chart facilitates the analysis of both gradual changes (trends) and sudden shifts in particular tests. It must then be determined whether changes represent an analytical, biological, pathophysiological, or other event. Even trends within the normal range may have profound clinical implications.

Validity

The data must be free from obvious sources of error or influences such as those described in Table 81.2. More importantly, they must meet tests of reliability and validity. *Reliability* is indicated by the consistency of a test over time. A reliable test (e.g., body temperature) has a high correlation between successive measures. *Validity* depends on correlation of that test with another index of the disease. To have validity it is necessary to have reliability, although to have reliability it is not necessary for the test to be valid.

Decision Levels

It is important to know how abnormal each test result may be before it is advisable to institute procedures to treat the abnormality. Although this decision is ultimately based on the individual patient, general guidelines have been published (see, for example, Statland, 1983). Clinical procedures are rarely all-or-none but reflect the degree of severity and the threat to the patient's well-being. Finally, the magnitude of change and the time scale over which change occurs are major considerations in reaching a decision on when to initiate a clinical response.

Other Abnormalities

The presence of other abnormalities can document a pattern that has been associated with a particular disease: When a diagnosis of most diseases and syndromes is considered, a range of abnormalities, usually of specific tests, is looked for. Abnormalities of several related test substances (i.e., analytes) usually strengthen the association of the abnormality with a particular disease.

Reference Population

Comparison with a reference population that is relevant to the patient in terms of demographic characteristics (e.g., age, race, sex) may be appropriate. There may be occasions when an individual with a different racial origin or genetic composition will have a different reference range of normal values and represent a distinctly different subpopulation.

Medical History

The patient's previous medical history is extremely important in understanding why some values are abnormal. Older medical records are also important in terms of comparing and evaluating the present set of data.

Duration of Treatment

An abnormal hematocrit and normal reticulocyte count, which indicates iron deficiency anemia, will not change immediately when treatment is begun. An increase in reticulocyte count, however, should be observed about 1 week after treatment has started.

Purpose

Tests may be used both to confirm and to exclude the presence of disease if the values of populations of normal and diseased patients do not overlap. If only a small degree of overlap occurs in certain tests, then those tests may also be used for both purposes.

Likelihood of Disease

It is important to estimate the likelihood of a disease being present in a patient prior to ordering a laboratory test. Although this is almost never done formally or in a written manner, it better enables one to interpret the results. If the likelihood of disease is high, then a positive result will tend to confirm the diagnosis, but a negative result will not generally rule out the diagnosis. If the likelihood of disease is low, then a normal value tends to exclude the diagnosis, but a positive value that was unexpected will not generally confirm the presence of the disease. This is an example of the philosophy underlying the Bayesian approach in statistics.

Size of the Abnormality

Does the abnormality require a clinical response? If so, then the abnormality is more serious than when no response is required. Increased observation or surveillance is a common clinical response.

Single Unconfirmed Value versus a Repeated Result

An abnormality that is based on a single unconfirmed value is more likely to have been a result of an error than is a repeated result.

Concomitant Medicines

Was the patient receiving concomitant medicine(s)? Is it known to elicit the abnormality or to interact with the test medicine?

Concomitant Treatments

Was the patient receiving a concomitant treatment (e.g., bed rest for muscle pain) that could have contributed to the improvement noted?

Concurrent Illness

Did the patient have other medical problems that contributed to the abnormality observed, either directly or indirectly?

Laboratory Errors

Table 81.2 lists many potential sources of laboratory error that may result in a purported laboratory abnormality.

Progression of Disease

Laboratory abnormalities often represent progression of the patient's underlying disease. This is particularly noteworthy in long-term chronic trials.

Pattern of Occurrence

The time after treatment initiation is particularly important to observe. Is the same pattern observed in different patients, and do values return to their baseline with continued treatment?

Pattern of Abnormalities

Well-known patterns exist for various types of gastrointestinal abnormalities and also for renal abnormalities.

How the Purpose of a Laboratory Test Affects the Interpretation of Results

Laboratory tests are conducted on patients for several different reasons described in the first section of this chapter. A test conducted to *confirm* or *exclude* a diagnosis will be interpreted at face value if the result is the one expected. If a different result is obtained, the test will be repeated and other tests possibly will be ordered. If the test is conducted for *screening* purposes, then most results are accepted. Results that are far outside the reference range will trigger a plan for additional tests to confirm the value obtained or to discover the patient's true diagnosis. Results within the reference range will be interpreted as normal and results outside but close to the reference range may or may not be repeated, depending on the patient and which specific test is involved.

When a patient who is believed not to have a laboratory abnormality has one, it is interpreted differently than when a patient believed to have the same abnormality has it. Tables 81.4 and 81.5 illustrate the

TABLE 81.4 *Consequences of laboratory results in a patient believed not to have a particular laboratory abnormality*

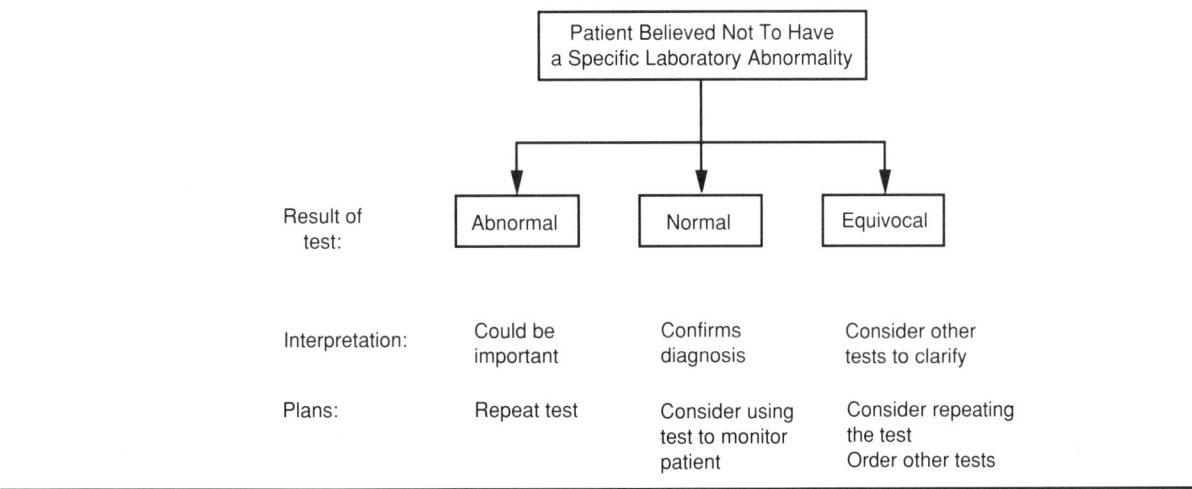

TABLE 81.5 *Consequences of laboratory results in a patient believed highly likely to have a particular laboratory abnormality*

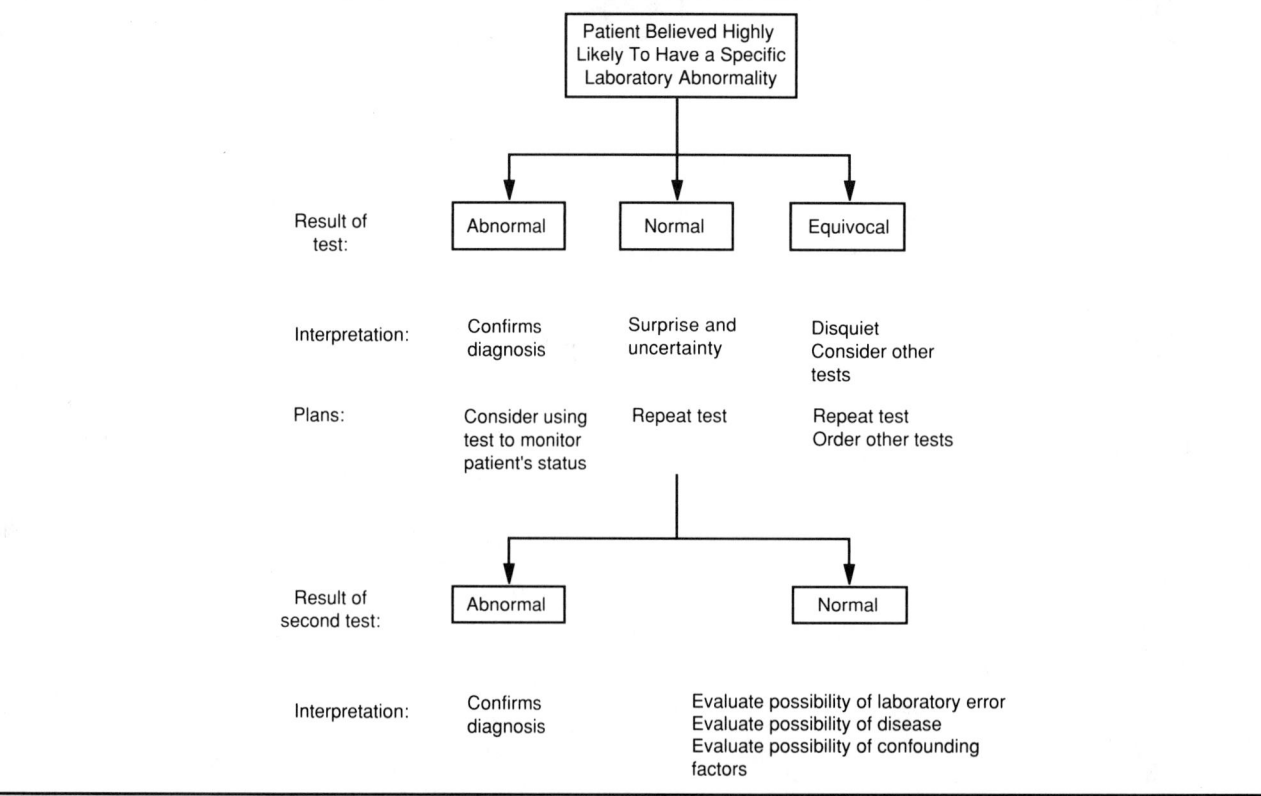

variety of interpretations and plans for follow-up that occur in these situations.

Sources of Information

Numerous sources of information on laboratory tests may assist in interpretation. Among the better works are *Effects of Diseases on Clinical Laboratory Tests* (Friedman et al., 1980), *Effects of Drugs on Clinical Laboratory Tests* (Young et al., 1975), *Interpretation of Diagnostic Tests* (Wallach, 1978), *Clinical Interpretation of Laboratory Tests* (Widmann, 1983), and a paper by Griner et al. (1981).

The Laboratory's Presentation of Results

A laboratory that presents data at a greater level of precision (i.e., with more significant numbers) than is justified by study methods does a major disservice to clinicians and others who must interpret the data. Values are often reported to more decimal places than appropriate, given the variability of the analyte measured and the ability of the equipment to detect small differences accurately. This leads clinicians to believe

that results are more accurate than is the case, and may result in misleading interpretations.

Practical Exercise for the Reader

Although this book intentionally avoids quantitative approaches to interpretation, there is a simple illustration of decision theory that will be presented. This particular example was described by Casscells et al. (1978), who referred to a previous publication, but there are many similar examples in the literature. The question they posed was:

> If a test to detect a disease whose prevalence is one per 1,000 patients has a false positive rate of 5%, what is the chance that a person found to have a positive result actually has the disease, assuming that you know nothing about the person's symptoms or signs?

The answer may be derived by using Bayes' theorem, but a common sense approach is preferred.

The reader of this book is requested to stop and calculate his or her answer. Twenty house officers, 20 fourth-year medical students, and 20 attending physicians at Harvard Medical School were asked the same question (Casscells et al., 1978). Of the 60 participants, only 11 gave the correct answer, so the reader should not feel bad if his or her answer is incorrect. Time is up! Write your answer here _____. The most common response was 95% (given by 27 participants), and the range of responses was 0.095 to 99%. The correct answer is that of 1,000 people studied, one will have the disease, and 5% of the remainder (999) will have false-positive responses. Therefore, roughly 50 false positives will occur and one true positive, so that the chance that a positive result actually represents a true positive is 1/51 or slightly less than 2%.

COMBINING DATA OBTAINED IN DIFFERENT LABORATORIES

Some of the considerations for combining data are listed in Table 81.6.

Interlaboratory Variability

Accurate interpretation of clinical laboratory data depends to a significant degree on having valid data to interpret. Many sources of errors and variability have been described, and they include a number of causes that relate to problems in the laboratory. The most common means to check for intralaboratory variability is to send repeat samples to the laboratory for analysis. When both results are suspicious to the investigator for any reason, it is worth comparing the results with data obtained in a different reference laboratory.

This procedure may be conducted by sending divided samples from a few patients to different laboratories (e.g., Spilker and Maugh, 1980) or by large-

TABLE 81.6 *Considerations for combining and evaluating data from different laboratories*[a]

A. Combining data
  1. Convert to common units
  2. Group data by type of units
  3. Classify data according to similar treatments
  4. Establish a range for times that samples were drawn
  5. Group data by tests that were conducted after administration of comparable doses (or dose ranges)
B. Evaluating data
  1. Evaluate the consistency of changes from baseline for groups of patients
  2. Evaluate the consistency or differences of changes from baseline between groups of patients
  3. Evaluate the differences observed between groups of patients on treatment
  4. Evaluate the differences, if any, at clinical trial termination versus baseline
  5. Evaluate the clinical significance as well as the statistical significance for all changes observed

[a] These concepts could be applied both to multiple sites of a single clinical trial (i.e., a multicenter trial) and to multiple clinical trials.

scale systematic evaluations of laboratories who receive known samples to measure from a central organization such as a society (Brosious et al., 1978) or the Centers for Disease Control (Hansen et al., 1985).

The results of evaluating the reproducibility of samples sent to multiple laboratories are generally not as reassuring as most people would like to believe. The variability in what is measured and in what is reported is often greater than desirable and sometimes is lacking in both consistency and in quality control. Most physicians do not rigorously critique the validity of the data they receive, which is one important reason to ensure that laboratories adhere to high standards in both their analytical measurements and reporting procedures.

EVALUATIONS OF NEW OR PROPOSED LABORATORY TESTS

There are extremely few systematic evaluations of new laboratory tests conducted in the way that clinical methods and medicines are evaluated. In many ways this is surprising, since there are studies on interlaboratory comparability in measuring standards, presentation of data, and occasional evaluations of factors that affect data obtained with laboratory tests (e.g., effect of air bubbles in syringes on blood gas determinations by Biswas et al., 1982).

Robertson et al. (1983) described a systematic approach to validating laboratory tests and suggested several procedures to formalize the evaluation of laboratory tests.

1. Choose subjects who are representative of the clinical population that will be the ultimate one evaluated with the test.
2. Perform all tests on all patients at the same point in their clinical course, since the validity of data obtained during the course of a disease may vary in terms of its clinical value (e.g., the MB isoenzyme of creatine phosphokinase is only present for a certain period of time in patients who have had a myocardial infarction).
3. Evaluate and determine the true answer to the clinical question posed through other methods that are considered reliable (i.e., the reference method) and are independent of the test being evaluated. The "gold standard" might include autopsy or a surgical biopsy.
4. Compare the test with the reference method through accepted statistical techniques and determine the relative rates of false-positive and false-negative results.

Evaluation of laboratory tests by this type of rigorous approach will enable investigators to utilize those tests that yield the most predictive data and therefore provide more accurate interpretations.

There are numerous pitfalls to avoid in evaluating new diagnostic tests (as for therapeutic modalities). Several of these are indicated by Lum and Beeler (1983). These authors also describe the type of public attention and hyperbole often accorded to new tests and suggest means of avoiding this potential problem.

OTHER TESTS OF SAFETY

In addition to laboratory tests to measure biochemical substances, electrolytes, and other analytes in blood, urine, and other body fluids, there are numerous other tests and procedures conducted in different laboratories that generate important safety data. These tests include pulmonary function tests and cardiovascular and other physiological tests. Data from these tests are generally interpreted in a similar manner as for other safety data.

Physical Examinations

There are numerous aspects of a physical examination, e.g., vital signs, weight, neurological, psychiatric, ophthalmological, and any of numerous other specialized examinations that may be performed. Safety data generated through conduct of physical examinations during clinical trials are usually evaluated in a straightforward manner. Whenever any data raise a suspicion or an actual problem is uncovered, all previously generated data that are relevant should be reevaluated. An index of suspicion allows the investigator and sponsor to evaluate carefully one or more particular aspects of an examination, to identify a problem more clearly, and to convince themselves that there is or is not a basis for the postulated problem.

Ophthalmological Lens Opacities

A complex series of problems rapidly arises if lens opacities are observed while a patient is receiving an investigational medicine, particularly if no opacities were observed at baseline. Apart from the real possibility that the opacities were caused by the medicine, it is also possible that the physician was not looking for the opacities as carefully at baseline, or that another physician conducted the earlier examination and applied different techniques or standards.

It is important to avoid a retrospective evaluation of patients' eyes to look for opacities that were not carefully looked for at baseline. Opacities are often both under- and overdiagnosed. After an alarm is raised about a potential adverse reaction, it is certain that some (or many) false positives will be diagnosed. This may attach a stigma to the medicine and may adversely affect its development, regulatory approval, sales, or ability to be marketed. This can be particularly damaging if the careful evaluation of patient's eyes during a clinical trial is triggered by the suggestions of possible cataractogenic effects of the medicine at extremely high doses in animals.

One means to avoid this situation is to require that most, if not all, patients on moderate to long-term therapy have a careful ophthalmological examination by the same physician at the start and end of the clinical trial.

PURPOSES OF INTERPRETING SAFETY DATA

Interpretation of safety data is intended to:

1. Identify trends in the data, even if the data lie entirely within the "normal" range. The clinical trial may not have lasted long enough for the value to drift into the abnormal range, but, for chronically used medicines, a trend may be quite important clinically.
2. Identify "red flags" in the data. Red flags are warnings of real or possible problems in the safety profile of the medicine. Red flags primarily indicate the identity of an area that should be carefully monitored. A more complete assessment of a potential (or actual) problem may be made at a later date when more data are obtained.
3. Establish the "denominator" for any problems that occur. This concept was discussed more completely in Chapter 80. The denominator relates to the total number of people exposed to a medicine, so that the number of patients with abnormal values (numerator) can be used to create an incidence figure (e.g., X number of cases per Y thousand exposures to the medicine, or one case per Z number of patients). This information allows a benefit-to-risk relationship to be assessed.
4. Identify groups at potentially high risk of developing safety problems resulting from medicine use.

Evaluations of tests by this type of rigorous approach will enable investigators to utilize those tests that yield the most predictive data and therefore provide more accurate interpretations.

USE OF CONSULTANTS

There are often questions raised about safety issues that require the services of a consultant who is a specialist in the field of interest. The consultant may be primarily concerned with diagnosis and treatment of a trial patient, but any potential problem should signal the investigator and sponsor about the possible need to enroll the help and assistance of competent specialists to consider nonaffected patients in the clinical trial. It is sometimes relevant to convene a panel of expert consultants to help interpret safety data and to advise on future plans for monitoring activities and designing trials regarding the potential (or real) "red flag."

CHAPTER 82

General Approaches to Interpreting Efficacy Data

ASSUMPTIONS

The same assumptions apply to the interpretation of efficacy data that were applied in the preceding discussions of safety data. Briefly, these assumptions are that (1) the clinical trial is complete, (2) the data have been analyzed correctly by statisticians using appropriate tests (although some additional comments will be made on this issue), and (3) the statistical report and data tabulations are complete and available to the individual(s) interpreting the results.

It is also assumed that the general concept of efficacy is understood, even though it is extremely difficult to evolve a totally satisfactory operational definition of this abstract concept. These same comments apply to the difficulty of operationally defining the concept of medicine safety. Both safety and efficacy are used as relative terms, and each involves input of clinical judgment.

BACKGROUND

A thorough knowledge of the therapeutic area investigated is mandatory to arrive at a well-developed and appropriate interpretation. The greater one's knowledge of an area of medicine, the greater is the likelihood that the interpretation will be well conceived, well developed, and well substantiated. Merely developing an interpretation of data is usually easy, but developing a meaningful interpretation is often difficult. Nonetheless, interpretation of data is sometimes like the story portrayed in the Japanese film "Rashomon." Four people describe the same tale, each from their own viewpoint, and there is little similarity between the four versions.

In order to interpret clinical data obtained in a trial adequately, the individual interpreter should have a thorough understanding of all of the basic aspects of the trial (e.g., objectives, design, conduct, tests, and parameters). This understanding includes both the considerations that influenced the planning of each step of the trial and the manner in which each aspect was implemented. Some important considerations of the basic aspects of the trial for interpreting data are described below.

Trial Objectives

The primary and secondary objectives of a clinical trial should be delineated in the protocol. Unless the objectives are clearly established prior to initiating the trial, the data obtained may not be useful, and the trial may have wasted valuable resources. The practice of establishing trial objectives after a trial is completed is below currently acceptable standards. Nonetheless, newly considered evaluations of data after a trial is complete may be used to develop a hypothesis or question to be evaluated carefully in future clinical trials.

Trial Design

The limitations and strengths of the component parts of the trial design (e.g., type of design, blind used, randomization used, dosage regimen) must be understood. Each component must be considered both in relation to the trial being interpreted (e.g., inherent weaknesses and limitations in the trial design) and in relation to the data that were obtained (e.g., were the data adversely affected or biased by weaknesses in the trial design).

Trial Conduct

The manner in which the clinical trial was conducted must be understood. This includes the degree of compliance to the protocol by both the patients and the investigator's staff. Any deviations from principles of good clinical practice in treatment of patients, collection of the data, or other aspects of trial conduct must be evaluated. Information on trial conduct comes from varied sources including (1) careful monitoring, (2) data generated on patient compliance, (3) rate of patient enrollment, (4) type and amount of missing data,

(5) number of patients who dropped out from the trial and the reasons for these dropouts, (6) number of patients who were discontinued from the trial by the investigator and the reasons for these discontinuations, and (7) patient interviews.

Trial Tests, Parameters, and Endpoints

Each of the tests and parameters used to measure efficacy, pharmacokinetics, and safety must be understood. The tests chosen to measure the outcome of the clinical trial must be understood both in terms of their validity compared with other possible tests (or parameters) and in terms of how predictive the tests are for the disease or target effect that is being diagnosed, treated, or prevented. This includes consideration of the likelihood that the trial produced either false-positive or false-negative data.

Endpoints are often described as being either objective or subjective and either hard or soft, although each of these extremes lies on a continuum. It is probably more accurate and useful to describe endpoints in terms of (1) hierarchy of discipline involved (e.g., clinical, pharmacological, biochemical), (2) degree of validity, (3) ease of measurement, (4) cost of measurement, (5) resources required to obtain, process, and analyze results, and (6) ability to interpret the results.

Although tests often measure efficacy in terms of pharmacological or therapeutic effects, the relationship between these effects should be considered when interpreting the data. Sometimes the pharmacological effect caused by a medicine is the same as the therapeutic effect desired (e.g., a neuromuscular blocking medicine causing relaxation of skeletal muscles prior to surgery). In most instances the pharmacological and therapeutic effects are different and are measured in different terms (e.g., a parasympathomimetic blocking medicine may relieve intestinal pain, an antihypertensive medicine will reduce the risk of stroke and renal failure).

INTERPRETATION: APPROACHES AND ISSUES

Overall Approach

Although most interpretations are performed by a single individual or a group of investigators, a number of consultants, staff members, or others may be assembled to assist or to develop an interpretation of a clinical trial's data. This is especially relevant if the trial is expected to have a major public impact. A meeting could be convened to (1) develop possible interpretations, (2) discuss possible interpretations, (3) reach final agreement on the proposed interpretation, or (4) plan follow-up trials. This group could discuss and, one hopes, resolve various issues related to an interpretation. For instance, in psychiatric trials, there is often a poor correlation between the clinical global impression rated by the treating physician and that rated by the patient. Reasons for this could be advanced, but in assessing medicine efficacy, it may be debated which measure is more meaningful.

It is possible to focus primarily on similarities between the data obtained and those of other clinical trials, or to focus primarily on differences. Usually the person interpreting the data knows if the clinical trial was conducted to support a particular view or as a challenge to another.

Major Steps

The major steps proposed in the overall approach to data interpretation are listed in Table 82.1. The process of interpretation begins after all or part of the data have been edited and compiled and initial (or final) statistical analyses have been performed. The process of interpreting clinical data after each of the background areas is understood often begins with assessing whether the data affirm or deny the primary objective(s) of the clinical trial.

Potential Problems in Reaching a Clear Interpretation

In many situations it is not possible to derive a clear interpretation, for many reasons. A few are listed below:

TABLE 82.1 Major steps in formulating and evaluating an interpretation of clinical data[a]

1. Compare treatment groups in terms of demographics and prognostic criteria
2. Evaluate whether the data affirm or deny the primary objectives
3. Evaluate whether the data affirm or deny the secondary objectives
4. Consider all factors that may have influenced or biased the data and the resulting interpretation
5. Consult with a statistician to review the interpretations and to determine any additional analyses or subgroup analyses to perform
6. Adopt the "devil's advocate" point of view and evaluate each point that is questioned
7. Compare the data and interpretation for the trial medicine with those obtained with standard medicines or treatments used in the trial and also compare trial data with results reported in the literature
8. Discuss the data and interpretation with colleagues and peers in the same field of research as well as with those from other disciplines
9. Extrapolate the conclusions to a larger population or to a different clinical situation (or conditions)
10. Develop hypotheses and plans to develop further or explore unanswered questions in the clinical program

[a] It is assumed that the trial has been completed and all data have been processed and analyzed by expert statisticians.

1. The data are equivocal and neither affirm nor deny the clinical trial objectives.
2. Different efficacy parameters or tests used to assess those parameters suggest different interpretations. If a hierarchical ordering of parameters or tests was made prior to the trial (i.e., from most important and predictive for assessing clinical significance to least useful or predictive), then this difficulty may not pose a significant problem. If no hierarchical ordering was made, or if the ordering does not resolve the dilemma (e.g., if the first and fourth parameters in importance indicate one interpretation, but the second and third parameters indicate a different interpretation), then a simple resolution may not be possible.
3. No clear definition of medicine activity was established prior to the trial, and the magnitude of patient response does not clearly indicate little activity or marked activity of the medicine.
4. The power of the statistical analysis was insufficient to allow a meaningful conclusion to be drawn.
5. The objectives of the trial may have been vaguely stated, and it is difficult to know whether the objective has been achieved. For example, an objective may be stated as "to establish safety of the medicine." This objective is too general and may lead to problems in reaching an interpretation.

When these problems occur the interpretation may only be suggestive, rather than conclusive. Given the enormous variation ascribed by physicians to terms of probability (see discussion in Chapter 72), a numerical score should be added, if possible.

Attention to Language

Differences within a language must be carefully considered to avoid ambiguity. The best approaches to this issue are the obvious ones of critiquing each sentence written, having multiple experts critique the text, or having one or more editors critique the material written.

Differences between languages, even American and English, greatly increase the possible number of problems. Literally hundreds, if not thousands of differences in meaning and usage can be given, not including spelling differences. For example, "to table" an issue means to place it on the table for discussion in the United Kingdom, and to temporarily take it off the table and not to discuss it in the United States. General statements such as "I am mad about my flat" can be interpreted as (1) the speaker is delighted about his or her apartment, (2) the speaker is angry about a puncture in his or her automobile's tire, or (3) as an unclear statement because it was possibly incomplete (e.g., I am angry about my flat note (in singing or playing an instrument), flat performance (in acting), and so forth.

Use of Multiple Types of Endpoints in a Single Clinical Trial

A clinical trial that includes measurements of multiple endpoints may lead to data that create numerous problems for interpretation. These problems include generation of an excessive number of statistical comparisons, which in turn leads to an increased number of false-positive results based on chance. Whether the endpoints chosen are clinical, biochemical, pharmacological, pathological, physiological, or related to another discipline, it is useful to prioritize their importance for addressing the objectives prior to the trial. One (or more) endpoint may clearly show a positive effect in most patients, whereas another may be unchanged or even show a negative effect in most patients.

Complex situations may arise when some patients improve according to one or a few of the measured efficacy parameters and other patients improve according to different parameters and show a different pattern of response. A total score or measure that considers some or all efficacy parameters evaluated may be developed. Evaluation of improvement may also be limited to the single most commonly accepted measure. Caution must be used in choosing the efficacy parameters because basing an interpretation of data on an unvalidated or less well accepted measure will undoubtedly be challenged within the medical community, especially if more widely accepted measures did not support the interpretation.

Utilizing multiple medical or scientific disciplines and types of endpoints (when possible) to evaluate efficacy usually represents a more comprehensive method to evaluate medicine responses. For example, when a new medicine is being evaluated for ulcerative colitis, it is possible to measure:

1. Clinical improvement on medicine (i.e., symptoms)
2. Pathological improvement on medicine (i.e., histological evaluation)
3. Endoscopic improvement on medicine (i.e., visual evaluation)
4. Biochemical improvement on medicine (i.e., laboratory evaluation)

Sometimes the overall improvement in each category may be high (e.g., 60 to 80% of all patients) but only a few patients may show improvement in all four areas. Although the interpretation of efficacy based solely on any single endpoint should be less convincing than when all four measures improve, it is not certain that the definition of medicine activity requires all four types of endpoints to improve. A further complication is that patients may improve in one or more of these areas based on either a placebo or nonspecific medicine effect.

Focus of the Interpretation

After the evaluation of a clinical trial's primary objective(s) is under way or completed, the secondary objectives of the trial should be examined. In evaluating the degree to which each primary or secondary objective is affirmed or refuted, the strength of the conclusion regarding each objective must also be assessed. The strength of the conclusion refers to how convincing it is to the medical community.

After the interpretations of the primary and secondary objectives indicated above are in progress or are complete, attention should be directed toward other possible interpretations of the data. In this context, it is useful to address scientific hypotheses that are outside the scope of the original objectives and to seek other possible analyses of the data that could (or should) be conducted. Data may be combined in a variety of new formats or according to different criteria. Interpretations of data presented in a different format may require new subgroup analyses. If these are moderately and cautiously performed and reported, one may avoid the charge of "data dredging" that is often raised when obscure relationships are shown to be statistically significant or relationships are found that are not part of the original trial objectives. The ten basic steps of interpreting data are listed in Table 82.1.

The types of conclusions that are usually reached in different phases of a medicine's development may differ markedly (Table 82.2). Some of the reasons that may be used to explain why a patient's response changes over time are listed in Table 82.3.

Assessing the Conclusions Reached

In order to evaluate the strength of the conclusion, it is often useful to adopt the "devil's advocate" position. This means that one assumes that the opposite or a different position is correct and questions the interpreter's conclusions. One means of adopting this approach is to consider each specific factor that could have influenced the data (many of these are described in Chapter 83). The investigator attempts to discern whether any single factor on its own or in combination with others could have had a significant influence on the data obtained or on interpretations reached.

After one has identified the specific factors that could possibly have relevance for the interpretation reached, it is important to evaluate these factors as

TABLE 82.2 *Selected interpretations that often evolve during different phases of medicine development*[a]

A. Phase I[b]
  1. Dose range of new medicine that is generally safe and well tolerated by normal volunteers (or by patients)
  2. Minimal dose leading to adverse reactions and the maximally tolerated dose
  3. Time course of the adverse reactions
  4. Identification of laboratory and safety parameters markedly or possibly affected by the medicine
  5. Initial pharmacokinetic profile for single and multiple doses and detailed pharmacokinetic characteristics at steady state
  6. Possible hints of efficacy in some situations, depending on the medicine, parameters of efficacy, and population studied
  7. Types of commonly noted adverse reactions characteristic of the medicine at different dose levels
B. Phase IIa[c]
  1. Early indications of the presence and magnitude of efficacy
  2. Duration of the biological effect(s) produced
  3. Doses of medicine that are effective
  4. Information on suitable dosage regimens and/or schedule(s)
  5. Relationship of pharmacokinetics to pharmacodynamics
C. Phase IIb[d]
  1. Definitive evidence of the extent and magnitude of efficacy in the indication(s) evaluated
  2. Detailed pharmacokinetic profile of the parent medicine and any metabolites
  3. Characteristics of patients in whom the medicine is active and development of the profile of patient response
  4. Better understanding of dosage regimens and clinical pharmacology of the medicine
  5. Development of a better-defined benefit-to-risk ratio
  6. Understanding of how the medicine affects the disease or condition evaluated
D. Phase III[e]
  1. Patterns of responses observed in larger patient populations
  2. Commonly observed medicine interactions
  3. Commonly observed "nonmedicine" interactions (e.g., with alcohol, cigarettes, caffeine-containing drinks, food)
  4. Unexpected benefits in the disease for which the medicine was used
  5. Unexpected benefits when the medicine was given to patients with a second clinical problem
  6. Profile of clinical activity in special populations
  7. Identification and characterization of less common adverse reactions and other safety abnormalities or issues
  8. Responses to final formulation, special dose forms, or other technical modifications (e.g., slow-release formulations)
  9. Comparisons with known medicine
E. Phase IV[f]
  1. Safety and tolerance of the medicine in the general population of patients given the medicine under "normal" conditions
  2. Early indications of unexpected or suspected beneficial activities
  3. Responses in specific populations studied[g]
F. During any phase
  1. Information on accidental or deliberate overdosage
  2. Idiosyncratic reactions (e.g., allergic manifestations)

[a] In general, each phase often includes trials that provide additional data that will strengthen or modify interpretations reached during the prior phase(s). Pharmacokinetic evaluations may be performed during any phase of medicine development but are often most closely associated with Phase I.
[b] Phase I: initial evaluation of safety in humans.
[c] Phase IIa: pilot trials of efficacy using either open-label or blind trial designs.
[d] Phase IIb: pivotal clinical trials (i.e., these are usually the most well-controlled trials performed on investigational medicines).
[e] Phase III: trials of the medicine in a broad or special population of patients plus special trials.
[f] Phase IV: postmarketing surveillance, epidemiology, and marketing studies.
[g] See Table 87.1 for listings of special populations.

critically as possible. This evaluation may take the form of (1) additional statistical analyses, (2) additional clinical trials that would have to be conducted, (3) additional questions to ask the patients, investigators, or others connected with the trial, or (4) conjecture and speculation about the most likely form or degree of influence that the factor had.

On the other hand, a completely rational and perfect argument often does not convince people and is not effective. To convince people you have to understand the emotions, prejudices, and fears of the group you are addressing, and you must direct the discussion or reasoning to these aspects.

Comparing Interpretations

Data obtained on the trial medicine or treatment should be compared with data obtained with standard medi-

cines or treatments in the same trial as well as with data from other trials. It is important to compare medicines that are related chemically and medicines of the same therapeutic class with the test medicine(s). In comparing data from two or more trials, all major differences in trial design, such as route of administration and other trial design factors, must be considered.

At this point in the process, it is usually beneficial to discuss the data and interpretation with knowledgeable colleagues and peers. It is quite likely that they will be able to question, challenge, or extend and expand the interpretations reached. If this occurs, then additional evaluations will often either reinforce or strengthen the original conclusions or lead to a revision of the interpretation. It is important to examine critically the results and interpretations and to ask whether they make sense. This simple question may provide a worthwhile perspective to examine one's own inter-

TABLE 82.3 *Selected reasons for changes in a patient's response to medicines over time*

A. Efficacy
1. Improved therapeutic response (e.g., antidepressant activity of tricyclic antidepressants requires up to 3 weeks on average for its effects to become clinically apparent)
2. Decreased efficacy resulting from enzyme induction in liver (e.g., a constant dose of barbiturates may elicit a smaller response over time as microsomal enzymes are induced and more rapidly metabolize the medicine)
3. Decreased efficacy resulting from classic tolerance (e.g., morphine's analgesic effect diminishes as tolerance to the medicine develops)
4. Decreased efficacy resulting from tachyphylaxis (e.g., frequent doses of ephedrine eventually elicit progressively diminished responses as stores of endogenous catecholamines are depleted)

B. Safety
1. Decreased safety when a medicine is suddenly withdrawn, resulting from addictive nature of medicine (e.g., morphine withdrawal)
2. Decreased safety when a nonaddictive medicine is suddenly withdrawn and the mechanism is either unknown (e.g., propranolol) or known (e.g., induced microsomal enzymes, which may affect other medicines)
3. Increased safety resulting from physiological adaptation (e.g., nitroglycerine-induced reflex tachycardia diminishes over time)

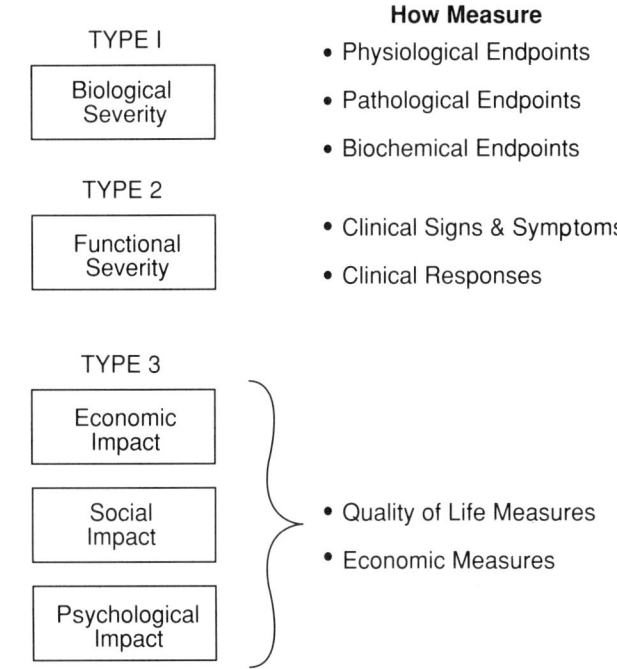

FIG. 82.1 Types of disease severity. The major types of measures used to assess each area are also indicated.

pretation with some degree of objectivity. It also may allow one to determine whether additional information is needed or would be useful to improve the interpretation.

Comparison of the conclusions reached with those obtained by other scientists is usually performed through reference to the medical literature. The manner in which one's interpretations fit with those of others is usually of great interest and importance. If significant differences in interpretation exist, it is essential to evaluate the reason for the differences. This problem arises frequently but is often extremely difficult to solve. There are a variety of reasons for this difficulty, and clues that may provide a basis for understanding differences should be sought in the trial design, trial conduct, and data analyses.

Characteristics and Examples of Poor Interpretations

Examples of poorly interpreted clinical trials may be found in most issues of all medical journals. Although the standards for both clinical trials and their interpretations are believed to have increased over the last few decades, many problems are still commonly found. A few representative examples follow.

1. Superficial interpretations are made and speculation, extrapolation, and comparisons are inadequate or absent.
2. Basic premises that should be questioned or at least discussed are not.
3. No real interpretation of the data is presented. The discussion section merely summarizes the results obtained.

4. Differences from expected results are inadequately addressed or are not addressed at all.
5. An excessively detailed or broad interpretation is made that is not supported by the data.
6. An excessively broad extrapolation of the data is made.
7. An interpretation is made that is illogical and no adequate discussion is given.

Poorly designed clinical trials that have fatal flaws (e.g., too few patients, incorrect endpoints measured) and that can never be saved by erudite interpretations unfortunately occur and their results are frequently published.

Types of Disease Severity

Although disease severity is traditionally considered in biological or clinical terms, various types of other scales or disciplines may also be used as measures. These include functional, economic, social, and psychological (Fig. 82.1). The major means of measuring each of these areas is summarized on the figure.

LEVELS OF INTERPRETATION

There are a number of levels in interpreting data. Three types of levels are:

1. *Levels of organization* in which each successive level includes all of the preceding ones: atom(s), molecule(s), subcellular particle(s), cell(s), tis-

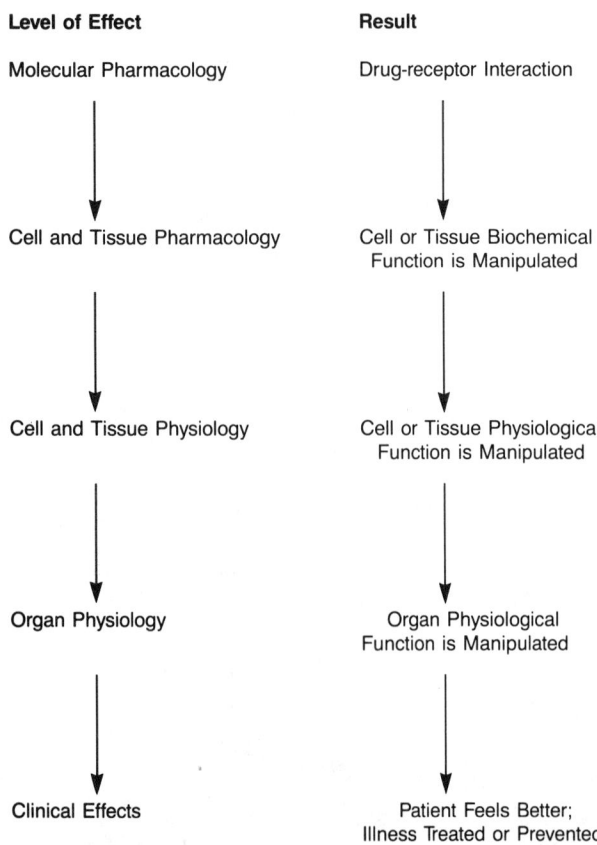

Level of Effect

Molecular Pharmacology

↓

Cell and Tissue Pharmacology

↓

Cell and Tissue Physiology

↓

Organ Physiology

↓

Clinical Effects

Result

Drug-receptor Interaction

↓

Cell or Tissue Biochemical Function is Manipulated

↓

Cell or Tissue Physiological Function is Manipulated

↓

Organ Physiological Function is Manipulated

↓

Patient Feels Better; Illness Treated or Prevented

FIG. 82.2 Hierarchies in the therapeutic process. The links between the pharmacological effects of a medicine and its therapeutic or toxic effects can be considered at the several different levels shown. (Reprinted from Grahame-Smith and Aronson, 1984, with permission of Oxford University Press.)

sue(s), organ(s), organ system(s), organism, groups of organisms, society of all organisms of one species (Fig. 82.2 and Table 82.4).

2. *Flow of pharmaceutic, pharmacokinetic, and pharmacodynamic processes* for a medicine. The list given does not represent a strict order of pro-

cesses: medicine ingested, medicine dissolves, medicine absorbed, medicine distributed, medicine present at site of action, medicine elicits pharmacological response, medicine elicits clinical response, medicine metabolized, medicine excreted. For example, if little or no efficacy is observed and a concomitant medicine is found that chelated the test medicine, it clarifies the step in this series of processes responsible for the lack of effect.

3. *The processes used to develop and extrapolate interpretations* may be viewed as levels: statistical level of data analysis; clinical interpretation of the data in the study; extrapolation of the clinical interpretation for diagnosis, prevention, and treatment of other patients with the disease evaluated; clinical understanding of the specific disease process; prognostication for other areas of medicine or for medicine development.

Most disciplines are associated with certain levels of organization. A given set of data obtained with a single parameter may sometimes be interpreted at several levels of biological organization. For instance, biochemical data are sometimes interpreted at molecular, subcellular, cellular, tissue, and organ system levels. In vitro pharmacological data are sometimes interpreted at the tissue, organ system, and complete organism levels. Physiological data are usually interpreted at the organ and organ system levels. A specific level may also be evaluated with numerous scientific disciplines. For example, it is possible to investigate the cellular level of isolated cardiac preparations using methods of histology, electrophysiology, pharmacology, and biochemistry.

Example: Cardiac Glycosides

In conceptualizing the actions of a medicine, it is generally useful to consider how these levels are linked and interact. One may often determine how effects at

TABLE 82.4 *Assignment of some attributes of Wilson's disease to hierarchical levels*[a]

Level	Disease attribute	Field
Patient as a whole	Malaise, bizarre behavior, labile affect, schizophreniform disorders, bipolar psychoses	Clinical medicine
Physiologic systems	Intention tremor, dysarthria, dystonia, choreoathetosis, rest tremor, chorea, drooling, masklike facies, fixed grin, Babinski sign	Physiology
Organs	Dysphagia, Kayser-Fleischer ring, ascites	Physiology
Cells	Opalski cells (brain), Alzheimer type II cells (brain), necrosis of neurons (brain), abnormal glycogen deposits (brain), Mallory bodies (brain)	Physiology, pathology
Biopolymers	Deceased serum ceruloplasmin, hypoalbuminemia, increased lactate dehydrogenase, increased serum levels of aspartate and alanine aminotransferases, increased alkaline phosphatase, proteinuria	Biochemistry
Molecules	Aminoaciduria	Chemistry
Atoms	Decreased serum copper, increased urinary copper	Physics

[a] Modified from Blois, 1988.

one level relate to and explain effects observed at the next higher level. As an example, the inhibition of the Na^+,K^+-activated ATPase pump on the surface of cardiac muscle cell membranes by cardiac glycosides at the molecular level leads to various intracellular biochemical events (Fig. 82.3). Intracellular Na^+ concentration increases in the cell since the ion can no longer be pumped out. This invokes another pump whereby calcium enters the cell in exchange for the sodium that has built up. Calcium is taken up in mitochondrial stores, and greater release of calcium may occur from mitochondria as a result of an action potential. Increased calcium leads to an increased force of cellular contraction, which leads to a positive inotropic response (pharmacological level), and physiologically, decreased hydrostatic pressure allows more edema fluid back into the circulation from extracellular spaces. Decreased edema in lungs, liver, legs, and

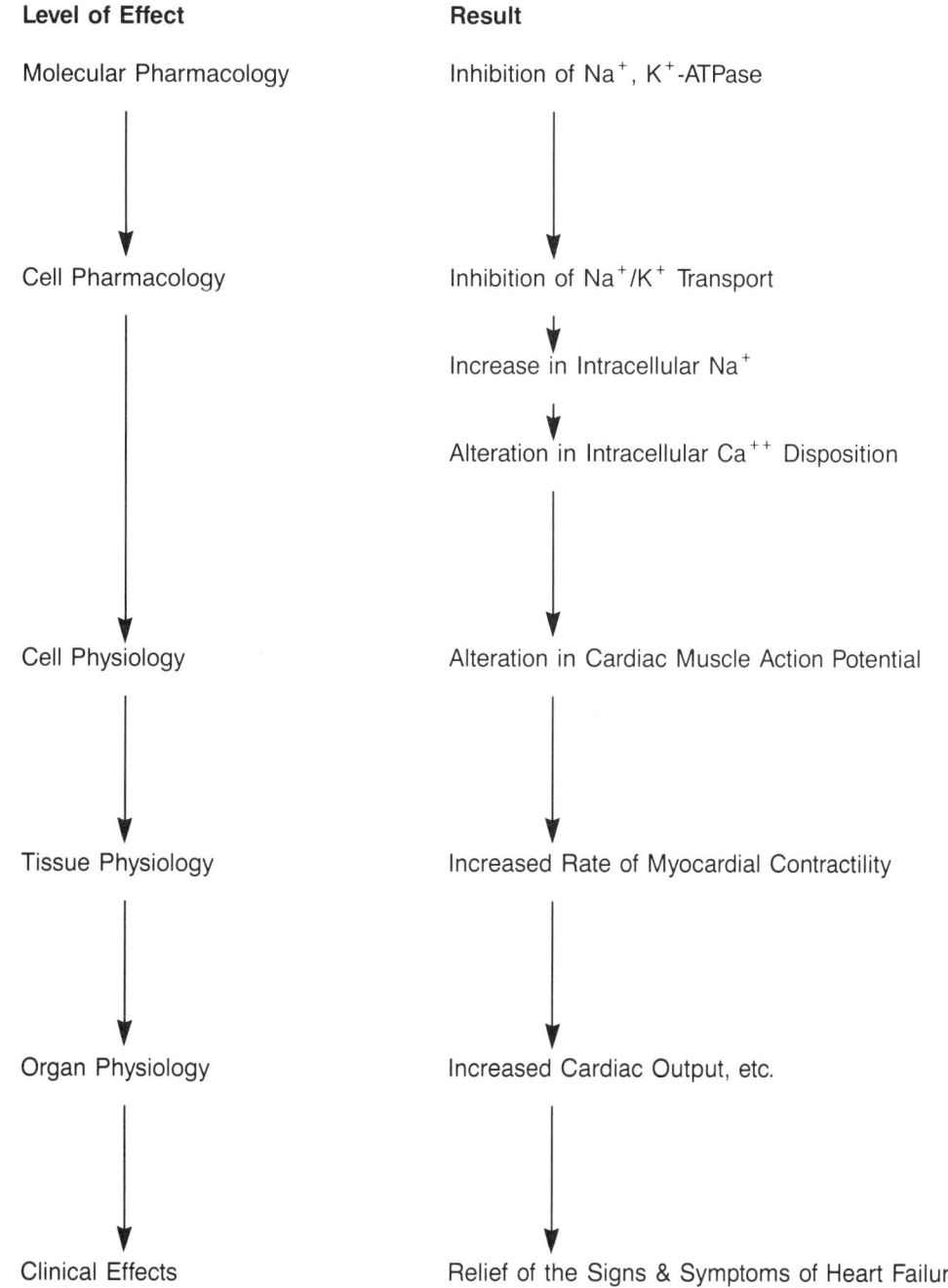

FIG. 82.3 Hierarchies in the therapeutic process: digoxin therapy in patients with heart failure. (Reprinted from Grahame-Smith and Aronson, 1984, with permission of Oxford University Press.)

other tissues allows the patient to breathe more easily and to be able to walk further (clinical level) and improves other signs and symptoms of congestive heart failure.

Clinical Levels

Clinical data may be interpreted at a number of different levels. These include the level of an individual patient, a small group of patients, a specific disease subpopulation, or all patients with the disease. The process of extrapolation is usually not straightforward, since data obtained in one type or group of patients are often extrapolated to a relatively more heterogeneous population, where many new and complex factors operate that were not previously considered or evaluated (see Chapter 90).

The process of considering multiple levels of interpretation is a generic one that may be applied in most situations, but because many effects sometimes occur at different levels, it cannot be assumed that they will always occur, especially if conditions vary. The types of interpretations reached in studies vary greatly according to the phase of clinical trial (for investigational medicines), type of blind used for many trials, and numerous other factors. Some of the types of interpretations that are appropriate depending on the phase of trial are listed in Table 82.2.

Relationship of Pharmaceutic, Pharmacokinetic, and Pharmacodynamic Processes

The various processes are illustrated in Fig. 84.1. The pharmacodynamic processes include not only the pharmacological effects that lead to beneficial therapeutic responses but also those that lead to adverse reactions or to no discernable clinical response. The connection between pharmacokinetic and pharmacodynamic effects is sometimes difficult to discern with precision.

The steps leading to the medicine–receptor combination involve the processes of pharmacokinetics. Those steps after the medicine has elicited a pharmacological response involve the processes of pharmacodynamics. The relationship between these two series of processes in terms of blood levels versus pharmacological effects may be either clear cut or difficult to separate. The pharmacological effects of some medicines rapidly wax and wane depending on the blood level of the medicine. In this situation, the medicine combines and dissociates rapidly from receptors (e.g., nitroprusside). Other medicines act differently and may elicit an effect that persists long after the medicine has disappeared from the receptor and even from the circulation (e.g., lowered blood pressure as a result

of catecholamine depletion caused by reserpine). Another group contains medicines that bind strongly to receptors and maintain their pharmacological effect even though their concentration is decreasing (e.g., monoamine oxidase inhibitors).

SURROGATE ENDPOINTS

Usefulness of Surrogate Endpoints

It is not always possible, practical, or appropriate to measure the clinical event that is of primary interest in a clinical trial. In many situations a surrogate endpoint is measured instead of the true endpoint. Surrogate endpoints are used to diagnose a disease and to evaluate patient response to therapy. In many clinical situations, use of a surrogate endpoint is so familiar (e.g., blood pressure) that we sometimes must remind ourselves that that is all it is.

Examples

A number of commonly used surrogate endpoints are listed in Table 82.5. The major reason for using surrogates is to get an earlier and less expensive assessment about the value of new treatments or medicines.

The Ideal Surrogate Endpoint

The ideal surrogate endpoint is a disease marker that reflects what is happening with the underlying disease. The relationship between the marker and the true endpoint is important to establish. After this is done, the validity of data based on how the marker is affected by a medicine or other treatment can be translated into a valid statement about the disease and true endpoint.

Validating a Surrogate Endpoint

The best method to validate the proposed surrogate endpoint is to conduct a clinical trial to evaluate both the marker (i.e., surrogate) and the final or true endpoint, even though this often requires a large amount of resources and a great deal of time. If a medicine does, in fact, show the desired effect on the true endpoint, then future clinical trials may utilize the surrogate endpoint. In addition, the surrogate endpoint may be used to study other medicines with the same mechanism of action.

Medicines with Different Mechanisms of Action

What about using a surrogate endpoint for evaluating medicines that have a different mechanism of action?

TABLE 82.5 *Examples of surrogate endpoints used to evaluate therapy in various diseases*

Disease	Surrogate endpoint	True endpoint[a]
1. Glaucoma	Intraocular pressure	Loss of vision
2. Cancer	Time to progression of tumor Tumor size changes Time to reappearance of disease	Survival
3. Myocardial infarction treated with thrombolytic therapy	Clot lysis, patency rate, reocclusion rate, left ventricular ejection fraction	Survival
4. Various types of mental illness	Score on a psychological test	Mental status
5. Diabetes mellitus	Glucose in blood	Survival
6. Hyperlipoproteinemia	Cholesterol in blood	Survival
7. Arrhythmias	Premature ventricular contractions	Survival

[a] Some patients and physicians are stating that improved quality of life should also be considered as the true endpoint in selected cases. Those cases are primarily when disease is severe and quality of life is compromised. See table 90.1 for other examples.

This use is not so certain. For example, if medicine X reduces end-organ damage (e.g., renal failure, cerebral strokes) and mortality through reducing blood pressure, does that mean that other medicines that reduce blood pressure by a different mechanism will also reduce end-organ damage and mortality? Literally speaking, the answer is no. Each class of antihypertensives must be evaluated to confirm the relationship with the final endpoint. Practically speaking, however, the assumption is usually made that it is possible to extrapolate results of one medicine's effect on a surrogate marker to other medicines that have the same clinical effect but act via a different mechanism.

When a Surrogate Is Uncertain

A complication arises when an appropriate surrogate is uncertain. For example, beta-receptor antagonists have been shown to decrease mortality after a heart attack, but the mechanism causing mortality to decrease is unknown. This mechanism could be related to effects on blood pressure, ischemia, platelet function, or arrhythmias. As long as a new beta-receptor antagonist had each of these activities, its reducing effect on mortality could be assumed, but if one of these activities were not present, then that assumption might not be valid.

It is usually necessary that the first medicine of a new type establish that the true endpoint is affected. Thereafter, all imitation ("me-toos") medicines can avoid the long and difficult clinical trials required to establish the value of the surrogate.

Surrogates for Surrogates

It is not always possible to measure the surrogate easily, or it is found to be easier to measure a surrogate for the surrogate endpoint. One example concerns measuring carcinoembryonic antigen as a surrogate for tumor response, itself a surrogate for the final endpoint of mortality (i.e., survival).

Markers Used to Diagnose a Disease

Many, if not most, diseases are diagnosed partially or entirely through laboratory tests in which specific analytes are used as markers of the disease.

ALTERNATIVE APPROACHES TO MEASURING AND DEMONSTRATING EFFICACY

In any particular field of study most of the standard measures of efficacy will be well known. There are occasions, however, when alternative parameters of efficacy are sought. This may be because established parameters are too restrictive or limited and may not or do not demonstrate an effect that the investigator is confident has occurred. A particular parameter or test may have been widely used simply because it has been available and has been used by others rather than because it has been shown to be valid. There are often a number of different approaches to consider in evaluating efficacy (Table 82.6).

Most (or all) of the measures described in Table 82.6 appear to be straightforward approaches to evaluating therapy, but these are usually not the traditional measures incorporated in most clinical trials. Even when it is possible to measure some of these parameters in a straightforward manner, they are not used. For example, the most common method of evaluating the therapeutic benefit of an epileptic medication is to count the number of seizures in a given time period and to compare this with an active or historical baseline. Global impressions of the investigator are also often used. A less common parameter is to measure the length of time between seizures. There is, how-

TABLE 82.6 *Possible parameters to evaluate efficacy in clinical trials*

1. Clinical global impressions of disease severity or the patient's clinical improvement rated in a double-blind manner by the investigator[a]
2. Clinical global impressions of clinical improvement or disease severity rated by the patient[a]
3. Clinical global impressions of clinical improvement or disease severity rated by a nurse (primarily for inpatient trials), a family member (especially if they are caring for the patient), or others[a]
4. Number of episodes of the disease per month, week, or other time period
5. Length of time between episodes (e.g., between seizures)
6. Time to onset of improvement after the treatment is initiated
7. Relapse rate while the treatment continues (i.e., is relapse prevented)
8. Relapse rate after the treatment is stopped
9. Functional measures of outcome suggested by patients in a prior trial
10. Partial responders may be defined in addition to all-or-none approaches
11. Prevention of further deterioration of disease
12. Reversal of specific signs or symptoms even though the overall disease remains stable
13. Failure to develop symptoms after exposure to disease (e.g., Retrovir given to asymptomatic patients who are antibody positive for HIV)
14. Number of patients requiring hospitalization or rehospitalization
15. Number of patients who died during treatment or follow-up
16. Duration of survival of treated and untreated patients
17. Number of times a patient has required ancillary therapy
18. Time period until a patient has requested ancillary therapy
19. Utilize a subset of a scale that is more appropriate to measure a disease than the entire scale (e.g., some aspects of the *Brief Psychiatric Rating Scale* are associated with schizophrenia and may be used as a subscale)
20. Rate of patient dropouts per month or other time period on test medicine, active medicine, and placebo
21. An index may be devised based on various measurements, tests, and scales, which must be validated and utilized in all trials of a similar type

[a] Clinical global impressions of a patient's improvement are not generally useful in clinical trials lasting for longer than approximately 3 months. After that period (or an even shorter one), it is difficult to recall accurately the original baseline. Disease severity can be assessed throughout a long-term trial, however, using other parameters.

TABLE 82.7 *Examples of presentations of efficacy data obtained in an antiepileptic medicine trial*

1. Average number of seizures in the active medicine group versus the placebo group during treatment
2. Average number of seizures in the active medicine versus placebo group at the end of treatment
3. Average number of seizures in the active medicine versus placebo group during the last 3 weeks of treatment
4. Average percent decrease in seizures for groups described in 1, 2, or 3 above
5. Number of patients who did better on active medicine versus those who did better on placebo
6. Number of patients on each treatment whose seizure frequency decreased by 0 to 1 seizure per month, 2 to 4 seizures per month, or more than 4 seizures per month
7. Number of patients on each treatment whose seizure frequency decreased by 0 to 25% per month, 26 to 50% per month, or greater than 50% per month
8. Total number of seizures during baseline minus those during treatment for each group of patients
9. Total number of seizure-free days during treatment for each group of patients[a]
10. Largest number of seizure-free days per patient during treatment for each group of patients[a]
11. Average intensity of seizures during treatment for each group of patients
12. Percent change from baseline in intensity of seizures for each group of patients
13. Quantity and type of concomitant seizure medicines used during treatment (above baseline) for patients in each group
14. Any of the above could be considered for specific types of seizures

[a] These comparisons are only relevant if each group had the same total days of exposure.

tween various medicines on the basis of their relapse rates even though their healing rates are equal.

Four alternative tools for describing clinical benefits are described by Laupacis et al. (1988) and consist of relative risk reduction, odds ratio, absolute risk reduction, and number of patients who must be treated to prevent one adverse event (e.g., death). These tools are discussed further in Chapter 99.

Resolving Differences between Initial and Final Baseline Values

A patient who has multiple baseline values may demonstrate changes among them. In comparing data, one must decide to use the first, intermediate, or final baseline value. Alternatively, all values may be averaged or some other combination created. Serious problems arise if there is a trend (either increasing or decreasing) during the baseline period, because effects during treatment may be influenced by whatever factors led to the unstable baseline.

FOLLOW-UP TRIALS TO CONFIRM OR EXTEND AN INTERPRETATION

Individual clinical trials are often stepping stones that the investigator follows either while moving in a

ever, no reason why additional measures cannot also be used. Not all of the measures need have equal weight in evaluating the overall effect of treatment. The relative importance ascribed to each should be established prior to initiating the clinical trial. Table 82.7 lists several types of evaluations that could be conducted on data obtained in an efficacy trial of an antiepileptic medicine.

Another example concerns the evaluation of antiulcer medicine therapy. Most antiulcer clinical trials evaluate measures of improvement (e.g., percentage of patients improved, rate of healing). There are a growing number of trials that are now evaluating the relapse rates of various medicines used to treat duodenal ulcers (e.g., Martin et al., 1981; Diaz, 1981; McLean et al., 1984). This parameter is especially interesting because it has been able to differentiate be-

TABLE 82.8 *Methods to confirm or extend an interpretation of efficacy data*

1. Reference other literature articles and compare both data and interpretations
2. Data from previous clinical trials may be pooled
3. Reinterpret previously reported data that apparently contradict the present data and interpretation. A new statistical or clinical approach may be used in reinterpreting the data
4. Obtain other viewpoints or arguments in support of the interpretation
5. Repeat the trial, double blind if possible, and improve the trial design to support and strengthen the validity of the data obtained
6. Encourage other scientists/clinicians to conduct the same or a similar trial
7. Establish a hypothesis, if possible, and attempt to challenge it with currently available data. Encourage others to challenge it through additional studies
8. Elicit ideas from consultants and others on how better to validate the interpretation
9. Adopt the "devil's advocate" viewpoint and attempt to disprove the original interpretation. Then seek to disprove the "devil's advocate" position

general scientific or clinical direction or while moving toward a specific clinical/scientific goal. After the process of reaching an interpretation has been completed, the next clinical step may be planned or implemented. Table 82.8 describes methods to confirm or extend an interpretation.

When the interpretation of a clinical trial is to be extended, the next step may be to:

1. Modify the clinical trial design to yield data that will provide stronger support for the conclusions reached or allow a clearer conclusion to be reached.
2. Conduct a new clinical trial specifically to evaluate one aspect or detail of the conclusions or to evaluate a hypothesis that was generated by the conclusions.

3. Conduct an entirely different clinical trial that will evaluate a new aspect in the investigator's overall plan that is not dependent on the interpretation or results obtained in the trial being analyzed.

In attempting to design a "tight," well-controlled trial that minimizes variability to confirm or extend an interpretation, many controls may be added to the design, and additional restrictions may be placed on the patients entered. There is a price to pay for this advantage. As one better defines and limits the clinical area studied, the ability to extrapolate the results to populations of other patients becomes more limited. It is analogous to the situation of knowing more and more about a smaller and smaller area. There is another price to pay. The more restricted the entry criteria for a trial become, the fewer patients are able to be found who will qualify to enter the trial.

Must All Well-Controlled Clinical Trials on a New Medicine Demonstrate Activity?

In designing and implementing additional trials to extend the results of an initial trial it should be remembered that every trial conducted on a new medicine or hypothesis does not have to be positive to demonstrate efficacy of a medicine treatment or the validity of a hypothesis. A few well-controlled positive trials usually provide evidence of true efficacy even though a number of other trials do not definitively distinguish between placebo and active medicine. There is also statistical support for this clinical view (Overall and Rhoades, 1984). This event is reasonably likely for medicines affecting the central nervous system, but not for all therapeutic areas, such as for antibacterial medicines.

CHAPTER 83

Specific Factors to Consider in Interpreting Efficacy and Safety Data

GENERAL CONSIDERATIONS

This chapter identifies many of the specific factors that affect the interpretation of clinical data and influence the planning of clinical trials. A pertinent issue is to identify and consider the most relevant factors that should be measured and controlled. There is no easy means to develop a definitive list of those factors. Once a list is developed, not all of the factors can be controlled or measured. It will probably be too expensive or impractical to control or measure some factors. Other factors may only be incompletely or even incorrectly measured, and yet others will probably be unknown or beyond the technical state of the art to measure. There may be factors that can be measured correctly and completely, but financial, social, political, or environmental conditions may prevent their measurement.

The specific factors described and discussed generally apply to both safety and efficacy data. Some of the examples given are clearly applicable primarily for interpreting either safety or efficacy data, but in most instances, examples relevant to either type of data could be given. No systematic attempt is made to identify factors that apply only to safety or to efficacy data. The tables in this chapter are not comprehensive but are meant to provide common examples for each of the factors described.

After all the data in a clinical trial are collected, they must be properly analyzed. At that point the influence of all relevant factors must be judged in order to reach an interpretation. If fully adequate information is not available on all relevant factors (which it rarely is),

then the interpretation must be considered as incomplete and even possibly as flawed. This is unfortunately the situation with almost all clinical trials. Interpretations are rarely perfect explanations of all data from a clinical trial.

Categorization of Factors

The factors presented in this chapter are heterogeneous in content and have been grouped into 12 broad categories for ease of discussion (Table 83.1). These categories are admittedly arbitrary and represent only one of many possible classification systems that could be created. Each of the broad groups is subdivided into separate tables listing the individual factors that make up each of the broad categories. Many of the specific factors discussed in each category are considered from two viewpoints: (1) selected ways in which the factor may influence or bias data or affect their interpretation and (2) how the influence of the factor on interpretation of clinical data may be controlled or measured. This approach is schematically diagrammed in Fig. 83.1.

It is certain that many factors may affect the interpretation of data from any single clinical trial, but it will virtually never be relevant to consider or investigate all of the factors listed in the tables in this chapter in any one trial. Some factors that are of minor or no importance in some trials are essential in other trials. A complete listing of potential factors to consider for all trials is virtually impossible to determine. The tables that follow present many of the most common factors that affect interpretation of data but represent a small fraction of the total number of possible factors.

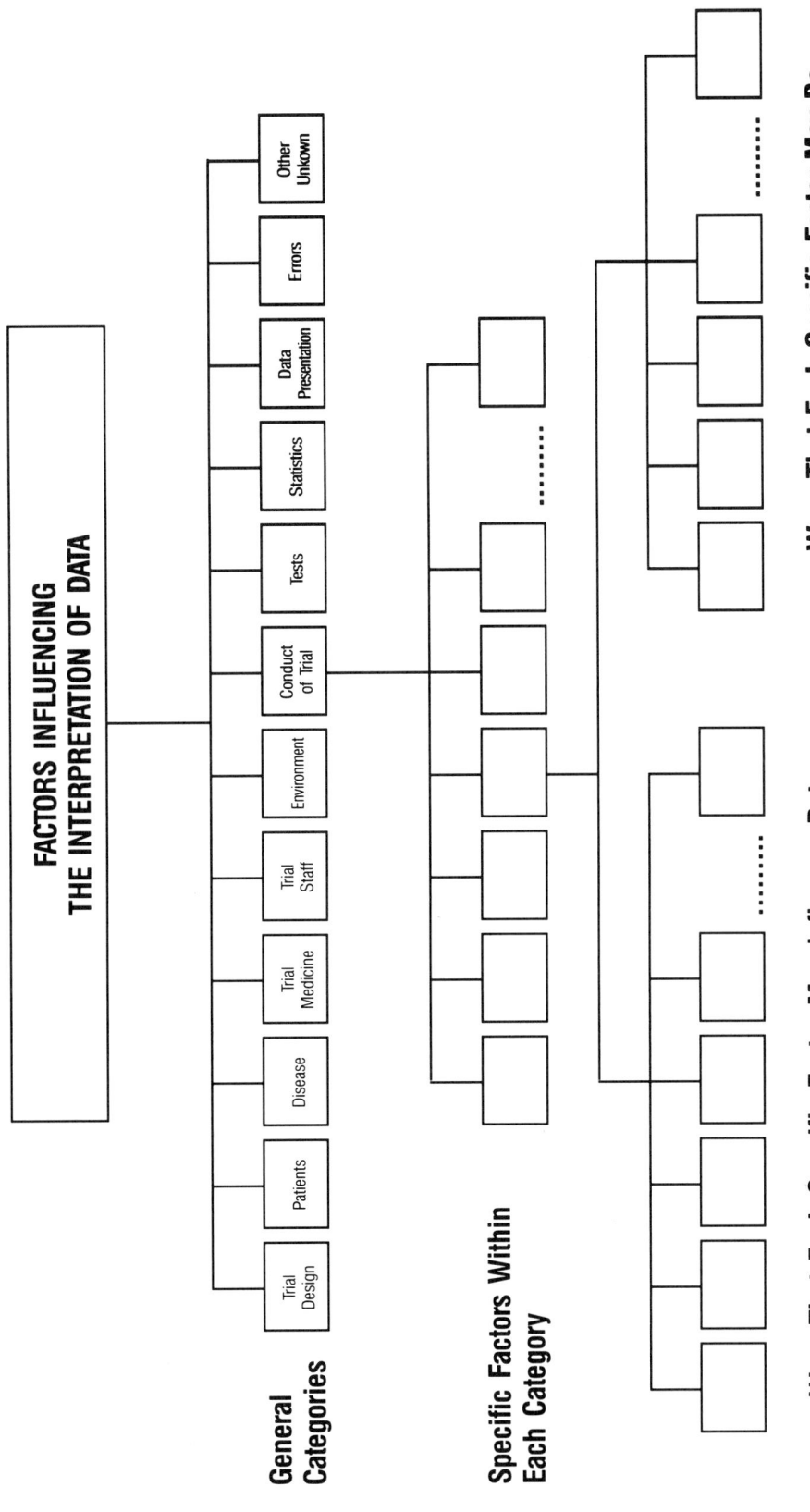

FIG. 83.1 Categorization of factors influencing the interpretation of data. Dotted lines represent from one to N additional boxes.

TABLE 83.1 *Classification of factors (sources of variability) that may bias data or affect their interpretation[a]*

1. Characteristics of the clinical trial design (see Tables 83.2 to 83.24)
2. Characteristics of patients (see Tables 83.25 to 83.51)
3. Characteristics of the disease or problem being evaluated (see Tables 83.52 to 83.54)
4. Characteristics of the trial medicine(s) (see Tables 83.55 to 83.74)
5. Characteristics of the investigator/trial staff (see Tables 83.75 to 83.77)
6. Characteristics of the environment (see Tables 83.78 to 83.80)
7. Conduct of the trial (see Tables 83.81 to 83.83)
8. Characteristics of the tests and measures used (see Tables 83.84 to 83.88)
9. Statistical factors (see Tables 83.89 to 83.91)
10. Characteristics of data presentation and writeup (see Tables 83.92 to 83.94)
11. Errors or deceit committed accidentally or purposely before, during, or after the trial (see Tables 83.95 to 83.98)
12. Other or unknown factors (see Tables 83.99 to 83.101)

[a] Almost any of the factors that make up any category may yield a false-negative or a false-positive interpretation. Each of these sources of variability represents groups of factors that are each broken down into various components in the following tables in this chapter.

Some factors that affect or bias the interpretation of data are more pertinent for individual patients, whereas other factors relate more to the entire group of patients enrolled in a clinical trial. No distinction is usually made in the tables between factors that are more pertinent for interpreting data from a single patient and those that mainly relate to a group of patients or all patients in a trial.

Combinations and Interactions of Factors

Tables 83.2 to 83.101 present ways in which specific factors may bias or influence the interpretation of clinical data. There are, however, many instances when two or more factors interact, and/or it is the combination that is responsible for the bias introduced. There are innumerable combinations of factors that may affect a particular patient's outcome in a clinical trial, and most of the specific factors and combinations are often never determined or known. If it appears, however, that one or more groups of patients in a trial yielded data different from what was expected, a rationally based evaluation of both single and combinations of factors should be considered. Even when the trial turns out to yield results that were expected, it is valuable to evaluate the influence of several specific factors to demonstrate that the results obtained were not spurious or related to a factor that should have been considered but was not.

A few examples of common factors that may be associated in combination with each other are:

1. Age of patient and degree of compliance (young patients may be less compliant unless supervised)
2. Severity of disease and degree of compliance (more severely ill patients are often more motivated to be compliant than mildly ill patients, but very severely ill patients may exhibit less compliance than others)
3. Type of referral center and general style of care and treatment (physicians in tertiary care referral centers often handle and care for patients differently than do physicians in primary care centers)

In reality, there are usually not one, two, or three factors that interact and influence data but many. The greater the number of factors involved, the greater will usually be the complexity of their interactions. Even after an attempt is made to control the most important factors, numerous others may not be controlled adequately. The importance of various factors may be evaluated by subgroup analyses or via other methods when the data are analyzed and interpreted.

The specific factors described in the tables may bias data, but this chapter does not indicate types of biases that may occur. A list or catalog of types of biases was published by Sackett and is presented in Chapter 5. Types of biases related to readers of clinical literature are presented by Owen (1982).

OVERVIEW OF SPECIFIC FACTORS

The following tables (83.2 to 83.101) indicate many of the factors that may be relevant or important to consider in planning clinical trials and interpreting safety and efficacy data. The various topics may be used as a checklist, reference source, or in other ways. The organization of these tables was described in the previous section of this chapter. It is important to note that not all of the specific factors are individually assessed. Several are grouped together or merely indicated as potentially relevant.

TABLE 83.2 *Specific factors related to trial design that may bias data or affect their interpretation[a]*

1. Type of design used (e.g., crossover, parallel)
2. Number, type, and size of comparison or control groups
3. Parameters chosen to evaluate and the number and timing of measurements
4. Type of randomization used
5. Type of blind used
6. Duration of trial
7. Use of placebo
8. Use of a washout period
9. Nature of baseline, screen, treatment, and follow-up periods
10. Inpatient versus outpatient trial

[a] Illustrations are given in the following tables of ways in which many of these factors may bias data or affect its interpretation and also how the factor may be controlled or measured.

TABLE 83.3 *How may the type of design used in a trial bias data or affect its interpretation?*

A. General comments
   1. If the overall trial design is inappropriate to achieve the trial objectives
B. Crossover design
   1. If all patients undergo one arm of the trial before being crossed over to the other arm of the trial, there may be a significant period effect
   2. Inadequate washout period between treatments, which allows a carryover effect from one baseline or treatment period to affect the next period
   3. Treatment or placebo periods that are inadequate in length to allow the full effect to be expressed
   4. Rules of crossover that allow patients to be crossed over based on clinical improvement rather than a fixed time period
   5. If the disease being evaluated does not return to the same baseline prior to initiation of each subsequent treatment period
   6. If the treatment or placebo periods are too long, there may be poor patient compliance, or the disease may not remain sufficiently stable
   7. If the design is too demanding and patient enrollment occurs slowly with many dropouts, an unacceptably large amount of missing data will occur
C. Parallel design
   1. This design may not be suitable if there are not enough patients to enter each arm of the trial
   2. The ratio of patients proposed to enter each arm of the trial may not allow an adequate power to be achieved if one arm has too few patients

TABLE 83.4 *How may the potential influence of the type of design on interpretation of clinical data be measured or controlled?*

1. Utilize a baseline period of adequate duration with a crossover design both prior to and between treatment periods to ensure stability of the disease and return of the most important parameters to a similar level prior to initiation of each treatment period
2. If a medicine-free baseline is impossible, then taper one medicine while the other is being added
3. If a carryover effect is suspected, consider repeating the trial with a parallel design
4. Confirm (insofar as possible) that the number of patients required to enter a trial is available

TABLE 83.5 *How may the number, type, and size of comparison or control groups used in a trial bias data or affect their interpretation?*

1. If the composition of the comparison group in terms of patient or disease characteristics is not "equal" to that of the test group(s), then a false negative or false positive or uninterpretable outcome may be achieved
2. If the comparison group receives a placebo or other treatment in a double-blind trial that is insufficiently designed to maintain the blind
3. If the investigator is able to break the double blind and communicates this information either directly or indirectly to patients, it will affect the integrity of the control group[a]
4. If the investigator is able to break the double blind and allows this to influence the evaluation and/or treatment of patients, even though the information is not communicated to the patients, it will affect the integrity of the control group[a]
5. If multiple doses of the trial medicine are not evaluated to yield a dose–response relationship, then an incorrect impression of a medicine's efficacy and/or safety may be obtained, especially if a placebo is not used
6. If an active medicine is used as a control without use of a placebo, then various misinterpretations may result[b]
7. If different types of hospitals or clinics are compared where there are differences in referral patterns, interests of the medical staff, methods used to diagnose patients, or other factors

[a] Blinds are discussed in Tables 83.11 and 83.12.
[b] See Chapter 94.

TABLE 83.6 *How may the potential influence of the number, type, and size of comparison or control groups on interpretation of clinical data be measured or controlled?*

1. Determine if the comparison or control groups chosen are the most appropriate ones possible
2. Determine if there are other comparison or control groups that might be equally or more appropriate to include (e.g., a "usual care" group,[a] hospital clinic versus general practice,[b] community-oriented versus hospital-oriented psychiatric care,[c] health maintenance organization members versus nonmembers,[d] home versus hospital treatment,[e] coronary care unit versus a general medical ward,[f] day hospital versus outpatient treatment,[g] university versus community hospital[h]
3. Use the techniques of stratification or minimization to allocate patients to treatment and comparison groups
4. Evaluate the integrity of the blind with an end-of-trial questionnaire, interview, or other technique directed at patients and/or investigator
5. The investigator may guess at the end of the trial which treatment each patient was on and state the reasons for his guess (e.g., adverse reactions, laboratory data, patient behavior, clinical improvement or deterioration) prior to breaking the blind. This could be one aspect of validating the trial blind and also help in designing better blinds in future trials
6. Include multiple dose evaluations of a trial medicine whenever possible, choosing doses with a high likelihood of demonstrating a difference in effects

[a] Luepker et al. (1984).
[b] Ellenberg and Nelson (1980), Hayes and Harries (1984), and Singh et al. (1984).
[c] Hoult and Reynolds (1984) and Reynolds and Hoult (1984).
[d] Kurata et al. (1982).
[e] Hill et al. (1978) and Mather et al. (1976).
[f] MacMillan and Brown (1971).
[g] Tyrer and Remington (1979).
[h] Gross et al. (1980).

TABLE 83.7 *How may the parameters chosen to evaluate safety and efficacy and the number and timing of measurements made in a clinical trial bias data or affect their interpretation?*

1. If all measurements are made before a lesion, event, or blood level of a medicine has reached its peak, the data may not represent the true maximal effects
2. If all measurements are made after most effects of a lesion have worn off, an event has passed, or blood levels have decreasd, the data may be inaccurate
3. If an excessive number of measurements are made, it may create patient fatigue, confusion, anger, or another symptom
4. If an inadequate number of measurements are made, it may not allow an adequate statistical approach to be used
5. If the parameters chosen are not the most appropriate ones to study
6. If too few or too many efficacy parameters are chosen to follow (one would expect one of every 20 independent statistical analyses to yield a $p < 0.05$ even if there were no true differences)

TABLE 83.8 *How may the influence of the parameters chosen to evaluate safety and efficacy and the number and timing of measurements be measured or controlled?*

1. Include an adequate number of repetitive measurements to obtain reliable data on the entire process being studied
2. Include an adequate number of measurements at different times during the process to capture data at both peak and trough levels of the medicine
3. Discuss the number of measurements with a statistician, other investigators, and staff. Conduct a dry run to ensure patient acceptability of the procedures and tests to be used in the trial
4. Discuss the number and type of parameters chosen with other investigators

TABLE 83.9 *How may the randomization used in a trial bias data or affect their interpretation?*

1. Unequal distribution of important patient or disease characteristics or parameters between groups may lead to a mistaken interpretation
2. Incorrect use of a randomization code by the investigator may lead to a flawed trial
3. Use of a simple randomization code (e.g., ABAB) or labeled bottles (medicine A and medicine B) in a double-blind study may allow the randomization code to be easily broken. Knowledge of the code may bias the investigator in favor of one treatment[a]

[a] There are numerous other ways for a randomization code to be broken.

TABLE 83.10 *How may the potential influence or bias of randomization used on interpretation of clinical data be measured or controlled?*

1. Calculate the magnitude of important patient and disease characteristics or parameters for each treatment group and compare the number of patients randomized to each treatment group with each important factor
2. Use a different randomization technique in a future trial (e.g., stratification, minimization) or randomize different groups (e.g., men versus women, 12- to 18-year-old versus 18- to 65-year-old patients)
3. Use randomization codes that are not easily broken
4. Do not provide bottles of medicine marked medicine A or medicine B to patients, which may readily unblind the clinical trial
5. Monitor a trial to ensure proper application of the randomization code

TABLE 83.11 *How may the type of blind used in a clinical trial bias data or affect their interpretation?*

1. Open-label trials have a greater tendency to yield positive data than do double-blind trials
2. Single-blind trials do not always yield more objective data and interpretations than open-label trials
3. A double-blind trial whose blind is broken by the investigator may not yield more objective data and interpretations than an open-label trial
4. If the blind in a double-blind trial is broken by a relatively small number of patients, it may not have a significant bearing on the interpretation of data. If a relatively large number of patients are able to break the trial blind, however, then the probability is also large that there is an effect on the data obtained and on its interpretation
5. Open-label Phase II pilot trials yield erroneous interpretations more often than large open-label Phase III or Phase IV trials. The latter two types of trials more closely approximate a normal clinical situation
6. Open-label Phase I trials are more likely to yield erroneous interpretations than double-blind Phase I trials utilizing a placebo treatment

TABLE 83.12 *How may the potential influence of the type of blind used in a clinical trial on interpretation of clinical data be measured or controlled?*

1. Measure the validity of the blind with (1) an end-of-trial questionnaire, (2) interviews of patients and investigator, (3) an investigator guess list, which requests the investigator to guess which treatment each patient received and to indicate the reason for each guess, or (4) other technique
2. Repeat an open-label or single-blind clinical trial utilizing a double-blind design while maintaining all other aspects of the design identical
3. Repeat a double-blind trial in which the blind had been broken with a modified design that will prevent (or minimize) the possibility of the blind being broken by patients or investigators

TABLE 83.13 *How may the duration of the clinical trial bias data or affect their interpretation?*

1. The trial's duration may not be long enough for the full effect of the medicine (or the placebo) to be manifested
2. The trial's duration may only permit investigation of the acute phase or exacerbation of a disease process rather than a chronic phase as well. Thus, information on the maintenance phase of a medicine's effect may not be achieved
3. A short trial duration may not allow an adequate number of measurements to be obtained for comparison with baseline
4. A trial duration that is excessively long may introduce extraneous factors such as concomitant medicines, changing baseline, other treatments, and personal, social, and/or psychological factors
5. The treatment period may have an adequate duration, but the dose ascension, dose taper, or follow-up periods may be too short either to obtain adequate information or to allow an appropriate time for the process to occur
6. The follow-up period may be too short to observe withdrawal effects of medicines or other rebound phenomena

TABLE 83.14 *How may the potential influence of the baseline on interpretation of clinical data be measured or controlled?*

1. Evaluate values of the endpoints (or parameters) measured periodically during baseline for their stability, variability, and trends
2. Discuss the appropriate length of a baseline with various experts in the particular field
3. Discuss the appropriate number of tests and measurements to obtain with a statistician

TABLE 83.15 *How may the influence of a placebo medication, placebo group, or placebo effect bias data or affect their interpretation?*

A. Placebo medication
   1. The color, size, shape, and other characteristics of a placebo[a] may not be identical to the trial medicine, allowing patients or the investigator to break the trial blind and bias results
   2. The color or other characteristics of the placebo may yield a greater or lesser placebo effect because of various psychological factors[b]
   3. The placebo may contain a substance (e.g., lactose) that will affect some patients (e.g., lactose-intolerant patients) and lead to adverse reactions
B. Placebo effect (response)
   1. In certain specific populations the effects of a placebo may be more or less marked than in the overall population
   2. An extremely large or small placebo response may indicate a significant problem in the trial design or conduct that should be evaluated
   3. The actual placebo response may be highly complex. If the data analysis consists of merely subtracting a determined value from the total effect, it may oversimplify and distort the conclusion
C. Placebo group
   1. Patients in the placebo group who were receiving other medicines that could have elicited their response may yield data that could bias interpretations reached
   2. Without a placebo group or placebo treatment period, effects may be attributed to medicines that were in fact spontaneous changes or related to the natural history of the disease

[a] See Table 25.1.
[b] See text for references.

TABLE 83.16 *How may the potential influence of a placebo medication, placebo group, or placebo effect on interpretation of clinical data be measured or controlled?*

1. Subtract the placebo response from the medicine response to obtain a net medicine-induced response.[a] This may be done on an individual patient basis (if the trial design permits)
2. Incorporate placebo in a trial to compare with an open-label or active medicine control and evaluate responses in absence of test medicine
3. Ensure that all physical characteristics of a placebo are identical to those of the trial medicine
4. Use a different substance than lactose as placebo in a trial in which some patients may be expected to be lactase deficient (i.e., certain studies involving patients with gastrointestinal diseases) and may react adversely to lactose

[a] This commonly used technique probably represents a simplification and rests on several unproven assumptions: (1) part of the medicine response results from a placebo effect, (2) the same amount of a medicine response results from a placebo effect as in the placebo group or placebo phase of the trial, (3) if the same patient has received both medicine and placebo, the baseline and conditions under which they were each taken were the same, (4) the placebo and medicine responses are linear, and (5) the placebo response is relatively constant in magnitude throughout the duration of the trial. The interaction of a trial medicine and placebo, however, is probably complex, and some of these assumptions are probably not valid.

TABLE 83.17 *How may the washout period in a clinical trial bias data or affect their interpretation?*

1. An inadequate washout period (or absence of a washout period) may allow previously administered medicines to influence the current trial (i.e., by creating a carryover effect)
2. An excessive washout period may lead to an unstable baseline and thus influence data
3. The clinical or ethical "impossibility" of having a complete washout period in some medicine trials may mean that the influence of carryover effect on the trial cannot be eliminated or that an add-on medicine trial must be performed

TABLE 83.18 *How may the potential influence of the washout period on interpretation of clinical data be measured or controlled?*

1. Evaluate the carryover effect
2. Initiate dose ascension of the trial medicine, and after it is partially or totally complete, withdraw the original therapy
3. Conduct an add-on trial and periodically remove one medicine at a time (every so many weeks, months, or at certain stages of improvement) to achieve an evaluation of the trial medicine as monotherapy
4. Evaluate a period of time each week (or month) when the patient is not given medicine (i.e., a medicine holiday)
5. Seek to develop a novel trial design when it is not considered ethically proper to include a washout in the clinical trial

TABLE 83.19 *How may the potential influence of the duration of a clinical trial on interpretation of clinical data be measured or controlled?*

1. Determine a suitable duration for a clinical trial by discussions with peers, colleagues, and statisticians[a]
2. Determine a suitable length for baseline, dose ascension, dose taper, and follow-up
3. Repeat the trial using a more appropriate trial duration
4. Develop continuation protocols for patients to enter after completing a trial of shorter duration

[a] Many trials utilize a duration thought to be suitable that later turns out to be unsuitable.

TABLE 83.20 *How may the nature of the baseline used in a clinical trial bias data or affect their interpretation?*

1. Historical (i.e., retrospective) baselines of other patients previously treated may be inappropriate or insufficiently documented to satisfy the requirements of the present trial
2. Historical baselines of the same patients being used in the treatment period may be inaccurate because data previously collected were generated and obtained according to different standards and techniques (i.e., retrospective recollection versus prospective recordings)
3. An active (i.e., prospective) baseline period may be too short in duration to capture the necessary range of variations in the parameters measured to compare with treatment data
4. An active baseline may be too long in duration in that the nature and/or measurements of the disease/problem are undergoing spontaneous change, so that the end of the baseline is quite different from the initial part
5. The number of tests and measurements during baseline may be too few or too many. The value of the baseline effect may be inappropriately chosen (e.g., it may be calculated as the average of all values, only the initial value, only the terminal value)

TABLE 83.21 *How may the potential influence of the baseline period on interpretation of clinical data be measured or controlled?*

1. Provide an optional extension period to the baseline to ensure that values of important parameters are relatively stable
2. In a crossover study, ensure that values return to the original baseline before initiating the second part of the treatment
3. Conduct an active (prospective) baseline instead of a historical (retrospective) one
4. Determine what data or documentation are required to substantiate reports of a historical baseline

TABLE 83.22 *How may the screen, treatment, and/or follow-up period in a clinical trial bias data or affect their interpretation?*

A. Screen
   1. A superficial screen may allow inappropriate patients to be enrolled
   2. A screen that is conducted once and not repeated may be insufficient because of variation in response and thus allow inappropriate patients to be enrolled
   3. A superficially designed or conducted screen may allow patients in a trial with conditions that may be detected during the trial and attributed to the trial medicine
B. Treatment
   1. An inadequate number of observations during treatment may not yield accurate data of responses to treatment
   2. A dose ascension of medicine that is too rapid may cause changes in the patient's disease state in addition to eliciting adverse reactions
   3. Medicine taper that is too rapid may cause withdrawal symptoms and exacerbate the patient's disease state
C. Follow-up
   1. A follow-up period that is inadequate in duration may not capture abnormal laboratory values or symptoms that occur after the trial is completed
   2. An inadequate duration of follow-up may not (1) allow sufficient time to observe regression of patient's disease, (2) observe long-term beneficial effects of patients off medicine treatment, and (3) observe the long-term benefits or waning of improvement after surgical interventions

TABLE 83.23 *How may the potential influence of screen, treatment, or follow-up periods on interpretation of clinical data be measured or controlled?*

A. Screen
   1. Conduct a double (i.e., repeated) series of screen tests for all patients. This helps to ensure that their values remain within a given range prior to enrolling them in the trial and is especially relevant if screen values fluctuate to a large degree
   2. Conduct a thorough examination at screen for all investigational medicines in Phases I and II even with tests that may only be repeated after the trial (e.g., electrocardiogram, ophthalmological examination). This will help prevent later abnormalities being attributed to the trial medicine when they might have been long-standing problems that the patient and investigator were not aware of
B. Treatment
   1. If some ineligible patients were enrolled, their data may be assessed separately and compared with those of eligible patients
   2. Values obtained at different times during treatment may be compared to determine the most suitable length for treatment periods in future studies
   3. Consider the appropriate number of measurements necessary to obtain at each time point of a trial from both a statistical and clinical perspective
   4. Evaluate different dosage ascension schemas if numerous adverse reactions occur during this period
   5. Evaluate different dosage taper schemas if withdrawal effects occur during dose taper
C. Follow-up
   1. Conduct a long follow-up period to determine the regression rate of patients when taken off a trial medicine and the time to return of their symptoms
   2. Determine the severity of symptoms that recur, especially in comparison with pretrial symptoms. Follow patients even if they are placed on alternate medicine therapy and measure their reactions to treatment when their symptoms return
   3. Institute a long-term follow-up program to track the whereabouts of surgical and/or selected medical patients

TABLE 83.24 *Factors related to inpatient or outpatient trial designs that may bias data or affect their interpretation*

A. Inpatient clinical trials
  1. Many patient factors may be controlled through the protocol, which will yield different data than an outpatient situation, when more variable patient behavior is likely to occur and is more difficult to standardize
  2. Certain subjective adverse reactions (e.g., fatigue) may be more likely in a tedious inpatient trial (the patient may be bored) than in an outpatient trial (patients are more active)
  3. More elaborate trial designs may usually be established for inpatient trials in terms of using elaborate dose regimens and sophisticated testing of clinical endpoints with patients who are more compliant than in outpatient trials. Data from inpatient trials may thus differ from outpatient

trials conducted in the "real world" using more limited testing measures

B. Outpatient clinical trials
  1. Outpatient trials may yield variable data because various factors (e.g., compliance, patient visits, social interaction) cannot adequately be controlled or practically implemented (e.g., controlled diet, elaborate dosage regimen)
  2. Either less or more social interaction, stress, and psychological stimulation may occur for a particular patient in an outpatient than an inpatient trial. This variation could affect degree of a patient's voluntary effort, cooperation, or performance on tests

TABLE 83.25 *Specific factors related to patient characteristics that may bias data or affect their interpretation[a]*

A. Inherent factors (see Tables 83.26 to 83.40)
  1. Age[b]
  2. Sex[b]
  3. Weight and body surface area
  4. Race and ethnic background[b]
  5. Genetic history[b]
  6. Circadian and other biological rhythms
  7. Menstrual cycle
  8. Blood type
B. Acquired factors (see Tables 83.41 to 83.46)
  1. Education
  2. Diet[b]
  3. Exercise and physical condition[b]
  4. Sleeping habits
  5. Pregnancy, lactation[b]
  6. Medical history[c]
  7. Allergies
  8. Periodic problems (e.g., seasonal diseases)
  9. Fever
  10. Gastrointestinal flora
  11. Immunization status
  12. Nutritional status[b]
C. Social and economic factors (see Tables 83.47 to 83.49)
  1. Social class
  2. Economic status
  3. Relationship of patient with family
  4. Relationship of patient with friends and acquaintances
  5. Relationship of patient with investigator and staff
  6. Personal habits: (1) alcohol, (2) cigarettes and other tobacco products, and (3) caffeine-containing beverages[b]
  7. Drug abuse[b]
  8. Techniques of patient recruitment
  9. Foreign travel by patients prior to or during the trial
  10. Occupation[b]
  11. Pets owned by patient, family, friends, or others
  12. Type and geographical location of residence
  13. Degree of crowding in the home, work, study, and other environments
D. Psychological factors (see Tables 83.50 and 83.51)
  1. Desire for treatment and benefit
  2. Desire to be in a clinical trial
  3. Compliance with trial requirements, excluding medicine ingestion

  4. Compliance with medicine ingestion
  5. Demands placed on patients by the trial
  6. Significant personal events occurring prior to or during the trial
  7. Personal and religious beliefs
  8. Nervousness or anxiety of patient during tests or procedures
  9. Relationship and behavior of patient with investigator and ancillary staff
  10. Propensity to augment or reduce the magnitude of external stimuli
  11. Blinded patient being inadvertently alerted to treatment being received, anticipated symptoms, and/or reactions of particular interest to the investigator
  12. Influence of informed consent on enrolling in trial
E. Factors relating to patient's disease (see Tables 83.52 to 83.54)
  1. Diagnosis of disease and any subtype
  2. Previous history of disease
  3. Degree and severity of present symptoms, signs, and illness (including physical examination)
  4. Prior medicine and nonmedicine treatment
  5. Concomitant medicines[b]
  6. Concurrent illnesses[b]
  7. Degree of refractoriness
  8. Alternative treatments available
  9. Presence and amount of transfusions
F. Factors relating to a patient's physiological state
  1. Risk factors for other problems
  2. Biochemical status of various organs, tissues, and/or cells
  3. Chemical status of various fluids (e.g., blood, urine)
  4. Physiological status of various organ systems (e.g., renal, hepatic, cardiovascular, pulmonary, hematological)[b]
  5. Immunological status and factors (e.g., amount and intensity of antibodies present or formed)
  6. Other physiological factors
  7. Functional disability of patient
  8. Acid–base status (e.g., P_{O_2}, P_{CO_2}, pH, bicarbonate)
  9. Fluid status (i.e., total balance of body fluids)
  10. Anamnestic responses (i.e., responses relating to previous medical history)
G. Inclusion criteria in a protocol that are not covered above

[a] Not all of these factors are individually described in the following tables.
[b] These factors are discussed in Chapter 87. Some are also described in this chapter.
[c] This is the part of the medical history that is not directly related to the patient's present illness. That part is listed under E.2.

TABLE 83.26 *How may the age of patients in a clinical trial bias data or affect their interpretation?[a,b]*

A. Neonates and infants (up to 2 years)
1. Dose must be adequately adjusted to account for size and other factors
2. Different physiological characteristics because of incompletely functioning symptoms may yield altered data
3. Different levels of enzymes, blood elements, or body chemicals may yield altered data
4. Inability to communicate adequately may yield altered interpretation(s)
B. Pediatric population (2 to 18 years)
1. Patients may be less likely to be compliant unless they have sufficient motivation
C. Adult (18 to 65 years)
1. No specific factors are listed since this group is the benchmark against which data from many other age groups are compared
D. Geriatric (over 65 yers)
1. Altered homeostatic mechanisms
2. Decreased renal function may delay excretion and lead to increased blood levels
3. Decreased muscle mass may affect medicine distribution and influence clinical effects
4. Decreased receptor density may affect ability of tissues to respond

[a] The age ranges given are quite arbitrary and may be modified as required for any trial.
[b] See Chapter 87 for additional details.

TABLE 83.27 *How may the potential influence of patient's age on interpretation of clinical data be measured or controlled?*

1. Conduct trials only in patients of defined age ranges
2. Measure critical factors (e.g., blood levels of a medicine, renal function) of the patients and create patient groups based on age for an analysis based on these physiological characteristics
3. Compare data obtained in a single trial for patients of different age groups
4. Conduct pharmacokinetic screens in different age groups

TABLE 83.28 *How may the sex of the patients in a clinical trial bias data or affect their interpretation?*

1. There may be a sex-linked genetic trait that has an influence on the data obtained
2. If all data are obtained in patients of only one sex, there may be an unknown potential influence of patient's sex on the results
3. If all patients receive a standard dose of a medicine and there is a large difference in the weights of males and females, then the females will receive a larger dose on a milligram per kilogram basis. This may lead to different responses in females than in males. Although the difference would be caused by dose of medicine it may be wrongly attributed to a sex-related difference
4. Differences in medicine absorption, distribution, metabolism, or excretion based on gender are sometimes observed in animals and may possibly be observed in humans
5. Behavior and/or social differences between males and females may alter how the medicine is used or how well the protocol is adhered to. In such circumstances there may be an apparent influence of the patient's sex on the outcome of the trial
6. Numerous diseases and adverse reactions occur at different rates in men and women[a]

[a] Batchelor et al. (1980).

TABLE 83.29 *How may the potential influence of the patient's sex on the interpretation of clinical data be measured or controlled?*

1. Analyze results separately for males and females and compare the data sets
2. Ensure that the number of males and females in each treatment group are approximately equal. This may be done by using a separate randomization code for males and females if it is believed that the patient's sex is a potentially confounding variable

TABLE 83.30 *How may the weight or body surface area of patients in a clinical trial bias data or affect their interpretation?*

1. Patients whose weight is greatly above or below their ideal weight may distribute medicine differently than patients whose weight is closer to the ideal
2. Patients whose weight is greatly above or below their ideal weight may have psychological problems relating to their weight, which may affect or bias the interpretation of data
3. Patients whose weight is greatly above or below their ideal weight will receive markedly different doses of the medicine (either "too low" or "too high") if doses are not given based on weight (e.g., milligrams per kilogram) or based on body surface area (e.g., milligrams per square meter)
4. Patients whose weight is greatly above or below their ideal weight may have eating habits or dietary intake that differs from other patients in the trial

TABLE 83.31 *How may the potential influence of patient's weight or body surface area on interpretation of clinical data be measured or controlled?*

1. Dose patients based on body weight or a close approximation (e.g., body surface area)
2. Exclude patients whose weight lies outside a specified range based on total weight
3. Exclude patients whose weight lies outside a specified range based on percent of ideal weight
4. Evaluate dietary histories and practices of all patients and exclude those whose history or practices are unacceptable
5. Evaluate psychological histories of all patients and exclude those whose history is unacceptable
6. Group patients based on weight and compare responses to medicines
7. Group patients based on weight and compare dietary practices or psychological histories of each group
8. Calculate percentage body fat of all patients and evaluate if this factor is related to medicine distribution

TABLE 83.32 *How may the race or ethnic background of patients in a clinical trial bias data or affect their interpretation?[a]*

1. A genetic factor that is more prevalent in one race may affect data collected [e.g., glucose-6-phosphate dehydrogenase (G-6-P-D) deficiency or sickle cell trait in blacks]
2. Skin pigmentation may create difficulties if skin tests or dermatological studies are being conducted (e.g., it is difficult in some blacks to measure the size of an erythematous reaction as in response to an intradermal histamine challenge)
3. A disease being evaluated may be more prevalent in one race or may have different manifestations in one race (e.g., hypertension)
4. Inclusion of all or almost all patients in a trial from one specific ethnic background or race may lead to a trial performed in only one social or economic group. This may influence data obtained and yield a biased interpretation relating to the race or ethnic background of patients
5. A certain race may have dietary preferences that influence treatment outcomes (e.g., incidence of coronary disease of Japanese living in Japan, Hawaii, and Los Angeles pointed to the importance of dietary influences on this disease)

[a] See also Chapter 87.

TABLE 83.34 *How may a patient's genetic makeup bias data or affect their interpretation?[a]*

1. Alterations in metabolism may occur as a result of a missing enzyme or aberrant form of an enzyme.[b] This may lead to accumulation and toxicity. Decreased absorption may lead to a failure to obtain a beneficial effect, whereas inadequate elimination may lead to toxicity
2. Genetic factors influence a patient's risk factors for several diseases
3. Patients may be more (or less) susceptible to a specific predictable side effect of the medicine
4. Patients may be more susceptible to an idiosyncratic or allergic reaction to the medicine (e.g., presence of an uncommon metabolite)
5. Patients may be less (or more) responsive to potential beneficial effects of the medicine because of altered absorption, distribution, metabolism, or excretion
6. Patients may be more susceptible to having an abnormal laboratory result or adverse reaction (e.g., via more rapid or slower metabolism of a medicine, presence of uncommon metabolites, rapid medicine buildup in blood)

[a] The influence of blood groups is described in Table 83.40.
[b] A list of some of these abnormalities is presented by Vesell (1978).

TABLE 83.33 *How may the potential influence of the patient's race or ethnic background on the interpretation of clinical data be measured or controlled?*

1. Conduct the trial only in patients of one race or of one ethnic background
2. Randomize patients of each race separately to treatment groups to ensure approximately equal number of patients of each race in each treatment group
3. Conduct a pilot trial prior to the major trial
4. Evaluate each patient for the presence or absence of specific markers (e.g., G-6-P-D deficiency, sickle cell anemia)
5. Evaluate only patients of the race with atypical results. In this group compare patients with and without a specific genetic (or laboratory) marker
6. Compare data obtained in patients of different races or ethnic backgrounds
7. Compare social, economic, education, and other factors between the groups studied

TABLE 83.35 *How may the potential influence of genetic history on the interpretation of data be measured or controlled?*

1. Exclude patients from the trial who have specific genetic characteristics that either place them at high risk or render them less responsive to treatment (e.g., blood types, inability to metabolize certain medicines rapidly)
2. Obtain a careful genetic history
3. Evaluate laboratory markers indicative of specific genetic characteristics
4. Evaluate groups of patients with and without the genetic characteristic in question
5. Perform a subgroup analysis after the trial is completed of patients with and without the genetic characteristic in question

TABLE 83.36 *How may circadian and circaseptan (7-day) rhythms bias data or affect their interpretation?*

A. Circadian rhythms may be related to or affect
   1. Pharmacokinetics, especially metabolism[a]
   2. Various chemical and endocrinological levels[b]
   3. Certain diseases[c,d] (e.g., rheumatoid arthritis, allergic diseases, asthma)
   4. Immunological parameters[d] (e.g., blood lymphocytes, immediate and delayed hypersensitivity responses, responses to antigen challenges)
   5. Responses of diseases to medicines (e.g., solid tumors,[e] diabetes,[e] adrenal insufficiency)
   6. Various physiological parameters[f] (e.g., heart rate, peak expiratory flow rate, body temperature)
   7. Perinatal death[g]

B. Circadian rhythms depend on or are influenced by
   1. Patients age[h]
   2. Medicines used to treat patients
   3. Psychiatric state of the patient

C. Circaseptan rhythms may be related to or affect human
   1. Kidney rejection[i]
   2. Recovering from postoperative swelling[j]
   3. Milk-binding activity[k]

D. Circannual rhythms may be related to or affect emergency room drug-overdose admissions[l]

[a] Vesell et al. (1977) and Reinberg and Smolensky (1982).
[b] Wisser and Breuer (1981).
[c] Wehr and Wirz-Justice (1982) and Moore-Ede et al. (1983).
[d] Dammacco et al. (1984)
[e] Stupfel (1975) and Focan (1979). Other related results obtained in animals are reviewed by Dammacco et al. (1984).
[f] Reinberg and Halberg (1971).
[g] Paccaud et al. (1988).
[h] Casale and de Nicola (1984).
[i] De Vecchi et al. (1979) and Besarab et al. (1983).
[j] Pöllmann (1983).
[k] Agrimonti et al. (1982).
[l] Morris (1987).

TABLE 83.37 *How may the potential influence of circadian rhythms on the interpretation of data be measured or controlled?[a,b]*

1. Compare data collected at different times of the day within patients and between groups of patients
2. Conduct all measurements at the same time of day
3. Perform subgroup analyses of factors that may have interacted with circadian rhythms (e.g., those listed in the preceding table) to evaluate the contribution of each factor

[a] Many more circadian and other inherent biological rhythms have been demonstrated in animals than in man (Reinberg and Halberg, 1971) This is not to suggest that humans differ from animals but that additional biological rhythms in humans will probably be demonstrated in time.
[b] Other biological and environmental rhythms are described in Tables 83.78 to 83.80.

TABLE 83.38 *How may a patient's menstrual cycle bias data or affect their interpretation?[a]*

1. Patients may have a changing baseline relating to trial measurements during the month, which may affect the activity of the medicine
2. Patients may experience behavioral or other adverse reactions related to the menstrual cycle, which could be attributed to medicine
3. Patients may have interactions of medicine and menstrual cycle leading to adverse reactions
4. Patients may be less compliant with trial medicine or trial protocol (e.g., keeping a diary, keeping appointments) because of adverse reactions from the menstrual period
5. Data obtained in various tests may be influenced by factors that are objective (e.g., hormonal blood levels) or subjective (e.g., patient's state of well-being)
6. Kinetics of medicines may be affected differently throughout the cycle[b]

[a] For example see Fourestié et al. (1986).
[b] Bruguerolle (1986); Wilson et al. (1982).

TABLE 83.39 *How may the potential influence of a patient's menstrual cycle on the interpretation of data be measured or controlled?*

1. Collect detailed information on the cycle, its periodicity, and subjective effects. Compare data obtained during different parts of the cycle
2. Exclude women who are still menstruating, particularly in pharmacokinetic trials
3. In acute trials (up to approximately 1 week), exclude women who are currently menstruating or who expect to begin their menstrual period during the trial
4. Evaluate the data for a 3- to 4-week periodicity that might be influenced by menstrual cycles
5. Conduct a separate trial in which menstrual cycles are examined in depth
6. Evaluate whether women with a history of clinically significant adverse reactions to their menstrual cycles perform differently in efficacy tests during peak or trough periods of the cycle or have clinically important adverse reactions on medicine. If so, is there a correlation between the time of occurrence of the menstrual cycle and either the adverse reactions or performance peaks (or troughs)?
7. Evaluate any influence the medicine may have on the duration or intensity of the menstrual period
8. Evaluate any influence the menstrual period has on the disease[a]
9. Evaluate women who use oral contraceptives separately from those who do not

[a] For example, see Newmark and Penry (1980).

TABLE 83.40. *How may the patient's blood group bias data or affect their interpretation?*

1. Certain blood groups may have importance as prognostic indicators of survival in specific diseases[a]
2. The presence or absence of blood groups from the surface of specific cells may be a prognostic indicator of how a disease will progress[b]
3. The type of blood group may relate to a patient's susceptibility to certain infectious diseases[c]
4. The type of blood group may relate to a patient's susceptibility to recurrent but not acute disease[d]

[a] For example, the type of blood groups are reported to be a prognostic indicator in patients with breast cancer (Holdsworth et al., 1985).
[b] For example, the presence of blood groups are reported to be a prognostic indicator in patients with bladder cancer (Lange et al., 1978).
[c] Kinane et al. (1982) describe recurrent urinary tract infections and have references to several other infectious diseases. Gupta and Chowdhuri (1980) describe malaria and have references to various diseases not referenced by Kinane et al.
[d] Sotto et al. (1983) describe a relationship of blood groups with recurrent but not nonrecurrent giardiasis.

TABLE 83.41 *How may the education of patients in a trial bias data or affect their interpretation?*

1. More patients who have a certain level of education may understand instructions, how to complete certain forms, perform certain tests, and take their medication as prescribed.
2. Only patients with a certain level of education may be treated in a positive interactive way by the investigator and staff
3. Compliance may differ in patients with a lower level of intelligence or education
4. Differences in education may be associated with differences in social/psychological behavior or other factors, which are the primary reasons why the data are influenced
5. Understanding patient package inserts may vary according to a patient's education (e.g., a package insert for patients that is only understood by well-educated individuals may lead to serious problems)

TABLE 83.42 *How may the potential influence of the patient's education (and/or intelligence) on the interpretation of clinical data be measured or controlled?*

1. Evaluate the trial participants' level of education and determine if it differs between treatment groups. If so, determine whether the difference is relevant to the study's outcome
2. Randomize patients according to their level of education or intelligence measured with a standard test either to balance all treatment groups or to create groups differing in terms of education
3. Conduct the trial only in patients with a narrow (or broad) range of education levels or intelligence

TABLE 83.43 *How may the diet of patients in a clinical trial bias data or affect their interpretation?[a]*

1. Interaction of a food or beverage with the medicine (e.g., alcohol interacts with diazepam)
2. Certain types of food or meals may decrease absorption of the trial medicine
3. Influence of dietary factors on some or all laboratory tests
4. Excessive amount of a food or beverage may lead to adverse reactions
5. Hypersensitivity reactions to food may occur that are attributed to the trial medicine

[a] See Tables 87.21 to 87.23 for additional information.

TABLE 83.44 *How may the potential influence of diet on the interpretation of clinical data be measured or controlled?*

1. Have all patients receive a standard diet
2. Provide information and/or counseling on acceptable diets
3. Provide information on appropriate times to take trial medicine relative to meals
4. Exclude patients who follow fad or unacceptable diets
5. Compare effects of medicine in groups of patients with and without the presence of food
6. Compare pharmacokinetic or medicine effects in patients receiving two or more types of diets (e.g., high or low protein, high or low fat, high or low carbohydrate)

TABLE 83.45 *How may the presence of patients who are pregnant or lactating bias data or affect their interpretation?[a]*

1. Physical condition of the mother may be affected (e.g., morning sickness, fatigue, emotional stress), which may affect data obtained
2. Distribution and blood levels of a medicine, especially in the third trimester (when the placenta and fetus are large), may differ between pregnant and nonpregnant women or between different medicines that are being compared
3. Many agents not generally considered medicines could differ between groups of women and affect the data obtained. These agents include alcohol, cigarettes, caffeine-containing drinks, vitamin and mineral supplements, diet, and laxatives. Other factors such as exercise, sleep, feeling of well-being, and level of physical activity may also affect data[b]
4. Women who are at one stage of pregnancy (or labor) may react differently to a medicine or intervention than women who are at a different stage

[a] See additional tables in Chapter 87.
[b] Pregnant women often differ from nonpregnant women with respect to these factors.

TABLE 83.46 *How may the potential influence of pregnancy or lactation on the interpretation of clinical data be measured or controlled?[a]*

1. Compare data obtained in lactating or pregnant women with and without the trial medicine or intervention
2. Compare a group of pregnant and nonpregnant women
3. Compare a group of lactating and nonlactating women
4. Evaluate each of the possible confounding factors in the groups of pregnant women given the trial medicine or intervention
5. Measure the amount of medicine in mother's milk at different periods after ingestion
6. Compare women who are at different stages of pregnancy (or labor) to evaluate the influence of the specific stage

[a] See additional tables in Chapter 87.

TABLE 83.47 *How may social or economic factors of patients in a clinical trial bias data or affect their interpretation?*

1. If patients of lower economic levels are required to provide transportation or meals they cannot afford (and are not reimbursed for), their compliance may markedly decline, which could bias data
2. Patients of different social classes have sometimes been reported to respond differently to treatment,[a] but the relevance of this factor has often been exaggerated[b]
3. The relationship of the investigator and staff with patients may be influenced by each of their social classes[c] and/or education.[d] This in turn could influence clinical responses and compliance by those patients
4. Patients who see the same physician at each visit may be more satisfied and have improved clinical reactions[e]
5. The personal relationships of patients with their family, friends, and others may influence the reactions of patients to treatment. Alternatively, adverse reactions of a medicine in patients may affect relationships with others and indirectly affect the willingness of patients to be compliant with the trial protocol
6. Personal habits such as use of alcohol, cigarettes and other tobacco products,[f] plus caffeine-containing beverages may have a significant impact on data obtained
7. Drug abuse or personal habits carried to extremes (e.g., some cases of dieting or exercising) may influence response to medicine and alter or bias data interpretation
8. The manner in which patients are recruited (i.e., methods and inducements used) may affect the motivation of patients and their attitudes toward the trial
9. If patient recruitment is too slow, there may be different types of patients entered in the trial in the early, middle, and late phases. Patients may be tested or treated differently depending on when they were enrolled
10. One method should be used to enroll patients in most situations, since patients enrolled in a trial may differ in their demographic, disease, or other characteristics when they are recruited by different techniques and may not be randomly allocated to treatment groups.
11. Patients may have allergies to pets or may acquire various diseases from pets
12. Patients may acquire a concurrent or confounding (1) disease or (2) undiagnosed problem during foreign (or domestic) travel
13. Lower-income patients tend to go to a university hospital rather than a community hospital,[g] which may influence the composition of patients recruited in a trial
14. Certain occupations have increased risk factors for specific diseases or problems[h]
15. Sanitation standards as well as crowding may influence infant mortality[j]
16. The incidence of some diseases and patient survival have been associated with social class[k]
17. Physical contact with the spouse may cause creams to transfer and lead to adverse reactions[l]
18. Marital status has been associated with survival from cancer[m]

[a] Snowden and Pearson (1984).
[b] Larson and Marcer (1984).
[c] This concept could be expanded to include any other patient characteristic (e.g., intelligence, religion).
[d] Waitzkin (1984).
[e] Wasson et al. (1984).
[f] Jusko (1978). See Chapter 87 for additional tables.
[g] Gross (1984) lists several additional demographic differences between university and community hospitals.
[h] Clarke and Mason (1985). See Chapter 87 for additional tables and references.
[j] Rahman et al. (1985).
[k] See Chapter 87 for references and additional details.
[l] Moore et al. (1988).
[m] Goodwin et al. (1987).

TABLE 83.48 *How may the type and geographical location of residence bias data or affect their interpretation?*

1. Patients living in apartments have been reported to have greater morbidity than those living in houses[a]
2. Patients living in smaller-spaced residences have been reported to have a higher incidence of respiratory infections
3. Patients in rural and urban locations may yield different responses as a result of stress or other reactions
4. Patients in a particular geographical location may have a reputation for social habits that differ from those in other areas (e.g., official rates of alcohol-related problems differ greatly in different areas, which in at least one situation was largely a reflection of admission policies in psychiatric hospitals),[b] which may influence the perspectives of physicians who interpret data
5. The number of physicians and/or surgeons may differ greatly between different areas and thus influence referral practices, amount and type of surgery practiced, and perspectives of physicians in treating patients[c]
6. Specific geographical locations may have a high percentage of patients with a particular heritage, race, or nationality

[a] Fanning (1967).
[b] Latcham et al. (1984).
[c] Bunker (1970), Vayda (1973), and McPherson et al. (1981).

TABLE 83.49 *How may the potential influence of the patient's social or economic factors on the interpretation of clinical data be measured or controlled?*

1. Compare data obtained in patients of different social or economic levels
2. Provide reimbursement or funds for transportation, meals, or other uses when absence of such money may affect patient motivation and/or participation in a trial
3. If the social or economic level of patients is believed to be a significant factor in influencing patient responses, then stratify patients according to this factor to create balanced groups or create groups based on social or economic factors
4. If personal relationships of patients with others are expected to have a large bearing on data obtained, conduct an inpatient study (if practical and possible) or else monitor the relevant relationships (e.g., with patient diaries) so that their potential influence may be assessed at a later date.
5. Measure amount and type of alcohol, cigarettes and tobacco products, or drinks containing caffeine consumed per day or week
6. Exclude patients from a trial if they consume more than a preset amount of alcohol, cigarettes or other tobacco products, or drinks containing caffeine
7. Patients who abuse drugs or follow certain diets or exercise more than a preset amount may be excluded.
8. If several methods of recruitment are used, evaluate the influence of recruitment by comparing data from groups recruited differently. Also compare the demographics and baseline parameters of groups recruited by different techniques
9. Compare data separately for patients with and without exposure to pets
10. Compare data from patients who live in different locations or types of dwellings
11. Include sites in a multicenter trial that represent different geographical locations and both rural and urban environments or only one particular environment
12. Evaluate the ethnic mix of the patients recruited and determine whether the factor played a role in the data obtained

TABLE 83.50 *How may psychological factors of patients in a clinical trial bias data or affect their interpretation?*

1. Patients with a strong desire for treatment and improvement often improve more than do patients who feel neutral or resist encouragement or actual attempts to have them improve
2. Patients who are compliant and cooperative with a trial protocol may yield different data than patients whose compliance and/or cooperation is less
3. Excessive demands placed on patients in terms of waiting time in an office, repetition of tests, unpleasantness of tests, and/or prolonged periods in the testing facility may influence data of each patient who experiences them
4. Significant personal events (e.g., death or illness of a person close to the patient, new or changed relationship, concurrent illness, or trauma of patient) may alter that patient's response in the trial. Several such events, especially in one treatment group, may bias group data and their interpretation
5. The quality of the physician–patient relationship and adequacy of communications are highly dependent on the sex of each and their economic background and status, education, prognosis, and social class.[a] This relationship may greatly affect the patient's responses to treatment
6. Patients who decline to enter a trial because of the informed consent may introduce a bias that causes either false-positive or false-negative results[b]
7. Historical controls did not sign an informed consent in most cases or undergo the psychological "stresses" of being in a trial and thus are not comparable to a group that has had these experiences
8. Stress may have various effects on immunological function, long-term survival in patients with cancer, hormonal levels, and other medical factors[c]
9. Patients who are nearing the end of a trial or the end of a particular day may be anxious to go home and may greatly increase or decrease their responses (e.g., on FEV_1)

[a] Waitzkin (1984).
[b] Edlund et al. (1985).
[c] Anonymous (1985b).

TABLE 83.51 *How may the potential influence of patients' psychological factors on interpretation of clinical data be measured or controlled?*

1. Evaluate each patient's desire for treatment and improvement and compare data obtained for those with strong versus little or no desire
2. Evaluate each patient's degree of compliance and compare data obtained for those with excellent, adequate, or poor compliance
3. Ensure that excessive demands are not made on patients and monitor relevant factors throughout the trial
4. Determine if any significant personal events may have affected the trial by conducting an interview at the end of the trial. This interview may be conducted during the trial if there is a reason to question this factor
5. Compliance is a measure not only of whether a patient takes medicines as prescribed but whether he or she adheres to the protocol and its spirit. There are important issues of compliance in some trials that relate to (1) adherence to scheduled visits, (2) making an appropriate effort on tests that require voluntary exertion, and (3) having a positive attitude toward the trial. These factors may be measured or rated
6. Standardize the methods used to motivate patients to perform well in all tests. Indicate what techniques were used and evaluate the effects of learning on performance in tests (as a result of repeated testing)
7. Evaluate the adequacy of communications between patients and physicians and determine the quality of the overall relationship and which factors (e.g., gender, class, economic status) may have influenced the data or should be controlled (if any)
8. Evaluate the relationship between patients and staff conducting the trial

TABLE 83.52 *Specific factors related to the disease or problem being evaluated in a clinical trial that may bias data or affect their interpretation*

1. The operational definition of the disease and its application in the trial by various investigators
2. True change in the incidence of the disease over a period of time (e.g., years or decades)
3. Spurious change in the incidence of the disease over a period of time (e.g., relating from increased or decreased reporting, improved diagnostic capabilities, confusion of prevalence and incidence)
4. Number of patients affected that are available for evaluation
5. Presence of subtypes of the disease
6. Ability to diagnose the disease with relative certainty
7. Etiologies of the disease or condition studied
8. Secondary problems resulting from the disease

TABLE 83.53 *How may factors related to the disease being evaluated bias data or affect their interpretation?*

1. Different diseases or subtypes diagnosed (or classified) as being the same will bias the data if patients with different subtypes respond differently to treatment
2. Etiologies of the disease may vary widely (e.g., for congestive heart failure), and different etiologies of the same disease that are diagnosed (or classified) as similar or the same may influence the response to treatment and bias interpretations of the data
3. Patients with many previous episodes or exacerbations of a disease may react differently than patients having no previous episodes or only a small number. Data that are predominantly from one such group may yield a different interpretation than data obtained in the other.
4. Patients with a severe intensity of a disease may respond differently (quantitatively or qualitatively) than patients with a mild form of a disease. Data that are predominantly obtained in one group may yield a different interpretation than data obtained in the other
5. Prior medicine and nonmedicine treatment of patients may affect their response or ability to respond to treatment in the current trial. An adequate washout period should be used prior to initiating a new treatment (whenever possible)
6. Concomitant medicines, either as part of the protocol in an add-on trial or taken outside the trial protocol, may have a marked influence on data obtained
7. Concurrent illnesses of either a chronic or acute nature may influence a patient's response to medicines or other treatment and bias the interpretation
8. Risk factors for either the disease being evaluated or other diseases may be a major influence on data obtained
9. Patients with compromised renal, liver, or other physiological function (e.g., immunocompromised patients) often respond differently to medicines
10. Various other manifestations of a disease may vary among the patients enrolled in a trial and may influence data obtained
11. If a rare disease is being studied, there may be numerous other factors to consider[a]
12. The controversial issue of whether obesity, alcoholism, and other "problems" are conditions or are diseases may influence the style and success of patient recruitment and treatment by investigators
13. The incidence of a disease or problem may change over time either depending on or independently of medicine use or other modalities.[b] This may especially be a problem if historical data are used as a control or if a retrospective study is conducted. The change may be real and based on a change in exposure to an etiologic or protective agent or a change in the presence or effectiveness of treatments. The change may be spurious based on differences in the accuracy and precision of the diagnosis made over time. This may occur as a result of new methodologies or new definitions
14. If trends in the severity of a disease are studied, they must be evaluated over a sufficient period of time for results to have validity[c]
15. Secondary medical problems resulting from a disease may affect a patient's responses to treatment

[a] See Spilker (1985).
[b] Taylor et al. (1984), Ikwueke (1984). Alderson (1974) illustrates this point quite convincingly for measles and diphtheria.
[c] Davis et al. (1983) and Nobrega et al. (1983).

TABLE 83.54 *How may the potential influence of a patient's disease factors on interpretation of clinical data be measured or controlled?*

1. The population of patients enrolled in a trial should be chosen extremely carefully. Nonetheless, the population of patients available for enrollment in a trial may differ markedly from those desired. The available population depends on what medicines or other treatments are currently available. This affects whether suitable patients or only resistant cases may be enrolled. Subgroup analyses may be performed to measure the importance of various disease factors
2. Changes in the incidence of a disease over time may be investigated through literature searches or through consultations with relevant government agencies, foundations, associations, or other groups
3. Evaluate the data both separately and together for patients who were misdiagnosed or for those who had a different disease subtype
4. Evaluate the data both separately and together for patients who have different etiologies of their disease
5. In trials in which a disease or condition is being evaluated that is controversial as to the patient's ability to control or influence its course (e.g., alcoholism, obesity), compare data obtained by investigators with different attitudes toward the "disease"

TABLE 83.55 *Specific factors related to a trial medicine that may bias data or affect their interpretation*

1. Dosage forms studied (e.g., tablet, elixir, solution, suppository)
2. Salt of medicine used
3. Promedicine versus parent medicine
4. Doses studied
5. Dosage regimen (e.g., frequency of dosing, time of dosing)
6. Routes of administration
7. Interactions with other medicines
8. Interactions with food
9. Interactions with nonmedicine factors (e.g., chemical contents of infusion solutions, walls of medicine container)
10. Excipients used in the formulation
11. Stability, storage, and preparation of medicine
12. Pharmacokinetic factors

TABLE 83.56 *How may characteristics of parenteral dosage forms used in a clinical trial bias data or affect their interpretation?*

1. Medicine may adhere to the walls of the container or tubing attached to patient (e.g., plastic, glass), and a smaller dose may reach the patient than intended or required
2. Medicine may be physically incompatible with the solution it is placed in and may form crystals, haze, globules, or other precipitates in an infusion side arm or syringe[a]
3. Medicine may be inactivated by the fluid or other medicines present in the i.v. tubing or syringe
4. The medicine may not be able to be mixed with blood without undergoing some deleterious chemical changes
5. The medicine may react with the contents of the stopper of the storage container
6. The medicine may be metabolized[b] by light during storage, preparation, or administration to the patient
7. The medicine may be metabolized if allowed to stand for too long a period after it is prepared
8. The medicine may be metabolized if the container is reused for a second or additional dose after a certain time period has elapsed
9. The medicine may only retain activity for a certain period after preparation even though it is kept on ice or at a suitable temperature
10. The medicine may require filters to be used before it can be administered to patients (to remove any particulates present above a certain size or number, which may cause phlebitis)[c]
11. The diluents used with the medicine may not be stable under all conditions

[a] Allen et al. (1977) and Johnston-Early et al. (1984).
[b] Medicines may be metabolized to inactive and/or active byproducts. Each of these will have its own profile of efficacy and safety.
[c] Falchuk et al. (1985). These authors reported that phlebitis associated with infusions is often related to this problem.

TABLE 83.57 *How may problems with parenteral dosage forms be measured or controlled?*

Most of the potential problems described in Table 83.56 may be evaluated in pharmaceutical tests prior to giving the medicine to humans. Steps to avoid each of those problems must be taken

TABLE 83.58 *Factors relating to the salt of the medicine or use of a promedicine that may bias data or affect their interpretation*

1. Salts of medicines often differ in their degree of absorption, which in turn may affect the peak blood concentration, degree and duration of therapeutic effect, plus incidence and severity of adverse reactions
2. Promedicines are often absorbed to a different degree than parent medicines, which may affect peak blood concentration, degree and duration of therapeutic effect, plus incidence and severity of adverse reactions

TABLE 83.59 *How may the doses used in a clinical trial bias data or affect their interpretation?*

1. If doses studied are at or below the threshold of the dose–response relationship, a false-negative response will occur
2. If doses studied are beyond those required to reach the peak of the dose–response curve, a higher incidence of adverse reactions and other problems (e.g., patient dropouts, lack of compliance, reduced overall efficacy) will probably occur
3. If concomitant diseases, medicines, or other factors prevent adequate doses from being tested, then a false-negative response may occur
4. If fixed doses of a medicine are used, they may not be appropriate to yield a positive response or dose response. In patients of widely different weights, the dose administered on a per-kilogram basis may vary enormously
5. If doses are titrated within fixed ranges, the ranges chosen may not be broad enough to elicit positive therapeutic responses

TABLE 83.60 *How may the potential influence of doses studied be measured or controlled?*

1. Determine a dose–response relationship in a pilot or separate trial to ascertain the appropriate range of doses to evaluate
2. Evaluate the influence of concomitant medicines, diseases, and other factors to identify pertinent interactions with the trial medicine or treatment
3. Consider dosing patients on a per-kilogram or other relative basis (e.g., milligrams per square meter) to avoid wide dosing differences in patients of different weights
4. Evaluate the effect of patient weight on responses if a fixed dose or fixed dose range is used

TABLE 83.61 *How may the dosage regimen[a] used in a clinical trial bias data or affect their interpretation?*

1. Patients taking medicines only during waking hours may not retain adequate blood levels during sleep to maintain a therapeutic effect (e.g., as with certain antibiotics)
2. Medicines taken either before or after meals may be absorbed to different degrees and thus yield different clinical effects. Diet may also affect medicine absorption
3. Medicines prescribed at convenient times for patients (e.g., morning and night) are taken as prescribed more often than when medicines are prescribed during the time that a patient is at work or away from home
4. Medicines that have an unpleasant odor, taste, or other characteristic will achieve less patient compliance than will a more neutral medicine
5. Children prefer certain flavors to others (e.g., grape flavor is usually preferred to licorice), and fluids with the preferred flavors are usually taken more as prescribed
6. Medicines given once a day are generally believed to have better compliance than medicines given more often
7. Dosages expressed in a form such as "20 mg/kg b.i.d." may be easily misinterpreted and lead to dosing errors, especially if more than one person doses patients for inpatient trials. The dose above may be interpreted as either 20 mg/kg per day split into two 10 mg/kg doses or as 40 mg/kg per day split into two 20 mg/kg doses

[a] The dosage regimen is defined as (1) the number of doses per given time period (usually days), (2) the time that elapses between doses (e.g., dose to be given every 6 hours) or the time that the doses are to be given (e.g., dose to be given at 8 A.M., noon, and 4 P.M. each day), and (3) the quantity of medicine or number of tablets (capsules, etc.) that are given at each specific dose.

TABLE 83.62 *How may the potential influence of dosage regimen on interpretation of clinical data be measured or controlled?*

1. Evaluate blood levels of medicine and/or its metabolites at numerous times after medicine administration
2. Evaluate if a minimum blood level is required to achieve a therapeutic effect
3. Evaluate the effect of food and diet on absorption of a medicine
4. Compare clinical effects of a medicine given at two (or more) different frequencies per day
5. Mask the flavor, taste, or other unpleasant characteristic of the medicine and reevaluate the clinical effect
6. Conduct a taste test using a panel of children or adults to evaluate patient preferences. A group of volunteers, patients, or professional tasters may be used
7. Evaluate patient compliance with two or more separate dosing regimens

TABLE 83.63 *How may the route of administration used in a clinical trial bias data or affect their interpretation?*

1. If less medicine is absorbed than is believed
2. If a route deemed unpleasant is used (e.g., rectal, intranasal, insufflation), that decreases patient compliance with the protocol
3. If patients are required to self-administer intramuscular injections, compliance may be less than if they are requested to inject themselves subcutaneously
4. A route that gives a high peak of medicine concentration in the plasma may yield a relatively high number of adverse reactions or abnormal safety results
5. A route that gives a rapid peak concentration of medicine often yields a plasma value and therapeutic effect that will not generally persist for as long a period as the effect resulting from the same medicine given by a route that reaches its peak concentration at a later time. This point assumes that the therapeutic effect results from the parent medicine and not from a metabolite, which could have a totally different time course from the parent medicine

TABLE 83.64 *How may the potential influence of the route of administration on interpretation of clinical data be measured or controlled?*

1. Compare data for patient compliance using two or more routes of administration
2. Measure amount of medicine absorbed with two or more routes of administration and follow the plasma concentrations over time. Compare various pharmacokinetic parameters

TABLE 83.65 *How may the interactions of a trial medicine with other medicines bias data or affect their interpretation?[a]*

1. Concomitant medicines may bind to proteins and displace the trial medicine, yielding elevated blood levels and increased toxicity or other effects
2. Concomitant medicines may be released from blood proteins by the trial medicine and lead to a wide variety of unanticipated effects
3. Concomitant medicines may affect the absorption, distribution, metabolism, or excretion of the trial medicine and cause falsely increased or decreased effects

[a] See Chapter 95 for additional information.

TABLE 83.66 *How may the potential influence of interactions with other medicines on interpretation of clinical data be measured or controlled?[a]*

1. Evaluate the absorption, distribution, metabolism, and excretion of a medicine in both the presence and absence of a concomitant medicine
2. Evaluate clinical effects of the trial medicine in groups of patients receiving specific (1) medicines, (2) doses of those medicines, and (3) medicine combinations

[a] See Chapter 95 for additional information.

TABLE 83.67 *How may the interactions of a trial medicine with food bias data or affect their interpretation?*

1. Patients who are fasted at the time they receive a medicine may behave differently than if they are fed
2. Patients who are always given a medicine either before, with, or after meals may behave differently than when a medicine is given at a different time relative to meals
3. Patients who take a medicine with or after meals may have different clinical effects depending on the content of the meal[a]

[a] See Chapter 87 for additional information.

TABLE 83.68 *How may the potential influence of interactions with food on interpretation of clinical data be measured or controlled?*

1. Evaluate medicines in both fasted and nonfasted patients
2. Evaluate medicine absorption in patients given medicine before, during, and after meals
3. Evaluate the content of meals on the absorption of medicines[a]
4. Evaluate interactions of food in patients with different genetic backgrounds or in patients of special populations

[a] See Chapter 87 for additional details.

TABLE 83.69 *How may the excipients in a medicine's formulation bias data or affect their interpretation?[a]*

1. Some excipients (e.g., color additives, preservatives) yield allergic and other adverse reactions[b]
2. Numerous excipients and formulation factors may adversely influence medicine availability and toxicity[c]
3. Identically named medicines may contain different excipients, which may affect various efficacy or safety parameters through differences in various properties (e.g., dissolution, dispersion, absorption) and thus yield different data and interpretations
4. The amount of excipients in a capsule, tablet, or other dosage form may affect medicine absorption[d]

[a] Excipients include binders, fillers, granulating agents, lubricants, antioxidants, wetting agents, disintegrants, dispersants, coatings, flavorings, coloring agents, diluents, suspending agents, and solubilizers (see Chapter 18 for a more complete list with examples).
[b] Pollock et al. (1989).
[c] Lach (1972).
[d] MacLeod (1972).

TABLE 83.70 *How may the potential influence of excipients on the interpretation of clinical data be measured or controlled?*

1. Ask the manufacturer for information on the identity and quantity of each excipient present in the medicine formulation
2. Compare lot and batch numbers of questionable lots and contact the manufacturer to inquire about the identity and amount of excipients used
3. Compare the amounts of excipients with those present in other medicine formulations[a]
4. Prepare formulations without specific excipients and compare them in tests with the original formulation
5. Dechallenge and rechallenge patients with questionable clinical responses. If the same marketed medicine with different excipients is available, it may be used as part of a rechallenge

[a] A list of antimicrobial preservatives by brand name and concentration or amount of preservative is given by Akers (1984). The article also lists the maximum acceptable concentrations for 11 antimicrobial agents.

TABLE 83.71 *How may the stability, storage, and preparation of medicines used in a clinical trial bias data or affect their interpretation?*

1. Outdated medicines (i.e., those whose expiration date has past) may have changed to a more toxic form (e.g., tetracyclines)
2. Outdated medicines may have partially or totally chemically degraded to inactive substances, and the smaller amount of an active medicine moiety may elicit a smaller clinical effect
3. Medicines that are inappropriately stored (e.g., outside of a refrigerator, exposed to light, on a hot water heating radiator) may lose their biological activity and yield a diminished clinical response
4. Medicines that are improperly prepared (e.g., thawed and refrozen, diluted, improperly mixed with the wrong diluent, mixed with another medicine or substance that inactivates the medicine) will usually yield false-negative data and may cause adverse reactions
5. Medicines that have been inappropriately stored by a wholesale distributor or retail store may have diminished biological activity before they reach the investigator or patient

TABLE 83.72 *How may the potential influence of stability, storage, and preparation of medicine on the interpretation of clinical data be measured or controlled?*

1. Inquire from the manufacturer about the precise methods that should be used to prepare and store the medicine
2. Carefully check the expiration date of medicines used in clinical trials
3. Send a sample of a questioned lot to the manufacturer for testing of its potency and to confirm that the medicine is what it is purported to be
4. Test a sample of a questioned lot in a suitable animal model, preferably in direct comparison with a sample from a lot known to be fully active

TABLE 83.73 *How may the pharmacokinetic factors of medicines used in a clinical trial bias data or affect their interpretation?[a]*

1. An adequate number of biological samples must be obtained from each patient to obtain adequate information for a suitable profile on the phenomenon under investigation (e.g., peak of concentration, rate of elimination, half-life, trough level for multiple doses)
2. The time that samples are drawn relative to the time of dosing, peak level, and trough level is important to consider in determining an appropriate number of samples to collect. Inappropriate sampling times may lead to determination of incorrect values of pharmacokinetic factors
3. Clinical events may be independent of pharmacokinetic parameters (e.g., when the clinical effects are not related to the presence of medicine in the body). For instance, hypotension resulting from reserpine depletion of catecholamines is present long after reserpine has been eliminated from the body
4. Pharmacokinetic parameters of a parent medicine may lead to an incorrect interpretation of pharmacokinetic data unless adequate information on the presence and pharmacokinetic parameters of significant active metabolites is known
5. The absorption, distribution, metabolism, or excretion of a medicine may be altered by a variety of factors (e.g., concomitant medicines, age, physiological function). The influence of each relevant factor may be important to determine
6. The relative concentration, biological activity, and pharmacokinetic parameters of parent medicine and each metabolite are all important factors to consider in evaluating the effects of a medicine in a trial

[a] The few points listed refer primarily to methodological factors. Additional factors are presented in Chapter 84.

TABLE 83.74 *How may the potential influence of pharmacokinetic factors on interpretation of clinical data be measured or controlled?[a]*

1. Discuss the appropriate number of samples to collect and when to collect them with a pharmacokineticist
2. Simulate the blood levels of upcoming experiments on a computer to plan and control the trial better
3. Evaluate biological fluids for metabolites of the parent medicine. Attempt to synthesize and then evaluate any metabolites identified
4. Measure the absorption, distribution, metabolism, and excretion of the medicine under carefully controlled conditions

[a] See Chapter 84 for additional information.

TABLE 83.75 *Specific factors related to the investigator, clinical trial staff, and sponsor that may bias data or affect their interpretation*

1. Adherence to the protocol
2. Adherence to "good clinical practice"
3. Quality and quantity of trial monitoring
4. Maintenance of the trial blind
5. Collection of data
6. Ability to solve problems that arise effectively
7. Relationship of investigator with the sponsor
8. Relationship of investigator and staff with patients
9. Relationship of investigator with his or her Ethics Committee/Institutional Review Board
10. Adequacy of investigator's equipment and physical facilities
11. Proximity of investigator to other facilities where data must be obtained in a timely fashion

TABLE 83.76 *How may the characteristics of the investigator/staff who plan or conduct a clinical trial bias data or affect their interpretation?*

1. Adherence of the investigator and staff to the protocol will exert a major influence on the data obtained
2. Adherence of the investigator and staff to the principles of "good clinical practice" will affect data obtained
3. Maintenance of the trial blind is important to ensure the integrity of the data
4. Collection of "all" necessary data is important to arrive at the proper interpretation
5. The nature of the relationship of the investigator and staff with patients, sponsor, and Ethics Committee/Institutional Review Board may influence how the trial is conducted and affect the data obtained.

TABLE 83.77 *How may the potential influence of investigator/staff characteristics on interpretation of clinical data be measured or controlled?*

1. The primary means of ensuring that the investigator and staff adhere to the protocol and to principles of "good clinical practice" is for careful monitoring to occur by the investigator(s), staff (internal monitoring), sponsor (external monitoring), FDA (regulatory monitoring), and Ethics Committee/Institutional Review Board (institutional monitoring)
2. The maintenance of the trial blind may be evaluated by various methods
3. Careful and periodic monitoring and troubleshooting will help ensure that data collection is progressing in a correct and timely manner
4. If an interview, questionnaire, or data collection form contains information or data that are not clear, follow up to clarify the point. In certain situations it may be useful to ask "What do you think the patient meant when he or she said. . . ."
5. The relationship of the investigator and staff with patients, sponsor, and Ethics Committee/Institutional Review Board may be assessed by carefully conducted interviews or by other techniques

TABLE 83.78 *Environmental factors in a clinical trial that may bias data or affect their interpretation*

A. Environmental factors that are primarily outdoors
1. Unexpected climatic variations, cycles, or extreme events
2. Weather conditions[a]
3. Air pollution in the outside environment
4. Barometric pressure
5. Amount of sunlight
B. Environmental factors that are primarily indoors
1. Quality of air inside the trial building(s)[b]
2. Airborne transmission of disease and infection[c]
3. Home or work environment, including physical and nonphysical hazards, and the "sick building syndrome"[d]
4. Whether one lives in a home or high-rise apartment[e]
5. Quality of light in the building or ward[f]
6. Design of the ward (for inpatient trials)[g]
7. Dampness in the building[h]
C. Other environmental factors
1. Biological rhythms influenced by the environment (e.g., lunar,[j] seasonal[k])
2. Composition of water used for drinking and cooking
3. Water in cooling towers and evaporative condensers[l]

[a] Anonymous (1985a) and Carey and Cordon (1986).
[b] Brundage et al. (1988).
[c] Ehrenkranz and Kicklighter (1972), Gundermann (1980), Imperato (1981), Ager and Tickner (1983), Remington et al. (1985), and Howorth (1985).
[d] Finnegan et al. (1984) and Riesenberg and Arehart-Treichel (1986).
[e] Fanning (1967), Moore (1976), and Cook and Morgan (1982).
[f] Ott (1976), Sterling and Sterling (1983), Glass et al. (1985), and London (1987).
[g] Whitehead et al. (1984).
[h] Martin et al. (1987).
[j] Vul (1976).
[k] Ransil et al. (1977), Khot et al. (1984), and Weiss (1990).
[l] Miller (1979).

TABLE 83.79 *How may environmental factors bias data or affect their interpretation?*

1. Various factors inherent in the environment may affect patient behavior, cooperation, symptoms, clinical responses, and other data obtained. These factors include pollution, climate, and amount of sunlight
2. Various factors concerning the patient's environment may be created or influenced by the specific medicine, surgery, or other treatment (e.g., hazards for driving because of medicine-induced adverse reactions)
3. Various biological rhythms may play a major role in the quality and type of data obtained and, if data are collected at various times in a biological cycle, may lead to an incorrect interpretation
4. The patient's home drinking water may contain high levels of specific substances (e.g., aluminum) or radiation, which could affect the data collected
5. The season of the year has been shown to be a relevant factor in influencing results obtained in various clinical situations[a]
6. Environmental exposure to toxins, such as heavy metals, insecticides, organic solvents, or other chemicals, may affect data
7. The number of cases of a disease may be influenced by airborne spread of infection even after the index case has left the site where infection was initiated[b]
8. The patient's work environment may cause a high incidence of symptoms that may be interpreted as trial-related adverse reactions[c]
9. It has been reported that young women and children who live in apartments require more primary health care than those living in houses[d]
10. Individuals who have a neurotic personality and live in apartments are at an increased risk of developing psychiatric symptoms[e]
11. Passive smoking (i.e., breathing air that contains tobacco smoke) may aggravate various diseases (e.g., angina pectoris,[f] asthma[g]) and represents a potentially serious form of air pollution[g]
12. Weather conditions may cause greater (or lesser) levels of pollens and fungal spores and affect patients with asthma[h]
13. The design of an inpatient ward may facilitate or deter social contact and interaction among patients, which would be especially important in a psychiatric ward[i]

[a] Ransil et al. (1977), Khot and Burn (1984), and Khot et al. (1984).
[b] Remington et al. (1985).
[c] Finnegan et al. (1984). See Chapter 15 for additional information.
[d] Fanning (1967).
[e] Moore (1976) and Cook and Morgan (1982).

[f] Aronow (1978).
[g] Sterling and Kobayashi (1977) and Weber and Fischer (1980).
[h] Anonymous (1985a) and Packe and Ayres (1985).
[i] Whitehead et al. (1984).

TABLE 83.80 *How may the potential influence of environmental factors on interpretation of clinical data be measured or controlled?*

1. Data may be subdivided and analyzed by groups according to various environmental factors or seasons of the year
2. Responses obtained at different parts of the day, lunar month, menstrual cycle, or according to other biological rhythms may be evaluated[a]
3. Responses that show regression to the mean or median of a measured event's frequency may be evaluated[b]
4. Patients may be removed from the environment responsible for a problem so that the issue may be evaluated
5. Conditions may be altered to improve the environment (e.g., remove allergens with air filters, eliminate parasites from the place where patients live) and new data collected
6. Suspected environmental factors (e.g., air, water) may be analyzed for composition and potential toxins
7. The building may be evaluated to determine if it is a "sick building." Postulated causes of this problem include (1) the presence of formaldehyde in insulation, furniture, and carpet adhesive, (2) excess number of airborne particles, (3) excess carbon dioxide, (4) bacteria in the air from contamination of the humidifiers, (5) cigarette smoke, (6) poor circulation of air, and (7) lack of negative ions[c]

[a] See Spilker and Segreti (1984) for references.
[b] Spilker and Segreti (1984).
[c] Finnegan et al. (1984).

TABLE 83.81 *Specific factors relating to the conduct of a clinical trial that may bias data or affect their interpretation*

1. Nature and source(s) of patient recruitment
2. Duration of time over which patients are enrolled
3. Location of site(s) where trial is conducted
4. Personal safety of patients in and near the site where the trial is conducted
5. Convenience of trial site for transportation, parking, access to laboratories, and other facilities
6. Requirements to move to various locations for trial tests, examinations, or procedures

TABLE 83.82 *How may factors related to the conduct of a clinical trial bias data or affect their interpretation?*

1. If the trial site is difficult to get to or has inadequate parking, it may compromise the compliance of patients with adhering to scheduled visits
2. If the trial site is relatively unsafe, it may compromise the compliance of patients with adhering to scheduled visits
3. If patient enrollment is too slow, the validity of the data may be questioned since conditions change over time and patients who enrolled early in the trial may differ from those who enrolled later
4. Methods used to enroll patients may change during a trial, and different types of patients may be recruited later in the trial who differ in significant characteristics from patients recruited earlier in the trial

TABLE 83.83 *How may the potential influence of factors related to conduct of a clinical trial on interpretation of clinical data be measured or controlled?*

1. A questionnaire or interview may be used to evaluate the degree of patient dissatisfaction with safety, parking, transportation, or other features of the trial site
2. The degree of patient compliance with attending all scheduled visits may be evaluated
3. The demographics and responses of patients enrolled in the first half of the trial may be compared with those enrolled in the second half (or other fraction) of the trial
4. The demographics and responses of patients recruited by various methods may be compared

TABLE 83.84 *Specific factors related to the tests and parameters used in a clinical trial that may bias data or affect their interpretation*

A. Factors related to the choice of tests and parameters
   1. Efficacy tests used (e.g., number of tests used, choice of specific tests, validation of tests used)
   2. Parameters chosen to follow in the efficacy tests used
   3. Safety tests used (e.g., number of different tests used, choice of specific tests, validation of tests used)
   4. Parameters chosen to follow in the safety tests used
   5. Ranking of efficacy parameters by importance in addressing trial objectives
B. Factors related to the conduct of the tests
   1. Time allowed between subsequent efficacy tests
   2. Time allowed between subsequent tests for ensuring patient safety
   3. Time required for data from various laboratory tests to be completed and for reports to be available to the investigator for interpretation
   4. Posture or position of patient while taking the test(s)[a]
C. Factors related to the data collected in the tests
   1. Number of measurements of efficacy tests conducted
   2. Number of measurements made of individual tests for patient safety

[a] An example of how arm position affects measurement of blood pressure was presented by Webster et al. (1984). Responses to diuretics are also dependent on posture (Ring-Larsen et al., 1986).

TABLE 83.85 *How may the efficacy tests used in a clinical trial bias data or affect their interpretation?*

1. Inappropriately chosen efficacy tests may yield biased or incorrect data. Too few efficacy tests may not yield adequate data to support an interpretation of efficacy. Inadequately validated tests may not yield data that are convincing to others
2. Using efficacy tests inappropriately, inconsistently, or incorrectly (e.g., improper calibration, incorrect use of equipment or instrument, incorrect data acquisition, variations in methods used by a patient to take a test)
3. Too few measurements obtained during baseline or treatment
4. Obtaining too many measurements in one test or repeating the test without an adequate rest period may have led to patient fatigue or frustration
5. Using tests just before or after a meal or when the patient is tired
6. Data that are not delivered to the investigator expeditiously from a laboratory or other facility may lead to delays in modifying or adjusting the patient's treatment according to a protocol

TABLE 83.86 *How may the potential influence of efficacy tests on interpretation of clinical data be measured or controlled?*

1. Discuss the choice of the most appropriate efficacy tests and parameters to measure with peers, colleagues, or consultants prior to a clinical trial
2. Rank efficacy parameters by their importance prior to a trial
3. Define standards of activity or success prior to a trial
4. Determine an appropriate number of efficacy evaluations to perform as well as appropriate methods to conduct the tests
5. Ensure that the staff operating the test(s) understand the proper methods for doing this, including calibrating equipment and standardizing means of instructing patients on how to take the test(s)
6. Confirm that all patients understand how to perform the test prior to its use. Confirm that patients actually perform the test or use the instrument in the correct manner
7. Conduct all tests at the same time of day unless it is known that this factor has no effect on results. Allow the same amount of time to elapse for all patients before and/or after medicine administration before conducting the test
8. Conduct tests at different times of day to evaluate the influence of this factor
9. Conduct tests when patients are fatigued and compare results with those obtained when they are alert
10. Conduct a different number of tests during a day and evaluate the optimal rest period before repeating a test or conducting a different one
11. Conduct several tests with patients to evaluate whether there is a learning effect that affects results

TABLE 83.87 *How may the safety tests used in a clinical trial bias data or affect their interpretation?*

1. Inappropriately chosen safety tests may not discern important safety problems for patients. Patients may be allowed to continue in a trial when they should be discontinued (or vice versa)
2. An inadequate number of safety tests may be used and miss observations on important events
3. The parameters chosen to follow (monitor) certain areas of potential problems may be inappropriate or less than optimal (e.g., using SGOT rather than SGPT to follow specific liver changes, CPK rather than the MB band of CPK to check for evidence of a myocardial infarction)
4. Too few measurements may be made during a trial, which allows long periods of inadequately monitored safety to elapse. This creates opportunities for potentially serious safety-related problems to develop and remain undetected
5. If too great a period elapses before data obtained in a test are returned to the investigator, it allows an opportunity for patient safety to be more seriously affected
6. Patients may take safety tests in different ways, and the lack of consistency may affect data (e.g., posture of patients during blood pressure measurements has an influence on results)[a]

[a] Webster et al. (1984).

TABLE 83.88 *How may the potential influence of safety tests on interpretation of clinical data be measured or controlled?*

1. Discuss the choice of the most appropriate safety tests and parameters to measure with peers, colleagues, or consultants prior to a clinical trial
2. Determine an appropriate number of evaluations of each safety test to perform during baseline, treatment, and follow-up
3. Ensure that the staff obtaining samples and operating any tests are well trained
4. Provide instructions to patients, encouraging them to report any specific or general observations that may be relevant for their safety
5. Provide instructions to patients or their families to conduct simple tests for safety
6. Conduct each test at the same time of day in a chronic trial unless it is known that this factor is not relevant to data obtained or is not possible to do
7. Conduct each test the same number of hours after the most recent ingestion of medicine in a chronic trial
8. Evaluate the influence of points 6 and 7

TABLE 83.89 *Selected factors related to statistics that may bias data or affect their interpretation*

1. Obtaining sufficient power in the clinical trial
2. Choice of valid statistical tests to analyze data
3. Conduct of interim analyses on data
4. Reporting the fact that interim analyses or peeks at the data were conducted
5. Consideration of patients excluded from data analysis
6. General trial design (e.g., parallel versus crossover)

TABLE 83.90 *How may statistical factors relating to data analysis bias data or affect their interpretation?*

1. Clinical trials with inadequate power have a higher likelihood of having false-negative or false-positive data. Even if the interpretation turns out to be validated by subsequent trials, the original data will not have demonstrated the result in a convincing manner
2. If tests used to analyze the data are not the most appropriate ones or were not previously validated, then the data may be misinterpreted
3. If the tests used to analyze the data are appropriate but are improperly used, then the data may be misinterpreted
4. If the data analysis excluded results obtained from patients who dropped out of the trial or were discontinued by the investigator, then the data may be misinterpreted. For example, patients often stop taking medicine when they feel improved and may discontinue a trial for that reason. If this occurs, then it is important to include their data in the analysis
5. The classification of patients as "responders" or "nonresponders" is not always clear, and patients are not necessarily either one or the other. The distinction between these categories may be somewhat arbitrary and/or controversial. Yet this definition may affect whether data are interpreted in a positive or negative manner

TABLE 83.91 *How may the potential influence of statistical factors on interpretation of clinical data be measured or controlled?*

1. Ensure that only studies with a high likelihood of attaining an adequate statistical power are initiated
2. Utilize only validated statistical procedures or tests to analyze data unless there are compelling reasons to the contrary
3. Conduct checks of the processes followed in data analysis to ensure accuracy
4. Determine which types of patients and data may be legitimately excluded from analysis prior to the trial. All other data must be included in analysis. Define a "completed patient" prior to the trial
5. Data for the group of "completed patients" and all patients may be analyzed separately
6. Define the criteria by which a patient is said to be a "responder" or "nonresponder" prior to the trial, i.e., define the criteria for medicine activity

TABLE 83.92 *Selected factors related to data presentation that may bias data or affect their interpretation*

1. Specific types of tables and/or figures chosen to illustrate data (e.g., histograms, pie charts, line graphs)
2. Specific headings used in tables (e.g., appropriateness, clarity, comprehensiveness)
3. Ordinate and abscissa used (e.g., choice of measures, scales used)
4. Level of detail (i.e., summary of clinical trial, subgroup, individual patient)
5. Degree of completeness of all data presented
6. Presentation of raw data versus derived data
7. Presentation of only summary data on all patients or of individual data as well
8. Presentation of the variability observed in important measurements

TABLE 83.93 *How may the report or presentation of results from a clinical trial bias data or affect their interpretation?*

1. Certain presentations of data may present a limited viewpoint
2. The ordinate and abscissa may have been constructed to make a given effect appear greater or smaller
3. The units used to express results may make the data appear larger or smaller in scale
4. Presenting only summary data may not present an adequate view of the events that occurred in the trial
5. Inadequate description of the variability (e.g., without standard deviation values) will not permit a proper interpretation
6. Presenting only derived data will not usually permit an adequate interpretation

TABLE 83.94 *How may the potential influence of the report or presentation of clinical data on its interpretation be measured or controlled?*

1. Discuss choices of format for data presentation with a statistician or other colleagues
2. In addition to a manuscript submitted for publication, send the journal other data that may be placed in a repository[a]
3. Prepare the data in different types of tables and figures and compare with the original ones to determine whether the choice of table (or figure) influences the interpretation of data
4. Prepare the data with different scales (e.g., semilog, log–log) or transformations of data (e.g., normalization) and assess the impact of the change
5. Review the statistical report to evaluate whether additional information could be presented that has not been included

[a] This practice is used by selected journals. Materials may then be requested by interested readers. A selected list of journals that utilize this system is given in Chapter 106.

TABLE 83.95 *Selected types of errors committed accidentally in a clinical trial that may bias data or affect their interpretation*

A. Investigator or staff related
   1. Equipment calibrated incorrectly or not at all
   2. Errors made by investigator in measuring an objective endpoint[a]
   3. Errors in transcriptions of results from tests, equipment, or reports to data collection forms[b]
   4. Reports attributed to the wrong patient
   5. Incorrect medicines given to or supplied to patient
   6. Patients inadvertently informed or alerted about certain responses or symptoms that are of particular interest, which are under voluntary control
   7. Patients inadvertently informed or alerted about investigator's desires or expectations
   8. Patients inadvertently informed or alerted about their expected behavior pattern
   9. Patients incorrectly diagnosed and do not meet entry criteria of the trial
   10. Patients admitted into trial before all of their screening data are available and the patient is later shown not to qualify for entry
   11. Investigators take "shortcuts" in conducting the trial
B. Patient related
   1. Patients inadvertently taking a nontrial medicine that compromises their data
   2. Patients inadvertently taking an incorrect dose of the trial medicine, which compromises their data
   3. Patients forget to mention an important point relating to entry criteria to the investigator, which makes them ineligible for entry in the trial (e.g., previous reactions to medicines, previous hospitalizations)

[a] Moertel and Hanley (1976).
[b] Monson and Bond (1978) reported that 62% of patient medical charts they examined contained inaccuracies regarding directions or dosage of medicines and 21% of charts omitted the name(s) of at least one prescribed medicine. The more medicines a patient was given, the less accurately the patient record was noted to reflect the therapy prescribed.

TABLE 83.96 *Selected types of errors, negligence, or deceit that may purposely be committed in a clinical trial*

A. Emanating from the investigator or staff[a]
　1. Data are fabricated by investigator or staff for a fabricated patient
　2. Data are "fudged" (i.e., altered) by investigator or staff for a real patient (e.g., some data points are ignored or discarded) to make the results fit a preconceived hypothesis or to look cleaner
　3. Investigators do not obtain Ethics Committee/Institutional Review Board approval to conduct the trial or do not use patient informed consents
　4. Investigator or staff follow unacceptable "shortcuts" in conducting a trial
　5. Investigator or staff do not adhere to protocol
　6. Patients are given unacceptable concomitant medicines
　7. Inappropriate patients are entered in a trial to boost enrollment figures or to obtain professional fees
　8. Patients are not requested to come to clinic at each visit scheduled in the trial or are not observed at each scheduled time for inpatient trials
B. Emanating from patients
　1. Patients alter responses to questions or tests to enroll or continue a trial
　2. Patients do not exert a full effort when required or requested to do so
　3. Patients do not properly complete tests in a trial
　4. Patients take medicines surreptitiously (and deny this), which creates problems for themselves or interferes with the trial
　5. Patients reenter a trial for a second or even third time when this is a protocol violation
　6. Patients enter another trial at the same time

[a] Numerous other examples are listed in Table 3 of Shapiro and Charrow (1985).

TABLE 83.97 *How may errors, negligence, or deceit in a clinical trial be detected?*[a-c]

A. Negligence or fraud on the part of the investigator or staff
　1. FDA type of audit[c]
　2. Careful trial monitoring and data editing
　3. Comparison of data written on data collection forms with laboratory and other original reports
　4. Comparison of data collection forms with patient medical records
B. Negligence or fraud on the part of patients
　1. Interviews with patients to evaluate their motivation, behavior, and attitudes toward the trial
　2. Analysis of trends in patient compliance and trial compliance
　3. Urine and/or blood screens to detect medicines that are unacceptable
　4. Room searches to seek unapproved medicines may be conducted[d]

[a] The NIH inquiry into the fabrication of scientific data by a Dr. Darsee was associated with "a pattern of lax supervision of Darsee's research, including the preparation of manuscripts" (Norman, 1984). The panel that conducted this inquiry listed recommendations that (if followed) should decrease the likelihood of this type of event occurring (see next table).

[b] Financial pressures and lures are possibly having a greater impact on the quality and slant of articles today than they had in the past. This results from conflicts of interest of scientists who have vested commercial interests in the outcomes and implications of their research (Maddox, 1984).

[c] Audits by the FDA from 1975 to 1983 showed that serious deficiencies were found in 6.3% of 964 audits (Shapiro and Charrow, 1985). The authors list the specific violations found and present five case studies.

[d] Cummings et al. (1974).

TABLE 83.98 *Suggestions of how to reduce the likelihood of fraud in scientific studies*[a]

1. Each trainee at a center should have a clearly designated sponsor, and the center's program director should be responsible for ensuring that this is the case
2. Publications and abstracts acknowledging the center should be approved in writing by all coauthors
3. Patient admission forms should be accompanied by a checklist to verify that clinical trials have been approved by relevant committees
4. Clinical trials performed by young investigators should be reviewed at regular intervals by the supervising physician, including raw data
5. The trainee should be encouraged to present findings at review sessions and seminars
6. Regular rounds should be conducted on a daily basis on all patients
7. Data for a given trial should be retrievable for at least 5 years after the work is completed

[a] These suggestions were made by the three-member panel of consultants to the NIH in 1984 (Norman, 1984).

TABLE 83.99 *Selected other clinical trial factors that may bias data or affect their interpretation*

1. Scheduling of patient visits at times that interfere with holidays, vacations, or weekends
2. Modifications of trial design or conduct during the course of the trial. In rare cases this may be done, and the changes must be considered when data are analyzed
3. Occurrence of a national event of great significance during the trial (e.g., assassination, war, influenza epidemic)
4. The sum of many individual patient complications that affect most or all patients' data may render the overall interpretation unclear or invalid
5. The type(s) of facilities used in the trial (e.g., Veterans Administration hospital, tertiary care referral center, primary care clinic, nursing home)
6. Different clinical practices in different countries[a]
7. Dose schedule of the medicine used. This is particularly important for anticancer medicines
8. Methods used to handle biological specimens (e.g., were they refrigerated or frozen appropriately)
9. Foreign travel by trial patients during or shortly prior to a trial

[a] Keirse (1984). See Chapter 40.

TABLE 83.100 *How may each of the factors described in the preceding table bias data or affect their interpretation?*

1. Patient visits scheduled at unsuitable times or close to major holidays usually diminish patient compliance with attending the clinic/office at the appointed time (e.g., most studies are therefore not scheduled to begin between Christmas and New Year)
2. Almost any modification of a trial design after its initiation (except for the most minor change) may have a significant impact on the data obtained and interpretations made
3. Unforeseen circumstances such as a national tragedy caused by a popular leader's violent death may lead to sorrow and grief reactions that could significantly affect data, especially subjective reactions
4. The influence of most of the factors described in this chapter is usually minor if only a small percentage of patients in a trial experience them. Nonetheless, if many separate events cause the data to be altered in a similar manner, they may exert a marked influence on interpretations
5. Pets may transmit diseases to humans or elicit allergic reactions, and their death may elicit a strong grief reaction
6. Patients may acquire diseases through foreign travel that may be difficult to recognize and diagnose but that may confound the trial data
7. Different clinical practices and beliefs in different countries may lead to different reporting practices on standard events (e.g., number of suicides, classification of infant mortality)[a]
8. Changes in a dose schedule often modify medicine toxicities and also affect a medicine's efficacy because the effect of some medicines depends on their cytokinetic and pharmacokinetic profiles
9. Specimens that are improperly handled may have a decrease in medicine viability and thus affect the perceived efficacy of treatment

[a] Keirse (1984).

TABLE 83.101 *How may clinical trial factors described in the preceding table be measured or controlled?*[a]

1. Measure the percentage of patient visits missed and assess the reasons for this
2. An end-of-trial questionnaire of factors that influenced patients during a trial may point out various factors previously not considered relevant or those that were not adequately controlled. A form that questions patients with numerous possible responses as well as allowing for unstructured responses should obtain maximal information from a relatively heterogeneous group of patients

[a] This table refers specifically to some of the points raised in the preceding table. It is clearly impossible to control most unknown factors through a systematic effort. Nonetheless, through the use of a relatively high degree of control in a trial it is assumed that many (if not most) unknown factors are controlled. In some circumstances the influence of unknown factors may be measured by subtracting the influence of all known factors.

PART VIII

Interpretation of Data from Special Trials, Modalities, and Populations

Learning, experimenting, observing, try not to stay on the surface of facts. Do not become the archivists of facts. Try to penetrate to the secret of their occurrence, persistently search for the laws which govern them.

—Ivan Pavlov

No human being is constituted to know the truth, the whole truth, and nothing but the truth; and even the best of men must be content with fragments, with partial glimpses, never the full fruition.

—William Osler, British physician

Interpretation of Pharmacokinetic Data

Pharmacokinetics is the quantitative analysis of the rate or extent of absorption, distribution, metabolism, and excretion of a medicine in a mammalian system. For the purposes of this chapter, the organism considered is human. Data may be obtained in normal volunteers or in patients but are usually obtained initially in volunteers. Volunteers usually provide cleaner pharmacokinetic data, but these data are also often less relevant to the "real world" than are data from patients.

This chapter presents a number of clinical factors that must be considered when interpreting pharmacokinetic trials. These factors are also important when planning clinical trials. Mathematical concepts are not presented or discussed in detail. There are numerous reviews and monographs for readers interested in more details of various aspects of this burgeoning field (e.g., Brodie and Heller, 1972; Koch-Weser, 1974; Gibaldi and Prescott, 1983).

The general processes that lead to a clinical response are illustrated in Fig. 84.1, which also shows which are associated with biopharmaceutics, pharmacokinetics, and pharmacodynamics. It should be noted that in most clinical situations the processes that lead to a clinical response do not depend on all of the four pharmacokinetic processes, although each may exert influences on the duration or nature of the overall response.

THE SPECTRUM OF PHARMACOKINETICISTS' ORIENTATION

The broad field of pharmacokinetics includes scientists with different orientations and perspectives in viewing problems. Broadly, one may describe scientists and clinicians in this field as either those who concentrate on metabolism of medicines or those who concentrate on the quantitative aspects and development of biomathematical models based on medicine concentration evaluations over time in various biological fluids (e.g., plasma, urine).

Metabolically Oriented Professionals

The scientists who are metabolically oriented focus on biochemical changes that occur in the medicine molecule. These scientists are often trained in medicinal chemistry and biochemical pharmacology and usually concentrate on the search and identification of metabolites. They conduct in vitro experiments in liver homogenates and other tissue preparations. After predicting the types of biochemical changes that may occur in a molecule, they will search for them in various types of experimental preparations or samples. They also search for the presence of and identify metabolites

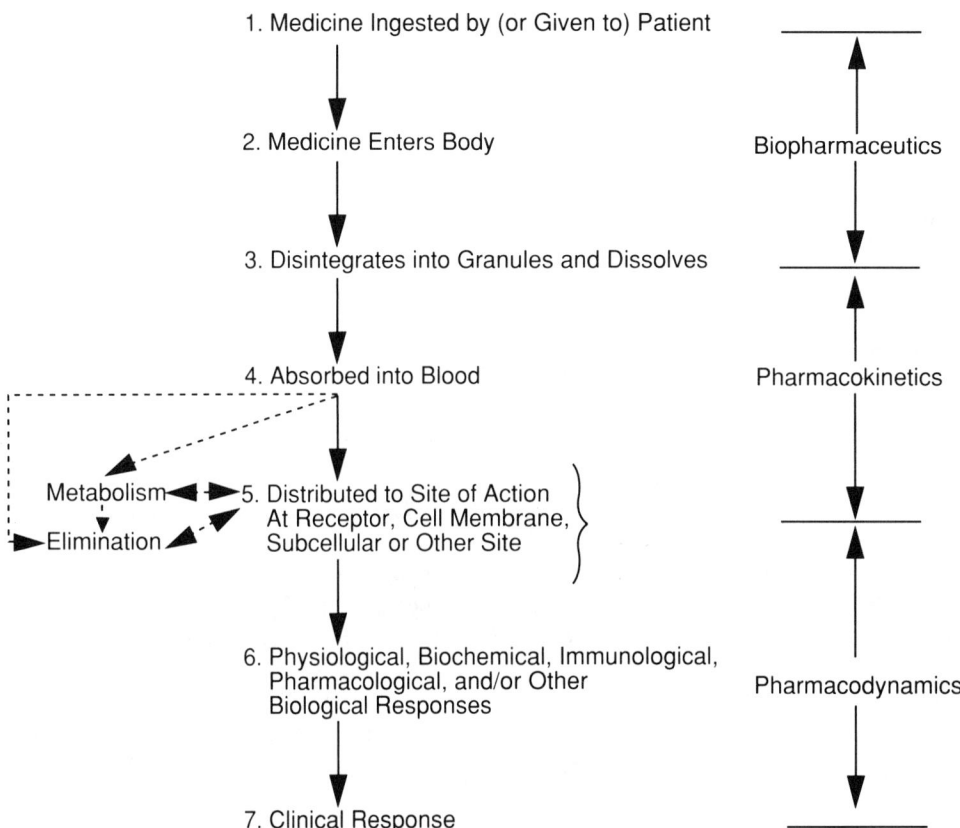

FIG. 84.1 Major stages leading to a clinical response after medicine ingestion, illustrating the general types of processes included in biopharmaceutics, pharmacokinetics, and pharmacodynamics. Biopharmaceutics includes processes until the medicine is available for absorption in a molecular dispersed form. Pharmacokinetics (medicine disposition in the body) includes processes up to the association of medicine and receptor plus processes of metabolism and excretion. Pharmacodynamics (medicine effects on the body) includes processes from medicine receptor combination to the clinical response.

that are present in biological samples collected in whole-animal experiments. This group is oriented toward conducting experiments.

Quantitatively Oriented Professionals

Scientists and clinicians who emphasize the quantitative approach are usually trained to use numerical analysis techniques to develop biomathematical models. They often monitor physiological events through collecting serial blood samples, which are then analyzed for medicine levels. They use these data to create a model of biological events that approximates the actual processes. They also develop simulations of hypothetical situations (e.g., simulation of blood levels during chronic usage of a medicine from single-dose data). These techniques are akin to the approach used by applied mathematicians (including engineers) who sample inputs and outputs from a system and then create a model that describes the raw data.

Bridging the Gap

Understanding these orientations helps individuals outside the field of pharmacokinetics appreciate the different perspectives of each group. In approaching the issues of absorption, distribution, metabolism, and excretion (ADME), each group sometimes defines these processes with different perspectives. There are also individuals who are trying to bridge the gap between the approaches used by these groups and thereby bring these two groups toward a common approach. Progress is slow, but there are indications that the two groups are slowly coming together.

It is clear that most clinicians have a different perspective on these issues and do not adhere to or follow either of these approaches. The clinician's perspective of ADME is usually oriented to understanding and improving the patient's overall response to a medicine such as the response that is related to therapeutic medicine monitoring (e.g., plasma level of an anticonvulsant).

ABSORPTION, BIOAVAILABILITY, AND BIOEQUIVALENCE

Bioavailability

Bioavailability relates to the rate of medicine absorption and the extent of administered medicine that reaches the systemic circulation. The extent of absorption is usually compared to a standard preparation of the medicine. For intravenously administered medicines this value is 100%. The term absolute bioavailability means that the bioavailability of a given dosage form is compared with the intravenous (i.v.) form. But many medicines are not available in an i.v. form, and it is often only possible to compare two other forms (e.g., two tablets of different salts, one tablet and one capsule, one tablet and a suppository). This comparison provides data referred to as relative bioavailability.

Bioequivalence

When the bioavailabilities of different preparations, salts, or forms of a medicine are compared at the same molar dose under similar experimental conditions and are found to be the same, the medicines are said to be bioequivalent. Bioequivalence of two medicines means that (1) the rate and extent of absorption are extremely similar, (2) the amount of each preparation reaching the bloodstream does not significantly differ, and (3) the preparations are chemically equivalent.

Medicines that yield the same plasma levels are bioequivalent and therefore considered clinically equivalent, as long as the dosage form is the same. Bioavailability of a medicine may be affected by many factors, the most important of which are formulation and physicochemical characteristics of the medicine. Other factors include (1) age of patient, (2) food ingested, (3) genetic history, (4) physiological capacity of the liver to metabolize, (5) diseases, (6) interactions with other medicines, (7) kidney function, and (8) other factors.

Factors 1 to 4 are discussed in Chapter 87 on special populations. Two chemically identical medicine dosage forms that have equal bioavailability and are pharmacokinetically bioequivalent in normal volunteers in an artificially controlled environment (i.e., clinical laboratory) should be therapeutically equivalent in usual clinical situations. An exception would be if the color of the medicine or its dosage form psychologically influenced the patient's response.

Therapeutic Equivalence

The term therapeutic equivalence has different meanings for a pharmacokineticist and a clinician. For the former it means that different doses of two (or more) medicine products yield the same blood levels. This may occur if one medicine is in a tablet and the other in a soft gelatin capsule (e.g., Lanoxin and Lanoxicaps). Therapeutic equivalence for a clinician means that two medicines yield equal clinical responses regardless of whether the dosage forms or quantities of medicine in the preparations are identical.

Relating Therapeutic Effects to Plasma Levels

There has been a growing trend to relate the therapeutic effects of a medicine with the blood or plasma medicine levels obtained rather than to the dose given to the patient. It has been reported that the doses of anticonvulsants in milligrams per kilogram vary considerably between animals and humans, although the effective plasma levels for anticonvulsant activity are closely related (Morton, 1984).

There is usually a linear relationship between the (log) plasma level of a medicine and the therapeutic (or toxic) effects. If this relationship is not apparent, it may reflect (1) an irreversible effect such as covalent binding, (2) presence of active metabolites, (3) a receptor in a compartment that is difficult for the medicine to reach, or (4) other pharmacodynamic effects that affect the desired response.

If only a small amount of medicine is observed in the systemic circulation, it may reflect (1) lack of absorption, (2) analytical problems, (3) poor choice of blood-sampling times, (4) noncompliance, (5) instability of medicine in biologic fluids, (6) enzyme induction, or (7) extensive first-pass metabolism. Tables 84.1 to 84.3 list factors relating to medicine absorption.

Data on medicine plasma levels may be used to answer questions oriented toward the past (e.g., whether medicine was taken, what medicine was taken, how much medicine was taken), the present (e.g., are the plasma levels of medicine too high or too low; how rapidly is elimination occurring?), or the future (e.g., how the dosage can be optimized). The answers to some of these questions require more than a single sample.

Dissolution of Medicines

Dissolution of solid dosage forms is a rate-limiting process that must occur to achieve absorption of a medicine. The major steps leading to dissolution of solid dosage forms are shown in Fig. 84.2. Absorption and bioavailability of solid medicines are generally facilitated by detergents and surfactants, which increase dispersion and aqueous solubility. Such agents are placed in capsules or tablets to improve dissolution properties. Dissolution can be controlled by the nature

TABLE 84.1 *Factors relating to patient characteristics that may influence medicine absorption*[a]

A. General and inherent characteristics
   1. General condition of the patient (e.g., starved versus well fed, ambulatory versus bedridden)
   2. Presence of concurrent diseases (i.e., diseases may either speed or slow gastric emptying)
   3. Age
   4. Weight and ponderal index (i.e., degree of obesity)
B. Physiological function
   1. Status of the patient's renal function
   2. Status of the patient's hepatic function
   3. Status of the patient's cardiovascular system
   4. Status of the patient's gastrointestinal motility and function (e.g., ability to swallow)
   5. pH of the gastric fluids (e.g., affected by fasting, disease, food intake, medicines)
   6. Gastrointestinal blood flow to the area of absorption
   7. Blood flow to areas of absorption for other dosage forms than those absorbed through gastrointestinal routes
C. Acquired characteristics
   1. Status of the patient's anatomy (e.g., previous surgery)
   2. Status of the patient's gastrointestinal flora
   3. Timing of medicine administration relative to meals (i.e., presence of food in the gastrointestinal tract)
   4. Body position of patient (e.g., lying on one's left side slows gastric emptying, and lying on one's right side speeds it)
   5. Emotional state of patient (e.g., stress increases gastric emptying rate, and depression decreases rate)
   6. Physical exercise of patient may reduce gastric emptying rate

[a] See Table 87.22 for a list of factors relating to characteristics of meals or ingested food that may influence medicine absorption. References for several of the factors in this table are listed in Mayersohn (1979).

TABLE 84.2 *Factors relating to medicine characteristics that may influence absorption of a medicine*[a]

A. Administration of medicine and its passage in body
   1. Dissolution characteristics of solid dosage forms, which depend on excipients present in addition to the properties of the medicine itself (e.g., excipients may decrease permeability of tablet or capsule to water and retard dissolution and diffusion)
   2. Rate of dissolution in gastrointestinal fluids. Medicines that are inadequately dissolved in gastric contents may be inadequately absorbed
   3. Medicines that are adsorbed onto food may have a delayed absorption
   4. Carrier-transported medicines are more likely to be absorbed in the small intestine
   5. Route of administration
   6. Medicine undergoes metabolism in the gastrointestinal tract
B. Physicochemical properties of medicines
   1. Medicines that chelate metal ions in food may form insoluble complexes and will not be adequately absorbed
   2. pH of medicine solutions. Weakly basic medicines are absorbed to a greater degree in the small intestine
   3. Salts of medicines used
   4. Hydrates or solvates
   5. Crystal form of medicine (e.g., insulin)
   6. Pharmaceutical form (e.g., liquid, solid, suspension)
   7. Enteric coating
   8. Absorption of quarternary compounds (e.g., hexamethonium, amiloride) is decreased by food
   9. Molecular weight of medicine (e.g., when the molecular weight of a medicine is above 1,000 absorption is markedly decreased)
   10. pK_a (ionization constant)
   11. Lipid solubility (i.e., a hydrophobic property relating to penetration through membranes)
   12. Particle size of medicine in solid dosage form. Smaller particle sizes will increase the rate or degree of absorption if dissolution of the medicine is the rate-limiting factor in medicine absorption. Medicines that have a low dissolution rate may be made in a micronized form to increase their rate of dissolution
   13. Particle size of the dispersed phase in an emulsion
   14. Type of disintegrating agent in the formulation
   15. Hardness of the tablet (i.e., related to amount of compression used to make tablet) or capsule if they do not disintegrate appropriately
   16. Other physical chemistry properties (e.g., pH, hydrogen binding, partition coefficients, solubility)
   17. Medicine subject to first-pass effect in the liver

[a] Many of these factors are reviewed by Bates and Gibaldi (1970), and some factors could be placed in both categories.

of the coating. For instance, an enteric coating prevents dissolution in the stomach and allows passage into the intestine, where it readily disintegrates. A light film coating or another coating will readily dissolve and not retard dissolution, but a film coat of many layers may retard dissolution. The film coat must dissolve (at least in part) before the medicine may dissolve. Essentially all tablets must be wet and disintegrate prior to releasing the active ingredients. The smaller the particle size of the medicine released, the more rapid is the rate of absorption. Solutions of medicines avoid the problems associated with dissolution. Suspensions may have better or worse dissolution profiles than solid dosage forms. In vitro dissolution data may not always predict how the medicine will behave in humans (e.g., a capsule shell may readily dissolve, but the medicine may form a hard plug when acted on by gastric fluids). In some situations, in vitro dissolution data may be sufficient to show bioequivalence between formulations without the need for a bioavailability trial (e.g., if there is a minor change in an excipient).

Time–Concentration Curves

Traditional time-dependent curves of medicine levels (i.e., plasma or serum concentration) are briefly re-viewed and illustrated in Chapter 16. Various pharmacokinetic parameters of these curves are used to establish bioequivalence between two different medicine products or formulations (or forms) of the same medicine. These are (1) the peak plasma concentration achieved (C_{max}), (2) the time to achieve this peak concentration (T_{max}), and (3) the area under the blood (or plasma) time–concentration curve (AUC_∞^0). Ideally the two curves should be superimposable, so one may conclude that the two medicines are bioequivalent. An important question to address is how much the curves may differ and the medicines still be considered bioequivalent.

TABLE 84.3 *Physiological and pharmacological principles that may influence the absorption of a medicine*

1. Food enhances gastric blood flow, which should theoretically increase the rate of medicine absorption
2. Food slows the rate of gastric emptying, which should theoretically slow the rate of passage to the intestines, where the largest amounts of most medicines are absorbed. This should decrease the rate of absorption for most medicines. Medicines absorbed to a large extent in the stomach will have increased time for absorption in the presence of food and should be absorbed more completely than in fasted patients
3. Bile flow and secretion are stimulated by fats and certain other foods. Bile salts may enhance or delay absorption depending on whether they form insoluble complexes with medicines or enhance the solubility of medicines
4. Changes in splanchnic blood flow as a result of food depend in direction and magnitude on the type of food ingested
5. Presence of active (saturable) transport mechanism places a limit on the amount of a medicine that may be absorbed

When the pharmacokineticist and statistician report that the amounts of medicine absorbed for two products vary by 30% within the therapeutic range it is important to know whether or not this difference is clinically significant. If all patients respond in a uniform manner to both products, the difference may not matter clinically, but if responses vary widely to both (or even to the one with the lesser bioavailability), then the additional medicine delivered to the circulation may be an important factor.

Rules of Bioequivalence

A number of authors have discussed whether it is possible to establish rules for bioequivalence. Dittert and DiSanto (1973) report that when the area under the time–concentration curve varies by 50% or more the two medicines are not equivalent, and when the difference between the two medicines is from 10 to 30%, the conclusion is a matter of clinical judgment. Clinical judgment is based on an evaluation of the safety and efficacy characteristics of the medicine (e.g., the therapeutic ratio) as well as on the characteristics of the disease treated. The Food and Drug Administration (FDA) defines bioequivalence as values within 20%. Other national regulatory agencies may have established different definitions. The definitions may also depend on the type of medicine studied.

Koch-Weser (1974) claims that there is no evidence to adopt any fixed figure from 10 to 50% as indicative of bioinequivalence. He indicates that the appropriate number (percentage difference) will vary for all medicines. He indicates eight factors relating to the medicines that should be considered to conclude that there is therapeutic inequality of the medicines (Table 84.4). Koch-Weser stated that up to 1974 "bioequivalence of different medicine products has been far more common than bioequivalence." The FDA usually requires that the blood levels of two medicines agree within 20% to consider the products bioequivalent. The FDA had a principle that 75% of patients should have plasma levels that are between 75% and 125% of the reference standard. This rule has been dropped because its statistical validity (basis) is questionable.

An alternate means of establishing bioequivalence relates to data on medicine concentrations measured in urine. The important parameters to measure are the rate and amount of medicine excreted in the urine. This

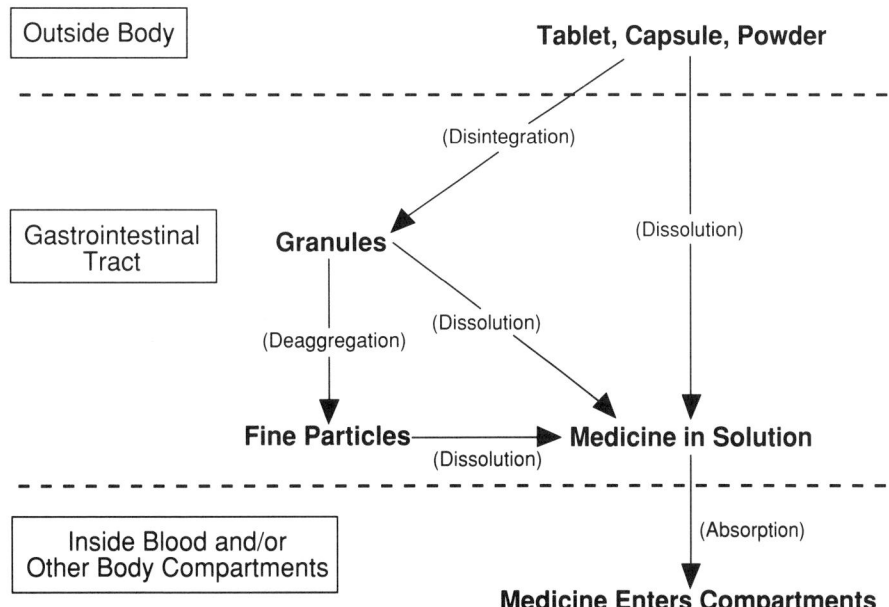

FIG. 84.2 Steps leading to medicine absorption of solid dosage forms ingested or placed in the gastrointestinal tract.

TABLE 84.4 *Factors to consider in determining bioequivalence of two forms of the same medicine*

1. The degree of non-formulation-related inter- and intraindividual variations in medicine bioavailability
2. The slope of the medicine's therapeutic and toxic dose–response curves
3. The part of the therapeutic dose–response curve on which the medicine is used clinically (i.e., threshold, rapid rise, plateau)
4. The medicine's therapeutic index
5. The relationship between medicine dosage and elimination kinetics (i.e., clearance)
6. The dosage schedule used
7. The disease being treated
8. The degree of illness of the sickest patients likely to receive the medicine

TABLE 84.5 *Selected factors that may affect medicine distribution to various tissues*

A. Factors relating to the medicine and its administration
 1. Degree of binding of medicine to plasma proteins (i.e., medicine affinity for proteins) and tissues
 2. Chelation of medicine to calcium, which is deposited in growing bones and teeth (e.g., tetracyclines in young children)
 3. Whether the medicine distributes evenly throughout the body (one-compartment model) or differentially between different compartments (two- or more compartment model)
 4. Ability of medicine to cross the blood–brain barrier
 5. Diffusion of medicine into the tissues or organs and degree of binding to receptors that are and are not responsible for the medicine's beneficial effects
 6. Quantity of medicine given
 7. Route of administration
 8. Partition coefficients (nonpolar medicines are distributed more readily to fat tissues than are polar medicines)
 9. Interactions with other medicines that may occupy receptors and prevent the medicine from attaching to the receptor, inhibit active transport, or otherwise interfere with a medicine's activity
 10. Molecular weight of the medicine
B. Factors relating to the patient
 1. Body size
 2. Fat content (e.g., obesity affects the distribution of medicines that are highly soluble in fats)
 3. Permeability of membranes
 4. Active transport for medicines carried across cell membranes by active processes
 5. Amount of proteins in blood, especially albumin
 6. Pathology of altered homeostasis that affects any of the other factors (e.g., cardiac failure, renal failure)
 7. Presence of competitive binding substances (e.g., specific receptor sites in tissues bind medicines)
 8. pH of blood and body tissues
 9. pH of urine[a]
 10. Blood flow to various tissues or organs (e.g., well-perfused organs usually tend to accumulate more medicine than less well-perfused organs)

[a] The pH of urine is usually more important than the pH of blood.

approach is not favored from a regulatory viewpoint because urine levels are less sensitive than plasma levels. Two overlapping curves establish bioequivalence. Nonetheless, this method is not currently favored by the FDA. Pharmacological effects may also be measured and used to establish bioequivalence.

DISTRIBUTION

The correlation of blood levels with efficacy of a medicine is best when there is a relatively small volume of distribution. When the volume of distribution is large, most of the medicine goes into tissues, so that only a small fraction of the dose remains in plasma, and the correlation with efficacy is therefore low. Factors relating to medicine distribution are listed in Table 84.5 and those factors that may increase the fraction of free medicine in the circulation are listed in Table 84.6.

METABOLISM

The field of metabolism (biochemical changes of a medicine) is too vast to delineate in a few tables and pages. This section merely highlights a few general concepts. Many of the specific factors that may influence medicine metabolism and the interpretation of plasma level data are shown in Table 84.7. Chapter 87 describes additional aspects of metabolism relating to food, ethnic background, cigarette smoking, and environmental factors.

Some of the therapeutic issues involving metabolism that may arise in clinical medicine are:

1. Is the therapeutic effect a result of the parent medicine or one or more metabolites?
2. If the therapeutic effect is a partial or total result of a metabolite, would there be advantages in giving patients the metabolite instead of the parent medicine?

3. If first-pass metabolism reduces systemic bioavailability after oral administration, can the medicine be given by another route? The first-pass effect, however, is not always an undesirable and negative effect.
4. If a medicine is partially or totally inactivated by

TABLE 84.6 *Selected factors that may increase the fraction of free medicine in the circulation[a]*

1. Renal impairment
2. Liver impairment
3. Hypoalbuminemia (plasma albumin concentration below a level of approximately 25 g/liter)
4. Other medicines that displace the test medicine from proteins in the circulation
5. Occupation of all of the available binding sites on the proteins by the same or other medicines
6. Last trimester of pregnancy

[a] Free medicine is defined as that medicine that is not bound by proteins.

TABLE 84.7 *Selected factors that may affect the rate of medicine metabolism[a]*

A. Interactions of patients with environmental factors
  1. Diet[b]
  2. Cigarette smoking[c]
  3. Exposure to insecticides[d]
  4. Alcoholism[e]
  5. Disease[f]
  6. Fever[g]
  7. Medications[h]
  8. Exposure to environmental toxins[i]
  9. Occupation
  10. Exposure to herbicides
  11. Exposure to household chemicals
B. Acquired or inherent patient factors
  1. Physical fitness[j]
  2. Age
  3. Ethnic background[k]
  4. Intestinal bacteria[l]

[a] It has been reported that cigarette smoking and chronic medicine ingestion have additive effects in enhancing hepatic medicine metabolism of antipyrine (Cooksley et al., 1979).
[b] Conney et al. (1977) and Pantuck et al. (1979). Alvares et al. (1979) list additional references.
[c] Vestal et al. (1975), Hart et al. (1976), Conney et al. (1977), and Jusko (1978).
[d] Kolmodin et al. (1969) and Poland et al. (1970).
[e] Iber (1977) and Rubin and Lieber (1968).
[f] Vesell (1978).
[g] Elin et al. (1975).
[h] Conney (1967)
[i] Alvares et al. (1975). Alvares et al. (1979) list additional references.
[j] Boel et al. (1984).
[k] Kalow (1982).
[l] Scheline (1972).

metabolism in the gastrointestinal tract, can this effect be blocked or prevented?

5. Is it possible to slow down the metabolism of a medicine and prolong its beneficial effects?
6. Is it possible to increase the rate of metabolism in cases of accidental or purposeful overdosage? This assumes that the medicine is converted to less toxic metabolites.
7. Is there evidence that the medicine can induce liver microsomal enzymes, and if so to what interactions might this lead?
8. Is there evidence that the medicine can inhibit metabolism of other medicines?
9. Is the hepatic clearance significantly altered in patients with compromised hepatic function?

EXCRETION AND ELIMINATION

Definitions

The terms *excretion* and *elimination* are used somewhat differently by pharmacokineticists and metabolism-oriented scientists. Elimination is used by pharmacokineticists to indicate that the medicine is taken out of action, since it may have been metabolized to metabolites, conjugated, or removed from the body in either a changed or an unchanged form. Excretion is used by pharmacokineticists to denote the mechanism whereby medicine is removed from the body or from the systemic circulation (e.g., via the bite, urine, feces). For metabolically-oriented scientists, excretion refers to the routes whereby a medicine and its metabolites are removed from the body. This section refers to excretion in this last context. Other scientists sometimes use an additional definition whereby excretion refers to waste products of tissues or organs that are removed from the body.

Issues

When the total amount of excreted medicine measured as parent and metabolites is calculated, it will usually be less than the amount of parent medicine administered. Complete or almost complete recovery is usually obtained when radiolabeled medicine trials are conducted. The major share of the remaining medicine is present as metabolites. Another portion of the dose may be stored in tissue compartments and released slowly. Finally, there are amounts of some medicines that are deposited for prolonged periods in various tissues (e.g., tetracyclines in bone, chloroquine in the retina). A variation of this issue occurs when a medicine triggers the synthesis of a substance that is normally absent or only present in small amounts. This new substance may remain long after the parent medicine and its metabolites are eliminated from the body. Examples include medicine-induced kidney stones and crystal deposits of certain poorly soluble medicines in the kidney. See Table 84.8 for a list of selected factors that affect elimination of a medicine.

Some of the therapeutic issues involving excretion that arise in clinical medicine are:

1. Is it possible to increase the clearance of a med-

TABLE 84.8 *Selected factors that affect elimination of a medicine*

A. Renal elimination
  1. Renal function
  2. Blood flow to kidneys
  3. Protein binding in plasma (protein-bound medicines cannot undergo glomerular filtration)
B. Hepatic elimination
  1. Hepatic function
  2. Blood flow to liver
    a. Flow-dependent hepatic elimination (metabolism of some protein-bound medicines depends on the rate of delivery to liver, e.g., propranolol)
    b. Flow-independent hepatic elimination (only unbound medicine is taken up by the liver, e.g., warfarin)
  3. Anatomical integrity of gastrointestinal tract

icine (i.e., accelerate a medicine's elimination) in cases of accidental or purposeful overdose?

2. Is there evidence of medicine–medicine interactions relating to elimination of usual doses?
3. Does the medicine behave the same in patients with compromised renal or hepatic function?
4. Is it possible to slow excretion processes to prolong the medicine's beneficial effect?

INTERPRETATION OF DATA ON BLOOD LEVELS

The following examples are of observations that require interpretation:

1. Blood levels of the medicine may not be detected after oral administration (see Table 84.9 for possible interpretations).
2. Blood levels may not be detected for parenterally administered medicines (see Table 84.10 for possible interpretations).
3. Blood levels may be unexpectedly high after medicine administration (see Table 84.11 for possible interpretations).

TABLE 84.9 *Possible explanations when diminished or absent blood levels are detected for orally administered medicines*

A. Factors related to medicine or patient
 1. The medicine did not dissolve
 2. The medicine dissolved but was metabolized prior to absorption
 3. No absorption occurred through the gastrointestinal tract (e.g., molecular weight was too high)
 4. Absorbed medicine was totally metabolized (e.g., first-pass effect through liver)
 5. Various considerations related to the patient's pathology (e.g., malabsorption syndromes) and compliance (e.g., "cheeking" and discarding the medicine, not taking the medicine)
B. Factors related to blood sample
 1. Blood samples were taken too soon or too late after medicine administration
 2. Blood sample was hemolyzed, which affected results
 3. The preservative in the tube used to collect the sample was inappropriate or was absent
 4. Blood samples were inappropriately stored (e.g., too long a period, at the incorrect temperature)
 5. Blood samples were inappropriately handled (e.g., too slow a freezing process, too rapid thawing, overheating)
 6. Medicine is unstable in plasma
C. Factors related to medicine assay
 1. Medicine assay was not sufficiently sensitive to detect medicine
 2. Other constituents in blood interfered with the medicine assay
 3. Assay was improperly performed
D. Factors related to data handling
 1. Computer error
 2. Error of laboratory reporting
 3. Error in transcribing data from laboratory report to patient's medical record or data collection form

TABLE 84.10 *Possible explanations when diminished or absent blood levels are obtained for parenterally administered medicines*[a]

1. Medicine was inactivated by other medicines given concomitantly in the same syringe or infusion set (i.e., medicine incompatibility)
2. Medicine adhered to the walls of the container when it was reconstituted, diluted, or withdrawn from the container
3. Insufficient medicine was given to the patient because of routine changing and discarding of i.v. sets
4. Binding of medicine to filter devices in the i.v. line
5. Errors in computing the amount of medicine to give
6. Medicine was improperly diluted, or dead space in the system was not adequately considered
7. Error of laboratory measurement
8. Error of laboratory reporting
9. Error in transcribing data from laboratory report to patient's medical record or data collection form

[a] Most of the considerations listed in Table 84.9 also apply but are not repeated.

TABLE 84.11 *Possible reasons for unexpectedly high blood levels of a medicine*

1. Dosage error (e.g., amount of medicine given or taken)
2. Sampling error (e.g., sample taken at the wrong time relative to dosing)
3. Overdose (intentional or unintentional)
4. Increased bioavailability (e.g., resulting from excipients)
5. Decreased metabolism
6. Decreased renal clearance and excretion
7. Error of laboratory measurement (e.g., interfering substances having same retention time during HPLC[a])
8. Error of laboratory reporting
9. Error in transcribing data from laboratory report to patient's medical record or data collection form

[a] HPLC, high-performance liquid chromatography.

TABLE 84.12 *A few pitfalls to consider in interpreting pharmacokinetic data*

1. If a pharmacokinetic model used for interpretation of data is assumed to be a first-order elimination and in fact elimination is zero order
2. If an incorrect rate-limiting step is assumed
3. Unknown metabolites may be present and have influenced the data
4. Biliary excretion may have occurred but has not been accounted for, and recycling of medicine occurs
5. Comparing results in different clinical trials in which different populations are evaluated
6. Comparing results in different clinical trials conducted under different conditions, such as with food intake versus fasting[a]
7. Comparing results obtained with different assay methodologies (e.g., steroids may be measured by (1) radioimmunoassay, (2) competitive protein binding, (3) gas–liquid chromatography, or (4) 17-hydroxycorticosteroid assay)

[a] Dittert and DiSanto (1973).

4. Blood levels may not correlate with either the magnitude or duration of clinical or biological activity.
5. Plasma levels may not correlate with brain levels of a medicine. This depends on penetration of the medicine into the brain and other factors.

A few selected pitfalls to consider in interpreting pharmacokinetic data are listed in Table 84.12.

When doses of two medicine products are stated to be equal based on equivalent blood levels, they may be equal in only one or in more than one of the following pharmacokinetic parameters: (1) half-life, (2) maximum blood (urine, or other sample) level, or (3) area under the curve. Clinical bioequivalence studies look for a lack of difference for two or more medicine products in these three parameters.

CHAPTER 85

Interpretation of Data from Surgical Trials

INTERPRETING SURGICAL DATA

Clinical trials conducted in surgery and medicine often differ markedly in a number of important aspects relating to design and conduct. Nonetheless, the type of data that are collected in surgical and medical trials usually do not differ. Furthermore, the general approach and methods used to enter data in a computer and to have it analyzed by a statistician and the general approach by the clinician who interprets the data do not differ. There is little that differentiates the processes used to develop interpretations of data obtained in surgical and medical trials.

There is, however, one area of great difference between medical and surgical interpretations that is of interest to discuss. This relates to some of the specific factors that may influence the interpretation of data. Many of the factors that influence the interpretation of data from surgical trials are similar or identical to factors that must be considered in interpreting data from medical trials. Many of these factors are listed in Chapter 83, but not all are directly relevant for any surgical trial. In addition, there are various considerations that primarily pertain to the interpretation of surgical trials.

The factors relating to interpretation of surgical data are divided into six broad groups:

1. Preoperative (Table 85.1)
2. Operative (Table 85.2)
3. Postoperative, prior to discharge (Table 85.3)

4. Postoperative, subsequent to discharge (Table 85.4)
5. Training and techniques of personnel (Table 85.5)
6. Data collection and analysis (Table 85.6).

The degree of enthusiasm shown by an investigator toward the patients who enter trials is important in both medical and surgical trials but may play a more important role in surgical trials. A number of authors have identified the importance of this factor in achieving a positive outcome in noncontrolled trials. Gilbert et al. (1977a) published data referring to the number of trials that were characterized by three degrees of enthusiasm and three degrees of control. It is clear that enthusiasm in this series is more characteristic of uncontrolled trials. The authors characterize a "statistical law" of Muench that states, "nothing improves the performance of an innovation as much as the lack of controls," and conclude that skepticism must be used in accepting the results of poorly controlled surgical trials.

The statistical concept of power is an important consideration in comparing and evaluating the clinical interpretation of multiple trials. If powers were reported for all trials, it would tend to diminish the widespread acceptance of results from trials with inadequate controls and numbers of patients. Multiple trials with the same outcome that are poorly controlled and have low power for detecting clinically meaningful differences have a tendency to acquire a greater impact on surgical practice than they deserve. This results from the il-

TABLE 85.1 *Preoperative factors that may affect the interpretation of surgical data*

1. Identity of preoperative medicines and dosages given to the patient
2. Reaction(s) to preoperative medicines after administration and prior to surgery
3. Medicines usually taken by the patient were withheld prior to (and/or subsequent to) surgery[a]
4. Previous surgical history[b]
5. Type and severity of condition requiring surgery
6. Level of patient's anxiety (stress)[c]
7. Enthusiasm of the surgeon
8. Manner in which patients were recruited

[a] See Wyld and Nimmo (1988).
[b] For example, multiple adhesions may make a routine surgical procedure a life-threatening and severely difficult one.
[c] Preoperative stress correlates with postoperative mood but not other measures (Johnston and Carpenter, 1980). Preoperative stress may affect some aspects of the surgery itself.

TABLE 85.2 *Operative factors that may affect the interpretation of surgical data*

1. Physical condition of patient
2. Concomitant medicines received during surgery
3. Type of anesthesia (e.g., local, general, epidural)
4. Occurrence of endotracheal intubation
5. Types and doses of anesthetics, neuromuscular blocking agents, and other medicines
6. Nature and severity of complications resulting from anesthetic or other medicines given during surgery (e.g., change in vital signs)
7. Duration of anesthesia
8. Duration of surgery
9. Complications resulting from the surgical procedures
10. Experience of surgeon and technical skills
11. Iatrogenically induced problems
12. Amount of blood transfused
13. Number and type of specimens and biopsies taken for examination
14. Surgical procedures followed that were outside the protocol
15. Quality of air in the operating room may be a factor in some situations[a]

[a] Haslam (1974) and Howorth (1985).

TABLE 85.3 *Postoperative factors (prior to discharge) that may affect the interpretation of surgical data*

1. Duration of time in recovery room (relative to the expected duration)[a]
2. Time required for all vital signs to return to normal levels
3. Presence of postoperative fever, infection, or respiratory or other problems
4. Treatment given for postoperative problems
5. Amount of blood transfused
6. Level of patient's anxiety (stress)
7. Quality of the pathological reports
8. Enthusiasm of the surgeon and relationship with patient

[a] There are many variables to consider that influence this period (e.g., change of nursing shift, number of nurses available, problems in the ward that delay transfers out of the recovery room).

TABLE 85.4 *Postoperative factors (subsequent to discharge) that may affect the interpretation of surgical data*

1. Photographic documentation used to illustrate the result of surgery (e.g., unless truly representative photos are used, an inaccurate interpretation may be drawn)[a]
2. Duration of follow-up (e.g., if patients are followed for a brief period, an inadequate interpretation of the results may be obtained)
3. Comparison of surgically treated and nonsurgically treated patients (e.g., when a medical and surgical treatment are compared, it is usually mandatory to collect data for a reasonable period after discharge to obtain a fair comparison)
4. Comparison of patients treated with each of the test surgeries (unless results are compared it will not be possible to determine the true value of most experimental surgeries)
5. Degree of relapse in each group (unless data on relapses are compared with a control or standard group, an accurate impression cannot be drawn)
6. The total cost of the surgery's follow-up subsequent to discharge as well as the cost up to the time of discharge (comparing the cost effectiveness of surgeries requires consideration of follow-up costs as well as hospital costs)
7. Trends observed during follow-up (e.g., effects may be observed postdischarge that were not apparent during the hospitalization)

[a] Photographs used to illustrate results should be examples of the median result or midscore unless otherwise indicated.

lusion that evidence is building up in support of a particular surgery, since "many" trials have reached the same conclusion.

PLACEBO EFFECTS AND SHAM OPERATIONS

Surgical procedures often include a placebo effect. The proof of this effect is perhaps best demonstrated by using a sham operation. The ethical basis for using a sham operation in a small number of patients is that it is far less ethical to subject many patients to an unproven or possibly harmful surgical procedure. The use of a relatively small number of patients given a sham operation in a carefully designed and controlled surgical trial (1) will probably save more people from

TABLE 85.5 *Factors relating to training and techniques of surgeons that may affect the interpretation of surgical data*

1. General training of surgeons (e.g., residents, board certified)
2. Experience of surgeons with each of the surgeries performed
3. Preference of the surgeons for one of the surgeries performed
4. Presence of a surgeon or a surgical review committee functioning as a monitor of the other surgeons
5. Number of surgeons involved
6. Personal interactions and relationship of surgeon(s) with patients to reduce their level of anxiety[a]
7. Consideration of whether the clinical trial was conducted during a period when a new operation was being developed and/or introduced or during a period when it was well established

[a] Johnston (1980).

TABLE 85.6 *Factors relating to a surgical trial that may bias data or affect their interpretation*

1. Whether the surgical results are assessed by a blinded interpreter
2. Whether the surgical outcomes and data are interpreted by a blinded interpreter
3. The magnitude of the variability observed in the data
4. The degree to which surgical data are supported by physiological, pathological, radiological, and pharmacological data
5. Results compared with those from other trials may differ in terms of mortality, morbidity, and demonstrated benefits
6. Whether each center in a multicentered trial obtained similar data
7. Data from outlier centers may disproportionately affect the interpretation
8. Data from outlier surgeons may disproportionately affect the interpretation
9. Data for patients with different severities of disease may differ
10. Data for patients from each social class may differ
11. Data from patients who were discontinued may differ from data from patients who completed the trial
12. Unpublished data may be available with which the trial data could be compared (e.g., hospitals in the United States are required under law to report their mortality)
13. The quality of life may have been affected by the surgery
14. In some trials the results are known by the time of patient discharge, but in others it requires 1 or more years after discharge before the effects may be fully evaluated

undergoing an unproven surgery, (2) will encourage more patients to have what will become a proven surgery, or (3) may be no less effective than the standard treatment (e.g., the internal mammary artery ligation studies of Cobb et al., 1959, and Dimond et al., 1960). Although this approach is ethically defensible if a carefully worded and reviewed informed consent is used, it is probably unrealistic to expect patients to agree to this type of study if a major incision and sham operation within the body cavity are involved.

Other sham procedures have involved (1) a trial of gastric freezing as a treatment of gastric ulcers (Ruffin et al., 1969; results from this method were shown to be no better than those from the sham procedure), (2) sham feeding in patients with duodenal ulcers (Feldman et al., 1980a,b), (3) sham hemodialysis for the treatment of psoriasis (Nissenson et al., 1979), (4) sham peritoneal dialysis for the treatment of psoriasis (Whittier et al., 1983), (5) sham laser photocoagulation in the management of central serous chorioretinopathy (Robertson and Ilstrup, 1983), (6) sham transcutaneous nerve stimulation for treatment of postoperative pain (Rooney et al., 1983), and (7) sham hemodialysis in schizophrenic patients (Schulz et al., 1981; Carpenter et al., 1983). Sham groups have also been used in clinical trials performed to evaluate apheresis (see Hamblin, 1984, for references), and electroconvulsive therapy (see Crowe, 1984, for references).

It is especially interesting that the magnitude of the placebo effect in several sham operations (approximately 35%) is exactly the same as that reported by Beecher (1962) for nonsurgical trials. Sham operations have been reported by Dimond et al. (1960) to elicit subjective improvement in all five patients with angina and by Cobb et al. (1959), who reported that the sham operation led to both objective and subjective improvement in patients with angina. Beecher (1961) stated that "the greater the subject's stress, the greater the effect of the placebo." This may account (at least in part) for the placebo effect noted in surgery, since stress is a well-known component of surgery. Stress occurs both prior to and after the day of the surgery (Johnston, 1980).

EXTRAPOLATING SURGICAL DATA

Direction of Extrapolation

To extrapolate data to a widespread patient population, it is important to characterize both the test population and the larger population. Inclusion and exclusion criteria, methods of patient recruitment, and procedures for patient enrollment are all important factors necessary to consider in characterizing a patient group in addition to their clinical outcomes.

There are also occasions when data from a broad patient group may be extrapolated to a smaller and more homogeneous population. This may occur as a result of a postmarketing study characterizing medicine use in a broad patient population. Data that indicate potential benefits or problems in a subset or in the entire population may be extrapolated and subsequently evaluated in a more narrow population. Adverse reactions that are observed in a broad population may be evaluated more closely in a subset of the larger patient group.

Quality of Life

Evaluations of therapy are based in large part on the patient's evaluation of how his or her quality of life has been (or is expected to be) improved. Measures of quality of life should be incorporated whenever possible into each medical and surgical protocol. At present, no single agreed-on test or tests can measure this parameter satisfactorily. Some tests are felt to be too objective, too subjective, inadequately validated, too broad, too narrow, and so on. Despite the controversies surrounding currently available methods, it is valuable to obtain data on the quality of life. These data have impact in encouraging physicians to present new therapeutic alternatives to patients and to discuss and consider functional improvement. This concept is discussed more fully in Chapter 97.

Survival Curves

Figure 85.1 is modified from a figure of Strachan and Oates (1977). If one assumes that interim reports on this hypothetical clinical trial are generated at yearly intervals, then the data obtained at the end of the first year suggest that the two treatments are equivalent. At the end of the second year, the conclusion is that medicine A is better than medicine B. The third year's report strengthens previous reports, and if the numbers of patients are sufficiently large, the trial may be published and could influence surgical practices. The fourth year's report would tend to add confusion unless the reasons for the switched positions of medicines A and B were known, and the final report at the end of year 5 would settle the study in favor of treatment with medicine B. Or would it? Is it more desirable for patients to undergo treatment with medicine B since the 5-year survival is superior to treatment with medicine A, or would treatment with medicine A be preferable because there is enhanced survival at years 2 and 3? The answer undoubtedly depends on many factors and cannot be made easily for all patients.

One variation of this problem would occur if the switchover from medicine A being better than medicine B occurred at year 3 instead of year 4 as in the current example. This variation would yield more clear recommendations, since at only one time point (year 2) would medicine A be better than medicine B. At all subsequent years (years 3, 4, 5), medicine B would be the preferable treatment.

Geographical Variations in Surgeries Performed

It has been reported that there are twice the number of surgeries performed in the United States (in proportion to population) as in England and Wales and that there are twice as many surgeons in the United States (Bunker, 1970). Bunker stated that (1) fee for service, (2) private practice, and (3) a more aggressive therapeutic approach contribute to the higher number of surgeries performed in the United States. He was unable to determine whether there are too few surgeries performed in England and Wales or too many performed in the United States. Vayda (1973) reported that the overall ratio of surgeries conducted in Canada compared with England and Wales is 1:8. The individual ratios varied widely between different types of surgeries. A list of 15 possible reasons to explain variations in rates of surgery based on geographic considerations was presented by McPherson et al. (1981). Surgical therapy is rationed for elective procedures in the United Kingdom, even though these procedures often influence the quality of life in a major way. Other

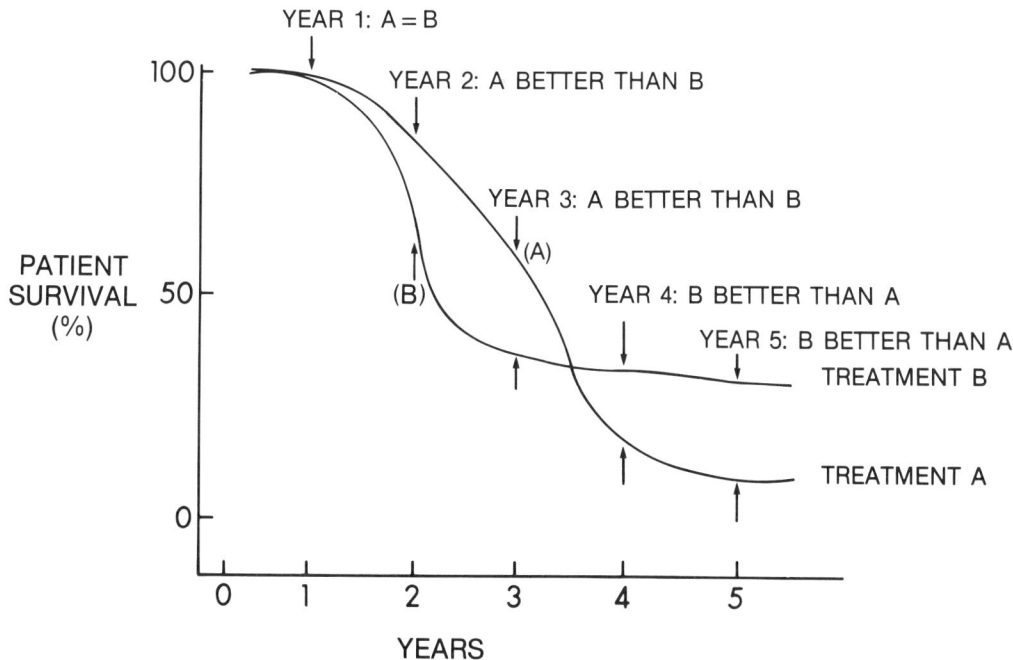

FIG. 85.1 Survival curves of patients treated with two hypothetical medicines (medicine A and medicine B) in a parallel trial. See text for discussion. (Modified from Strachan and Oates, 1977, with permission of the publisher, Blackwell Scientific Press.)

authors have described geographic variations in number of surgeries (Leape et al., 1989). It is often uncertain whether one area is receiving too many surgeries and another is receiving too few, or whether both areas are receiving too many, too few, or the correct amount.

COMPARISON OF SURGICAL AND MEDICAL PARAMETERS IN A SINGLE TRIAL

Therapeutic Areas Where Surgical and Medical Outcomes Are Compared

A few medical areas in which a comparison of surgical and medical treatments may be evaluated in the same clinical trial are:

1. Bleeding duodenal ulcer
2. Unstable angina pectoris
3. Brain abscess
4. Juvenile laryngeal papillomatosis
5. Bilateral carotid stenosis

Trial Designs

Parallel trial designs are usually used, since patients treated with surgery (e.g., for brain abscess or for coronary artery disease) are not then suitable for medical treatment. One exception is for patients with juvenile laryngeal papillomatosis, where recurrent surgeries are required and crossover designs may be employed if a long baseline is used between treatments to prevent carryover effects from occurring. In some situations it is possible to compare medical treatment versus combined surgical plus medical treatment (EI/IC Bypass Study Group, 1985). Patients who fail one treatment and are crossed over to the other therapy may have that event (i.e., failure) serve as an endpoint.

Problems

Comparisons of medical and surgical treatments create numerous problems and biases that must be addressed. One potential dilemma is how to handle patients who are randomized to the medical treatment group but deteriorate and require surgical treatment. If that patient is withdrawn from the medical group, it would bias the resulting data. One convention might be to define that patient as a "death" following medical treatment, but this may overstate the situation and bias the data in the opposite direction. In some situations the switch per se may be used as an endpoint. Various solutions may be reached, but it is important to consider as many possibilities as one can prior to initiating the trial.

CONCLUSIONS

When examining surgical data it is important to use the same standards in interpreting data as when examining medical trials. Caution and even skepticism must be used in accepting results of poorly controlled surgical trials. The standards for conducting surgical trials appear to be increasing, and there are a gradually increasing number of well-controlled trials in the literature.

CHAPTER 86

Special Modalities: Biofeedback, Radiation Therapy, Hyperthermia, Hypnosis, Electroconvulsive Therapy, Apheresis, and Hyperbaric Oxygen

There are numerous preventive, diagnostic, and therapeutic modalities used in clinical medicine apart from pharmacological (i.e., medicine) approaches. Data obtained in clinical trials using nonpharmacological evaluations are generally processed, analyzed, and interpreted in much the same manner as described for medicines in the other chapters of this book. There are a number of special considerations, however, that enter the process of data interpretation in clinical trials utilizing other modalities.

This chapter does not describe or evaluate any of these techniques in detail. Instead it discusses a number of factors that are often considered in interpreting data from clinical trials using nonpharmacological modalities. The modalities mentioned in this chapter represent only a few of those that are commonly used.

BIOFEEDBACK

Types of Biofeedback

Biofeedback refers to the process by which an individual gains voluntary control to increase, decrease, or modify a physiological activity or an involuntary function. He does this through subjective trial-and-error techniques via immediate use of sensory input (visual or audio). This technique began to be applied when computers were widely introduced in science in the 1960s. Patients are trained to modify their thoughts, feelings, or other inward efforts to obtain the desired change in function and to train themselves with internal cues. Biofeedback may be presented to the patient via headphones or speaker as (1) a continuous tone whose pitch changes or (2) a click whose frequency changes. Patients may also observe a visual display on an oscilloscope whose amplitude or color changes according to the patient's physiological response. Daily (or periodic) practice is usually encouraged at the patient's home, and a series of training sessions is held.

Uses of Biofeedback

Biofeedback was originally used to train volunteers to modify a physiological function, such as decreasing their heart rate or increasing or decreasing α waves in their electroencephalogram (Spilker et al., 1969). Although these particular physiological responses were not specifically targeted to a disease, the biofeedback process often helped patients to relax.

More recently, biofeedback has been widely used to treat many different diseases. Spinally injured patients have been trained to activate motion in their limbs, and patients who have had a stroke, head trauma, or cerebral palsy have been partially rehabilitated (Goldsmith, 1985). The role of biofeedback in treating migraine is controversial, and no conclusions can be drawn (Johansson and Ost, 1982; Holmes and Burish, 1983; Masek et al., 1984). It appears to work in treating tension headache (Ford, 1982; Holmes and Burish, 1983); however, it does not appear to be more effective than methods of relaxation training, with which it is often combined. It is also combined with relaxation training in treating patients with asthma (Kotses and Glaus, 1981).

Biofeedback techniques have been used to treat patients with various ophthalmological problems (strabismus, nystagmus, blepharospasm, elevated intraocular pressure, and myopia; Rotberg and Surwit, 1981). These authors have concluded that biofeedback techniques have most promise in the treatment of blepharospasm and strabismus. Patients with amblyopia have also been shown to benefit from biofeedback therapy (Ciuffreda and Goldrich, 1983).

Electromyographic signals have been used to assist patients in learning to relax their skeletal muscles. This approach is used to treat muscular contraction headache, spasmodic tortocollis, dyskinesia, muscular pain, asthma, insomnia, anxiety, and elevated blood pressure (Hatch, 1982). Other diseases treated with biofeedback techniques include Raynaud's disease, Raynaud's phenomenon, irritable bowel syndrome, essential hypertension (reviewed by Ford, 1982), seizure disorders, cardiac arrhythmias, hypotension, and fecal incontinence (references listed in review by Steiner and Dince, 1981).

Clinical trials of heart rate control in treating premature ventricular contractions and sinus tachycardia, plus hypertension, coronary artery disease, and Raynaud's disease are reviewed by Blanchard and Miller (1977), and summary tables are provided.

Use of Cues

In certain disease/problem areas, patients have been trained with biofeedback to focus on cues that are not related to their symptoms. For example, patients with migraine headaches have been trained to increase blood flow to the finger, therefore increasing finger temperature. The rationale for this treatment is that peripheral vasodilation increases blood flow to the periphery and decreases flow to the extracranial vessels, which are at least partly responsible for the headaches. In addition, peripheral vasodilation is associated with diminished sympathetic tone and presumably is consistent with a more relaxed state. Patients have also

been trained to decrease the amplitude of the blood pressure pulse in the temporal artery (Holmes and Burish, 1983).

Issues in Interpretation

Several authors have identified methodological problems such as the lack of adequate controls as a major reason for the equivocal evidence of efficacy noted throughout the biofeedback literature (Hatch, 1982; Thompson et al., 1983; see the latter paper for additional references). Various types of control groups for biofeedback trials are discussed by Hatch (1982). These include (1) a sham biofeedback group, which Hatch refers to as a "pseudofeedback" group, and (2) a placebo group who are not told that the stimulus is biofeedback and are similar to a no-treatment group except that they go through the various processes in the laboratory. This group is called an "attention placebo" group by Hatch. A third type of control is referred to as "altered contingency" by Hatch. This group receives altered feedback. For instance, Hatch quotes trials in which subjects were given feedback when electromyographic (EMG) signals were increasing although they were led to believe they were decreasing. Another control group received EMG feedback from forearm muscles when they believed it was from their foreheads, and a third group were given biofeedback when they stabilized their EMG at baseline levels rather than by reducing EMG levels. A list of selected factors to consider in interpreting data from biofeedback trials is shown in Table 86.1.

Visual Evoked Responses

Visual evoked response has been used as a research tool in both animal and clinical research for several decades. The medical usefulness of this method has been rather limited, although it has been used in the diagnosis of multiple sclerosis. When the visual evoked response data from patients suspected of having multiple sclerosis were combined with the presence of oligoclonal bands in the cerebrospinal fluid (Kempster et al., 1987) the false-positive rates were zero. False-positive rates with either test alone were 10% for visual evoked responses and 12% for the cerebrospinal fluid test.

RADIATION THERAPY

The state of the art in radiation therapy is probably more advanced than that of the other modalities discussed in this chapter. The doses to be used in treating patients with cancers have been established, and there is a large quantity of data that document the value of

TABLE 86.1 *Factors to consider in interpreting data from biofeedback trials*

A. Factors related to training of patients
1. Training and skills of the therapist[a]
2. Duration of training and number of sessions required to achieve a satisfactory response
3. Amount of effort required by patients to learn the biofeedback method
4. Percentage of patients who succeed in learning the technique
5. Determination of how well patients maintain their physiological target without external feedback as compared with results obtained with external feedback
6. Whether patients are tested for voluntary control at the start of a session or at the end of the session, after receiving training[b]
B. Factors related to a patient's therapeutic benefit from the technique
1. Therapeutic benefit obtained in daily life
2. Duration of therapeutic benefit after biofeedback training stops
3. Comparison of therapeutic benefit with that obtained with conventional therapy
4. Assessment of the degree to which patients are able to maintain their physiological target without feedback after their training was complete
5. Duration of time to retrain patients who have lost the ability to control the physiological target
6. Whether concomitant techniques are being used after the biofeedback training is stopped
C. Factors related to the trial design
1. Whether a sham group or sham period is incorporated in the trial
2. Ability to control the physiological parameter or target with external feedback.
3. Ability to control the physiological parameter or target without external feedback
4. Whether patients can be identified who have a high likelihood of learning this procedure
5. Whether concomitant techniques are being used in addition to feedback (e.g., relaxation training for headache relief)

[a] Taub and School (1978) found that an impersonal therapist could train only 2 of 22 subjects, whereas a friendlier therapist succeeded at the same task with 19 of 21 subjects.
[b] A proposed scheme for training and assessment of self-control is presented by Thompson et al. (1983).

TABLE 86.2 *Factors related to the interpretation of data obtained after radiation therapy[a]*

A. Factors related to the dose, equipment, and administration of the radiation
1. Dose of radiation (i.e., number of rads used)
2. Radiation modality: photons or electrons
3. Calibration of equipment
4. Target volume (i.e., primary volume, regional nodes, size of portal)
5. Fractionation schedules (i.e., amount of radiation applied at each session)
6. Tolerance doses for sensitive structures
7. Allowable photon energy
8. Minimum target-to-skin distance
9. Definition of prescribed dose (e.g., midplane, isocentric)
10. Total central-axis dose
11. Doses delivered to desired target
12. Number of fractions given per week
13. Total duration of treatment
14. Variation in total dose
15. Daily dose or total dose dependence on age of patient
16. Homogeneity of dose delivered
17. Number and duration of rest periods between treatments
B. Factors related to concomitant treatment
1. Use of oxygen concomitantly
2. Use of calcium perfusion
3. Prophylactic radiation of lymph nodes
4. Concomitant modalities
C. Factor related to clinical outcome
1. Duration of tumor control

[a] Modified from Perez et al. (1984).

TABLE 86.3 *Factors related to the interpretation of data obtained with hyperthermic techniques*

A. Factors related to the equipment
1. Device used to produce hyperthermia[a] (e.g., ultrasound, microwave, radio-frequency generator) and the type, size, shape, number, and placement of applicators
2. Temperature range used (41°C to 43°C is common)
3. Calibration of all equipment
B. Factors related to the method of application
1. Hyperthermia applied to the whole body, to a general region, or localized to area of the tumor
2. Size of the area heated
3. Hyperthermia may be applied to the skin surface or channeled under the skin to a tumor
4. Cold spots observed during treatment
5. Depth to which the heating extended
6. Types of implanted catheters used that were heated (e.g., blind ended, either rigid or flexible)
7. Method used to immobilize the catheters (e.g., buttons, beads, sutures)
8. Method used to shield nontargeted areas from heat (e.g., absorbing versus reflecting materials)
C. Factors related to the clinical trial design
1. Method used to measure the temperature at and near the test site
2. Number of times the patient was treated per week or month
3. Duration of each treatment
4. Other modalities used concurrently (e.g., radiation therapy, chemotherapy)
5. Number of sites at which temperature was measured
6. Medicines given concurrently (e.g., mild sedatives)
D. Factors related to the patient
1. Tissue type of the tumor, its perfusion, size, anatomic location
2. Degree of improvement noted
3. Time to occurrence of remissions
4. Adverse reactions observed

[a] Special considerations apply to each of the methods used.

this modality. A set of guidelines exists for assuring quality of radiotherapy in clinical trials (Perez et al., 1984). The factors listed in Table 86.2 are those that may influence the interpretation of data from trials using radiation therapy.

HYPERTHERMIA

The modality of hyperthermia (using heat that is above body temperature) is becoming established in the field of oncology. Hyperthermia is sometimes combined with radiation therapy or chemotherapy, but the optimal methods for this use, as well as the optimal techniques for hyperthermia alone, are not yet resolved. The methods of administering hyperthermia have been presented by Nussbaum (1984). Table 86.3 presents many of the general factors relating to hyperthermia that should be considered in interpreting data. Highly technical criteria have not been included in this table.

HYPNOSIS

The validity of hypnosis as a therapeutic modality in medicine has been strongly questioned by some people for many years. Serious questioning has primarily occurred because there have been few well-controlled clinical trials and a plethora of extravagant claims. There is substantial evidence that hypnosis can play a role in treating patients with numerous diseases or conditions, especially those in which psychological factors are involved. These diseases include asthma (Maher-Loughnan, 1970; British Tuberculosis Association, 1968), migraine (Anderson et al., 1975; Andreychuk and Skriver, 1975), irritable bowel syndrome (Whorwell et al., 1984), smoking cessation (Rabkin et al., 1984), sleepwalking (Reid et al., 1981), insomnia (Anderson et al., 1979), and phobias (Marks et al., 1968). Other physiological processes reported to be responsive to hypnosis include lowering of high blood pressure (Deabler et al., 1973) and establishment of analgesia (McGlashan et al., 1969; Stephenson, 1978).

Some of the many factors that may influence the interpretation of data obtained with hypnotic methods are listed in Table 86.4.

ELECTROCONVULSIVE THERAPY

There are numerous reviews of electroconvulsive therapy (ECT), and a bibliography (Crowe, 1984). The medical value of this modality cannot be challenged in terms of its general efficacy in treating severe depression (Janicak et al., 1985), although ECT has a number of drawbacks regarding safety (e.g., muscle pain, reactions to anesthetics, headaches, memory distur-

TABLE 86.4 Factors related to the interpretation of data obtained as a result of hypnotic techniques

1. Concomitant medicines
2. Number of hypnosis sessions
3. Duration of each hypnosis session
4. Length of time over which the sessions occurred
5. Test used to demonstrate that the patient was hypnotized (e.g., arm catalepsy)
6. Technique(s) used to induce hypnosis
7. Training and experience of hypnotist
8. Number of sessions prior to the start of the trial
9. Controls used[a] (e.g., psychotherapy hypnosis without suggestions)
10. Evaluation of patients by an investigator blind to patient assignment to treatment group[a]
11. Use of diary card to evaluate symptoms on a daily or weekly basis

[a] These factors are relevant for all of the tables on special modalities but are only listed here because of their particular relevance for hypnosis.

TABLE 86.5 Factors related to the interpretation of data obtained by electroconvulsive (ECT) therapy

1. Number of treatments (8 to 12 are usually given)
2. Frequency of treatments (two to three are usually given per week)
3. Diagnosis for which ECT is given (severe depression accounts for most cases)[a]
4. Level of electrical energy used (low-energy stimulation appears to be less effective than higher levels)[b]
5. Concomitant medicines given immediately prior to ECT (e.g., short-acting anesthetic, oxygen, atropine, succinylcholine)
6. Nature and degree of adverse reactions
7. Medical history of patients who had severe adverse reactions
8. Concomitant medicines patient has been receiving
9. Unilateral or bilateral electrode placement (unilateral is usually placed on the nondominant hemisphere)
10. Electricity delivered by a continuous sinusoidal wave versus a brief pulse of electricity

[a] Other indications include manic–depressive illness, schizophrenia, and catatonic stupor.
[b] Crowe (1984).

bances). Table 86.5 lists some of the considerations in interpreting or evaluating data obtained with this technique.

PLASMAPHERESIS AND OTHER FORMS OF APHERESIS

Apheresis refers to removal of a constituent of blood from a patient and replacement by exchange with the patient's own fluid or that from a donor. The most common type of apheresis is the exchange of plasma (plasmapheresis), but patients have also been treated by erythrocytopheresis (exchange of red blood cells), leukocytopheresis (exchange of white blood cells), lymphocytopheresis (exchange of lymphocytes), and thrombocytopheresis (exchange of platelets).

The field of apheresis has been developed over the last two decades, and its role as a therapeutic modality is still in a state of flux. The technique is primarily investigational at present. Although many great successes and failures have been reported, there has been a paucity of well-controlled clinical trials. Better-controlled trials are being designed and conducted in a wide variety of diseases at present, and a clearer evaluation of this modality should be available within a few years (AMA Panel on Therapeutic Plasmapheresis, 1985). Until that time, claims for therapeutic success should be viewed with the same skepticism afforded uncontrolled trials (see Chapter 4).

Factors to consider in interpreting data obtained using apheresis techniques primarily relate to the specific disease, type of apheresis, and group of patients studied and are not described in detail. Techniques and schedules used will undoubtedly have at least some influence on the data obtained as well as the answers to the standard question of who should have it, how much material should be removed, and at what point during the disease process it should be removed.

HYPERBARIC OXYGEN

There were numerous reports that hyperbaric oxygen was beneficial in patients with multiple sclerosis. It is interesting to observe that clinical trials followed the same pattern with this modality as with most others; i.e., early trials were uncontrolled and highly positive, and these were followed by controlled trials that had mixed results (Fischer et al., 1983; Barnes et al., 1985). A well-conducted double-blind trial (Wiles et al., 1986) showed no beneficial medical value of this modality in treatment of multiple sclerosis.

The complications (analogous to adverse medicine reactions) of hyperbaric oxygen include barotrauma (of sinuses, teeth, middle ear), visual blurring, nausea, headache, and claustrophobia while patients are in the chamber. This field was recently reviewed (Grim et al., 1990).

Special Patient Populations

This chapter describes a number of special patient populations that may be evaluated in clinical trials. Factors that are relevant to consider when data are interpreted are listed or described for each group. Thirty-six types of "special" populations are described in Table 87.1. These have been arbitrarily divided into four groups:

1. Populations based on chronological age
2. Populations based on inherent characteristics of each patient
3. Populations based on physiological characteristics of each patient
4. Populations based on acquired characteristics of each patient

It is understood that some populations described could fit into more than one of the four groups, depending on the specific objectives and conditions of the clinical trial. Nonetheless, each group was placed in the broad category that appeared most logical. Although group 1 is really a subset of group 2, it is separated because of the importance of this one characteristic in establishing special populations for study. Each of the four major groups of populations is discussed separately.

POPULATIONS BASED ON AGE

Most clinical trials are conducted on adults between 18 and 65 years of age. These individuals do not constitute a special population. Many considerations that are generally applied to adults are not listed in this chapter.

Neonatal and Pediatric Age Groups

The neonatal period is arbitrarily defined as the first month of life. Although absorption of medicines in the neonatal period is generally governed by the same mechanisms as in children and adults, there are a number of highly significant differences in the appropriate dose (per kilogram or per square meter) in the newborn as compared with infants, older children, and adults. Several of the differences in physiological function of neonates are listed in Table 87.2, and selected factors to consider in reaching an interpretation of medicine data from newborn babies and those in the neonatal period are listed in Tables 87.3 and 87.4. Readers are referred to *Drug Therapy in Infants—Pharmacological Principles and Clinical Experience* by R. Roberts

TABLE 87.1 *Selected examples of special patient populations*

A. Populations based on age
   1. Neonates[a]
   2. Infants[a]
   3. Children[a]
   4. Adolescents near puberty
   5. Retirees
   6. Geriatrics[a]
B. Populations based on inherent patient characteristics
   1. Genetic history[a]
   2. Race or ethnic background[a]
   3. Congenital diseases or conditions
   4. Sex[a]
   5. Social class[a]
   6. "Normals"
C. Populations based on physiological characteristics
   1. Decreased hepatic function
   2. Elevated microsomal enzymes
   3. Decreased renal function
   4. Patients on hemodialysis
   5. Immunocompromised patients
   6. An elevated risk factor(s) for a specific disease
D. Populations based on acquired characteristics
   1. Pregnancy[a]
   2. Lactation[a]
   3. Special diet or food[a]
   4. Tobacco use
   5. Alcohol use
   6. Drug abuse
   7. Place of work
   8. Type of work
   9. Exposure to an accident or to environmental or other hazards
   10. Prior treatment or response to treatment (e.g., history of refractoriness to medicine therapy)
   11. Specific concomitant medicines
   12. Education[a]
   13. Special body weights[a]
   14. Use of caffeine-containing drinks
   15. Exercise or fitness habits
   16. Special sexual habits or preference
   17. Undergoing general anesthesia or surgery
   18. In an intensive care unit

[a] Additional details are presented in Chapter 83.

TABLE 87.2 *Selected physiological differences in the neonatal period[a]*

A. Related to the gastrointestinal system
   1. Gastric contents are less acidic
   2. Gastric emptying time is slower
   3. Intestinal transit time is slower
   4. Greater ratio of gastrointestinal tract weight to total body weight
B. Related to body tissues and fluids
   1. Body fat content is low
   2. Body water as a percentage of total body weight is high
   3. Extracellular water as a percentage of total body weight is high
   4. Elevated free fatty acid concentration in blood
   5. Lower blood pH
C. Related to medicine distribution
   1. Blood–brain barrier is more permeable
   2. Decreased amount of protein binding (i.e., lower albumin concentration in plasma)
   3. Decreased affinity of albumin for medicines
   4. Increased volume of medicine distribution
D. Related to metabolism
   1. Microsomal enzymes are immature (i.e., not fully developed)
   2. Various biochemical processes are deficient (e.g., acetylation, conjugation with amino acids or glutathione)
   3. Presence of β-glucuronidase (this enzyme can convert glucuronide-conjugated medicine to the free form of the medicine and thus allow reabsorption to occur)
E. Related to excretion
   1. Decreased glomerular filtration
   2. Decreased tubular secretory rate in kidneys
   3. Decreased tubular reabsorptive rate in kidneys

[a] Many of these factors may influence medicine dosing.

ics) suggest that it may behave differently in the elderly patient. Under these conditions it is essential to understand the most important factors to consider in regard to the elderly patient that may bias data or affect its interpretation. These factors are indicated in Tables 87.6 and 87.7.

(1984) for additional details. Some of the relevant considerations in interpreting data from older pediatric age groups, including adolescents, are listed in Table 87.5. Parents who agree to enroll their children in clinical trials were reported to be more socially disadvantaged than parents who refused (Harth and Thong, 1990).

Elderly Patients

Factors to Consider in Geriatrics

Developing an interpretation of data from elderly patients is not different in the methods used from any other subgroup analysis. Special considerations relating to the elderly exist for interpreting data if the patients differ significantly from a control population or if the medicine's characteristics (e.g., pharmacokinet-

TABLE 87.3 *Selected prenatal or birth factors that may bias or affect interpretation of pharmacokinetic or pharmacodynamic data in newborns*

A. Prior to delivery
   1. Medicines given while in utero (including dose and duration of exposure)
   2. Genetic history and predisposition
   3. Family's medical history
   4. Nutritional status
B. At the time of delivery
   1. Type of delivery
   2. Apgar scores
   3. Complications of birth
   4. Resuscitation methods used during delivery and after birth
   5. Gestational age in weeks
   6. Birth weight
   7. Rh status
   8. Acid–base status
   9. Birth defects
   10. Need for isolation

TABLE 87.4 *Selected postnatal factors that may bias or affect interpretation of pharmacokinetic or pharmacodynamic data in newborns*[a]

1. Rate of growth
2. Feeding ability and type of feeding (e.g., breast or bottle feeding)
3. Assessment of behavior
4. Enhanced penetration of many medicines into brain
5. Altered metabolism (e.g., change in bilirubin)
6. Maternal disease
7. Development of pulmonary surfactant
8. Oxygen-carrying capacity of blood
9. Glucose homeostasis
10. Medicines given, including dose, basis for calculation of dose, and duration of exposure
11. Passage of medicines and/or their metabolites from mother through breast milk to neonate

[a] Many of the factors listed in Table 87.3 are relevant but are not repeated.

Cognitive Function

One of the most overlooked problems in interpreting data from this population relates to cognitive function. The occurrence of confusion or forgetfulness in this group is often attributed to old age rather than to a partially reversible adverse reaction. This problem is especially prevalent when patients receive numerous medicines at the same time. It is usually not possible merely to stop all medicines and observe the patient for signs of improvement. Because of withdrawal effects and return of disease symptoms, it is almost impossible to discern a stable medicine-free baseline in most patients who take multiple medicines. Probably

TABLE 87.5 *Selected factors that may bias data or affect their interpretation in children (1 to 18 years) and adolescents (12 to 18 years)*[a]

A. Inherent characteristics
1. Age
2. Sex
3. Weight, height, body surface area
4. Growth history
5. Current growth rate
6. Intelligence
7. Genetic endowment
B. Acquired characteristics
1. Motivation to improve clinically
2. Motivation to participate in clinical trial
3. Medical history related to disease or condition under study
4. Medical history related to other conditions
5. Allergies
6. Performance in school and at other activities
7. Social behavior
8. Self-image
9. Illicit drug use
10. Nutritional status
C. Other factors
1. Basis on which dose amounts were calculated
2. Attitudes of parents (or guardians) toward the trial[b]

[a] Adolescents are arbitrarily considered as a subset of children.
[b] Especially in outpatient trials.

TABLE 87.6 *Selected factors relating to elderly individuals that may bias data or affect their interpretation*

A. Inherent characteristics and physical status
1. Age
2. Degree of physical disability
3. Degree of dependence on others for performance of daily activities
4. Underlying physical state of the function(s) measured
5. Concurrent diseases
B. Physiological characteristics
1. Status of renal and hepatic function
2. Function of other organ and physiological systems
3. Nutritional status (e.g., albumin concentration available for protein binding)
4. State of hydration
C. Social, psychological, and other characteristics
1. Degree of emotional and psychological disability
2. Location of patients (e.g., nursing homes, outpatients, inpatients in Veterans Administration hospitals, community hospitals, and other types of hospitals)
3. Economic status (i.e., patients who cannot afford to fill prescriptions will tend to be noncompliant)
4. Social status (e.., support systems, friends, family, community status)
5. Concomitant medicines (e.g., medicine interactions may occur)
6. Adverse reactions present but not detected or identified during baseline
7. Use of medicines that some patients do not consider to be "medicines" (e.g., antacids, laxatives, vitamins, mineral supplements, diuretics)

TABLE 87.7 *Factors that may affect pharmacokinetics in the elderly*[a]

A. Absorption
1. Diminished acid secretion by stomach
2. Reduced gastric motility and increased gastric emptying time
3. Decreased splanchnic blood flow
4. Decreased intestinal surface area
5. Decreased active transport system for monosaccharides
6. Increased duodenal diverticula
B. Distribution
1. Decreased lean body mass
2. Decreased total body water
3. Smaller total body mass
4. Plasma albumin decreases
5. Increased fat is present
6. Decreased cardiac output
C. Metabolism
1. Decreased liver size
2. Decreased ratio of liver weight to body weight
3. Decreased hepatic blood flow
4. Decreased number of functional liver cells
5. Decreased clearance of highly extracted medicines given i.v.
6. Decreased enzyme activity for some medicines[b]
7. Enzymes may be "resistant" to induction
8. Decreased first-pass effect
D. Renal elimination
1. Glomerular filtration rate decreases (creatinine clearance falls)
2. Decreased renal blood flow
3. Renal tubular excretory function decreases
4. Renal tubular secretory function decreases
5. Renal mass decreases

[a] Most of these points are discussed further in Crooks et al. (1976), Vestal (1978), Ouslander (1981), and Shand (1982).
[b] Greenblatt et al. (1982).

the most realistic approach is gradually to withdraw medicines one at a time through progressive lowering of the dose. Clinical signs and symptoms that emerge may not allow this process to be performed for all medicines that the patient is taking. Another approach is to substitute alternative medicines for those that are most likely to be responsible for the patient's diminished cognition.

Physiological Changes and Diseases Associated with the Elderly

There are physiological changes in the elderly that affect how they react to certain medicines. For example, their total muscle mass decreases (Grimby and Saltin, 1983), which affects the distribution of some medicines. Numerous other age-related changes in physiological processes are listed in Table 87.8. These factors may play an important role in interpreting data from clinical studies. In addition to physiological changes, there are a number of chronic diseases/conditions that have a high incidence in the elderly. These include (1) cataracts, (2) anemias, (3) osteoarthritis, (4) osteoporosis, (5) arteriosclerosis, and (6) diabetes. In several well-recognized diseases, the elderly often present a quite different clinical profile than does the younger adult (see Rowe, 1977, for examples).

Impaired Homeostasis

The concept of impaired homeostasis in the elderly must be considered in interpreting data. This factor may be related to medicine-induced cases of hypothermia, orthostatic hypotension, and confusion. Decreases in the homeostatic capabilities of various organs (e.g., kidneys, lungs) to function normally lead to a decreased overall homeostatic capacity (Rowe, 1985). The aging of one organ or physiological function cannot be used to predict the aging of another. Although chronological age is far from being a perfect indicator of overall age, there are no better parameters available.

Receptor sensitivity and number of receptors have been reported to change in the elderly (Lamy, 1982). This may be one reason why homeostasis often differs between adult and elderly patients. The elderly are generally more sensitive to some medicines (e.g., warfarin) and less sensitive to others (e.g., propranolol).

Pharmacokinetics in the Elderly

The general consensus of pharmacokinetic observations of medicines in the elderly are summarized in Table 87.7 and in the points listed below:

1. With most medicines there is no age-related change in either the rate or extent of absorption. With a few medicines (e.g., digoxin) there may be decreased absorption in older patients.
2. The volume of distribution of lipophilic medicines (e.g., diazepam) often increases with age because of a relative increase of body fat. There is no consistent pattern of change in either the extent of plasma protein binding or volume of distribution for most medicines.
3. Medicines affected by conjugation processes are not generally metabolized differently in older patients, but medicines that undergo oxidation may have reduced hepatic clearance.
4. Renal excretion of medicines decreases with age.

Clinical Trial Designs

There are various pitfalls to avoid in interpreting data obtained with each clinical trial design. In the longitudinal design there may be minor variations over time in how measurements are obtained and laboratory tests performed that may affect the data. A learning effect on various tests may occur, and this could be a problem in parallel cross-sectional trials as well. Rowe (1977) illustrates situations in which the interpretation of data from trials with an elderly population is dependent on the trial design used. He describes the Framingham Study data on the effect that age has on a patient's weight. Cross-sectional data indicate a decline in weight with advancing age, whereas longitudinal data obtained over an 18-year period illustrate the opposite trend.

An important consideration in interpreting data from all clinical trials is that elderly patients over 75 years

TABLE 87.8 *Selected physiological and physical changes in the older population*

1. Decreased lean body mass
2. Increased body fat
3. Menopause in women
4. Decreased flexibility of the lens, which is manifested as a decreased ability to accommodate to near vision
5. Increased opacity of the lens, which leads to cataract formation
6. Arteriosclerosis (i.e., hardening of the arterial walls) with accompanied increases in systolic blood pressure
7. Decreased pulmonary function (e.g., maximal breathing capacity, vital capacity)
8. Decreased renal function (e.g., glomerular filtration rate, renal plasma flow)
9. Decreased maximum heart rate achieved with exercise
10. Changes that mimic disease (e.g., decreased glucose tolerance, decreased plasma renin levels)
11. Dcreased hepatic blood flow
12. Decreased immunological function[a]
13. Decreased cardiac output and cardiac index
14. Decreased gastrointestinal motility

[a] See King and Fenoglio (1983) for table of specific changes.

of age are a biologically different group of individuals than younger adults. The older group has experienced at least 75% mortality, and most biologically weaker members have been culled from this population.

POPULATIONS BASED ON INHERENT CHARACTERISTICS

Genetic Factors

Pharmacogenetics is defined as "the study of genetically controlled variations in drug response" (Vesell, 1984a). The general methodological approach used is to compare medicine responses in different groups of patients. Medicine metabolism and clinical responses (both beneficial and adverse) are aspects of clinical pharmacology that are most affected by genetically linked differences in the population. Clinical responses sometimes occur in patients that result from differences in metabolism or from other genetic related causes.

A number of pharmacogenetic issues facing investigators in this field were presented by Vesell (1984a):

1. Patients who are genetically unable to metabolize a medicine, either because of a lack or diminished quantity of an enzyme, will usually experience toxicity from an accumulated quantity of medicine.
2. Patients who metabolize a medicine more rapidly than the general population because of genetically controlled mechanisms may need larger or more frequent doses of the medicine to achieve equitherapeutic effects.
3. Patients with structurally altered receptors because of genetically controlled mechanisms may have either enhanced or diminished biological responses.

Detecting Pharmacogenetic Differences

If a genetically influenced mechanism is suspected of being responsible for differences in data obtained, there are two major techniques that can probe this possibility. The first is to measure the activity of the enzyme that is responsible for metabolizing the medicine. If this activity differs in a well-controlled clinical trial conducted in two different populations, there is evidence in favor of the hypothesis. Specific examples of this type of genetic difference relate to (1) a variant form of pseudocholinesterase that leads to prolonged muscular paralysis in some patients treated with suxamethonium (a skeletal muscle relaxant), (2) a variant form of glucose-6-phosphate dehydrogenase in some patients, which leads to hemolytic reactions after treatment with sulfonamides or several other medicines,

and (3) a variant form of hepatic N-acetyltransferase in some patients, which leads to differences in metabolism of isoniazid, hydralazine, procainamide, dapsone, various sulfonamides, and others. "Slow acetylators" of these medicines generally attain higher serum concentrations, which sometimes leads to serious toxicity.

Medicine Probes

The second technique that is widely used to discern genetic differences in human metabolism of medicines involves the use of medicine probes. The most widely used model medicine in this regard is antipyrine. Other medicine probes include acetaminophen, caffeine, phenacetin, and theophylline.

Medicine probes are used in pharmacokinetic trials to determine whether there are any interactions with the test medicine. Medicine probes such as antipyrene are highly metabolized in the liver and any interaction with a test medicine will indicate an increase in metabolism. In these metabolic trials, either urine or plasma levels of antipyrine and its metabolites are monitored as a baseline. Patients are placed on test medicines for 2 to 3 weeks and the antipyrene challenge is repeated to check for any differences in metabolism. A shorter half-life of antipyrene would relate to microsomal enzyme induction (i.e., stimulation) caused by the test medicine. Inhibition of microsomal enzymes in the liver is more complex and difficult to test. Inhibition may be a result of many processes, including conjugation. Some people use acetaminophen as a medicine probe to test for conjugation.

Polymorphism

Metabolic profiles resulting from administration of these medicines have revealed many cases of polymorphism in the population. Polymorphism denotes an inherited trait that is controlled by one genetic locus with two alleles. Moreover, the gene frequency of both alleles in the population must be 1% or more (Weinshilboum, 1984). This frequency is assumed to be greater than that resulting from spontaneous mutations. As shown by protein electrophoresis, approximately 25% of all human enzymes studied were polymorphic (Weinshilboum, 1984). Thus, there is enormous theoretical potential for marked interhuman variation in the metabolism of medicines and an increased incidence or severity of adverse reactions or a decreased medicine efficacy resulting from genetic differences. Debrisoquine hydroxylation polymorphism has been associated with personality differences (Bertilsson et al., 1989). The investigators reported that poor hydroxylators had higher vitality, alertness, efficiency, and ease of decision making. The authors speculate that debrisoquine hyroxylase is also involved in the metabolism of endogenous substances important for central nervous system function. Monoamineoxidase activity in platelets has also been associated with personality traits (Schalling et al., 1987).

Clinical Implications of Pharmacogenetic Testing

It is anticipated that future determinations of genetically related predispositions to medicine toxicity will enable physicians to avoid many adverse reactions in genetically susceptible patients. This is already occurring in some patients who are to receive suxamethonium during surgery, through preoperative measuring of plasma cholinesterase activity. Other in vitro assessments of pharmacogenetic susceptibility to toxic medicine metabolites are being explored (Spielberg, 1984).

The field of pharmacogenetics overlaps the area of ethnic differences in metabolizing medicines. Some of the genetic differences in the population (relating to metabolism of medicines) are highly correlated with race and are described in the following section. Tables 83.34 and 83.35 present additional information on how genetic makeup may bias data or affect their interpretation.

Racial and Ethnic Factors

Metabolic Differences between Races

There are several areas of medical research such as metabolism and genetics in which racial and ethnic factors are important considerations in interpreting data and planning studies. In addition, there are factors relating to social and behavioral differences between some racial groups primarily because of cultural or environmental factors that may affect the interpretation of data. It was recently reported (Svensson, 1989) that American blacks are underrepresented in clinical trials of investigational medicines. They reported that only 10 of 50 clinical trials reported in *Clinical Pharmacology and Therapeutics* provided data on race. This is particularly noteworthy because the majority of articles in that journal deal with pharmacokinetics, the area where the particular importance of race is expected to be present.

Various clinical trials have demonstrated that racial and ethnic factors may play a role in how medicines are metabolized (Kalow, 1982; Pelikan, 1989). The ability to understand racial factors requires careful consideration of both genetic and environmental influences. Environmental factors may appear to be based on race or ethnic heritage, whereas genetic factors may

constitute the primary reason(s) that account for differences between racial groups. It is not always possible to determine whether differences in metabolism between races relate to genetic or environmental causes. There are also cases in which both causes may be involved. For example, the inheritance of a trait that involves several genes is often modified in its expression by environmental factors.

Genetic factors may account for major qualitative differences that are observed between races (e.g., sickle cell disease) or for minor quantitative differences that are observed in the distribution of enzyme variants. Differences in metabolism between races were reviewed by Kalow (1982), who operationally defined the terms "racial" and "ethnic" as "virtually interchangeable." Kalow described several examples of racial differences including (1) distribution of acetyltransferase deficiency and (2) alcohol and aldehyde dehydrogenases. These enzymes were measured in several different populations.

Differences in metabolism among races may markedly affect a medicine's efficacy or safety (e.g., medicine toxicity may occur from elevated blood levels resulting from slow metabolism and cumulation, disease exacerbation may occur from diminished blood levels resulting from rapid medicine metabolism). Tables 83.32 and 83.33 present factors related to racial or ethnic background that may bias data or affect its interpretation.

Mechanisms

The biological basis of intrinsic differences between races in their metabolic capabilities may be related to (1) differences in the quantity of enzymes, (2) differences in the molecular structures of metabolizing enzymes, since it is now known that the liver contains a mixture of isoenzymes of cytochrome P450, or (3) differences in the effects of modifiers of enzyme activity. Modifiers of enzyme activity include cofactors, inhibitors, and activators.

Pitfalls in Interpretation

There are various pitfalls to avoid in interpreting data from a metabolic trial if the two population groups being compared live on different continents. Even when the two groups live within the same city, there are numerous confounding factors that may affect the results, such as (1) diet, (2) body weight, (3) socioeconomic status, (4) other social factors, (5) use of concomitant tobacco, (6) alcohol, (7) oral contraceptives, and (8) use of various other medicines. These factors must be carefully controlled to achieve data that will yield a meaningful interpretation.

Clinical Aspects

It was reported that Chinese patients responded more strongly to the beta-receptor antagonist propranolol than did Western patients (Zhou et al., 1989), in reducing both heart rate and blood pressure. The precise reasons for this finding have not yet been elucidated, and these results should be confirmed.

Congenital Disease/Condition

A few factors that may influence the interpretation of data from patients with congenital diseases/conditions are listed in Table 87.9.

Normals

The term normal may be narrowly or broadly defined, but in most clinical situations, a narrow definition (e.g., including the requirement that all laboratory values must be within the normal range) is usually too restrictive and excludes at least part of society that is normal. A population of medical students who volunteer for a clinical trial would be considered normal. Nonetheless, they are a select population in terms of age, physiological function, psychological health, and other factors and usually do not represent a valid control group to compare with patients or with the rest of society. There are occasions (e.g., some pharmacokinetic trials) when use of this particular population would be acceptable.

"Normal Ranges"

In pharmacokinetic trials involving a few individuals who are carefully and thoroughly evaluated, a narrow definition of normals may be more appropriate than a broad definition. Part of the inclusion criteria will focus

TABLE 87.9 Selected factors relating to patients with congenital diseases/conditions that may bias data or affect their interpretation

1. Specific congenital disease/condition
2. Genetic association with the disease/condition
3. History of maternal medicine use during pregnancy, labor, and delivery
4. History of other maternal exposures during pregnancy, labor, and delivery (e.g., radiation therapy, X-rays)
5. Family history of the disease/condition or of possible causes
6. Previous treatment(s) given to the patient for the disease/condition
7. Present treatment(s) being given to the patient for the disease/condition
8. Severity of the disease/condition

TABLE 87.10 Selected factors relating to patients classified as normals that may bias data or affect their interpretation[a]

Normals are individuals whose physical and laboratory examination values are within a generally accepted range in terms of

1. Age
2. Weight, height, body surface area
3. Past medical history, especially as it may relate to potentially serious risks posed by the medicine (e.g., seizures, bone marrow suppression)
4. Physical examination and vital signs
5. Neurological examination
6. Psychiatric examination
7. Ophthalmological examination
8. Laboratory examination (e.g., urinalysis, clinical chemistry, renal function tests, hepatic function tests, complete blood count)
9. Physiological tests relating to the trial protocol (e.g., pulmonary function tests, exercise tests)
10. Electrocardiogram
11. Other laboratory measures or other aspects of the physical examination (e.g., urological, gynecological) pertinent to the particular protocol in which these parameters may be described in general or specific detail

[a] The concept of "normal" usually indicates that the patient's values are within a specified range. Many (if not most) normal volunteers have at least one laboratory value that lies outside the reference range. These values often fluctuate over time and may represent variations in the patient, laboratory measurement, or both.

on whether a patient is acceptable if any of his or her control laboratory values lie outside the "normal" (i.e., reference) range. There are numerous reasons why insisting that all laboratory values must be within the "normal" range is not generally useful or necessary. There are also circumstances when values that are classified as normal may actually be abnormal in certain groups. For instance, a clinical trial of 50 elderly patients found that their normal mean temperature was 97.9°F (Thatcher, 1983), and another trial of 60 elderly patients reported a mean temperature of 97.7°F (Higgins, 1983). Whatever type of definition is derived, the criteria that are used to define the normal population should be described in all reports.

Classifying Patients as Normals

If a normal population is to be compared with a treated group of patients, then every attempt should be made in the normal population chosen to duplicate the treated group in distribution of age, sex, race, and other relevant factors. If a normal population is to be evaluated on its own or divided into subgroups that will be assigned different treatments, then a decision must be reached as to the desired homogeneity of the population studied. Table 87.10 lists selected factors that may influence the interpretation of data from patients classified as normal.

POPULATIONS BASED ON PHYSIOLOGICAL FUNCTION

Patients with Compromised Hepatic Function

Liver disease may have a major effect on the body's ability to metabolize medicines. This may lead to elevated concentrations of the parent medicine (or metabolites) or to the medicine's presence in the body for a longer period than expected. These effects will often increase the medicine's toxicity and may also have an adverse effect on the efficacy of the medicine. Liver disease such as cirrhosis may lead to shunting of blood through anastomoses from the portal to the systemic circulations, thus bypassing the principal site of initial medicine metabolism. In some cases, the hepatic metabolite is the active medicine, so that decreasing the ability of the liver to metabolize the parent medicine may decrease effective blood levels and diminish efficacy. When microsomal enzymes are induced, this leads to increased metabolism of the parent medicine. If the parent medicine is active, the decreased blood levels lead to decreased activity.

Induction of Microsomal Enzymes in the Liver

The metabolism of many medicines is related to hepatic microsomal enzymes. The activity of microsomal enzymes in the liver may be increased by medicines (e.g., phenytoin, barbiturates), substances in foods (e.g., xanthines, flavones, indoles; Conney et al., 1977), or by smoking (Vestal et al., 1975). As a result of the greater activity of these enzymes, there is a more rapid metabolism (i.e., increased hepatic clearance) of various medicines, including the medicine that initially induced the enzymes (e.g., carbamazepine). As a result of enzyme induction, large doses of medicines may need to be given to patients to obtain the same therapeutic effect as that obtained prior to the induction. The process of induction usually requires from 3 to 10 days to be observed clinically. Discontinuation of the inducing agent may result in increased levels of other medicines whose administration is continued. Various environmental chemicals (e.g., ozone, carbon monoxide, carbon tetrachloride, certain organophosphorous insecticides) inhibit the activity of these enzymes (Conney et al., 1977).

Factors affecting hepatic medicine metabolism are sometimes evaluated in clinical trials through the use of specific test medicines (e.g., antipyrine, aminopyrine). Some of the factors shown to influence the interpretation of data in patients with altered hepatic function are listed in Table 87.11. Table 87.12 lists factors related to patients with increased hepatic microsomal enzymes that may influence the interpretation of data.

TABLE 87.11 *Selected factors relating to patients with altered hepatic function that may bias data or affect their interpretation*

1. Nature of hepatic disease or problem (e.g., is it a result of a direct or indirect effect of a lesion or problem with the liver? Is it biopsy proven?)
2. Severity of hepatic disease or problem
3. Duration of hepatic disease or problem
4. Nature of metabolic pathways of the trial medicine, metabolites, and any control medicines
5. Ability of the liver to metabolize the trial medicine, metabolites, and any active control medicines
6. Concomitant medicines that affect hepatic function or interact with the trial medicine (e.g., by inducing microsomal enzymes)
7. Concurrent illnesses or problems that affect hepatic function
8. Multiorgan involvement (e.g., cardiovascular compromise)
9. Laboratory evaluation of enzymes and other blood constituents related to hepatic function

Patients with Compromised Renal Function and Those on Hemodialysis

Some of the specific factors that may influence the interpretation of data from patients with decreased renal function are summarized in Table 87.13, and those from patients who are receiving hemodialysis in Table 87.14. Other factors are discussed in Chapter 83.

TABLE 87.12 *Selected factors relating to patients with increased hepatic microsomal enzymes that may bias data or affect their interpretation*

1. Cause of elevated microsomal enzymes
2. If the elevated microsomal enzymes are medicine induced:
   a. Name of medicine(s)
   b. Dose of medicine
   c. Duration of treatment
   d. Is patient currently receiving the treatment that elevated the microsomal enzymes?
   e. Adverse reactions caused by the medicine that induced the microsomal enzymes
3. Effect of elevated microsomal enzymes on the trial medicine

TABLE 87.13 *Selected factors relating to patients with decreased renal function that may bias data or affect their interpretation*

1. Identity and nature of renal disease or problem (e.g., acute or chronic)
2. Severity of renal disease or problem (e.g., based on creatinine clearance, biopsy results)
3. Duration of renal disease or problem
4. Type of excretion (e.g., tubular secretion, active reabsorption) of trial medicine and any active control medicines
5. Multiorgan involvement (e.g., cardiovascular compromise)
6. Change in systemic pH (e.g., acidosis of uremia or alkalosis after severe potassium depletion)
7. Trend in values of blood urea nitrogen (BUN) and creatinine
8. Hypoalbuminemia leading to altered protein binding (e.g., in nephrotic syndrome)
9. Composition of urine (e.g., electrolytes, protein, casts, red blood cells) and trends in these constituents
10. Site of action of trial medicine (i.e., is it renal? If so, where?) and any active control medicines

TABLE 87.14 *Selected factors relating to patients undergoing hemodialysis that may bias data or affect their interpretation*

1. Nature and extent of renal problem
2. Duration on dialysis
3. History of past and present complications on dialysis (e.g., hypotension)
4. History vis-à-vis renal transplants
5. Allergies

POPULATIONS BASED ON ACQUIRED CHARACTERISTICS

Pregnancy and Lactation

Numerous physiological changes that may occur during pregnancy are summarized in Table 87.15. When clinical trials are conducted in pregnant women, there are a number of specific factors that must be considered (Table 87.16) both in designing the trial (Table 87.17) and interpreting the data.

After birth there are many medicines given to the mother that may influence a nursing baby. Factors that affect the excretion of medicines in human milk have not been studied thoroughly. Most clinical trials involving lactation in humans measure the concentrations of medicine in human milk at a single time point or evaluate medicines designed to suppress lactation. Tables 87.18 and 87.19 present some of the factors to consider in designing trials in newborns and interpreting data in which lactation is being suppressed.

Some of the factors that affect the composition of human milk are listed in Table 87.20. The transport of medicines into human milk depends on its physicochemical properties (e.g., ionization, molecular weight, and lipophilicity) and pharmacokinetic properties. Although the quantities of medicines that appear in a mother's milk vary, it has been reported that "virtually every medicine appearing in the maternal circulation will also appear in the milk" (Janas and Picciano, 1984). Nonetheless, the percentage of the dose administered to the mother that can be consumed by the infant is very small, usually less than 1% (Welch and Findlay, 1981).

The potential for infants to experience adverse reactions to medicines obtained through breast milk depends on a number of factors including:

1. The degree to which the medicine passes from the maternal circulation to milk

TABLE 87.15 *Selected physiological changes that may occur during pregnancy*

1. Edema	5. Increased platelet turnover
2. Hypertension	6. Hyperuricemia
3. Weight gain	7. Activation of coagulation factors
4. Proteinuria	

TABLE 87.16 *Selected factors relating to pregnant women that may bias data or affect their interpretation[a]*

1. Trimester or week of pregnancy or stage of labor
2. Distribution of medicine between mother and embryo or fetus
3. Physical condition of the mother relative to exercise tolerance, morning sickness, general discomfort, weight increase, emotional status, and other factors
4. Number of prior pregnancies, live births, miscarriages, abortions (i.e., pregnancy and birth order)
5. Genetic history
6. Health and overall status of previously born children at the time of their birth
7. Medical history of previous pregnancies
8. Age of the mother
9. Existing physical and emotional support system for the woman and her family
10. Attitude of the mother toward the unborn child

[a] See also Tables 83.45 and 83.46.

2. The amount of milk consumed
3. The amount of medicine in the milk
4. The ability of the neonate, infant, or child to metabolize the medicine
5. The ability of the neonate, infant, or child to excrete the medicine

Influence of Dietary Factors and Food

Background

The evaluation of how food influences medicine absorption is not a theoretical exercise. Welling (1977) has reviewed the literature and found that absorption

TABLE 87.17 *Special considerations in designing protocols and interpreting data from trials conducted on pregnant women[a]*

1. Involve the patient's obstetrician in the trial via direct participation (if possible and convenient) or through frequent feedback of information
2. Ensure that demands on the patients are commensurate with their physical and emotional abilities
3. Determine patient's expected date of delivery as accurately as possible
4. Determine the duration of pregnancy (in weeks) permissible at patient entry
5. Determine whether sonograms, amniocentesis, fetal monitoring, or other procedures are acceptable or mandatory
6. Determine if any special restrictions on diet or activity during pregnancy, labor, and delivery are relevant
7. Conduct appropriate follow-up of the mother and of the newborn to evaluate any possible effect the trial may have had
8. Involve the spouse and other family members to assist in the trial (e.g., to observe the patient for any relevant signs and symptoms)
9. Provide arrangements for transportation to and from the trial site and, if the patient is near term, to and from the hospital where delivery will take place

[a] Additional toxicology studies may also be performed (e.g., transplacental carcinogenicity studies) prior to the studies beyond those usually done to ensure medicine safety in this group of women.

TABLE 87.18 *Special considerations for designing protocols and interpreting data from clinical trials on newborn babies and infants*

A. For the mother near and during the time of birth
 1. Previous reproductive history of mother
 2. Type of birth (e.g., cesarean, forceps)
 3. Type of anesthesia
 4. Medications used by the mother
 5. Details of labor (e.g., duration of each stage, complications)
 6. Details of delivery [e.g., presentation (breech, cephalic), complications (nuchal cord, shoulder dystocia)]
 7. Smoking and illicit drug use
B. For the newborn just before and after birth
 1. Fetal heart rate tracings
 2. Apgar scores at 1 and 5 minutes
 3. Resuscitation efforts
 4. Examination of newborn
 5. Length and weight
C. For the infant during the first year of life
 1. Events at birth (e.g., prematurity, Apgar scores, type of birth)
 2. Breast or bottle feeding
 3. Percentile of length and weight
 4. Changes in growth performance over time
 5. Time of initiation of solid food
 6. Type of solid food eaten
 7. Family situation (e.g., mother's employment status, number and age of siblings)
 8. Amount and type of stimulation given to the infant

TABLE 87.20 *Factors reported to have an influence on the composition of human milk[a]*

1. Age of the mother
2. Number of previous children
3. Number of previous children who were breast fed
4. General nutrition of the mother
5. Specific diet of the mother
6. Time that lactation has been in process (days, weeks, months)
7. Time of day (relative to diurnal variation)
8. Time at which a sample is taken within a single feeding

[a] Janas and Picciano (1984).

minor role in any particular medicine trial, but they should be considered during the trial design phase so that adequate controls may be introduced and also during the data interpretation phase so that the relevance and importance of specific factors may be evaluated. An evaluation of clinical trials assessing adverse reactions to foods is given by Atkins (1986).

Types of Interactions

There are two major aspects to consider in interpreting how dietary factors may influence a medicine trial. These are (1) how food may affect medicines and (2) how medicines may affect food. This section concentrates entirely on the first aspect. The second aspect includes consideration of medicine-induced malabsorptive states for certain vitamins, minerals, and nutrients (e.g., isoniazid-induced vitamin B_6 deficiency). The reader is referred to a discussion of this topic by Roe (1984). Another related topic of how medicines may affect food relates to how medicines affect appetite.

Pharmacokinetics: Overall Level

Most of the important clinical influences that food has on medicines may be viewed in terms of the overall concept of absorption, distribution, metabolism, and excretion (ADME). These influences on ADME in turn affect blood levels, physiological responses, and clinical effects. The importance of this topic has grown in recent decades, especially because of improved pharmacokinetic evaluations of medicine bioavailability and the many factors that influence this. Food and medicines are often found in close physical proximity in the gastrointestinal tract at the same time. It may be for this reason that the influence of food on medicine absorption is the most important of the four characteristics (ADME) to evaluate. Although food may influence distribution, metabolism, and excretion, the effects of food on these processes often result from chronic long-term dietary practices rather than acute effects of a single meal. Effects of food on distribution

of 51 of 55 medicines studied was influenced by food, and it is well known that a number of medicine-induced clinical responses are affected by food. In discussing the influence of food on medicines, one may consider either the pharmacologically active chemical in the medicine product or the entire medicine product, which includes excipients. The latter use is the preferred one in this section, although most effects are probably related to the active moiety in the medicine product.

It has been known for a long time that taking certain medicines with food lessens the propensity of those medicines to cause adverse reactions. It has been recognized that many dietary factors exist that may affect medicine absorption, distribution, metabolism, and excretion. These dietary factors may have a major or

TABLE 87.19 *Factors to consider in interpreting data from clinical trials on the inhibition of lactation by medicines*

1. Plasma prolactin levels
2. Amount of breast milk and secretions (per day and cumulatively)
3. Degree of breast pain
4. Degree of breast engorgement
5. Occurrence of rebound lactation
6. Time to onset of menstruation following delivery
7. Amount of analgesics required
8. Composition of breast milk
9. Time to cessation of breast secretion from onset of medicine administration
10. Time of medicine administration relative to delivery
11. Amount of medicine given (total dose and individual doses)
12. Number of doses of medicine given

are probably least important and are not presented. The types of influences of food on medicine absorption (Table 87.19) are discussed first.

Pharmacokinetics: Absorption

Many of the diet-related factors and other factors that either increase or decrease absorption of medicines are listed in Tables 84.1 to 84.3 and in Tables 87.21 to 87.23. General influences that food may have on medicine absorption are listed in Table 87.21. Specific factors are arbitrarily divided into those that relate to patient characteristics (Table 84.1), medicine characteristics (Table 84.2), physiological and pharmacological principles (Table 84.3), and characteristics of meals or ingested food (Table 87.22). Many of the factors that may influence the interpretation of data in patients on special diets are listed in Table 87.23. Additional information on how food may affect data is presented in Tables 83.43 and 83.44.

Pharmacokinetics: Metabolism

Metabolism of medicines may be affected by numerous dietary factors. These factors have generally been identified and measured in well-controlled clinical trials usually lasting from several days to 2 weeks. Although a single meal may definitely affect the metabolism of a medicine, most effects result from established dietary habits or practices. An important consideration in this regard is that intrapatient variability is often as great as interpatient variability. Thus, the clinical significance of many of the observations obtained in a small number of patients must still be established for large groups or populations. Moreover, the ability to extrapolate data from tightly controlled pharmacokinetic trials conducted in a small number of homogeneous patients to a heterogeneous group of patients is usually fraught with potential problems.

TABLE 87.21 *Possible influences of food on medicine absorption[a]*

1. Medicine absorption reduced (e.g., ampicillin, tetracycline, levodopa)
2. Medicine absorption delayed (e.g., most cephalosporins, most sulfonamides, digoxin tablets)
3. Medicine absorption unchanged (e.g., theophylline, prednisone, digoxin elixir)
4. Medicine absorption increased (e.g., griseofulvin, nitrofurantoin, riboflavin)
5. Medicine absorption variable, depending on time interval between eating and drug ingestion (e.g., penicillin V, alcohol)
6. Medicine absorption dependent on the specific components in food (e.g., acetaminophen, alcohol, propoxyphene)[b]

[a] Data obtained from Welling (1977).
[b] See Table 87.22 for some specific components.

TABLE 87.22 *Factors relating to characteristics of meals or ingested food that may influence medicine absorption[a]*

1. Chemical composition of the meal (e.g., percentage of protein, fats, and carbohydrates)
2. Form of food (i.e., liquid or solid)
3. Quantity of food (e.g., a large quantity may prevent medicine reaching the mucosal surface)
4. Caloric content of the food
5. Temperature of the food (e.g., hot food delays gastric emptying)[b]
6. Viscosity of the food (e.g., high-viscosity foods delay gastric emptying)[c]
7. Time between the ingestion of the meal and medicine
8. Rapidity with which food is consumed
9. Types and quantity of fluid ingested with medicine
10. pH of the food
11. Buffering capacity of the stomach as influenced by the pH of food

[a] See Table 84.1 for a list of factors related to patient characteristics that may influence medicine absorption. Published references to the influence of these factors are given by Mayersohn (1979).
[b] Davenport (1961).
[c] Levy and Jusko (1965).

A number of test medicines have been evaluated to determine the influence of a specific dietary factor. The test medicine (e.g., antipyrine, caffeine, phenacetin, theophylline) is given before, during, and after the dietary change being evaluated. Numerous factors and substances have been shown to affect the metabolism of one or more of these medicines. These factors and substances include (1) malnutrition, (2) cruciferous vegetables such as brussels sprouts and cabbage, (3)

TABLE 87.23 *Selected factors relating to special diets that may bias data or affect their interpretation*

1. Type of diet
   a. Gluten-free (e.g., cystic fibrosis patients)
   b. Replacement therapy of congenitally absent enzymes or other chemicals
   c. Low sugar (e.g., diabetic patients)
   d. Low protein (e.g., patients in hepatic coma)
   e. Vegetarian (e.g., patients with specific philosophical and/ or religious beliefs)
2. Duration on diet
3. Degree of adherence to diet
4. Frequency of meals
5. Rapidity with which food is consumed
6. Quantity of food consumed at each meal in terms of calories and weight
7. Dietary supplements used (e.g., vitamins, minerals)
8. Type and quantity of beverages used (e.g., caffeine-containing drinks, alcohol)
9. Composition of diet: fats, proteins, carbohydrates
10. Types of fats (e.g., animal or vegetable, saturated or unsaturated)
11. Type and quantity of snacks consumed; time of day they are eaten
12. General concepts or beliefs about food, meals, eating (e.g., pleasure, boring)
13. Food hypersensitivity[a]

[a] Metcalfe (1989).

charcoal-broiled beef, and (4) ratio of carbohydrates to proteins. It is likely that numerous additional factors will be identified in future years that affect metabolism of one or more of these medicines. The clinical importance of each dietary factor that affects metabolism must be assessed individually, since it is usually not easy to extrapolate results from the clinical laboratory to clinical practice.

The metabolism of antipyrine was found to be under genetic control (Vesell and Penno, 1984). This indicated that genetic factors in addition to dietary ones are responsible for antipyrine metabolism. Vesell and Penno (1984) proposed a general methodology to identify other polymorphisms of medicine oxidation.

Pharmacokinetics: Elimination

The rate of elimination of some medicines by renal mechanisms may be decreased in patients who are fasting or starving for a prolonged period. Fasting decreases the rate of urine flow and causes a fall in urine pH, which favors diffusion of the medicine from the renal tubule back to the blood. Free fatty acids increase in plasma as a result of fasting, and these acids tend to displace highly bound medicines from albumin in plasma. The increased free concentration of medicine is then available to produce greater pharmacodynamic responses and for more rapid elimination (Reidenberg, 1977; Vesell, 1984b). This would tend to transiently increase clearance until steady state is reached. At that point, the total level is lower, but the free concentration is the same. Starving patients have greatly altered pathophysiological changes (Table 87.24) and must be viewed as a highly specific patient population whose responses to medicines and treatments should be interpreted with caution.

Cigarettes and Tobacco Products

Tobacco smoke reportedly contains over 3,000 chemicals (Dawson and Vestal, 1982); hence, it is not surprising that one or more pharmacokinetic parameters of a medicine often differ between smokers and nonsmokers. The effects of different medicines given to patients often differ on any single pharmacokinetic parameter (e.g., increased metabolic rates of some medicines and no change or decreased rates with other medicines). There appears to be no effect of smoking on liver blood flow in humans (Vestal et al., 1979) or on liver size (Lewis et al., 1972). There are numerous evaluations of the influence of smoking on medicine metabolism (Jusko, 1978; Dawson and Vestal, 1982) and also the interactions observed between smoking and age, caffeine, and alcohol (Vestal et al., 1975). Nonetheless, there are few examples of clinically im-

TABLE 87.24 *Pathophysiological changes in malnutrition likely to alter medicine kinetics and metabolism[a]*

A. Gastrointestinal changes
  1. Anorexia, vomiting, diarrhea
  2. Hypochlorhydria
  3. Mucosal atrophy, atony, gastric and mucosal dysfunction
  4. Delayed emptying and increased/decreased transit time
  5. Pancreatic dysfunction
  6. Changes in intestinal microecology
B. Body composition, body fluids, electrolytes, and minerals
  1. Decrease in total body protein, fat
  2. Increase in total body water, extracellular fluid, plasma volume, and intracellular hydration
  3. Decrease in potassium, magnesium, and other electrolyte changes
C. Plasma and tissue proteins
  1. Hypoalbuminemia, decreased albumin turnover
  2. Increase in γ-globulins
  3. Decrease in tissue proteins (muscle)
  4. Decrease in lipoproteins and other carrier proteins
D. Hepatic changes
  1. Fatty infiltration, decreased apolipoprotein synthesis, ultrastructural alterations (e.g., mitochondrial damage)
  2. Reduction in endoplasmic reticulum, ribosomal dispersion
  3. Decrease in phospholipids, adaptive changes in protein synthesis
  4. Reduced BSP excretion
E. Renal changes
  1. Hypotonic urine, acidic urine
  2. Decrease or no change in renal plasma flow and glomerular filtration rate
  3. Poor concentrating ability
F. Cardiac changes
  1. Bradycardia, hypotension, myocardial damage (electrocardiographic changes)
  2. Reduction in cardiac output, prolonged circulation time
G. Hormonal changes
  1. Adaptive changes (e.g., increased cortisol and growth hormone levels)
  2. Decreased binding of cortisol
  3. Reduced insulin and depressed thyroid function
  4. Increase in antidiuretic hormone and aldosterone levels
H. Metabolic changes
  1. Changes in intermediary metabolism
  2. Carbohydrate, protein, and fat metabolism
I. Immunological changes
  1. Impaired cell-mediated immunity, impaired humoral immune mechanism
  2. Altered phagocytic and complement system

[a] Reproduced by permission of ADIS Health Sciences Press, Inc., from Krishnaswamy (1983).

portant interactions between medicines and tobacco smoking (D'Arcy, 1984). D'Arcy mentions four medicines (insulin, propoxyphene, propranolol, and theophylline) for which evidence exists of clinically important interactions between medicines and smoking.

One reason for the few examples of clinically important interactions of medicines and tobacco is that the influence of smoking on taking most medicines has not been extensively studied. This is partly because there are many other patient-related factors that could confound the trial and data analysis. The relative ease of conducting controlled clinical trials on the influence of smoking on medicine metabolism and absorption

TABLE 87.25 *Differences between populations of smokers and nonsmokers*

1. Metabolic rates[a]
2. Risk factor for disease (e.g., lung cancer, chronic obstructive pulmonary disease, myocardial infarction)
3. Accumulation of chemicals in body (e.g., cadmium)[b]
4. Risk factor for reproductive disorders (e.g., increased incidence of abortions, preeclampsia, and neonatal mortality; decreased number of pregnancies and birth weight of newborn)

[a] Vestal et al. (1975) and Cooksley et al. (1979).
[b] Lewis et al. (1972).

TABLE 87.27 *Selected factors relating to a patient's consumption of alcohol that may bias data or affect their interpretation*

1. Type of alcohol consumed (e.g., beer, wine, various types of hard liquor)
2. Frequency of consumption
3. Amount of alcohol used per day, week, or month
4. Blood level achieved
5. History of consumption prior to the clinical trial
6. Consumption during the trial
7. Interactions with trial medication
8. Use of branded alcohol versus "moonshine" alcohol

accounts for the extensive literature in this area. Table 87.25 lists some of the differences between smokers and nonsmokers and Table 87.26 the factors that may influence the interpretation of data from patients who use tobacco products.

Passive smoking (i.e., inhalation by nonsmokers of tobacco smoke) is becoming more widely recognized as a potential health hazard for patients with allergies (Zussman, 1974) and angina (Aronow, 1978), as well as for normal individuals (Speer, 1968; Weber and Fischer, 1980; Jarvis et al., 1985). Passive smoking may alter pharmacokinetics of medicines. Matsunga et al. (1989) report that passive smokers metabolize theophylline more rapidly than nonsmokers.

Alcohol and Drug Abuse

It is generally desired to eliminate patients from a clinical trial who abuse alcohol or drugs unless one of these groups is specifically desired as a trial population. There are several reasons for their exclusion, including (1) potential medicine interactions that may occur and could yield data incorrectly attributed to the study medicine; (2) difficulty in obtaining an accurate medical history; (3) unreliability of many patients in terms of protocol compliance; (4) increased likelihood of subclinical as well as clinically apparent signs, symptoms, and physiological abnormalities (e.g., hepatic enzyme elevations); (5) increased likelihood of subclinical dis-

eases, psychological problems, or behavioral abnormalities, which may be exacerbated by illicit drugs or alcohol taken during the study; and (6) lack of cooperation in keeping clinic appointments as scheduled.

There are numerous clinical trials that are specifically conducted in one of these populations. For example, a group of drug abusers may evaluate the abuse potential of a new medicine in a double-blind manner with a relevant control drug (e.g., morphine, amphetamine). Clinical trials designed to wean patients off alcohol or drugs require the target patient population to evaluate efficacy. Virtually all such clinical trials should be conducted in a double-blind manner. Viamontes (1972) has reported that 95% of 72 uncontrolled trials of alcohol withdrawal treatment have reported successful outcomes, whereas only 1 of 17 controlled trials had a successful outcome.

Whether clinical trials are conducted in populations of alcohol and drug abusers or in other populations that include patients who may use alcohol or illicit drugs, it is often important to obtain precise data on the extent of patient alcohol and drug use. A number of factors related to alcohol and drug use that may affect data or bias its interpretation are indicated in Tables 87.27 (alcohol) and 87.28 (drugs).

Occupations

In most studies the population of patients enrolled have various occupations, and any influence on the clinical

TABLE 87.26 *Selected factors relating to tobacco products that may bias data or affect their interpretation*

1. Type of tobacco used (e.g., cigarette, pipe, cigar, chewing)
2. Frequency and amount used
3. Brand of tobacco used
4. Amount of tar and nicotine present in the tobacco
5. Amount of tobacco inhaled
6. Presence or absence of a filter
7. History of use prior to clinical trial
8. History of use during the trial
9. Influence on patient's metabolic function[a]
10. Interactions with trial medicine
11. Influence on patient's clinical state
12. Degree and nature of enzyme induction

[a] Jusko (1978).

TABLE 87.28 *Selected factors relating to patients who abuse drugs that may bias data or affect their interpretation*

1. Identity of drug(s) being abused
2. Type of abuse
3. History of abuse
4. Previous types of treatment
5. Previous results of treatment
6. Recent history of abuse
7. Complications from abuse
8. Motivation to stop abuse
9. Reason(s) for enrolling in clinical trial
10. High incidence of underlying physical abnormalities (e.g., liver enzyme elevations)
11. High incidence of underlying psychological abnormalities (e.g., compliance may be poor, prevarication may occur)

TABLE 87.29 *Selected factors relating to a patient's type of work that may bias data or affect their interpretation*

1. Number of people who report directly to the patient
2. Total number of people who report to the patient
3. Level of challenge experienced by the patient
4. Level of job satisfaction
5. Level of stress experienced by the patient
6. Opportunities for career growth perceived by the patient
7. Degree of authority used by the patient's supervisor(s)
8. Amount of personal contact with other individuals
9. Amount of creativity allowed or encouraged
10. Demands and requirements placed on a patient
11. Amount of hard physical work
12. Length of work day and number of hours worked per week
13. Exposure to biological toxins, noxious fumes, chemicals, radiation, other electromagnetic waves[a]
14. Degree of danger associated with the position

[a] Tomlin (1979). See text for additional references.

trial relating to their occupation is nullified because most of the other patients will have different occupations. Nonetheless, there are trials that are conducted either purposely or by chance in patients predominantly or entirely of one occupation. In these situations it is important to consider whether there is any influence of the occupation or specific place of work on the data obtained. A list of various factors relating to a patient's type of work that may affect data and influence the interpretation of data is given in Table 87.29. A list of factors that relate to the patient's place of work is given in Table 87.30. If factors relating to either the type or place of work are considered to be potentially important influences on data, then the methods of patient recruitment should be appropriately modified.

Many occupations are associated with conditions that present medical hazards to workers. Even families of workers may be affected by medical problems relating to the occupation of the spouse (Tomlin, 1979). Apart from occupations that are hazardous because the person is occasionally risking his life (e.g., soldier, po-

liceman, specialist in bomb disposal), there are many occupations in which a higher incidence of specific hazards is known to occur than in the general population (e.g., carpenters often are physically injured, farmers and textile workers often contract pulmonary disease, animal breeders often contract various diseases). Numerous occupations also have either vague or specific reports of medical problems, and occupational risks have not yet been fully determined. Examples chosen from the medical area include operating room personnel (*Ad Hoc* Committee on the Effect of Trace Anesthetics on the Health of Operating Room Personnel, 1974) and dental workers (Schneider, 1974), plus nurses exposed to antineoplastic medicines (Selevan et al., 1985; Bingham, 1985). The field of occupational medicine was recently reviewed (Cullen et al., 1990).

Medical risks associated with some individual professions have been known for many decades [e.g., hatters who became insane from mercury poisoning (this is the origin of the term "mad as a hatter"), coal miners who acquired various pulmonary diseases, radiologists who had numerous problems from excessive exposure to radiation, uranium miners who had high rates of lung cancer (Roscoe et al., 1989), agricultural workers who suffered from herbicides (Hoar et al., 1986)]. A summary of various medical risks of fatality associated with different occupations is presented by Pochin (1975). People who must stand or sit for excessive periods often develop various muscle problems in their backs and/or legs. A number of the factors that may affect data or its interpretation from patients exposed to hazardous occupational conditions or to industrial or environmental accidents are listed in Table 87.31. A method that may be used to estimate a person's history of occupational exposure to chemical

TABLE 87.30 *Selected factors relating to a patient's place of work that may bias data or affect their interpretation*

1. Geographical location (e.g., city, farm)
2. Location either outdoors or indoors
3. Environmental factors (e.g., quality of air, presence of natural light)
4. Floor or location in building
5. Physical conditions at work (e.g., temperature, square feet)
6. Psychological conditions of work (e.g., stress, intensity of work)
7. Type of lighting (e.g., sunlight, incandescent, full-spectrum fluorescent lights, narrow-spectrum fluorescent lights)
8. Noise level
9. Relationship with co-workers, superiors, individuals reporting to person (e.g., degree of harassment)
10. Length of time spent at current place of work (in months or years)

TABLE 87.31 *Selected factors relating to patients exposed to hazardous occupational conditions or to an industrial or environmental accident that may bias data or affect their interpretation*

1. Whether the patient is in the primary group of people affected
2. Whether patient was directly affected; if so (1) how, (2) to what degree, and (3) for what length of time
3. Presence of other physical, emotional, or other preexisting conditions in the patient that may exacerbate or mitigate the results
4. Presence of any physical, emotional, or other conditions in the patient that occurred after the event and are probably or definitely a result of exposure
5. Direct or indirect evidence that associates the accident with other health-related problems in the patient
6. Current exposure of the patient to the hazard
7. Evaluation of the patient's previous medical reaction to the accident or hazard
8. Previous treatment of the patient for exposure or hazard
9. Status of the patient vis-à-vis any possible litigation or workman's compensation

TABLE 87.32 *Selected factors relating to a patient's prior treatment or response to treatment that may bias data or affect their interpretation*

1. Prior treatment with one modality (e.g., radiation, surgery) may render patients less (or more) responsive to other treatment modalities
2. Prior treatment with certain medicines will have an effect on a patient's response to other medicines (e.g., patients treated with medicines that induce microsomal enzymes in the liver)
3. Lack of response to certain treatments, which indicates that a patient is a nonresponder or at least less responsive than expected to standard therapy
4. Hypersensitivity in response to a given treatment may indicate that the patient has a high likelihood of having a similar response to other treatments

TABLE 87.34 *Selected factors relating to patient consumption of caffeine-containing drinks that may bias data or affect their interpretation*

1. Type of drinks consumed (e.g., coffee, tea, colas)
2. Frequency of consumption
3. Amount of caffeine consumed per day, week, or month
4. History of consumption prior to the clinical trial
5. Consumption during the trial
6. Interactions with trial medicine

TABLE 87.35 *Selected factors relating to special exercise programs that may bias data or affect their interpretation*

1. Type of exercise
2. Frequency and duration of exercise at each session
3. Level of exertion and elevation of heart rate obtained
4. History of activity during the clinical trial
5. Adherence to prescribed program
6. Reason for patient's participation in the program (e.g., obesity, cardiac disease)

agents is presented by Gérin et al. (1985), and a standard method for conducting research on reproductive effects of occupation is presented by Joffe (1988).

Social Classes

The incidence of several types of cancers has been associated with social class (Anonymous, 1988a), although several logical reasons have been given in most cases (e.g., influence of diet in causing stomach can-

TABLE 87.33 *Selected factors relating to concomitant medicines that may bias data or affect their interpretation*

1. The identity of the concomitant medicine(s) the patient is taking
2. The reason the patient is taking concomitant medicines
3. The dose that is being taken
4. The frequency of taking the medicines
5. Whether the concomitant medicines are allowed by protocol (e.g., unacceptable medicines may yield responses attributed to trial medicine; acceptable medicines may interact with the trial medicine to influence results)
6. Whether concomitant medicines are interacting with the trial medicine. If so, how
7. Whether concomitant medicines are treating the same condition as the trial medicine
8. Whether concomitant medicines are acting by the same mechanism as the trial medicine
9. Whether the trial is an add-on trial (i.e., one in which patients receive medicines that may or may not be controlled by name and dose in the protocol and the trial evaluates the effects of a medicine added to the patient's regimen)
10. Whether concomitant medicines approved by the protocol are taken with greater, lesser, or the same compliance as the trial medicine
11. Whether there are adverse reactions resulting from the concomitant medicines[a]
12. Trial medicines are sometimes evaluated for their ability to treat adverse reactions resulting from a concomitant medicine. In those trials, the adverse reactions of the concomitant medicine must be of sufficient magnitude (i.e., intensity) and character to qualify the patient for enrollment

[a] It is often difficult, if not impossible, to differentiate between adverse reactions resulting from a trial medicine, a concomitant medicine, or their interaction.

cer, smoking in causing lung cancer). Reye's syndrome (Morris and Schapiro, 1986) is another disease whose incidence is reportedly related to social class, as is coronary heart disease (Rosengren et al., 1988). Mortality from coronary heart disease and cystic fibrosis (Britton, 1989) are both reported to be related to social class.

Social class has also been correlated with length of hospital stay (Epstein et al., 1988) and with rates of cesarean section (Gould et al., 1989). But these and other medical service differences probably occur for logical reasons that could be evaluated.

Other Patient Populations

There are several other special patient populations that may be evaluated in separate clinical trials or assessed as factors (e.g., by a subgroup analysis) in a trial in which the population issue is a secondary consideration. Table 87.1 lists several of these groups, and Tables 87.32 through 87.36 describe factors related to several of these populations.

TABLE 87.36 *Selected factors relating to sexual habits or preferences that may bias data or affect their interpretation*

1. Heterosexuality, homosexuality, or bisexuality
2. Nature of sexual habits
3. Frequency of sexual activities
4. Types of sexual dysfunctions (e.g., decreased libido, impotence, dyspareunia)
5. "Selective recall" may readily bias data because of the sensitive nature of the topic for many or most patients

PART **IX**

Issues and Problems of Clinical Data Interpretation

Overinterpretation is an effort to compensate for underplanning.

—Jerome Cornfield, American statistician

True Science teaches, above all, to doubt, and to be ignorant.

—Miguel de Unamuno

I seem to have been only like a boy playing on the seashore and diverting myself in now and then finding a smoothe pebble or a prettier shell than ordinary whilst the great ocean of truth lay all undiscovered before me.

—Isaac Newton

CHAPTER 88

Extrapolation of Safety (i.e., Toxicological) Data from Animals to Humans

INTRODUCTION

Degree of Risk

Before it is legal to test any new chemical compound in humans toxicological studies must be performed in laboratory animals. These studies are intended to characterize adverse effects and ensure that the risk for humans is minimal or at least acceptable. The consequences of failing to conduct adequate toxicology studies prior to exposure of the medicine to humans can include severe adverse reactions that could have been prevented. A series of eight case histories of this type of occurrence with sulfanilamide elixir, pronethalol, triparanol, hexobendine, triflocin, cinanserin, ethynerone, and chlormadinone acetate are presented by Nestor (1975). Other similar studies are reported by Fraumeni and Miller (1972) and Thiede et al. (1964). The degree of risk that is allowed by regulatory agen-

cies varies, depending on (1) the target disease or condition for which the medicine will eventually be tested, (2) availability of other medicine or nonmedicine treatments for the target disease, (3) the relative safety and efficacy of the alternative medicine or nonmedicine treatments, (4) the general degree of safety of chemicals related to the class of study medicine, and (5) any other factors deemed relevant. If the test medicine is intended to prevent a disease (or problem) from occurring, less risk would generally be acceptable and preclinical testing would be more rigorous.

Types of Extrapolation

The primary assumption underlying toxicological studies is that the data obtained are predictive for effects that would (or could) be observed in humans. This chapter focuses on the evidence that supports the extrapolation of animal toxicological data for predicting human adverse reactions. Readers interested in the scientific basis underlying extrapolation of animal data to humans are referred to *Principles of Animal Extrapolation* (Calabrese, 1983). Extrapolations of toxicological data are primarily of two types. The first is between species, and the other is from effects noted at high or moderate doses to dosage levels that are at or below levels that may be of interest for clinical trials.

The most direct approach for determining the extrapolatability of toxicological effects for humans is to measure retrospectively the correlation between results obtained in animals and humans. Even the best possible data, however, will not enable one to predict whether the next compound tested will yield false-negative, false-positive, or correct data about effects that will be observed in humans.

One of the biases against the direct comparison of animal and human data is that most medicines that are highly toxic in animals are never tested in humans. This bias makes it difficult to study the predictive value of preclinical toxicology studies. Before exploring this topic, let us look at the types of toxicological studies.

TYPES OF TOXICOLOGICAL STUDIES

Toxicological studies are usually performed with the objective of either (1) predicting potentially serious toxicity that may occur in humans or (2) clarifying and examining in detail suspected or documented toxicities previously observed in humans or in animals (if considered relevant for humans). Only the first of these functions is considered in this chapter. The types of toxicological studies discussed are dose-ranging studies, acute studies, subchronic and chronic studies, and specialized studies (e.g., mutagenicity, carcinogenicity, teratogenicity, reproduction, and fertility studies).

Dose-Ranging Studies

Dose-ranging studies are high-dose preliminary studies that provide an initial toxicologic characterization of test materials and provide data used to select doses of a medicine suitable for evaluation in future toxicological studies. Species are chosen on the basis of (1) similarity of absorption, distribution, metabolism, and/or excretion to humans, (2) evolutionary level of animal, (3) sensitivity of the species to the medicine, (4) sensitivity of the species to demonstrate an effect of interest (e.g., rats do not vomit), (5) economic factors, and (6) time constraints and other practical factors. Doses chosen are usually multiples of the anticipated

human dose. Although most patients and physicians would be better able to assess a medicine's safety when toxicology studies were conducted at several doses up to 100 times the maximum human dose than when a single dose of only twice the maximum human dose is given, using large multiples of the human dose often creates practical problems. Large doses may compromise study interpretation. There may be physical difficulties with administering large quantities of medicines to animals, and there may be problems relating to pharmacokinetic processes (e.g., saturation of enzymes or elimination mechanisms). Some of these problems are listed in Table 88.1.

Dose Levels Evaluated in Toxicology Studies

Standard toxicology studies use three dose levels at arithmetic intervals (e.g., $\times$, $2\times$, $4\times$; $\times$, $3\times$, $9\times$). Alternatives include using two dose levels and unequal dose intervals, but international guidelines require the former approach.

Low-Dose Level. One hopes not to see any adverse effects at a low-dose level. This dose may be as low as the human dose, but is chosen as the highest dose for which no toxic effects are anticipated in animals. One exception occurs when dose-ranging studies have failed to demonstrate any toxicological effects. In that situation, the highest doses practical to test at equal dose intervals are usually chosen.

Mid-Dose Level. The mid-dose is a multiple (e.g., twofold, threefold) of the low dose that is chosen to see some toxic effects in animals. Effects observed may be minimal.

High-Dose Level. The high dose is usually a three-, four-, or sixfold increment of the low-dose level, chosen to observe clear toxicity short of death of all animals. It is not surprising to observe a few deaths at high-dose levels.

TABLE 88.1 *Reasons why high-dose toxicological testing does not usually mimic human bioavailability or metabolism*

1. Solubility of the compound may be limiting
2. Kinetics may be nonlinear (e.g., an enzyme may be saturated), and absorption may be decreased
3. Michaelis–Menten kinetics may be applicable, and the blood levels may be greater than predicted[a]
4. Metabolites formed may reach much higher blood levels than in a clinical trial. These metabolites may cause toxicity that would not occur with lower doses (e.g., this is observed with high doses of phenacetin)
5. Detoxification mechanisms in the liver may be depleted or saturated (e.g., this is observed with high doses of acetaminophen)

[a] The Michaelis–Menten equation gives the initial rate of the reaction between an enzyme and a substrate.

Acute, Subchronic, and Chronic Studies

Acute studies include the now discontinued LD$_{50}$ test (i.e., determining the dose of the medicine that kills 50% of the test species). The LD$_{50}$ of a single medicine varies according to experimental conditions and has limited use in predicting adverse reactions in humans (Heywood, 1984). It is now the practice to perform only limited acute testing. Determination of a precise LD$_{50}$ value has no necessary role in the development of new medicines (Dayan et al., 1984) and is generally believed to be a waste of animal resources. Subchronic and chronic toxicological studies usually last from 2 weeks to 2 years. Most regulatory authorities require data from two species before approving a new compound for sale.

Carcinogenicity Tests

One of the most critical aspects of extrapolation of toxicological data relates to assessing the potential of medicines to cause cancer in humans. Few toxicological findings will terminate development of new medicines as rapidly as carcinogenicity. One of the few exceptions is for anticancer medicines, some of which also actually cause cancer.

Before one attempts to determine how well rodent carcinogenicity bioassays predict the ability of medicines to cause cancers in humans, it is valuable to determine if such data can be extrapolated from one rodent species to another. Two authors have studied this question in detail (Purchase, 1980; Di Carlo, 1984). In evaluating data on 230 bioassays conducted on 221 substances, Di Carlo found extremely poor interspecies correlation and concluded that "Carcinogenesis in the mouse cannot now be predicted from positive bioassay data obtained from the rat and vice versa." In evaluating 250 compounds, Purchase found fewer discrepancies (17%) between results obtained in the two species, but concluded that "extrapolation from results in a single animal study to man may be subject to substantial errors."

Bioassays in animals were compared with in vitro tests in terms of costs and considering false-positive and false-negative results. Lave and Omenn (1986) supported the approach of in vitro testing, but these authors were examining toxic chemicals from society's viewpoint of evaluating a large number of untested versus poorly tested chemicals.

Two types of tests are used to try to detect potential of medicines for causing malignant tumors: short-term mutagenicity tests described under genetic toxicology and lifetime in vivo exposure of rats and mice to the medicine. Carcinogenicity bioassays of chemicals or new medicines are usually conducted in rats and mice

dosed for their natural lifespan (approximately 2 years). Both false-positive and false-negative results have been reported (Schein et al., 1970; Salsburg, 1983). Although the correlation between animal and human data for carcinogenic effects is variable, it is assumed that carcinogenicity in animal studies is generally predictive of human risk. Few patients would be willing to take a medicine that may be carcinogenic (unless of course the benefit-to-risk ratio dictated otherwise).

An important consensus of most toxicologists is that extrapolation of data from animals to humans for carcinogenesis is more valid for data obtained from intact animals exposed to the chemical than for data obtained from various in vitro tests. Nonetheless, as rodents age, they experience a high incidence of endocrine disturbances and tumors not frequently found in humans (Goodman et al., 1979), indicating that untreated control animals are not totally representative of unexposed humans. In addition, these animals are overfed and are celibate. The practice of testing high doses of chemicals in the bioassay may further limit the utility of this method in the safety evaluation process. There are also important species differences in pharmacokinetics, metabolism, and response to the medicine. Although the carcinogenesis bioassay has never been validated, it is still considered the definitive and most useful technique for addressing questions about the carcinogenic potential of new medicines. Toxicologists currently are engaged in extensive debates about the future of the bioassay.

The dose of a medicine (relative to human exposure) that causes cancer in animals, the type of cancer, the number of animals involved, and time to occurrence are all important features in assessing the relevance of the data for humans. Most cancers that occur as a result of medicines would be difficult to detect in epidemiological studies unless they affected a relatively large percentage of exposed patients with a relatively short period. If a small number of patients treated with a specific medicine developed a common cancer several years later, it would be extremely difficult to identify the cancer as being medicine related. Thus, animal studies will probably remain the mainstay of predicting medicine-induced cancers in humans until there are major changes in technology.

Developmental Toxicology Studies

Several basic types of developmental toxicity studies are performed in toxicological testing. Teratologic tests involve giving the medicine to female rats, mice, and rabbits during the period of their pregnancy (organogenesis) when their fetuses are most vulnerable to teratogenic effects. Their fetuses are evaluated for the presence and type of congenital malformations. General reproductive studies involve dosing parental animals during oogenesis and spermatogenesis. Both the females and offspring are observed at various times to evaluate fertility and development. Separate studies on spermatogenesis are sometimes conducted. Finally, peri- and postnatal studies involve dosing females through the last quarter of pregnancy and during lactation to evaluate effects on both mother and offspring (Table 88.2). The predictive ability of these tests for the human situation has not been explored extensively.

The number of known teratogens in humans is relatively small. Although chemicals reported to produce malformations in laboratory animals number in the hundreds, Shepard (1986) lists only 29 pharmaceuticals as known human teratogens and another five that are considered questionable.

Genetic Toxicology Studies

The field of genetic toxicology is directed primarily toward detection of agents that may affect genetic material. Such effects can be limited to certain cancers or fetal malformations. The predictability of most of the tests for human events is unknown but is presumed to be relevant, because many of the tests are based on a study of DNA damage and repair. There are over 100 tests available, and they are ordered in a hierarchy from those studying subcellular components in vitro to other in vitro tests involving tissues and to in vivo animal tests. Each test can only indicate that a potential exists to induce a particular kind of genetic damage in humans. For this reason, various combinations (i.e., a battery) of tests are used to evaluate investigational or marketed medicines. A common strategy for testing medicines is to start with highly sensitive and artificial tests. The actual specificity, predictability, and validity of such tests are not yet established, although in vivo tests are believed to have greater relevance for human effects (von Wittenau and LeBeau, 1982).

Not all carcinogens are mutagens, and vice versa.

TABLE 88.2 *Selected measures of behavioral change in animals born to mothers exposed to medicine[a]*

1. Psychological tests
2. Learning
3. Short- and long-term memory
4. Reproductive behavior
5. Passive avoidance for shocks
6. Fine motor control
7. Sight
8. Extinction (i.e., how long does it take for a learned response to disappear)
9. Social behavior
10. Emotionality (e.g., spontaneous activity)

[a] These studies are primarily conducted in rats.

The carcinogenicity bioassays described above are the major tests used to identify potential human carcinogens. Additional evaluations are required to understand which systems and endpoints (e.g., molecular alterations of DNA, cytological observation of gross chromosomal damage, point mutations) are most predictive of human response. At present, many false positives and negatives are believed to result from evaluations such as the Ames test.

Many people loosely use the terms *mutagenicity* and *genetic toxicology* interchangeably. However, mutagenicity and genetic toxicity are not identical. Mutagenicity does not include the concept of risk assessment that is part of genetic toxicology, nor does mutagenicity strictly include the study of chromosomal damage.

Types of Differences in Pharmaceutical Effects Observed within Species

Many pathological effects observed in animals as they age are dependent on the species studied. Toxicological effects for a specific medicine may differ depending on the strain and species as well as environmental factors.

Type I Intraspecies Effects. These depend on factors relating to the species, such as strain, sex, metabolism, genetic breeding, weight, age, or other factors.

Type II Intraspecies Effects. These depend on factors relating to the environment, such as temperature, housing conditions, humidity, type of diet, amount of food, number and proximity of animals, amount of light, and amount of handling.

Overall differences observed for a medicine may be:

1. No effect in one species and an effect in another
2. Opposite effects in two species
3. Different effects in the same system in two species (e.g., white blood cells affected in one species and red blood cells in another)
4. Same effect in both species, but of a substantially different magnitude or time of occurrence

PREDICTING ADVERSE HUMAN EFFECTS FROM TOXICOLOGICAL DATA

In most situations there are greater difficulties in interpreting clinical data than animal data. The basis for this, in large part, is related to the simple fact that human test populations are not as well defined and uniform as the laboratory animals toxicologists study. In most instances animals will have been bred to be similar in genetic composition (Festing, 1990) and possibly even to share certain physiological characteristics such as risk factors for developing a certain disease. One noteworthy exception to this concept occurs when the interpretation of data is dependent on direct (or even indirect) communications between the subject (animal or patient) and investigator. It is more difficult to obtain reliable data from animals in these situations, such as evaluating the presence and degree of pain or stress.

Questions to Address

When a deleterious effect is noted in animal toxicological studies, it is important to investigate whether the effect is:

1. Observed in animals at both high and low doses (i.e., is the effect dose related or idiosyncratic?)
2. Observed in other animal species
3. Observed at low or high multiples of the maximum human dose
4. Reversible when the medicine is stopped (or continued)
5. Observed in humans, resulting from the trial medicine
6. Observed in humans, resulting from other medicines. If the effect occurs with other medicines, how is the effect related to the other medicines? If patients who enter a trial previously have been treated with the other medicine, how can the effect accurately be attributed to the correct medicine, especially if the effect may be noted after medicine treatment is stopped?
7. Able to be followed with a biological marker

Published Evaluations

Other types of toxicologic data have been evaluated to assess their predictive value for humans. Retrospective data from five animal species (mouse, rat, hamster, dog, and monkey) tested with 18 compounds were used with two different models to determine which model and species was best able to predict the maximum tolerated dose (MTD) of anticancer medicines in man. The MTD in humans (in milligrams per square meter) was about the same for the compounds tested as that observed in each animal species (Freireich et al., 1966). Retrospective data for 25 anticancer compounds tested in dogs and monkeys were found generally to predict toxicities observed in humans, but a high percentage of false-positive toxicities was observed in animals (Schein et al., 1970). Wilbourn et al. (1986) reported that tests of known and suspected carcinogens were quite sensitive (about 84%).

Heywood (1984) reported that for 42 compounds evaluated in both the rat and dog there was an extremely poor correlation of the target organs affected. Litchfield (1962) evaluated six compounds studied in humans, rats, and dogs and calculated the likelihood that (1) adverse reactions would be found in humans if they were found in both rats and dogs and (2) adverse reactions would not be found in humans if they were only found in one animal species. He found that 68% of the toxic effects observed in both rats and dogs were found in humans and 79% of the toxic effects observed in either rats or dogs (but not in both species) were not found in humans. He found that for the specific medicines tested the dog yielded better data than did the rat for predicting human responses (Litchfield, 1961). The best correlations between animals and human data were reported for gastrointestinal complaints, especially vomiting. Schein et al. (1970) reported that Litchfield's analysis overstated the results by not accounting for the large number of false negatives in animals, which accounted for 68% of the toxicity observed in humans. Fletcher (1978) reported that for any medicine (of the 45 in his sample), 25% of the toxic effects noted in animals could occur as adverse reactions in humans. Also see discussions by Garattini (1985), Griffin (1985), Ruelins (1987), and Calabrese (1988).

Could Toxicology Studies Designed in Hindsight Predict Actual Human Adverse Reactions?

Heywood (1984) evaluated many of the major clinical adverse reactions reported in the literature since 1961 and evaluated whether animal toxicological tests (in hindsight) would have been predictive of the clinical problem. These data are shown in Table 88.3. Fourteen specific medicines or types of medicines are listed as causing 13 adverse reactions in humans. Of the 13 adverse reactions, 6 were not observed in animal testing. Of the seven cases in which confirmatory animal results were observed in hindsight (after the human toxicity was known), several involved either uncommon testing procedures (e.g., experimental lactic acidosis induced in dogs infused with phenformin) or use of uncommon species for routine toxicological studies (e.g., Syrian hamsters were used to demonstrate a lethal enterocolitis from clindamycin or lincomycin). Issues relating to the predictive utility of preclinical toxicological testing for various medicines (e.g., bethanidine, bromocriptine, cimetidine, tamoxifen) are explored in a book (Laurence et al., 1984).

Three reasons were given by Johnsson et al. (1984) to explain why it is difficult to relate human adverse reactions to animal data: (1) subjective adverse reac-

TABLE 88.3 *Major medicine-induced adverse reactions observed clinically on marketed medicines since 1961[a]*

Medicine	Adverse reaction in humans	Results of animal toxicity testing[b]
Practolol	Oculomucocutaneous syndrome	Not predictive
Oral contraceptives	Thromboembolism	Not predictive
Phenacetin (analgesics)	Nephropathy	Confirmatory—rat[c]
Phenformin	Lactic acidosis	Confirmatory—dog
Sympathomimetic aerosols	Asthmatic death	Not predictive
Clioquinol	Subacute myelo-opticneuropathy	Confirmatory—dog
Diethylstilbestrol	Vaginal cancer in female offspring	Confirmatory—mice, cebus monkeys
Chloramphenicol	Aplastic anemia	Not predictive
Halothane	Jaundice	Predictable in rats, mice, dogs, monkeys
Methysergide	Retroperitoneal fibrosis	Not predictive
Lincomycin, clindamycin	Pseudomembranous colitis	Confirmatory—hamster
Phenylbutazone	Aplastic anemia	Not predictive
Phenothiazines	Dyskinesia	Predictable in dogs, monkeys

[a] Reproduced by permission of Almqvist and Wiksell from Heywood (1984).
[b] These tests were conducted after the adverse reactions were observed, in an attempt to mimic the finding in animals.
[c] High doses and physiological modification.

tions are not detectable in animals (e.g., dizziness, headache, nausea), (2) medicine doses (and plasma levels) are often excessive in animal studies, and (3) immunological effects are difficult to detect in animals. A detailed discussion of this topic for a single hepatotoxic medicine is given by Clarke et al. (1985).

The Scaling Factor

A principle that underlies extrapolation of toxicological data to humans has been referred to as the "scaling factor." Certain mathematical relationships of body weight are consistent in many animal species (Calabrese, 1983). This is the basis whereby doses calculated per square meter of surface area can often be compared across species. A clear example of this is shown in Table 88.4 for the anticancer medicines methotrexate and mechlorethamine. Doses on a milligram per square meter per day basis are quite consistent across species and different sized humans, although the other measures shown in the table are quite variable.

Comparisons of doses based on body surface area have been most useful for identifying starting doses for cancer chemotherapeutic agents. The endpoints in laboratory animals are prominent (e.g., death) and generation of a reactive metabolite is characteristic of this work. There is no evidence that for routine toxicologic purposes extrapolation is better when doses are expressed on the basis of body surface area than when expressed on the basis of body weight (e.g., mg/kg).

ISSUES AND CONTROVERSIES IN TOXICOLOGY RELATING TO EXTRAPOLATION OF DATA

Duration of Long-Term Tests

A few controversies in the field of toxicology that relate to extrapolation of animal data to humans can be mentioned. Some toxicologists claim that chronic tox-

TABLE 88.4 *Dosages of methotrexate and mechlorethamine in several species[a]*

Subject	Weight (kg)	Surface area (m^2)	Dose/day (mg)	Dose (mg)/kg per day	Dose (mg)/m^2 per day
			Methotrexate		
Mouse	0.018	0.0075	0.027	1.5	3.6
Rat	0.25	0.045	0.125	0.5	2.8
Infant	8.0	0.4	1.25	0.15	3.1
Older child	20.0	0.8	2.5	0.12	3.1
Adult	70.0	1.85	5.0	0.07	2.7

Subject	Weight (kg)	Surface area (m^2)	Total dose (mg)	Total dose (mg/kg)	Total dose (mg/m^2)
			Mechlorethamine		
Mouse	0.018	0.0075	0.072	4.0	9.6
Hamster	0.050	0.0137	0.15	3.0	10.9
Rat	0.25	0.045	0.5	2.0	11.1
Human	70.0	1.85	21–28	0.3–0.4	11.3–15.1

[a] Reprinted by permission of *Cancer Research* from Pinkel (1958).

icology tests that last for more than a certain duration (about 3 to 6 months) yield little meaningful data or information beyond that obtained in the first 3 to 6 months. John Griffin (1986) writes "I came to the personal conclusion that with most NCEs [New Chemical Entities], little new data on the toxicology was revealed after 3 months, and that no significant new toxicological manifestations were revealed by prolonging the repeated-dose toxicity tests beyond 6 months. . . . Apart from the investigation of carcinogenic potential, little seems to be gained by conducting repeated-dose toxicity studies beyond 6 months." McNamara (1976) quotes numerous references that discuss this point.

Doses to Use in Toxicology Studies

Another issue relates to the magnitude of the doses that should be evaluated in animals to seek information about potential human toxicity. Some toxicologists believe that very large doses should be used in animals to elicit as many potential human toxicities as possible (Schein et al., 1970). Other toxicologists stress the fact that extremely high doses may saturate various pharmacologic, metabolic, or elimination mechanisms and lead to altered pharmacokinetic processes and irrelevant toxicity in animals that would never be observed in humans. Moreover, when animals are given extremely high doses, new metabolic routes may be used, and new metabolites may be formed. These new compounds could then elicit their own toxicities, which again would be unrelated to effects encountered with human exposure.

Assessing Clinical versus Toxicological Endpoints

Another difficulty in extrapolating toxicological data to humans relates to the clinical endpoints measured. Many relevant endpoints in humans (e.g., subjective feelings) cannot be measured in animals, and others measured in animals are not relevant for humans (e.g., anatomical structures only found in animals). Rare events in humans will generally be rarely observed in animals. This is noteworthy because few animals are evaluated in comparison with human exposure to most medicines.

Threshold Doses in Carcinogenicity Studies

A particularly strong controversy exists about whether currently used carcinogenicity tests in animals are the best designed studies to use for predicting potential for human cancers. Certain critics of the current methodology (e.g., Salsburg, 1983) have been strongly at-

tacked by proponents who believe that "there is clearly a strong positive correlation between human carcinogens and adequately designed laboratory animal carcinogenicity studies" (Haseman et al., 1983). One of the basic issues concerns the question of whether there is a safe level of exposure below which there is no risk to humans or if no threshold of the dose–response relationship exists and there is always some degree of risk, even with minute doses. Although pharmacological dose–response relationships are sigmoidal for chemical substances, some scientists believe that these relationships are linear for carcinogenic substances starting at the origin of the curve (i.e., it is necessary to go to zero dose to eliminate the risk of cancer). Another way of stating this issue is that when effects are observed at high doses, what is the likelihood that they will be observed with usually prescribed doses? This is shown in Fig. 88.1.

Circadian Effects

Circadian fluctuations in toxicologic and pharmacologic effects of medicines have been reported for many medicines that affect the central nervous system (Nagayama et al., 1981). The relevance that this may have for future toxicological studies is uncertain but is probably small.

Species Specificities

Species that are higher on the evolutionary scale are usually considered to give better data for human predictability than do lower animals. Nonetheless, there are numerous exceptions. The single most important factor causing differences among species in their susceptibility to toxic agents is metabolism (Calabrese, 1983, page 577). Other important factors include (1) absorption, (2) protein binding, (3) intestinal flora, and (4) biliary excretion. There are also differences between species in the way that they maintain homeostasis in the presence of toxic chemicals by protecting, stabilizing, and repairing mechanisms.

Background Incidence of Lesions and Tumors. All strains of rodents develop a substantial incidence of spontaneous tumors beginning at approximately 16 months. This means that it becomes more difficult to differentiate a medicine's effects from background effects as time extends beyond 1 year. In addition, there are marked species differences between tumors that occur in mice, rats, and humans. There is also a difference in the incidence of numerous tumors observed in males versus females. These points are ironic, because long-term effects are of particular importance in evaluating the carcinogenic effects of most medicines.

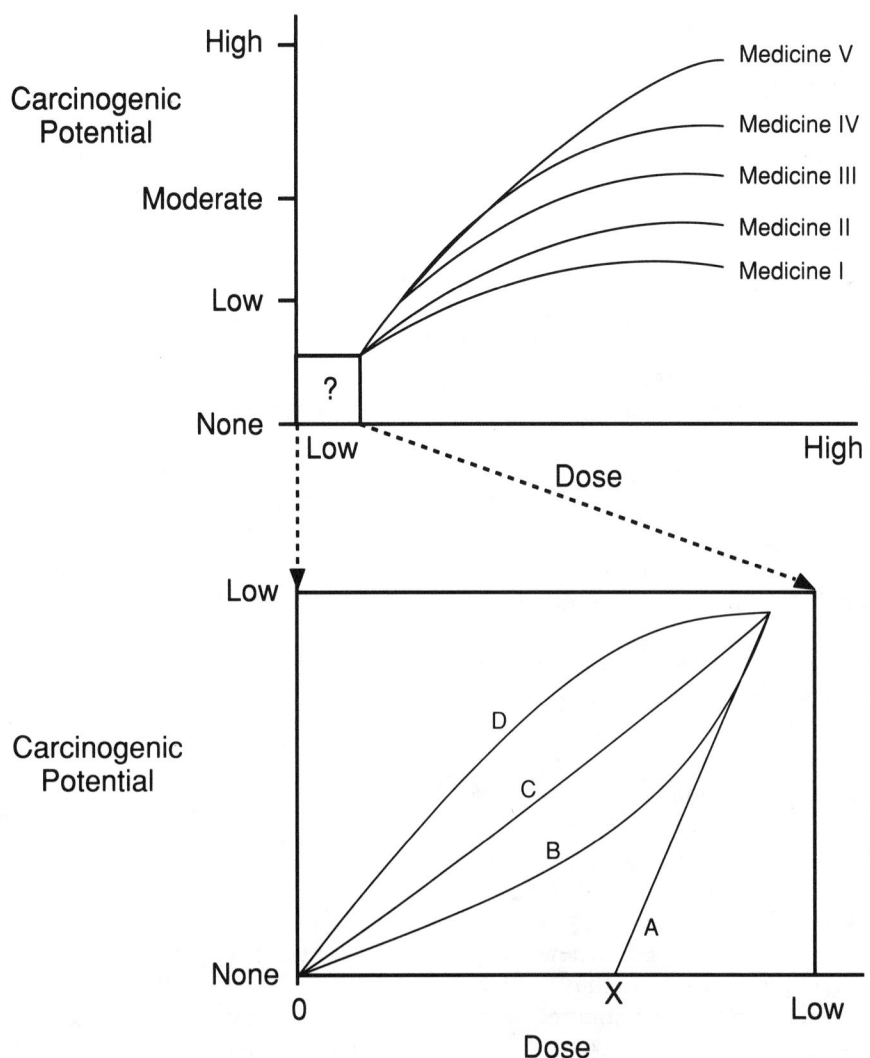

FIG. 88.1 Upper graph: Dose–response relationship for five hypothetical carcinogens. **Lower graph:** Four possible models (A to D) of the boxed area shown with the "?" in the upper graph. Model A represents the concept of a medicine with a threshold effect, with no carcinogenic potential at doses below X. Model C represents the concept of a linear relationship without any threshold back to the origin (i.e., zero dose), and models B and D are nonlinear relationships of supralinear and sublinear types, respectively.

Choice of Species

There are various pressures in society at this point to use the lowest phylogenetic species possible and to conduct in vitro studies in lieu of sacrificing animals. There is a balance that must be achieved by all groups conducting toxicological studies to provide the best evidence of medicine safety for humans while avoiding unnecessary sacrifice of animals.

The author considers it most prudent to consider each animal species and evaluation as providing independent data, but similar findings in two or more species must be taken even more seriously. Toxicological findings raise questions of deleterious or potentially deleterious effects that must be considered and looked for in humans. Pharmacokinetics of various anticonvulsants illustrate that these parameters should be viewed as species specific (Morton, 1984).

Should Pathologists Read Tissue Slides Blind or Unblind?

There is an old joke among pathologists that if you get five pathologists together, you get eight separate opinions. No consensus exists as to whether pathologists should read slides and interpret specimens blinded or unblinded. The unblinded argument states, in part, that knowledge of the clinical diagnosis helps the pathologist interpret the data, since numerous types of interpretations could usually be made. An ultradefensive editorial in support of unblinded slide reading (Society of Toxicologic Pathology, 1983) does not present objective evidence to support its actual position, but ironically presents reasons to support blinding (e.g., "The long-standing practice of open or non-blinded slide reading is based on the fact that morphologic diagnostic pathology is a highly subjective and complex discipline) and even fails to consider various types of blinding (e.g., blinding only to treatment group). The argument for blinded reading relates to minimizing the biases that readily enter data analysis and interpretation. The author agrees with this latter approach of blinding in almost all situations.

Should a Toxic Medicine Be Studied in Humans?

Even if an animal model is validated for providing data that are similar to effects observed in humans, there will probably be some false-positive and false-negative results. These exceptions usually do not challenge the validity of a model, since virtually no model predicts with 100% accuracy. The exceptions do provide a measure of the degree of reliability or predictability of the model. Models may also be validated for some chemical or biological classes of medicines and not for others. Some of the reasons for false-positive and negative results are shown in Tables 88.5 and 88.6.

If a medicine is intended for treatment of a disease with high morbidity or mortality and there are no ef-

TABLE 88.5 *Selected reasons for false-positive results in toxicology[a]*

1. Excessive dosage
2. Creation of metabolites in animals (but not in humans) that lead to toxicity
3. Environmental factors favor the lesion, but these factors would not occur in humans
4. Species-specific effect
5. Physiological or anatomical differences
6. Differences in metabolism
7. Microbial status of the animals differs
8. Animal housing inappropriate
9. Diet of animals (e.g., sterile distilled water versus tap water, autoclaved food versus normal animal food)
10. Technician errors

[a] Many other reasons discussed in this chapter also apply.

TABLE 88.6 *Selected reasons for false-negative responses in toxicology studies*

1. Species difference (e.g., genetic factors)
2. Poor absorption
3. Differences in metabolism or elimination[a]
4. Physiological or anatomical differences
5. Enzyme induction
6. Failure to observe subjective signs or symptoms
7. Failure to observe most skin reactions
8. Failure to observe hypersensitivity reactions
9. Absence of the disease and its pathological effects
10. Failure to measure the effect later found to occur in humans
11. Differences in microbial status

[a] Target organ may not have received sufficient exposure.

fective treatments available or no effective treatments with minimal risk, then it may be suitable to take a compound even with a questionable toxicological profile to the clinic for evaluation. A well-known example is in the field of cancer chemotherapy. As soon as less toxic medicines possessing at least equivalent activity to currently used therapy are developed, standards that a new medicine must meet are raised.

Paradoxical Effects in Toxicology among Species

Three types of paradoxical effects may arise when data from two (or more) species are compared:

Type I Paradoxical Effects. The compound or medicine affects one aspect of an organ or system (e.g., hematological system) in one species and affects a different aspect of the same organ or system in another species. Examples include compounds that affect white blood cells in one species and red blood cells in another.

Type II Paradoxical Effects. The compound causes opposite effects on the same organ or system in two different species. An example would be a compound that elevated white blood cells in one species and decreased them in another.

Type III Paradoxical Effects. The compound affects an organ or structure in one species that is not present in another (Schiavo et al., 1984). This is not literally a paradoxical effect, but illustrates a type of species difference considered in toxicology studies.

CHAPTER 89

Extrapolation of Efficacy (i.e., Pharmacological) Data from Animals to Humans

It is almost always essential to consider animal data on a compound in deciding whether to test the agent in human trials. Animal data are used to predict human efficacy. It is also relevant to consider data obtained in animals when interpreting results of clinical trials. For instance, biochemical and pharmacological effects observed in animals are often invoked to interpret clinical signs, symptoms, and effects of treatment. Therefore, it is relevant in this section on interpreting clinical data to examine how data obtained in animal studies correlate with human results. This involves a discussion of animal models of human disease and ways in which new animal models are developed and validated.

This chapter complements the preceding one of extrapolating preclinical safety data to humans and the following one of extrapolating clinical data from one situation to another.

ANIMAL MODELS OF HUMAN DISEASE

Animal data provide preclinical evidence that a compound may have clinical use in the practice of medicine. The Registry of Comparative Pathology (1973) describes many models of human diseases in which the gross pathological and/or histological lesions produced in animals yield data that are in close agreement with similar results in human disease. Numerous pharmacological references also provide information on animal models of human disease (Table 89.1). Nonetheless, many human diseases develop slowly over a protracted period, and this facet is rarely duplicated in the animal models discussed.

Animal models are created to evaluate medicines for many purposes, including the medicine's (1) activity, (2) safety, (3) pharmacokinetics, (4) mechanism of action, or (5) interactions with other medicines. Some models are developed to observe characteristics of the disease itself and to evaluate how changes in various conditions affect the progression or nature of the disease. Models created in any therapeutic area may involve methodologies of biochemistry, pharmacology, physiology, immunology, or other disciplines. The choice of the best disciplines to use in developing a new model depends on current knowledge of the pathophysiology of the disease, availability of resources,

TABLE 89.1 *Selected books that present information on animal models using pharmacological methodologies*[a]

1. *Pharmacological Experiments on Intact Preparations:* University of Edinburgh Department of Pharmacology Staff and L.J. McLeod (1970)
2. *Pharmacological Experiments on Isolated Preparations:* University of Edinburgh Department of Pharmacology Staff (1968)
3. *Animal Models for Oral Drug Delivery in Man:* In Situ *and in* Vivo *Approaches:* W. Crouthamel and A.C. Sarapu (eds.) (1983)
4. *Spontaneous Animal Models of Human Disease,* Vols. 1 and 2: E.J. Andrews, B.C. Ward, and N.H. Altman (eds.) (1979)
5. *Animal Models for Biomedical Research IV:* Symposium sponsored by Institute of Laboratory Animal Resources, the National Research Council, and the American College of Laboratory Animal Medicine (1971)
6. *Methods of Animal Experimentation,* Vols. I to IV: W.I. Gay (ed.) (1965 to 1973)
7. *Textbook of* In Vitro *Practical Pharmacology:* I. Kitchen (1984)
8. *Animal Models in Psychopathology:* N.W. Bond (ed.) (1984)
9. *Methods in Pharmacology,* Vol. 1: A. Schwartz (ed.) (1971)
10. *Animals for Medical Research: Models for the Study of Human Disease:* B.M. Mitruka, H.M. Rawnsley, and D.V. Vadehra (1976)
11. *Principles of Animal Extrapolation:* E.J. Calabrese (1983)
12. *Screening Methods in Pharmacology:* R.A. Turner (1965)
13. *Screening Methods in Pharmacology,* Vol II: R.A. Turner and P. Hebbom (eds.) (1971)
14. *Evaluation of Drug Activities: Pharmacometrics,* Vols. 1 and 2: D.R. Laurence and A.L. Bacharach (eds.) (1964)
15. *Animal and Clinical Pharmacologic Techniques in Drug Evaluation:* J. Nodine and P. Siegler (eds.) (1964)
16. *Animal Experiments in Pharmacological Analysis:* F.R. Domer (1971)
17. *Animal Models: Assessing the Scope of Their Use in Biomedical Research:* J. Kawamata and E.C. Melby Jr. (eds) (1987)

[a] Complete references are given in the bibliography. Books that include primarily biochemical, microbiological, or other models are not included in this list, nor are the many books that describe pharmacological methods in a particular therapeutic field.

and a sound scientific rationale for developing a suitable model.

Types of Animal Models Used to Evaluate Compounds or Medicines

The large variety of in vitro, in vivo, and other types of animal models may be summarized as belonging to a few general types.

Type I Animal Models. The animal species (or strain) naturally has (or spontaneously develops) a characteristic that would be of interest to study or evaluate, such as a lesion similar to that found in a human disease. Such characteristics may sometimes be bred into the animal. Examples include spontaneously developed hypertension in rats and spontaneous congestive heart failure in Syrian hamsters.

Type II Animal Models. Animal models are experimentally induced to create characteristics of interest

to study or evaluate. The lesion may or may not be similar to that found in the analogous human disease. Examples include steroid-induced hypertension in rats, and pulmonary artery banding in dogs or cats to create a state of congestive heart failure.

Type III Animal Models. Animals are normal but are used either in vitro, in vivo, or in situ as models of the disease state in humans. Measurements made and effects of compounds are found to correlate to some degree with effects in the human disease. Examples include normotensive rats or cats in vivo, and papillary muscles from cats that are used to measure cardiac contraction as a model for inotropic agents for congestive heart failure in humans.

Figure 89.1 shows several models in a schematic manner. In model A one measures the effect of a response or activity of the animal model as influenced by a medicine (*). The medicine usually blocks or enhances an effect of the animal model. In model B something is done to the model to influence the effect observed. The test medicine or compound may be given either before or after the action on the animal model. If the medicine is given beforehand, it usually is intended to prevent the occurrence of the effect. In addition, the medicine or compound may be given simultaneously with the action usually to prevent the effect. Finally, the medicine may be given after the effect occurs to reverse it (model C).

General Principles Relating to Animal Models

How well do animal models predict clinical response to medicines? It is not possible to provide a simple answer to this question but only to indicate a number of principles.

Ability to Mimic Human Disease

Although most animal tests are imperfect models of human disease, some models mimic human disease more closely than others. For example, spontaneously hypertensive rats are a better model of hypertension than merely injecting a normotensive animal acutely with a pressor agent. Animals that are normotensive yield relatively poor data about antihypertensive effects of medicines compared with data obtained in hypertensive animals. It is preferable to select compounds for initial testing in humans based on the most predictive models available.

Predictability

The predictability of data obtained from animal models for humans varies enormously, from those models

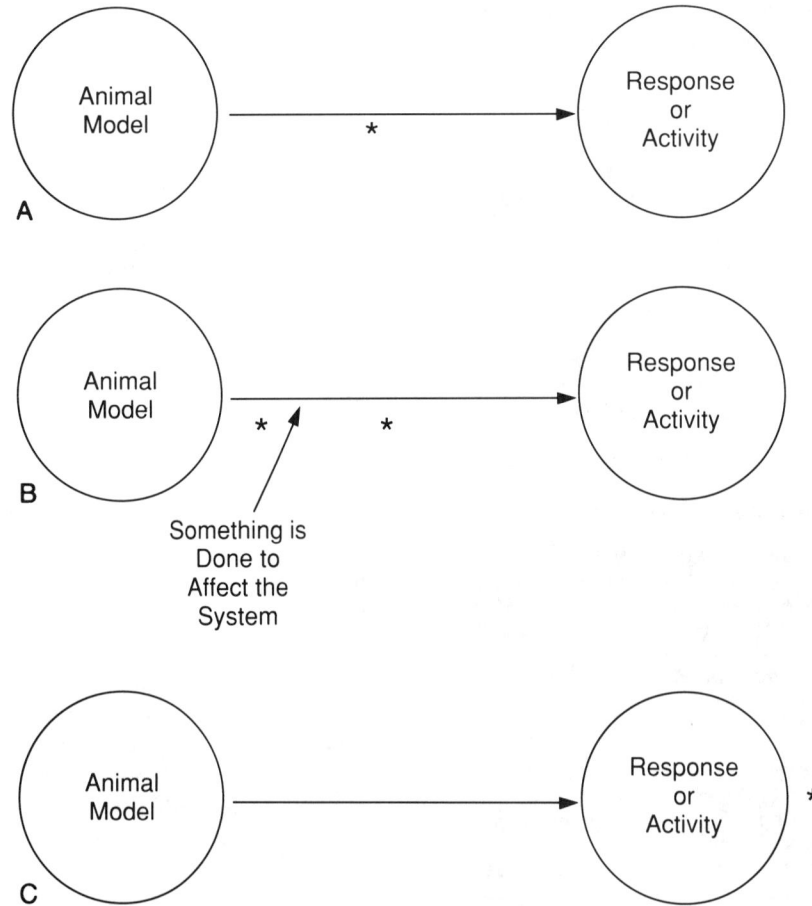

FIG. 89.1 Various periods when test compounds or medicines (*) may be evaluated in an animal model. **A:** The period during which a response or activity (either acute or chronic) is being generated. **B:** Something is done to the system. The test may occur either before or after something is done to affect the animal model. **C:** Test compound is given after the response or activity occurs in an attempt to reverse it.

whose results have a high correlation with clinical data to those models for which the correlation is extremely low. One potential problem with animal models is that they invite overgeneralization of results. Most models are gross oversimplifications of human disease and may only represent one aspect of the disease. Some of the reasons why data obtained in animals do not always predict responses in humans are listed in Table 89.2.

Animal models used to evaluate compounds in some therapeutic areas generally have great predictability for efficacy in humans (e.g., antiinfectives), whereas the predictability in other therapeutic areas is weak (e.g., compounds affecting the central nervous system).

Sensitivity and Specificity

Both the sensitivity and specificity of different animal models vary. Both false-positive and false-negative re-

TABLE 89.2 *Selected reasons why data obtained in animals do not always predict clinical efficacy*

1. The animal species chosen differ in response from humans. The same model in a different animal species may have yielded more predictive results
2. Differences in absorption, distribution, metabolism, or excretion may occur in some (or all) animal species and humans
3. The anatomy relating to the test model in animals may differ from that in humans
4. Different animal strains of the same species may yield different results
5. The pathological nature of the lesions may differ at a macroscopic or microscopic level between the animal species and humans
6. There may be important differences between the species at a subcellular, cellular, receptor, or physiological level that lead to different pharmacodynamic responses
7. No appropriate animal models may exist
8. Various experimental conditions in the animal model(s) may yield qualitatively different data, and it is uncertain which set of data relates most closely to humans
9. The dose required to elicit the effect in animals is never able to be achieved in humans (e.g., because of toxicity)
10. Paradoxical effects sometimes occur between different species

sults occur in these models and are expected to occur in humans (see Chapter 96: "False-Positive and False-Negative Results"). Accuracy of animal-derived data may be improved if all evaluations and scores are made by personnel who are unaware of the medicine (or nonmedicine) treatment. This is especially important if there is any possibility of a subjective element entering the evaluation.

Use of Multiple Models of One Disease or Activity

A single animal model rarely provides an adequate basis for determining that a clinically beneficial response will be observed. Rather, multiple models are generally utilized to obtain a profile of characteristics that will, one hopes, provide confidence for investing adequate resources to test a new compound in humans. Using multiple models to evaluate compounds is essential, since an agonist in one model may be a partial agonist or even antagonist in another. Also, some models may yield data on either affinity or efficacy (or both). Both in vitro and in vivo animal models are important to study when such models are available.

Use of Multiple Models of Multiple Diseases or Activities

Many animal models of diseases other than the disease targeted are important to use with experimental medicines. This helps ensure that undesirable effects will not be encountered in humans. General screening tests as well as detailed evaluation of pharmacological, biochemical, or other biological activities may provide clues of potential clinical uses that had not been considered.

When multiple animal models are used, there is a tendency in some therapeutic areas to use broader screens initially and to progress to those that evaluate more specific biological questions (e.g., evaluating antibacterials). In other therapeutic areas or for other reasons, specific biological activity is screened for initially (e.g., when a specific biochemical activity is desired).

Pharmacokinetics

Although some animal models may accurately reproduce the pathological lesion of the human disease, the data obtained with test compounds will differ from human responses if both species absorb, distribute, metabolize, or excrete the compound differently. Differences at the receptor site and in pharmacodynamic effects may also account for species differences.

Mechanism-of-Action

New animal models sometimes evolve from a better understanding of previously unexplained mechanisms of active medicines. Some animal models are highly selective for determining activity of compounds that act via a single specific mechanism, and others will show activity for compounds acting via any one of many mechanisms.

In addition to providing data that may be extrapolated to humans, animal models help scientists learn abut underlying mechanisms or other aspects of a particular disease and also help discern new relationships and details that may be searched for or evaluated in humans.

Types and Degrees of Artificiality

Many animal models of human disease consist of extremely artificial test systems to evaluate medicines. It is important to note that there are various types and degrees of artificiality. If one considers injecting carbon tetrachloride in animals as a model of hepatic injury in humans, then this is an artificially induced injury. After an actual clinical event has occurred (e.g., hepatic injury), a patient would be given a medicine to treat or counteract the injury. This clinical approach is also theoretically possible to mimic with the animal model described, i.e., carbon tetrachloride may be given to produce an injury, and then a test medicine is given to treat the injury produced. A different type of artificiality occurs when an animal is pretreated with a test medicine and then carbon tetrachloride is injected. The extent to which the test medicine prevented the occurrence of the expected hepatic injury is measured. This example uses an artificial animal model in an artificial way, since in clinical situations patients do not usually take a medicine to prevent an injury that has not yet occurred. If hepatocytes are cultured in vitro and are used to evaluate the effects of carbon tetrachloride, this represents a different type of artificiality.

The pharmacological, physiological, and biochemical literature contains many examples of each of these approaches as well as others (e.g., giving the agent that causes the problem simultaneously with the test medicine that may effect a cure in order to determine whether the combination prevents the problem from developing). Other approaches include giving multiple doses of the "treatment" prior to causing the lesion. This is probably the most artificial approach described. Finally, giving a compound or medicine both prior to and subsequent to the lesion has been used as a technique to measure biological activity. Several of these models are shown in Figs. 89.2 and 89.3. Artificiality in clinical models is discussed in Chapters 12 and 90.

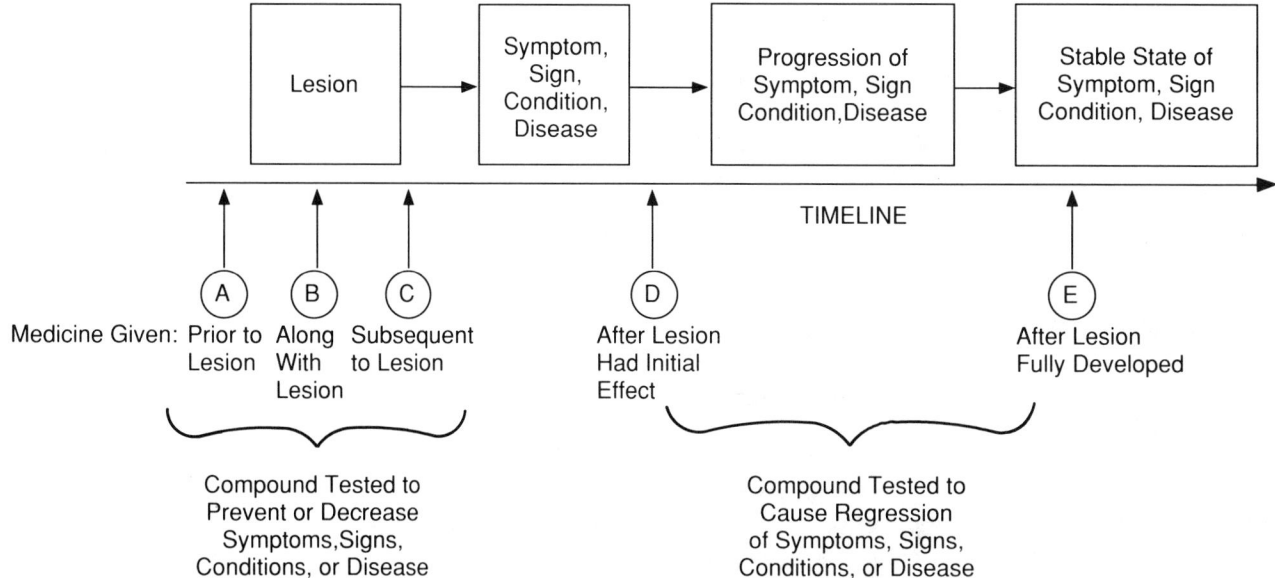

FIG. 89.2 Testing of compounds or medicines in an animal model illustrated in more detail than in panel B of Fig. 89.1.

Comparison of Data Obtained in Animals and Humans

Relative Potencies in Multiple Models

One method used to validate animal models as predictors of human efficacy data is to evaluate a series of different medicines in an animal test and to compare the relative potencies with data derived in human trials. The medicines evaluated may represent closely related structures, but it is often preferable (and usually necessary) to choose a variety of standard medicines to compare. Ideally, the medicines should be evaluated in the animal model and the clinical trials under identical experimental conditions. Animal data are often obtained under nearly identical conditions,

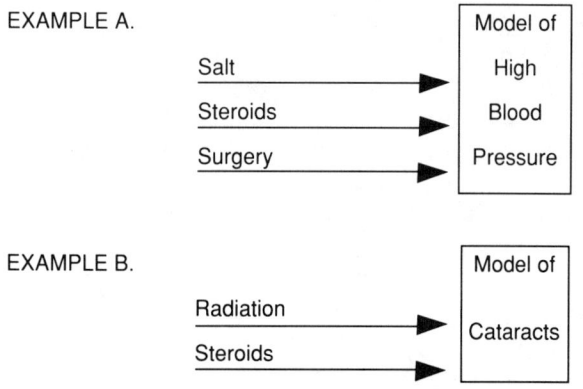

FIG. 89.3 An animal model may be produced by different lesions. It is necessary to assess whether each model produced is the same or different.

but the human data may of necessity be derived from several separate trials using a variety of protocols. In comparing animal and human data, it is preferable if more than one animal model is used to generate the data and if more than one animal species is studied. Examples of this approach are studies that compare (1) relative potencies, (2) rank order of potencies, or (3) models of pharmacokinetic parameters in multiple species.

Relative potencies of the intravenous, oral, and aerosol routes and in vitro tests of bronchodilators were compared in guinea pigs, dogs, and humans (Spilker et al., 1975a). The rank order potency of a series of medicines was compared in a variety of tests in several species with results obtained in humans (Pearl et al., 1976). Pearl et al. compared the activities of eight psychoactive medicines in four animal models with the activities of the same medicines for producing extrapyramidal effects in humans by using a rank order of medicine potency in the various tests Some important issues and questions of extrapolation are illustrated in Fig. 89.4.

Mathematical Models

Mathematical models of biological events may be created using data from animals and humans. One example is a mathematical model created to predict tissue distribution of methotrexate (Zaharko et al., 1971). Another method used to create, as well as validate, animal models is to demonstrate that the lesions observed in animals are similar (or identical) histologically and at

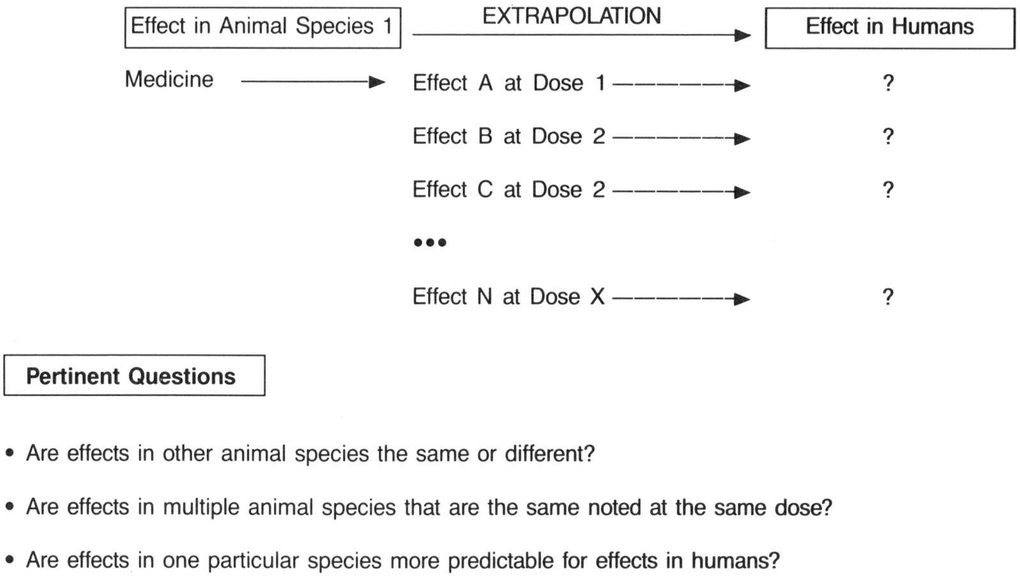

FIG. 89.4 Extrapolating the effects observed in an animal species to humans.

a gross morphological level to those observed in humans.

Extrapolating In Vitro Human Data to Clinical Situations

A variety of in vitro tests utilize human cells or tissues. Examples include human cell lines, human blood cells (e.g., for platelet aggregation studies), and isolated human tissue removed during surgery or autopsy. The relevance and validity of extrapolating data from studies on these human tissues to the clinical situation still must be established, as for all animal models. Evaluations on biological materials removed from patients, such as hair samples, must also be validated, since there are numerous reasons why such samples may not yield clinically meaningful results (Spilker and Maugh, 1980).

ESTABLISHING AND VALIDATING A NEW ANIMAL MODEL

Purposes

Animal models of human disease are used for several purposes. Among these are to evaluate new compounds for their potential efficacy (or safety) in humans and to investigate the nature of the disease process as well as its etiology, progression, and prevention. Some animal models test normal cells, tumors, organs, or entire organisms. Some animal models evaluate one time point in the progression of

a disease (e.g., many in vitro tests in which a tissue is removed at a specific time after the animal is pretreated or affected in a desired manner). Other models mimic the entire progression of the disease (e.g., Japanese quail model of atherosclerosis). A standard goal in many disciplines of preclinical research is to establish a battery of models that can evaluate different aspects of a disease or utilize methodological approaches from different scientific disciplines to evaluate one or more aspects of the overall disease. A summary of many common pharmacological activities produced by medicines is given in Table 89.3.

TABLE 89.3 *Selected types of pharmacological activities produced by medicines*

1. Receptor stimulation (e.g., dopamine receptor stimulation by bromocriptine, β-adrenergic receptor stimulation by isoproterenol)
2. Receptor inhibition (e.g., histamine-2 receptor inhibition by cimetidine) of competitive or noncompetitive type
3. Transport processes enhanced (e.g., insulin enhances the inward movement of glucose into cells in diabetic patients)
4. Transport processes decreased or blocked (e.g., thiazide diuretics decrease reabsorption of sodium in the distal tubules)
5. Enzymes stimulated (e.g., catecholamines stimulate adenylate cyclase)
6. Enzymes inhibited competitively (e.g., allopurinol inhibits xanthine oxidase) or noncompetitively (aspirin inhibits cyclooxygenase)
7. Replacement therapy for a missing or decreased chemical, vitamin, or hormone (e.g., iron salts for iron deficiency anemia, thyroxine replaces low thyroid hormone)
8. Medicines may affect foreign or undesired invaders (e.g., bacteria, tumors, viruses) through various mechanisms
9. Medicines may affect membranes (e.g., antiarrhythmics, general anesthetics)
10. Various other mechanisms (e.g., chelation, osmotic diuretics, false neurotransmitters)

Generating Ideas for New Models

If a scientist is seeking ideas of how to develop new models, it is often useful to draw schematics of the known physiology, biochemistry, and pharmacology of the therapeutic or scientific area in question. Evaluate each of the places in the system where a medicine could act. Determine how to test the hypothesis with one or more animal models.

Few animal models, if any, are exact duplicates of human disease. Scientists usually attempt to create models that are as close as possible to the clinical situation. There are many reasons for the inability to create exact models, including incomplete knowledge of most diseases, the highly complex nature of many diseases, and technical difficulties in creating complex models. Animal models must be compared with the human situation in regard to the lesion or condition that is created and the predictability of the data that the model yields. It is clearly the latter consideration that is of primary importance, since a pathologically lesioned animal that exactly mimics human disease but provides spurious or inconsistent results is of little predictive value. Reasons for poorly predictive models of this type may relate to differences in absorption, distribution, metabolism, or excretion between species.

It is important to develop a list of both required and desired characteristics for a new model. The required characteristics should include both aspects that must be present and those that must be absent.

Characteristics of Animal Models

Characteristics that are often required of a new animal model are to be able to (1) yield predictive data for humans, (2) obtain statistically treatable data, (3) conduct a certain number of tests that can be performed each day, week, or month, (4) demonstrate activity of treatments that work in humans with an acceptable rate of false-positive and -negative responses, (5) utilize a given amount of compound per test, and (6) cost no more than a specified amount per test. Desirable characteristics include the ability to obtain (1) objective data that may be tested statistically, (2) a dose–response relationship, (3) a preliminary estimate of toxicity, (4) reproducible results from experiment to experiment, (5) an indication of the duration of effect, (6) data that are relevant to study both cause and treatment of a specific disease, (7) a similarity of symptoms in the model and humans, and (8) underlying pathology, physiology, and biochemistry that are similar in animals and humans. The model should be able to be reproduced by other investigators. Required characteristics for some models would only be desirable characteristics for other models (and vice versa). Another approach to creating criteria for a new model is to develop a set of ideal, realistic, or minimally acceptable criteria. An example of describing characteristics of an ideal method is given by Spilker (1987c) for inducing pruritus and evaluating antipruritics.

Validating a New Model

The model should be tested to determine the rate of both false-positive and false-negative responses. If a series of models is being used or developed, the initial ones used should have a higher rate of false positives and a lower rate of false negatives than the later tests. If no suitable agents are available to test in the model, it may be a long time before the validation of a model may be performed. Until the time of validation, the model will probably provide data of only limited value.

There are several ways in which a new animal model can be validated. These potentially include techniques from all biological disciplines, including histology, pathology, physiology, pharmacology, biochemistry, immunology, virology, and microbiology. In most cases, utilizing techniques of multiple disciplines will more firmly establish the model as valid. Within each discipline, numerous techniques may be applied (e.g., relative potencies in multiple models, false-positive rate, false-negative rate). The use of multiple techniques will generally yield more convincing data than a single test and will help validate the model. See Chapter 43, "Validation of Clinical Tests and Measures" for details about validation techniques.

There are animal models that are not developed for their similarity to a human disease but for the predictive value they yield for explaining how a medicine will react in patients with the disease. For instance, in vitro preparations of cat papillary muscle are not a facsimile of congestive heart failure, but this model yields predictive data of how patients with the disease will react to medicines. This type of animal model is usually validated by evaluating effects of medicines known to be both active and inactive in human disease as well as through evaluation of various biological "research tools" (i.e., compounds that have known biological effects in animals but are not used as medicines for the target disease). The rates of false-positive and false-negative results using the animal model are important to determine. A number of possible explanations are given in Table 89.4 for situations when in vivo data do not confirm in vitro results.

Validation of an Animal Model to Mimic a Human Disease versus Validation to Predict Treatment Effects

A pharmacological model of a human disease may be created to mimic exactly the human histology, physiology, or even symptomatology of the disease. There is a wide gap from this model to the point at which a

TABLE 89.4 *Possible interpretations when in vitro data do not predict results of in vivo studies*

1. Medicine is not absorbed at all or is poorly absorbed in in vivo studies
2. Medicine is well absorbed but is subject to first-pass effect in liver
3. Medicine is distributed so that less (or more) reaches the receptors than would be predicted on the basis of its absorption
4. Medicine is rapidly metabolized to an active or inactive metabolite that has a different profile of activity and/or different duration of action than the parent medicine
5. Medicine is rapidly eliminated (e.g., through secretory mechanisms)
6. Species of the two test systems used are different
7. Experimental conditions of the in vitro and in vivo experiments differed and may have led to different effects than expected. These conditions include factors such as temperature or age, sex, and strain of animal
8. Effects elicited in vitro and in vivo by the particular medicine differ in their characteristics
9. Tests used to measure responses will probably differ greatly for in vitro and in vivo studies, and the types of data obtained may not be comparable
10. The in vitro study did not use adequate controls (e.g., pH, vehicle used, volume of drug given, samples taken from sham-operated animals)
11. In vitro data cannot predict the volume of a medicine's distribution in central or in peripheral compartments
12. In vitro data cannot predict the rate constants for medicine movement between compartments
13. In vitro data cannot predict the rate constants for medicine elimination
14. In vitro data cannot predict whether linear or nonlinear kinetics will occur with a specific dose of a medicine in vivo
15. Pharmacokinetic parameters (e.g., bioavailability, peak plasma concentration, half-life) cannot be predicted based solely on in vitro studies

model does not share any characteristics with the human disease. The place that a specific animal model lies on this scale does not necessarily predict how well the model is able to predict the effects in humans of compounds tested in the model. Some models that closely mimic human disease are notoriously poor predictors of the activity of medicines in humans. Likewise, some models that do not mimic human disease at all are excellent predictors of activity of medicines in humans.

Many animal models do not reflect the histology, pathology, physiology, or symptomatology of a human disease, but are good predictors of medicine activity in humans with the disease. Many in vitro tissue preparations (e.g., guinea pig electrically driven left atria, cat papillary muscle) fit this category for congestive heart failure (Spilker, 1973a). Many in vivo preparations of normal anesthetized dogs are excellent predictors of certain classes of antiasthmatic medicines when given compounds that antagonize respiratory effects of histamine (Spilker et al., 1975a). Many biochemical tests also are in this category.

The opposite category—of excellent physiological and pathological models that are poorly validated for predicting human effects of compounds—include many models developed for studying the histology of diseases.

All animal models of Alzheimer's disease currently represent a large question mark because they cannot be validated. No medicine for Alzheimer's is effective in humans, making it impossible to know whether any of the currently used models have any predictive ability. When one or more medicines are found that are active, the tests that they do and do not work in will be determined. Those tests will then be available to test for more active, more potent, and safer medicines. Of course, activity in a test does not mean that other models in which the medicine is inactive are also not valid. A different chemical class of medicine may be required, however, to validate a different model.

Using Clinical Data to Improve Animal Models

One of the most important means of developing improved animal models is to obtain clinical pharmacological profiles of a new medicine being evaluated in humans. The comparison of the profile obtained in humans with that previously obtained in various animal models allows the most predictive model(s) to be ascertained. The strengths and weaknesses of each model may be assessed when data on the new medicine are compared with the predictability of other medicines evaluated in the same animal model. Once a new animal model is validated, the presence of new false-positive or -negative results does not invalidate a model, although the model may become less predictive or less valuable in terms of data generated.

Compounds that Are Active in Animals but Not in Humans

If a compound that was active in all standard animal models in a given therapeutic area was found to be inactive in humans, possible interpretations are that (1) the dose tested in humans was insufficient, (2) the pharmacokinetics are different, and (3) the experimental conditions used in the animal tests were inappropriate, or (4) other reasons for species difference were present. It is important to determine (if possible) whether the animal data yielded false-positive results or whether the human data yielded false-negative results.

USING ANIMAL MODELS TO EVALUATE COMPOUNDS AND MEDICINES

Developing a Scheme for Using Multiple Animal Models

There are no perfect animal models that provide all of the data required to determine if a given compound will be effective in humans. In addition to providing efficacy data, animal models must be used to derive safety and other types of data. Thus, a wide variety of animal models must be used. The pros and cons for each must be understood to interpret the data in a meaningful way.

In developing multiple tests, it is possible to use, or to combine, them in different ways, depending on the purpose(s) of the models and the nature of the scientific or therapeutic area being studied. Figure 89.5 illustrates five common patterns. In this figure each box with a letter from A to J represents a separate test and may yield different types of data. Each test from A to J may also be conducted with techniques of one or multiple scientific disciplines. The purpose of choosing

a number of tests (i.e., boxes) and of ordering them in one of the five patterns shown (or a different one) is to test compounds and to advance only those of interest (i.e., those with the type of activity desired). Thus the choice and pattern of tests establishes a series of hurdles for compounds to pass. These tests represent a "weeding out" or screening process.

For one test (e.g., test A) it may be necessary for compounds to:

1. decrease a certain effect by Z%
2. increase a certain effect by Y%
3. prevent a certain effect occurring for X hours by another compound used as part of the test
4. reverse the effect of another compound used as part of the test within W minutes

Once a compound passes this test (test A) it is then evaluated in test B (pattern 1), both tests B and C (pattern 2), or tests B, C, and D (patterns 3 and 4), or compared with data obtained in tests B and C to determine whether or not it should be advanced to tests D and E (pattern 5). Criteria must be established for a compound to progress to the next test in the series. A series of models used to screen and characterize compounds' inotropic activity is shown by Spilker (1973a). Many of the tests, in which standard medicines have different activities, can be used to characterize new compounds (Spilker, 1970).

The tests in boxes A to J (Fig. 89.5) may represent different animal models or may represent the same model with different conditions or objectives. In one box, for example, the test may be to measure the effects of a single fixed dose or concentration of a compound. In another box, the same animal model may be used to conduct a dose–response relationship and measure the dose that yields a 50% response (EC$_{50}$ or ED$_{50}$). Many variations of a specific test are possible (e.g., test a single dose and then test a single dose after 3 days of pretreatment in the same model).

Panel 1 in Fig. 89.5 illustrates a simple sequential ordering of models, whereas panel 2 illustrates a pyramid type of ordering. Panels 3, 4, and 5 illustrate more complex patterns. These are the more usual systems used by pharmacology departments in the pharmaceutical industry. Each system is used to screen or evaluate properties of medicines in a given therapeutic area or with a specific targeted objective.

Often one primary model is relied on more than others to evaluate the efficacy of a compound. This model is rarely the first one used to screen compounds because a high rate of false positives is generally desired in the initial screen(s). In addition, lower animals in an evolutionary sense are usually used at that early stage, and the primary model may involve a higher species.

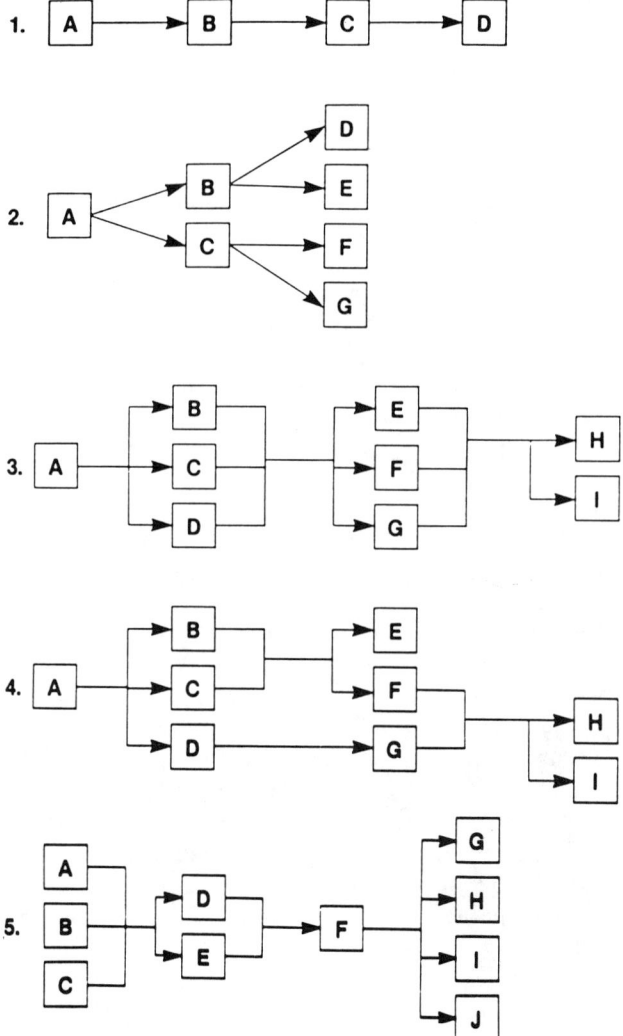

FIG. 89.5 Hypothetical formats for organizing multiple animal models and tests to screen for and study medicine activity. Each letter represents a separate model or test. One pattern would be chosen to progress compounds per disease area, with each box representing a sort of hurdle that the compound must clear.

Blood Levels of Test Compounds

Blood levels of the test compound are often measured in these animals, especially at the dose that yields about 50% of the total response. When humans are eventually tested with the same compound, the blood levels obtained in animals are often used as an approximate indicator of levels to be anticipated in humans. Thus, if these blood levels are obtained in humans and the medicine is ineffective, there is a rationale for not increasing the dose further to determine if the medicine is effective in humans. On the other hand, if significant toxicity has not been observed in humans, higher doses may be carefully explored for efficacy. If the blood level achieved with a medicine in humans is found to be less than that observed in animals, then a lack of effect in humans may represent an inadequate dose or another factor(s) and should not be used as evidence that the animal model is not valid. There are many factors to consider in evaluating the relationship between efficacy and blood levels in humans and animals. These factors include possible differences in absorption, distribution, metabolism, or excretion profiles.

Evaluating the Profile of a Compound

It is usually not possible to use only one animal model to evaluate compounds for choosing those that are most suitable to test in humans. A battery of tests is often established in which standard medicines may have a variety of different activities. It is sometimes possible to profile the activities of several standard medicines in multiple tests so that a compound may be sought that mimics a known profile. The relevant series of animal models to use could be chosen based on the types of activities desired. The profile of standard medicines can also be used for comparison with an investigational drug. For example, profiles of eight standard inotropic agents were obtained using 15 tests, and their activities were compared (Spilker, 1973a). Desirable characteristics of an animal screen are listed in Table 89.5.

TABLE 89.5 *Desirable characteristics for an animal screen*

A. Biological properties
1. The biological basis should be understood and scientifically sound
2. Rates of false positives and false negatives should be acceptable
3. The screen can differentiate between activities of compounds with closely related chemical structures
4. Reproducible results are obtained on different occasions
5. Genetic uniformity of organisms used is present

B. Practical aspects
1. Small amounts of compounds are required for early screens in a series
2. The time to run the screen should be minimal
3. The cost to run the screen should be minimal
4. The number of compounds tested in early screens should be large
5. Conditions for operating the screen may be standardized
6. An acceptable standard to pass or fail compounds at a desirable rate may be established
7. This standard may be titrated to pass either fewer or more compounds
8. Data handling may be automated or otherwise dealt with efficiently
9. Random positive controls may be submitted in a blind manner
10. The test fits into a series of screens to extrapolate data effectively

C. Ethical aspects
1. Animals as low as possible on the evolutionary tree are used
2. The fewest numbers of animals possible are used
3. Tests treat all animals in a caring and humane manner
4. A protocol for animal use is written, reviewed, and approved by relevant people or committees
5. Standard operating procedures are established to obtain, handle, and care for animals in an acceptable and humane manner

CHAPTER 90

Extrapolation of Data from Clinical Trials

INTRODUCTION

Environment and Facilities

Interpretations and medical opinions that are relevant for treating patients in one clinical setting are sometimes totally inappropriate for treating patients in another. The clearest example of this is to consider how patients are treated in different countries. Sophisticated techniques and procedures, especially those that utilize expensive equipment in developed countries, are limited in their relevance and applicability for patient care in underdeveloped countries. The opposite is also true, in that techniques that improve patient treatment in rural underdeveloped areas often have no relevance in modern urban hospitals or medical centers.

Types of Medical Practice

Current medical practices differ to some degree between countries, but in the highly industrialized countries there are more similarities than differences in fundamental clinical approaches used by most physicians. In less developed countries there are often enormous differences in approach followed by medical personnel, and there is often a dual system whereby both folk and "Western" medicine are practiced. There are also major differences in underdeveloped (and some developed) countries in the practice of medicine between many rural and urban areas and among primary, secondary, and tertiary care centers. Knowledge of the existence and nature of these differences is essential for accurately extrapolating clinical interpretations of data obtained from one of these groups to another.

The "Real World"

The term "real world" is used to include the manner in which a particular medicine or treatment is usually used, given, or administered. Although this term is used as if it represented a single entity, this is obviously not true. Except in rare circumstances, the "real world" includes an incredible diversity and complexity of factors that may interact with any medicine or treatment prescribed and influence a patient's clinical outcome. It is this diversity, in part, that has led to the need for controlled clinical trials to evaluate treatments.

TYPES OF EXTRAPOLATIONS

Most medically oriented individuals have either questioned or wondered about the relationship between the results from a clinical trial and the "real world" in which patients are treated. The extrapolation of data from a clinical trial to the society in which patients are treated requires knowledge of the practices with which patients are treated in clinical practice, the validity of various aspects of the trial, and the group for which the data are being extrapolated.

Types of extrapolation are shown in Fig. 90.1. This figure illustrates that the major categories of factors to be considered are (1) patients, (2) physicians, (3) settings, and (4) times at which the extrapolation is made. A fifth category, levels of organization, is also described.

Extrapolating Across One or More Dimensions

Extrapolations are usually more conservative when only one of these five types of factors i.e., dimensions is involved. When data are extrapolated both to a new patient population and to a different setting, the probability of the conclusion being correct is usually less than when the extrapolation is made only to a different setting within the same patient population. The greater the number of dimensions that differ from the index trial, the less is the likelihood that the results may be extrapolated with confidence.

Extrapolating Across One or More Levels of Organization

Extrapolations are often made to different levels of organization. In the direction toward larger units, data are sometimes extrapolated from the individual patient to social groups, diagnostic groups, national groups, or all patients with the disease. In the direction toward smaller units, data from a patient or trial are extrapolated to organ systems, physiological and pharmacological effects, or biochemical and other subcellular effects. Data that are interpreted at any specific level are sometimes extrapolated to both larger and smaller levels. Examples are given in Chapter 82.

Types of Clinical Models of Disease

Figure 90.2 shows a simple model (model I) of a diseased patient who has a response or activity that is measured. The medicine may be studied by giving it to normal subjects at point A, prior to their having a disease (e.g., vaccines, antibiotics given prophylacti-

cally in surgery). Medicines can also be given at point B to patients with a disease to prevent recurrences or new episodes. These medicines are often referred to as suppressive or prophylactic in nature. Examples include propranalol to prevent recurrences of migraine, acyclovir to prevent recurrences of genital herpes, and steroids for the prevention of asthma. Most medicines are given at point D to help treat the patient's symptoms. In model II something is done to the patient that causes a response that may also be measured at points A and C. In addition, it is possible to evaluate the patient either before or after the event marked "Something is Done."

In model IV, some of the common conditions that can be artifically created in a laboratory in normal volunteers and then evaluated with medicines are (1) cough with citric acid, (2) diarrhea with castor oil, (3) pain with various models, and (4) emesis with syrup of ipecac or cis platinum. Some of the conditions that may be evaluated in normal volunteers without doing anything special (i.e., model III) include anesthesia and evaluating diuresis in water- and saline-loaded hydrated patients.

RELATIONSHIP OF AN ARTIFICIAL CLINICAL SETTING OR MODEL TO DIAGNOSIS AND TREATMENT OF PATIENTS

Artificial clinical settings are defined as settings that are not representative of the actual environment in which actual patients with the disease are diagnosed or treated. If inpatient clinical trials are conducted to obtain information on medicines that will later be used on an outpatient basis, the inpatient setting represents an artificial environment. The inpatient setting may be an accurate (i.e., not artificial) setting for patients in an institution who will be treated with the medicine. Data generated on patients in an artificial setting may not be representative of data obtained in real-world environments, and interpretations may not be extrapolatable to patients treated in actual clinical situations. Studies on volunteers are always, by definition, conducted in artificial clinical settings.

Types of Differences Between Clinical Trial Settings and the "Real World"

The concept of artificial clinical models applies to almost all clinical trials conducted on investigational medicines, since it is rare that usual clinical practice is mimicked in investigational trials. Differences may be minor, such as having the patient sign an informed consent, but in most trials more tests are run and data collected than are obtained in usual clinical situations.

EXTRAPOLATION OF DATA FROM ONE PARTICULAR TRIAL TO:

1. **Other Patients Who May Have Different:**

   - Diagnoses
   - Disease Subgroups
   - Concurrent Disease
   - Concurrent Medicine and/or Nonmedicine Treatments
   - Cultures and Social Customs
   - Behavioral Characteristics
   - Psychological Characteristics
   - Ages
   - Dose Regimens, Dosage Forms, or Dosages
   - Personal Habits (Tobacco, Alcohol, Caffeine-Containing Beverages)
   - Disease Severity
   - Ability to Pay For Treatment
   - Risk Factors

2. **Other Investigators or Physicians Who May Have A Different:**

   - Training
   - Specialty
   - Type of Practice
   - Physical Facility for Seeing Patients
   - Set of Equipment
   - Relationship With Patients
   - Approach to Treating the Same Disease
   - Referral Pattern
   - Motivation to Spend Time With Patients

3. **Other Settings Which May Be Present:**

   - "Real World" Versus "Artificial Setting"
   - Inpatient Versus Outpatient
   - Different Type of Practice (e.g., group, solo, clinic)
   - Different Type of Hospital (e.g., primary, secondary, or tertiary care)
   - Different Environmental Conditions (e.g., desert, tropical forest)
   - Different Population Density (e.g., rural, town, metropolis)
   - Different Socioeconomic Conditions

4. **Patients Treated At Other Times:**

   - Different Medical Practices and Treatments
   - Different State of the Art in Available Equipment
   - Different Ethical Standards

5. **Other Levels of Organization:**

FIG. 90.1 Extrapolating data from a specific clinical trial: types of extrapolations and various considerations of each.

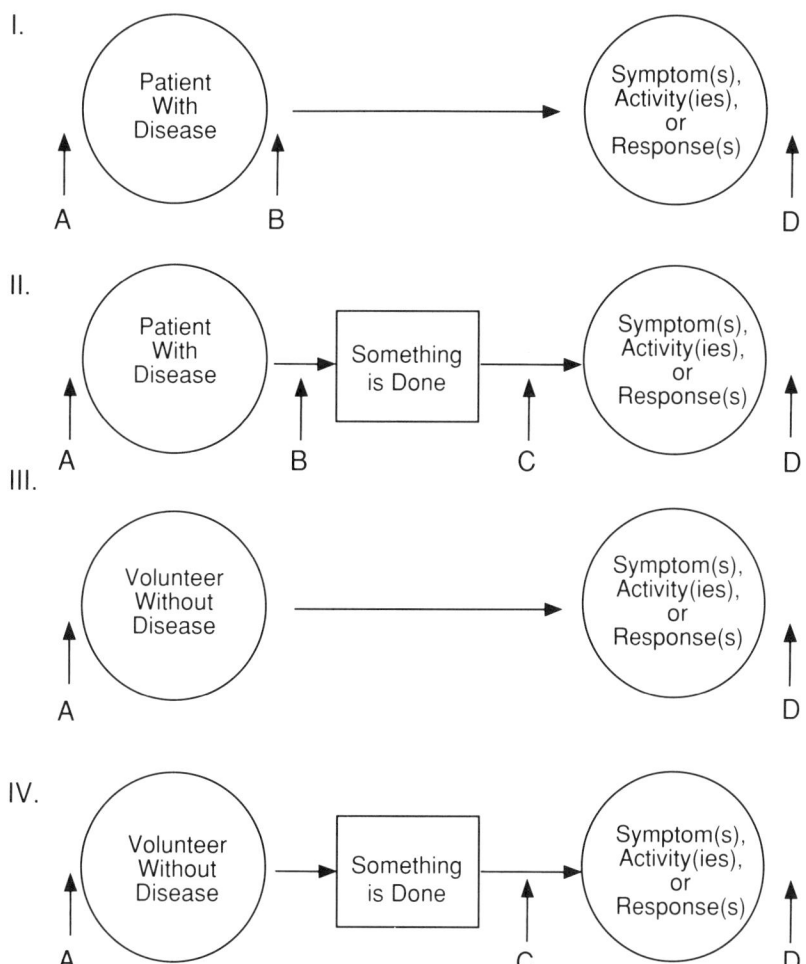

FIG. 90.2 Four models for studying medicines in humans. *A, B, C,* and *D* are the time points when patients may be evaluated. *A* represents a test of a prophylactic or preventive medicine. *B* represents a test after initial signs or symptoms of an episode are present. *C* represents a test after a challenge or something else is done to the patient or volunteers. *D* represents the time after full effect of the symptoms, activities, or responses have occurred. Not all models can be used to study each disease.

Phase I and Phase II trials are almost all conducted using artificial models or environments, although the degree of artificiality will vary enormously. Even in Phase III and many Phase IV trials, in which medicine evaluations are often performed under "usual conditions," there are numerous differences between this setting and the "real world." These include such factors as (1) increased physician attention and observation, (2) patient awareness of the special nature of the trial, (3) increased staff attention, (4) increased number of tests and evaluations, (5) prohibitions against various activities or medicine uses, and (6) informed consent.

Clinical Models of Disease

Certain clinical models of human disease come closer to reproducing the actual target disease than do others.

There are also clinical models that are at a lower level of organization and are often considered artificial and only indirectly related to human disease. These models include evaluation of biochemical markers such as measuring cholesterol levels to obtain data relating to myocardial infarctions. Table 90.1 lists a few additional examples of this phenomenon whereby the effect measured in clinical trials is not the therapeutic goal for the medicine's use. Other models use an artificial stimulus to induce a clinical condition/problem/lesion. An example of this is to induce diarrhea in normal patients by administering castor oil and then treat it with the test medicine. Each test or model yields both false-positive and false-negative results (e.g., the model of exercise-induced myocardial ischemia). The magnitude of these potential problems for data interpretation should be known so that data may be interpreted in the most meaningful way.

TABLE 90.1 *Selected examples in which the clinical effect measured is not the therapeutic goal for the medicine's use[a]*

Medicines	Patients treated	Clinical effect measured	Reason for therapy (i.e., clinical effect desired)
1. Diuretics, β-blockers, vasodilators	Hypertensives	Change in blood pressure	Decrease risk of stroke, renal failure, and myocardial infarction
2. Hypolipidemics	Hypercholesterolemics Hyperlipidemics	Change in various lipid levels	Decrease risk of myocardial infarction
3. Antiarrhythmics	Those with premature ventricular contractions (PVCs)[b] or ventricular tachycardia	Changes in number of PVCs and other arrhythmias	Prevention of sudden death from cardiovascular causes

[a] See Chapter 82 for a discussion on surrogate endpoints.
[b] Above a given frequency.

Artificiality of Major Parts of a Clinical Trial

Each clinical trial consists of numerous parts that have differing degrees of artificiality. There is a highly complex series of questions to consider in evaluting the degree of artificiality of a clinical trial. Moreover, the relationship of clinical trial tests and environment to those in clinical practice must be evaluated separately for each situation.

Five parts of the clinical trial are described, and general comments and examples are given, including specific comments relating to antidiarrheal trials. These parts of a trial were chosen to illustrate issues relating to artificiality and differ somewhat from the four parts of a trial described in Chapter 82.

Design of the Clinical Trial

The clinical trial design chosen often mimics the clinical process in which patients seek treatment or treat themselves for a specific problem or condition. Some studies, however, pretreat the patient with a medicine and then apply a test lesion or intervention to determine whether the result is ameliorated or prevented. The data are thus obtained using an artificial model and may or may not be relevant for actual clinical situations. This type of artificiality is most often seen in animal studies and was discussed in Chapter 89.

If a medicine is to be tested for its acute antidiarrheal effect, the clinical state may be mimicked by giving the medicine after diarrhea occurs. If the diarrhea is induced with castor oil or another substance, it represents an artificial stimulus. The data from this type of trial, however, will better reflect the eventual clinical situation if the treatment is initiated after the diarrhea has occurred than if the medicine is tested by determining if pretreatment prevents diarrhea from occurring.

Subjects Enrolled in the Clinical Trial

The degree or magnitude of extrapolation of data to actual treatment of patients is greater if animals rather than patients are used as subjects. Within the universe of animal studies there is a general rule that higher species (in an evolutionary sense) yield data that are more closely applicable to humans. There are many exceptions to this rule, and factors relating to the particular model or aspect of the experiment must also be considered. Patients with the disease eventually to be treated yield more authoritative data than do normal volunteers without the disease. There are numerous instances, however, when "clean" data, uncompromised by various concurrent medicines, previous treatments, and other factors, make volunteers generally preferable to use as subjects in a study. One example is of measuring a medicine's bioavailability profile under a variety of different conditions (e.g., diet, smoking, fasting).

If an antidiarrheal effect is eventually intended to help patients receiving chemotherapy, it still may be useful to demonstrate efficacy initially in otherwise normal people. These volunteers could have either spontaneous (i.e., acute) diarrhea or artificially induced diarrhea.

Environment of the Clinical Trial

Clinical trials are performed in environments that vary from an artificial laboratory setting where most factors are controlled to the other extreme where the environment is that of usual clinical practice and efforts are made not to disrupt what naturally occurs but merely to observe and monitor certain events. This latter type of study includes observational Phase IV studies. Between the two extremes are a variety of possible environments with different degrees of artificiality.

An investigator may choose to do an inpatient trial, since that will be the site of usual clinical practice in which the medicine or modality will eventually be used. An inpatient trial may also be conducted since more factors may be controlled in that environment, even though the results will eventually be applied to outpatients. Medicine trial designs may simulate an environment to make it closer to clinical practice. Alternatively, a usual clinical practice environment may be modified by the investigator, who understands that this intervention changes the environment to some degree and introduces an element of artificiality.

Evaluating acute diarrhea induced in a laboratory setting differs markedly from evaluating patients who are on a foreign trip or are in a hospital setting. Studying travelers on a foreign trip in a clinical setting is an example of introducing a modification into the usual clinical practice environment (assuming that the medicine was designed to be used eventually without contacting a physician). There are obviously many permutations that may be considered that will affect the magnitude of extrapolation necessary to include all potential patients.

Tests Used in a Clinical Trial

Tests used in clinical trials to measure the effects of treatment may or may not be the same as those used in actual clinical practice. Even if the same tests are used, the clinical manner in which patients take the tests may differ. The tests used to measure efficacy may be primarily described as being used in either an artificial or actual clinical practice manner.

Examples of an artificial efficacy test used in an artificial manner would be experimentally induced pain. A real-world evaluation used in an artificial manner would be dental pain evaluated in a clinical laboratory, and a real-world test used in a real-world setting would be dental pain evaluated in a dentist's office.

In the case of diarrhea, the test situation of artificially inducing diarrhea in patients in an artificial (laboratory) environment offers certain advantages in being able to elicit and measure the condition in a relatively standardized manner. This approach should not totally replace evaluation of patients with natural causes of diarrhea in separate studies.

Parameters Measured

Most efficacy tests have a variety of parameters that may be measured. Some relate closely to clinical symptomatology and clinical practice, whereas others are more artificial. In the electroencephalogram (EEG), the presence or absence of certain patterns (e.g., 3-Hz spike and wave) usually correlates strongly with clinical symptoms, but other potential parameters (e.g., frequency distribution, height of waves) usually have less of a clinical correlation. Some EEG techniques such as photic stimulation at 10 Hz are somewhat artificial, since this frequency of flashing lights does not often occur in nature and it may precipitate a seizure in patients who otherwise would not have had one.

In an antidiarrheal trial, improvement is usually measured in terms of decreasing number of bowel movements (per day) and improvement in the consistency of the stool (formed versus fluid). These are the same parameters that would be evaluated by both patients and physicians in the "real world."

Clinical Evaluation of Artificial Environments

In a few clinical trials investigators have attempted to discern the difference in response between two environments, one of which was more artificial. Riley et al. (1981) found that the seizure rate of epileptic patients decreased when they were admitted to hospital for observation. Riley et al. (1981) did not suggest that there was fabrication of the preadmission seizure data and believe that there is clearly an important psychological component behind the differences observed. It has also been reported that patient response to pain is greater in a clinical than in a laboratory setting (Dworkin and Chen, 1982). Even the effects of placebos as well as medicines will vary in different environments. Beecher reported (1962) that placebo is 10 times as effective in improving natural pathological pain as in affecting experimentally induced pain.

After a period of time, most patients acclimatize well to initially unfamiliar or even uncomfortable environments. This issue should be considered by the investigator prior to the trial. If this creates a potential problem, then efforts may be made to increase the patient's familiarity and comfort, not only with the trial environment, but with the protocol's requirements as well. In some situations a dry run should be conducted so that patients are more comfortable and will be more likely to give reliable data. A *training effect,* which influences results and their interpretation, however, may occur in a trial. Consideration of this potential bias will help to prevent it from influencing the trial.

Several other clinical trials that compare patient responses in different environments are listed in Table 83.6.

ISSUES INVOLVED IN EXTRAPOLATING DATA

The Hawthorne Effect

The Hawthorne effect, as applied to medicine, refers to the influence on patient behavior of the process of conducting an evaluation (i.e., research). The change in a patient's behavior brought about by his/her participation in research is defined as the Hawthorne effect, which may be described as having three components. These are the patient, the environment, and the research process.

The Patient

Patients who are participating in research may consciously modify their behavior to achieve a personal goal. This effect occurs most strongly in patients with emotional problems or in normal patients who are aware of being evaluated and are displeased or wish to create problems. Questions that could be evaluated include:

1. Which patients change?
2. How do they change?
3. How may the change be measured?
4. Why do they change (e.g., some patients want to please the investigator)?
5. What are the implications for the clinical trial's interpretation?

The Clinical Trial Environment

The research environment of a clinical trial varies and includes one or more of the following: the patient's real world at home, work, or both; hospital wards or operating rooms; medical clinic; clinical laboratories; research laboratories; and others. Some of these settings make patients more uncomfortable and tend to influence their behavior. Ensuring that patients are acclimatized to the clinical trial environment will tend to decrease the Hawthorne effect.

The Research Process

The third component of the Hawthorne effect is the research process, which is the design or protocol of the clinical trial. The major elements of the research process that influence the magnitude of the Hawthorne effect are the degree of artificiality of the clinical trial and the types of requests made of patients. Artificiality of a clinical trial includes whether the problem evaluated is induced (e.g., citric-acid-induced cough, castor-oil-induced diarrhea) or is natural. Other aspects of artificiality include the research environment, number of tests, amount of time required for a clinical trial, degree of fasting, and so forth. The types of requests made of patients vary from none, to requests that greatly modify their normal behavior, and may also be requests that the patient finds objectionable or even unethical.

Given the importance and complexity of these three components, it is clear that the Hawthorne effect may compromise the ability to extrapolate data obtained in a clinical trial.

Data from Dropouts and Discontinued Patients

Extrapolation is an extremely difficult procedure to implement fully and accurately. In most clinical trials, data are obtained with a sample of patients who are generally compliant with the protocol, although some patients drop out (i.e., withdraw) on their own or are discontinued by the investigator for a variety of reasons. Thus, in extrapolating the data from this select sample to a larger group, there will generally be inherent biases if data and experiences of the dropouts and discontinued patients are not considered. Even patients who were eliminated from participation in a trial for a variety of methodologically sound reasons should be considered (insofar as possible) in the process whereby trial data are extrapolated to a broader population.

The demographics and relevance of the dropouts and patients who did not qualify for the trial will be at least partially unknown, their reactions to treatment will be partially unknown, and the characteristics of the larger population involved in the extrapolation will also be partially unknown. Table 90.2 lists important information on a trial that will be useful if the data are to be extrapolated. The influence of dropouts and discontinuers, plus dropins, patient refusers, and nonqualifiers is discussed in Chapter 31.

Importance of Assessing the Representativeness of the Clinical Trial Population

For the results of most clinical trials to be extrapolated with confidence, an adequate number of patients must have been enrolled in a trial. This number is determined by sound statistical techniques in addition to experience, clinical judgment, or other factors. When a trial enters only a small proportion of the total number required to achieve adequate power, it is usually difficult to place credence in the ability to extrapolate the data. Also, when a trial enters only a small proportion of those patients screened or eligible for admission, its ability to be extrapolated may be compromised even if the trial entered sufficient patients to have adequate power. That is because the characteristics of those patients who were not entered are rarely

TABLE 90.2 *Important information to obtain for the optimal extrapolation of data*

1. Methods of patient recruitment and selection
2. Demographics of the patient population and comparison with other standard populations
3. Identity of any special characteristics that the treatment group(s) did (or did not) have
4. Determination of whether patients with various disease subtypes reacted differently to known treatments
5. Evaluations of whether one can predict which patients are responders and nonresponders
6. Evaluation of whether the therapeutic modality, medicine, or intervention has clinically important interactions with other known medicines
7. Assessment of how convincing available data are on the new treatment
8. Assessment of how homogeneous the group is to which the data will be extrapolated

known. It might be that the patients who did not enter the trial differed clinically or demographically from those who did. If a careful record were maintained of patients who were not entered into the trial, then a better case could be made for the validity of the extrapolation (see Charlson and Horwitz, 1984). Rosengren et al. (1987) evaluated the nonparticipants in a large clinical trial they were conducting. Nonparticipants had a higher rate of both social and alcohol problems than did participants. Although this result is an important demonstration of a type of study that should be done more often, there are various reasons why the results could have been expected and cannot be extrapolated widely.

Methods of Assessing the Representativeness of the Clinical Trial Population

Investigators who wish to extrapolate their results to other groups should attempt to evaluate whether their population is representative of a larger population. There are several different techniques whereby information on the representativeness of a population may be assessed or estimated.

1. Include all patients in a clinic, hospital, or other setting with a particular disease/problem who were observed (or treated) between two specified dates. These patients should be representative of those patients who receive treatment in similar settings.
2. Indicate how all patients who were eligible for the clinical trial were winnowed down to the number who eventually entered the trial. If the characteristics of those entered and those who were not admitted are compared, it may provide data on how representative the former group is (see Fig. 90.3).
3. When patients are recruited (rather than winnowed from a total population), clearly state and discuss the selection criteria and, if possible, determine the clinical status and demographics of those patients who did not enter the trial and compare with those patients who did enter the trial.
4. Compare the clinical characteristics and demographics of the group of patients who (1) dropped out of their own volition, (2) were discontinued by the investigator during the trial, (3) remained in the trial and completed it, (4) did not pass the screen, (5) dropped in to one group from another, (6) refused to enroll after passing the screen, or (7) fit another category.
5. Provide the number of patients who were eligible for the trial, completed the screen, consented to enter, completed baseline, and completed treatment. Discuss the reasons why the number of patients decreased from step to step.

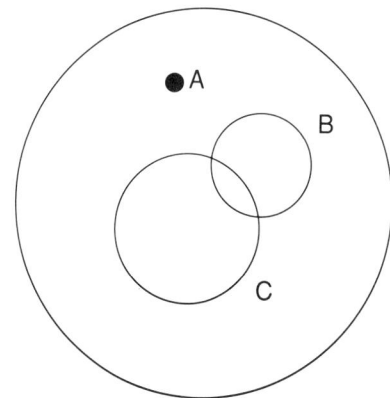

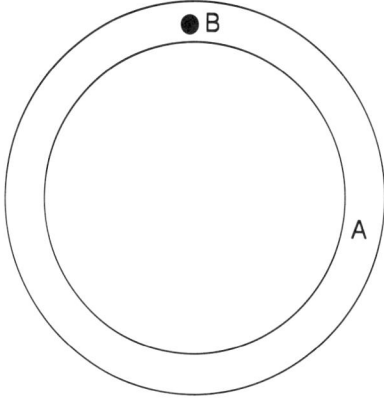

FIG. 90.3 Schematic illustration of the representativeness of patients in a clinical trial to the entire patient population with the same disease. A, B, and C are the relative range of patients enrolled in a single clinical trial. The outside circle represents the scope of the entire patient population. The diameter is controlled by the inclusion criteria, and the larger the diameter, the greater is the ability to extrapolate the data. The **upper figure** represents most Phase II clinical trials in which narrow (A) or somewhat broader patient populations are evaluated. The **lower figure** represents most Phase III clinical trials in which extremely broad (A) or very narrow patient populations are usually studied.

6. Analyze all clinical data available from patients who dropped out or were discontinued and compare with results of those patients who completed the trial.
7. The authors of a publication should state to which populations of patients their results do and do not apply.

It is interesting to note that a well-known painkiller evaluated in thousands of patients during the 1960s revealed no problems of abuse. The sponsor was certain that the medicine was free of abuse potential. After the medicine was marketed, however, this problem began to surface. After marketing the medicine was used by an entirely different population, i.e., habitual drug abusers, who had been systematically excluded from all of the clinical trials.

Formal Evaluation for Generalizability

In some cases it may be important to test formally the extrapolatability of data from a clinical trial. If resources are available, an external committee of experts should have the clinical trial audited. The audit will provide information on the conduct of the trial (e.g., were randomizations conducted as planned?, were patient exclusions appropriate?), design of the trial (e.g., was the power adequate?), and data processing and statistical analyses. The group can then determine how representative the patients are of all patients with the disease. This would involve a comparison with patients not enrolled in the clinical trial as well as with refusers, dropouts, nonqualifiers, and discontinued patients. The checks on extrapolatability that could be conducted are listed in Table 90.3.

Homogeneous versus Heterogeneous Trial Populations

Investigators sometimes choose between conducting a clinical trial in a narrowly defined homogeneous population or a broadly inclusive heterogeneous group of patients. The former group may yield data that are hard to extrapolate to a wider group of patients. The other extreme is to conduct a trial in a broad heterogeneous group of patients, which will be more variable but will provide data of more widespread clinical applicability (Fig. 90.3).

The solution to this issue relates to the objectives of the clinical trial. In Phases I and II of medicine development, a narrow homogeneous population is almost always preferable, whereas in Phases III and IV more heterogeneous populations have many advantages. When specific objectives are posed, the group

TABLE 90.3 Aspects to evaluate in assessing extrapolatability

1. Baseline characteristics of prognostic variables
2. Demographics
3. Results and patient profiles across clinical research centers
4. Subgroup analyses of apparent relevance
5. Comparison with patients who refused entry[a] or did not qualify for entry
6. Hypotheses of suspected problems
7. Sensitivity of results for analysis deviations
8. Literature results

[a] This is sometimes called a *volunteer effect*, because patients who volunteer to enter a clinical trial are usually different from those who do not.

TABLE 90.4 Ability to predict therapeutic efficacy of various types of medicines based on data from normal volunteers

Disease or condition	Parameter used	Usefulness
Hypercholesterolemia	Cholesterol	Fair
Hypertension	Blood pressure	Fair
Insomnia	Sedation	Good
Anxiety	Sedation	Good
Beta blockade	Heart rate	Excellent
Anticoagulants	PT/PTT[a]	Excellent

[a] PT, prothrombin time; PTP, partial thromboplastin time.

chosen should be the population that will best address the objectives and provide the "extrapolatability" desired. Table 90.4 lists the ability to extrapolate data from normal volunteers to patients.

Another perspective is to view all individuals as differing from each other and conclude that we can only know and evaluate some of the pertinent factors in any clinical trial. Summary data of an adequate-sized group of dissimilar people will be obtained. It is reasonable to expect that another similar or slightly different group will react in a similar manner.

In some diseases there is a continuum of patients with differing types of the disease or with differing severity of illness. One treatment may be best for one type of disease and another treatment best for those with a different type. How should one determine the midrange, and what treatment should be given to those patients? It is not possible to extrapolate data from patients with one type of disease to another without at least some evidence that this procedure is likely to be clinically meaningful.

Direction of the Extrapolation

Another issue relating to extrapolation concerns the direction of extrapolation. This means that one may extrapolate results from an entire group or population to one patient or extrapolate results from a single patient to an entire population. Most of the foregoing discussion assumed that the results of a single clinical trial are being extrapolated to the entire population of patients with the particular disease. This is mainly a theoretical consideration, since extrapolation by practicing physicians usually goes in the opposite direction, i.e., toward the single patient they are treating. Clinical relevance for specific patients with the disease is based on interpretations of data obtained in trials using a larger patient population. Extrapolation to an entire population from a single patient usually represents a pitfall to be avoided.

CHAPTER 91

Data That Are Difficult to Interpret

REASONS WHY DATA MAY BE DIFFICULT TO INTERPRET

Despite the most assiduous attention to detail in designing a clinical trial and adhering to high standards in its conduct, situations will still arise in which the data obtained are difficult to interpret. When this situation occurs, the initial step is to ascertain the primary reason for the difficulty. A few common reasons are listed in Table 91.1.

Seeking Clues

In analyzing data one must often seek clues that might help to explain the results. Clues such as changes in important staff personnel, clustering of data, and changes in the protocol may all be important in this process. Unfortunately, a single factor is often not able to unravel the complexities of difficult data on its own. With many complex clinical situations and trials, it is often not possible to tease out a single thread.

If an entire clinical trial yields data that are difficult or "impossible" to interpret, the reason(s) may be primarily factors relating to the protocol or trial design, patients entered in the trial, or the investigator and

staff who conducted the trial. Almost any aspect of the trial may be responsible, and it is not possible to present a simple checklist to determine how this problem may have occurred. A list of some methods that can be used to identify why a set of data is difficult to interpret is presented in Table 91.2.

Nonresponders

Data may be difficult to interpret if there were a relatively large number of nonresponders in the clinical trial. The data may be broken down and analyzed by degree of patient response. If two groups of patients receiving treatment may be identified as responders and nonresponders, various clues may be considered and evaluated as possible reasons why some patients were nonresponders. This technique is useful for hypothesis generation but is not suitable for drawing a definitive interpretation. Specific factors that may be evaluated include (1) duration of illness, (2) severity of illness, (3) response to previous medication, (4) reason for current exacerbation, (5) compliance with trial, (6) differences in blood levels, and (7) differences in dosages given or taken. Chapter 98 discusses the concept of responders and nonresponders in more detail.

TABLE 91.1 *Selected reasons why a specific data set may be difficult to interpret*

A. Reasons related to the protocol
 1. Too few patients entered
 2. Too many patients entered (overpowered tests will detect small, clinically unimportant differences)
 3. Trial design flawed (e.g., blinding, randomization, efficacy measures, or controls used were inappropriate)
 4. Inadequate methodology exists to measure the endpoints accurately and reproducibly
 5. Inappropriate statistical tests used to analyze the data
B. Reasons related to the investigator not following the protocol
 1. Errors in patient assignment to treatment
 2. Trial blind not maintained
 3. Unacceptable biases entered the trial
 4. Irregular compliance with protocol
C. Reasons related to the patient
 1. Patients were not compliant and did not take medicine as instructed or missed numerous appointments so that insufficient or inaccurate data were collected
 2. Patient characteristics that related to the response differed in different treatment groups
 3. Patients may not have been accurately diagnosed or may have represented different subgroups of the population
 4. A large number of nonresponsive patients were entered in the trial
D. Reasons related to the disease or problem being evaluated
 1. The disease process is particularly complex or not well understood
 2. The disease process was too advancd in some patients or too mild in others
E. Reasons related to the outcomes of the trial
 1. The placebo response may have been much larger than anticipated
 2. The active control response may have been much smaller than anticipated
F. Other reasons
 1. Only one or a few case studies are available for interpretation
 2. Only retrospective data are available
 3. Large gaps exist in the data collected (i.e., the data are incomplete)
 4. Too many anecdotal observations, hearsay, or conjecture were included in the data collected

Dirty or Noisy Data

One of the most common reasons why some data are difficult to interpret concerns the concept of "clean" and "dirty" data. Dirty or noisy data have that term applied because the data (1) are incomplete and fragmentary (see discussion of incomplete data sets in this chapter), (2) were obtained under suboptimal conditions and have a great deal of variability, inconsistency, or lack of ascertainment (i.e., the validity is questionable), or (3) were obtained under close to optimal conditions but still have a great deal of variability, inconsistency, or lack of ascertainment.

TECHNIQUES TO USE IN DIFFICULT SITUATIONS

Prevention and Approaches

A number of approaches can help to prevent situations in which data are difficult to interpret or to deal with

such situations after they have occurred. Most of the situations that lead to collecting data that are difficult to interpret may be avoided through careful planning of the design and conduct of the clinical trial and careful data editing. The reason(s) for difficulty in data interpretation may also relate to problems in data analysis or to another factor that can be corrected or reconsidered without requiring duplication of the entire trial. A few approaches to consider are listed in Table 91.3.

Developing New Hypotheses or Interpretations

Dividing the data according to new factors (e.g., age, sex, weight of patient) and reanalyzing the data of the new groups obtained may lead to new hypotheses or interpretations. If an attempt to demonstrate the positive association between two or more events, medicines, or effects is unsuccessful, it might be useful to evaluate whether qualitative differences among the test parameters may be demonstrated. It is also sometimes possible to focus on the inverse of what is being examined as a means of achieving an adequate interpretation of previously "uninterpretable" data. See Chapter 76 on Developing Hypotheses.

Creating a Differential Diagnosis

There is a clinical analogy in the approach to be followed in solving problems of interpretation. The per-

TABLE 91.2 *Techniques or approaches to identify reasons why certain data are difficult to interpret*

1. Evaluate the difficulty in an overall manner and systematically attempt to identify techniques that may resolve the difficulty
2. Consult with statisticians, consultants, colleagues, and peers in your own clinical field and occasionally in a different one
3. Use techniques of "lateral thinking"[a]
4. Use a "devil's advocate" approach
5. Repeat the statistical analyses
6. Evaluate each of the individual factors that might have affected and complicated the data, including steps conducted in data collection, editing, processing, and analysis
7. Consider various pitfalls that may have occurred and could have created problems
8. Consider various biases that may have influenced the data
9. Reanalyze the data with new methodologies or by subgroups and attempt to create hypotheses based on the new results
10. Evaluate the trial design for possible flaws that led to the problems in developing a suitable interpretation
11. Use flow diagrams, algorithms, and other related techniques to analyze one's thought processes and to identify new questions or relationships
12. Evaluate the conduct of the trial for possible problems that led to the difficulties in interpretation
13. Determine whether interpretation at a different level (e.g., molecular, cellular, physiological, pharmacological) is more appropriate
14. Determine whether subclassifications of the disease, receptors, or activities are more useful to consider than broader classifications

[a] See text and references by de Bono (1967a, b; 1969).

TABLE 91.3 *Techniques or approaches to interpret difficult data*[a]

1. Use appropriate caveats in the interpretations reached
2. Present an interpretation of "grays" even though a "black-and-white" (e.g., all-or-none) answer was sought
3. Modify the problem to make it even more difficult to solve. For example, the use of an extreme case or situation may suggest an approach or interpretation not previously considered
4. Discuss only those parts of the data for which a reasonable interpretation may be achieved. Comment on data where a reliable interpretation is not possible
5. Discuss the interpretation in terms of the degree of association between two events (i.e., is a cause and effect highly unlikely, possible, probable, almost definite, unknown, or virtually impossible)
6. State what the data do not mean. This may be a useful starting point in developing the interpretation, especially for subjective data
7. Suggest what additional information would be required to reach a more definitive interpretation and then attempt to obtain that information
8. Utilize an "if–then" exercise whereby a point of view, hypothesis, or statement follows "if." The consequences of the statement are then developed starting with the term "then." These consequences are then looked for, to determine their existence, nature, and/or validity

[a] See Table 91.2 for additional methods.

son who is interpreting the data should establish a differential diagnosis of the possible interpretations or problems preventing the interpretation and then systematically evaluate each until the correct one(s) is identified. The old clinical cliché applies that "when you hear hoofbeats think of horses, not of zebras" (i.e., common reasons rather than esoteric ones are usually the true cause of the problem).

Questions to Pose

When data are difficult to interpret, a concerted attempt should be made to identify the source of the problem. One approach to identifying the specific factors involved is first to identify (if possible) whether the problem is related to the (1) patient, (2) tests used, (3) measurements obtained, (4) investigator, (5) professional and ancillary staff, (6) environment, (7) test medicine itself, or (8) concomitant treatment. Other possible categories may also be considered. After the broad category is identified, a search for more specific factors may be considered and conducted.

Another approach is to identify any unusual aspects of the data. One should attempt to determine why these aspects occurred and focus on those elements that may provide a basis for interpreting the data. This type of analysis may demonstrate the need to conduct a new clinical trial that is better designed and/or better conducted.

The number of specific questions to pose is almost without limit. A small sample of the types of questions to ask that relate to any aspect of the trial (the medi-

cine, the patients, or the data) is presented in Table 91.4. Finally, after consultation with peers and consultants, one may reluctantly have to conclude that no suitable explanation or interpretation of the data is possible.

Statistical Considerations

The individual who is interpreting data should have a collaborative and interactive relationship with a statistician. They should review the data analyses to ascertain that the appropriate methods were used to address the clinical questions. It may be decided that it is relevant to perform additional statistical analyses. This situation may occur if statistical tests that were not used to analyze the data are equally valid as those tests that were used. It is also possible that the original data may be analyzed with different statistical tests to evaluate the data from a different perspective. For example, trials are often conducted in which a medicine is given to patients and data are obtained each hour for a given number of hours. The data obtained may be analyzed in several ways. A few of the more straightforward methods are shown below. For between-treatment evaluations:

1. Data obtained at each individual hour of the trial may be compared for two or more groups.
2. Algebraic differences between a baseline and each individual hourly result may be compared for two or more groups.
3. Data obtained at the average of all trial hours after

TABLE 91.4 *Specific questions to pose when an interpretation of difficult data is sought*

1. Do data include different lengths of treatment for different patients?
2. Are patients remaining in the clinical trial for different lengths of time in different groups?
3. Are blood levels different in different groups of patients?
4. Is the chemical stability of the medicine known with assurance?
5. Are impurities or different isomers present in some batches of medicine?
6. Did each patient receive the correct medicine? Has this been confirmed with analysis of a sample of their medication?
7. Are all medicines getting to the site of action?
8. Does the medicine act differently in different species?
9. May animal studies be conducted to address questions about the problem (e.g., does medicine cross the blood–brain barrier)?
10. How did the patient's behavior change as a result of being in the trial?
11. Are many patients nonresponders?
12. Can a more detailed knowledge of all patients medical history provide clues?
13. Can a detailed analysis of one patient's history provide hints for the entire trial?
14. If the medicine does not cause an effect of its own, perhaps it modulates the same effect caused by other medicines?

treatment may be compared for two or more groups.

4. Algebraic differences between the baseline and the average of all trial hours after treatment may be compared for two or more groups.
5. Analysis of variance or other more sophisticated tests may be used to evaluate the data.

For within-treatment evaluations, each of the five processes described may be conducted with data of one treatment group. Variations include (1) only choosing a single or a few representative time points to evaluate, such as the initial or final response, (2) averaging all baseline values or only averaging the last *n* values, (3) averaging baseline with posttreatment follow-up values as a control, or (4) defining baseline in a different manner.

Use of Lateral Thinking

Use of lateral thinking in interpreting data should be considered, although this approach is often difficult to implement effectively. The four major principles of lateral thinking (de Bono, 1967b) are:

1. Recognize dominant polarizing ideas
2. Search for different ways of looking at situations or problems
3. Relax the rigid control of vertical (i.e., logical) thinking
4. Use chance in arriving at a solution

These concepts cannot be adequately summarized in a few sentences, and interested readers are referred to de Bono's books, in which he describes four types of thinking: natural thinking, logical thinking, mathematical thinking, and lateral thinking. Edward de Bono has described lateral thinking as a low-probability sideways thinking. He presents its use in *The Five-Day Course in Thinking, The Use of Lateral Thinking,* and *The Mechanism of Mind* (see references). Lateral thinking may enable a person to search for novel solutions to a problem or to rephrase the question being asked in a way that would allow a solution to be achieved.

The second principle may be approached by intellectually viewing the data in a different perspective that allows an answer to be achieved. One example is when a specific relationship is consciously reversed. For example, a glass of water may be viewed as being either half full or half empty. Another example is to view the walls of a building as suspended from the roof rather than viewing the walls as supporting for the roof. Finally, an object could be viewed as moving in a curve through space, or space itself may be viewed as curved. One must be cautious when using this ap-

proach, because a measure such as pain intensity may not simply be the inverse of pain relief.

Use of the Delphi Technique

This technique is applicable to many disciplines but should be carefully evaluated before it is used. It may be most useful if it is desired to have a group, rather than a single individual, address the problem of interpretation. Interested readers are referred to a concise review article by Duffield (1988) for details.

Situations in which There Are Both Positive and Negative Responses in Efficacy

A potentially difficult situation in interpretation of data may arise if some parameters measured are positive and others either do not change or are negative. In this situation it is almost impossible to rank order the importance of parameters after a clinical trial is complete without bias, to determine whether the overall interpretation is more positive than negative or vice versa. There are, however, a few choices to consider. One is to present all of the data and results without attempting to compare the importance of parameters that are positive with those that are negative. This is an "objective" approach, but clearly it is unsatisfactory to most people.

Creating a Hierarchy of Parameters

The most satisfactory approach is to anticipate this potential dilemma prior to the clinical trial and initially to decide which specific tests and parameters are most important. Additional parameters or tests may be identified that will be used for objectives of secondary importance or as supportive data. A variation of this approach is to establish a definition of medicine activity prior to the trial. Then, if the primary parameter is negative but other parameters are highly positive and the medicine achieves the definition of activity, a convincing overall interpretation may be possible.

A situation may occur in which two parameters were rated (prior to the clinical trial) of primary importance and two others of secondary importance. The data may indicate that only one parameter of each group was positive and the other from each group negative. If both parameters that were negative in this example were neutral (i.e., unchanged), then the trend of the trial would probably be viewed as positive. But every situation encountered will present a unique set of data and analyses and therefore will have to be judged in the context of many factors. This approach often raises the problem that various efficacy variables can often not be ordered or directly compared.

Apples versus Oranges

Parameters evaluated often differ from each other, and it may be difficult to compare them adequately. For example, some efficacy parameters that may be difficult to compare accurately and rank in an arthritis trial are (1) patient's clinical global impression, (2) swollen joints, (3) physician's assessment of a patient's functional ability, (4) quality of life, (5) various biochemical tests, and (6) number of painful joints. The most satisfactory solution in many cases is to create an overall index that includes consideration of several parameters.

INCOMPLETE DATA SETS

Why Do Incomplete Data Sets Occur?

Data are usually difficult to interpret when only fragments of interpretable data are available. This situation may arise (1) when a retrospective trial is conducted, (2) when an excessive number of patient dropouts or missed appointments have occurred, or (3) when an interim analysis is being conducted.

An interim analysis of data that is difficult to interpret should not present a serious problem to the investigator, who will either be blinded to the outcome of the analysis or will continue the clinical trial regardless of the results. If the interim analysis suggests that real or potential issues have arisen in the trial that must be considered, then these should be addressed with the assistance of a statistician. The most common reason for occurrence of fragmented data is when a trial has been conducted that is markedly flawed for some reason (e.g., too few patients, too many dropouts, too great a quantity of missing or flawed data).

Data may be incomplete because of an excessive number of dropouts, noncompliers, poorly randomized patients, incorrectly diagnosed patients, or many other problems that sometimes arise in clinical trials. There are statistical conventions and techniques for dealing with such trials.

Another source of data fragments is when an event is observed in a single or small number of patients or in a single clinical trial (e.g., a published report that medicine Z caused toxicity X in Y number of patients), but the background information and sequence of events that led to the adverse reaction (or other problem) are unknown or unreported. The data will be incomplete and may not indicate how long the event has occurred, whether it had a gradual, sudden, or stepwise onset, whether it was worse in the past and is now being measured or observed during a phase of gradual or rapid improvement, or if a cycling phenomenon of improvement and subsequent deterioration is present. A great deal of caution is needed in interpreting fragments of data without knowledge of the natural history and resolution of the event in question.

Publication of Fragments

Publication of fragments of a large clinical trial (e.g., one site's data from a multicenter trial) is counterproductive when it is not possible to develop an adequate and accurate interpretation. Thus, any interpretation of such data presented will introduce bias in the literature and lead to a situation that may create significant problems for others to explain or resolve. This type of clinical data is usually best kept out of the medical literature through high standards of publication adhered to by journal editors. A statistician may provide advice to investigators prior to a clinical trial that will help prevent this type of data from being generated. For example, if the power of a trial is extremely low, then the possibility of the data representing a false-negative or -positive event becomes high.

Many individual and multicenter clinical trials with insufficient power to address the clinical objectives are published in the literature. These trials contain a generally unreliable set of data and may inadvertently provide false information on a topic and also may mislead medical thought for many years.

The opposite perspective also has merit and should be noted. Case reports or incomplete data may present clinical information that has clinical significance even though the clinical trial is incomplete or only a few patients were involved. Publication of such data may also alert other clinicians and scientists of adverse reactions that should be sought, monitored, and evaluated.

A Complete Clinical Trial That Yields Fragments: The Jigsaw Puzzle Problem

Even clinical trials that are perfectly conducted may be difficult to interpret for reasons other than those listed in Table 91.1. The most common reason would be that the data cannot all be gathered together in a neat grouping to evaluate the treatment effects, and the data therefore consist of many fragments, possibly analogous to pieces of a jigsaw puzzle. Dealing with only a few pieces of a jigsaw puzzle is difficult because they can often be arranged in several different ways. The interpreter often has to fill in the missing pieces. If most or all of the important pieces of a puzzle are available, then the missing ones may be recreated with relative assurance of little bias. On the other hand, if

TABLE 91.5 *Pertinent questions to ask about data fragments*[a]

Will the data fragments be more clear if:
1. More patients are entered in the clinical trial
2. The trial is continued for a longer duration
3. A higher dose of trial medicine is added
4. An additional control group is added
5. The trial is conducted double blind instead of single blind or open label[b]
6. The protocol is adhered to more closely by the investigator or patients[b]
7. New measurements or tests are incorporated into the trial[b]
8. The trial design or trial conduct is modified in a different manner[b]

[a] Data fragments are incomplete data sets from a clinical trial.
[b] Note that these changes in the trial must generally be adjusted for in the analyses.

only a few of the major pieces are present, then creating the entire picture will require an excessive amount of conjecture and educated guesses, and the result will probably be more open to challenge. When the data appear to be highly fragmented, there are several questions to ask. Some of these are presented in Table 91.5. A major question relates to the importance of data obtained in a flawed trial. The nature and degree of all significant flaws in a trial are essential to determine. At that point it is possible to assess whether the trial is mildly compromised or whether its interpretation will have virtually no validity. Discussions with statisticians or consultants may offer possible paths out of this dilemma.

ANECDOTAL OBSERVATIONS

Most clinical trials elicit a number of anecdotal comments from both patients and investigators, and these are often placed on the data collection forms or in various reports. These comments or observations are often tidbits of information that may (1) assist in the interpretation of data, (2) clarify results obtained, or (3) provide information that may have usefulness at a later time. All anecdotal comments should be collected and reviewed at some point during or after a trial for possible insights or suggestions.

Observations and Comments from Patients

It may be extremely difficult for the investigator to interpret anecdotal observations and comments from patients in a clinical trial. If the patient's comments fit a well-established pattern, then additional questioning may develop a better understanding of the report. But if the report is unusual, then it is often best to describe it succinctly under "Investigator's Comments" in the data collection forms for consideration at a later time.

Observations and Comments from Investigators

Anecdotal observations from investigators who have conducted a clinical trial may be indicated in the appropriate place in the results and possibly discussion sections of a published report. If a brief or full communication is published describing experiences with only one or a few patients, then it is extremely important to consider summarizing or describing the anecdotal comments or observations and to place them in proper perspective. Anecdotal observations often relate to adverse reactions.

When novel adverse reactions to a medicine begin to appear in the literature, additional case studies may provide extremely valuable data and a better perspective on the clinical significance of the potential problem. This is especially so when an understanding of the incidence of the adverse reaction is discussed along with details of clinical severity, degree of association with the medicine, and other factors.

Interpreting Anecdotal Observations

In preparing reports on limited clinical trials, anecdotal observations and comments may be informative in gaining clues that will help understand the nature of a medicine's clinical profile. On the other hand, all anecdotal (i.e., testimonial) information and data must be viewed with at least some skepticism. Recall the often quoted comment that if testimony could establish a fact, then one of the best established facts in the Middle Ages was the existence of the devil, since he was frequently seen and was carefully described by many individuals.

CHAPTER 92

Reconciling Different Interpretations from Different Trials

TYPES OF DIFFERENCES

Among Animal Experiments

Many investigators who conduct scientific studies in animals often attempt to replicate previous experiments conducted by themselves and others. Despite careful attention to even the most minute detail and experimental condition, many animal experiments are not easily replicated. Even when one attempts to follow identical conditions, results often turn out differently on different occasions. Evaluating the reason(s) for the differences in the results obtained is usually extremely difficult. This often makes it impossible to choose the "correct" interpretation of the experiment. The experiment is sometimes repeated a third time in the belief that if two of the three studies reach a similar conclusion, the probability is that the majority interpretation is correct. A fourth or even larger number of studies may be conducted to search for and confirm the correct interpretation. The rationality of this approach may be questioned.

Among Clinical Trials

Clinical trials are also often repeated, but they rarely utilize the same experimental conditions or the identical protocol. Each investigator who wishes to repeat a trial usually adds variations to the protocol that either

(1) are designed to "improve the trial" or (2) serve to obtain data of particular interest. The variations commonly introduced in developing clinical trial designs and protocols are only one aspect of the many differences between animal studies and clinical trials. The use of awake, active humans in most trials rather than inbred (often anesthetized) animals or in vitro studies creates many other significant differences. There are even more differences between chronic studies conducted in humans and animals, since many additional factors may influence the data. Chronic studies represent a minority of animal studies conducted but a relatively large percentage of human clinical trials. These considerations indicate that it is rare for multiple clinical trials, but not for animal studies, to be conducted under similar experimental conditions.

FACTORS TO EVALUATE

Who Is Doing the Reconciliation

The first factor to examine in reviewing different interpretations is clarification of the relationship between the investigator(s) and the person who is evaluating the interpretations. Although differences in clinical interpretation may arise when a single investigator has performed two or more related clinical trials, differences in interpretation are more common when trials have been performed by two or more investigators or groups of investigators. The person attempting to reconcile the interpretation may be:

1. An investigator whose interpretation of his or her present clinical trial differs from a previous trial
2. An investigator whose interpretation of his or her trial differs from the interpretation of one (or more) trials conducted and reported by others
3. A "third party" who is attempting to reconcile two (or more) published trials that differ in interpretation

Perspective and Aims of the Clinical Trial

The second factor to evaluate is to determine the point of view or perspective expressed within each clinical trial. If one trial was reported by regulatory agency personnel, it might be slanted toward a view reflecting their mission to protect the nation's health. A trial from certain academicians might reflect a highly theoretical perspective, and at least some industrial physicians use a practical perspective for developing an interpretation. If one trial report presented data without attempting to propose or defend a hypothesis, whereas another trial proposed a hypothesis, and a third trial defended one, these varying orientations might well have had a marked influence on the interpretations advanced.

The Myriad of Details

Other differences in interpretations relate to the myriad of factors that make up the design, conduct, and analysis of the clinical trial. Whenever a trial is conducted, it means that many factors and conditions will differ from those in a trial conducted at an earlier time, even when an attempt is made to keep conditions constant. Differences are usually difficult to delineate fully and will often affect data collected and interpretations reached.

Obtaining information on many of the relevant factors to evaluate (see Chapter 83 for identification of many of these factors) will prove exceedingly difficult if the individual conducting the evaluation was not the investigator of all clinical trials being compared. If one must rely on published reports for some or all of the information needed to compare interpretations, one is at a marked disadvantage. Although one may write or telephone the original investigators to obtain relevant information, the response to this approach is generally limited.

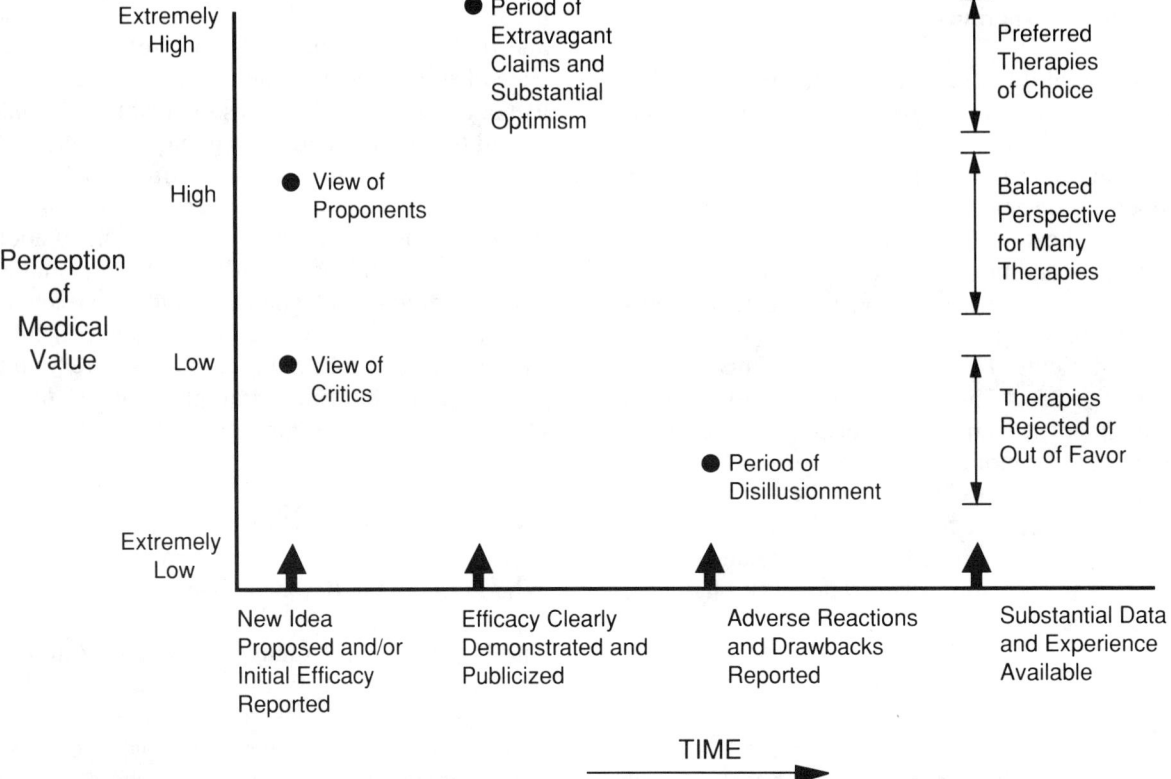

FIG. 92.1 Perception of a new medical treatment's value and the change of that perception over time. Although there are always various perceptions of the medical value of a treatment at any time, only the major consensus points are shown.

Lazarus Phenomenon

One reason why different clinical trials yield different responses is that nonresponders are entered in some trials (sometimes in large numbers). Expecting patients who have been unresponsive to all other medicines to respond to the latest one is expecting the Lazarus phenomenon. Fortunately for some patients, this does occur from time to time. However, even when one or two examples of the Lazarus phenomenon occur, the clinical trial itself may still be negative if many other "burned-out" patients were entered or if the medicine itself is relatively inactive in most patients.

Examples of Different Interpretations

Horwitz (1987) collected 36 topics in gastroenterology and cardiology for which conflicting results were obtained in over 200 randomized clinical trials. The interested reader is referred to his paper for details. He found nine major methodological sources of variation to account for differences that were related to either clinical trial design or interpretation. His results are summarized in Table 92.1.

Horwitz purposely avoided clinical trials in which differences were a result of small sample size or obvious bias, the two most common reasons for incorrect outcomes reported in the literature of clinical trials.

PERCEPTIONS OF NEW MEDICAL THERAPIES

There are often wide swings in the medical literature in how a new medicine, modality, diagnostic test, or technique is viewed. An illustration of this phenomenon is shown in Fig. 92.1. Initial reactions tend to be skeptical, but almost unbridled enthusiasm often occurs at a later time, often followed by a period of disbelief and almost sarcasm. Finally a more balanced evaluation is achieved. Some of these swings are a result of the changing views of the organization's leaders, plus the project's proponents. Media involvement (if present) also plays a major role. Another factor is the time necessary before sufficient data and experience are collected to allow a balanced perspective to be obtained.

The faddish nature of therapeutics is not a recent phenomenon. Osler has been reported to have said "Make haste to use a new remedy before it is too late" (quoted by Alderson, 1974). Miller and Melmon (1972, p. 409) also describe this phenomenon and briefly discuss the "wild swings of popularity and debasement" experienced by dimethylsulfoxide (DMSO). Lum and Beeler (1983) observe that this phenomenon is also seen with new diagnostic tests, such as carcinoembryonic antigen, α-fetoprotein, and acid phosphatase

TABLE 92.1 *Variations that accounted for differences in clinical trial results in a survey conducted by Horwitz[a]*

1. Eligibility criteria and selection of study groups (e.g., some clinical trials in hypertension included high-risk patients with evidence of end-organ damage)
2. Baseline state differences in patient population evaluated (e.g., in evaluating recurrent gastrointestinal bleeding in patients with cirrhosis, one group had a much larger population in which alcoholism was responsible)
3. Protocols for use of the principal therapy (e.g., large variations in dose and treatment duration may explain different results of the use of steroids to treat alcoholic liver disease)
4. Protocol requirements (e.g., corticosteroids in patients with septic shock work best when given early, but some clinical trials required time-consuming tests prior to enrollment that delayed administration of the medicine and affected results)
5. Use of concomitant therapy (e.g., diuretic treatment as concomitant therapy in one of two nitroprusside clinical trials is believed to have accounted for differences in outcome)
6. Managing patients in more artificial versus realistic protocols (e.g., hypertension is often studied by withholding treatment from the control group, which tends to enhance the difference from the treated group; when control patients are treated if their diastolic blood pressure exceeds 105 to 110 mmHg, the treatment strategy more closely resembles actual practice)
7. Regulatory requirements in data analysis and interpretation (e.g., intention-to-treat analyses that are *de rigueur* at regulatory authorities are often unacceptable to clinicians)
8. Poorly blinded double-blind trials (e.g., decreases in blood pressure or cholesterol in one treatment group effectively unblind many clinical trials, even if adverse reactions or laboratory data do not)
9. Use of different efficacy endpoints (e.g., use of overall mortality or prevention of ventricular fibrillation to assess efficacy in lidocaine prophylaxis trials in patients with acute myocardial infarction)

[a] From Horwitz, 1987. The wording of his nine categories has been modified.

(by radioimmunoassay). Laurence (1973) and Steiner and Dince (1981) also discuss this topic.

This kind of evaluation occurs when investigational medicines are proceeding through the phases of development, as well as after they are marketed. In the former case, opinion within the company often changes radically, whereas in the latter case opinion within the larger medical community changes.

APPROACHES TO A SOLUTION

General Approaches

This section describes both broad general approaches and a few specific steps that may be used in reconciling interpretations of two different studies. A few of the broad approaches are:

1. Evaluate and compare the quality of the clinical trial designs.
2. Evaluate and compare the quality of the conduct of the trials.

4. Combine (pool) data from all (or most) comparable trials to obtain an overall interpretation of results from trials other than those being compared.
5. Evaluate each possible interpretation of the data and choose the most reasonable single interpretation.
6. Look for both general and specific differences between patients.
7. Look for both general and specific differences between trials.

In regard to the last two approaches, it is necessary to go through the protocol, data, analyses, and other details of each trial step by step, looking for differences in trial design, methodology, results, patient management, and other areas. After important differences are identified, one must attempt to determine which trial or trials yielded the most reliable data.

Specific Approaches

In establishing a specific approach to use with problem situations, a number of the following questions may be relevant to address:

1. Do the trials meet current standards of design and conduct? Those that do not probably should be deleted from serious consideration, or they should be considered in a separate group.
2. Can the reasons for the differences be identified? This usually involves consideration of many specific factors.
3. Are the differences in interpretation irreconcilable, or do they represent minor variations?
4. If a resolution is impossible at this time, is it possible to design a new trial that will resolve the differences between or among the trials?
5. If a solution is not apparent, see the approaches listed in Chapter 91 on Data That Are Difficult to Interpret.

Group meetings may be held to attempt a resolution. These may be large or small, informal or formal, private or public. Whatever type of meeting is adopted, it is useful if discussions are held ahead of time to determine people's views and the types of arguments, beliefs, and reasons they will advance to support their view or to challenge others. This is analogous to discovery depositions used by lawyers in advance of a trial. One difference from legal depositions, however, is that the premeetings are excellent opportunities to lobby for one's cause.

Finally, if desired, the Delphi technique may be used. This approach is nicely summarized by Duffield (1989) and may be used to resolve many types of issues arising in medicine and science.

CHAPTER 93

Interpreting Placebo Data

TYPES AND USES OF PLACEBO

Placebo Medication or Treatment

The term *placebo* has been applied to many types of substances used in a variety of different ways. The most common definition refers to a material that does not contain any active medicine and is pharmacologically inert. Various materials may be used to make a placebo in the form of a tablet, capsule, or other dose form. This type of placebo has sometimes been called a "pure placebo." An "impure placebo" refers to any substance used as placebo that is not believed to be totally inert. For example, a homeopathic dose of an active medicine is an impure placebo. A list of various types of placebos is given in Table 93.1 and includes nonmedicine placebos and sham techniques.

Uses of Placebo

The major uses of a placebo medication in a clinical trial are (1) to serve as a control for psychological factors, (2) to maintain the double-blind design of the trial,

(3) to evaluate spontaneous variations in the disease, (4) to control the sensitivity of the measurements, and (5) for deception. This last practice cannot be condoned except in exceptional circumstances and when the patient's rights have been carefully considered by an Ethics Committee/Institutional Review Board (IRB).

Placebo Effect

Deception by Physicians

The effect observed after a placebo is given or used is referred to as the *placebo effect*. Placebos are sometimes given by physicians to their patients to simulate a therapeutic medicine and to evaluate the placebo effect. The physician's intention is to deceive the patient into believing that an active medicine is being given. Although the physician's purpose is often to differentiate between a "real" problem and an "imagined" or "functional" problem, this distinction is often not possible to make and may represent an artificial characterization (Goodwin et al., 1979).

TABLE 93.1 *Types of placebo treatments*

A. Medicine-like substance
  1. Active medicine given to a patient for its placebo effect in treating a different disease
      a. Knowingly (e.g., many cases of antibiotics given to patients for viral illnesses)
      b. Inadvertently (e.g., patient has been incorrectly diagnosed)
  2. Homeopathic dose of an active medicine given to a patient for a correctly diagnosed disease
  3. Blank medicine given as a control in a clinical trial[a]
  4. Blank medicine given to "treat" a patient in a medical practice outside of a clinical trial[a]
B. Nonmedicine placebo
  1. Care given patient by physician and the interaction between physician and patient
  2. Interactions between patient and nonphysician health personnel
  3. Additional care and attention given by physicians to patients in a clinical trial above that provided in the "usual" practice of medicine[b] (e.g., more frequent clinic visits, longer clinic visits, more careful patient evaluation, training, and personal discussions)[c]
C. Other techniques
  1. Sham surgical operations
  2. Sham procedures[d]

[a] Lactose-filled placebos may cause adverse reactions in some patients with lactase deficiency (Havard and Pearson, 1977). A blank medicine is one without an active ingredient to treat the condition for which the medicine is used. Ideally, and in most cases, it also does not have any ingredient that would be active in other conditions.
[b] This is related to the "Hawthorne effect," where increased efficiency was observed in factory workers as a result of the increased attention provided during a study.
[c] Wilhelmsen (1979) and Reiser and Warner (1985).
[d] See Chapter 85 for a listing of several sham procedures.

TABLE 93.2 *Factors that influence the placebo effect of the physician–patient interaction*

1. Attitude of the physician (or other health personnel) toward the patient. This refers to the degree and nature of a physician's interest, warmth, friendliness, liking, sympathy, empathy, neutrality, disinterest, rejection, and hostility[a]
2. Attitude of the physician (or other health personnel) toward the treatment. This refers to factors such as faith, belief, enthusiasm, conviction, commitment, optimism, positive and negative expectations, skepticism, disbelief, and pessimism[a]
3. Attitude of the physician (or other health personnel) toward the results. This refers to the introduction of observer bias that often affects the data, usually caused inadvertently by the physician (or other health personnel).[b] Factors include (1) the bandwagon effect, (2) nonverbal behavior and communication between investigator and patient, (3) expectations, (4) motivation, (5) prestige, (6) visual and verbal cues, (7) sex and personality characteristics of patient and investigator
4. Attitude of the patient toward the physician or other health personnel[c]
5. Attitude of the patient toward the treatment[c]
6. Attitude of the patient toward the results[c]

[a] Shapiro (1969).
[b] Examples of this effect are discussed by Shapiro (1969).
[c] These include the influence of outside individuals and events on the patient, which in turn affect the patient's attitude. The patient's attitudes are a reflection of fears, hopes, previous experiences, expectations, prejudices, ideas, and concepts.

In some hospitals, physicians sometimes give a small syringe full of saline to a patient complaining of pain as a test of the objectiveness of the pain. A positive response (i.e., benefit to the patient) is seen as evidence of the patient's either falsifying symptoms or having psychologically induced (i.e., functional) symptoms. If the patient has no response to the saline, it supposedly confirms the authenticity of the patient's pain. Apart from the arguments given above against this interpretation, the enthusiasm of a physician as well as other factors of the physician–patient relationship described in Table 93.2 often lead to a positive response in the patient.

Objective Changes Elicited by Placebo

Many authors have demonstrated objective physiological changes in patients given placebos. There appear to be few responses in conscious individuals that have not been observed to occur to some degree after a placebo is given. Beneficial effects caused by placebos have frequently been shown as changes in objective efficacy parameters relating to the disease, not just subjective feelings of improvement. Some of the objective parameters of efficacy that have responded to placebo include lowering of blood pressure in a double-blind clinical trial (Gould et al., 1981), relief of ulcer symptoms (Sturdevant et al., 1977), decreased exercise-induced bronchospasm in 40% of asthmatics, and a 50% reduction of the rapid eye movement phase of sleep (Vogel et al., 1980).

Adverse reactions caused by placebo have also been shown to be related to those caused by the active medicine. Schindel (1968) reviewed the literature and quoted references reporting the following adverse reactions (among others) attributed to placebo: (1) watery diarrhea, urticaria, and angioneurotic edema of the lips after a mephenesin placebo, (2) loss or impairment of hearing and eosinophilia after a streptomycin placebo, and (3) hallucinations, loss of vision, paresthesias, constipation, and stuffy nose after a reserpine placebo. Schindel (1968) has reported that the frequency of placebo-induced adverse reactions in the literature ranges from 1% to 61% and averages about 10% to 20%. Thus, both safety and efficacy responses to placebo often demonstrate objective changes of the type expected with an active medicine.

It is impossible to state that the 35% of patients who are believed to respond to placebo (Beecher, 1962) are not experiencing a genuine physical response. In a specific patient given an active medicine it is usually not possible to differentiate between that part of the response caused by the pharmacological properties of the medicine and that part of the response that would have occurred if the patient had only been given a placebo. Figure 71.2 illustrates that the overall clinical response observed is usually a combination of several factors.

Because the concept of placebo effect is so intertwined with both the patient's and physician's belief system, a full understanding of the nature and magnitude of the placebo effect requires at least some data on this topic. This information is not easily obtained.

An Ideal Clinical Trial in Which to Evaluate the Placebo Effect

One approach to obtaining a full understanding of the placebo effect is to obtain clinical data in a trial from four groups of patients:

1. Patients given a placebo who believe they received a placebo
2. Patients given a placebo who believe they received the active medicine
3. Patients given the active medicine who believe they received a placebo
4. Patients given the active medicine who believe they received the active medicine

This approach is only a hypothetical goal since it is not ethically acceptable to deceive patients in clinical trials unless there are special extenuating circumstances that are approved by an Ethics Committee/IRB (see Chapter 64).

Placebo Control Group and No-Treatment Control Group

A control group in a clinical trial that receives no treatment differs from a control group that receives a placebo medication. The no-treatment approach fails to account for the pill-giving ritual and any effects that this event may have on efficacy. Effects from taking placebos have often been shown to be greater than effects in a no-treatment group. The concept of the placebo control group is discussed in several chapters.

FACTORS AFFECTING THE PLACEBO RESPONSE

There is a placebo response relating to efficacy measures in a clinical trial and also a placebo response relating to safety measures. The most complex safety measures relating to the placebo effect concern adverse reactions. The number, intensity, nature, and other characteristics of adverse reactions are highly subject to wide variation and depend on many factors. A few of the more important factors to consider are listed in Table 93.3. These factors are based on char-

TABLE 93.3 *Selected factors to consider in interpreting placebo data on adverse events*

1. Determine who obtained the adverse event data. It is widely believed that the incidence of adverse events varies depending on whether a physician, nurse, or other individual obtains the data as well as on the manner in which the information is obtained[a]
2. Determine if a list of possible adverse events was read to the patient, or if a general probe was used, or if the patient spontaneously volunteered all information. There is general consensus that the incidence of adverse events is greater when a specific list of possible adverse events is read to patients than when patients respond to a general probe
3. Determine if the data were obtained from a clinical trial (Phase I to Phase IV) or from monitoring of usual clinical practice. It has been reported that the incidence of adverse events is greater during a clinical trial than in a routine monitoring of the usual practice of medicine (e.g., postmarketing surveillance)[b]

[a] It is not agreed, however, whether physicians usually obtain a larger or smaller number of adverse events than their staff.
[b] Rossi et al. (1984).

acteristics of the patient, the investigator, and the medicine.

Placebo responses relating to efficacy measures are also dependent on many factors. Those relating to the physician–patient relationship are summarized in Table 93.2. Many other factors that may affect placebo responses are identical or similar to those that affect responses to active medicine (see Chapter 83).

Personal Contact and Interaction with Physicians as a Basis of the Placebo Response

A study of 97 patients demonstrated that those assigned to intensive contact with anesthesiologists both pre- and postoperatively were prescribed about 50% less analgesics by surgeons who were unaware of the clinical trial than the group who only received routine pre- and postoperative procedures (Bourne, 1971). In addition, the patients who had more contact with physicians were sent home by the surgeons an average of 2.7 days earlier than their counterparts. It would be interesting and potentially important to evaluate this hypothesis in other clinical situations.

Effect of Color, Dosage Form, and Size of the Capsule on Patient Perception and Response to Placebo

There have been several clinical trials to evaluate associations of medicine color, form, and size with expectations of effect. Capsules are generally perceived as being stronger than tablets, larger capsules are perceived as stronger than smaller ones, and certain colors are associated with expectations of certain effects (Buckalew and Coffield, 1982a). A second trial by these authors demonstrated some marked differences in how different racial populations associate colors with anticipated clinical activity (Buckalew and Coffield, 1982b).

Although these clinical trials revealed interesting results that relate to a patient's race, they were inadequately controlled and cannot eliminate the possibility that environmental factors were responsible. It is the author's opinion that larger and better designed trials must be conducted if their conclusion is to be supported. Factors such as socioeconomic status, age, medicine experience, and environmental factors must be included to arrive at more definitive data. Even then, the results will probably vary from group to group within any country and will depend on numerous cultural factors. Any conclusions reached will also be likely to change as environmental, social, and other conditions change.

Color of the Placebo

Other investigators have conducted clinical trials in which the color of the placebo (and active medicine) was evaluated in actual clinical studies (as opposed to an experiment conducted in a clinical laboratory setting). Lucchelli et al. (1978) evaluated a standard hypnotic (hepabarbital) versus placebo in 96 hospitalized insomnia patients using two colors of each medication. They observed a significant interaction of color and sex of the patient. The same group of authors evaluated the sedative effects of different color placebos (no active medicine was given) and observed significant differences in the color preferences of each sex (Cattaneo et al., 1970). Schapira et al. (1970) performed a different type of experiment in which they gave patients oxazepam to treat anxiety. The medicine was prepared and dispensed in different colors (green, yellow, and red), and each color was used for 1 week in a Latin-square design. Patients and physicians were asked to rate the effectiveness of each "medicine." Color preferences were noted for treating anxiety with green medicine and for treating depressive symptoms with yellow medicine, but these differences did not reach statistical significance. Other studies have also confirmed the influence that color has on patient responses to placebo (Huskisson, 1974) or patient perceptions of their activity (Jacobs and Nordan, 1979).

EVALUATING THE MAGNITUDE OF THE "TRUE MEDICINE" RESPONSE

How is the True Medicine Effect Obtained?

The complexities of assessing a placebo response have never been adequately described, nor have all of the possible interactions been evaluated. It has conveniently been assumed in most clinical trials that medi-

cine-induced clinical effects and placebo-induced clinical effects are simply additive. This means that the response obtained by the placebo group (or during the placebo period) may be subtracted from the active medicine response to derive the "true" magnitude of the medicine response. This assumption has not been proven. Moreover, it defies common sense and clinical judgment for several reasons.

Efficacy: Are Placebo and Efficacy Responses Simply Additive?

The process of subtracting the placebo response from the total response to yield a "true" medicine effect has been questioned by Lindahl and Lindwall (1982). They provide a number of examples that demonstrate an interaction between the placebo and the "real" effect of a medicine. Some of the factors that may interact with placebo and thus may invalidate the assumption that the placebo and "real" effects are additive are (1) carryover of previous treatment, (2) continuation of other concomitant medicines, (3) continuation or initiation of nonmedicine modalities, (4) withdrawal effects of previous treatment, and (5) changes in magnitude of the placebo response over time.

Understanding Placebo Responses

If an investigator reports that placebo elicited a 50% response, this value must be qualified in several ways to indicate the following:

1. What is the variation among patients (i.e., did some patients have a 100% response and others a 0% response, or did most cluster around 50%)? A standard deviation, range of values, and confidence limits are all methods of illustrating the variability observed.
2. How did the placebo response change with time? At what point in the clinical trial did it develop, for how long a period during the trial did it persist, and did the effect wear off?
3. Did the changes in placebo response with time mirror the changes in efficacy noted with the trial medicine? What are the implications for the interpretation of the data and for data from other trials (as well as for designing future trials)?
4. Was the magnitude of the placebo response related to a factor of the trial (e.g., age or sex of patient, severity of disease)?

Ceiling Effect

One can consider circumstances in which a placebo gives an all-or-none effect. One example is in evaluating an analgesic, when pain relief may be graded as 100% with placebo. In this situation no additional activity is possible to elicit with the active medicine, and a "ceiling effect" has been reached.

Safety

Some specific adverse reactions are more closely associated with placebos than others. It was reported that of all symptoms, nausea and vomiting were most closely associated with placebo in a well-designed crossover trial of women receiving oral contraceptives (Goldzieher et al., 1971). All other symptoms reported with the oral contraceptives decreased markedly in occurrence when placebo was initiated. Nonetheless, there is a large background frequency of adverse reactions in the general population who are not receiving medicines. A survey of over 400 university students and hospital staff who were without illness and who had not taken any medicines within at least 3 days found that only 19% were symptom-free over the preceding 3 days. The median number of symptoms reported was two (from a predetermined list of 25 symptoms), and 30 people reported six or more symptoms (Reidenberg and Lowenthal, 1968). Similar results were reported by Spilker and Kessler, 1987).

The reasons why patients receiving placebos experience adverse events characteristic of the test medicine or the active control are several. The most common reason may be that the adverse reaction was listed in the informed consent. This could heighten patient awareness and anticipation of that particular reaction and somehow lead to its occurrence, or the belief that it occurred. A second reason may be that the adverse reaction is characteristic of an entire class of medicines and the patient had previously experienced the adverse reaction while on a related medicine. A third reason could be a *contact reaction* that the patient on placebo experienced in a waiting room (for an outpatient trial) or anywhere in a clinic or hospital (for an inpatient trial). A contact reaction occurs when close proximity to another patient experiencing an adverse reaction leads through the power of suggestion or psychological contact to the elicitation of reaction in another patient. Fourth, the patient on placebo may learn about the adverse event of trial patients on the active medicine in a clinic or elsewhere. Finally, the adverse event may be part of the disease itself.

PLACEBO RESPONSES THAT ARE LESS OR GREATER THAN EXPECTED

Placebo responses may be less than expected for many reasons, some of which are presented in Table 93.4. Reasons for this occurrence can be grouped into two

TABLE 93.4 *Possible interpretations of a placebo response that is less than expected*

1. Patients were extremely ill and less responsive to medicine therapy in general
2. Patients had a high frequency or number of nonresponders, and a placebo response was expected based on previous data
3. Disease/problem is not likely to improve substantially with treatment, and thus a larger placebo effect should not have been expected
4. Small response observed represents the lower end of normal variation
5. Trial blind was not effective, and patients knew they were receiving the placebo
6. Placebo medication was not identical to the trial medication, and patients knew they were receiving the placebo
7. Inadequate period was allowed in the trial for the placebo response to develop
8. Excessive period was allowed for the trial and the placebo response wore off
9. Patients in the placebo group were receiving concomitant medication that was partially effective, and patients had diminished ability to show any medicine (or placebo) effect
10. The placebo was always given after medicine in a crossover trial[a]
11. No placebo response should have been expected (e.g., a placebo effect is not believed to be present in comatose patients)

[a] See Cormia and Dougherty (1959) for data that support this conclusion.

basic categories. The first is that the actual placebo response was less than expected or was less than previously observed in other studies. The second category relates to spurious conclusions about the placebo response that were based on operational definitions, ambiguities in the study, or other reasons unrelated to the placebo effect itself. A few of the reasons from the second category relating to small placebo responses can be described in more detail.

Ceiling Effect

It is assumed that there is a sigmoid-shaped dose–response relationship for most measured medicine effects on efficacy. The plateau of this curve represents the maximal response (activity) possible. Response to placebo is measured in terms of the same efficacy parameter. As the placebo response increases toward 100% effect, there is a decrease in the ability of an active medicine to demonstrate its effect. It is assumed that it is easiest to demonstrate an effect of a medicine's activity either near the threshold or lower part of the dose–response relationship and that it becomes progressively more difficult to demonstrate positive activity as the plateau is approached. This is also referred to as the "ceiling effect," which indicates that the plateau of the dose–response curve represents a maximum or near-maximum level of activity above which it is (usually) not possible to go.

Placebo Responses That Are Greater Than Expected

If a placebo response occurs that is greater than expected, it is usually an unwelcome occurrence because of the increased difficulty in differentiating between active and placebo treatments. A number of reasons for this situation are presented in Table 93.5.

Do Placebo Effects Wear Off?

It is difficult and often impossible to evaluate the presence or magnitude of interactions between the placebo effect and true medicine effect in any one individual, let alone an entire group of patients. When an initially dramatic clinical effect wears off in time, it is possible to speculate that the residual effect is the true medicine effect, but there is little evidence to support this view. There is, however, evidence that demonstrates the development of tolerance to medicine effects, which is another possible interpretation when diminished efficacy is observed over time.

TABLE 93.5 *Possible interpretation of a placebo response that is greater than expected*

1. Most patients who were entered into the clinical trial had mild (or moderate) disease and were more sensitive to a placebo response
2. Patients entered the trial with severe disease, and as a result of the natural variations in the course of chronic disease (i.e., phenomenon of regression to the mean), the disease yielded an apparently large placebo effect
3. Expectations for a smaller placebo response were not justified
4. Patients were more responsive to treatment than previously studied groups and were at the upper end of the normal variation observed
5. The population studied was different from previously studied groups in an important manner (e.g., they were more susceptible to psychological suggestion)
6. The blind was better maintained than in previously conducted trials, and a more accurate placebo response was observed
7. The optimal time points for measuring placebo response were used, whereas previous trials had missed detecting the peak response and had observed a smaller placebo effect
8. Patients had been withdrawn from all treatment for a relatively long period and were especially sensitive to "treatment"
9. Patients in the placebo group were receiving concomitant medicines unbeknownst to investigator
10. Patients in the placebo group received active medicine as a result of a packaging error
11. Placebo was always given prior to medicine in a crossover study, and a greater response (relative to the medicine effect) was observed[a]
12. Environmental settings may influence the magnitude of the placebo effect

[a] See Cormia and Dougherty (1959) for a discussion on the order of medicine and placebo presentation and data that support this conclusion.

Interpretation When a Medicine Is Not Better Than Placebo

A failure to differentiate statistically between the effects of a trial medicine and placebo in a clinical trial may seem to indicate that the trial medicine is not clinically useful. This failure generally should not be viewed as positive evidence against the possibility that the trial medicine is active. Rather, the trial's outcome is not evidence in favor of the medicine being active. Such a perspective is especially applicable in clinical trials of psychoactive medicines. There are many logical and sound clinical and scientific reasons why a trial medicine may fail to demonstrate activity: (1) the dose studied was too low, (2) the trial was too short, (3) the patients were noncompliant, (4) the patients did not have the disease they were supposed to have, (5) the patients were nonresponders, and (6) the patients improved on both treatments, illustrating the phenomenon of regression to the mean. Thus, a study failing to demonstrate medicine activity for an explainable reason should not adversely affect the interpretation that a medicine is active, provided that the view is supported by findings in well-designed, well-controlled, and relevant clinical trials.

Possible Interpretations When Placebo Is Found to Be More Effective Than Active Medicine

A number of controlled trials have reported that patients receiving placebo responded better than patients receiving active medicine treatment. Results were statistically significant. What are the possible interpretations of these incidents? In some cases the data interpretation was simply that the patients on active medicine did less well than those on placebo and that the medicine should not be used in those patients. An example is idoxuridine for herpes simplex encephalitis (Boston Interhospital Virus Study Group, NIAID-sponsored cooperative antiviral clinical study, 1975). Other interpretations are listed in Table 93.6. In a clinical trial evaluating whether dexamethasone shortened

TABLE 93.6 *Possible interpretations if placebo responses are statistically significantly better than the active treatment*

1. The medicine and placebo supplies were reversed
2. The active medicine makes the disease worse
3. There is a difference between the two groups, either in baseline values or in inherent differences
4. There is confounding by other factors (e.g., surgery, prior treatment)
5. The sample size used was too small
6. The parameters measured were inappropriate
7. The clinical trial was conducted over too short a period
8. Adverse reactions influenced the results of treatment
9. Results occurred as a chance event

the duration of coma in patients with malaria, it was found that the effect of dexamethasone was significantly worse than that of placebo (Warrell et al., 1982). This finding should lead to cessation of that treatment in medical practice, since the trial was apparently well designed, conducted, and analyzed. This conclusion is not always warranted when a placebo is statistically better than active medicine treatment. In some situations a placebo may be better than active medicine in one trial but not in others using the same trial design (e.g., comparison of placebo and ketanserin in intermittent claudication; Bounameaux et al., 1985).

CHAPTER 94

Interpreting Data from Active Medicine Control Groups

TYPES OF ACTIVE MEDICINE CONTROL GROUPS

A number of types of active medicine control groups may be used in clinical trials. The strength of the interpretations drawn varies to a large degree and depends on the specific type of active medicine trial used. Within either the parallel or crossover category of trial design, the most common types of active medicine trials may be divided broadly into two groups. These categories may be used to describe clinical trials conducted in any clinical phase of development.

1. Two-arm trial. Comparison of (1) a test medicine with (2) an active medicine control in an open-label, single-blind, or double-blind manner
2. Three-arm trial. Comparison of (1) test medicine, (2) placebo, and (3) active medicine control in a single-blind or double-blind manner

Within parallel trials a fourth or additional arm is often used. This usually involves either a second or third dosing group, whose members receive the test medicine or a combination medicine. This type of trial is included in the discussion of a three-arm trial. The term *group* could be substituted for *arm* in this operational definition. Interestingly, some authors use the term *leg* instead of *arm*.

In general, there are more problems in interpreting data from two-arm than from three-arm clinical trials. In three-arm trials, especially when conducted in a double-blind manner, data from the active medicine group can be compared with placebo responses to confirm that the active medicine control yielded a positive response. This avoids one of the major problems associated with two-arm studies, i.e., the difficulty of demonstrating that either medicine was effective if they gave statistically indistinguishable results. This assumes that one is not evaluating a clinical problem in which the evidence of efficacy is absolutely incontrovertible, such as when a test medicine immediately brings patients out of a coma.

DOSE–RESPONSE RELATIONSHIPS

It is possible to develop variations of clinical trial designs for most active medicine trial comparisons that avoid the problem of not being able to demonstrate that the active medicine was actually effective. A good example is when a dose–response relationship of the trial medicine is determined and one dose of an active medicine control is evaluated. If the doses chosen for the dose response are able to elicit a wide range of efficacy responses (i.e., from a small response at low doses to a greater response at a higher dose), it would provide a framework against which the active medicine could be compared. Moreover, there would be relatively high assurance (if the clinical trial were well designed, performed, and analyzed) that the comparisons between active and test medicine were valid. It is also possible to perform dose–response evaluations for the active medicine instead of the test medicine or for both the active and study medicines. Although not strictly two-arm trials because of multiple treatment groups, these variations still utilize just two medicines to arrive at a potentially strong conclusion.

COMBINATION MEDICINES

Another example in which assurance of the validity of a clinical trial's interpretation could be achieved in evaluating an active medicine versus a trial medicine involves combination medicines. Each component of the combination could be tested separately in a parallel trial design. A crossover trial design, though rarer, could be used in certain diseases wherein each patient would receive during separate periods in the trial the test medicine as a combination, each of the entities that make up the combination, and the active medicine control (which could either be a single entity or combination medicine). In this situation it is assumed that either one or more than one of the separate medicines in the combination being tested would demonstrate less efficacy than the combination (or no efficacy). Thus, there would be a possibility of confirming that the active medicine possessed activity through comparison with the single entities and combination.

These alternatives (e.g., a third or fourth arm) would also address the concern that using an active medicine control (in the absence of placebo) does not provide adequate incentive to the investigator and sponsor to have the clinical trial succeed (i.e., show a difference between treatments). A statistically significant difference between at least two groups in the trial would be important to strengthen the conclusions reached. If the response to an active control is less than anticipated, a number of interpretations are possible (Table 94.1).

PROBLEMS WITH A TWO-ARM ACTIVE MEDICINE CONTROL TRIAL

Temple (1982) has pointed out three major categories of problems with the two-arm type of active medicine control (i.e., in the absence of a placebo treatment):

1. It is more difficult to prove statistically that two

TABLE 94.1 *Possible interpretations when the response to an active medicine control is smaller than expected*

1. Inadequate dose given
2. Inadequate compliance by patient
3. Medicine was not biologically active because of chemical decomposition (e.g., medicine was photosensitive, medicine sat on a heated radiator, medicine was left out of the refrigerator)
4. Medicine was not effective in population studied, possibly because it was distributed or metabolized or eliminated in an atypical manner, perhaps resulting from inclusion of an unusual patient population
5. Medicine was not adequately absorbed (e.g., resulting from interactions with food)
6. Patients were relatively nonresponsive (i.e., because of normal variation)
7. Patients had mild disease and did not have much of a therapeutic range in which to demonstrate improvement
8. The placebo response was much greater than expected (or usual), and the magnitude of the response caused by the active medicine control was thus proportionally less

results are the same than to prove that they are different. If both treatments yield the same effect, there is no test to establish that a statistically significant similarity exists. If the test medicine is statistically better than the active control (or vice versa) in a two-arm clinical trial, then this issue does not arise.

2. Since the investigator does not wish to observe a difference between treatments, there is no incentive to conduct the trial well. In fact, the more poorly it is conducted, the more likely the data will be the same with both medicines. Thus, poor technique represents an inadvertent means to obtain data that demonstrate that the test medicine is as efficacious as the standard medicine.

3. There is no accepted statistical means of demonstrating that either medicine worked if there is no statistically significant difference between them in the results obtained. If both medicines are approximately equal in the effect they elicit, it does not prove that either medicine is truly efficacious. Either both medicines were efficacious in the trial or neither was. Temple points out that in any particular study a standard medicine may be inactive even though it is generally well established to be an active medicine for treating patients. Many active medicines have been shown to be no better than placebo in at least some well-controlled clinical trials in analgesia and other areas.

Although Temple's third point is that both medicines were efficacious in the trial or neither was, the real situation is more complex, and many interpretations are possible (see Table 94.2 for selected examples).

TABLE 94.2 *Possible interpretations when the average clinical response is equal for a group of patients on study medicine and active control medicine[a]*

A. Both medicines are clinicaly effective[b]
   1. Each medicine was active in the same types of patients
   2. One medicine was highly active in a few patients, and the other medicine was less active in a larger number of patients
   3. One medicine was active in one type of patient, and the other medicine was active in different types of patients
   4. One medicine had a false-positive response and the other medicine was actually active
   5. Both medicines had false-positive responses
B. Neither medicine is clinically effective
   1. Clinical changes were nonspecific and resulted from a placebo-like effect
   2. One medicine caused a false-negative response, and the other medicine was actually ineffective
   3. Both medicines had false-negative responses
C. It is impossible to evaluate whether the medicines elicited a clinical response

[a] This table assumes that only a single dose of each medicine is tested and no placebo group is included.
[b] The conclusion of "effectiveness" depends on well-established historical data demonstrating activity of the active control medicine or clear clinical evidence of activity.

WHEN MAY TWO-ARM ACTIVE MEDICINE TRIALS BE CONDUCTED?

The author agrees with the validity of Temple's points in most cases. Nonetheless (as Temple agrees), two-arm active medicine control trials cannot be avoided in certain situations. For example, in patients with terminal cancer, severe bacterial infections, or numerous other severe conditions for which adequate therapy currently exists, it would not be ethically acceptable to test a new medicine against a placebo. Active controls are not the only solution to designing a trial in these situations, however, since a historical control group could be used, but active controls are often preferable. Likewise, in situations in which a test medicine is being evaluated for its value in long-term therapy in a chronic disease, it is often unethical to use a placebo medication. In these situations an active control has some value. Some of the techniques to overcome the limitations of two-arm trials were previously mentioned, and are also described at the end of Chapter 6.

Patient-Specific Differences

An additional issue that may arise in either two- or three-arm active medicine trials is that two medicines may yield equivalent overall effects, but the responses they cause in specific types of patients may differ enormously. This issue may be addressed by a subgroup analysis of the data. A variation of this issue is that if medicine X is statistically superior to medicine Y, there still may be a group of patients who will respond to medicine Y, and not to medicine X. This possibility should be considered, although it is not always straightforward to test for this. If a crossover trial design is used in a chronic disease, it should be possible to evaluate this possibility. A parallel design could also address this issue by evaluating subgroups of patients, although this approach is not as efficient as using a crossover trial when that design is suitable. This type of potential problem may be particularly prevalent in some clinical trials of psychotropic medicine. For example, the characteristics of groups of schizophrenic patients often vary widely between different trials, as do their responses to specific medicines (Chassan, 1979).

Choosing an Active Medicine to Use as a Control

Finally, the choice of an active control medicine may be based on many factors including (1) therapeutic category, (2) mechanism of action, (3) chemical class of the medicine, (4) regulatory considerations, (5) medical reputation of the medicine, (6) medical use of the medicine, and (7) marketing considerations.

Interactions Among Medicines

Medicines interact with numerous factors or substances both within and without the body. Outside the body medicines may interact with air, light, water, heat, and humidity in the environment or with part of the container in which the medicine is stored. These reactions often inactivate the medicine, although they sometimes lead to the formation of a more active (or toxic) metabolite(s). There are also physical interactions that occur when mixtures of two or more medicines are put in solution or when a single medicine is put in solution. These interactions may cause precipitation or otherwise inactivate or modify the medicine through physicochemical changes. Within the body innumerable types of interactions are possible. These include interactions both with other medicines (i.e., medicine–medicine interactions) and with nonmedicine factors (e.g., foods).

MEDICINE–MEDICINE INTERACTIONS

Classification of a Medicine's Interactions with Other Medicines

Classifications may potentially be based on (1) mechanism-of-action, (2) types of sequelae, (3) clinical significance of the outcome, (4) degree of assurance that the interaction is well established, or (5) other categories. The first approach (mechanism-of-action) is important in understanding the event, but the mechanisms of many interactions are unknown and others are speculative. The second approach is difficult to use because various sequelae could occur for even a single interaction, depending on many factors, not all of which are known. The third approach is reasonable, but the significance of many interactions is unknown. The fourth approach raises many questions because it is often uncertain that a real interaction has occurred, or if it did, that it will recur on a regular basis.

Assurance that an interaction has occurred can be described in three major categories: (1) definite association, (2) probable association, and (3) anecdotal reports. It is difficult without conducting one or more controlled clinical trials to demonstrate an association adequately.

The discussion above illustrates the difficulty of deriving an acceptable basis for classifying the types of interactions among medicines.

When Do Interactions Occur?

The term *medicine–medicine interaction* is usually applied to antagonistic or synergistic (potentiation) interactions between two medicines, and this is the major focus of this chapter. Interactions occur during various processes, including (1) absorption, (2) distribution, (3) transport (active or passive), (4) combining of a medicine with receptors, (5) eliciting a biochemical, pharmacological, or other effect, (6) conversion of the biochemical, pharmacological, or other effect to a clinical effect, (7) inactivation of the medicine through reuptake or other processes at or near the receptor site, (8) metabolism, and (9) elimination. Brodie and Feely (1988) divided interactions between medicines into those caused by the pharmacokinetics of the affected medicine and those influencing the pharmacodynamic response to it.

Results of Interactions

A medicine–medicine interaction may result in either synergistic (potentiated) effects or a diminution of response. The two medicines that interact may each have the same therapeutic effect and may be combined purposely or used together to take advantage of their interactions. Their mechanism of action may differ, and this factor may allow for a synergistic action (e.g., use of multiple hypotensive medicines). Several mechanisms that may lead to synergistic effects are listed in Table 95.1 and those that may lead to diminished effects are listed in Table 95.2. Some mechanisms (e.g., receptor blockade) may lead to either enhanced or diminished responses. Some medicine–medicine interactions do not affect responses.

Clinical Sequelae of Interactions

Medicine–medicine interactions may affect efficacy or safety. In terms of safety, adverse reactions are often the primary area of interest. Many factors are known that may influence adverse reactions resulting from medicine–medicine interactions. These factors relate primarily to the patient, medicines, or trial design, and a few are listed in Table 95.3.

Intended Interactions

The two medicines that interact may be combined purposely so that one medicine prevents or slows a process such as renal elimination or metabolism that would inactivate or eliminate the other medicine (e.g., penicillin and probenecid). In this situation only one of the two medicines produces a therapeutic effect, although the effect is enhanced by the presence of the other medicine. It is generally important to differentiate in the interpretation of data between those interactions that were a result of a purposeful step and those that occurred inadvertently.

Other Factors to Consider

The time between the administration of two (or more) medicines that interact is usually important in determining the magnitude and clinical significance of the response. Evaluating doses of the two medicines that interact is also essential to understanding the clinical significance (if any) of the purported interaction. Many hundreds or even thousands of medicine–medicine interactions have been reported, but the number that have been established as probably true is far smaller,

TABLE 95.1 *Mechanisms involved in medicine–medicine interactions that may lead to synergistic clinical activities*[a]

1. Displacement of one medicine by another from protein binding sites in plasma (e.g., salicylates may displace phenytoin, thus increasing the concentration of free phenytoin in plasma)
2. Inhibition by one medicine of an enzyme that normally metabolizes and inactivates the other (e.g., inhibition of an enzyme's synthesis or activity)
3. Competition of two medicines for the same enzyme (e.g., noncompetitive inhibition)
4. Modifying the pH of urine can increase or decrease excretion of certain medicines (e.g., aspirin and sodium bicarbonate)
5. One medicine may cause biochemical or pharmacological changes, leading to conditions that increase the effect of another medicine (e.g., hydrochlorothiazide leads to decreased potassium levels, which render patients receiving cardiac glycosides more liable to have a toxic reaction)
6. Medicines with similar biochemical, pharmacological, or physiological effects may produce synergistic clinical actions
7. A medicine may affect a pharmacological receptor so that another medicine's action is enhanced
8. A medicine may prevent reuptake of another medicine into a storage site (e.g., cocaine's potentiation of sympathomimetics)
9. A medicine may prevent metabolic inactivation of another medicine
10. A medicine may modify gastrointestinal absorption of another medicine

[a] Resulting effects may be beneficial or toxic.

TABLE 95.2 *Mechanisms involved in medicine–medicine interactions that may lead to a diminished therapeutic effect*[a]

1. Physicochemical inactivation prior to absorption (e.g., chelation of one medicine by another, adsorption of one medicine by another)
2. Modification of gastrointestinal absorption
3. Physicochemical inactivation subsequent to absorption (e.g., protamine sulfate reacts with heparin in the vasculature)
4. Microsomal enzyme formation may be induced in the liver by one medicine. The liver then more rapidly metabolizes and inactivates another medicine
5. Specific or nonspecific receptor antagonism by one medicine may prevent or diminish the action of a second medicine. The receptor antagonist may elicit an opposite effect, no effect, or may be a partial agonist[b]
6. Alterations in urine pH may increase the excretion of certain medicines or may lead to crystalluria (e.g., methenamine plus sulfonamides)
7. Displacement of one medicine by another from plasma proteins. The displaced medicine is then more rapidly distributed to tissues, metabolized, or excreted
8. Direct physical action of one medicine on another (e.g., a topical medicine that prevents a second medicine from penetrating the skin)
9. Direct chemical action of two medicines (e.g., mixture of two medicines in a syringe or infusion apparatus)

[a] Resulting effect(s) may be beneficial or toxic.
[b] Numerous types of receptor antagonism may occur (e.g., competitive or noncompetitive, reversible or irreversible).

TABLE 95.3 *Selected factors that may influence adverse reactions resulting from medicine–medicine interactions*

A. Factors relating to the medicines
1. Dose of each medicine. Larger doses are more likely to cause adverse reactions
2. Dosage form (e.g., sustained-release forms usually yield lower peak plasma concentrations than immediate-release forms of a medicine and may be less likely to interact with other medicines)

B. Factors relating to trial design
1. Route of administration. This parameter can best be evaluated in the context of each medicine's mechanism of action
2. Time of administration. Interactions relating to medicine absorption are more likely to occur when the time between administration of the two medicines is reduced
3. Order of administration. This may be important to consider depending on the mechanism of the interaction

C. Factors relating to the patient's physiological function
1. Renal function often has a major role in affecting the occurrence and magnitude of medicine–medicine interactions via effects on the excretion of medicines
2. Hepatic function insofar as metabolic capacity and capabilities are concerned may influence adverse reactions

D. Factors relating to the patient's inherent and acquired characteristics
1. Genetic history
2. Disease state(s)
3. Age
4. Diet
5. Smoking

and the number with clinical significance is smaller still.

NONMEDICINE INTERACTIONS

A few of the nonmedicine interactions with medicines that may occur outside the body were indicated in the introduction (e.g., decomposition as a result of air, water, or other environmental factors). Within the body, nonmedicine interactions include effects on medicines resulting from (1) the pH of fluids the medicine encounters, (2) food that is ingested, (3) cigarette smoke, and (4) various other factors.

Another area that might be considered as a medicine interaction is the effect of a medicine on diagnostic laboratory tests. Alterations in laboratory test results may occur either as a result of the medicine affecting the patient or from interactions resulting from interference by the medicine with a step in the analytical laboratory test procedure.

In interpreting data it is often difficult to identify each of the unanticipated interactions that may have occurred in a clinical trial. An index of suspicion to consider interactions when unanticipated events occur will help uncover these events.

CHAPTER 96

False-Positive and False-Negative Results

This chapter discusses definitions and general concepts of false-positive and -negative responses as well as methods to probe for why they are there and why they occur. Related concepts of rates, specificity, and sensitivity are also described. False-positive and -negative results occur with diagnostic tests (e.g., laboratory measurements) and with efficacy tests used to evaluate medicines. Occasionally, the results of an entire clinical trial may be reported as yielding data that are either falsely negative or positive.

RATES

Rates are used to present both safety and efficacy data and are determined on a response-per-unit basis. Thus, both a numerator and denominator are required. The numerator is usually the number of times an event occurred or the number of patients who are affected by or otherwise involved in a particular issue. The denominator could be presented in terms of patients, problems, physicians, or medical practices. Patient populations can be viewed in terms of a single clinical trial, group of trials, all trials on a medicine, or in terms of a patient characteristic or characteristics. Within a single trial the denominator may refer to patients who (1) are potentially available to enter the trial, (2) are considered for entry, (3) complete screens successfully and are eligible, (4) sign an informed consent, (5) enter the baseline, (6) enter the treatment period, (7) complete treatment, (8) are analyzed, or (9) have completed adequate follow-up.

A detailed discussion of incidence and prevalence is given in other chapters.

SENSITIVITY AND SPECIFICITY

The Ideal World

In measuring a medicine's efficacy or safety many different types of tests are used. The ideal test would have a 1:1 correlation in accuracy with the desired results. There would be no positive results obtained that were truly negative (false-positive response) and no negative results obtained that were truly positive (false-negative response).

Statistical and Clinical Definitions

Since the ideal situation is not observed, it is important to know what the rate is of false-positive and of false-negative results. This information allows one to determine how much reliance should be placed on results from a particular test. A statistical definition of sensitivity of a test is the true positive rate. A clinical definition is that sensitivity relates to how finely detailed data may be and still be recognized as positive, i.e., if one test can discern responses of 1 cm and another test can discern responses of 1 mm, the latter test is much more sensitive than the former. Definitions are shown in Table 96.1.

The true negative response is known in statistics as the specificity of a test. Clinically, specificity relates to how well the test can differentiate between the test medicine and other medicines. If one test can distinguish among five separate medicines and identify only the test medicine as positive and note the others as negative, then it has a higher degree of specificity than

TABLE 96.1 *Definitions of various terms relating to false positives and false negatives*

Sensitivity	= Probability of correctly classifying a diseased patient as diseased
Sensitivity (%)	= $\dfrac{\text{number of diseased persons with a positive test}}{\text{total number of diseased persons tested}} \times 100$
Specificity	= Probability of correctly classifying a nondiseased patient as nondiseased
Specificity (%)	= $\dfrac{\text{number of nondiseased persons with a negative test}}{\text{total number of all nondiseased persons tested}} \times 100$
False-positive rate	= Probability of incorrectly classifying a nondiseased patient as diseased
False positives	= $\dfrac{\text{number of false positives}}{\text{total number of all nondiseased persons treated}}$
False positives[a]	= 1 − specificity
False-negative rate	= Probability of incorrectly classifying a diseased patient as nondiseased
False negatives	= $\dfrac{\text{number of false negatives}}{\text{total number of all diseased persons tested}}$
False negatives[a]	= 1 − sensitivity

[a] Assume that all diseased patients are classified either correctly or incorrectly. The probability of being correct in the diagnosis plus the probability of being incorrect = 1.0. The probability of being correct in the classification of diseased patients = sensitivity. Therefore the probability of being incorrect (i.e., a false negative) = 1 minus the sensitivity. A similar description can be used to illustrate that the false positives = 1 minus the specificity.

a test that cannot distinguish among any of the five medicines. One means of categorizing positive and negative results is shown in Table 96.2.

There are numerous publications that evaluate the sensitivity and specificity of (1) a particular test performed by different methods (e.g., see Steinberg et al., 1985), (2) groups of clinical trials using different types of controls (e.g., see Sacks et al., 1983), and (3) reports of diagnostic tests (e.g., Sheps and Schechter, 1984).

TYPES OF FALSE-POSITIVE AND FALSE-NEGATIVE RESULTS

False-positive or false-negative results generally fit one of three types. The occurrence of a false result may be (1) known, (2) unknown, or (3) suspected. If it is unknown, then this brief chapter will not provide definitive or even likely means to reveal this fact. If the problem is suspected, one immediate goal will be to determine whether the suspicions are correct or not.

If the problem is known to exist, then further steps toward uncovering the reason(s) for its existence should be undertaken.

The suspicion of a false-negative (or -positive) result is extremely common during some parts of many clinical trials. Steps that may be followed to evaluate this possibility are outlined in Table 96.3. Some of the reasons for false-positive results occurring in a trial are listed in Table 96.4, and reasons for false-negative results are listed in Table 96.5. These tables list only a small portion of the reasons that may affect data obtained in a trial in either a positive or negative direc-

TABLE 96.2 *Categorization of positive and negative results*

Test results	True state	
	Disease is present	Disease is absent
Positive	True positive	False positive
Negative	False negative	True negative

TABLE 96.3 *Possible actions and considerations if a false-positive or false-negative result is suspected*

1. Identify the suspected factor(s)
2. If the identity of the suspected factor(s) is not totally clear, discuss with colleagues which methods could be used to identify and evaluate possible factors
3. After suspected causes are identified, list and evaluate possible reasons why those causes could have led to false-positive or -negative results
4. Discuss the suspicion with a statistician
5. Conduct appropriate reanalyses of data
6. Develop algorithms or a decision tree that may be tested
7. Evaluate relevant articles in the medical literature
8. Determine if any additional laboratory, efficacy, or other tests on some (or all) of the patients in the clinical trial could resolve the issue
9. Determine if a protocol modification for ongoing or future trials could resolve (or address) the issue
10. Discuss the suspicion with colleagues, peers, and consultants

TABLE 96.4 *Selected reasons for false-positive data*[a]

A. Patient related
1. Patients were not as ill as the investigator believed, and the medicine was more effective in mildly ill patients than in moderately or severely ill patients
2. Patients were much more ill than the investigator believed, and the medicine was more effective in severely ill patients than in mildly or moderately ill patients
3. A number of patients had unsuspected renal or liver disease, which prevented rapid metabolism and/or elimination. Blood levels were maintained at a therapeutic level for a longer period than in patients who had normal renal and liver function
4. Too few patients were evaluated, and activity was noted by chance
5. A few patients had a large response, which skewed the overall data
6. Patients tend to enroll in clinical trials when they are most severely ill and often gradually improve independent of any therapeutic interventions. This illustrates the phenomenon of regression toward the mean and when not controlled gives an impression of a beneficial effect
7. Patients are sometimes more easily recruited for a clinical trial when they have a high risk of developing a disease that is not the primary focus of the trial but is being evaluated. This yields a falsely elevated incidence value for the disease[b]
8. More medicine was absorbed than anticipated or would normally occur (e.g., because of the presence of food, which delayed gastric emptying)
9. Patients were not compliant with the trial protocol and took an excessive amount of trial medicine or concomitant medicines
10. Patients may feel a strong allegiance to the investigator or feel stong pressure to demonstrate a positive medicine effect
11. Patients received concomitant nonmedicine treatment modalities, which were responsible for improvement noted (e.g., bed rest in patients with lower back pain)
B. Trial design and medicine related
1. The blind used in the trial was broken or was ineffective, and the physician or patients inadvertently biased the results in favor of the test medicine
2. In an open-label trial a larger response occurred than was anticipated, but there was no placebo control group to interpret properly the magnitude of the apparent placebo response
3. The medicine decomposed to a more active metabolic product
4. An error occurred in dosing patients, who received a greater dose than intended
5. Inadequate washout period was used, and patient's previous treatment had a carryover effect
6. Inappropriate clinical endpoints, tests, or parameters were used
C. Investigator and staff related
1. The investigator and staff demonstrated great enthusiasm and stimulated the expectations of the patients
2. The investigator and staff used an aggressive therapeutic approach
D. Results and data related
1. The data illustrated "clumping," where a preponderance of events occurred in a nonrandom manner
2. A high percentage of nonresponders and partial responders dropped out of the trial, leaving a relative preponderance of responders
3. Data analysis did not appropriately account for all patient dropouts
4. Only a portion of the baseline or treatment period data were analyzed

[a] Data demonstrated a statistically significant effect of the medicine, whereas more convincing data obtained subsequently or prior to the trial clearly demonstrated inactivity. Most factors listed in Chapter 83 may be responsible for false-positive data.
[b] Lavori et al. (1983) reported this effect in a 15-year follow-up trial of patients who were evaluated for developing breast cancer, even though that was not the primary objective of the trial.

TABLE 96.5 *Selected reasons for false-negative data*[a]

A. Patient related
1. Patients were either much less or much more ill than the investigator believed and did not respond to the medicine as would patients with severity of disease intended as the trial group
2. The patient group included a relatively large number of nonresponders
3. The patients had unsuspected renal or hepatic problems, which caused rapid excretion or inactivation of the trial medicine
4. The patients were not compliant with the trial design and did not take their doses as directed
5. Patients took concomitant medicines that interacted with the test medicine and prevented full expression of its activity
6. Patients were persistently exposed to conditions that prevented improvement (e.g., bacteria or protozoa that continually reinfected the patients)
B. Medicine related
1. The medicine had lost its potency through (1) lack of chemical stability, (2) improper storage, (3) improper preparation, (4) exposure to light, or (5) for other reasons
2. The medicine was not adequately absorbed
3. The medicine's metabolism was different in the study population than in other patient groups
C. Trial design related
1. Too few patients were entered to demonstrate a medicine effect (i.e., there was a lack of power)
2. An inappropriate trial design was chosen (e.g., efficacy was measured at the wrong time, in the wrong manner, with the wrong equipment)
3. An insufficient dose of the medicine was tested
4. Efficacy tests or parameters were used that were unable to demonstrate a medicine effect
5. Inadequate washout period was used, and previous treatment interacted with the trial medicine, preventing full expression of efficacy to be observed
6. Concomitant nonmedicine therapy interfered with full expression of the trial medicine's efficacy
D. Investigator related
1. The investigators may have used a too conservative approach to patient treatment or to the data (e.g., data analysis, clinical interpretation)
2. Patients were given the wrong medicine or wrong size tablet or insufficient quantity of medicine, or the label on the medicine container was incorrectly printed
E. Results and data related
1. Patients who improved dropped out of the trial, and a higher percentage of nonresponders remained
2. Data analysis did not appropriately account for all patient dropouts

[a] Data did not demonstrate a clinical effect that was shown in previous or subsequent trials. Most factors listed in Chapter 83 may be responsible for false-negative data.

tion. It is important to evaluate as many factors as possible in attempting to determine which ones were responsible.

If the presence of false-negative or -positive results is detected, then different mechanisms should be utilized to discern the reason(s) for their existence. Once the causes are discovered and dealt with, then the factors can be eliminated and the data reanalyzed. In a worst-case scenario, the clinical trial may have to be repeated utilizing an improved methodology that eliminates or minimizes the likelihood of obtaining a false-negative or -positive result.

CHAPTER 97

Interpreting Quality of Life Data

MEASURES OF QUALITY OF LIFE

Since the primary goal in treating most patients with chronic disease is to improve their function and quality of life, it is important to measure and interpret this concept. The difficulties of interpreting subjective quality of life data are generally much more complex than those involved in interpreting more objective data. There are many controversies in this area, and identifying a few will indicate the types of difficulties and complexities encountered. A number of factors that may be measured with quality of life scales are listed in Table 97.1.

Is It Important to Measure Quality of Life?

An important controversy in the past was whether or not it is worthwhile to measure quality of life. Proponents stress that it is the major goal of health care and that placing attention on a patient's functional outcome is important. Opponents used to stress the scientific value of objective tests and treatments for obtaining new data on major (and minor) diseases and the rigorous (and objective) scientific approaches that led to these medical advances. Another argument concerned the vagueness and difficulty of assessing and interpreting quality of life measures. The importance of quality of life assessments is now generally accepted.

Definition

Another controversy is how the term *quality of life* is defined. There is no universally accepted definition of this term. A definition should include consideration of physical, psychological, economic, and social well-being plus a measure of a patient's ability to perform daily activities. See Chapter 52 and Spilker (1990a).

Quality versus Quantity of Life

The balance between the value of therapeutic measures that increase a patient's life by a short period at the expense of its quality is becoming more widely debated both within and without the medical profession, especially in terms of terminally ill patients who sometimes choose not to be treated or who choose hospice care. More patients and physicians are stating that it is essential to consider life's quality in addition to its duration when a therapeutic regimen is established.

Spectrum of Measuring Instruments

A patient's quality of life and its change as a result of treatment may be evaluated with subjective parameters (e.g., how a patient feels) or with objective parameters (e.g., the number of days worked per year or per month). Some authors and tests focus on objective criteria to define and measure quality of life, whereas others stress the measurement of subjective aspects of this concept. Using both approaches is best.

Choosing Tests and Scales

There are many different tests and scales used to measure the quality of life. Although some are better validated than others, it is generally difficult to compare data obtained with different scales. Numerous scales are described in *Quality of Life Assessments in Clinical Trials* (Spilker, 1990a), plus the *Bibliography on Health Indexes* (U.S. Dept. of Health and Human Services, Public Health Service, 1983). This bibliography was issued several times. See also Spilker et al. (1990).

It is possible to measure the patients' ability to function in their daily activities in terms of either their actual behavior or their potential ability. Many types of problems may act as variables to confound the data. These problems may arise from many of the factors described in Chapter 83 (e.g., social environment, physical environment, genetic inheritance).

Parameter measures may be weighted or unweighted. The use of *unweighted parameters* means that each parameter is considered to be equal. *Weighting* means that the parameters are not considered equal, making it desirable (or necessary) to create an imbalance in their relative importance to make their combination together more fair or correct. For example, assume there are three measures (A, B, C); A is twice as important as B and a third (C) is only one-half as important as B. The weighting of the values prior to combining them means that A is 4 times C, B

TABLE 97.1 *Factors that may be measured or assessed with quality of life scales*

A. Function in daily life
 1. Ability to bathe, dress, and feed oneself
 2. Ability to control physiological functions (e.g., urine, bowel movements)
 3. Ability to ambulate and move in and out of furniture and/or cars
 4. Ability to achieve satisfactory sleep and rest
B. Productivity and economic status
 1. Ability to work productively at the patient's desired (or other) vocation
 2. Ability to support oneself, family, and/or others at a satisfactory standard of living
C. Performance of social role
 1. With relatives, friends, and others
 2. Family relationships
 3. Community relationships
 4. Recreation and pastimes
D. Intellectual capabilities
 1. Memory
 2. Ability to communicate
 3. Ability to make decisions
 4. Overall ability to think, act, and react
E. Emotional stability
 1. Mood stability and swings
 2. Beliefs about the future
 3. Emotional levels
 4. Religious and philosophical beliefs
F. Assessment of satisfaction with life
 1. Level of well-being
 2. Perception of general health
 3. Outlook for the future
G. Signs and symptoms of illness
 1. Nature of problems
 2. Severity of problems
 3. Duration and frequency of problems
 4. Amount of treatment required
 5. Adverse reactions

TABLE 97.2 *Potential methods and approaches to combining data from three or more separate tests*[a]

1. Present raw data for all patients and sum all scores so that the contribution of each test depends on the potential range of that test plus actual score achieved.
2. Transform raw data for all patients to a scale of 1 to 100 for each test and then sum all scores so that each test contributes one-third of the total.
3. Weight the results of each test by a numerical factor that is based on its importance in the overall total score achieved or on another basis described in a footnote (or in the text).
4. Instead of transforming or weighting individual patient scores, conduct these statistical tests on the overall scores for each treatment group.
5. Use other methods to transform data (e.g., see Chapter 81) before combining them.

[a] It is assumed that all tests were conducted in a single clinical trial and that the possible range of raw scores that could be achieved differs among the tests.

is 2 times C, and C is unity. Another way to view it is that 7 Cs in value (4 plus 2 plus 1) equal 100%, and of the total, A is 57%, B is 29%, and C is 14%. Methods for combining and presenting data from multiple tests are given in Table 97.2 and Fig. 97.1. Zimmerman (1983) reported that there was a high correlation (0.94) between weighted and nonweighted totals across 18 studies that evaluated the stress–illness relationship. Of course, other weighting procedures would generate different results and may be useful in other types of quality of life scales.

Relevance for National Policy

The rapidly escalating cost of national health care services is one reason why greater attention is directed toward quality of life measures. Evaluation of expensive medical therapies and procedures sometimes requires that an assessment of quality of life be made. This assessment is often conducted as part of an economic analysis of the costs and benefits of such procedures to the whole society as well as to the individual patient. For example, an evaluation of quality of life in patients with end-stage renal disease was reported (Evans et al., 1985).

The personality of the patient evaluated, his or her disease severity, and prognosis will each affect quality of life scores obtained. Demographic characteristics may also be important. If these factors are not controlled or evaluated, then data obtained with any test may prove to be difficult to interpret.

Relevance of Disease and Personality Types

Popular beliefs relating to the psychosocial aspects of disease and coping mechanisms are beginning to be analyzed more systematically than in the past. The hypothesis that the psychological status of chronically ill patients does not differ according to specific diagnoses was tested by Cassileth et al. (1984) in patients with

QOL PARAMETER [+]	CAPOTEN (N = 181)	METHYLDOPA (N = 143)	PROPRANOLOL (N = 162)
General well-being	○	◍	◍
Physical symptoms	◍	●	●
Sexual function	◍	●	●
Work performance	○	●	◍
Sleep dysfunction	◍	◍	◍
Cognitive function	○	○	○
Life satisfaction	◍	●	●
Social participation	◍	◍	○

FIG. 97.1 A revised form of the data from Croog et al. (1986) illustrating comparative quality of life (QOL) data for three medicines in eight categories. *White circle,* improved; *gray circle,* stable; *black circle,* worsened.

arthritis, depression, diabetes, cancer, renal disease, and nonmelanomatous dermatologic disorders. Their data supported this hypothesis. They observed that patients with recently diagnosed disease (in all groups) had poorer scores of mental health than did those patients who had had their diagnosis made at least 4 (or more) months previously. These results challenge the once popular view that individuals with certain specific personality types or emotional traits are more at risk of becoming ill with a particular disease or problem. Older patients (above 60) had better mental health scores than did those in the 40- to 60-year range, whose scores in turn were better than those who were still younger (below 40).

Quality of life measures in some illnesses may need to be tailored to the disease/illness measured. Although Cassileth et al. (1984) reported similarities in responses of six groups of patients with different chronic diseases, specific aspects of each disease may be relevant. A number of articles have evaluated the quality of life as it relates to cardiovascular disease (Wenger et al., 1984), oncology (Edelstyn et al., 1979; Sugarbaker et al., 1982), renal disease (Evans et al., 1985), and lung disease (McSweeny et al., 1982). These papers and those in Spilker (1990a) point out the wide variety of ways in which this subject is currently interpreted.

Reference Time of the Measurement

Measurements of the patient's quality of life may be made in reference to the precise moment the test is being completed. In addition to or in lieu of this time

frame, it is possible to measure the previous day, week, or some other time period. Another approach is to compare the present instant, day, or week to the pretrial baseline. A third approach is to measure both the present time and the best previous point during the trial (or the previous week, month, or other time). If the quality of life is determined for a cancer patient, it may be debated whether the measurements should be made at the time of treatment, a few weeks later, during remission, or at a different time or times.

When Should Quality of Life Be Measured?

It is generally not necessary to measure and evaluate the quality of life when a medicine is life saving or has a much higher benefit-to-risk ratio than other medicines for the same disease. The question of quality of life measurements becomes important when a treatment or medicine (1) has a small or moderate benefit-to-risk ratio, (2) is only partially curative, (3) is extremely expensive, or (4) relieves disease symptoms but elicits moderate or severe adverse reactions. The field that is concerned with these issues is growing rapidly, and attempts to validate various tests and measures will continue.

CRITERIA TO EVALUATE QUALITY OF LIFE TESTS

Six criteria were described by Deyo (1984) to evaluate tests used to measure quality of life. These should be considered by investigators and sponsors who must choose tests to include in clinical trials.

1. Applicability to the purpose and group being tested
2. Practicality in terms of effort and cost to conduct the tests
3. Comprehensiveness of the questions posed as related to each important area
4. Reliability of the test in terms of its reproducibility from time to time
5. Validity of the test. There are various types of validity and means of establishing this. Deyo (1984) describes some of these issues
6. Sensitivity of the test to detect important changes or differences in magnitude

QUALITY OF LIFE ASSESSMENTS IN CLINICAL TRIALS

The discussion above touches briefly on a few issues relating to the interpretation of quality of life data. Sixty authors recently contributed to a book entitled *Quality of Life Assessments in Clinical Trials* (Spilker, 1990a), which presents a detailed discussion on these and other topics. The book is organized into five sections: (1) introduction to the field (chapters discuss concepts, choosing approaches, validating models); (2) standard scales, tests, and approaches to quality of life assessments (individual chapters discuss the various domains—economics, social interactions, psychological well-being, and physical function); (3) special perspectives (e.g., ethics, culture, marketing, industry, regulatory); (4) special populations (e.g., pediatrics, geriatrics, substance abuse, rehabilitation, chronic pain, cardiovascular surgery, gastrointestinal surgery); and (5) specific disease (e.g., cardiovascular, neurologic, psychiatric, inflammatory bowel, renal replacement, pulmonary disease, cancer, and chronic rheumatic disease).

PRESENTING RESULTS

The results of a complex quality of life test that has several parts may be expressed with a single number, whereas a more simple test with multiple parts may yield multiple numbers (i.e., one for each part). Batteries of tests invariably lead to multiple numbers/results that cannot be combined. The major approaches to use when comparing medicines with multiple tests are to (1) create a hierarchy of test importance prior to a comparative trial, (2) express summaries of all data (e.g., medicine A had a higher score in 4 of 6 tests), or (3) merely list results obtained in each test. In the first case, an indication should be given of how much of a change in the major test(s) would be considered clinically significant, in addition to stating which test(s) is most important. In the second case, sufficient data would have to be presented so that readers could determine if they agreed with the implicit interpretation suggested by stating that 4 of 6 tests showed medicine A to be superior. The data in Fig. 97.1 lend themselves to this type of presentation. Merely listing results of each test enables readers to make their own comparisons and interpretations and to reach their own conclusions. The first method is the best approach because it minimizes bias while indicating which test(s) is deemed most important. The question of which medicine leads to a better quality of life depends on its attributes, the specific patients studied, and the test(s) chosen to use in a clinical trial. Numerous presentations of data on quality of life are given by Spilker and Schoenfelder (1990).

CHAPTER 98

Responders and Nonresponders

DEFINITIONS AND BACKGROUND

The operational definitions of a responder and a non-responder are often arbitrary in many diseases, especially chronic diseases for which a complete cure is not expected. A *nonresponder* may be operationally defined as a patient who has not responded sufficiently (or adequately) to treatment whether the treatment was a study medicine, active medicine, placebo, no treatment, or a specific previous treatment. Criteria may be established to define a positive response more specifically. This may include reference to the duration of response. In some areas of medicine (e.g., oncology), the term *partial responder* (i.e., incomplete responder) is often used in addition to the other two terms. This may help clarify the definitions in some situations, since responses of chronic diseases are rarely all or none.

An investigator may be asked to rate a patient as being either a responder or nonresponder, and to record that rating on the data collection forms. The sponsor may overrule the investigator's decision if the sponsor's action is based on objective criteria that it established or decided to use prior to initiating the clinical trial.

In certain clinical situations (e.g., many acute problems), responses occur in an all-or-none manner. All patients who have received treatment in this type of clinical situation may be classified as being either responders or nonresponders.

Partial Responders

The definition of *partial response* in oncology is usually based on either improvement in nonmeasurable lesions for at least 1 month or a 50% decrease in *size* of measurable lesions. Measurable refers to a direct physical measurement of a patient's lesion(s).

Unfortunately, there is a wide disparity in how this definition is applied. In some clinical trials size refers to volume, and a 50% decrease is reflected by a 21% reduction in a linear dimension. In other clinical trials size refers to area, and a 50% decrease is reflected by a 29% reduction in a linear dimension. Moreover, some investigators apply the definition to each measurable lesion and others apply it to the sum of all lesions.

REASONS FOR NONRESPONSE

The nonresponder's lack of response may have resulted from a high degree of refractoriness that was present prior to the clinical trial, although this may only be known in hindsight. In refractory patients, it is sometimes concluded that virtually no treatment with the characteristics of the trial medicine could have elicited a positive response. On the other hand, patients entered in a trial may have been able to respond to therapy with the characteristics of the trial medicine but for some reason(s) did not. It is not always possible to determine which category of nonresponse a specific patient fits. In some cases a high degree of refractoriness may be predictable based on a patient's clinical history. The main method to eliminate such patients from a trial is through carefully developed inclusion criteria. It is, however, generally impossible to eliminate all nonresponders of the first type (those who will not respond to any treatment) prior to the trial.

When results of a clinical trial are negative or are

TABLE 98.1 *Selected reasons for a patient being classified as a nonresponder*[a]

A. Patient is noncompliant because of dissatisfaction related to
1. Time taken away from job to attend clinic
2. Cost of meals and transportation to get to clinic
3. Excessive demands of the clinical trial in terms of time, effort, or other factors
4. Lack of dramatic clinical benefit
5. Lack of rapid onset of clinical benefit
B. Problems related to trial medicine or protocol
1. Dose of medicine is inadequate
2. Duration of treatment is inadequate
3. Medicine composition has deteriorated as a result of storage, handling, or method of preparation
4. Definition of response is narrow
5. Measurements of response are taken at inappropriate times
6. Inadequate or unclear directions are given to patients, many of whom then take the medicine improperly
C. Patient characteristics or responses
1. Patient develops tolerance to the medicine's effect
2. Patient eats a diet containing food that inactivates the medicine
3. Blood levels are inadequate (e.g., variable absorption between patients)
4. Patient stores the medicine improperly

[a] The reasons given for a false-negative result (Table 96.5) include reasons why a patient may be classified as a nonresponder. Also see Chapter 15.

less significant than anticipated, it may be that an excess number of nonresponders were entered. A number of reasons why a patient may be classified as a nonresponder are listed in Table 98.1 and Fig. 98.1.

Ceiling Effect

When the difference in response is small between placebo and treated groups, more patients in the treated group will be considered as nonresponders than when the difference between the groups is great. If patients receiving placebo have a much larger response than expected, the number of patients receiving active medicine who will be defined as nonresponders may be increased artificially. One reason is that there is often a maximum response possible ("ceiling effect"), and this limit is being approached by patients in the placebo group, allowing less potential for medicine recipients to demonstrate a greater effect. This concept is discussed further in other chapters.

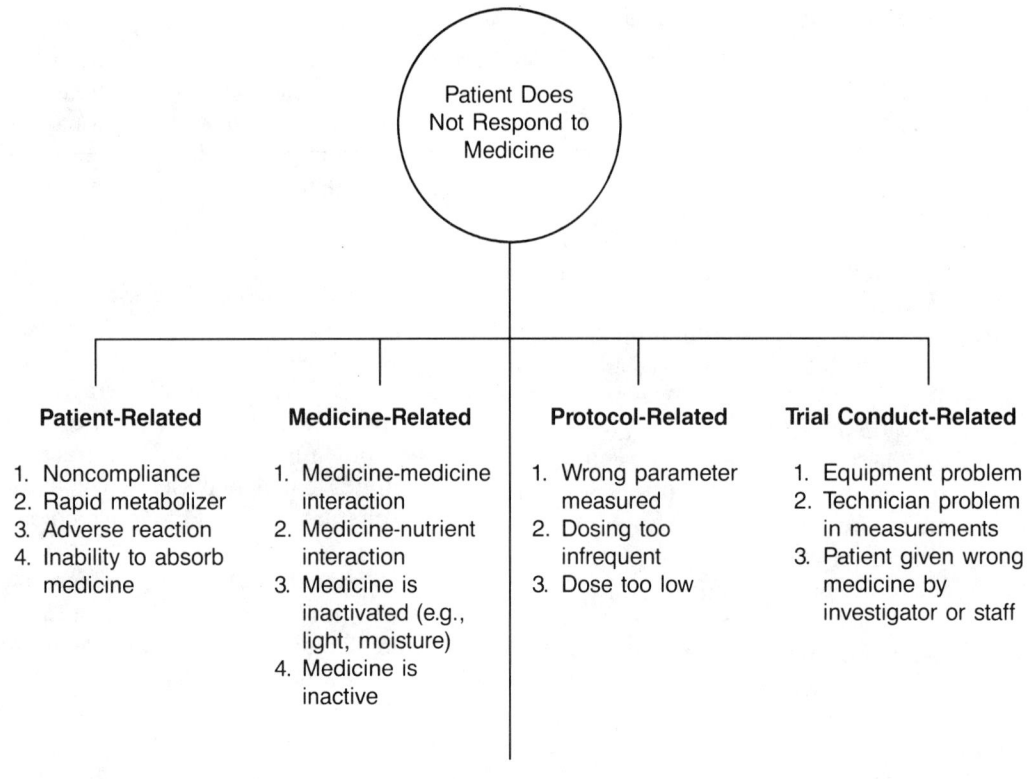

FIG. 98.1 A number of reasons why a patient may not respond to the active medicine in a clinical trial. Other reasons include: wrong type of disease diagnosed, inappropriate clinical trial design used, incorrect data analysis conducted, and parameters measured incorrectly, and patient given wrong medicine because of a packaging error.

Influence of Time

Although the above concepts are described as if they are independent of time, that is generally not true. Clinical responses may be permanent, but especially with chronic diseases, many symptoms and problems tend to recur in a fixed or variable cycle. Problems usually recur either with a waxing and waning pattern or with discrete episodes, although other patterns exist.

Some examples are described below as methods that can help determine the basis of a patient's response and thus differentiate between responders and nonresponders. These examples focus on blood levels of a trial medicine and survival curves.

RESPONSES AND PLASMA LEVELS

It is usually straightforward to determine whether responders and nonresponders may be differentiated on the basis of a medicine's blood level rather than dose. The most direct approach to this issue is to graph the blood level (or concentration) versus clinical response to determine if higher blood levels are associated with superior responses. A positive correlation suggests a relationship, although toxicity may affect this relationship for patients who have higher blood levels. Additional evaluations should be made if data suggest a possible relationship. A negative correlation may also be observed. For instance, if a medicine's bioavailability differs widely between different individuals at the same dose level, some may have a blood level in the therapeutic range and be classified as responders, whereas others may have lower blood levels and be termed nonresponders. This pattern may suggest a relationship between response and blood level if the numbers of nonresponding patients with a blood level in the therapeutic range and of responding patients with a blood level below the therapeutic range are relatively small. Other clues that may be useful in differentiating responders and nonresponders are listed in Table 98.2.

A detailed description is given below of the process through which it can be evaluated if patient responses are related to the blood level of the trial medicine. All patients who have received medicine in the groups to be compared should be classified as responders or nonresponders. If a relatively small number of patients cannot be easily classified, they may be omitted from this analysis, placed in a separate category, or divided as responders or nonresponders based on other criteria established. Patients who have received placebo should be omitted from this analysis, since whether or not they were responders is not pertinent to an evaluation of blood levels. If the medicine's bioavailability at one (or more) dose is highly variable, then blood

TABLE 98.2 *Selected characteristics to differentiate between responders and nonresponders*

1. Patients studied in the morning versus afternoon
2. Patients evaluated by Dr. A versus those evaluated by Dr. B
3. Patients entered in the clinical trial at its inception versus those entered toward the end of the trial
4. Differences in blood level peaks or troughs of the trial medicine or its metabolites
5. Differences in various pharmacokinetic parameters (e.g., areas under the curve, half-life of medicine)
6. Differences in physiological function
7. Differences in metabolites or concentrations of metabolites
8. Differences in past medical history or any specific patient characteristic[a]

[a] See patient characteristics described in Chapter 83 and listed in Table 83.25.

levels will probably be related to individual patient bioavailability. Patients receiving different doses may have equivalent (or divergent) blood levels.

A Practical Example

It is desirable to examine blood levels of responders and nonresponders separately at each dose or dose range studied. A simple hypothetical example to illustrate the reason for this approach is given below. Assume that the following data are obtained in a clinical trial.

1. Responders ($n = 21$) average 100 units of medicine/ml of blood.
2. Nonresponders ($n = 21$) average 40 units of medicine/ml of blood.

These patients received doses from 80 to 400 mg/day. Although these data make it appear as if the patients' responses are related to the blood levels, when the data were subdivided on the basis of dose of medicine the following were obtained:

1. Patients ($n = 21$) who received medicine in the dose range of 80 to 150 mg/day average 31 units of medicine/ml of blood.
2. Patients ($n = 21$) who received medicine in the dose range of 200 to 400 mg/day average 109 units of medicine/ml of blood.

These data make it appear as if blood levels are related to the dose of medicine. If the responders and nonresponders are then evaluated separately at each dose range:

1. At a dose range of 80 to 150 mg/day, responders ($n = 3$) average 40 units of medicine/ml of blood, and nonresponders ($n = 18$) average 30 units of medicine/ml of blood.
2. At a dose range of 200 to 400 mg/day, responders

($n = 18$) average 110 units of medicine/ml of blood, and nonresponders ($n = 3$) average 100 units of medicine/ml of blood.

Thus, the apparent relationship that was initially shown between blood levels and patient response was shown to be false when the data were examined on the basis of dose ranges the patients received.

HOW TO TURN NONRESPONDERS INTO RESPONDERS

Most investigators attempt to determine and understand the reasons why patients improve. This allows the investigator to continue effective therapy in that patient and possibly to try the same techniques in others. One of the most common reasons for therapeutic improvement in some patients but not in others relates to a medicine's blood level. It is often a useful exercise to attempt to correlate clinical efficacy with the blood level of a therapeutic medicine. If a strong correlation is achieved, then it is possible that a range of medicine levels in blood or plasma may be specified within which the therapeutic response should occur. In this situation, it would allow physicians to dose patients to a given blood level in seeking a therapeutic effect and should prevent underdosage of patients imparting a falsely negative label to the medicine's therapeutic potential. Another advantage of this approach is that toxic effects of a medicine should be minimized, since physicians would not dose patients to blood levels above the therapeutic range. A number of mechanisms that may turn nonresponders to responders are listed in Table 98.3.

TABLE 98.3 *Selected mechanisms that may turn nonresponders into responders[a]*

1. Change the definition of the terms *responder* and *nonresponder* in relation to the degree or duration of improvement
2. Add a category of *partial responder* and define this term
3. Provide counseling to patients to improve motivation, attitude, or desire to improve
4. Utilize mechanisms to turn poor compliers into better compliers[b]
5. Raise dose of medicine or modify dosage regimen within the limits of the protocol or modify the protocol (or initiate a new clinical trial)
6. Involve the patient's family in the trial to a greater degree
7. Improve investigator and staff relationships with the patient

[a] Each approach initially involves the determination of the reason(s) why a patient or group of patients are not responders and addressing that particular reason. Patients or staff may be interviewed to elicit possible reasons for lack of adequate patient response.
[b] See Chapter 15.

CALCULATING PATIENT SURVIVAL CURVES

Several authors (Weiss et al., 1983; Oye and Shapiro, 1984) make a strong case that patient survival in cancer trials should not be compared between groups of patients defined as "responders" or "nonresponders" based on tumor shrinkage after a trial is completed. These articles present a variety of reasons to support the conclusion that comparison groups should be created prior to the trial, since responders may primarily include patients with the most favorable prognosis.

1. Many pretreatment factors influence patient survival (e.g., extent of disease, functional status, histology of the cancer), and these would not be expected to be evenly distributed in patients classified as responders and nonresponders.

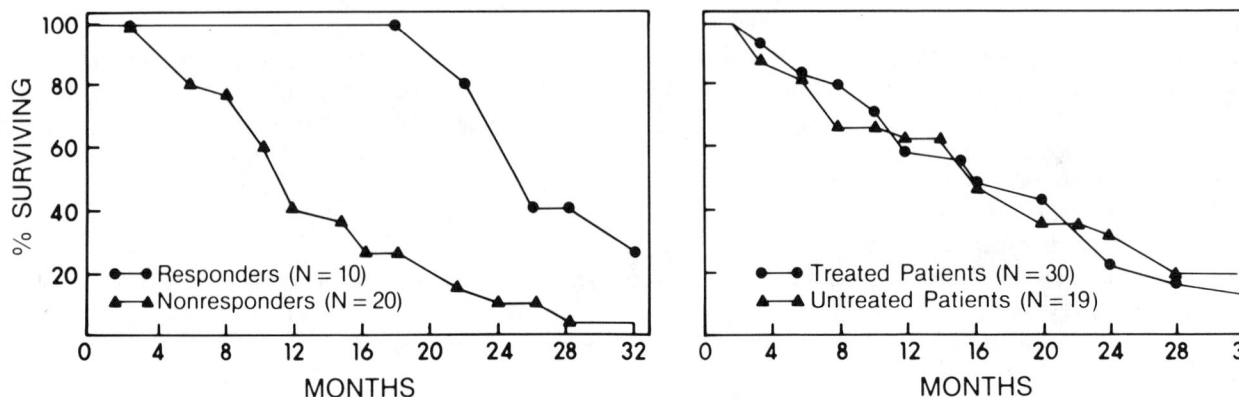

FIG. 98.2 Survival rates of cancer patients in a clinical trial (Payne et al., 1981) evaluating 5-fluorouracil. Data in the **left panel** compare responders and nonresponders. Data in the **right panel** compare treated and untreated patients. (Reprinted by permission of the *Journal of the American Medical Association* from Oye and Shapiro, 1984. Copyright 1984 by the American Medical Association.)

2. Individual variation occurs and may not yield equivalent groups when selection occurs based on patient response.
3. A preponderance of the most severely ill patients would be expected to be in the nonresponder group, and thus this group would have the poorest prognosis for survival.
4. Radiation, surgery, or additional chemotherapy would be expected to be more prevalent in non-responders and may shorten their survival.

Data from a study by Payne et al. (1981) comparing survival of responders and nonresponders to chemotherapy (Fig. 98.2) apparently demonstrated improved survival of responders to chemotherapy (left panel), and that is what the authors concluded (Payne et al., 1981). A concurrent group of untreated patients was included in this clinical trial, and Oye and Shapiro (1984) compared the survival of all treated patients with all untreated patients (right panel of Fig. 98.2). It is clear that the supposed advantage of treatment disappears when this more appropriate comparison is made. This same point was illustrated by Tannock and Murphy (1983) with data from a different trial.

Benefit-to-Risk Assessments and Comparisons

It would be desirable if the assessment of benefits and risks could be readily quantitated and expressed as a single overall number to be compared between medicines. This is unfortunately impossible today. To achieve this goal both benefits and risks would have to be measured in the same units. It is currently necessary to assess independently numerous types of both benefits and risks for a single medicine, each of which may be expressed differently. Then, it is necessary to weigh these factors using a global introspection technique in a manner that depends on the use to which the data are being applied. Multiple perspectives may be considered, including those of the patient, physician, and society.

Benefits that are often imperfectly understood must be compared to the universe of risks and hazards, both known and unknown, to create a relative concept of benefit to risk for a single medicine. This theoretical concept for a single medicine is usually complex, and comparisons with other medicines usually raise additional complexities.

The comparison of benefit-to-risk considerations for two or more medicines in actual medical or economic situations is often much simpler and straightforward than the discussion above might suggest. This is because most factors that affect benefits or risks are either not major considerations in specific situations or are so similar between alternative therapies that they do not greatly impact the overall benefit-to-risk concept or decisions based on this concept. A single factor may represent the total basis for choosing a medicine for a particular patient. For example, in choosing among similar medicines for a patient with renal failure, it is possible that only one medicine is excreted by the hepato-biliary route and would not be expected to lead to toxicity for a specific patient. Benefit-to-risk considerations would thus favor choosing that medicine. Another example would be a patient whose bacterial infection was sensitive to four antibiotics, and the patient was allergic to three of them. Benefit-to-risk considerations suggest choosing the fourth medicine, unless other extremely important factors must also be considered that could override the potential risks.

ASSESSING BENEFITS AT DIFFERENT LEVELS

Types of Benefits

The term *benefits* includes numerous concepts beyond that of a medicine's efficacy. Efficacy relates to how well a treatment achieves its objectives, in a comparative way (e.g., medicine A improves symptoms 40% better than medicine B) or in a noncomparative way (medicine A improves patients' disease measures by 25%). Benefits also include quality of life considerations at the individual patient level or at the collective patient level of various groups [e.g., patients in a Health Maintenance Organization (HMO)]. For a society at the city, province, country, or world level, benefits are often considered in terms of improved public health and improved utilization of resources (e.g., efficient allocation of money to the health care of a population).

Certainty of Benefits

Benefits may be either *predictable* (almost definite), *probable, possible,* or *unlikely.* Each of these four types is described below, and arbitrary probabilities in terms of percent likelihood are assigned to each category.

Predictable benefits relate to clinical effectiveness of a medicine that is almost certain to occur in a patient or group of patients (e.g., for preventing disease). A greater than 95% likelihood of the predicted response is expected.

Probable benefits refer to a situation in which a medicine has not yet been given to a specific patient or has been given, but it is too early in the treatment period for a positive effect to be observed. Based on previous clinical data and experiences, the likelihood of a benefit is judged to be excellent or highly probable (i.e., greater than 50% likely). Giving a diuretic to a volume-overloaded patient who previously responded to diuretics is an example in which the probability of clinical benefit is extremely high.

Possible benefits are those in which the degree of uncertainty of patient response is greater than in the two previous situations, and the chance of benefits is less than 50%. One example is of a new medicine tested in animals, shown to be safe in humans, but not yet demonstrated to be efficacious in humans. Even though the new medicine might eventually save human lives, the benefit-to-risk ratio often requires a cautious approach in early testing, because the benefits are only possible or potential. Because of the many factors that influence a patient's response, almost all medicines can only be said to offer possible benefits in most clinical situations. The number of situations in which a predictable (i.e., almost definite) benefit is expected are much fewer than those situations in which benefits are judged probable or possible.

Benefits may be judged as *unlikely* (i.e., less than 5%) in certain situations when clinical judgment dictates that use of the treatment is still worthwhile. This sometimes occurs in life-threatening situations or with severely ill patients, when alternative therapy is either not available or has been used without success. The risk of the treatment may range from negligible to substantial, and the benefit-to-risk ratio may be unsatisfactory. Nonetheless, the "long-shot" treatment in such situations may be entirely justified on both a medical and an ethical basis.

Levels of Benefits

At each of the levels discussed in this section there are numerous perspectives that are often applied. As one moves from the level of individual patients to the level of society as a whole, the perspective and role of the individual patient becomes progressively less important, while the importance of health policy planners and administrators becomes greater. The impact of physicians and other medical professionals is greater at the individual and group level than at the society level. Specific perspectives are those of (1) the patient, (2) the medical professional, (3) the health policy planner, and (4) various types of administrators.

Level One: An Individual Patient

At the level of an individual patient, defined as level one, the term benefit refers to improvements in both efficacy and quality of life. Although it is theoretically possible to describe benefits as a decrease in adverse reactions of one treatment versus another, this topic is usually discussed in terms of risks. Improvement in symptoms relating to a disease, however, are described as a benefit of treatment. One special caveat applies to medicines developed primarily to decrease adverse reactions caused by other medicines. One example is a new medicine designed to decrease emesis caused by cis platinum and another example is a medicine that is used to decrease anticholinergic effects of some antiparkinsonian agents. In these or other examples, the degree to which the test medicine diminishes or eliminates the target adverse reactions is a measure of its efficacy (benefits).

Level Two: Groups of Patients

The same types of benefits described above also apply at the level of groups or subsets of patients with a disease (level two). The way in which an HMO, hospital, or other medical organization allocates resources to different treatments depends on how aggregate data of these treatments compare in benefit-to-risk terms, as well as on a consideration of costs and utilization of the group's resources (e.g., health care professional time required, equipment needs).

Level Three: All Patients

The level of society as a whole (level three) considers benefits in various public health terms for all patients. This includes judgment of which medicines and therapies are best for present and future patients. A major difference between this level and the other two is that at this level benefit-to-risk ratios, costs of treatment, and utilization of overall health care resources are usually compared across many, if not all, diseases, rather than within a single disease. This means that a society must decide how much of its available money and resources to place on research and treatment for each specific disease and problem, and not just among the different treatments for a single disease. This allocation of money is largely determined by which treatments are available for use, and their benefits and risks, plus pressures placed on decision makers by various groups. It is at this third level that the greatest impact of nonobjective factors occurs in decision making. These factors and pressures are often referred to as politics. The choices that a society must make in allocating its health care money (or funds within other areas) is sometimes sarcastically referred to as determining whose ox gets gored.

Measuring Benefits

To determine and measure clinical benefits objectively, the most common and accepted approach is to conduct clinical trials. Two other methods used to evaluate clinical benefits are to conduct Phase IV observational studies and meta-analyses. At the society level, government agencies, large trade associations, foundations, institutes, and other organizations conduct many surveys in which they collect data that are relevant for these assessments. Social, health, and economic data and statistics obtained are most often utilized at the third level.

Unintended medical or nonmedical benefits may occur with medicines or other treatments. For example, if aspirin is being compared with nonsteroidal antiinflammatory medicines, the additional benefits of aspirin in decreasing the incidence of myocardial infarctions is an unintended benefit that should be considered. If different modalities used to treat cancer (e.g., radiotherapy, surgery) are being compared and greater use of one modality would also help alleviate an unemployment problem, then that impact may be considered as an unintended benefit for society.

RISKS

The public is being barraged with information about risks, often without the proper perspective to understand these important concepts (e.g., news coverage by certain media of risks of immunizing children). Although society is increasingly informed that there are no totally safe medicines or medical treatments, many individuals appear to be intolerant of and unwilling to accept risk. Many of these (and other) people are requesting more information about risks of treatment and a greater role in choosing their own treatment. This is a positive event because each treatment involves some degree of risk, and it is usually important for physicians and patients to compare and discuss the magnitude and possible severity of a treatment's risk along with its anticipated benefits.

There is an enormous difference between risks that people voluntarily accept (e.g., smoking cigarettes, abusing drugs, sunbathing, drinking alcohol) and risks that are involuntary (e.g., cosmic rays, depletion of ozone). There is increasing discussion in the scientific literature about assessment of both involuntary and voluntary risks (Dinman, 1980; Spilker and Cuatrecasas, 1989), but this topic cannot be explored in this book.

Definition

In medicine the term *risk* usually refers to the probability that a given patient will experience a deleterious reaction to the specific treatment under study or, more generally, that something bad will happen. It is the "bad" aspect that differentiates risk from uncertainty, since it is usually uncertain whether a pregnant woman will have a boy or girl, but this is not bad. The deleterious reaction of which there is a risk could be an adverse reaction, physical sign or symptom, laboratory or physiological abnormality (e.g., abnormal electrocardiogram, pulmonary function test), or other problem. Risk may relate to (1) a single patient, (2) a group of patients (such as those in a clinical trial), (3) the entire population of patients who have been given a medicine, or (4) all patients who may be given a medicine.

The risk of an event may be described in terms of the probability of a future problem occurring if the patient takes a medicine, or it may be the probability of a future problem resulting from the fact that the patient already took the medicine. In both situations the event is a potential one, but in the first case the probability of the event's occurrence and its severity will be used to reach a decision as to whether the medicine should be taken. The two spectra, therefore, along which a risk is judged are the probability of the undesirable event occurring, and the severity of the event or its occurrence.

Types of Risk

There are several different types of risks, and not all can be accurately measured. For example, an idiosyncratic reaction such as an allergic or anaphylactic reaction cannot be predicted with accuracy for a patient with limited prior exposure to the medicine, and incidence figures for these events are often difficult to acquire. Some medicine risks are dose related, and different incidence figures must be obtained for individual doses or dose ranges. Even a patient's failing to improve on an experimental treatment could be viewed as a type of risk, since an alternative treatment might have provided the patient with a greater likelihood of achieving a therapeutic benefit. A different type of risk is incurred by patients who refuse treatment.

Risks to Populations of Patients

During the course of a medicine's development, progressively more information is gathered to help determine its risk assessment profile. At the time of a medicine's initial marketing, however, there is usually little estimation available on population risks. This is a result of the small number of patients evaluated at the time when a new medicine is approved (see Chapter 119). This information is either gathered or becomes available during Phase IV when the medicine is given to larger numbers of patients.

Baseline Risk and Excess Risk

There is almost always a baseline risk of a specific adverse event, even if a patient is not treated with a medicine. This is estimated by determining the incidence of the event in the general population. The additional risk related to a medicine is called the *excess risk*. The excess risk may be estimated from Phase IV cohort studies, large field studies, or by evaluating large multipurpose automated data bases with record linkage. This last method is rapidly gaining favor as the method of choice. However, the cardinal rule of

validating patient diagnoses must be followed, regardless of the specific method adopted.

Risk Factors

Risk factors usually relate to specific characteristics of populations, which are by inference sometimes reflected to patients. Risk factors relate to the increase of the patient's probability of experiencing an adverse reaction, disease, or other medical problem as a result of medicine treatment. Risk factors are also used to describe some nonmedicine treatment situations (e.g., risk factors exist and may be identified for having a myocardial infarction or developing hypertension). There is no acceptable manner of accurately calculating the magnitude and/or interaction of two or more risk factors for different diseases. Clinicians are often in the dilemma of trying to use overall population risk data and relating this to a specific patient.

Most diseases or syndromes have risk factors associated with them. These factors may be (1) well established, (2) incompletely established, (3) unknown, and/or (4) controversial. Standard medical textbooks and references enumerate and describe many of these factors. The importance of particular risk factors is described in different ways. They may be presented on a high-to-low risk scale or broadly classified as major or minor (e.g., for having a myocardial infarction). Some risk factors are well known and well researched, such as those for hypertension or myocardial infarction, whereas others are speculative or are unknown.

Deriving the risk factor in benefit-to-risk and other analyses may be straightforward or extremely complex. Major factors to consider in identifying and assessing risk are (1) the probability of the risk occurring, (2) the magnitude or clinical severity of the event if it occurs, (3) the ability to reverse the problem if it occurs, (4) whether any residual effects will remain, and (5) potential effects in the specific patient being considered.

Risks associated with medicines may sometimes be described in absolute terms (e.g., X grams of medicine A will always cause a fatal reaction, Y tablets of medicine B will always make the patient unconscious). Almost all risks for medicines, however, are relative. These may be defined as the risk for patients in a specific treatment group (or those exposed) divided by the baseline risk (or the risk in those unexposed). A relative risk of approximately 1.8 to 2.0 and above is considered clinically significant. This means a twofold greater risk exists. A relative risk of 2 to 4 is usually described as moderate and risks above that as strong. Examples of relative risks include the association of maternal use of diethylstilbestrol and vaginal cancer in the offspring (relative risk about 250), smoking and lung cancer (about 10), and reserpine and breast cancer (2 or less) (Stolley, 1990).

Each treatment group may have different risk factors that usually increase their chance of having a specific problem, i.e., increase their risk of the event(s) in question. Risk factors determine the degree of risk. Risk factors often include evaluation of age, sex, weight, genetic makeup, physiological function, and numerous factors related to the disease, plus characteristics of past and present treatment (e.g., total number of courses of therapy, total dose). Risks for specific patients of adverse events differ depending upon the particular subgroups to which they belong and their particular risk factors. Basic questions to pose about risks are listed in Table 99.1.

Therapeutic Index

A single number that partially expresses the overall risk of a medicine is the therapeutic index. This is also known as the therapeutic ratio. In general terms this number is an approximation of the relative safety of medicines. A large number denotes greater safety and vice versa. However, the therapeutic index may vary widely for individual patients, because of unknown or known (e.g., genetics, risk factors, disease severity) factors. The value does not provide sufficient information about either risks or benefits. For example, a large therapeutic index for a potentially highly toxic medicine (if misused or overdosed) may create more anxiety in physicians and patients than a small therapeutic ratio for a relatively safe medicine.

This ratio should be as large as possible for all new medicines. In reality, the lowest ratio acceptable for new medicines depends on the seriousness of the disease and also on the ratio for existing treatments for the same indication. In the therapeutic area of cancer, the ratio may even be less than unity for some treatments. This means that toxicity is virtually always observed at the same or at lower doses than those necessary to produce benefits. For cardiac glycosides the ratio is about 2, and for a relatively safe medicine (e.g., aspirin) the ratio is quite high for most patients.

TABLE 99.1 *Questions to consider about risk*

1. Is the risk well established?
2. Is the risk's outcome immediate or delayed?
3. Is exposure to the risk voluntary?
4. Is the risk related to the dose of a medicine?
5. Are specific risk factors known?
6. Is the risk avoidable?
7. Are the outcomes fixed or variable?
8. How severe is the outcome?
9. Is the risk associated with strong emotions?

Two Essential Questions to Address

In considering risks it is often important to address and differentiate between the following two questions:

1. What is the likelihood that a specific adverse event experienced by a patient was related to a specific medicine?
2. What is the likelihood that a particular patient will experience a specific adverse reaction if treated with a specific medicine?

The first question is one of cause and effect attribution and looks to the past. It may be discussed at all three levels described under benefits, while the second question looks to the future and is only appropriate to consider at the first level (i.e., the individual patient). One may compare both questions only at the first level. The major issue in question one is to establish whether or not the event was caused by the medicine. This is discussed at length in Chapter 73. The answer to the second question depends on previous data gathered in that patient in particular, and on the medicine in general. Other questions to consider are listed in Table 99.1.

Offsetting Risks with a Single Medicine

One seldom simply weighs benefits and risks to arrive at an overall assessment. Most risks that accompany a medical treatment do not simply increase or decrease with its use. Rather, some may be increased at the same time others are decreased, or those of one medical therapy may be immediate or short-term, while others are longer-term (i.e., do not occur for a long time).

Two types of offsetting risks are described below, based on their time of occurrence.

Type 1. Risk A is decreased and risk B is increased at the same time. This is observed with many medicines, particularly when comparing risks of the disease itself (i.e., risk A), which are presumably decreasing while the risks associated with therapy (i.e., risk B) are increasing. To evaluate how the two balance each other, one must compare the overall benefit-to-risk ratio of the treatment versus other treatments or no treatment. In determining this aspect it is usually desirable to evaluate quality of life issues, as well as certain practical issues (e.g., costs). Examples would include the risks of not treating certain fungal diseases versus risks of the medicine used (e.g., amphotericin); or, the risk of not treating a urinary tract infection versus risks of the antibiotic used.

Type 2. The treatment causes risk A to decrease in the present and risk B to increase at a later time in the patient's life. For example, assume that the risk of death from cardiovascular disease is decreased with therapy and patients are shown to live longer; however, a number of patients develop a specific type of cancer at a later stage in their life if they are given the treatment.

Risk Perception

A substantial amount of psychological research has demonstrated that the ways in which risk is perceived depends on the way in which problems are presented. Presenting the same problem requiring a decision in different ways (i.e., emphasizing either negative or positive attributes of the outcome) elicits different responses (Tversky and Kahneman, 1981; Slovic et al., 1982). People usually make decisions to avoid present risks and choose a sure thing over a probability. McNeil et al. (1982) reported that preferences of both lay people and physicians depend on whether probabilities are expressed in terms of death rates or survival rates. Patient perceptions of risks of prescription medicines are generally low (Slovic et al., 1989), which should influence their compliance plus attitudes about accepting adverse reactions. These data were obtained in Sweden and it is uncertain if the same results would be obtained in most other countries.

The public is often confused because of media hype (either playing up small risks, or ignoring relative large risks). As a result people often overestimate the likelihood of rare events (e.g., death by tornados, vaccines, or lightning) and underestimate the likelihood of frequent events (e.g., death from heart attacks). Another issue is that the public is often given information about suspected risks when no one knows the true magnitude, and known risks when the magnitude is known. Many adverse reactions exist of both types (i.e., suspected and known risks).

It is difficult to combine and often to compare data on *voluntary* risks (i.e., those risks an individual person accepts and brings on him- or herself), such as smoking cigarettes, driving a family car, or driving a racing car, and *involuntary* risks (i.e., those beyond a single person's control) such as living in an area with nuclear power plants, cosmic rays, or disappearance of ozone.

Assessing Risks in Six Steps

The process of assessing risks of medicines may be divided into six separate steps, as follows:

1. Identify known risks and also potential risks.
2. Quantitatively assess known and potential risks in terms of their probability of occurrence (i.e., along the spectrum from 0 to 1).
3. Determine the degree of exposure of patients to each relevant risk.
4. Assess the known and potential risks in terms of their severity (i.e., along a spectrum).
5. Determine which risks are additive, synergistic, mutually exclusive, or otherwise interact.
6. Derive an overall assessment of both individual and collective risks for one or more patients, considering data from the first four steps and information from the fifth. This assessment may include determining whether for a specific treatment (1) the severity of risks is low and probability of occurrence is also low, (2) the severity of risks is low, but the probability of occurrence is high, (3) the severity of risks is substantial, but the probability of occurrence is low, or (4) the severity of risks is substantial and the probability of occurrence is also high.

DETERMINING BENEFIT-TO-RISK RATIOS

Definition

The benefit-to-risk ratio for a particular patient is really the answer to the question: what is the value of giving a specific treatment to a specific patient at a specific time under a defined set of conditions? A comparable definition of benefit-to-risk ratio exists for a group of patients or for all patients with a specific disease.

Describing the Benefit-to-Risk Concept

The benefit-to-risk ratio relates the potential or actual benefit that a patient derives from a medicine to the risks incurred by the patient through using the medicine. A medicine that is life saving provides an enormous benefit. If the medicine is relatively safe and thus has a low risk, the patient will have a high benefit-to-risk ratio. If, on the other hand, the risk of severe adverse reactions is also high, then the ratio may be low. The risks may be so great that even the potential life-saving qualities of the medicine may make its use unacceptable (e.g., a terminally ill patient who does not want a medicine that may prolong life a short period but with major adverse reactions). The benefit-to-risk ratio is not expressed as a finite number but in qualitative terms such as high, low, equal, very low, and so forth.

The benefit-to-risk concept includes consideration of multiple types of risks. There is the type of risk of adverse reactions described above. The likelihood of one of these deleterious events occurring may often be quantitated. The data base for this is derived from both pre- and postmarketing studies. The likelihood of the adverse reaction's occurrence will assist a decision as to whether possible clinical benefits appear to be sufficiently greater than risks involved in undergoing treatment. This judgment is based on both the severity of the potential risks that may be anticipated and their likelihood of occurring. Among those risks that may be anticipated, many (if not most) will be minor or moderate in importance. If potentially serious or life-threatening risks are possible, then consideration must be given to the expected frequency of their occurrence. It is clear that the more severe the potential complication is, the less likely that it will be acceptable, unless the potential benefit derived by the patient is expected to be even more substantial.

Use of Benefit-to-Risk Ratios

The concept of the benefit-to-risk ratio is often used by physicians as part of their decision-making process to determine the precise therapy to use in a particular situation. A medicine with potential for both high benefits and high risks is often less desirable than a medicine with moderate benefits and low risks because the benefit-to-risk ratio is greater in the latter case. Clinical judgment must be used when choosing among multiple medicines or nonmedicines, all of which involve risks and benefits that cannot easily be compared. A common medical practice is to initiate therapy with medicines or nonmedicine treatments that have the least risk and to switch to other medicines or treatments if the initial ones are ineffective, in a manner that progressively increases the risks to the patient. This approach has the advantage that a medicine with a low risk may have greater efficacy than anticipated in the particular patient being treated.

High-Risk Groups

Some patients have elevated risks because of one or more characteristics that place them in a high-risk group. Common factors that place many patients in a high-risk group are compromised renal, hepatic, or immunological function; age (e.g., infants, children, elderly); pregnancy; and other factors described in Chapter 87. High-risk groups for a specific medicine may be identified on the basis of medical history or laboratory findings. The identification of specific risk factors is usually made during clinical investigations, either through a systematic evaluation or serendipitously. Some of the risk factors identified will probably be related to the characteristics of the patient's disease, whereas others will depend on the biochemical, phar-

macological, and other activities of the medicine. Risk factors may also be based on a patient's previous or current clinical treatment as well as most of the patient factors listed in Table 83.25.

Establishing the Ratio for Different Groups of Patients

Benefits must be determined in the context of a patient's clinical condition or disease and the availability of alternate forms of treatment. Thus, the benefit-to-risk ratio is usually established for each patient based on his or her particular medical history and present medical situation. Alternatively, benefit may be established for a given group of patients based on the total range and characteristics of their situation. This evaluation is usually in the province of epidemiology. Finally, the benefit-to-risk ratio may be established at the level of an entire society and/or at all levels of the health care system (e.g., formularies, practicing physicians). This is usually in the province of health policy planners, legislators, and regulatory agencies.

How Benefit-to-Risk Ratios Change Over Time

As new information about a medicine emerges during a patient's treatment, in terms of increased risks or anticipated clinical improvement, it may be necessary to reassess the benefit-to-risk ratio. If a particularly severe and serious adverse reaction or safety problem occurs, then the benefit-to-risk ratio may be questioned for all patients in a clinical trial and not solely for the patient receiving the medicine. In the clinical trial environment, revising the informed consent for all patients or even discontinuing the trial may be necessary. In the environment of clinical practice, the physician must disclose substantial new information on risks to the patient, especially in our litigious society. In some cases it may be possible to assess the best treatment for a particular patient through using an N of one ($n = 1$) clinical trial design (see Chapter 38).

A benefit-to-risk ratio often changes over time for a single patient, all patients, or a society. For a single patient, prior to ever receiving a medicine the ratio might be positive and the physician may decide to give the medicine to the patient. Assume that the patient experiences a mild adverse reaction, but it is not as bad as the response the patient experienced with other related medicines. The benefit-to-risk ratio falls, but remains positive (i.e., in favor of using the medicine). Now, the adverse reactions become worse, and the benefit-to-risk ratio becomes negative. The patient is therefore switched to another treatment. Assume another patient takes the same medicine and a skin rash develops. If the medicine is intended for a serious disease and no other medicines of equal efficacy are available, the physicians may decide to (1) continue treatment and watch the patient carefully, (2) lower the dose, (3) stop the medicine and begin desensitization procedures, (4) switch to another medicine, (5) treat the problem and continue the medicine, or (6) follow another treatment plan.

The benefit-to-risk ratio usually depends on the severity of an individual patient's disease and its prognosis. The more severe a disease and the more negative its prognosis, the greater the risks that most patients and physicians are willing to take.

When a much safer new medicine is introduced the benefit-to-risk ratio changes for all patients with the disease and in some cases most patients will receive the new medicine. For an entire society the information on benefit-to-risk ratios of many medicines and treatments for many diseases is often used to help make decisions on allocating limited health care resources. Improved benefits for patients through discovery of new treatments that have greater benefit-to-risk ratios encourages more resources to be allocated to those treatments.

COMPARING BENEFIT-TO-RISK RATIOS FOR DIFFERENT MEDICINES

As indicated in the introduction, benefit-to-risk ratio comparisons for two or more medicines may focus on a single factor or multiple factors. The comparison may be simple or complex, easy or difficult to conduct, or may be impossible because of lack of sufficient information. The results of a specific comparison may or may not have importance in medical practice. If there is to be an impact on medical practice it is essential to express this information in a way that practicing physicians can easily understand.

Expressing Measurements Relating to Benefit and Risk

Laupacis et al. (1988) reviewed four methods of measuring the consequences of treatment and recommended one (i.e., number needed to be treated) as providing the clearest information for practicing physicians. The four measures are described below.

Relative Risk Reduction

Relative risk reduction is an expression of the amount of reduction of adverse events. This term is presented as a proportion of the control rates (i.e., control rate

minus treatment group rate, divided by the control rate). The major disadvantage of this approach is that it does not reflect the magnitude of the risk without therapy, and this may be misleading or, at best, incomplete in the information provided. Relative risk reduction is often expressed as a percent (e.g., medicine X reduces the risk of stroke by 32%).

Odds Ratio

The odds ratio expresses the relative likelihood of an outcome. It is frequently used in meta-analyses, but for expressing risks it has the same disadvantages as relative risk reduction. An odds ratio of 6, 11, or 15 means that a target outcome (e.g., adverse reaction) is 6, 11, or 15 times more likely to occur than is the other possibility.

Absolute Risk Reduction

Absolute risk reduction is the difference in adverse event rates for two groups, usually control and treatment. The number is usually a decimal and does not make inherent sense to practicing physicians as a basis for making a choice among therapies (e.g., medicine X reduces the risk of stroke by 0.14 compared with placebo).

Number Needed To Be Treated

Mathematically, the number of patients who must be treated to prevent one major adverse event is the reciprocal of the absolute risk reduction. This number has a readily understood meaning to physicians and has numerous statistical advantages over the other expressions described above (Laupacis et al., 1988). For example, for every seven patients treated with medicine X one fewer patient will have a stroke.

CONCLUSIONS

In reaching a decision on which treatment (1) a physician should use for a particular patient, (2) an HMO should keep on their formulary, or (3) a health policy advisor should recommend for their society, three questions should be considered.

1. Is the net benefit [i.e., sum of all benefits (including quality of life) minus the sum of all risks] greater than zero? If not, then giving no treatment may be the preferable choice.

2. Is the net benefit of the treatment in question greater than the net benefit of other alternative therapies (or no therapy)?
3. If both of the answers to these questions are "yes," then is the net benefit worth the cost in terms of additional money, equipment, profes-sional time, and administration associated with the treatment?

Additional discussions on benefit-to-risk ratios are presented in references by Pochin (1981), Lowrance (1988), and von Wartburg (1988).

CHAPTER 100

Coordination and Integration of Statistical Analyses with Clinical Interpretations

INTRODUCTION

Roles of Statisticians and Clinicians

There have been many comments throughout this book on the collaborative activities of a clinician and statistician in planning clinical trials and analyzing results. The analyzed results are interpreted by the clinician, who may request additional analyses to be performed. It is the author's contention that the role of the statistician is not usually to interpret data clinically or extrapolate data, although statisticians may provide valuable advice to the clinician who has these roles. Clearly, the statistician does provide the analyses on which much or all of the interpretation(s) and extrapolation(s) are based.

One of the differences in approach between statisticians and clinicians is that statisticians usually discuss the methods of treating large numbers of patients in a clinic, whereas physicians treat a single patient at a time. This difference is often reflected in different attitudes toward individual patients and groups of patients.

May a Single Professional Fill Both Roles?

Some individuals have been trained in the disciplines of both statistics and medicine. This does not affect the preceding comments, since it is possible for an individual to fulfill both roles adequately. When an individual is not adequately trained in both disciplines, a variety of problems may arise, involving both "in-

vasion of the other's turf" and a failure to plan clinical trials or interpret data adequately. An incorrect application of statistics in the trial design or data analyses is also possible.

Integration in an Ideal Situation

In an ideal situation, no formal integration process of statistical analyses with clinical interpretations should be necessary. All of the necessary statistical analyses should be completed prior to initiation of the clinical interpretation of a trial. The process of interpretation may be conducted immediately after the analyses are complete. The major point is that they are two separate processes, even if performed by one individual in a sequential manner. Various clinical hypotheses or questions may be posed, which may suggest further exploratory analyses or additional evaluations of the data. Nonetheless, if there is one set of accepted statistical analyses and they are generated prior to development of their clinical interpretation, the two processes should be able to be conducted without the need for formal integration of efforts beyond clinical input into the format and presentation of results.

SITUATIONS IN WHICH INTEGRATION IS REQUIRED

General and Specific Types of Examples

Sometimes the two processes require a large degree of integration, as illustrated by a few hypothetical situations. In the first example, only one type of standardized and validated statistical technique is suitable for analyzing the clinical trial data, but two or more different types of clinical interpretations are possible. Each interpretation can be supported to some degree by the statistical analysis. The second example is the (opposite) situation in which two or more statistical approaches to the data are possible but only one clinical interpretation is plausible regardless of which set of statistical analyses are used. The final example is one in which both multiple statistical analyses and multiple clinical interpretations are possible.

Specific examples include:

1. A one- or two-tailed t-test may be used, but data are clinically interpreted as positive regardless of which test is used.
2. Data may be analyzed by last observation carried forward or by simply using actual data obtained. Data may be analyzed by using intent-to-treat or by defining an "efficacy population." The clinical interpretation will be positive only when one (or two) of these analyses is used.
3. Data are only analyzed one way, but depending on whether a global clinical impression of improvement or a global clinical impression of disease severity is used, the outcome will be positive or negative.
4. Data are only analyzed one way. The clinical interpretation of the most important test narrowly misses statistical significance, but the second, third, and fourth tests in order of importance are positive. Is the trial positive?
5. Data are only analyzed one way, but can support two or more clinical hypotheses to explain the results.

Practical Approaches

In order to evaluate whether any of these situations exist, it is often necessary to conduct what the statistician and clinical interpreter believe to be the most reasonable analyses of the data and then to examine the statistical results from a clinical perspective. It should then become clear whether the analyses support more than one interpretation, hypothesis, or model. If the answer to this question is uncertain, then additional statistical analyses may be performed, and a subsequent evaluation made of whether an alternative clinical interpretation may be supported. It should be noted that the present discussion refers to an interpretation of data in regard to the primary and secondary objectives of the clinical trial. Various subgroup analyses may be useful and important for developing hypotheses to test in future studies, but

these are not part of the primary clinical interpretation of data described in this section.

Once it has been established that multiple statistical analyses or clinical interpretations are possible, it becomes important to integrate the analyses and interpretations. If there is either a single clinical interpretation (and multiple statistical analyses) or a single statistical analysis (and multiple clinical interpretations), there is a straightforward means of integrating them. That procedure is to choose the best clinical or statistical possibility among the multiple possibilities and to marshal all arguments in support of this choice. Reference to the other possibilities should be made, but strong arguments in favor of the chosen possibility will serve to tie together and integrate the statistical analyses and clinical interpretation. In the process of choosing one statistical analysis among many, reference may be made to reasons based in either the field of statistics, clinical medicine, or both. Insofar as a choice of statistical procedures is supported with clinical arguments or vice versa, there will be a strong connection between the two.

The other situation occurs when both multiple statistical analyses are possible to conduct and multiple clinical interpretations are possible to defend. A prioritization within each group may be a useful means of identifying which analyses and interpretations are most reasonable. Alternatively, the single set of data analyses and interpretations may be chosen that fit best with each other. The question may be raised as to whether the analyses (or the interpretations) are actually the best within their own group and also when considered as a pair. In substantiating the choices made among analyses or interpretations, references to published literature are often useful, as is evidence showing that the other choices (or other pairs) lead to less meaningful interpretations of data.

When the sample size in a clinical trial is large, there is a greater likelihood that differences will be observed that are statistically but not clinically significant. This occurs because the large statistical power allows the trial to detect small differences between two groups. One means of avoiding this potential dispute is to determine criteria of clinically meaningful medicine activity prior to the trial.

ESTABLISHING AND MAINTAINING EFFECTIVE RELATIONSHIPS BETWEEN STATISTICIANS AND CLINICIANS

Some of the most important techniques for effective collaboration between statisticians and clinicians are for them to discuss and agree on (1) goals, (2) work assignments to achieve these goals, (3) providing information in both directions, and (4) eschewing use of jargon in favor of clear and open communications. These procedures should be operational before, during, and after a clinical trial if optimal data analyses and interpretations are to result.

Finally, statisticians and clinicians who are working as part of a team on one project should not operate totally independently but should communicate frequently. It is generally useful after the clinical trial is completed for the statistician to describe what happened in the trial from a statistical perspective in addition to providing tables of raw data and analyses. This information will assist the clinician in interpreting the data. Furthermore, the statistician should review the interpretation(s) and any extrapolations reached by the clinician to ensure that they are properly supported by the best possible analyses of the data. Statisticians should help clinicians distinguish between the statistical and clinical significance of data.

CHAPTER 101

Misinterpretation of Data

Misinterpretation of data is a common event that pervades most aspects of one's existence. Just open the pages of any newspaper or magazine and there are innumerable examples of data being distorted, mispresented, and misinterpreted. Most examples result from naïveté, inexperience, incomplete reviews, or poor presentation of data, rather than deliberate attempts to distort data. Two hypothetical examples from the world of education (based on actual reports) are briefly described to illustrate this point.

MISINTERPRETATION OF DATA IN DAILY LIFE

Example One: Student Test Scores

State A's average scores for a national college entrance examination are reported in the newspaper to have fallen compared with their neighboring states. State A now ranks 45th out of 50, compared with its previous ranking of 43rd. Articles and editorials are written in many state newspapers about declining educational standards and results within the state. Loud calls are heard from politicians for more money to be spent on education and for the quality of the schools to improve. Many other strong statements are made at public meetings, in the state legislature, and elsewhere.

These comments are primarily based on conclusions that usually represent a misinterpretation of the data (apart from the insincere posturing that usually occurs among certain political groups and individuals). A few representative questions that should be asked about the data before drawing any firm conclusions include:

1. What is the percentage of high school students taking the test in each of the states? A state in which poor or borderline students are directly or indirectly discouraged from taking the test will have higher average scores than a state in which a greater percentage of the students are encouraged take the test.

2. Did the percentage of students who took the test in the state increase or decrease compared with the previous year? A concerted effort by teachers to encourage more students to go to college would result in more borderline and poor students taking the test. This would lead to lower scores, although more students might attend college and potentially have a more productive future (which is clearly a major goal of education).

3. Did the absolute values on the test increase or decrease? A state's position relative to other states could decrease because (1) its scores increased, but to a lesser degree than did other states, (2) its scores did not change, but those of other states increased, or (3)

its scores decreased, but those of other states increased, did not change, or decreased to a lesser degree.

4. Are other states designing their educational curriculum to help students do well in the tests? "Teaching to the test" is becoming a more common practice. If the neighboring states are doing this and their scores surpass those of state A, it does not necessarily indicate that the standards of education in state A have changed.

5. Are more students in other states taking preparatory courses outside of school to help with their tests? If there is a large economic difference in the population of the states and state A is poorer (or wealthier), this factor would be important.

6. Are a greater percent of students enrolled in private schools in one state than another? There are various reasons why educational tests should not always be compared between public and private schools, without caveats.

7. What social groups of students are taking these tests? If the often quoted fact is correct that black children and poor children are at a significant disadvantage in taking the test because it includes words and knowledge that are more familiar to the middle class rather than being class neutral or balanced, then this factor could have great impact on the state's scores. Have more poor and blacks entered the state? Is a higher percentage of this category of students taking the test compared with other states?

If other states' scores are rising faster than state A's scores, it is necessary to determine the reasons before making interpretations about the conclusion. This rational approach usually is drowned out by reports in the media and at meetings by a loud chorus of charges, defenses, and entrenched positions. Each side in an argument often focuses their efforts on reaching decision makers who have political clout, rather than discovering and presenting an objective view based on logic and reason. The public seldom learns enough details (without hard work) to reach an independent judgment based on all available data on an issue. Even motivated individuals are seldom able to obtain sufficient information on any topic to reach a truly informed decision.

Many additional questions and issues should be considered for almost any item reported in the news. That is probably why so few reasonable interpretations are provided by the media for world news events, statistical results, or other information one is exposed to in daily life. Few people want to ask continually the pointed questions necessary to achieve a better interpretation of the events presented. Those that do make a great effort usually learn that the answers received

to their appropriate questions are unclear or may be viewed in various ways.

Example Two: Quality of Education

The second example concerns a school system that is always bragging about how fine the education is that their students receive, because more students become National Merit Finalists each year than from any other school in the entire state.

It is unreliable to reason backwards from an event to its purported cause in this manner. A more likely reason that the school leads the state in the number of finalists relates to the pool of students from which the school system draws. In this case it was observed that the parents of the students are primarily highly educated professionals, who are associated with one of two fine universities in the area, work at a nearby research park, or provide professional services to the community. This pool of students would be highly motivated and educated at home. They would make any school system look like a winner based on standardized tests, almost independently of the level of the education provided by the school.

It is possible, however, for a school or school system to test the hypothesis that it has the best educational program in a region or state. Students in most grades are currently given national standardized tests. The differences in each student's score from year to year could be easily calculated.

If a school offered superior education, then the differences in a longitudinal educational trial over the 12 years of public education for each baseline strata of student (e.g., students with high, medium, and low scores at the start of first grade) should be greater in that school system than in others. Even then, it would be impossible to conclude that the education those students received was outstanding. For instance, the teachers could be "teaching to the test," particularly in the higher grades, when students (and schools) are thinking more about entrance into universities and colleges. Second, tests are an imperfect measure of education, although relative improvements (in percentiles) from year to year over a 12-year period might be expected to have some relationship to the quality of education. Third, both social and economic factors would have to be considered in comparing different school systems. Other questions and issues involve possible assessment of (1) the percent and number of students graduating, (2) the number who attend or eventually graduate from college, and (3) all students or just a subset (e.g., those intending to go on to college).

Major and minor decisions must often be made on a medical issue without answers to most of the important questions necessary to interpret the data fully. Nonetheless, it is essential that attempts be made to obtain answers to major questions.

MISINTERPRETATION FROM ACCEPTING STATEMENTS IN ABSTRACTS

Functions of Abstracts

Abstracts published in reputable journals as part of professional meetings serve several valuable functions. First, by reading them prior to a meeting, people can decide whether or not to attend. Second, they enable people at the meeting to decide which talks to attend, which poster sessions to visit, and which people to contact. Subsequent to a meeting they allow people to obtain a flavor of what transpired or to refresh their memories if they attended the meeting.

Variety of Abstracts

The relationship between the contents of abstracts and scientific truth is often tenuous. Many abstracts are written before experiments or clinical trials are complete and abstracts often present interim data or are even written without any actual results. Others project what the authors anticipate will be found in their clinical trials or experiments. This practice is clearly unethical. Still others create or round out stories or experimental results to develop a whole picture that contains various distortions. Interpretations reached are often inadequately supported by the data.

Interpretation of Abstracts

Readers almost never have sufficient data to agree with or challenge the results and interpretation reported in an abstract. This issue is not a major problem when the full results are published within a year or so in a peer-reviewed journal. At that point the reader may more completely judge the quality of the work conducted, its presentation, and interpretation.

Abstracts should be viewed as having the functions mentioned above. If the data are important the authors have a responsibility to publish a complete paper. The failure to find a full paper in the literature within 3 or so years after an abstract with important results is published is definitely not proof that the abstract was false, or that later results went in a different direction. Nonetheless, suspicions will be raised. Many authors freely admit that some of their abstracts were prepared prematurely in that initial results were not confirmed, or that final results were not worthy of full publication.

References to Abstracts in the Medical Literature

Another problem regarding abstracts is that they are sometimes quoted as equal references to full papers in support of, or to refute, a certain point. The author is aware of several abstracts that have been widely quoted to support claims of a medicine's efficacy, but efficacy has not been supported by data in full publications. Specific examples are not quoted to avoid embarrassing those authors. The conclusion is that abstracts should be used for purposes described and not as references to scientific truth.

MISINTERPRETATIONS BASED ON PUBLICATION OF PILOT TRIAL DATA

It is unfortunately true that many (if not most) pilot trials are generally viewed as "quick and dirty" trials (i.e., designed, conducted, and possibly analyzed at a lower standard than that applied to controlled trials). Thus, the data obtained are often considered to be useful to apply to subsequent (better controlled) trials but are rarely convincing on their own. Pilot trials have a higher incidence than controlled trials of arriving at false-positive or false-negative conclusions and thus may mislead clinicians into believing that a given therapy has less or greater value than it truly has.

The proper responses to this dilemma are to (1) improve the standards of pilot trials so that data obtained are more reliable, (2) view reports of pilot trials with some skepticism, and (3) understand what types of data can validly be obtained from pilot trials.

PARADOXES, MISCONCEPTIONS, AND DISTORTIONS OF NUMBERS

There are many paradoxes about numbers, logic, statistics, and other areas that may sometimes influence, affect, or interfere with the interpretation of clinical data. A humorous collection of paradoxes is presented in the book *aha! Gotcha* by Martin Gardner (1982), the author of *Scientific American*'s "Mathematical Games column." Many of the points he makes about statistical concepts are important to consider when one is interpreting data. A few of these will be summarized.

Averages

When there are a few extreme values, information about the "average" (arithmetic mean) may be highly misleading. If 100 patients have two lesions each and 5 patients have 200 lesions each, the average number of lesions is 11.4. This number can be a misleading figure if only the average number of lesions is stated in a report or publication.

If a study on drowning incidents reports that one person drowned in a river that has an average depth of 15 centimeters, it may conjure an image of someone who was inebriated, toxic, or had a heart attack and fell face down in a shallow pool of water and died. If it turns out that the person drowned in a place where the river is 10 meters deep, this information will assist in developing a more accurate overall impression.

The word *average* is sometimes used to denote the median (the middle value in a list in which all values are placed in order of their magnitude) or mode (the value that appears most often).

The average value given may be imaginary and not denote a possible situation. A well-known example describes the average number of children in an American household as 2.4.

Thus, the term average is ambiguous primarily because it may have three definitions, mean, median, and mode, and also because it does not provide any indication of variance of the numbers used to generate the average.

Jumping to Conclusions

Assume that it is reported that more people proportionally die of cancer in Florida than in any other state. Does this mean that there are environmental factors in Florida that predispose patients to contracting cancer? The answer is that many elderly people go to Florida because of the environment, and since the overall incidence of cancer is related to age, Florida has a higher incidence of cancer than other states. Similarly, patients with tuberculosis often move to certain states because of their climates. This makes it appear that the incidence is highest in those states and may incorrectly raise the suspicion that something about that state contributes to the disease.

Many events, major, minor, and even trivial, change over time, and if two or more events are each measured and compared, the changes observed in each may appear to be related. This does not necessarily mean that there is a true connection between the two events. Assume that the annual number of patients in a state who die from a particular type of cancer had been increasing over a number of years. If one also measured the consumption of chewing gum, the number of bingo halls, or hours of television watching, and one or more of those events also showed a similar increase over the same period, no one would seriously associate the increase in cancer with the other event(s) as cause and effect. As an aside, it is possible that there could have been an additional factor such as increased radiation

emitted by defective television sets or toxins found in the chewing gum that might raise questions about their association with cancer. Even then, however, a true connection with increased numbers of cancer cases in the short term would probably be far fetched. If, however, there was a prolonged increase in pollution levels, radiation leaks from a nuclear power plant, chemical additives in foods, or changes in a factor that had been previously related to cancer, the association with the increased number of cancer deaths would be more likely to be related as cause and effect. Murphy (1982) described a number of bizarre associations that turned out to be true. Acquiring adequate information prior to reaching a conclusion is essential but difficult if the issue is one of great public interest and there is pressure for a rapid resolution of a problem. The point of this discussion is that it is important to avoid jumping to a conclusion.

MISINTERPRETATION BASED ON MISPRESENTATIONS OR CONFUSING PRESENTATIONS OF DATA

Chapter 105 discusses mispresentation of clinical data and Chapter 13 in *Presentation of Clinical Data* (Spilker and Schoenfelder, 1990) illustrates a number of overly complex and confusing presentations. An index of suspicion is often the only clue that the presentation contains flaws. The golden rule to follow in this area is that interpretations should be based on actual raw and tabulated data whenever possible, rather than graphical presentations (unless a complete set of data are graphically presented) or data summaries. The reader should be satisfied that all major questions about the data have been addressed before accepting an interpretation as valid.

MISINTERPRETATION BASED ON PRESENTING DIFFERENT ANALYSES AND DATA THAN THOSE DESIGNED TO ADDRESS THE PRIMARY OBJECTIVE

Most, if not all, clinical trials generate data that are analyzed in a variety of ways. Even when a single statistical test is planned to be used for the analysis, a variety of other tests and approaches are often explored. This is generally acceptable. However, some authors find that the data are more interesting when new clinical questions (i.e., trial objectives) are asked after the trial is completed, rather than simply analyzing the data that address the primary objective. If these results are published and no mention is made of the original objective, then it is unethical.

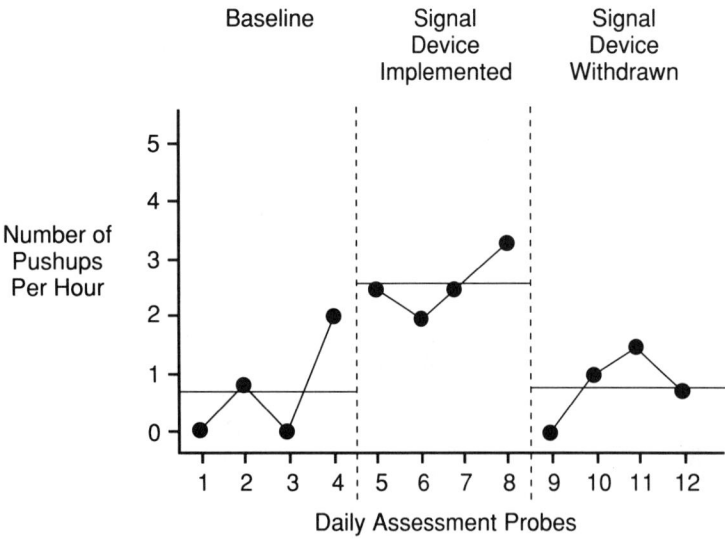

FIG. 101.1 Frequency of pushups per hour and mean values for each of the three phases. (Reprinted from Gouvier et al., 1985 with permission of the American Congress of Rehabilitative Medicine.)

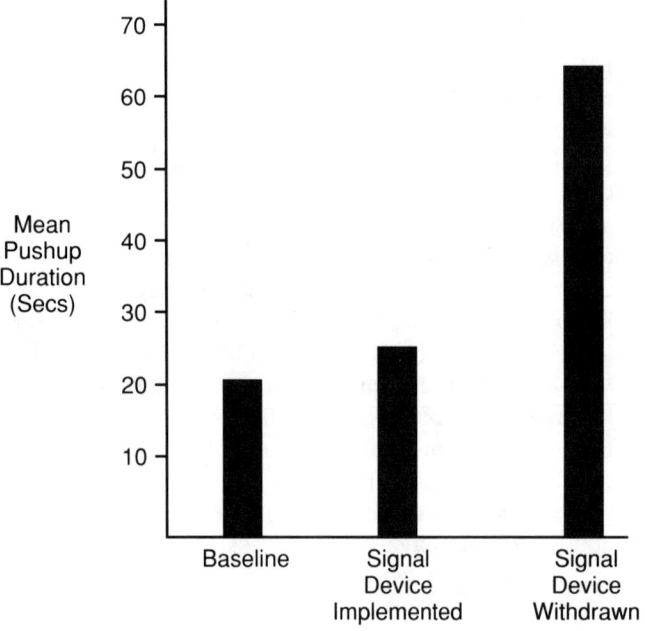

FIG. 101.2 Mean duration of pushups within each experimental phase. (Reprinted from Gouvier et al., 1985, with permission of the American Congress of Rehabilitative Medicine.)

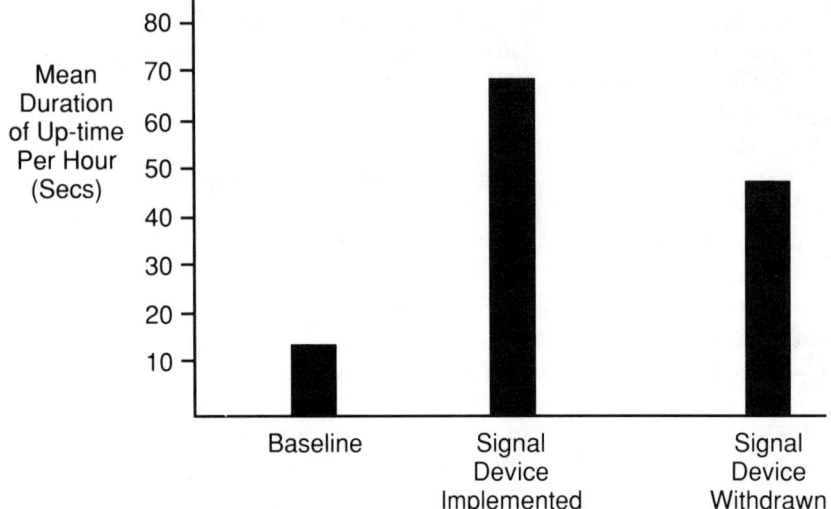

FIG. 101.3 Mean duration of up-time per hour within each phase. (Reprinted from Gouvier et al., 1985, with permission of the American Congress of Rehabilitative Medicine.)

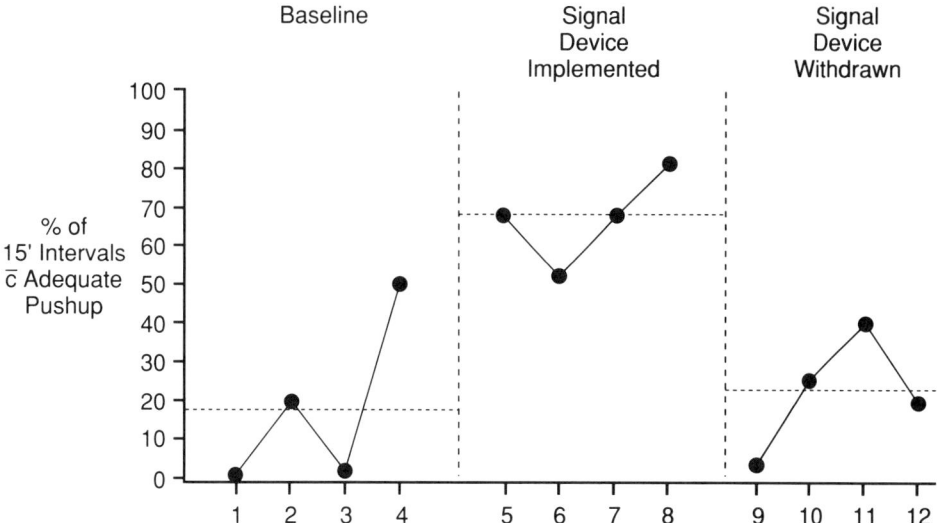

FIG. 101.4 Percentage of 15-minute time periods across conditions in which a pushup of adequate duration occurred. $\bar{c}$ means "with." (Reprinted from Gouvier et al., 1985, with permission of the American Congress of Rehabilitative Medicine.)

A classic paper by Gouvier et al. (1985) describes how the data of a single patient trial gave one interpretation when the original objective was addressed, but totally different interpretations when variations of the original objectives were assessed. This is shown in Figs. 101.1 to 101.4 below. Imagine how much distortion is possible in a more complex clinical trial.

Plotting the number of pushups per hour at each session (Fig. 101.1) shows an effect of the timing device but no lasting effect after it was removed. Plotting the mean duration of pushups (Fig. 101.2) shows that there was a lasting effect, but it was only observed after the intervention was stopped. The mean time per hour spent doing pushups combines aspects of frequency and duration and shows different results (Fig. 101.3). This shows a dramatic improvement when the signal device was implemented that partially persisted after it was withdrawn and implies a training effect.

The primary objective of the clinical trial was to train the patient to do pushups of at least 10 seconds duration every 15 minutes. When these data were plotted (Fig. 101.4) the results show an effect while the signal device was implemented, but no training or lasting effect occurred.

PART X

Publishing Clinical Data and Evaluating Published Literature

A man's judgment cannot be better than the information on which he has based it. Give him the truth and he may still go wrong when he has the chance to be right, but give him no news or present him only with distorted and incomplete data, with ignorant, sloppy or biased reporting, with propaganda and deliberate falsehoods, and you destroy his whole reasoning processes, and make him something less than a man.

—*Arthur Hays Sulzberger, American journalist*

I equate the function of critical journals of opinion with the spirit and method of science. Dissent is the journalist's way of asking the scientist's question: "Who says so?" "Can you prove it?" or, simply, "I don't believe it." It is the way by which individuals and societies protect themselves not only against oppressive orthodoxies but against foolish fallacies.

—*Carey McWilliams, American writer, editor*

Preparing Articles for Publication

At some point after data have been interpreted, it is often desirable to prepare an article for publication. In addition or alternatively, a summary report may be written for distribution to a limited group of individuals, or an extremely detailed final medical report may be prepared as part of a regulatory submission. The detail and scope of a report (as opposed to an article) vary enormously, from a cursory synopsis to a highly detailed report that includes most (or all) of the raw data obtained plus detailed statistical analyses. This chapter considers the example of an article that is prepared for publication, and Chapter 125 discusses final medical reports.

Many different types of articles may be prepared to present or discuss data and/or results from clinical studies. A number of types of published articles are listed in Table 102.1. Although most comments in this chapter are applicable to most categories listed in this table, the specific example used is an article that presents data or new information.

Before preparing the article, all data to be presented, interpretations, and extrapolations should generally have been worked out and should be clear to the author(s). Some parts of the article (e.g., introduction, methods) may be prepared while the clinical trial is still progressing. If more than one person prepares the actual document, a meeting to review each step in the process is usually essential. Assignments may be made at that time so that each individual understands and accepts his responsibilities in helping to prepare the final draft. It should be stressed that the basic approach, as well as contents and conclusions of the article, should be clear to all authors before they start to write the first draft. It is important to agree on the order of authorship or at least to identify the primary author to prevent problems from developing.

CHOOSING A JOURNAL

It will be advantageous to have chosen the specific journal that will be receiving the article prior to writing the article. This allows the author to fit the format and sometimes even the style to match the journal's requirements. Many biomedical journals have agreed to review articles prepared according to a standardized format (see International Committee of Medical Journal Editors, 1982, for a complete description). This convention has been accepted by more than 150 journals and should save a great deal of time for authors in revising manuscripts. Another alternative is initially to write the article in a general standardized format and to revise it after one or more drafts have been completed to accommodate the desired format of a specific journal.

The choice of journal usually involves many factors, some of which are listed in Table 102.2. Any one of these factors may be paramount in influencing an author to choose a particular journal, or a combination of factors may be involved.

Once a prospective journal or journals are chosen, it is useful to obtain their "instructions to authors." These are usually published in each issue or in selected issues of a journal. A document titled *A Compilation of Journal Instructions to Authors* (U.S. Department of Health and Human Services, Public Health Service, 1980) is a collection of many such guidelines to authors from biomedical journals.

TABLE 102.1 *Categories of published articles in clinical medicine[a,b]*

1. Article on methodology or procedure (new or previously described)
2. Article on a hypothesis (new or previously proposed)
3. Article on a mathematical model to describe events (e.g., ideal or real model that is new or was previously proposed)
4. Report to present an observation
5. Report to present data or new information[c]
6. Report on case study or studies, with or without substantial commentary
7. Review of a specific or general area or issue
8. Discussion of pros and cons about a current controversy or issue of medical interest
9. Editorial or commentary
10. Surveys of various groups (e.g., investigators, Institutional Review Boards, regulatory agencies, pharmaceutical companies)
11. Discussion from professional meetings, presented either verbatim or summarized
12. Proceedings of a professional meeting (e.g., symposium)
13. Abstracts and/or posters to be presented at a professional meeting
14. Discussion of public policy
15. Letter written to a journal (1) to present data on a hypothesis or proposal, (2) to comment on an article, or (3) to respond to another letter written to the journal
16. Theses

[a] The articles in most of these categories may support or challenge previous publications or provide new information or interpretations. Numerous other types of medical reports that are published do not generally present original data and are not described (e.g., book reviews).
[b] Various combinations of these types of articles are often published.
[c] This is probably the most common type of clinical publication.

PREPARING AN ARTICLE

Order of Writing Sections

There are many different approaches used by authors. An individual author's approach will often vary from article to article, depending on the particular data, type of article to be prepared, mood of the author, and other factors. There is no ideal method of "where to start" and "how to proceed," but a few general comments are relevant about the usual order in which sections are written:

1. The introduction, methods, and results sections may be written in any order, but the results must be presented in a way that addresses the objectives of the clinical trial as described in the introduction.
2. The discussion section is usually not written until after the above three sections are complete or close to completion.
3. The summary and/or abstract may be written at any time during preparation of the manuscript but is often prepared at or near the end of the process.

Use of Checklists

It is often helpful to use a checklist to ensure that all relevant information is included in an article that is being prepared. This may be utilized either before, during, or after a draft is prepared. Even experienced investigators and writers who may not have any difficulties in "dashing off" a polished manuscript may fail to include information that would be useful to the reader, especially in the methodology section. At present, it is relatively uncommon for journal editors or reviewers to utilize checklists to ensure that articles submitted for publication contain all of the elements that should be included.

Word Choice

The choice of words used in any scientific publication may vary from those with highly specific, concrete meanings to those with broader or more general denotations. Words or expressions that are vague should be expurgated from any draft. The most precise word or phrase should be chosen to convey the most specific meaning possible with the fewest connotations. Words

TABLE 102.2 *Selected factors to consider in choosing a journal to publish a medical paper*

1. Authors' assessment of the importance of the article
2. Reputation of journal
3. Circulation of journal[a]
4. Nature of the audience who read the journal (i.e., is it primarily a general audience with varied scientific interests or a specialized audience with highly focused interests)
5. Previous publications on the same topic by other authors in the journal
6. Previous publications by one or more of the current authors in the same journal
7. Journal's reputation for rapidity of reviewing manuscripts
8. Time required to communicate with the editors (e.g., a journal with offices on another continent may slow communications to an unacceptable degree)
9. Journal's reputation for rapidity of publishing manuscripts after an article is accepted
10. Cost of each page published and whether these charges may be waived if the author(s) cannot afford them
11. Desire to choose the journal of a particular society
12. Requirements posed by submitting an abstract on the same material to a society that requires that the full article first be sent to a specific journal
13. Desire to present the material at a specific meeting or conference, the proceedings of which will appear in a predetermined journal
14. Relationship of one of the authors with the editor or others associated with a particular journal
15. Desire for widespread publicity for the article, since certain journals are carefully read each week by news services
16. Frequency of publishing (e.g., quarterly, monthly, weekly)

[a] Journals published in the United States include this information in one issue each year (usually toward the end of the year).

with numerous connotations are more likely to be misinterpreted. In choosing the words to describe the interpretation of data, it is not always possible to use the most precise terms that one would like to choose, because the data may be uninterpretable, incomplete, or subject to more than one interpretation.

Choosing Tenses

In many aspects of article preparation, a few simple rules generally suffice to guide an author successfully through the maze of potential problems. For example, the question of which tense to use may readily be addressed in most situations with the following few rules.

1. Use the past tense to present your results.
2. Use the past tense to attribute results to others.
3. Use the present tense to refer to parts of your article.
4. Use the present tense to state facts originally reported by others.

Sources of Guidance

There are a number of excellent books that present details and approaches used to write a scientific article. Some of the best are by Huth (1982), CBE Style Manual Committee (1983), and Day (1983). The book by Day presents numerous practical suggestions for dealing with journal editors and reviewers.

SUMMARY AND INTRODUCTION OF AN ARTICLE

The relevant components of a summary are given in Fig. 102.1. The terms abstract and summary often have specific and distinct meanings but are also often used interchangeably and may refer to a variety of different types of synopses. If a separate abstract and summary must be written for an article, it is best to consult the instructions to authors as well as examples in the journal to distinguish accurately between the two.

A clear description of the clinical trial objectives and rationale for conducting the trial are the most important parts of the introduction. If the objectives are not clearly and adequately presented, it will be impossible for readers to know whether the trial design was appropriate and whether the data obtained are relevant. It is unfortunately true that the background and rationale for conducting trials are sometimes created "after the fact." This technique makes it appear that the authors were "clever fellows" when, in reality, the trial was conducted for totally different reasons and the explanation given in the article is a purely teleological and convenient explanation. The rationale for conducting many trials is not necessarily of central importance to the data obtained. The important point is whether the objectives were reasonable and were satisfactorily addressed by the trial design and protocol.

A checklist of the relevant components that may be included in an introduction is given in Fig. 102.2. Some authors prefer long introductions, but the current vogue in most journals is for short ones. The introduction should present a synopsis of background information that allows readers to understand the results without having to refer to other articles. It is generally worthwhile to include mention of important results in the introduction rather than trying to build suspense through the paper until the reader reaches the conclusion.

MATERIALS AND METHODS SECTION

Most shortcuts are taken in the materials and methods section. Every scientist and clinician who has tried to reproduce the work of another scientist (or clinician)

TOPICS FOR SUMMARY OR ABSTRACT

_____ Name and doses of medicine(s) studied plus route(s) of administration
_____ Essential background information
_____ Number of sites and number of patients studied
_____ Major objective(s) of trial
_____ Major method(s), techniques, apparatus used to obtain data
_____ Major parameter(s) used
_____ Synopsis of results
_____ Important findings or conclusions that are described in the article
_____ Major interpretation(s) and hypotheses
_____ Major implications and extrapolations of results

FIG. 102.1 Checklist of topics to consider for inclusion in the summary or abstract of a publication.

TOPICS FOR INTRODUCTION

_____ Historical background and pertinent literature
_____ Statement of the problem
_____ Methodological approach taken in this trial
_____ Rationale for the approach taken
_____ Previous experience with the medicine, medical device, or other treatment
_____ Description of the primary and secondary objectives
_____ Major results of the trial
_____ Reference to any preliminary publication or abstract

FIG. 102.2 Checklist of topics to consider for inclusion in the introduction of a publication.

based solely on information in the methods section knows how woefully inadequate it often is. It is rare for authors to include the necessary amount and level of detail required to explain fully the results and discussion and/or to repeat the clinical trial if desired. Of course, when authors send a manuscript to journal editors with detailed methodological descriptions, it is likely that a great deal of material will be cut. This issue is discussed in Chapter 106.

The specific information that is often helpful to include in the methods section is listed in Fig. 102.3. The ten categories are subdivided to indicate better the specific types of information that may be included. Several of these categories are rarely presented in currently published articles but would allow readers to evaluate better the quality of the trial and data obtained. Subheadings are often useful to divide this section into smaller parts for ease of reference. The number of patients who are described as "entered" in a clinical trial or who are involved at different stages should be defined clearly in either the materials and

methods or results section. A number of possible categories are listed in Table 79.3 for types of involvement and in Table 79.4 for definitions of enrollment (see Chapter 79).

RESULTS SECTION

Problems

Two major problems often encountered in the results section of publications are insufficient quantity of data on both safety and efficacy parameters and inadequate quality in terms of the data presentation. These problems may be addressed by critiquing one's own work and by discussing this issue with statisticians or clinical peers.

Expressing Results as Percent Change

An example of the latter problem is observed when data are only presented as "percentage change" or in other vague terms that do not provide sufficient detail to convert the percentage figures to values with real units. There are occasions, however, when expressing data as percentage change is acceptable (e.g., decrease in neuromuscular twitch tension). It is also relevant to indicate the percentage (or number) of patients who improved according to established criteria. If a report fails to provide these data and only presents average changes of the groups, it may be difficult to understand the clinical significance of the results. Summary tables and figures should be presented in the units measured, and a careful description of all manipulations of these data should be provided.

Quantitating Results

Authors should generally quantitate all important results presented (e.g., inflammation) even if only a qual-

TABLE 102.3 *Representative types of illustrations*

1. Drawings	10. Maps with various identifications
2. Photographs	11. Four-quadrant distribution charts
3. Line graphs	12. Gantt charts
4. Histograms	13. Computer graphics
5. Pie charts	14. Three-dimensional line graphs
6. Flow charts	15. Three-dimensional histograms
7. Decision trees	16. Scatter diagrams
8. Algorithms	17. Vector analyses
9. Schematic diagrams	

TABLE 102.4 *Parameters usually plotted along the X or Y axis*

Parameters that are usually plotted along the X axis	Parameters that are usually plotted along the Y axis
Dose of medicine versus	Response to medicine (i.e., activity)
Time versus	Concentration measured
Time versus	Response to medicine

TOPICS TO INCLUDE IN A MATERIALS
AND METHODS SECTION

Trial Design

_____ Basic design (parallel, crossover) and length of each period (baseline, dose ascension, treatment, taper, follow-up)

_____ Type of blind used and how it is defined (e.g., in a double-blind trial were the pharmacist, monitor, statistician, and other staff also blind?)

_____ Verification of the blind

_____ Type of randomization used

_____ Number of trial sites

_____ Number of patients planned per group

_____ Number of clinic visits per patient

_____ Type(s) of control groups used

_____ Conditions where concomitant medicines or other therapies were allowed or required

_____ Doses of medicines studied and route of administration

_____ Frequency and time of medicine administration

_____ Method(s) to adjust doses during ascension or taper, for adverse reactions, or for other reasons

_____ Frequency of allowing dose adjustments

Inclusion Criteria (includes "exclusion criteria")

_____ List or description of all pertinent inclusion criteria including the methods and criteria used to establish the diagnosis

_____ Replacement criteria for patients discontinued by investigator

_____ Replacement criteria for patients who drop out of their own volition

Efficacy Measurements

_____ Parameters that were measured

_____ Was global impression evaluated by the investigator and/or patient

_____ Frequency of measuring each efficacy variable

_____ Method(s) of measuring each efficacy variable

Safety Measurements

_____ Parameters that were measured

_____ Frequency of measuring each safety parameter

_____ Method(s) of measuring each safety parameter

Equipment

_____ Identification of all equipment used

_____ Type, manufacturer, manufacturer's address of relevant equipment

_____ Model number(s) of relevant equipment

_____ Number of tests, samples, or repeated determinations at each session

_____ Information on calibration of equipment

Medicines and Chemicals Used

_____ Identification of all medicines and chemicals, including the type of salts used

_____ Source or supplier, location

_____ Relevant chemical information (e.g., molecular weight of the heparin used)

_____ Storage conditions

_____ Dispensing techniques

_____ Methods used to modify dosages

_____ Concurrent medicines allowed or required

_____ Characteristics of placebos evaluated, to demonstrate that they were "identical" to trial medicines

FIG. 102.3 Checklist of potential topics for inclusion in the materials and methods section of a publication. Consult the instructions of the journal for additional information that may be required.

Pharmacokinetics/Medicine Levels
_____ Parameters that were measured and evaluated
_____ Methods used to collect and store samples, measure and evaluate the parameters
_____ Frequency of collecting samples, measuring and evaluating the parameters
_____ Influence of pharmacokinetic values on patient treatment or trial design (e.g., did medicine levels above a certain value require dosing to be modified?)
_____ Assays used to measure medicine levels

Trial Management
_____ Dates of the trial (initiation and completion)
_____ Location(s) of the trial (especially if different from sites listed for authors)
_____ Operational definitions used. Confirm that important terms are defined and used the same way as in the literature, unless there are reasons to use different definitions
_____ Individuals who participated in the trial (i.e., investigator's staff, sponsor, consultants, others)
_____ Discussion of any pretrial roundtable meetings
_____ Description of the major roles of staff who assisted in the trial
_____ Relevant qualifications of the staff (e.g., did anesthesiologists, board-certified anesthesiologists, or nurse anesthetists participate?)
_____ Description of monitoring procedures used
_____ Indicate if the trial monitor was blind to patient randomization
_____ Methods of data collection, processing, and quality assurance
_____ Measurement(s) of patient compliance
_____ Measurement of investigator compliance
_____ Method(s) of handling patient and/or investigator deviation from acceptable compliance
_____ Method(s) used to verify the trial blind
_____ Instructions given to patients
_____ Indicate whether a written informed consent was obtained from every patient
_____ Indicate whether monitors were blind to patient randomization and results of any interim analyses
_____ Indicate if and how the protocol changed during the trial
_____ Indicate if an identical protocol was followed at each site. Describe any differences
_____ Indicate if an end-of-trial questionnaire was used
_____ Indicate if the protocol was approved by an Ethics Committee/Institutional Review Board

Patient Demographics and Related Factors
_____ Number of patients screened, accepted, enrolled (plus reasons for failing screen or refusing to enter trial), and completing each period of the trial
_____ Number of patients discontinued from the trial by the investigator (plus reasons for discontinuation and demographic summary)
_____ Number of patients who dropped out of the trial (of their own volition) and demographic summary
_____ Source(s) of patients
_____ Number of patients in each treatment group at each site
_____ Summary statistics of demographics for (1) all patients entered, (2) all patients completed, and/or (3) all patients to be evaluated
   1. Age of patients enrolled of each sex (plus range or standard deviation)
   2. Sex of patients enrolled
   3. Pertinent physical characteristics (e.g., weight, height, race)
   4. Pertinent social, political, or economic characteristics (e.g., education, marital status, place of residence, income)
   5. Pertinent baseline/screen characteristics (e.g., vital signs)
_____ Compliance of patients with taking medicines as prescribed
_____ Compliance of patients with other aspects of the trial (e.g., keeping scheduled visits)

Data Analysis
_____ Describe how data were processed (e.g., double entry, quality-assured procedures) and analyzed
_____ Indicate power of the trial
_____ Describe which statistical tests were used
_____ Describe how the statistical tests were applied
_____ Discuss how data were handled for patient dropouts
_____ Discuss how data were handled to account for protocol violations
_____ Provide criteria used for patient improvement and/or medicine activity
_____ State number and type of any interim analyses performed
_____ Discuss any effect of interim analyses on the trial

FIG. 102.3 (*continued*)

itative scoring system is used (e.g., one plus to four plus). Relying on vague descriptive terms (e.g., inflammation was generally improved) is less meaningful to readers. Another alternative is to specify the number of patients with improvement or deterioration in addition to presenting means or other values. It is well known that mean values can be quite misleading even when standard errors or standard deviations are included. Median values are often more appropriate to use and often provide information that is meaningful clinically.

Information To Include

A number of specific types of information and data that may be included in the results section are listed in Fig. 102.4. When only a small number of patients are studied, the presentation of raw data is usually particularly helpful in understanding the results. It would be beneficial to interested readers if more data than could be included in a paper were sent to a group that would serve as a repository and provide these data to interested readers for a reasonable fee. This concept is discussed further in Chapter 108.

Patients Who Were Discontinued or Who Dropped Out

The interpretation of a clinical trial may be entirely different if the data of all patients who were discontinued from a trial are included. An example of this is illustrated by the Department of Clinical Epidemiology and Biostatistics, McMaster University (1981). On the other hand, there are a large number of reasons for patient dropouts, and the investigators may believe that it is not scientifically correct to include any (or all) of the dropouts in the analyses. The statistician may be in agreement. One solution is to analyze and present (or discuss) the data both including and excluding patient dropouts and discontinuations. It is important to state what decisions were made regarding dropouts and discontinuations and why they were made. Chapter 31 discusses this topic in detail.

Protocol Violations

An additional complication in presenting the results concerns patients who took doses that were protocol violations or were inappropriate: (1) the dose prescribed was inadequate to elicit the desired effect fully, (2) the dose given violated the protocol by being given at the wrong time or in the wrong amount, or (3) concurrent medicines were given that were protocol violations and were believed to contaminate the data. Approaches to these issues and presentation of other protocol violations should be discussed with a statistician.

A movement away from p values and toward the use of confidence intervals is apparent in numerous medical journals (Braitman, 1988; Gardner and Altman, 1988). This is a positive step because it provides readers with more information for interpreting results. For example, merely stating that a comparison is not significant does not tell you whether the p value is 0.055 or 0.20; illustrating confidence intervals gives a still better view of how different the data are that are being compared.

TOPICS FOR RESULTS SECTION

_____ Patient accountability (number entered, dropped, completed; reasons for patient dropout and for investigator discontinuation)
_____ Modifications of the protocol
_____ Violations of the protocol
_____ Safety data (e.g., laboratory examinations, adverse reactions, electrocardiograms, physical and plasma examinations, plasma levels of medicine)
_____ Efficacy data (analyses of data from all completed patients and from other defined groups of patients)
_____ Pharmacokinetic data
_____ Placebo data (e.g., magnitude of the response, effects observed)
_____ Data from other control groups
_____ Problems encountered in the trial
_____ Missing data (e.g., quantity, areas where it occurs)

FIG. 102.4 Checklist of potential topics for inclusion in the results section of a publication.

DISCUSSION SECTION

Purposes

From the perspective of presenting the interpretation of data, the discussion is the most important part of an article. This is the section where (1) data are interpreted, (2) interpretations are extrapolated, (3) additional hypotheses are presented or modified, (4) other clinical trials are critiqued, and (5) speculation (within limits) is presented. Some authors propose other experiments or trials that are suggested by their outcomes and may even indicate which trials they will undertake next.

Responsibilities To Readers

Regardless of the many possible directions and approaches an author may adopt in the discussion section, the author(s) have certain responsibilities to readers of the article. Some of these are:

1. Findings in the present clinical trial should be compared with those of previous studies that are related, and significant points of difference (and agreement) should be noted and discussed.
2. If the objectives of the trial were not achieved, the reason(s) for this should be described.
3. In addition to the interpretations discussed, alternative reasonable and plausible interpretations should also be presented. The pros and cons of each may be included.
4. Data from all treatments and groups evaluated should be compared and any unexpected findings discussed.

Methods To Create a Discussion Section

Various aspects of a discussion are presented in Fig. 102.5. A few techniques that may be helpful in developing discussions are described below.

TOPICS FOR DISCUSSION SECTION

Within This Trial
_____ Brief summary (but not a recapitulation) of the major result(s)
_____ Discuss which aspects are of statistical significance
_____ Discuss which aspects are of clinical significance (both theoretical and practical)
_____ Discuss which aspects have statistical significance but do not have clinical significance
_____ Discuss how the data might affect future scientific/clinical trials
_____ Discuss how the data might affect future clinical practice of medicine
_____ Present conclusions and interpretations
_____ Present exceptions to the interpretations or conclusions
_____ Present aspects of the trial that are unclear or questionable

Comparison with Other Trials
_____ Discuss how major results compare with those reported by others
_____ Comment on reports that do not agree with the present trial and indicate possible reasons for differences
_____ Trace historical development of an idea, model, hypothesis, treatment, or other aspect relating to the trial
_____ Relate the current trial to the relevant field of medicine
_____ Comment on the methodologies and equipment used by others versus those used in the present trial (e.g., validation, state-of-the-art, limitations)
_____ Comment on the statistical analyses used by others versus those used in the present trial (e.g., power, number of patients, types of tests used)

Implications
_____ Discuss questions raised that cannot be answered
_____ Propose new hypotheses, models, or questions to be studied in the future
_____ Identify which comments reflect the author's view and which reflect "general consensus." Reference the latter views (if possible)
_____ Present any extrapolations

Conclusion(s)
_____ Present pros and cons of all major conclusions as fairly as possible
_____ End the article with a brief synopsis

FIG. 102.5 Checklist of potential topics for inclusion in the discussion section of a publication.

1. Develop algorithms to sort mentally through complex trial objectives, results, interpretations, possible hypotheses, or extrapolations.
2. Utilize "if, then" exercises in which the author begins a statement with "if" and then adds a phrase beginning with "then." This encourages speculation about various alternative or more detailed (or broad) interpretations.
3. Determine if other trials can be envisioned that would either confirm or deny a new hypothesis or interpretation.
4. If the current interpretation differs from previous results, evaluate possible reasons for the discrepancy. Examine each of the experimental conditions, parts of the trial design, and manner in which the trial was conducted.
5. If comparing one's results with other trials appears to be difficult or complex, consider presenting a table of all other published trials (or a selected subset) with pertinent parameters, results, conclusions, interpretations, and other information.
6. Present a table of various possible interpretations of the present trial with the pros and cons of each.
7. Present a table with pertinent details on each of the methods used in the present or other trials. Choose categories that highlight important similarities and differences. Other aspects of a trial may also be presented in this type of comparative framework.

ILLUSTRATIONS

The basic type of illustrations used in medical articles are generally well known. Most published illustrations are examples of the types shown in Table 102.3. Many other types of illustrations are used in special circumstances. Cleveland and McGill (1985) describe many newer statistical methods that may be used to present data, such as box plots, two-tiered error bars, scatterplot smoothing, dot charts, and graphing on a log-base-2 scale. An informative reference on creative illustrations of data was written by Tufte (1983). A recent book, *Presentation of Clinical Data* (Spilker and Schoenfelder, 1990), presents over 650 figures, graphs, and tables that are intended as prototypes of major formats. Variations of most of these formats are illustrated and the reason why each is included is clearly indicated.

Selected Conventions

There are usually conventions as to which parameters should be on the abscissa (horizontal or X axis) and which should be along the ordinate (vertical or Y axis) in a line graph. A few examples are shown in Table 102.4.

Figures must be used judiciously to illustrate results accurately in an optimal manner. Care should be taken to avoid putting too much information in an illustration, or it will confuse rather than enlighten the reader. Inappropriate types of illustrations or inappropriate scales along the ordinate or abscissa will tend to distort the data and make reader comprehension more difficult. Most individuals are familiar with the cliché of "Figures don't lie, but some liars figure." Yankelowitz (1980) showed in a humorous manner how data may be distorted in figures prepared for publication.

REVIEWING A MANUSCRIPT

A simpler checklist than those described in this chapter was proposed by Dixon et al. (1983). Their list is shown in Fig. 102.6. After a completed draft of an article is prepared and reviewed with (or without) checklists for completeness, there are usually a number of additional steps to follow before it is submitted to a journal. In addition to seeking critiques from peers, there are a number of considerations related to content and format that are described in Table 102.5.

TABLE 102.5 *Criteria to use in reviewing a manuscript draft*[a]

A. Related to content
  1. Consider overall flow and content in terms of the article's objectives
  2. Evaluate each section of the article to ensure that it contains sufficient information and attains an appropriate balance of specific information, interest, and readability
  3. Evaluate each paragraph in terms of its content and placement within the section
  4. Confirm that sufficient data and measurements of variability are included
B. Related to format
  1. Evaluate the format and organization of the overall article and within each section. Consider the use of subdivisions within each section
  2. Determine if there should be additional (or fewer) tables or figures
  3. Determine if some tables could be made into figures (or vice versa)
  4. Confirm that all tables and figures are referred to and adequately described in the text
  5. Confirm that all references are listed in the text and that they are listed in a consistent manner according to the journal's requirements
  6. Confirm that all references in the text to other publications are listed in the bibliography and that they are all in the same format. Confirm exact details with original sources
  7. Review tenses of all words and confirm that the correct tenses were used
  8. Confirm that all tables, figures, footnotes, and references adhere to the journal's requirements
  9. Confirm that marginal notes are included to indicate where tables and figures should be inserted in the article
  10. Confirm that all pages are numbered consecutively

[a] It is advantageous to reread some articles several times, each time concentrating on different criteria or issues.
[b] A number of general considerations in writing and polishing a draft protocol are listed in Table 34.1.

A CHECKLIST OF DATA THAT SHOULD BE CONSIDERED FOR INCLUSION IN A CLINICAL TRIAL REPORT

TITLE
Indicate design of study and drug(s)
Incorporate indexible words
Maintain a balance between detail and attention-seeking qualities

SUMMARY
First sentence should catch the reader's attention
Must be factual

INTRODUCTION
Why do the study? (background)
What is the principal question being asked?

PATIENTS
Entry criteria (disease and disease activity)
Numbers
Exclusions
Methods of randomization
Source
Ethics committee approval, patient consent

DRUGS
Dosages
Duration
Times of administration
Additional therapy allowed

METHODS
Clinical measurements—objective, subjective, reproducibility, monitoring of side effects, radiology
Laboratory measurements—hematology, immunology, routine clinical biochemistry, specialized biochemistry, reproducibility
Drop-outs—replacement criteria, handling of data from drop-outs
Escape clauses
Statistics—tests to be used, power

RESULTS
Changes in clinical and laboratory assessments
Drop-outs—numbers, reasons
Report other side effects
Statistics—pretreatment matching of groups, treatment group comparisons, improvement within each treatment group, power
Individual patient responses to therapy
Was 'blindness' maintained?

DISCUSSION
Advantages and disadvantages of the therapy under investigation
Side effects—serious, minor, unusual
Future work?
Therapeutic implications

CONCLUSIONS
Answer the question set out in the introduction

ACKNOWLEDGEMENTS

REFERENCES
Include references for non-routine methods
Refer to review articles in preference to a series of papers

FIG. 102.6 Checklist for preparation of articles for publication by Dixon, Smith, and Evans. (Reprinted by permission of *British Journal of Rheumatology* from Dixon et al., 1983.)

Common Deficiencies

In reviewing one's own manuscript, it is important to confirm that common problems are not present. A 10% sample of English language clinical papers published in 1980 were analyzed (Meinert et al., 1984), and the major deficiencies found were:

1. The rationale for the sample size used was not stated.
2. The primary outcome measure was not designated.
3. There was an inadequate description of the method of treatment assignment.
4. There was a discrepancy in the number of patients enrolled with the number used in analysis.
5. The source of support was not stated.

Each of these deficiencies occurred in over half the clinical trials analyzed.

Many stylistic rules differ from journal to journal, but must be considered and followed before the manuscript is sent for editorial review. Failure to do this may bias the editor or reviewer against the paper.

TABLE 102.6 *Selected details to check in a manuscript and cover letter sent to a journal for publication*

A. Overall
  1. Name of journal listed in cover letter
  2. Pages are numbered consecutively
  3. All typing is double spaced
  4. The appropriate number of copies is sent
  5. A copy is kept by the author
  6. Any sections to be set in small type should be marked
  7. Running title and key words included
  8. Footnotes included with indications in text of where they belong
  9. All measurements are provided in appropriate units
B. Tables and figures
  1. Each is on a separate sheet
  2. Each is numbered consecutively using appropriate numbers (e.g., arabic, roman)
  3. Appropriate formats are used according to journal's style
  4. Places to insert each are shown in text
  5. High-quality photographs are enclosed with the first author's name written on the back along the edge. Consider putting a small piece of tape over the name to prevent smudging or transfer of ink
  6. Top of photographs are marked, if necessary
  7. Color figures or photographs are discussed with editors before mailing
  8. All technical details in the Instructions to Authors are followed
  9. Separate figure legends are prepared and all symbols and marks are explained
  10. Permission for reproduction is obtained and indicated in the text, and a copy is enclosed with the manuscript
C. References
  1. Correspondence of names and years with those given in the text, or, all numbers in the text correspond with correct reference citations
  2. No references are listed that are not cited and vice versa
  3. Abbreviations of journal titles follow the journal's policy
  4. Sequence and style of references follow journal's policy

Some of the points usually described in the Instructions to Authors are indicated in Table 102.6.

PROOFING MANUSCRIPTS

Proofing the final copy of an article prior to printing is an activity that requires concentration and attention to detail. Therefore, it should be done in a suitable environment. For most people, this means relative quiet and freedom from distractions or other competing thoughts.

Objectives

The objectives of proofing an article are to confirm (and correct if necessary) that (1) nothing is deleted, (2) sentences flow smoothly and achieve the desired clarity, (3) incorrect words or typographical errors are

TABLE 102.7 *Objectives and techniques of reading galley proofs*

Objectives	Techniques to achieve objectives
1. Confirm that all paragraphs, tables, figures, titles, and major sections are included and are sequenced in the correct order	1. Skim original and proof to confirm that all parts of the article are included
2. Confirm that all sentences, words, and specific details (e.g., footnotes, table legends, references) of the original manuscript are included in the proof	2. Read proof for content (meaning) and compare with original after every few lines or sentences
3. Determine that the placement and size of tables and figures are acceptable	3. Review layout of tables and figures for appropriateness and suitability
4. Confirm that there are no typographical errors present	4. Read galley proof line by line. Pronounce each word out loud or silently, mentally dividing multisyllable words into individual syllables to confirm that their spelling is correct[a]
5. Determine if any modifications are required to the proof	5. Add clarifications, information, references, "notes added in proof," or modify statements[b]

[a] It is often useful to cover all galley proof lines that are either above or below the line being read. Read each line of the galley proof forwards and/or backwards (i.e., read the words in each line from right to left) or alternate between lines, reading one forwards and the other backwards. Reading the lines forward should not give the reader any meaning of the words read that relate to the subject of the text. This reading should be of isolated words or groups of words. If this type of reading is not possible or easy for the reader to achieve, then it is preferable to read each line backwards.

[b] Publishers desire to keep changes by the authors to an absolute minimum.

not present, (4) tables and figures are inserted in the correct place and are of appropriate size, and (5) there is consistency throughout the article in punctuation, grammar, and details of format. Under exceptional circumstances, a "Note Added in Proof" is appropriate. This should only be included if it provides important new information for understanding the article.

Three useful approaches to proofing are described:

Method A: Thrice Through

Read the proof three times using a different technique each time. The first time the proof is read, confirm inclusion of all paragraphs, sentences, tables, and figures. The second time, read each sentence for meaning and inclusion of all words, confirming that punctuation is correct. The third time read each word individually or in groups of two to three words, checking only for spelling. This last reading may be performed by reading each line of the text (and tables) either forwards or backwards. Ensure that if the words are read forward the person proofing the manuscript focuses on the spelling of isolated words rather than on the meaning or context of the words. One of the most effective means of ensuring that each word is spelled correctly in the proof is to read each line backwards, mentally dividing multisyllable words or even reciting the words out loud. This time-consuming technique is not usually necessary in most situations.

Method B: Twice Through

Read the proof twice. During the first reading think about both of the objectives described above for the first two separate readings. During the second time through the proof, read each word or pair of words as described in the third reading described above.

Method C: Twice Through

Read the proof twice. The initial two readings described in the first approach listed should be followed, and the third approach for reading the proof is omitted.

As indicated above, there are various techniques used for proofing an article, and it is usually advantageous to use several of them. Different types of articles often benefit from use of different proofing techniques or other combinations of these techniques. Several are listed in Table 102.7. Many authors regard proofing as a bothersome chore that should be handled by their assistant, secretary, or publisher. This process is certainly also performed by publishers, although the quality of their proofing varies. More importantly, proofing is a final opportunity for the author to confirm that each word chosen is correct and appropriately conveys each thought with clarity and accuracy. Large parts of an article should not be rewritten during proofing, but changing a single word or phrase where necessary may substantially improve the clarity of an important point.

EDITING (i.e., COMPILING) A BOOK

Although most medical books identify one or more editors, their major function is to compile chapters written by various authors. The editors serve as content

TABLE 102.8 *Forms for tracking progress of a book project*

A. Soliciting authors

Chapter number	Chapter title	Prospective authors (in order of desirability)	Telephone number	Called (date)	Issues	Date to respond	Letter with prospectus sent?

B. Handling draft manuscripts (or chapter outlines)

Chapter number	Chapter title	Senior author	Draft received	Status of draft	Status of chapter	Editor's to do	Date to complete

C. Handling final manuscript

Chapter number	Final manuscript rec'd (date)	Acknowledgement sent (date)	Name and title OK? (date)	Is the content OK?	Are the references OK?	Communication with authors	Is style OK for publisher?	Copy made for publisher

editors in that they review and evaluate the content of each chapter and may request changes in content or even style. Even though some editors correct grammatical errors, this function is appropriately handled at a later stage by copy editors.

Many approaches may be used to compile a book including (1) collecting manuscripts presented at a conference, (2) transcribing talks presented at a conference, (3) asking one's friends and colleagues to contribute manuscripts on a general or specific theme, and (4) creating a table of contents and single approach to

be used in organizing and writing each chapter before approaching prospective authors. If the last method is being considered, then obtaining an outline from each author is strongly advised. It is easier for authors to modify their approach if they have only written a one- or two-page outline than if they have already prepared a 20- or 30-page typewritten manuscript.

To expedite progress on the preparation of a book, a number of forms may be created to follow the progress of various components. Three related forms are shown in Table 102.8.

Systems to Evaluate Published Data

There are several reasons why most individuals closely involved with clinical trials read and evaluate publications of other clinical investigators. These reasons include the desire (1) to evaluate how reliable and relevant others' data and conclusions are, (2) to learn new information, hypotheses, and developments, and (3) to determine how other trials may affect the interpretation of his or her own trials that have been previously conducted or may be conducted in the future. Other trials may provide information on problems to avoid, methods to use, pointers to consider, and possible hypotheses or interpretations to test. It is therefore important to judge the quality of trials and to differentiate between trials that are well and poorly conducted, interpreted, and reported.

USING PERSONAL VERSUS STANDARD APPROACHES

Most people who read the medical literature develop individual skills in evaluating articles through direct experience, discussions with colleagues, and information acquired in other ways. Few individuals ever approach this topic in a systematic manner. With time, experience, and practice, the need for formal training on this subject usually disappears. Nonetheless, there are occasionally reasons why experienced individuals desire to perform a systematic evaluation of published reports. This chapter presents a series of published systems to evaluate medical reports. Proposals that relate to a coding system for clinical trials (e.g., Bellamy, 1984) or to a classification of clinical trials (e.g., Bailar et al., 1984b) are not discussed. The approaches presented can be used by newcomers to medical science in critiquing the literature. It is hoped that this presentation will also provide pointers to experienced readers.

Critiquing One's Own Data versus Those of Others

There are two major differences between critiquing one's own interpretation of data and critiquing the published results of another investigator. The first is the bias one usually has when evaluating one's own work and the difficulty of viewing it objectively. The second concerns the limitation in quantity of data and ancillary information that is available about published trials. Apart from these factors, the approaches one uses are generally similar. As a result of the general similarity, most of the techniques, methods, and checklists presented in previous chapters about how to develop and critique one's own interpretation, plus how to prepare an article for publication, are also relevant for this chapter on evaluating published data and results.

COMMON PROBLEMS

In reading articles in any area of medicine, it is helpful to be familiar with common problems that occur in publications. Since there are an extremely large number of possible problems that could be discussed, only a few broad areas are mentioned. Serious shortcomings may be found in any section of a publication and often reflect an absence of information rather than a distortion, bias, or error in what was presented. Table 103.1 lists problems that begin when the authors initially decide to prepare an article. Few problems are

TABLE 103.1 *Common problems with clinical publications that relate to their preparation*

A. Introduction
 1. Insufficient description of the objectives
 2. Excessive amount of background information
B. Methodology
 1. Insufficient detail or inadequate description of information presented
 2. Omitting information on certain topics (e.g., trial management)
C. Results
 1. Presenting derived data without adequate information on actual numbers or raw data
 2. Presenting data in an ambiguous manner
 3. Presenting insufficient efficacy data to allow the reader to arrive at his or her own interpretation
 4. Presenting insufficient data on adverse reactions to address many basic questions
D. Discussion
 1. Some discussions lack conciseness and a clear organization
 2. Results may only be compared with other papers that are favorable to the author's interpretation
 3. All of the factors expected to influence the results obtained may not be considered
 4. Data may be extrapolated to patient populations with an insufficient basis for such statements
 5. Too many tangential issues may be presented

described that relate to clinical trial design (e.g., inadequate power) or to the conduct of a trial (e.g., excessive amount of missed patient visits and data). Problems relating to data analysis are not presented in this table. The types of trial designs published in prestigious journals have been shown to include a high percentage of weak trial designs (Fletcher and Fletcher, 1979).

It is crucial to differentiate the quality of a clinical trial's *design* from the quality of its *conduct* and also from the quality of the *interpretation* of data obtained. Any one or two of these elements may be excellent, but unless all three are at a high standard the clinical trial results will not be completely convincing. Various permutations of the adequacy of a clinical trial are possible, based on assessment(s) of the components of these three elements.

INFORMAL APPROACHES TO EVALUATING PUBLICATIONS

Most people who read the medical literature follow an informal approach. Each clinical trial requires that a different set of questions be kept in mind by the reader. Many of these questions are basic ones that the reader brings to any article, and others are suggested by the nature of the article itself. This section comments only on the former (generic) type of questions.

Each reader has probably formulated a personalized series of generally similar questions that are posed (either consciously or not) before, during, and after reading an article. In fact, reaching a decision to read

(or even skim) an article means that it has already passed a significant hurdle, since scientists and clinicians are only able to read a relatively small number of available articles. Most readers use multiple systems to decide which articles to read. There are many sources of information listing which articles are available. Some of these sources also present abstracts of the articles.

Questions To Pose

When reading an article, most readers will pose questions, and this may also occur after they have finished reading the article. A list of some general questions that apply to most papers is listed in Table 103.2. These questions refer both to the evaluation of the article's contents, how the article affects the reader, and to a decision about the procedures that the reader will follow after completing the article.

The most general aspects of a clinical trial to evaluate are:

1. What is the value of the trial in terms of new knowledge?
2. What is the overall quality of the data obtained?
3. Is the quantity of data obtained sufficient to address the objectives and to support the conclusions?
4. Were the analyses appropriately chosen and performed?
5. Are the interpretations and conclusions justified?
6. Are the extrapolations reasonable?
7. Will this article affect the reader's research, clinical practice, or other activity?

To obtain the answers to these questions each person develops their own approach. Rennels et al. (1987) developed a computer-based model. In this approach an expert was asked to think aloud as he read an article. He related certain basic elements to the context in which the clinical trial was conducted. For example, (1) "what type of patients seek care at the hospital where the research was done? (2) what is the track record of the author? (3) how qualified are the allied specialities that are involved in patient care but are not the subject of investigation, for example, postoperative nursing care? (4) what are the exact technical details for the treatments being compared (e.g., two trials may compare the same medicines but the dose and dosing schedules might differ)?"

SYSTEMS TO EVALUATE PUBLICATIONS

Numerous systems have been proposed and used to evaluate published articles. These systems vary greatly in complexity, intended purpose, and useful-

TABLE 103.2 *Selected questions to consider while reading and evaluating clinical publications*

A. Relating to the clinical trial design, methodology, and conduct
 1. What type of trial was reported (e.g., case report, historical control, double-blind randomized control)?
 2. Was the primary objective reasonable and worthwhile to evaluate?
 3. Was the trial design appropriate to address the primary objective?.
 4. Was the protocol well conceived?
 5. Were the assumptions reasonable?
 6. Were the definitions used acceptable?
 7. Were the endpoints used clinically relevant?
 8. Is the method measuring what it claims to have measured?
 9. Were the methods and research tools used validated, and are they well accepted?
 10. Were the methods and research tools used appropriately, and was their degree of variability presented?
 11. How was the trial conducted (e.g., careful attention to detail, sloppily), and can the technical quality be assessed?
 12. Were there any glaring problems in the trial?
 13. What was the magnitude of protocol violations, and how much influence does it have on the interpretation(s)?
 14. Was the trial protocol changed during its conduct?
B. Relating to the data collection, analysis, and interpretation
 1. Were the data collected, processed, and analyzed well statistically?
 2. If some data were collected from two or more sources, did they differ, by how much, and why? What are the probable reasons for this, and are values for variability given?
 3. Were sufficient data collected, and were the data well presented in the article?
 4. Is there agreement between results obtained by various techniques, people, and methods?
 5. Are the results similar to those from other trials?
 6. Are there any significant omissions in the data collected?
 7. Were positive results related to the major trial objective(s) or only to secondary ones or to a subgroup analysis?
 8. Were reasonable interpretations considered, and do they make sense clinically?
 9. Were the extrapolations that were made reasonable?
 10. Overall, was the paper convincing?
C. Relating to the reader
 1. Are there findings that impact on the reader's previous trials?
 2. Are there findings that impact on the reader's planned (or current) trials?
 3. Are there conclusions or findings in the paper that should affect the reader's present medical practice or other activities?
D. Relating to the reader's processing and storage of the paper
 1. Is there anyone I know who should read this material? If so, send a copy with a note or letter or merely identify the reference in a letter
 2. Do I want to have a copy of this paper in my files? If so, make a photocopy, tear out the article, or request a reprint
 3. Do I want to write comments on my copy or elsewhere?
 4. What is the best way to file this paper? Is it necessary to cross index this reference for ease of later retrieval?

ness; they are described here as simple and more formal systems. A spectrum is shown in Fig. 103.1. It is useful to use one (or more) systems to judge or evaluate publications when:

1. It is done as a learning experience and the goal is to familiarize oneself (or one's students) with one or a few scales.
2. One (or more) scales are used to evaluate grants.
3. One is interested in placing a few codes or comments on each paper or report to assist in filing or to help remember one's assessment at a later date.
4. The purpose is to judge the quality of the papers to be included in a meta-analysis or traditional type of review.
5. Editors of journals wish to evaluate manuscripts submitted.

All scales used should be validated. Validation methods are discussed in Chapter 43.

Simple Systems

There are a few simple systems that can be used to review papers qualitatively. These approaches may be used informally, or they may be printed on separate forms, written in the margins of the paper itself, or entered in a computer file.

The specific checklists presented in Chapter 102 to plan one's own publication may also be used in evaluating published data to ensure that all relevant parts are included. Journal reviewers could be provided with checklists if journals establish a policy to include certain types of information or presentations.

1. A few simple types of evaluations that may be used in reading the literature include an assessment of the overall value of the paper for the reader based on a scale of (1) "relevant" or "not relevant" (i.e., a two-point scale), (2) "great importance, some importance, little importance, no importance" (i.e., a four-point scale), or (3) "1 to 10" (i.e., a ten-point scale). Other scales may be used. The score may be written on the front of the paper, on index cards, or entered in a computer. Scores may be categorized and then filed by the article's title, subject, author, or another category. Computer filing systems allow rapid cross indexing through use of multiple key terms, whereas filing in drawers or cabinets usually restricts an individual to use of only the single most appropriate term chosen at that time.

2. A few comments may be handwritten on the article or on a separate card, or comments may be filed on a computer disk, without any reference to a scoring system.

3. A simple evaluation form may be preprinted on blank pages. This approach may be useful to some authors who wish to retrieve information when preparing or reviewing an article or for other purposes. Two examples of a simple form that may be used in conjunction with a computer (or without one) are:

A. Reference
 Key terms

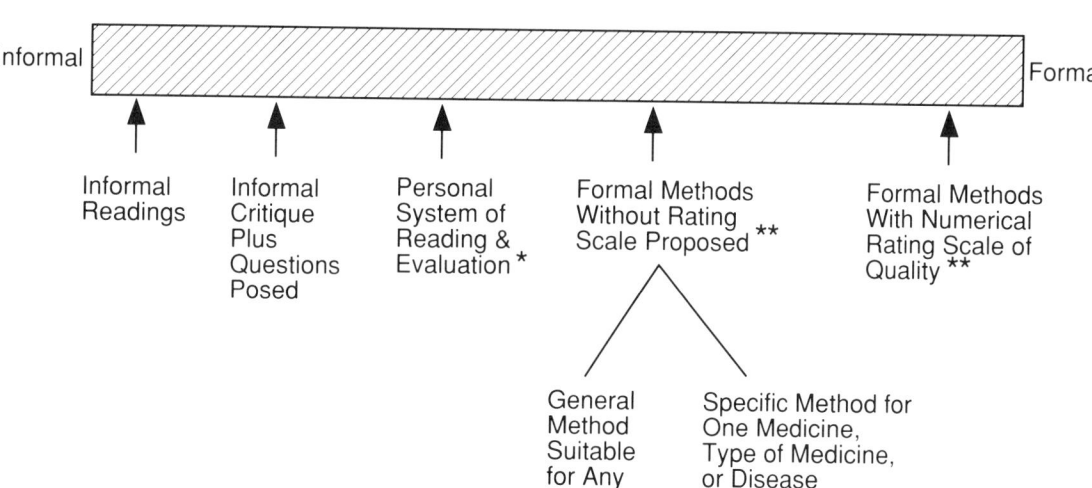

FIG. 103.1 Spectrum of methods used to evaluate articles in the medical literature. *, also varies along a similar continuum from informal to formal approaches; **, these methods may or may not be validated. The degree of validation also varies along a continuum.

Objectives of clinical trial
Were objectives achieved?
Implications for my research
Implications for my medical practice
Implications for medical practice (in general)
Problems with paper
How important is the paper for me?
Category used for filing
B. Area (aspect) of study reviewed
   Key terms
   Points made
   Problems/shortcomings/qualifications
   Impression(s)

Among the most common problems encountered in the literature are clinical trials in which the number of patients enrolled is too small to have adequate power. Young et al. (1983) have published sample size nomograms that easily allow someone who is interpreting clinical data to determine whether negative clinical studies have enrolled an adequate number of patients.

More Formal Systems

There are numerous published checklists, series of questions, or criteria that various authors have used or proposed for use in evaluating the clinical literature. A number of these systems (see Table 103.3) are presented in their entirety.

Method of Mahon and Daniel. Mahon and Daniel (1964) proposed a four-step method to evaluate reports of medicine trials. Their process consists of applying the following four criteria:

1. Were adequate controls used?
2. Were treatments randomized?

3. Were medicine effects measured objectively? This usually involves double-blind techniques.
4. Were results analyzed statistically?

Their publication states that these questions are meant to provide a simple method for practicing physicians and others who are relatively unskilled in analyzing clinical publications. They used this straightforward approach to evaluate 203 articles published in the *Canadian Medical Association Journal* over a 5-year period. Their method has been used by others in assessing the quality of clinical publications (e.g., Reiffenstein et al., 1968).

Method of Lionel and Herxheimer. Lionel and Herxheimer (1970) presented a checklist (Fig. 103.2, pg. 779) that they used to evaluate 141 clinical trials in four medical journals. The conclusion of their checklist provides a final assessment of whether the article is definitely acceptable, probably acceptable, or un-

TABLE 103.3 *Selected authors who have proposed criteria, checklists, or other methods to evaluate clinical studies[a]*

1. Mahon and Daniel (1964), see text
2. Lionel and Herxheimer (1970), Fig. 103.2
3. Horwitz and Feinstein (1979), Table 103.4
4. Levine (1980), Fig. 103.3
5. Chalmers et al. (1981), Fig. 103.4
6. University of Rochester Clinical Pharmacology Group (Weintraub, 1982), Fig. 103.5
7. DerSimonian et al. (1982), Table 103.5
8. Haynes et al. (1983), Fig. 103.6
9. Bailar et al. (1984a), Table 103.6
10. Evans and Pollock (1985), Table 103.7
11. Meinert (1986), Table 103.8

[a] Suggestions are also presented by the author in this chapter and in the checklists shown in Chapter 102. Other checklists and methods to evaluate published trials are discussed in the text.

acceptable. This method has been used by others (e.g., Ravikiran et al., 1980).

Method of Horwitz and Feinstein. Horwitz and Feinstein (1979) proposed a set of 12 standards to apply to retrospective case-control research. These standards are listed in Table 103.4 and were used to evaluate 85 clinical trials.

Trial Assessment Procedure Scale (TAPS) Method of Levine. This method was proposed by Dr. J. Levine in 1980 to evaluate the quality of a study (J. Levine, *personal communication*). The form used is more detailed than most of the others and is one of the few that contains a scoring system. It is relatively easy and rapid to use, especially after some practice. This form is shown in a slightly abridged form (Fig. 103.3, pg. 780) and may readily be used to rate protocols as well

TABLE 103.4 *Methodological criteria of Horwitz and Feinstein for judging case-control research*

1. Predetermined method (i.e., the established method should be chosen prior to obtaining and analyzing the data)
2. Specification of the agent (i.e., the precise definition of what constitutes exposure to the purported causal agent must be identified, and this should be done prior to obtaining and analyzing the data)
3. Unbiased data collection [i.e., the individual who collects the data should be unaware of the objective(s) of the clinical trial as well as the identity of the patient as case or control]
4. Anamnestic equivalence (i.e., the differences in a patient's ability or incentive to recall previous exposure to the purported causal agent should be minimized between the cases and controls)
5. Avoidance of constrained cases (i.e., bias is to be prevented in the choice of cases by applying standards that may affect the makeup of cases more than controls. Criteria for exclusions should be applied to both cases and controls)
6. Avoidance of constrained controls (i.e., bias is to be prevented in the choice of controls by applying standards that may affect the makeup of controls more than cases. Criteria for exclusions should be applied to both cases and controls)
7. Equal diagnostic examination (i.e., diagnosis of the disease should be made with similar procedures and criteria in both cases and controls)
8. Equal diagnostic surveillance (i.e., diagnosis of the disease should be made in patients who have been exposed to similar prehospital surveillance procedures and criteria in both cases and controls)
9. Equal demographic susceptibility (i.e., confirmation should be made of comparable demographic characteristics in both cases and controls)
10. Equal clinical susceptibility (i.e., confirmation should be made of equal number or magnitude of risk factors for the disease in both cases and controls)
11. Avoidance of protopathic bias (i.e., it is possible that a disease is present in a subclinical and unrecognized form prior to use of the suspected causative agent. This agent may be wrongly associated with the disease at a later date. Alternatively, if an early, unrecognized manifestation of the disease leads to a certain treatment, then the eventual manifestation of the disease may be blamed on the treatment)
12. "Community control" for Berkson's bias[a] (i.e., this bias occurs because people who are both exposed and diseased are more likely to be admitted to hospital than other groups)

Headings are reprinted by permission of *American Journal of Medicine* from Horwitz and Feinstein (1979).
[a] This criteria was stated to be optional.

as published clinical trials. Copies are available from Dr. Jerome Levine, Maryland Psychiatric Research Center, University of Maryland, P. O. Box 21247, Catonsville, MD 21228.

Method of Chalmers, Smith, Blackburn, Silverman, Schroeder, Reitman, and Ambroz. A checklist was proposed by Chalmers et al. (1981) that can be used to evaluate clinical trials (Fig. 103.4, pg. 787). This checklist is more detailed than that of Lionel and Herxheimer (Fig. 103.2). In addition to this list, the authors proposed an index of a randomized clinical trial (RCT) quality that yields a single number that is indicative of the overall quality of the trial evaluated. This score is based on the checklist answers for their forms numbered 2, 3, and 4. Readers are referred to their paper for information on their detailed method. A variation based on this approach by Poynard et al. (1989) uses fewer items (n = 14) and fewer responses for each item (n = 3).

Method of The University of Rochester Clinical Pharmacology Group. The checklist of the University of Rochester Clinical Pharmacology Group (Weintraub, 1982) is shown in Fig. 103.5, pg. 790 and provides a column for evaluation/comment on most items. The overall assessment of an article is in terms of four important questions: (1) are there any "fatal" errors that invalidate results? (2) are the conclusions justified? (3) are results "significant" or "extrapolatable"? and (4) do benefits outweigh risks? This checklist was originally based on that of Lionel and Herxheimer (Fig. 103.2) but was greatly modified.

Method of DerSimonian, Charette, McPeek, and Mosteller. DerSimonian et al. (1982) selected 11 specific criteria by which to evaluate published clinical trials. These criteria are listed in Table 103.5 and are directed toward assessing the methods sections of clinical reports, in particular the design of the trial and the analyses performed.

DerSimonian et al. reviewed 67 trials published in four journals within an 18-month span. This method has been used by others (Emerson et al., 1984). The major point about this method is that it is limited to evaluating the methodology of a clinical trial and does not evaluate the manner in which a trial was actually performed, nor does it evaluate the data interpretations themselves.

Method of Haynes, Sackett, and Tugwell. Haynes et al. (1983) published a flow diagram of various steps involved in evaluating a clinical trial (Fig. 103.6, pg. 792). Their approach is directed toward busy practitioners and academicians who must rapidly process and sift through many articles and can only read a small number.

Method of Bailar, Louis, Lavori, and Polansky. There are often sound reasons why some clinical trials cannot include adequate or even any internal controls.

TABLE 103.5 *Criteria proposed by DerSimonian, Charette, McPeek, and Mosteller to evaluate the design and analysis of clinical trials*

1. Eligibility criteria (i.e., information explaining the criteria for admission of patients to the clinical trial)
2. Admission before allocation (i.e., information used to determine whether eligibility criteria were applied before knowledge of the specific treatment assignment had been obtained)
3. Random allocation (i.e., information about random allocation to treatment)
4. Method of randomization (i.e., information about the mechanism used to generate the random assignment)
5. Patients' blindness to treatment (i.e., information about whether patients knew which treatment they were receiving)
6. Blind assessment of outcome (i.e., information about whether the person assessing the outcome knew which treatment had been given)
7. Treatment complications (i.e., information describing the presence or absence of adverse reactions or complications after treatment)
8. Loss to follow-up (i.e., information about the numbers of patients lost to follow-up and the reasons why they were lost)
9. Statistical analyses (i.e., analyses going beyond the computation of means, percentages, or standard deviations)
10. Statistical methods (i.e., the names of the specific tests, techniques, or computer programs used for statistical analyses)
11. Power (i.e., information describing the determination of sample size or the size of detectable differences)

Reprinted by permission of *New England Journal of Medicine* from DerSimonian et al. (1982).

Such trials often rely on external controls from outside the trial (e.g., historical controls). Bailar et al. (1984a) proposed a series of five questions to be used in assessing the value (i.e., strength of evidence) provided by externally controlled trials. Their questions, which were used to evaluate a group of 20 publications in *The New England Journal of Medicine,* are listed in Table 103.6.

Method of Evans and Pollock. This method was based on that of Chalmers et al. (1981) and utilizes a score system with 100 points maximum. Evans and

TABLE 103.6 *Method of Bailar, Louis, Lavori, and Polansky for evaluating clinical trials with weak or absent internal controls*

1. Does it appear that the intervention was applied with the primary intent of affecting the outcome reported, such as cure, survival, or the incidence of complications?
2. Is it clear that the authors' intent to analyze and report their findings preceded the generation of the data (though the data may have been gathered for a different primary purpose)?
3. Have the authors shown that they had a plausible rationale for their interpretation of the data before the data were inspected or the analysis was undertaken?
4. Would the results have been interesting (i.e., publishable) if they had been different in some important sense from those actually obtained? Would "negative" findings have had a chance of being reported?
5. Do the authors present reasonable grounds for generalizing their results?

Reprinted by permission of *New England Journal of Medicine* from Bailar et al. (1984*a*).

Pollock (1985) used their method to rate 56 randomized controlled clinical trials and found that only 16 papers scored over 70 points. Their system of 33 rules is shown in Table 103.7.

Method of Meinert. Meinert's (1986) method poses "questions to consider when assessing a published report," and is less formal than some of the other recent methods. No rating scale is proposed (Table 103.8).

Other Methods. A number of other forms and checklists have been proposed to evaluate clinical studies. Some of these systems have been proposed or used to evaluate a particular type of clinical trial, such as trials concerned with contrast media (Andrew, 1984), perinatal medicine (Tyson et al., 1983), or lung cancer (Nicolucci et al., 1989). Other checklists are general (Hines and Goldzieher, 1969; Nyberg, 1974).

A series of 29 separate reviews of the quality of clinical trials was presented by Hemminki (1982). Of these 29 reviews, 10 were general in regard to overall quality,

TABLE 103.7 *Method of Evans and Pollock for evaluating controlled clinical studies*

	Yes	No
Design and conduct		
Is the sample defined?	2	0
Are exclusions specified?	2	0
Are known risk factors recorded?	3	0
Are therapeutic regimens defined?	5	0
Is the experimental regimen appropriate?	5	0
Is the control regimen appropriate?	5	0
Were appropriate investigations carried out?	2	0
Are endpoints defined?	5	0
Are endpoints appropriate?	5	0
Have numbers required been calculated?	2	0
Was patient consent sought?	1	0
Was the randomization blind?	3	0
Was the assessment blind?	4	0
Were additional treatments recorded?	4	0
Were side effects recorded?	2	0
Analysis		
Withdrawals: Are they listed?	3	0
Is their fate recorded?	4	0
Are there fewer than 10%?	4	0
Is there a comparability table?	3	0
Are risk factors stratified?	3	0
Is the statistical analysis of proportions correct?	3	0
Is the statistical analysis of numbers correct?	3	0
Are confidence intervals reported?	2	0
Are values of both test statistics and probability given?	1	0
In negative trials, is the type II error considered?	4	0
Presentation		
Is the title accurate?	2	0
Is the abstract accurate and helpful?	3	0
Are the methods reproducible?	3	0
Are the sections clear-cut?	2	0
Can the raw data be discerned?	2	0
Are the results credible?	3	0
Do the results justify the conclusions?	3	0
Are the references correct?	2	0

Reprinted by permission of *British Journal of Surgery* from Evans and Pollock (1985).

TABLE 103.8 *Questions to consider when assessing a published report*

A. General
  1. Does the manuscript indicate the purpose of the trial and rationale for the treatments studied?
  2. Does the trial address a relevant question?
  3. Is the paper in a peer review journal?
B. Investigators
  1. Have the investigators done any previous work related to the trial being reported? If so, do you consider the work to have been of good quality?
  2. Does the paper indicate the location and institutional affiliation of the various members of the team responsible for carrying out the trial?
  3. Does the team include people with appropriate training and expertise for conduct and analysis of the trial?
C. Sponsorship and structural
  1. Does the paper indicate how the trial was funded?
  2. Is the role of the sponsor in designing, directing, or analyzing the trial indicated? (especially important in trials involving proprietary products)
  3. Are the key investigators, especially those responsible for analyzing the results and for writing the paper, independent of the sponsor?
  4. Did responsibility for data collection and analysis in the trial reside with a group of people who were independent of the sponsor?
  5. Did the authors recognize the possibility of conflicts of interest for study members (especially important if the report concerns a proprietary product) and do they indicate steps taken to avoid such conflicts?
  6. If the trial involved multiple centers, does the paper list all affiliated centers and the functions performed by each?
  7. For multicenter trials, does the paper list committees, along with their membership and a brief description of their functions?
D. Trial design
  1. Outcome measure
    a. Is the primary outcome measure identified?
    b. Does it have clinical relevance?
    c. If multiple outcomes are used, is it clear which one is of primary importance in the trial?

2. Treatments
    a. Is there a defined test treatment?
    b. Is the test treatment of any interest and does the administration of it correspond roughly to the way it would be used in general practice?
    c. Is there an appropriate control treatment?
  3. Trial population and sample size
    a. Are the eligibility and exclusion criteria for patient entry into the trial stated?
    b. Is there a discussion of the types I and II error protection provided with the observed sample size?
  4. Allocation
    a. Is the method of treatment allocation described?
    b. Does it appear to have been free of selection bias?
    c. Does it meet the general conditions specified in Section 8.4 of the book?[a]
  5. Data collection procedures
    a. Is the data collection schedule described?
    b. Are the patients in the test and control-treated groups enrolled and followed over the same time frame?
    c. Does the design include adequate provisions to protect against bias in the administration of the treatment and in measurement of the outcome, as evidenced by the use of appropriate masking procedures or other safeguards?
E. Trial performance
  1. Was a recruitment goal for the trial stated? Was it achieved?
  2. Was the missed examination rate low?
  3. Was the dropout rate low?
  4. Was the dropout rate among the treatment groups about the same?
  5. Was it possible to locate all patients, including dropouts, at the end of the trial to update key morbidity and mortality data? If not, was the number who could not be located small and about the same for each treatment group?
  6. Did all the patients enrolled meet the eligibility criteria of the trial? If not, was the number who did not small?

Reprinted from Meinert (1986) with permission of Oxford University Press.
[a] Section 8.4 of Meinert's (1986) book.

6 were specific to a particular disease(s), 6 were specific to a particular medicine(s), and 7 to a particular medicine(s) in a given disease or group of diseases. Some of these reviews utilized their own systems for reviewing the literature.

Hines and Goldzieher (1969) concluded their article with the statement "The Romans had a motto for the marketplace: *Caveat emptor*. The reader of reports of clinical investigation can have one, too: *Caveat lector*."

CHECKLIST FOR ASSESSING A THERAPEUTIC TRIAL REPORT

Author and Journal reference

Title

Y = Yes
N = No, or not clear
D = Doubtful

1. *AIM:* specific ☐, or not clear ☐; single ☐, or multiple ☐

2-4. *DESCRIPTION OF SUBJECTS, DRUG ADMINISTRATION, ETC.* — ARE THE FOLLOWING SPECIFIED?

2-1	Healthy subjects or patients?	Y	N
2-2	Volunteers or not?	Y	N
2-3	Age	Y	N
2-4	Sex	Y	N
2-5	Race	Y	N
2-6	Criteria of selection	Y	N
2-7	Contraindications	Y	N
2-8	Presence of disease other than that treated	Y	N
2-9	Whether additional treatments were given	Y	N
	If they were, are they described?	Y	N
3-1	Daily dose	Y	N
3-2	Frequency of administration	Y	N
3-3	Hour(s) o'clock when given	Y	N
3-4	Route of administration	Y	N
3-5	Source of drug (e.g., name of manufacturer)	Y	N
3-6	Presentation (e.g., tablet, syrup, etc.)	Y	N
3-7	Timing of drug administration in relation to factors affecting absorption (e.g. meals)	Y	N
3-8	Checks that drug was taken	Y	N
3-9	Other therapeutic measures (if drug was not used)	Y	N
	If yes, are they described?	Y	N
3-10	Total duration of treatment	Y	N
4-1	Persons who made the observations	Y	N
4-2	Inpatient/outpatient	Y	N
4-3	Setting (e.g., one or several hospitals/clinics/wards)	Y	N
4-4	Dates when trial began and was completed	Y	N

5. *METHODS AND DESIGN*

5-1	Are the methods of assessing therapeutic effects clearly described?	Y	N
5-2	Were these standardized methods?	Y	N
5-3	Were control measures used to reduce variation that might influence the results	Y	N

If *yes*, specify:

Concurrent controls ☐   Run-in period ☐   Identical ancillary
Stratification or   Patient his own   treatment ☐
  matched subgroups ☐   control ☐   Other ☐

5-4	Were controls used to reduce bias?	Y	N

If *yes*, specify:

"Blind" observers ☐   "Blind" patients ☐
Matching dummies ☐   Random allocation ☐

6. *ASSESSMENT OF THE TRIAL*

6-1	Were the subjects suitably selected in relation to aims (see sections 1 and 2)?	Y	N
6-2	Were the methods of measurement valid in relation to the aim?	Y	N
6-3	Were they adequately standardized?	Y	N
6-4	Were they sufficiently sensitive?	Y	N
6-5	Was the design appropriate?	Y	N
6-6	Were enough subjects used?	Y	N
6-7	Was the dosage appropriate?	Y	N
6-8	Was the duration of treatment adequate?	Y	N
6-9	Were carry-over effects avoided or allowed for?	Y	N
6-10(a)	If no controls were used were they unnecessary?	Y	N
(b)	If controls were used were they adequate?	Y	N
6-11	Was comparability of treatment groups examined?	Y	N
6-12	Are the data adequate for assessment?	Y	N
6-13(a)	If statistical tests were not done were they unnecessary?	Y	N
(b)	If statistical tests are reported		
	(i) Is it clear how they were done?	Y	N
	(ii) Were they appropriately used?	Y N	D

ARE THE CONCLUSIONS JUSTIFIED?   Is the trial ACCEPTABLE?

Completely ☐   Partially ☐   No ☐   Definitely yes ☐   Probably yes ☐   No ☐

COMMENTS

FIG. 103.2 Checklist of Lionel and Herxheimer to evaluate published articles. (Reprinted by permission of *British Medical Journal* from Lionel and Herxheimer, 1970.)

STUDY	TYPE	TREATMENT	STATUS	PHASE	RATER

DEPARTMENT OF HEALTH AND HUMAN SERVICES
PUBLIC HEALTH SERVICE
ALCOHOL DRUG ABUSE, AND MENTAL HEALTH ADMINISTRATION
NATIONAL INSTITUTE OF MENTAL HEALTH

TRIAL ASSESSMENT PROCEDURE SCALE
(TAPS)

NAME OF RATER	DATE

AFFILIATION

ADDRESS

PHONE

Trial Title and/or Identification Number: _____

Type, Source and Date of Report: _____

Name of Investigational Drug(s) or Treatment(s): _____

Trial Status: ☐ Planned   ☐ Completed

Trial Phase: ☐ I   ☐ Early II   ☐ Late II   ☐ III   ☐ IV

No. of Treatment Groups: _____   No. of Subjects in Trial: _____

INSTRUCTIONS

OVERVIEW. The Trial Assessment Procedure Scale (TAPS) is a systematic technique for evaluating the quality of a clinical trial. The technique involves an analysis of the report (e.g., protocol, completed study report, or journal article) in terms of many descriptive characteristics or attributes which reflect trial quality. The attributes are logically clustered into eight categories so that the quality of various components of the trial can be independently assessed. The intent is to rate the quality of the trial without regard to findings concerning treatment efficacy or safety.

Each category is composed of two to five related attributes. For example, the first category, RESEARCH PROBLEM, is composed of two attributes labeled Background and Rationale and Objectives and/or Hypothesis. A separate rating page is provided for each attribute category, which lists the constituent attributes, along with examples of the kinds of factors that should be taken into account in evaluating each respective attribute. Examples are representative and do not exhaust all of the factors that may be considered when rating a given attribute.

RATING PROCEDURE. The TAPS rating procedure is identical for all attributes. The rating is made on a five-point scale: Totally Satisfactory, Satisfactory, Marginal, Unsatisfactory, or Totally Unsatisfactory. For each attribute, the rater is asked to check the appropriate box in the QUALITY RATING column, reflecting how well the trial under evaluation measures up on that attribute. The rater is encouraged to comment on the basis for the rating of any attribute, and space has been provided for this purpose.

RATING PROBLEMS. Because of differences in the nature and content of clinical trial reports, it may be difficult to meaningfully rate a given attribute. Thus, under the column heading RATING PROBLEMS AND EXPLANATION, two boxes are provided. The first box, Not Applicable, pertains to the applicability of the attribute with respect to either the type of trial or type of report (e.g., protocol, journal article) through which the trial is being evaluated. This box is checked only when the attribute does not have meaning either in the context of the given trial or type of report, and therefore a quality rating should not be made. The second box, Poor Documentation, concerns the availability and clarity of the written description needed to make a meaningful judgment about the given attribute; this box should be checked when the appropriate information is either lacking or inadequate. Even after making a quality rating in response to the attribute, this box can be checked to indicate that the relevant documentation is poor.

Raters are advised to keep the following rules in mind. Lack of confidence about expertise in a specific area should not prevent the rater from making a rating. If the rater is having difficulty because the attribute is not applicable to the trial itself or to the type of report, the Not Applicable box is checked and explanation made in the space provided. No quality rating is given to that attribute. If the rater is having difficulty because no information is given in the report to permit a judgment on a given attribute (when it would have been applicable), the Poor Documentation box is checked. If the information given is unclear, incomplete, or has to be inferred, a quality rating is made and the Poor Documentation box is checked. Thus, whenever an attribute quality rating cannot be provided, either the Not Applicable or Poor Documentation box must be checked and an explanation given. If a quality rating is made, and the rater wishes to indicate that the documentation is poor, the box Poor Documentation is checked.

GLOBAL RATING. Once ratings have been completed for all attributes, a global rating is made indicating the rater's assessment of the OVERALL QUALITY or "goodness" of the entire trial. The overall rating should take into account all the individual ratings across the attribute categories, as well as any other considerations that may have been noted. For example, if the quality rating of an attribute is so unacceptable that the trial is "fatally flawed," then a very low global rating would be given even though other attributes had been judged Satisfactory or better. As shown on the global rating sheet, the rating is made on a 0-to-100 scale, where 0 is "Very Poor" and 100 is "Very Good." Any number between 0 and 100 can be assigned. Below the global rating scale, space is available for comments about the overall rating for the trial. This area can also be used for additional comments about the trial, any of the ratings, or other relevant considerations.

RATING THE TRIAL REPORT. After the rater has become familiar with the format and content of TAPS, it is recommended that the report of the trial to be rated first be read in its entirety. Then, the attributes should be rated in the sequence presented in TAPS referring back to various sections of the trial report as often as necessary.

SCORING TAPS. After ratings have been completed a series of numerical scores can be derived according to the SCORING INSTRUCTIONS.

FIG. 103.3 Trial Assessment Procedure Scale (TAPS) system of Dr. Jerome Levine to evaluate published articles.

I. RESEARCH PROBLEM

ATTRIBUTE	QUALITY RATING	RATING PROBLEMS AND EXPLANATION	
A. Background and Rationale —appropriate presentation of previous relevant research findings; justification of research need and basis/rationale for hypothesis to be tested.	☐ Totally Satisfactory ☐ Satisfactory ☐ Marginal ☐ Unsatisfactory ☐ Totally Unsatisfactory	☐ Not Applicable	☐ Poor Documentation
B. Objectives and/or Hypothesis —clarity of objectives, meaningfulness and precision of research question; relevancy of hypothesis for claims to be made.	☐ Totally Satisfactory ☐ Satisfactory ☐ Marginal ☐ Unsatisfactory ☐ Totally Unsatisfactory	☐ Not Applicable	☐ Poor Documentation

COMMENTS:

II. RESEARCH MANAGEMENT

ATTRIBUTE	QUALITY RATING	RATING PROBLEMS AND EXPLANATION	
A. External Review/Monitoring —adequacy of scientific and ethical review by a qualified independent group; use of external monitoring of research practices, conditions, and progress.	☐ Totally Satisfactory ☐ Satisfactory ☐ Marginal ☐ Unsatisfactory ☐ Totally Unsatisfactory	☐ Not Applicable	☐ Poor Documentation
B. Site Selection —explicitness and objectiveness of clinical site selection; appropriateness of treatment and assessment setting.	☐ Totally Satisfactory ☐ Satisfactory ☐ Marginal ☐ Unsatisfactory ☐ Totally Unsatisfactory	☐ Not Applicable	☐ Poor Documentation
C. Personnel —appropriateness of staff organizational structure, e.g., adequacy of supervision; professional skill of staff members for performing patient care, assessment ratings and data analysis functions.	☐ Totally Satisfactory ☐ Satisfactory ☐ Marginal ☐ Unsatisfactory ☐ Totally Unsatisfactory	☐ Not Applicable	☐ Poor Documentation
D. Trial Period —appropriateness of length of planning phase, data collection period and analysis period, as well as the appropriateness of the intervals between completion of data collection and initiation of analysis.	☐ Totally Satisfactory ☐ Satisfactory ☐ Marginal ☐ Unsatisfactory ☐ Totally Unsatisfactory	☐ Not Applicable	☐ Poor Documentation

COMMENTS:

FIG. 103.3 (*continued*)

III. DESIGN CHARACTERISTICS

ATTRIBUTE	QUALITY RATING	RATING PROBLEMS AND EXPLANATION
A. Independent Variables —choice of factors included in the design, e.g., treatments and choice of drugs within treatments (experimental drug, standard drug, placebo), patient diagnosis, periods of administration, etc.	☐ Totally Satisfactory ☐ Satisfactory ☐ Marginal ☐ Unsatisfactory ☐ Totally Unsatisfactory	☐ Not Applicable ☐ Poor Documentation
B. Design Configuration —appropriateness and precision of experimental design, e.g., use of a crossover or independent groups design, as required; avoidance of effects which may be confounded with the treatment factor, e.g., treatment order, time, setting, etc.	☐ Totally Satisfactory ☐ Satisfactory ☐ Marginal ☐ Unsatisfactory ☐ Totally Unsatisfactory	☐ Not Applicable ☐ Poor Documentation
C. Subject Assignment —adequacy of sample size (within each treatment group) for testing hypothesis; appropriate assignment of subjects to treatment groups by proper randomization, matching, sequential procedures, etc.	☐ Totally Satisfactory ☐ Satisfactory ☐ Marginal ☐ Unsatisfactory ☐ Totally Unsatisfactory	☐ Not Applicable ☐ Poor Documentation
D. Control of Treatment-Related Bias —adequacy of treatment and assessor blinding (e.g., double or triple blind); comparability of dosage schedule, dosage form, time of administration; provision to break blind for individual patient without breaking blind for all patients; utilization of explicit rules or criteria for dealing with marked improvement or worsening of subject illness, or occurrence of treatment-emergent side effects of toxicity.	☐ Totally Satisfactory ☐ Satisfactory ☐ Marginal ☐ Unsatisfactory ☐ Totally Unsatisfactory	☐ Not Applicable ☐ Poor Documentation
E. Control of Extraneous Variables —suitability of research environment, e.g., absence of marked investigator bias, "Hawthorne Effect," hopeless atmosphere, etc; reduction of pretreatment bias by, e.g., the use of stratification, avoidance of carry-over effects, etc.; limitation or control of other concurrent therapies including drugs other than those under study; utilization of explicit rules or criteria for dealing with such problems as intercurrent illness, change of residence, etc.	☐ Totally Satisfactory ☐ Satisfactory ☐ Marginal ☐ Unsatisfactory ☐ Totally Unsatisfactory	☐ Not Applicable ☐ Poor Documentation

COMMENTS:

FIG. 103.3 (*continued*)

IV. TREATMENT CHARACTERISTICS

ATTRIBUTE	QUALITY RATING	RATING PROBLEMS AND EXPLANATION	
A. Description —specification of relevant characteristics of experimental and control treatments, e.g., presumed clinical actions, side effects, duration of actions, pharmacological profile; rationale for choice of comparison agent, i.e., standard drug or placebo.	☐ Totally Satisfactory ☐ Satisfactory ☐ Marginal ☐ Unsatisfactory ☐ Totally Unsatisfactory	☐ Not Applicable	☐ Poor Documentation
B. Dosage —adequacy of dosage levels, equivalence of dosage across standard and test drugs, criteria for dosage adjustment; appropriateness of schedule and pattern (fixed or variable) of administration with respect to duration of action, research design and phase of the trial; appropriateness of form or route of administration, degree of consistency with pharmacological properties.	☐ Totally Satisfactory ☐ Satisfactory ☐ Marginal ☐ Unsatisfactory ☐ Totally Unsatisfactory	☐ Not Applicable	☐ Poor Documentation
C. Duration —necessity for, and appropriate length of, drying-out (pre-treatment) period, drug administration (treatment) period, and follow-up (post-treatment) period.	☐ Totally Satisfactory ☐ Satisfactory ☐ Marginal ☐ Unsatisfactory ☐ Totally Unsatisfactory	☐ Not Applicable	☐ Poor Documentation

COMMENTS:

V. SUBJECT CHARACTERISTICS

ATTRIBUTE	QUALITY RATING	RATING PROBLEMS AND EXPLANATION	
A. Selection Criteria —clarity, explicitness, appropriateness and general acceptance of criteria used to diagnose patients and to include or exclude them in study.	☐ Totally Satisfactory ☐ Satisfactory ☐ Marginal ☐ Unsatisfactory ☐ Totally Unsatisfactory	☐ Not Applicable	☐ Poor Documentation
B. Sample Representativeness —correspondence between sample and population in terms of illness-related characteristics (e.g., pattern and severity of psychopathology) and demographic/situation-related characteristics (e.g., age, sex, acuteness of illness, inpatient/outpatient status, etc.)	☐ Totally Satisfactory ☐ Satisfactory ☐ Marginal ☐ Unsatisfactory ☐ Totally Unsatisfactory	☐ Not Applicable	☐ Poor Documentation
C. Subject Induction —appropriateness and consistency of subject recruitment procedure, and degree of adherence to requirements for obtaining informed, voluntary subject consent.	☐ Totally Satisfactory ☐ Satisfactory ☐ Marginal ☐ Unsatisfactory ☐ Totally Unsatisfactory	☐ Not Applicable	☐ Poor Documentation

FIG. 103.3 (*continued*)

V. SUBJECT CHARACTERISTICS (CONTINUED)

ATTRIBUTE	QUALITY RATING	RATING PROBLEMS AND EXPLANATION
D. Subject Compliance —adequacy of techniques to check for and assure medication ingestion as well as compliance with assessment procedures and schedule.	☐ Totally Satisfactory ☐ Satisfactory ☐ Marginal ☐ Unsatisfactory ☐ Totally Unsatisfactory	☐ Not Applicable ☐ Poor Documentation

COMMENTS:

VI. DATA COLLECTION

ATTRIBUTE	QUALITY RATING	RATING PROBLEMS AND EXPLANATION
A. Scope of Assessment —adequacy of breadth of measures for assessing areas such as: sample (identification and recording of degree of illness, demographic information, etc.); efficacy (assessment to demonstrate improvement or worsening of patient illness); side effects (assessment to detect expected and unexpected treatment-emergent symptoms); dosage (recording of dosages actually administered); safety (use of appropriate laboratory tests which are specific to drug under study, general for assessing bodily functions, etc.); other relevant areas (depending upon illness, drug, or special assessment techniques, e.g., EEG, blood levels, behavioral measures, etc.)	☐ Totally Satisfactory ☐ Satisfactory ☐ Marginal ☐ Unsatisfactory ☐ Totally Unsatisfactory	☐ Not Applicable ☐ Poor Documentation
B. Assessment Measures —appropriateness of measures and instruments selected with respect to areas being assessed; extent that rating scales and recording forms have been previously shown to be sensitive, reliable, and valid; degree to which measures have been generally used and accepted.	☐ Totally Satisfactory ☐ Satisfactory ☐ Marginal ☐ Unsatisfactory ☐ Totally Unsatisfactory	☐ Not Applicable ☐ Poor Documentation
C. Assessment Schedule —appropriateness of frequency and schedule of ratings, collection of baseline measures prior to start of trial, etc.	☐ Totally Satisfactory ☐ Satisfactory ☐ Marginal ☐ Unsatisfactory ☐ Totally Unsatisfactory	☐ Not Applicable ☐ Poor Documentation
D. Conduct of Assessment —consistency throughout trial of application of rating and assessment techniques; attempt to maintain same rater for any given patient throughout trial; evidence to establish interrater reliability and rating validity within context of this trial.	☐ Totally Satisfactory ☐ Satisfactory ☐ Marginal ☐ Unsatisfactory ☐ Totally Unsatisfactory	☐ Not Applicable ☐ Poor Documentation

COMMENTS:

FIG. 103.3 (*continued*)

VII. DATA ANALYSIS

ATTRIBUTE	QUALITY RATING	RATING PROBLEMS AND EXPLANATION
A. Data Preparation • —adequacy of data collection techniques (case report and recording forms, etc); data checking, editing, and verification techniques; use of standard computer analysis program vs. hand calculations, checking of intermediate data processing steps.	☐ Totally Satisfactory ☐ Satisfactory ☐ Marginal ☐ Unsatisfactory ☐ Totally Unsatisfactory	☐ Not Applicable ☐ Poor Documentation
B. Data Presentation —clarity, meaningfulness and utility of data description, organization, and display; appropriate level of data detail or summarization.	☐ Totally Satisfactory ☐ Satisfactory ☐ Marginal ☐ Unsatisfactory ☐ Totally Unsatisfactory	☐ Not Applicable ☐ Poor Documentation
C. Statistical Analysis —correctness of application of statistical procedures, e.g., data transformations, pooling of data, handling of dropouts and missing data, etc.; use of statistical model appropriate to research design, e.g., parametric vs. nonparametric, analysis of variance vs. analysis of covariance, etc.; degree of statistical follow-through, e.g., use of multiple comparisons after finding a significant F-ratio, etc.	☐ Totally Satisfactory ☐ Satisfactory ☐ Marginal ☐ Unsatisfactory ☐ Totally Unsatisfactory	☐ Not Applicable ☐ Poor Documentation
D. Data Synthesis —demonstration of systematic approach to answering research question; appropriate analysis of functional relationships (e.g., dose-response curves).	☐ Totally Satisfactory ☐ Satisfactory ☐ Marginal ☐ Unsatisfactory ☐ Totally Unsatisfactory	☐ Not Applicable ☐ Poor Documentation

COMMENTS:

VIII. CONCLUSIONS AND INTERPRETATION

ATTRIBUTE	QUALITY RATING	RATING PROBLEMS AND EXPLANATION
A. Focus —degree that conclusions (findings) and interpretation (explanation) presented are specific and clear; meaningful correspondence between conclusions and research hypothesis.	☐ Totally Satisfactory ☐ Satisfactory ☐ Marginal ☐ Unsatisfactory ☐ Totally Unsatisfactory	☐ Not Applicable ☐ Poor Documentation
B. Logic —extent that conclusions are unambiguously supported, both logically and statistically, by the data collected in the study.	☐ Totally Satisfactory ☐ Satisfactory ☐ Marginal ☐ Unsatisfactory ☐ Totally Unsatisfactory	☐ Not Applicable ☐ Poor Documentation

FIG. 103.3 (*continued*)

VIII. CONCLUSIONS AND INTERPRETATION (CONTINUED)

ATTRIBUTE	QUALITY RATING	RATING PROBLEMS AND EXPLANATION
C. Application —appropriateness of generalization of conclusions from sample in study to the larger population (i.e., claims are not over-stated or over-generalized beyond the sup-porting data); appropriateness of inter-pretation with regard to other published findings.	☐ Totally Satisfactory ☐ Satisfactory ☐ Marginal ☐ Unsatisfactory ☐ Totally Unsatisfactory	☐ Not Applicable ☐ Poor Documentation

COMMENTS:

OVERALL QUALITY OF TRIAL

— 100 Very Good

— 75   Good

— 50   Borderline

— 25   Poor

— 0   Very Poor

Assign any number between 0 and 100 in accordance with the scale at the left.

GLOBAL RATING

COMMENTS:

SCORING INSTRUCTIONS

This page provides instructions and space to derive numerical scores from the TAPS ratings. The specific scoring procedures are as follows:

CATEGORY SCORES These are derived from the attribute Quality Ratings previously recorded.

(1) Convert each attribute Quality Rating in every category (I-VIII) into an equivalent numerical Attribute Score as follows: Totally Satisfactory = 100; Satisfactory = 75; Marginal = 50; Unsatisfactory = 25; and Totally Unsatisfactory = 0. Record these scores on the appropriate lines in the table below.

(2) Sum the Attribute Scores for each category and enter in the table. Note and enter the number of attributes rated in each category. Divide the Attribute Score Sum by the Number of Attributes Rated and record the resultant Category Score on the designated line in the table. (If no attributes were rated in a given category, there would be no Category Score).

ATTRIBUTE	I	II	III	IV	V	VI	VII	VIII
						CATEGORY		
A	___	___	___	___	___	___	___	___
B	___	___	___	___	___	___	___	___
C		___	___	___	___	___	___	___
D		___	___		___	___	___	___
E			___					
Attrib. Score Sum	___	___	___	___	___	___	___	___
No. Attrib. Rated	___	___	___	___	___	___	___	___
Category Score	___	___	___	___	___	___	___	___

TOTAL SCORE Sum all Category Scores derived above and divide by the number of Category Scores (usually eight):

Sum of Category Scores _____ ÷ Number of Categories _____ = Total Score _____ .

DIFFERENCE SCORE Compute the numerical difference (i.e., absolute value) between the Global Rating and the Total Score. Record the Difference Score _____ .

POOR DOCUMENTATION SCORE Count the total number of attributes where the Poor Documentation box was checked and write the number _____ .

FIG. 103.3 (*continued*)

Form 1: BASIC DESCRIPTIVE MATERIAL

ID # _____ Study # _____ Reader _____

Title _____

_____

Journal or publication _____

_____

Peer reviewed: Yes____ No____ Unknown____

Year of publication_____

1.1 Biostatistician
  ____1. Author
  ____2. Credits
  ____3. Neither
  ____4. Unknown

1.2 Country
  ____1. U.S.
  ____2. U.K.
  ____3. Scand.
  ____4. Other
  ____5. Unknown

1.3 Center status
  ____1. Single Center
  ____2. Cooperative study <5 grps.
  ____3. Cooperative study >5 grps.

1.4 Source of financial support (multiple items possible)
A. N.I.H. or M.R.C.
  ____1. Yes
  ____2. No
B. V.A.
  ____1. Yes
  ____2. No
C. Drug Co.
  ____1. Yes
  ____2. No
D. Other
  ____1. Yes
  ____2. No
E. None given ____

1.5 Source of patients (multiple items possible)
A. University
  ____1. Yes
  ____2. No
B. Public
  ____1. Yes
  ____2. No
C. Private
  ____1. Yes
  ____2. No

D. Clinic (no hosp.)
  ____1. Yes
  ____2. No
E. Industry
  ____1. Yes
  ____2. No
F. None given ____

1.6 Number in Controls
  Tr. grp. 1
  Tr. grp. 2
  Tr. grp. 3

1.7 Type of trial
  ____1. Simple comparative
  ____2. Restricted (blocking)
  ____3. Stratified
  ____4. Crossover
  ____5. Factorial
  ____6. Other
  ____7. Unknown

1.8 Significance of findings
A. Major endpoints
  ____1. + + Statistically significant (treatment)
  ____2.   + Trend (treatment)
  ____3.   0 No difference
  ____4.   — Trend (control)
  ____5. — — Statistically significant (control)
  ____6.   Significant in author's opinion but no statistical test with probability stated.
B. Minor endpoints
  ____1. + + Statistically significant (treatment)
  ____2.   + Trend (treatment)
  ____3.   0 No difference
  ____4.   — Trend (control)
  ____5. — — Statistically significant (control)
  ____6.   None

1.9 Side effects, statistical finding
  ____1. + + Statistically significant
  ____2.   + Trend
  ____3.   0 No side effects
  ____4.   N.A.

FIG. 103.4 Checklist of Chalmers, Smith, Blackburn, Silverman, Schroeder, Reitman, and Ambroz to evaluate published articles. N.I.H., National Institutes of Health (US); M.R.C., Medical Research Council (UK). (Reprinted by permission of Elsevier North Holland, Inc., from Chalmers et al., 1981.)

Form 2: THE STUDY PROTOCOL

ID # _____ Study # _____ Reader _____

2.1 Selection description
_____1. Adequate
_____2. Fair
_____3. Inadequate

2.2 Number of patients seen and reject log
_____1. Yes
_____2. Partial
_____3. No
_____4. Unknown

2.3 Withdrawals
_____1. List given
_____2. No withdrawals
_____3. No list
_____4. Unknown
_____5. >15% withdrawals for long-term
  studies and >10% for studies
  lasting less than 3 months

2.4 Therapeutic regimens definition
_____1. Adequate
_____2. Fair
_____3. Inadequate

2.5
A. Control regimen (placebo) appearance
_____1. Same
_____2. Different
_____3. Unstated
_____4. N.A.

B. Control regimen (placebo) taste
_____1. Same
_____2. Different
_____3. Unstated
_____4. N.A.

2.6 Randomization blinding[a]
_____1. Yes
_____2. Partial
_____3. No
_____4. Unknown

Method of random blinding
_____1. Envelope
_____2. Pharmacy
_____3. Other
_____4. Unknown
_____5. N.A.

2.7 Blinding of patients[a]
_____1. Yes
_____2. No
_____3. Unknown
_____4. N.A.

2.8 Blinding of physicians re therapy[a]
_____1. Yes
_____2. Partial
_____3. No
_____4. Unknown
_____5. N.A.

2.9 Blinding of physicians and patients re results
_____1. Yes
_____2. Partial
_____3. No
_____4. Unknown

2.10 Prior estimate of numbers (endpoints selected, diff.
  of clinic interest α and β estimated)
_____1. Yes
_____2. No
_____3. Unknown

2.11 Testing randomization
_____1. Yes
_____2. Partial
_____3. No
_____4. Unknown

2.12 Testing blinding
_____1. Yes
_____2. Partial
_____3. No
_____4. Unknown
_____5. N.A.

2.13 Testing compliance
_____1. Yes
_____2. Partial
_____3. No
_____4. Unknown
_____5. N.A.

2.14 Biological equivalent
_____1. Yes
_____2. No
_____3. Unknown
_____4. N.A.

FIG. 103.4 (continued)

Form 3: STATISTICAL ANALYSIS

ID # _____ Study # _____ Reader _____

3.1 On major endpoints
_____1. If possible, test statistic and observed probability value are stated
_____2. If observed probability level given, but test statistic value not stated
_____3. If test statistic but not observed probability value given
_____4. If neither test statistic nor observed probability level given

3.2 Posterior β estimates of observed difference for negative trials
_____1. Yes
_____2. Mentioned and necessity for more patients
_____3. No
_____4. N.A.

3.3 Statistical inference
A. Confidence limits
_____1. Yes
_____2. No
_____3. N.A.

B. Life-table or time-series analysis
_____1. Yes
_____2. Shown but incorrect
_____3. No
_____4. N.A.

C. Regression analysis correlation
_____1. Yes
_____2. No
_____3. N.A.

3.4 Appropriate statistical analysis
_____1. Excellent
_____2. Good
_____3. Poor
_____4. Inadequate

3.5 Handling of withdrawals
_____1. Analyzed several ways
_____2. Included in original randomization
_____3. Counted as end result at time of withdrawal
_____4. Discarded
_____5. Changed groups
_____6. Unknown
_____7. No withdrawals/N.A.

3.6 Side effects, statistical discussion
_____1. Adequate
_____2. Fair
_____3. Poor
_____4. N.A.

3.7 Proper retrospective analysis
_____1. Good
_____2. Partial
_____3. None

3.8 Blinding of statistician or analyst re results
_____1. Yes
_____2. No
_____3. Unknown
_____4. N.A.

3.9 Multiple looks considered
_____1. Yes
_____2. Fixed sample size, no look
_____3. No

Form 4: PRESENTATION OF RESULTS

ID # _____ Study # _____ Reader _____

4.1 Dates of starting and stopping accession
_____1. Yes
_____2. No

4.2 Results of prerandomization
A. Data Analysis
_____1. Adequate
_____2. Fair
_____3. Inadequate

B. Prognostically favoring
_____1. Treatment
_____2. Control
_____3. Equivocal
_____4. Unknown

4.3 Tabulation of events employed as endpoint for each treatment
_____1. Presented
_____2. Not presented

4.4 Timing of events
_____1. Complete
_____2. Available to reader
_____3. Neither

FIG. 103.4 (*continued*)

CHECKLIST FOR ASSESSING CLINICAL DRUG TRIALS

Title, author, and journal (or book) _____

General Aspects

Aim: Efficacy, toxicity, both: _____

           Explanatory or pragmatic: _____

Phase: ☐I   ☐II   ☐III   ☐IV   ☐Other

Type: ☐Experiment
           ☐Survey: prospective or retrospective (case-control)
           ☐Therapeutic
           ☐Prophylactic
           ☐Symptomatic

Design: ☐Within patient (crossover, Latin square, randomized blocks)
           ☐Between patient (non-crossover, one way, parallel groups)

Objective: Major _____

            Subsidiary _____

Specific Characteristics

	Discussed	Evaluation/Comment
Population		
Type (patients, healthy subjects)	___	___
Criteria for inclusion	___	___
Criteria for exclusion	___	___
Comparability of treatment groups:		
Demographic (age, race, sex)	___	___
Prognostic criteria	___	___
Stage of disease	___	___
Response to therapy	___	___
Associated disease	___	___
Generalizability (on basis of similarity of participants to patient population)	___	___
Consent	___	___
Treatments compared		
Rationale for dose:		
Based on weight, amount/time	___	___
Fixed or flexible (If flexible, what is rule of dosage adjustment?)	___	___
One dose level or dose-response?	___	___
Dosage form and/or route of administration	___	___
Interval between doses and/or hours of administration	___	___
Ancillary therapy (Forbidden? Or if permitted, standardized, measured?)	___	___
Duration of therapy	___	___
Setting (hospital, home)	___	___
Source of drug (ie, lot, bioavailability, changed formulation of standard medication, resemblance of control and test preparation)	___	___

FIG. 103.5 Checklist of The University of Rochester Clinical Pharmacology Group to evaluate published articles. (Reprinted by permission of *Drug Therapy* from Weintraub, 1982.)

Experimental design details	Discussed	Evaluation/Comment
Controlled?		
Controls: Active or inactive	_____	_____
Concurrent or historical	_____	_____
Assignment of treatments:		
Randomized (balanced?)	_____	_____
Matched	_____	_____
Stratification or minimization	_____	_____
"Run-in" or "washout" period	_____	_____
Timing (schedule of visits, laboratory tests, assessments)	_____	_____
Starting and stopping of treatment	_____	_____

Compliance

Participant (with treatments)	_____	_____
Investigators (with protocol)	_____	_____

Data collection

Measurements used to assess goal attainment (Appropriate type? Sensitive enough? Done at appropriate time?)	_____	_____
Observers (Who? Same or variable?)	_____	_____
Method of collection (Standard? Reproducible?)	_____	_____
Adverse effects		
Subjective (Volunteered or elicited?)	_____	_____
Laboratory tests for toxicity (Done at appropriate time?)	_____	_____

Control of bias

"Blind" observers	_____	_____
"Blind" subjects	_____	_____
Evaluator blind but physician treating participant not blind	_____	_____
Statistician blind (analysis done with treatment groups unidentified	_____	_____

Data analysis

Comparability of treatment groups (at beginning and at end of study)	_____	_____
Missing data	_____	_____
Drop-outs (drop-ins)	_____	_____
Reasons	_____	_____
Effect on results	_____	_____
Compliance taken into account?	_____	_____
Statistical tests		
If differences observed, are they clinically meaningful?	_____	_____
If no difference shown, is this due to statistical power of study?	_____	_____

Overall Assessment

Any "fatal" errors that invalidate results?	☐Yes	☐No	
Conclusions justified?	☐Yes	☐No	
Results significant or extrapolatable?	☐Yes	☐Perhaps	☐No
Do benefits outweigh risks?	☐Yes	☐Perhaps	☐No

General comments: _____

_____

_____

_____

_____

_____

FIG. 103.5 (*continued*)

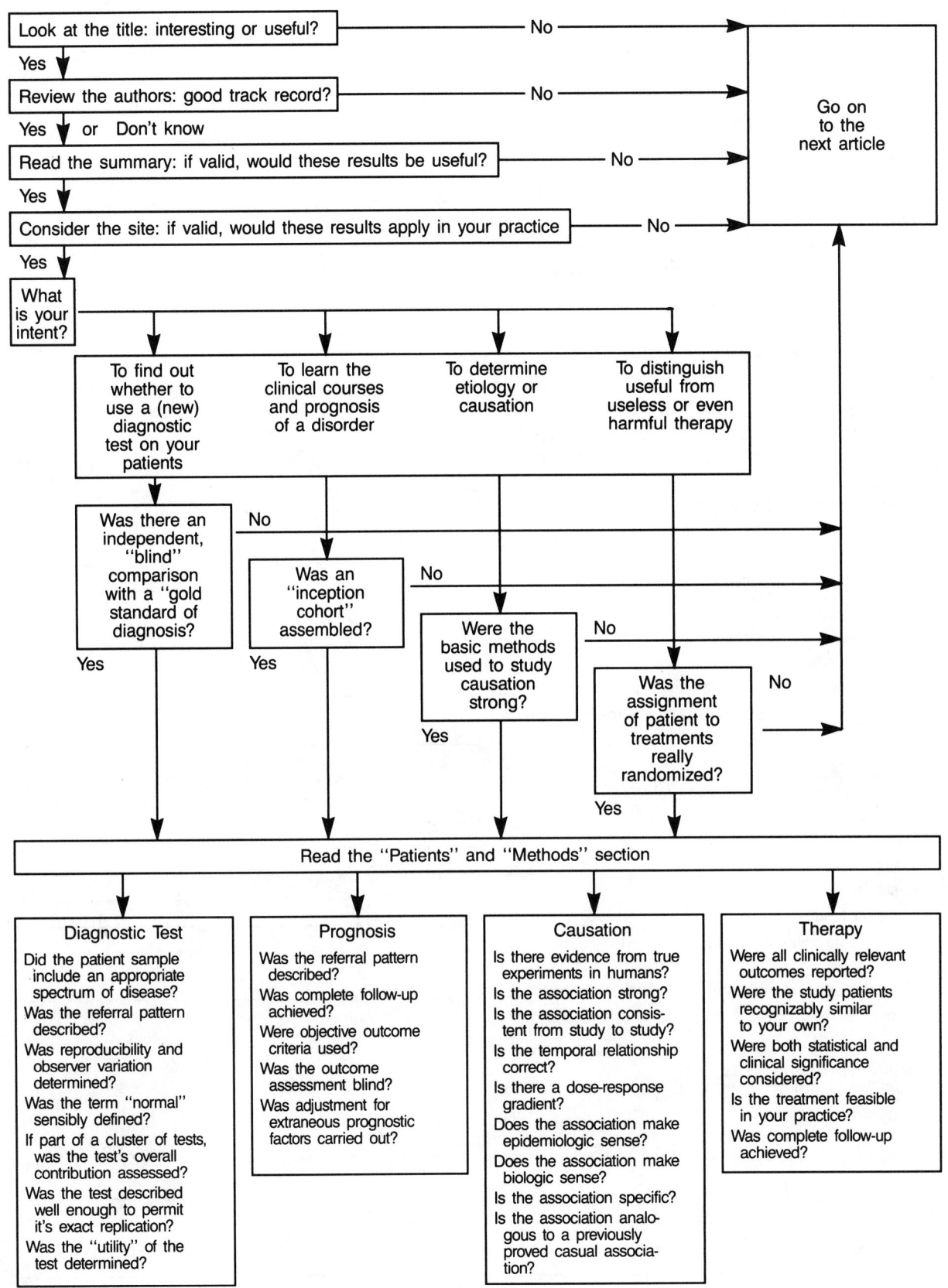

FIG. 103.6 Flow chart of Haynes, Sackett, and Tugwell to evaluate published articles. (Reprinted by permission of *Archives of Internal Medicine* from Haynes et al., 1983.)

CHAPTER 104

Meta-Analysis

INTRODUCTION

Meta-analysis is a relatively new method for reviewing and combining results from multiple clinical trials. Whereas other review methods usually involve narrative discussions of individual trials, a meta-analysis systematically aggregates and quantifies results.

Definitions

Meta-analysis is described (Sacks et al., 1987) as "a new discipline that critically reviews and statistically combines the results of previous research." A meta-analysis, therefore, is the process of systematically combining and evaluating the results of clinical trials that have been completed or terminated. A further simplification states that meta-analysis is a quantitative summary of research.

Types of Data Pooling

The term "pooling" is often observed in the meta-analysis literature, but it is used with two separate meanings. One refers to combining actual raw data, so that the combined numbers have more power and are more convincing. The second meaning refers to combining the conclusions (e.g., odds ratios) of individual trials to create an overall averaged odds ratio. The author proposes that there is an intermediate level of pooling data that relates to combining summary data of specific groups of patients from multiple trials. Thus, the first level of pooling is that of individual patients' raw data, the second level is that of summary data of specific groups of patients, and the third level is of overall trial results. Saying that eight of ten clinical trials show medicine A is more effective than placebo is a type of pooling at level three.

Purposes of Meta-Analysis

A scientist or clinician who conducts a meta-analysis may have one or several purposes in mind. These include:

1. To answer research or clinical questions in a systematic way that have not previously been posed. To allow examination of interstudy variations as well as any patterns that may be present in the results.
2. To increase the statistical power for addressing important research or clinical questions. Individual trials with a small sample size are often characterized by low power for detecting meaningful differences; the overall power is increased when data are pooled. This approach also allows subgroup analyses to be conducted with higher power.
3. To serve as a tool to address research or clinical questions when controversy or conflicting data exist. This may take the form of looking at old trials or planning new clinical trials that have the best possibility of addressing an important question using the best methods. A meta-analysis helps determine whether new clinical trials are warranted, and if so, the sample size required to answer definitively the research question.
4. To quantify better the magnitude of certain clinical or nonclinical responses.
5. To decrease biases in addressing specific clinical issues by being more objective, thorough, and systematic.
6. To learn more about which treatments are optimal for different types of patients.
7. To strengthen regulatory submissions for new indications of older medicines or to support an old indication.

Meta-analyses are relevant to conduct when ethical reasons preclude the conduct of additional placebo-controlled clinical trials to address an important research question. Practical reasons, including cost factors also encourage use of a meta-analysis in selected situations.

STEPS TO FOLLOW IN CONDUCTING A META-ANALYSIS

Meta-analysis takes place in the following twelve steps, which will be described in greater detail below.

1. Develop a protocol for conducting the meta-analysis that specifically identifies the objective and describes the methods to be used throughout the study.
2. Identify sources of materials to be searched for relevant clinical trials (e.g., computerized data bases, ad hoc searches, bibliographies from the first two sources). Also determine whether specific scientists or clinicians will be contacted to provide information on unpublished trials or trials published in nonindexed journals.
3. Define the criteria for selecting trials to be included in the meta-analysis. Then develop a checklist to score papers for possible inclusion. When the quality of papers or trials will be rated, choose a scale for this rating.
4. Have two or three independent readers read, classify, code, score, and finally evaluate and choose the group of trials that will be included in the meta-analysis.
5. Adjudicate any differences between readers on whether specific trials should be included in the meta-analysis.
6. Develop a checklist of questions, procedures, and analyses to which papers included in the meta-analysis will be subjected. This step is often conducted as part of step 1 (i.e., protocol development) and the methods to be used are included in the protocol. This step differs from step 3, which is the evaluation of trials for inclusion in the meta-analysis.
7. Have two or three independent readers read the papers and answer questions listed on the checklist that was developed in step 6. These readers are extracting the data to be used in the meta-analysis and should be either all the same as or all different from those who conducted step four.
8. Adjudicate any differences between readers (if appropriate) on their quantitative measurements in their specific trials.
9. Combine results obtained and quality-assure the data.
10. Analyze results of the meta-analysis. Create odds ratios if appropriate.
11. Interpret results.
12. Report results. Adequate documentation should be included to help readers of the report interpret the results, and also to enable future reviewers to repeat the meta-analysis, if desired.

A number of these steps will be described in more detail.

Step 1: Develop a Protocol for Conducting the Meta-Analysis

It is essential to identify specifically the question(s) to be addressed and to determine which measures will be used to address those questions. If any data are to be pooled at levels one or two, the parameters involved must be identified. Creating a protocol for a meta-analysis will help to minimize the introduction of biases into the procedure. Determine, insofar as possible, the statistical tests that will be applied to the data obtained. The protocol should provide general information on many of the subsequent steps.

Step 2: Identify Sources of Information To Be Used

Major sources used to identify potential studies are (1) literature searches of computerized data bases, (2) colleagues, (3) references included in published trials, and (4) unreferenced reports and fugitive literature from academic, private, and government authors (e.g., pharmaceutical company files, government reports). If colleagues or others are contacted, determine if this will be via telephone, letter, or by formal written request sent to members of one or more societies. A published request may also be made either as a letter to the editor or as an editorial in an appropriate journal(s).

Some professionals who conduct a meta-analysis want to fine-comb the medical community to locate all possible studies and data for inclusion in the meta-analysis, including unpublished results. Their reasoning is based on the well-known publication bias toward positive studies. Other professionals choose to limit meta-analyses to published data. A third approach (favored by the author) is to obtain as many trials (published and unpublished) as may be obtained without "superhuman" efforts. All studies (both published and unpublished) should be rated as to quality and then stratified into low- and high-quality categories. Separate meta-analyses of each group of trials should be conducted as well as combined meta-analyses to determine any influence of trial quality on outcomes.

Step 3: Define the Criteria To Be Used for Selecting Trials to Include in the Meta-Analysis

There are several approaches to judging the quality of clinical trials for possible inclusion in a meta-analysis. Choose a scale for rating quality of papers and trials or develop a checklist for identifying trials to include in the meta-analysis. The simplest approach is to use a scale that has been derived ahead of time. Several standard scales have been proposed as valid indicators of a trial's quality (see Chapter 103 for examples of many of these scales). Scales may be disease specific, medicine specific, or general.

These scales may yield descriptive or general assessments, or a specific numerical value. There is no consensus that one type of scale or any specific scale is best. Nonetheless, it is important to determine if the scoring system used to evaluate a clinical trial's quality is validated.

1. Does the scale give reproducible results when different people use it to evaluate the same paper?
2. Can the scale pick up differences both within papers or trials and between papers or trials that correlate with accepted differences in medical treatments?
3. How does the scale compare on the above points with other scales used to rate clinical trials?

A drawback of the rating scale approach is that some or many of the trial characteristics that the scale is rating are presented in papers in an extremely brief manner, or not at all. Journals often cut large amounts of material from the very parts of a paper (i.e., methods and results) that are mainly used to judge the quality of a paper. This means that the factor(s) being rated might have been cut from a paper and a rating of "not present" could be made in many categories. Alternatively, the authors may not have submitted adequate details on their trial for it to be fairly judged.

If a scale is used to rate papers, it should be established beforehand whether only papers achieving a score of X will be included in the meta-analysis. Alternatively, the top Y% of papers may be included or the top Z number of papers.

A further approach to quality rating is to speak to the authors of each published paper or to write them a letter indicating those questions that are unanswered in their publication. This approach requires a substantial effort and responses are usually returned slowly, making this method impractical for obtaining additional data on more than a few studies. It is possible to conduct a meta-analysis both with and without poorer quality trials, to see if the outcome is affected.

Typical criteria used in a checklist for determining which clinical trials to include in a meta-analysis are:

1. Published in a journal
2. Published in specific journals
3. Original research
4. Human research
5. Minimum number of patients
6. Minimum age of patients
7. Minimum duration of treatment
8. Minimum dose of medicine
9. Minimum quality score of publication or unpublished report
10. Type of blind (e.g., double blind)
11. Type of clinical trial design (e.g., randomized controlled trial)

Reasons why each rejected paper was not included should be tabulated. This information is often important in interpreting the results of the meta-analysis, as well as in understanding the quality of the trials conducted in a particular therapeutic area.

If one combines a class of medicines in a specific

meta-analysis it may increase any bias present. For example, if anticoagulants are being evaluated, they vary in activity, safety, and other effects. Anticoagulants include aspirin, dipyridamole, warfarin, and ticlopamide.

Step 4: Read, Classify, Code, Score, Evaluate, and Choose Papers for Inclusion

People who rate clinical trials and decide on whether or not to include them in a meta-analysis should be blind both to the identity and type of institution of authors and to the source of funding for the reported research. Such information could bias those who are evaluating papers. Strict criteria for inclusion of trials in the meta-analysis must be established prior to acquiring and reviewing the papers.

Two (or more) independent readers of the papers should use a checklist for each step. When they are not in agreement about whether to include the paper in the evaluation, either one of them is incorrect, or the paper is vague on a particular point(s). The lack of complete information in most published trials is one of the greatest obstacles to conducting an accurate meta-analysis. Any differences between readers should be settled by adjudication.

Ensure that the number of articles evaluated at each part of step 4 is indicated in the final report. This could be accomplished by presenting data for each of the following.

1. Total number of papers read:
2. Number of papers ineligible for inclusion because of X, Y, Z reasons:
3. Total number of papers scored for quality:
4. Total number discarded for A, B, C, reasons:
5. Final number of papers included in the meta-analysis:

Step 5: Adjudicate any Differences Among Readers

The one person (usually) chosen to fulfill this role should be chosen ahead of time and be acceptable to all readers whose differences may require adjudication. An alternative is to have the readers themselves settle any differences that arise.

Step 6: Develop Questions, Procedures, and Analyses to Pose of Trials Included in the Meta-Analysis

This step relates to the methods that are used to address the objective of the meta-analysis. The methods may be simple or complex, loose or rigorous, involve subjective judgment or be totally objective. The methods chosen depend on the nature of the objective and the state of the art in the therapeutic area being evaluated. A typical assessment relates to whether active medicine or placebo is preferable and by how much.

Step 7: Read Papers and Answer Questions Listed on the Checklist

This step should be done by two or three people who work independently. Some or many papers will not furnish answers to all of the questions used in the meta-analysis. In some cases this may be because the clinical trial did not obtain data to address those questions, but in many cases it will be because the data were not published. Therefore, a table or answer sheet of extracted data plus unanswered questions are often sent to the authors, who are requested to confirm data extracted and to provide missing data.

Step 8: Adjudicate Differences Among Readers on Quantitative Measurements

Guidelines may be created so that only differences greater than a specific amount (or percent) require adjudication. This process may be conducted by one or more independent professionals unassociated with the meta-analysis, or it may be conducted by the readers themselves.

Step 9: Combine Results Obtained and Quality-Assure the Data

Numerous approaches to combining data may be considered. The correct approach depends on the protocol, the specific questions posed, and the nature of the data obtained for the meta-analysis.

One common analytic approach is to pool all data and evaluate the combined results. Data pooling may be in terms of raw or averaged data from individual patients, groups of patients, or individual studies. However, saying that 9 of 13 clinical trials had negative results and 4 of 13 had positive results ignores the number of patients in each trial and the quality of each trial. Pooling individual patient data is usually impossible because of marked differences between trials in patient inclusion criteria, treatments offered, and trial design.

Another approach is to pool the mean results of numerous trials. The following formula may be used for this purpose:

$$\text{effect size} = \frac{\left(\begin{array}{c}\text{mean size in}\\ \text{the treat-}\\ \text{ment group}\end{array}\right) - \left(\begin{array}{c}\text{mean size in}\\ \text{the control}\\ \text{group}\end{array}\right)}{\text{standard deviation in the control group}}$$

Step 10: Analyze the Results

Analyses may vary greatly between meta-analyses. If studies utilizing different doses or other design aspects are pooled, there probably will be a bias in the type and number of adverse reactions reported. Thus, aggregating adverse reactions (or other outcomes of a trial) may introduce biases or confounding factors.

Many published papers claim either positive or negative results, but careful evaluation by the readers participating in the meta-analyses may define outcomes differently. Another factor to consider in analyzing results is that two separate analyses used for one (or more) trial could yield different results.

Confidence intervals are often used to present results of multiple clinical trials. This method has the advantage that confidence intervals illustrate the degree of agreement among the trials. This perspective is not obtained when outcomes of clinical trials are described as statistically significant, nonsignificant, or even highly statistically significant.

Is it appropriate to average the means of the incidence reported for adverse reactions in different clinical trials (even if weighting is used to consider the numbers of patients evaluated)? Such pooling is impossible if the quality (or design) of each trial is different. How does one include consideration of the quality of each trial when combining results? It is possible to test whether poorer quality trials had different outcomes than better quality trials, in which case the poorer ones can be discarded. It may be, however, that some trials were rated as having a lower quality because the data desired could not be extracted from the publication or report, and not because the trials were poorly designed or conducted.

Step 11: Interpret the Results

The clinical interpretation of meta-analyses has sometimes been almost impossible. For example, if all clinical trials are grouped together regardless of their quality, there may be major problems in interpretation. There are a number of commonly encountered reasons for difficult interpretation. Treatment dosages may have been inadequate to yield an effective response. Clinical trials may have been uncontrolled. Combining results from open-label and double-blind controlled trials often obfuscates the overall results. Patients may not have been stratified by either the nature or the severity of their disease. Treatments often work differently in severely ill and mildly ill patients. Furthermore, patients may not have been stratified by their degree of risk for events being measured (e.g., risk of having myocardial infarction). It would not be possible to combine myocardial infarction results from a clinical trial of patients who had a low risk of myocardial infarction with those from a trial where patients had a high risk.

A more general problem is that trial designs may have been poor. Obviously, such trials tend to generate invalid data. The endpoints evaluated in the included trials may have been inappropriate or did not represent state-of-the-art measurements. Also, different endpoints may have been used in different trials.

Finally, it may also be important to attempt to determine how much data are missing from the meta-analysis that might influence the results.

Step 12: Report the Results

Reporting involves traditional methods of publication and dissemination of information.

THE CASE AGAINST META-ANALYSIS

Meta-analysis is a sound concept with many practical applications. The following comments are not made as an attack on meta-analysis, but as a statement about its limitations.

Heterogeneity of Clinical Trials

Assume that someone who wishes to conduct a meta-analysis works extremely hard and locates all clinical trials ever conducted on the research question (i.e., the objective of the meta-analysis), both published and unpublished. Examination of those trials reveals that they are quite heterogeneous and addressed different questions. Combining their results may be less valid than identifying the single (or two or three) best clinical trials and accepting its (their) data as the answer to the question. The counterargument is that the best trials cannot always be identified, and even if one or more are identified as best by one person or group, others will not necessarily agree with this assessment. Moreover, the counterargument states, lack of agreement about which is best (i.e., highest validity) is the very reason to do a meta-analysis.

Approaching the Truth

A fallacy pervading this field is that an answer closer to "the truth" will be achieved by combining data from all existing clinical trials on a specific question or issue. The value and validity of a meta-analysis in addressing a specific question has more to do with the quality of the meta-analysis and the quality of the trials combined than with the number of trials, patients, or any other factor.

Can Tons of Garbage Yield a Single Diamond?

Given the great inaccuracies within clinical trials in methods, presentations, and interpretations, it is absurd to believe that combining poor or mediocre trial results will yield summaries that approach the truth. Combining garbage does not yield diamonds. However, quality is only one factor and one would not want to include extremely high-quality trials in a meta-analysis, regardless of other criteria. A good example is the assessment of the operative mortality of coronary artery bypass grafts. The standards of surgical technique have improved over the last 20 years, so that older surgical trials should be excluded from a meta-analysis even though the trials may have been extremely well done. However, these trials would be important to include if one was comparing current and older results or was plotting mortality trends.

POTENTIAL AND ACTUAL PROBLEMS OF META-ANALYSIS

Most criticisms of meta-analyses in the literature are directed toward the inherent problems of combining data from multiple trials. Some of these problems are listed in Table 104.1, and others are briefly mentioned below. A more complete discussion of methodological issues is given by Furberg and Morgan (1987) and in other articles presented at the same conference (Workshop on Methodologic Issues in Overviews of Randomized Clinical Trials), whose proceedings are published (Yusuf et al., 1987). Boissel et al. (1989) also present a major review of various issues.

Publication Bias. Investigators are less likely to write up negative than positive results of clinical trials. A survey of 58 investigators who conducted 921 ran-

TABLE 104.1 *Potential problems in conducting a meta-analysis*

Important differences may exist among trials combined in terms of the:

1. Question posed in the clinical trial
2. Diagnosis of patients
3. Severity of the patients' problem(s)
4. Concomitant medicines and diseases
5. Prior treatment of the patients' problems
6. Doses of medicines used
7. Dosing schedules of treating patients
8. Duration of treatment
9. Quality of the clinical trials' design (e.g., open-label versus double-blind)
10. Quality of the clinical trials' conduct
11. Quality of the clinical trials' statistical analysis
12. Quality and completeness of the clinical trials' publication or report
13. Parameter(s) used to measure efficacy
14. Definition of a successfully treated patient
15. Types of statistical analyses used

domized controlled trials found that 96 (21%) of the trials were unpublished and that their positive studies were more likely to be published (77% vs. 42%, $p = 0.001$ (Chan et al., 1982). Journals, too, are less likely to publish negative trials. Simes (1986, 1987) proposed that this bias could be eliminated by establishing an international registry of all clinical trials that could serve as a primary source of data for future meta-analyses. This subject is discussed further in Chapter 106.

Selection Bias of Articles for Review. Clinical trials excluded from the meta-analyses may be critical to addressing the question posed. Some individuals advocate including only randomized clinical trials, whereas others are not as adamant on this point.

Retrospective Approach. The nature of meta-analysis is retrospective, and such research is less likely to lead to valid results than is prospective research.

Incomplete Data in Source Documents. Few reports or papers of clinical trials have sufficient information to answer fully the questions posed for conducting the meta-analysis. One approach to solve this problem is to contact the authors directly to supply missing data.

Observer Bias. Those who read and evaluate papers may introduce their own biases.

Quality of Data. If any data or analyses are substandard, then the quality of the meta-analysis will be affected

Interpretation Bias. Reviewer's bias may affect quality.

Nonindependence of Results. Nonindependence is a statistical issue.

False Sense of Security. The fact that a mathematical approach has been used to combine data across clinical trials makes some people believe that the outcome has greater validity than it truly does.

Data from Abstracts. Given the relatively lower validity of abstracts in general compared with full papers, data from abstracts should not be included in meta-analyses. If included, the meta-analysis should be conducted both with and without those data.

Although some authors have challenged the processes and concepts of meta-analyses, this approach is a significant advance toward reaching answers to major medical questions. The procedures used to conduct meta-analyses will undoubtedly change and improve, but the process is here to stay.

A study of pooled results was conducted by Baber and Lewis (1982) to address a specific question relating to the time of initiation of β-receptor blocker treatment after a myocardial infarction. The authors pooled clinical trial results separately for those authors who initiated treatment "early" or "late" after onset of pain. They observed a greater reduction in mortality in clinical trials in which treatment was initiated "late."

There are a number of arguments against the practice of pooling data from separate clinical trials. Some of these reasons are listed in Table 104.2. Each of these points has some validity, and they should be considered when this type of exercise is conducted. Nonetheless, each of these points may be strongly debated, and it is the author's view that the balance is often on the side of pooling and reanalyzing data, providing that the potential drawbacks are considered. Pooling data from clinical trials that consider important therapeutic questions may eliminate ineffective therapies from medical practice more rapidly than would otherwise occur. Nonetheless, many interesting medical questions are not amenable to this approach.

EXAMPLES OF META-ANALYSES

Two specific examples are used to illustrate the methodologies and approaches used in tertiary interpretations. These examples involve the questions:

1. Should antibiotic prophylaxis be used in patients during surgery of the colon?
2. Should anticoagulants be used in patients who have had a recent myocardial infarction?

The question addressed in the first example was considered by Baum et al. (1981). They found that pooling mortality data (one of their two endpoints) from multiple trials enabled them to improve on the original analysis of the data. Each of the individual trials had too few deaths to conduct a valid statistical analysis. They examined 26 trials published from 1965 to 1980. In the most recent publications in these series (14 from 1976 to 1980), three advocated against the use of pro-

TABLE 104.2 *Potential problems in pooling data from clinical trials that used different protocols*

1. Definitions of important terms may differ between clinical trials
2. Inclusion criteria and the types of patients enrolled may markedly differ between clinical trials
3. Clinical trial designs or particular aspects of the design (e.g., medicine dosages, medicine regimens, controls, concomitant medicines) differ between clinical trials, and it is difficult to combine data from differently designed trials
4. Endpoints used may differ between clinical trials in the disciplines and methods used to measure effects (e.g., clinical, biochemical, physiological, pathological)
5. Even when the same endpoint is used, the definition of that endpoint may differ, or the tests and parameters used to evaluate the same endpoint may have differed
6. Unpublished clinical trials may have been performed that gave negative results and were not included in the pooled data. This tends to skew combined results in a positive direction
7. The quality of published clinical trials varies, and unless an evaluation is made of each, there is a risk of having one or more substandard trial have too great an influence on the pooled data
8. Combined data obtained at different points in time may invoke an additional confounding factor

phylactic antibiotics, whereas 11 advocated the use of prophylactic antibiotics.

The other endpoint they evaluated was abdominal wound infection. They observed that 19 of the 26 trials defined the criteria for wound infection but that differences existed in the operational definitions used. Sixteen trials required the presence of pus in the wound to state that the wound was infected, 5 trials required a positive culture, and 12 specified the time period during which wound infections could be detected.

An example in which all available articles on a topic are collected but the data are not pooled is in the same area of antibiotic prophylaxis in surgery (Di Piro et al., 1984). These authors listed trials that presented data on 13 parenteral cephalosporins, but they did not pool and reanalyze the data.

The second example involves the evaluation of anticoagulant medicines in patients who have had a recent myocardial infarction. The efficacy of this treatment was said to be unsettled in 1969 (Gifford and Feinstein, 1969). Between 1969 and 1973, four randomized controlled trials were conducted and demonstrated a lower rate of deaths in treated patients, but only one of these trials had a difference that was statistically significant (see Chalmers et al., 1977). These four trials plus 28 other controlled trials were reexamined, and all data from randomized control trials were pooled. Pooled data on fatality rates were statistically significant in favor of using anticoagulants (Chalmers et al., 1977).

FUTURE OF META-ANALYSIS

A meta-analysis differs from the traditional narrative review article of a field of medicine or of a particular scientific topic. The popularity of meta-analysis has grown substantially during the 1980s and is expected to continue to grow during the 1990s. The method, unfortunately, can be easily applied to inappropriate questions or may be poorly executed. Either problem will result in a poor meta-analysis—one that could mislead and certainly would not enlighten. This potential pitfall can be avoided through use of appropriate standards by journal editors.

Journal editors are interested in the topic of meta-analysis and several have written editorials on the topic (e.g., Simon, 1987b; Cunningham, 1988; Naylor, 1988). Other journals have had "special communications" (Thacker, 1988) or "perspectives" (Wachter, 1988) on this topic. Reviews of meta-analyses are given by Sacks et al. (1987) and by Gerberg and Horwitz (1988). A symposium on meta-analysis was published in an edition of *Statistics in Medicine* (Yusuf et al., 1987).

If, in the future, more investigators provide data on individual patients to archives, the pooling of raw data from different clinical trials will be possible. This would be an almost ideal way to conduct meta-analyses. Additional details on patients could be provided through archives, publications, or by authors who are contacted directly.

Interpretation of meta-analyses requires a great deal of common sense and a careful judgment of the clinical significance of the results. Results may be statistically significant, but one should question whether the difference in efficacy parameters presented is large enough to justify altering (or confirming) a clinical practice.

Mispresentation of Clinical Data

Correct presentations of data are shown in *Presentations of Clinical Data* (Spilker and Schoenfelder, 1990). This chapter illustrates a number of presentations that misrepresent the data, whether done purposely or inadvertently. Additional examples are given by DeJonge (1983). Many other methods that illustrate how statistics may be used to deceive intentionally rather than enlighten were presented in the books *How to Lie with Statistics* (Huff, 1954), *Flaws and Fallacies in Statistical Thinking* (Campbell, 1974), and *aha! Gotcha* (Gardner, 1982).

METHODS USED TO MISPRESENT CLINICAL DATA

Format Used

Inappropriate formats (i.e., table, graph, figure) are sometimes used. If the reader should be shown details of the data to support a conclusion and only a summary graph is shown, it may be concluded that the wrong format was used.

Transformation Used

Data are transformed (e.g., to percent change), the raw data are not shown, and there is no method for the reader to determine the values of actual data obtained. This is a common error in the medical literature. See Chapter 117.

Choice of Scales or Omitting Error Measurements

This type of misrepresentation involves the use of graphs to illustrate data that have an obviously inappropriate scale (e.g., logarithmic scale for time), or an inappropriate scale that is less obvious (e.g., a logarithmic scale for certain variables that should be expressed arithmetically). The comparison of trends in two different groups may be greatly distorted if a logarithmic scale is used, or if two separate scales are used for either the abscissa or ordinate (Fig. 105.1).

1. A histogram without error bars or confidence limits can give the appearance of a large change having occurred that is probably significant. Nonetheless, not all histograms require error bars or confidence limits.
2. A narrow scale (e.g., diastolic blood pressure graphed from 90 to 95 mmHg to show medicine effects) can exaggerate minor changes.
3. A broken scale can also exaggerate minor effects.
4. A scale of clinically unimportant values can make a meaningless effect seem important.
5. A scale of values that are never observed clinically may make an unrealistic effect seem relevant.

A graphic illustration of how the presentation of data may influence interpretation is shown in Fig. 105.2. The plot of deaths from diphtheria using a logarithmic scale makes it appear as if the introduction of diphtheria immunization led to a rapid and major decline in childhood deaths. The arithmetic plot on the right illustrates that the death rate was markedly falling at the time when immunization was introduced and that

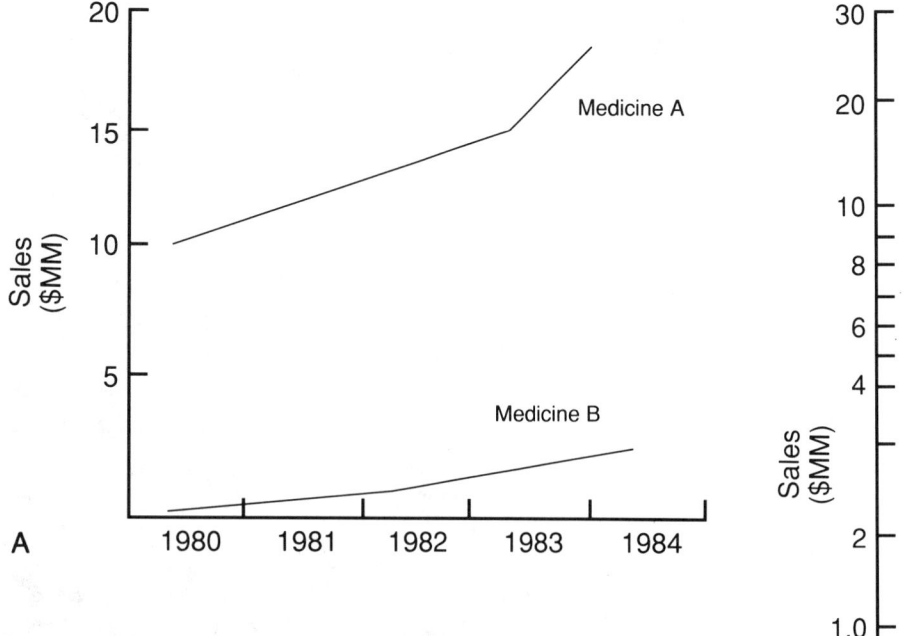

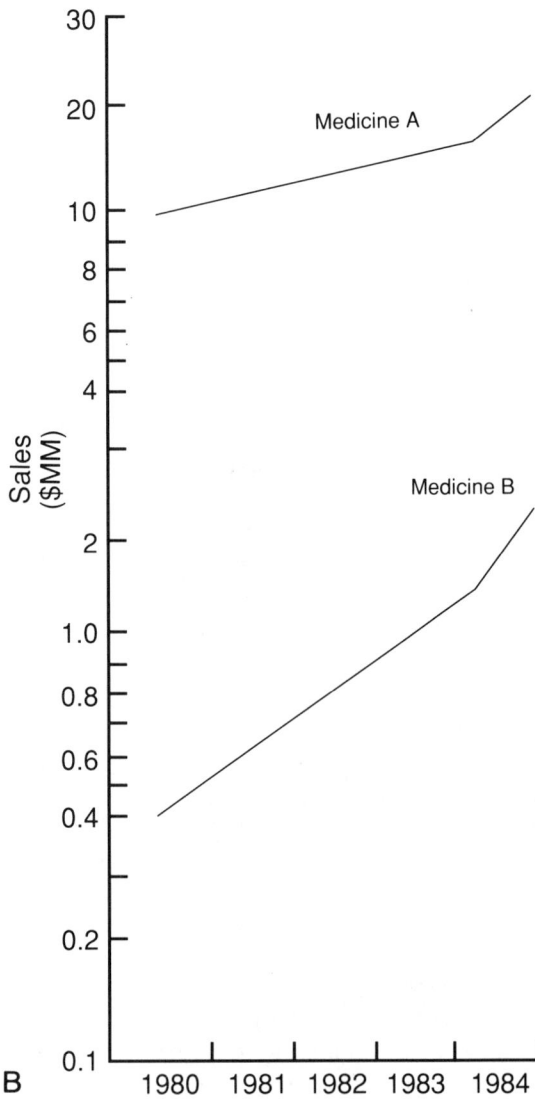

FIG. 105.1 Illustrating the same data using arithmetic (A) or logarithmic (B) scales.

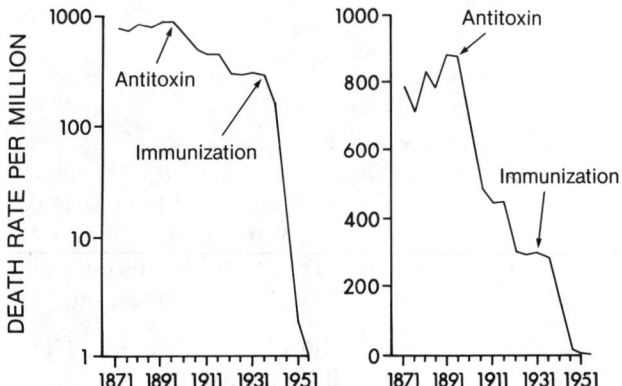

FIG. 105.2 Death rate per million in children under 15 years from diphtheria from 1871 to 1951. The same data are plotted using a log scale (A) and an arithmetic scale (B) on the *ordinate*. (Reprinted by permission of the *British Medical Journal* from Altman, 1980.)

immunization probably played a minor role in influencing the already declining death rate. Alderson (1974) presents these data (using the logarithmic scale) and superimposes a graph of the death rate for measles over the same time course, which was prior to the discovery and use of a vaccine against measles. The plots of deaths from diphtheria and measles are remarkably similar, illustrating that the incidence of deaths from some diseases changes markedly over time.

Complexity and Confusion

A complex graph, figure, or table may be presented that is difficult (or even impossible) to understand. Chapter 13 of *Presentation of Clinical Data* (Spilker and Schoenfelder, 1990) illustrates several examples of this type of mispresentation of data.

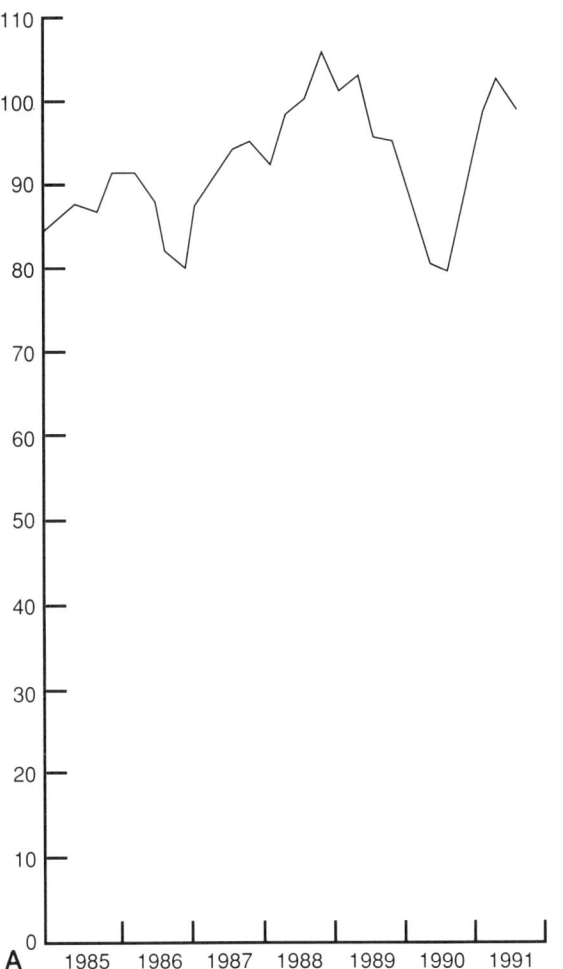

FIG. 105.3A–F Variable presentations of identical data, with various scales. Data from the last full year have been deleted in some presentations to emphasize a given trend.

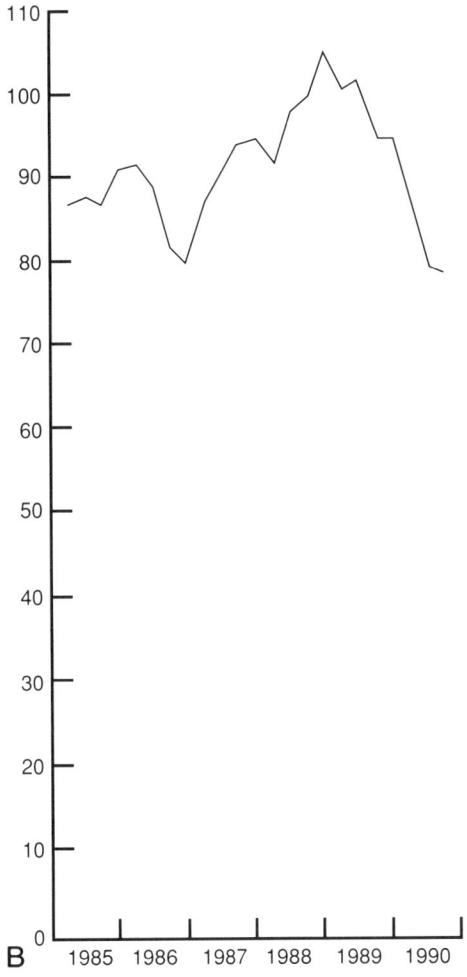

FIG. 105.3 (*continued*)

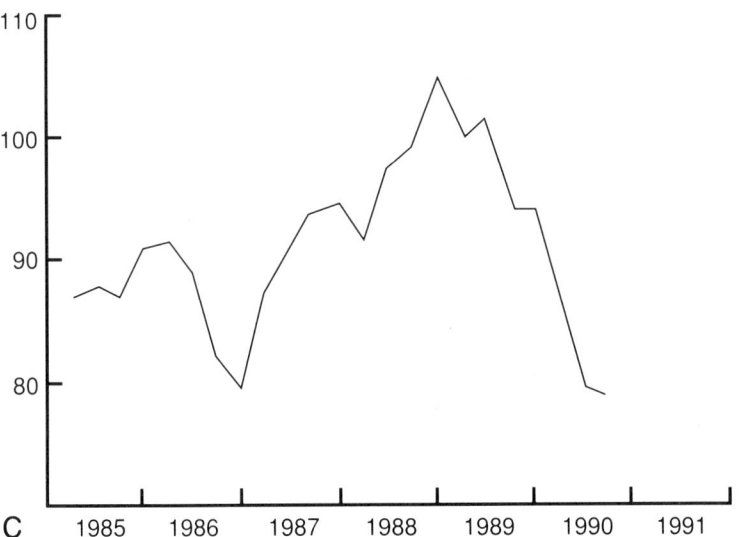

FIG. 105.3 (*continued*)

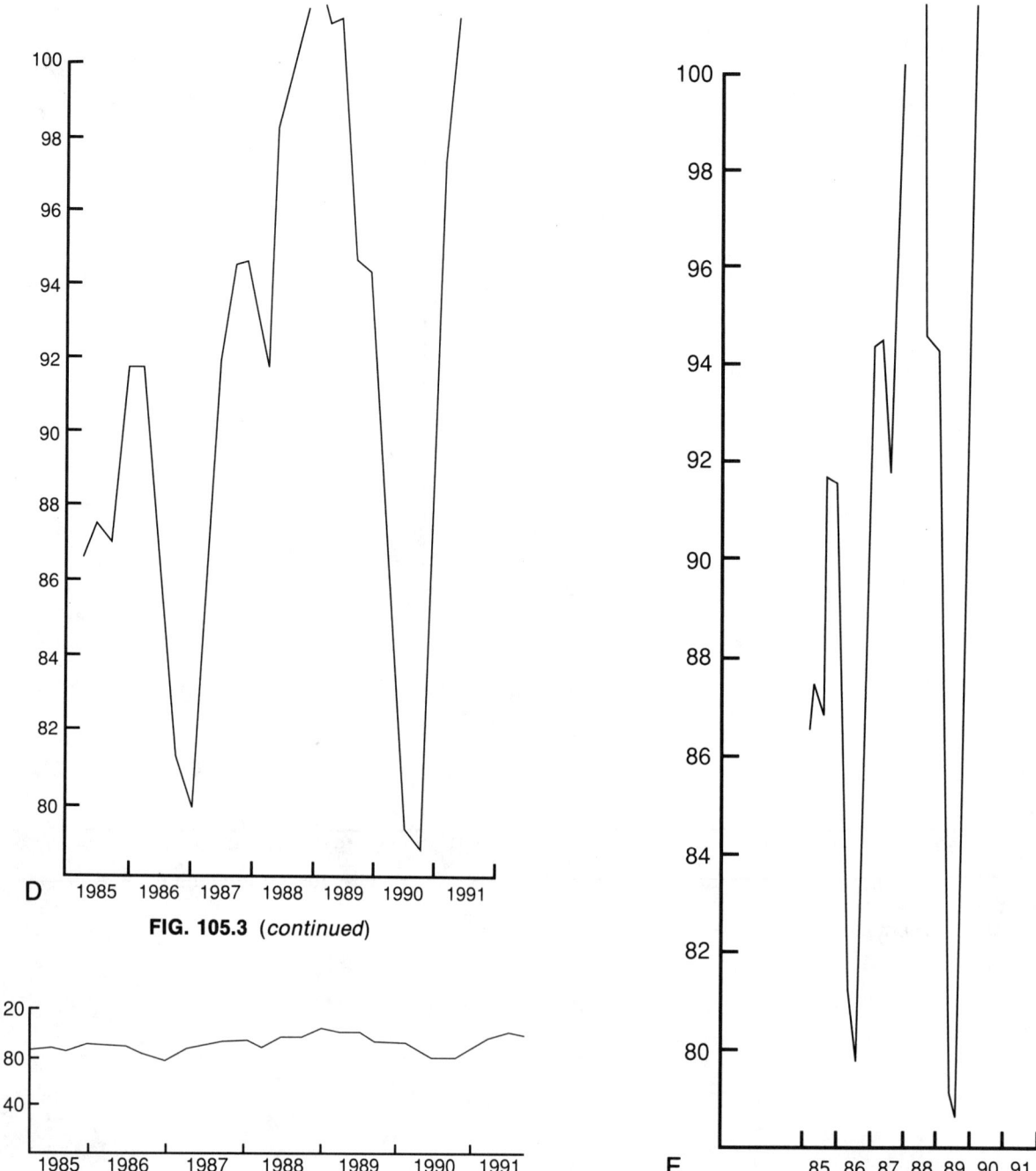

D

FIG. 105.3 (*continued*)

F

FIG. 105.3 (*continued*)

E

FIG. 105.3 (*continued*)

Using Nonconventional Presentations

Clinical improvement is usually shown in graphs as values move farther from the origin along either the ordinate or abscissa. It becomes confusing if one of these principles is changed and improvement occurs as values move closer to the origin for only one axis. If both axes are switched it is generally less comfortable to view and interpret the graph, but this type of graph is usually not as confusing as when a single axis is shifted.

Illustrating Part of the Data

If the presenter chooses to show only selective parts of the data available (e.g., selected years), it may indicate an effect that was not apparent in a more complete data base (Figs. 105.3A–F).

Labeling Scales

Showing axes without values is unacceptable, since it permits great distortions to occur. Condensing or elon-

TABLE 105.1 *Selected types of misrepresentation of graphed clinical data*

1. Inappropriate type of axis scale used (e.g., logarithmic)
2. Inappropriate parameters graphed
3. Inappropriate groups of patients graphed
4. Inappropriate part of the scale shown or omitted
5. Inappropriate elongation or condensation of scale used
6. Inappropriate data shown (e.g., different number of patients in each group compared, when that difference is relevant)
7. Failure to indicate error bars or confidence limits on graphs (when they can assist interpretation)
8. Inappropriate use of a broken scale to exaggerate a minor effect
9. Use of a scale showing clinically unimportant values
10. Use of a scale showing values that cannot be realistically achieved clinically

gating a scale may readily distort any set of data. This method is used to make data appear to be either more variable or more constant than they truly are (Figs. 105.3A–F). Note that some parts of Fig. 105.3 do not begin at 0, but at a higher number. Other graphic elements used to mispresent clinical data are listed in Table 105.1.

Incomplete Expressions

The literature is replete with statements similar to "50% of patients studied had a complete response and 20% had responses lasting over 1 month." It is unclear whether the second number is a percent of the first,

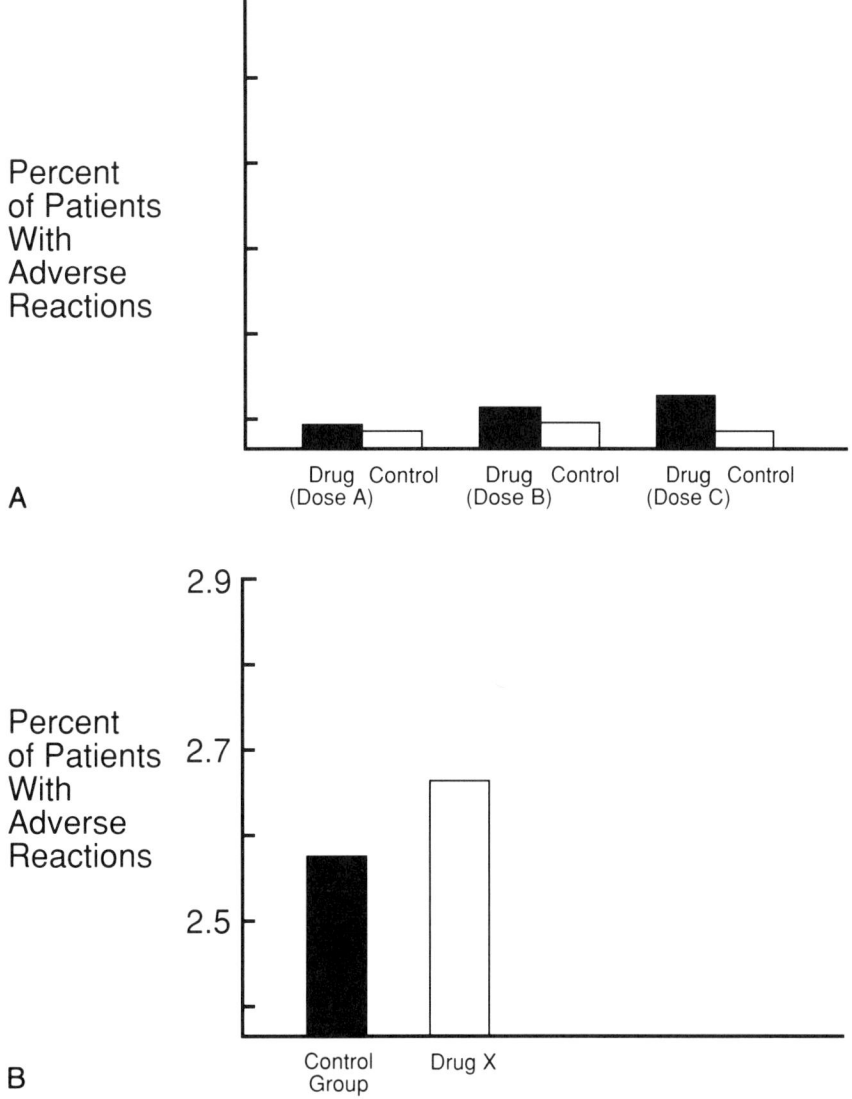

FIG. 105.4A: This approach to presenting adverse reaction data conveys the impression of a relatively small increase. This approach may readily mask a large increase in the incidence (e.g., a doubling or tripling) that is clinically significant. **B:** This approach may exaggerate differences between groups.

20% of 50% (i.e., 10%) or if it is 20% of the entire group of patients (i.e., 20%).

Additional examples of these and other mispresentations are found in articles by Hailstone (1973) and DeJonge (1983), and in the book *The Visual Display of Quantitative Information* (Tufte, 1983).

MOTIVATION OF INDIVIDUALS WHO MISPRESENT DATA

Motives of individuals who mispresent data vary greatly. Some are naive, others want to bolster a scientific or clinical theory, and others are attempting to deceive the reader.

PRESENTING A SINGLE SET OF DATA IN SEVERAL WAYS

A few examples are given of the same data presented in different ways, each leading to a different interpretation. The primary lesson is that interpretations of data must not be made based solely on the appearance of a graph or figure. (See also Figs. 105.1–105.3.)

Example 1. A map of a country may have a number of its states or provinces shaded to illustrate the total number of people in the country who have a particular medical problem. If the person preparing the graph wants to dramatize the importance of the medical effect he or she may shade those states or provinces that have small populations and a very large area, i.e., using an area of less densely populated provinces to represent the true number. If the purpose is to downplay the significance or impact of the data, then only the smallest sized, but most populated areas may be shaded, again proportionally to the total number of patients with the problem. This latter approach would lead to a small area being shaded. Trends may also be either magnified or minimized using this same approach.

Example 2. Using an appropriate scale a 100% in-

crease in the incidence of an adverse reaction may be minimized. Figure 105.4A illustrates this point and gives the impression of a small increase. The opposite approach (Fig. 105.4B) exaggerates small differences between groups.

Example 3. Gouvier et al. (1985) present actual data obtained with one patient in a rehabilitation study, using an ABA study design (i.e., baseline, experimental period, baseline). After a baseline period of 4 days a signal device was attached to the patient's wheelchair that beeped when 15 minutes passed without the patient doing a wheelchair push-up of at least 10 seconds. The third (and last) phase of the study was a second baseline. Each period of 4 days had daily sessions.

Data were presented in four figures in Chapter 101 (Misinterpretation of Data). The interpretation of Fig. 101.1 (based on number of push-ups per hour) is that the timing device led to a threefold increase in push-up frequency, but its withdrawal led to a prompt return to baseline and no lasting improvement. The interpretation of Fig. 101.2 (based on mean push-up duration) is that the intervention had a lasting effect that was only observed after the intervention trial was complete. The interpretation of Fig. 101.3 (based on mean duration of push-up time per hour) shows a marked effect when the device was introduced, a persisting effect, although at a reduced level after it was withdrawn, and a lasting training effect. The last figure (Fig. 101.4) illustrates the original objective of the study, to increase the proportion of 15-minute intervals during which an adequate push-up (defined in the paper and their protocol) occurred. This figure is interpreted similarly to Fig. 101.1.

This is a classic example of how results of even a single straightforward test conducted in one patient can yield three different interpretations depending on how data are presented. It illustrates the absolute need to specify in advance what the exact objectives are of a clinical trial, and preferably how they will be assessed. If multiple measures of efficacy (or other endpoints) are to be used, it is critical to give a hierarchy of their importance.

CHAPTER 106

Methods for Authors and Journals to Improve the Quality of Clinical Publications

TYPES OF PROBLEMS WITH PUBLISHED ARTICLES

Specific problems that exist in the medical literature as a whole are somewhat different from those that exist in specific journals. The following comments are general and are meant to apply to most biomedical journals. No specific journal or small group of journals is being especially criticized. All journals are assumed to have lacunae where additional attention would improve their quality.

The problems listed include some that are primarily the responsibility of authors and others that are primarily the responsibility of journals.

Problems Attributed to Authors

1. Problems in the quality of statistical analyses in published articles.
2. Investigators do not write enough papers about methodological aspects of conducting clinical studies (e.g., recruitment, relative advantages and disadvantages of different tests to assess a particular result, manner of interviewing patients). Lasagna (1979) described these and other deficiencies in the literature in relation to testing of clinical analgesics. Bigby et al. (1985) observed that methods used in dermatological trials were poorly reported. A list of potential topics and information to include about methodological details is given in Fig. 102.3.

Problems Attributed to Journals

1. Failure of most journals to publish an adequate number of well-designed and well-conducted clinical trials with negative results.
2. Failure of most journals to publish sufficient information in the materials and methods section and also in the results section.
3. Failure of some journals adequately to support attempts to improve the quality of clinical trials conducted in certain fields (e.g., surgery).
4. Failure of some journals adequately to support at-

tempts to improve the quality of clinical trials conducted with therapeutic modalities that are not totally established (e.g., biofeedback, hypnosis).

Although each author generally claims the right to choose the quantity of data, references, and other material included in a publication, journals have established standards on how much detail they are willing to publish. Current publications rarely print sufficient information for interested readers to obtain answers to many reasonable questions, especially concerning information generally placed in the methods and results sections. Increasing the amount of information allowed (and required) in these sections would increase the length of each publication and thereby the costs to the journal, subscribers, and advertisers. It is possible, however, that publishing fewer articles, but those that adhere to higher standards, would prevent a number of poorly designed or conducted clinical studies from entering the medical literature.

ON THE NEED TO IMPROVE THE QUALITY OF PUBLISHED STUDIES

Reviews of Published Trial Quality

When one reads reviews of clinical methodologies, it is striking that the authors of these reviews are almost universally critical of the overall quality. They state that investigators can design and conduct clinical trials that adhere to higher standards. Many of the papers that evaluate clinical methodologies conclude that more data would be beneficial to readers who wish to evaluate critically and understand a particular trial (e.g., Lavori et al., 1983; Louis et al., 1984).

Responsibilities of Journals

There are also statements from journals that the methods used in clinical trials could be reported more completely (Munro et al., 1983, reporting for *Lancet*). Although journal editors may respond that authors do not generally submit more data or better analyses, it is this author's position that journal editors are in a position to establish requirements for publication and to insist on authors supplying this information. It is understood that each journal has significant problems and issues of its own. Many of these relate to viability (e.g., circulation, escalating costs), and others, to various practices that journals wish to control (e.g., repetitive publication; Lock, 1984).

Benefits of Improving Publication Standards

A protocol usually requires and contains more details about a clinical trial's methodology than the publication describing the trial in the clinical literature. However, it is difficult to judge a paper fully and adequately when important or relevant details from the protocol are not published. There is a need to increase the amount of detail in published trials so that more relevant questions about each trial may be addressed and answered by the readers.

Readers may ask why standards for publishing articles should be increased, since the overall quality of clinical trials conducted is not as high as it could be. The major answer is that the standards of journals (as well as agencies giving grants) greatly influence the quality of trials that are conducted.

Some ineffective treatments may be used on patients today because they were found to be effective in poorly designed or uncontrolled trials. These treatments will probably continue to be used until well-designed trials show them to be of marginal or no benefit. Ineffective treatments usually have both a morbidity and mortality, and without high standards in both conducting and reporting clinical trials, hazardous or unproven treatments will continue to be used. Examples of this point are given in Chapter 85 on surgery and in the following chapter.

If journals adhered to high standards of publication and presented more details of well-designed trials, it would tend to diminish extreme examples of the effect shown in Fig. 92.1. One of the justifications for markedly increasing the standards by which works are judged for publication is that improperly designed or conducted trials may mislead readers and may mislead medical opinion in general. There may be far-reaching consequences in terms of improper or inadequate treatment of patients.

Baar and Tannock (1989) dramatically illustrated how abbreviated reporting of a clinical trial presented data as positive, while more complete reporting of the same data demonstrated a negative response. The errors of reporting and omissions used in the positive report were the same ones that they found in recent issues of major oncology journals.

IMPORTANCE AND BENEFITS OF PUBLISHING NEGATIVE DATA

Avoiding Duplication of Effort

Publication of negative data from well-designed and well-conducted clinical trials is both desirable and medically important for several reasons. One is that it informs investigators and sponsors who were considering the same or a similar type of trial that it has already been conducted. This will result in a substantial savings of time, effort, and money in many cases. Publication may encourage other investigators to conduct a trial that has greater potential to obtain more meaningful results.

Improving Data on Adverse Reaction Incidence

Publication of negative data relating to adverse reactions would allow a better perspective to be used in evaluating the importance of individual cases of severe adverse reactions. Without some means of attaining information on the numbers of patients exposed (denominator of the incidence ratio), the clinical significance of one or a few severe cases (numerator) cannot easily be assessed in most situations. The incidence rate (numerator over denominator) is one important aspect of evaluating and comparing the clinical significance of adverse reactions.

Impact in Academia

Moreover, the fact that more negative data would be published would presumably relieve some of the pressure experienced by investigators in academia who are concerned about the numbers (and quality) of publications. This in turn might minimize the data dredging conducted in some clinical trials in which a positive result is vigorously searched for and exploited to justify publication of the trial. As a result of these pressures, there are articles in which essentially negative data are presented in a way that demonstrates a positive effect. It is sometimes difficult to gain an accurate perspective of a trial's interpretation, since the author may have deliberately or unintentionally omitted conflicting data that would have raised questions about the conclusions.

Relieving Pressure on Investigators

Investigators who spend their efforts and resources on achieving an optimal design and exceptional conduct of a clinical trial could be more confident about its eventual publication if there were less pressure to publish positive data. They would know that regardless of the trial's outcome, the high standards they adhered to would ensure publication in a reputable journal. Interpretations would in some cases become more objective, since investigators would have less pressure to demonstrate positive results and interpretations. An extreme hypothetical example is one in which 20 groups of investigators independently conduct a similar trial and by chance alone one of the 20 groups (each using $p < 0.05$ as evidence of a beneficial effect) finds a positive effect and publishes it. Without publication of at least some of the negative trials, a wrong (and misleading) conclusion may become established in the literature and clinical practice.

The term *negative trial* has been used in several ways. These include:

1. Trials where no statistically significant difference is observed between treatment and placebo.
2. Trials where no statistically significant difference is observed between two active treatments.
3. Trials that are never completed.
4. Trials where results challenge currently accepted theories.
5. Trials where differences observed are statistically but not clinically significant.

These differences emphasize the importance of clarifying precisely what is meant by a negative trial whenever the term is used.

The Counterargument

On the other hand, many clinical trials in which negative data are reported may simply have missed finding a positive response because the sample size was inadequate. Freiman et al. (1978) examined 71 negative clinical trials and found that 67 of them had more than a 10% chance of missing a true 25% improvement and that 50 of these trials had more than a 10% chance of missing a true 50% improvement.

ROLE OF JOURNALS IN IMPROVING STANDARDS OF CLINICAL TRIALS

The universal demand for "news," new data, and short succinct articles creates pressures that strongly counter the suggestions made to publish negative data. For instance, it is not difficult to imagine a difficult commercial situation for a journal if only one or a few journals started to print longer articles and included numerous studies of negative results. The circulation of a popular weekly medical journal might rapidly decline. Therefore, a significant number of major journals would have to initiate this practice in order for it to have a strong likelihood of success.

The degree to which journals are willing to accept the responsibility to increase standards varies, and there is certainly great potential for improvement. The emphasis placed by the author on journals does not relieve investigators of responsibility. To the contrary, individuals who conduct clinical trials constitute the primary group who must actually improve their standards. Journals are viewed as an important source that can exert pressure to bring this about. Some of the techniques that journals may utilize to influence standards are described in the next section.

POSSIBLE TECHNIQUES FOR JOURNALS TO IMPROVE STANDARDS OF CLINICAL TRIALS AND PUBLICATIONS

Points in the Clinical Trial Process at Which Standards May Be Influenced

During the process of planning and conducting a clinical trial and publishing results, the quality may be influenced and controlled at several points, including (1) the approval or disapproval of the reviewing or funding agency that provides money for the trial (e.g., National Institutes of Health, private foundations), (2) the interface between an investigator and sponsor (often a pharmaceutical company) that pays for many clinical trials, (3) input of professional societies that must decide whether to accept a paper, abstract, or poster for a meeting, (4) journals that review manuscripts to determine whether or not to publish the article, and (5) comments and reviews of a paper by one's peers.

Many of the suggestions that follow will not be possible for most journals to implement immediately, nor would each suggestion be appropriate for all journals. Nonetheless, it is hoped that some of the suggestions are viewed by journals as desirable goals. Most of these ideas have already been expressed numerous times in the literature and are not presented as original suggestions. Although they focus on publications, it is clear that they would in turn put increased pressure on investigators and sponsors to improve standards of designing and conducting clinical trials.

Enlarge Methods and Results Section

Include important and relevant data that are presently excluded from articles. This is the exact opposite of the current trend towards progressively shorter articles (Smith, 1984). It is primarily in the methods section that this need is greatest, but it is also present in the results section of some papers. This author has not observed any overall problems in the length of introductions or discussions and agrees with those who claim that these sections are already too long in many articles.

Increase the amount of material required (or allowed) to be included in the methods section. Several authors have stressed that editors should not delete important methodological details and should require more (e.g., Lionel and Herxheimer, 1970; Mosteller, 1979; Mosteller et al., 1980; Andrew, 1984). There are various types of information that are rarely found in methods sections (see Fig. 102.3). It would be useful to have a separate subsection called "Study Management" (or even a totally new section) that contained some of the information listed in Fig. 102.3 that is not currently included in publications.

Provide Checklists to Authors and Reviewers

Provide checklists (or guidelines relating to each part of a clinical trial) to reviewers and potential authors via Instructions to Authors. Alternatively, indicate that such checklists (or guidelines) may be obtained

by writing to the journal, or publish such lists in the journal and then refer to that issue. Several authors and groups have endorsed this concept for either journals or authors to follow (e.g., Mosteller et al., 1980; Epidemiology Work Group, 1981; Emerson et al., 1984). Many authors desire clearer details or even lists from journals on criteria necessary for inclusion of a paper and favor increasing the standards for publication (DerSimonian et al., 1982; Dixon et al., 1983; Zelen, 1983; Gardner et al., 1983; Tannock and Murphy, 1983). *The British Medical Journal* has published a number of checklists and one is reprinted at the end of this chapter.

Define and Improve the State of the Art

If the journal concentrates on a specific field or modality, it should identify and describe the state of the art in clinical trial design, conduct, and data analysis to potential authors. This may be done through discussion, reference to other articles, inclusion in Instructions to Authors, or through other means. Encourage publications dealing with innovation and alternative methodologies. This policy will clearly contribute toward advancing the state of the art.

Establish a policy that all clinical trials whose results are published, regardless of the field of endeavor or modality used, must incorporate appropriate controls and use an appropriate trial design.

Provide Access to Additional Data

Encourage authors of approved publications to submit additional results or raw data (not published) to the National Auxiliary Publications Service or another repository service. Some of the journals presently following this practice are: (1) *New England Journal of Medicine*, (2) *Journal of Pharmacology and Experimental Therapeutics*, (3) *Federation Proceedings*, (4) *American Journal of Clinical Nutrition*, (5) *Cancer Research*, (6) *American Journal of Physiology*, and (7) *Journal of Applied Physiology*.

Alternatively, the author could put a footnote on the front of all appropriate articles, "More detailed information is available from the author about sections marked (*)." This technique, which is used by the *European Journal of Clinical Pharmacology* (Hemminki, 1981), should be a responsibility of all authors of relevant works.

The *Uniform Requirements for Manuscripts Submitted to Biomedical Journals* (International Committee of Medical Journal Editors, 1982) states that "an editor, on accepting a manuscript may recommend that additional tables . . . too extensive to publish be deposited with the National Auxiliary Publications Service or made available by the author(s)." As Mosteller has stated (1979), "Later use of the data cannot be anticipated. It is time to consider ways to make data available for those who request it."

Publish Less Exciting Results

Be willing to publish negative data from well-controlled and -designed clinical trials. This recommendation has been proposed by numerous authors (e.g., Southam, 1973; Evans, 1982; Tannock and Murphy, 1983). Reasons for this are presented in another section of this chapter.

Be willing to publish data from confirmatory trials if they are well controlled and well designed. H. Tilson (*personal communication*) has suggested that journals should require authors of case reports on adverse reactions to confirm in a letter prior to publication that they have submitted the reports to appropriate regulatory authorities.

Improve Standards in Surgical Journals

Apply steadily increasing standards to surgical trials and those of other modalities for which standards are not presently at as high a level as for medical trials. The author agrees with the principle espoused by Spodick et al. (1978): "There is no scientific or humanistic reason why standards for acceptance should not be equal for all treatments." They were referring primarily to surgical trials. On the other hand, it will take a period of several (or many) years to reach that stage, and it is not realistic to expect that these standards will be instituted immediately. Nonetheless, it should be a clearly stated goal of all relevant journals, and efforts should be enacted to achieve this goal in an expeditious manner.

Provide More Details on Patient Numbers

Information on the numbers of patients available, screened, available for entry, refused entry, entered, dropped out, discontinued, and so on should be provided. Edlund et al. (1985) reviewed 232 articles for information on informed consent. They noted that of 61 articles that mentioned informed consent, 14 listed the numbers of "refusers" and "nonrefusers," and only four noted the characteristics of the "refusers." A similar scenario exists for the other numbers relating patients who are "in" a clinical trial at different milestones and the reasons why they are not, as well as the patients' makeup. These data are important for both interpretation and extrapolation.

Access to Raw Data

Require authors to provide access to the raw data used to create the manuscript while it is being reviewed if reviewers pose questions.

Quoting References

Require authors to affirm that they are quoting original sources and not secondary reports, unless each is clearly identified. Many errors in the literature are perpetuated by this method (Dickersin and Hewitt, 1986).

Illustrations of Practical Lessons

Encourage publication of discussions of actual problems encountered in clinical trials that provide practical lessons.

Prior Commitment to Publication

Protocols could be submitted to a journal prior to conducting a clinical trial and the editors asked for an assurance that the results could be published in their journal, even if negative. The problem with this concept is that many problems might arise during the course of the trial that would make the results unsuitable for publication, even if the data processing, statistical analyses, and clinical interpretation were all done appropriately.

Providing Clear and Complete Definitions

Ensure that all diseases that are characterized or defined differently in various countries (e.g., hypotension, hyperkinetic children, irritable bowel syndrome) are clearly defined in the article. The same comment applies to adverse reactions. Reference diagnostic criteria promulgated by a specific society whenever appropriate.

Providing Dates When the Patients Were Tested

Including the actual dates when patients were treated may help readers differentiate between prospective and retrospective clinical trials if the authors have tried to gloss over this point.

Providing Information on Financial Conflicts of Interest

Authors with positions, stock, or other arrangements that may present a conflict of interest should state this in their article (Relman, 1989).

Providing Structured Abstracts

A number of well-respected journals are now providing structured abstracts (i.e., using subheads) that identify objective, design, settings, patients, intervention, measurements, results, and conclusions. Other categorizations are possible. This approach provides much more information on clinical trials than most nonstructured abstracts.

IMPROVING JOURNALS' STATISTICAL REVIEWS

It has been claimed that about one-half of all published medical trials contain errors in statistics (Freiman et al., 1978; Glantz, 1980; Altman, 1981; Gardner et al., 1983; Bland et al., 1985). These references list many additional references with similar findings and conclusions. Moreover, it is widely stated that there are too few patients in many trials to demonstrate an effect, even if one were present. In the statistical vernacular, there is often inadequate power to detect the desired difference between treatment groups.

Although the focus of this book is on clinical rather than statistical concepts, there are suggestions in the literature for guidelines on improving the quality of published statistical analyses (O'Fallon et al., 1978; Altman, 1981). Their suggestions are summarized in Tables 106.1 and 106.2. O'Fallon et al. also described numerous problems relating to the use and misuse of statistics. Gardner et al. (1983) published a checklist (Fig. 106.1) that they claim is suitable as an aid in preparing and reviewing manuscripts. Some common statistical problems found in reviews of the literature have been presented (Schor and Karten, 1966; Pocock et al., 1987; Smith et al., 1987; McKinney et al., 1989; Altman and Doré, 1990). Pocock et al. present a list of ten recommendations to enhance the statistical quality of published data.

The current checklist used by reviewers of the *British Medical Journal* is shown at the end of this chapter. The journal *Cancer Treatment Reports* published guidelines (Simon and Wittes, 1985) that represented a major step in the direction of improving the standards of their methodology section, and they are to be commended. Many other journals such as *Journal of the American Medical Association* and *Circulation* (Glantz, 1980) conduct a statistical review at some stage of their review process, but not all of those journals describe to authors what is considered a necessary checklist of acceptable statistical requirements. Without such a list, a rejection from a journal usually means that an unaltered or slightly modified version will eventually find its way into the literature. With a list, it is more likely that the rejection will encourage authors to aim at a higher standard.

TABLE 106.1 *Suggestions of O'Fallon et al. to improve the quality of statistics in medical journals*

A. To improve the medical trials being done
  1. Editors should give publication preference to well-documented reports of controlled clinical trials instead of reports of exciting data from poorly controlled trials
  2. Statisticians should be involved at the very beginning of research projects
B. To improve the documentation in medical research papers
  1. Standards governing the content and format of statistical aspects should be developed to guide authors in the preparation of manuscripts. These standards should be made part of the publication policy and should be enforced by reviewers and editorial boards[a]
  2. All raw data should be made available for examination by interested readers
  3. In publishing reports of uncontrolled clinical observations, editorial boards should either print a warning section or insist that the author(s) explicitly spell out the limitations of the trial
  4. A system for classifying medical articles based on the quality of their scientific evidence should be developed. The classification criteria should be printed in the journals
  5. Editors should refrain from cutting material that critical readers need to evaluate the paper, and editors should reproduce in great detail those papers that are concerned with areas of controversy or uncertainty
C. To improve the editorial review process
  1. Journals should recruit biometrically sophisticated people as manuscript reviewers and editorial board members
  2. Authors should prepare a detailed exposition concerning methodology, which would not appear in print but would be available to the editor and referees when evaluating a manuscript
  3. Editorial boards should carefully consider the quality of the trial design, conduct, presentations of results, and analysis when evaluating a manuscript

Reprinted by permission of *Biometrics* from O'Fallon et al. (1978).
[a] See Vaisrub (1985).

TABLE 106.2 *Suggestions of Altman to improve the quality of statistics in medical journals[a]*

1. Statisticians should help referee manuscripts submitted for publication
2. All papers using any statistical procedure should be refereed by a statistician
3. Revised papers should be returned to the same referee for reappraisal
4. Journals should state clearly what their refereeing policy is
5. There should be statistical guidelines for contributors
6. All research papers should include a separate section on statistical methods
7. Journals should give priority to well-executed and well-documented clinical trials
8. Authors should be encouraged to supply additional information (especially on methodology) to help the referees but not for publication
9. Authors should be encouraged to include raw data in their papers
10. Journals should employ editorial staff with some understanding of statistics

[a] See Altman (1981). He indicated that many of these suggestions have been made before, and he lists five references.

EVALUATION OF STATISTICAL ASSESSMENT — PILOT STUDY

Paper number_____ (If any answers are "No" please make comments in Section 11 below.)

Name of assessor _____

1. Is the objective (purpose) of the study sufficiently described? .... Yes   No

2. Is an appropriate study design used to achieve the objective?.............................. Yes   No

3. Is the selection of study members adequate in:
   (a) its description? .... Yes   No
   (b) the source of patients? .... Yes   No
   (c) sample chosen? .... Yes   No
   (d) response rate?... Yes   No

4. (a) Is the reason for the sample size used discussed? .... Yes   No
   (b) Does the sample size seem adequate?... Yes   No

5. (a) Is there a statement describing or referencing all statistical tests used? .... Yes   No
   (b) Are the tests used appropriate? .... Yes   No

6. Is the presentation of statistical material clear in the:
   (a) text?.. Yes   No
   (b) tables? .... Yes   No
   (c) figures? .... Yes   No

7. Is an appropriate/correct conclusion drawn from the statistical analysis? .... Yes   No

8. Was a statistician involved as:
   (a) author? .... Yes   No
   (b) acknowledged help? .... Yes   No

9. From the statistical viewpoint is the paper of acceptable standard to have been
   published? .... Yes   No

10. Other remarks.. Yes   No

11. Comment on questions 1-9 where answer was "No"

FIG. 106.1 Checklist of the *British Medical Journal* to evaluate statistical aspects of articles submitted for publication. (Reprinted by permission of the *British Medical Journal* from Gardner et al., 1983.) Their current checklist is shown at the end of this chapter.

Should Reviewers for a Journal Be Blind to the Identity of Authors of Manuscripts?

The advantage of blinded reviewers is that manuscripts without the author's names or professional affiliation would theoretically be reviewed more impartially. Blind reviews have been shown to be successful (McNutt et al., 1990). However, most reviewers who are familiar with the types of research being conducted in a scientific area will be able to guess whose work is being reviewed. Their guess may be based on what experiments or clinical trials are being conducted, what is said in the introduction and discussion, and the specific references quoted. Blinding the manuscript sent for review also means that the copy sent to reviewers must not contain paper watermarks that can be identified, or photographs that state which university or organization was responsible for their preparation.

PUBLICATION BIAS

The simplest definition of publication bias is that a greater proportion of clinical trials that contain positive results than those that contain negative results are (1) written as manuscripts, (2) submitted for publication, and (3) published. This occurs because of biases of investigators, journal reviewers, and journal editors, each of whom are responding to a variety of influences and pressures. The subject has been discussed and reviewed at some length by several groups (e.g., Dickersin et al., 1987; Begg and Berlin, 1989). The review by Begg and Berlin discusses numerous studies of this phenomenon, particularly as it occurs in the field of cancer therapy, and also describes numerous issues that relate to this topic. It is apparent that clinical journals could play a major role in altering publication bias, particularly if they act in concert.

Is Publication Bias Applied Equally to All Types of Clinical Trials?

Several authors believe that there is a greater bias against publishing negative clinical trials that are historically controlled than there is against publishing randomized controlled clinical trials that are negative. Data that would be completely convincing on this point are unavailable. There is a sound reason for journal editors to have this bias. Because uncontrolled and poorly controlled clinical trials are more likely to yield positive data, it is more likely that historically controlled clinical trials will yield false-positive results than will well-controlled clinical trials. However, it is also more common to observe false-negative results in uncontrolled and poorly controlled clinical trials than in well-controlled trials. As a result, if negative results are observed, they will be less convincing to readers if they are observed in a historically controlled trial than in a well-controlled trial.

Suggestions To Reduce Publication Bias

One author's suggested approach to reducing publication bias—to create an international registry of clinical trials (Simes, 1986)—holds promise. Simes presents the rationale and value of this approach clearly, as well as examples in two areas of cancer research. More practical issues of identifying sources of funding and determining who would operate this system are still major hurdles.

Hetherington et al. (1989) support the concept of prospective registration of clinical trials. They described in detail what was probably the largest effort ever mounted to obtain information retrospectively on unpublished clinical trials in a specific therapeutic area (i.e., perinatal medicine).

Another way to reduce publication bias is to obtain peer review of protocols at the planning stage by funding bodies and journals (Newcombe, 1987). The major issue to resolve here is which groups should have this responsibility. The responsibility really belongs to the authors of the protocol. A related issue is whether Ethics Committees/Institutional Review Boards should use checklists and other methods to ensure adequate standards for all clinical trials conducted. This latter approach is sound, whether or not international (or other) registries are implemented. After all, registries

per se do not improve standards, they only collect data on clinical trials that are, or have been, conducted.

Finally, journals could publish short reports of negative clinical trials (Higginson, 1987). Other suggestions are given by Begg and Berlin (1989).

Reducing Publication of Fraudulent Material

Several proposals are being pursued to reduce the publication of fraudulent research. These proposals include (1) establishment by academic, government, and other institutions of guidelines for scientists conducting research; (2) reducing and limiting the number of publications reviewed when scientists are considered for tenure (e.g., five publications for assistant professor, seven for associate professor, and ten for full professor); and (3) acceptance of full responsibility for a paper's content by all authors instead of the "partial" responsibility many authors claim today (e.g., "I only did. . . ."). Changing the incentives of authors from the number of publications to the quality of publications should have a major positive effect on the medical literature. See Chapter 64 for guidelines issued by the University of North Carolina Medical School at Chapel Hill, North Carolina.

CHECKLIST AND GUIDELINES FOR AUTHORS

Clinical Pharmacology and Therapeutics is one journal that provides a checklist for authors, and *Cancer Treatment Reports* has provided methodological guidelines for several years (Simon and Wittes, 1985).

CHECKLIST FOR STATISTICIANS

This last section illustrates a journal's checklist for statistical review, plus an excerpt from the Instructions for Authors in the *British Medical Journal*.

Statement to Authors on Statistical Assessment from the *British Medical Journal**

"The comments made by referees are considered by the 'hanging' committee, which decides whether each paper should be published, perhaps after revision, or rejected. If the paper seems promising, the committee may decide to send it for statistical assessment. In this case a statistician looks at the paper, completes a checklist, and probably also writes a report, which as with the scientific referee's report, may be sent to the author. The statistician completes one of two checklists: one is for general papers and the other, which is

---

* *Guidelines for Writing Papers*, 1987;294:36–38.

more detailed, is for papers on clinical trials. For each question under the headings 'Design features' and 'Conduct of study/trial' the statistician is asked to circle the reply Yes, Unclear, or No; for each question under the headings 'Analysis' and 'Recommendations' he or she is asked to circle the reply Yes or No."

Checklist for Statistical Review of General Papers

Design features

1. Was the objective of the study sufficiently described?
2. Was an appropriate study design used to achieve the objective?
3. Was there a satisfactory statement given of source of subjects?
4. Was there a power-based assessment of adequacy of sample size?

Conduct of study

5. Was a satisfactory response rate achieved?

Analysis and presentation

6. Was there a statement adequately describing or referencing all statistical procedures used?
7. Were the statistical analyses used appropriate?
8. Was the presentation of statistical material satisfactory?
9. Were the confidence intervals given for the main results?
10. Was the conclusion drawn from the statistical analysis justified?

Recommendation on paper

11. Is the paper of acceptable statistical standard for publication?
12. If "No" to question 10, could it become acceptable with suitable revision?

Checklist for Statistical Review of Papers on Clinical Trials

Design features

1. Was the objective of the trial sufficiently described?

2. Was a satisfactory statement given of diagnosis criteria for entry to the trial?
3. Was there a satisfactory statement given of source of subjects?
4. Were concurrent controls used (as opposed to historical controls)?
5. Were the treatments well defined?
6. Was random allocation to treatment used?
7. Was the method of randomization described?
8. Was there an acceptable delay from allocation to start of treatment?
9. Was the potential degree of blindness used?
10. Was there a satisfactory statement of criteria for outcome measures?
11. Were the outcome measures appropriate?
12. Was there a power-based assessment of adequacy of sample size?
13. Was the duration of posttreatment follow-up stated?

Conduct of trial

14. Were the treatment and control groups comparable in relevant measures?
15. Were a high proportion of the subjects followed up?
16. Did a high proportion of subjects complete treatment?
17. Were the dropouts described by treatment/control groups?
18. Were side effects of treatment reported?

Analysis and presentation

19. Was there a statement adequately describing or referencing all statistical procedures used?
20. Were the statistical analyses used appropriate?
21. Were prognostic factors adequately considered?
22. Was the presentation of statistical material satisfactory?
23. Were confidence intervals given for the main results?
24. Was the conclusion drawn from the statistical analysis justified?

Recommendation on paper

25. Is the paper of acceptable statistical standard for publication?
26. If "No" to question 25, could it become acceptable with suitable revision?

CHAPTER 107

Prospective Registration of Clinical Trials

PURPOSES OF A REGISTRY

A registry is a listing of clinical trials. For each trial it may contain any amount of information, from a general title to a large amount of data. Numerous people have suggested that some or all clinical trials should be registered at the time of their initiation (see Meinert, 1988, for a list of eight references). This chapter refers primarily to registries created prospectively. The major purposes of a clinical trial registry are to:

1. Enhance communications and increase the number of collaborations between clinical researchers. Interested professionals could determine who is initiating activities in a specific area at an earlier time than is possible without a registry.
2. Help clinical researchers who are planning new clinical trials avoid unnecessary duplication.
3. Assist clinical researchers who are conducting meta-analyses of clinical trials. A relatively complete prospective registry would minimize or prevent publication bias. After a period of time, all clinical trials would be listed, and completed unpublished trials that were negative could be included in a meta-analysis.
4. Assess information on national or regional research activities (i.e., what is ongoing within a specific country or region). Policymakers and health planners could use this information to influence grant expenditures and allocation of their resources.

TYPES OF REGISTRIES

A number of registries of clinical trials currently exist (Table 107.1). These are primarily disease oriented, although the specific discipline of medicine (e.g., perinatal medicine) and type of approach (e.g., thrombosis and hemostasis trials) have also been used as a basis of creating clinical trial registries. A registry could be designed on the basis of other characteristics of clinical trials (e.g., those conducted in country X, those involving over 1,000 patients). Pharmaceutical companies usually maintain registries of clinical trials conducted on their medicines, even after a medicine is marketed. Complete information about these registries usually is not available to outside requests, although most pharmaceutical companies would probably answer specific questions of a nonproprietary nature.

Prospective registries are created from information obtained prior to conducting the clinical trial, whereas retrospective registries are created from published results. The latter group do not include unpublished trials and thus have a publication bias (discussed in more detail in Chapter 106). Another problem with retrospective registries is the time lag involved in identifying clinical trials.

A relatively complete clinical trial registry encompassing all therapeutic areas would be extremely complex and expensive to develop and maintain, and it is doubtful that it would be given sufficient priority to receive adequate funding. Even if a national agency endorsed and financially supported this concept, it is

TABLE 107.1 *Selected list of current registers of clinical trials*

Register	Location	Inclusion criteria	Methods of identification of new trials	Source of information
International thrombosis and hemostasis trials register	France	Thrombosis and hemostasis trials, multicenter, randomized	Mailing list, voluntary submission	Journal of Thrombosis and Hemostasis
Oxford Database of perinatal trials[a]	United Kingdom	Perinatal trials, randomized	Survey of obstetricians, journal advertisements	Classified bibliography, floppy diskette
U.K. coordinating committee on cancer research	United Kingdom	Cancer trials, Phases I–III, discontinued and suspended trials	Mailing lists, voluntary submission	Publication
Physician Data Query	United States	Cancer trials, Phases I–III	Mailing lists, voluntary submission	Computer database (CLINPROT)
EORTC[b] register of cancer trials	Belgium	Cancer trials, multicenter	Database of EORTC-sponsored trials, voluntary submission	Computer database
AmFAR[c] register of AIDS trials	United States	Randomized, trials in all stages	Database of NIH-sponsored trials, voluntary submission	Publication with three monthly updates

This table was provided by Dr. Phillippa Easterbrook and is reprinted with permission. Numerous registries exist of patients with rare diseases, and of information about rare diseases.

[a] Chalmers et al. (1986).
[b] EORTC, European Organization for Research and Treatment of Cancer.
[c] AmFAR, American Foundation for AIDS Research.

unlikely that international cooperation would be sufficient for the registry to obtain all needed and desired information.

Specific disease or therapeutic area registries appear to be more practical and realistic goals for the next decade. Such registries currently are being promoted, although a broader effort, possibly even organized and supported by professional societies or other groups with specific interests, is really necessary. Surveys (to establish the degree of interest) combined with pilot programs would help determine if registries are feasible in areas where they do not exist. Another practical type of registry is one maintained by a single Ethics Committee/Institutional Review Board (IRB) or group of Ethics Committees/IRBs. The value of these registries would have to be assessed over time, because their usefulness would not cover all of the purposes described above.

PROCEDURES TO CREATE AND MAINTAIN A REGISTRY

A complete registry should clearly indicate which clinical trials are published (and provide the references), unpublished, ongoing, and planned. The specific procedures for creating and maintaining a registry are varied. Nonetheless, a few systems appear to be workable. The first is for each IRB in the United States or Ethics Committee in other countries to collect appropriate information on all studies they approve. A prototype list of data that could be collected is shown in Table 107.2. Additional data suggested by Meinert (1988) are listed in the footnote to this table. Collecting

data on even the 11 basic items in Table 107.2 may be found to be impractical. Collecting the additional data suggested by Meinert could raise yet more problems.

IRBs and Ethics Committees could submit sheets with this type of information (one sheet per study) to a national or international group that would collate and disseminate the information or make it available to interested people. The national group could be a government agency, professional society, professional association, foundation, or private organization. The international group could be the World Health Organization or any of the groups mentioned above. There are pros and cons for each type of organization, but secure funding plus a long-term commitment are two

TABLE 107.2 *Types of data that should be collected for a prospective registry of clinical trials[a]*

1. Investigator's name(s), affiliation(s), and address(es)
2. Site(s) at which the clinical trial is being conducted
3. Disease or condition being treated or evaluated
4. Clinical trial design (e.g., parallel, crossover)
5. Projected sample size for each treatment group
6. Medicine(s) or treatments being evaluated and dosage regimen
7. Blinding (e.g., open-label, single-blind, double-blind)
8. Projected duration of trial
9. Projected starting date
10. Sources of funding
11. Procedure for assignment of treatment (e.g., randomization in blocks of six)

[a] Other data that could be requested, as suggested by Meinert (1988), include: (1) patient demographic characteristics, (2) patient eligibility criteria, (3) purpose of trial, (4) primary and secondary outcomes, (5) projected length of patient follow-up, (6) administration procedures, (7) specifics of proposed methods of analysis, (8) list of data collection sites, and (9) list of coordinating centers, central laboratories, and data reading centers.

important requirements for any organization involved in a registry.

Funding of registries is an important issue, but is not addressed in this chapter.

Use of Ethics Committees/IRBs

All clinical trials and studies approved by an Ethics Committee or IRB theoretically should be included in a registry if a complete data base is a goal. However, there are additional trials that could (or should) also be included.

Clinical Trials That Are Not Reviewed by an Ethics Committee/IRB

Some clinical trials are conducted without being submitted to an Ethics Committee for review and approval. These include surgical studies, retrospective studies, case series, and single patient trials. A voluntary system whereby investigators would be encouraged to submit information from these types of trials to the registry would partially address this issue.

Some clinical trials are not required to be approved by an Ethics Committee (e.g., volunteer trials in the United Kingdom). Most volunteer trials are submitted to Ethics Committees in the United Kingdom, but there are a few that are not. New laws requiring all human trials to be reviewed by Ethics Committees could readily close this loophole.

Ethics Committees/IRBs That Do Not Wish to Participate

Some Ethics Committees may not wish to participate in a registry program. A national law or regulation mandating participation might remedy this situation, but it is doubtful that appropriate legislatures would agree to mandate participation.

Local, Regional, or Disease-Specific Registries

A totally different approach would be to create a local register of clinical trials, which could be maintained by each Ethics Committee that chose to do so. These registries would primarily be for local or regional use, and for others with a specific interest in the registry. Another approach is for groups of Ethics Committees (e.g., of a hospital chain, of certain universities) to join to establish and maintain common registries, or for specific government agencies to do so.

Meinert (1988) has proposed that various registries could be created for specific treatments, diseases, or medical specialties. If such registries were assembled, participation by most if not all Ethics Committees would be necessary to achieve the goals described.

Alternatively, individual investigators could accept responsibility for sending the requested information to the relevant center. Unfortunately, this last approach is impractical because many investigators either will not cooperate at all, or will lose their good intentions and not follow through after a period of time. There is inadequate incentive for most investigators to participate.

SECURITY OF INFORMATION IN A REGISTRY

Competitive Value of Information During Each Phase of a Medicine's Development

Although the general concept of prospective registration of clinical trials appears relatively simple and straightforward, there are several potential problems of great magnitude that must be addressed. First, the information in Table 107.2, or even a subset of that information, would have enormous competitive value for some new medicines in Phases I, II, and III. A few of the many uses of such information by competitive companies would include:

Phase I. The registry would identify the type of new medicines being developed by a potential competitor and might identify a specific medicine. Depending on the design of the clinical trial used, it could also identify specific or general problems that had occurred and how these problems were being approached.

Phase II. Information in the registry would identify which new indications for a marketed (or investigational) medicine are being evaluated in a pilot trial or are being actively pursued in multiple trials. The endpoints or clinical trial design used could provide extremely valuable information for competitors.

Phase III. Information would be readily apparent on any problems that developed (e.g., an unexpected clinical trial of a medicine in patients with compromised cardiac function). The types of clinical trials in Phases II and III would clearly indicate the development strategy being followed.

The rate of a competitor's progress could be easily measured from Phases I, II, and III clinical trials. This information would allow a competitor to modify or redirect the course of its own medicine's development or to change priorities and resources applied to any specific activity. Even the names of investigators in all phases would provide important competitive information.

Confidentiality

It is readily apparent that major safeguards must be built into any system of prospectively registering trials. One such safeguard would be to give the sponsor the option of maintaining confidentiality on a clinical trial for a period of time (e.g., 2 to 5 years). While a clinical trial's confidentiality is often essential to a sponsor at the early stages of a drug's development, it is often in the company's interests to promote important clinical trials later in the medicine's development. Nonetheless, companies often wish to protect the data and even titles of certain trials for several years after they are conducted. One reasonable guideline would be for sponsors of investigational medicines to provide information on all clinical trials conducted with a specific medicine after it is approved for marketing or after all work on it is terminated. Even these guidelines would create numerous other questions and issues. Work may continue on new dosage forms or indications after initial marketing approval and, also, marketing of a new medicine does not occur simultaneously in all major countries at the same time. There is usually a period of 5 to 10 years between the time a sponsor's dossier is first submitted to a regulatory authority and when regulatory approval is received to market a new medicine in all major countries.

A second major problem is that the media could use information in a registry prematurely, to praise or severely criticize a clinical trial that is just getting started. This could place public pressure on sponsors to terminate clinical trials that are of medical value. Stockbrokers, analysts, and consumer advocate groups could literally chart every company's development activities and the progress on each of their individual new (and old) medicines. Finally, many of the issues of competition and confidentiality described for the pharmaceutical industry are also felt by government and academic clinicians and scientists. A number of additional problems are listed in Table 107.3. These issues must be considered to determine if the usefulness of each registry is worth the investment of effort and money.

TABLE 107.3 *Selected issues and problems in establishing a prospective registry of clinical trials*

1. Identifying a funding source willing to make a long-term commitment of adequate magnitude
2. Degree of commitment by each Ethics Committee/Institutional Review Board to participate at an acceptable level
3. Confidentiality of the data
4. Security of the data
5. Investigators' interest in participation
6. Investigators' interest in using the data base created
7. A means of easy access for clinicians to use the registry

The only registry that would probably obtain the pharmaceutical industry's endorsement is a purely voluntary one. Whether this approach would prevent useful registries of medicines from being established is uncertain. Many types of registries would not be greatly affected by lack of industry participation.

IMPLEMENTATION OF A CLINICAL TRIAL REGISTRY

The best approach toward implementing this concept, in part or in toto, is for interested people to develop a proposal that is widely acceptable to most relevant groups. Professional disease- or discipline-oriented societies, associations, and foundations could debate and discuss this issue at their meetings. They could determine whether their involvement is justified based on the anticipated returns. A survey and pilot study could be conducted to confirm such a project's practicality and feasibility. At that point a plan should be developed to implement this idea. This plan will probably require input and backing from government, academic, and industry representatives. It would be ideal if the plan were international, but even a modest start toward a national (or even regional) plan would represent a major accomplishment.

CHAPTER 108

Archiving Clinical Trial Data

At the conclusion of a clinical trial a report or publication is usually written and the data are either stored or discarded. At a certain stage almost all data are discarded. These data represent a valuable reservoir of information that could be used for several different purposes. Various ways of storing these data in centralized or decentralized locations and making them available to others for legitimate uses have been considered. This chapter describes some potential types of data archives, their purposes, and issues surrounding their establishment.

PURPOSES OF ARCHIVES

To Conduct Meta-Analyses

Archives of data would allow scientists to conduct meta-analyses more accurately than they can at present. Using raw data obtained from archived clinical trials would enable a greater degree of pooling of results than is now possible. This approach should lead to more meaningful meta-analyses.

To Address Clinical Research Questions Without the Need to Conduct a New Clinical Trial

If clinical data already exist, but were not originally analyzed to address a specific question, it would be cost effective, and could be scientifically valid, to use them to address a new research question.

To Address Clinical Research Questions That Would be Difficult to Answer in Other Ways

There are clinical questions that can only be answered by analysis of raw data from multiple clinical trials.

For example, how do the numbers of seizures for individual patients compare during an active baseline versus a placebo period in multiple clinical trials? This question was addressed by Spilker and Segreti (1984) using raw data obtained from the published literature.

To Understand a Published Paper Better or to Answer Particular Questions About It

The limitations on space set by most publications prevent authors from presenting a sufficient amount of their methods or results. If tabular data and a protocol were available from an archive, interested readers could obtain data of particular interest and thus reach a more definitive interpretation.

To Assist in Teaching Others About Clinical Trials or the Subject Archived

Many lessons could be gleaned from perusing archived clinical data, including a better understanding of why a particular clinical trial was successful or unsuccessful. These lessons could be incorporated in courses, lectures, or books.

TYPES OF ARCHIVES

Archives of clinical trials are a relatively new concept. Thus their definition is still open to refinement. There is a great heterogeneity in type and size of clinical trials and in the nature of data collected as well as in formats used to create a data base. Thus any archive created would probably contain a heterogeneous collection of information in multiple formats. Indexing and providing these data to interested parties would probably present major difficulties. Future efforts might be targeted on one or more of these problems.

Whether an archive was a profit or not-for-profit enterprise would be expected to impact on many aspects of the archive's initiation and functioning. Ideally, any archive formed would be well funded, relatively complete for certain categories of data, and easily accessible.

PROBLEMS OF ARCHIVES

Misuse and Misinterpretation of Data

Many current owners of data that could be placed in an archive will have few incentives to participate in a voluntary scheme. They will be concerned about (1) what sceptical or even hostile critics may find in the archive, (2) how their data may be misinterpreted or misused, and (3) how their data may provide scientific or commercial help to academic researchers, commercial researchers, or other competitors. In addition, they may resent the loss of ownership of the data and its use by others.

Funding

Ideally an archive should be self-supporting, receiving its revenue from people who are interested in obtaining access to data in the archive, and for receiving information from the archive. If funds are insufficient to support this type of facility, it could readily go out of business, unless backed by a long-term government grant or philanthropic organization. Investigators who submit data to an archive should not be charged, as that would be a major disincentive to contribute clinical data.

Submission of Data

Data could be submitted in a number of different formats. Electronic data (on tape or disk) are currently created utilizing multiple systems of hardware and software. It would be ideal, though difficult, for an archive to adopt a single system and insist on receiving electronic data in that format. A preferable system, from the contributor's perspective, would be for the archive to change all data received to a previously agreed-on format. Patient or volunteer names must not be left on data deposited in an archive. A procedure should be instituted to ensure confidentiality.

Accessing the Data

An index to data contained in an archive is essential. The price of the archive service would be related to the quantity of data requested; if someone was uncertain about what specific data to request, it could be difficult, frustrating, and expensive to order and view a large segment of archived data.

Retaining Data

Each archive should determine how long to retain data after they are received, or after the data have been published. This could be a fixed amount of time (e.g., 6 years) or it could vary based on the assessed value of the data, possibly having a renewal period at the end of a fixed term.

The author has attempted to use two private archives referenced in medical journals with little success. One group was willing to provide information on specific archived studies, but had no index of data in their collection for identifying which clinical trials had submitted data. This group was identified by a reference in a medical journal stating that additional data could be submitted by authors to a central repository. The other group never responded to numerous letters and presumably went out of business.

ALTERNATIVES TO A CENTRALIZED ARCHIVE

The problems that would arise in attempting to archive data from all clinical trials in a single centralized repository is daunting. Alternatively, smaller archives could be created that could contain data from:

1. Clinical trials in a specific disease, therapeutic area, or modality
2. Clinical trials on a specific medicine
3. Clinical trials with particular social or political impact
4. Clinical trials with particular medical or scientific impact
5. Phase IIb clinical trials (the most well-controlled clinical trials conducted on a new medicine)
6. Phase IV clinical studies
7. Selected clinical trials voluntarily submitted by investigators (i.e., a voluntary system)

Government agencies could initiate or fund archives if they considered this to be a worthwhile activity. Alternative groups that could establish archives are large medical libraries, institutions, professional societies, or private businesses.

The amount of space required to house a large archive would be substantial. One simple alternative to an archive would be for all investigators to agree to maintain all data from their own clinical trials for a period of time (e.g., 5 years) and to make some or all of these data available to other scientists for legitimate purposes. Journal editors and professional societies could explore how this approach would be perceived in the medical community.

AN EXISTING ARCHIVE

There is an existing data archive at the National Technical Information System (NTIS). The NTIS (5285 Port Royal Road, Springfield, VA 22161, USA) contains selected reports of research sponsored by the United States Government. NTIS keeps a microfiche of all records sent to them. The archive is funded by sales of documents. Clinical data come from universities, state agencies, federal agencies, and other sources.

This group's activities could, in theory, be expanded to service a larger function.

CONCLUSIONS

In view of the overwhelming problems inherent in creating a total archive of clinical trials, that possibility is not considered feasible. A limited system of selective archives would be more efficient and cost effective. Given the reluctance of many people to part with their data (for a variety of reasons), the most practical concept would initially involve a voluntary contribution of selected data by authors to either a national center or to a specific type of archive. If the pressures to initiate one of these systems are not sufficiently strong, then even more modest archiving activities must be considered.

CHAPTER 109

Models of Clinical Research

DEFINITION OF CLINICAL RESEARCH

A commonly held view by those outside the field of medicine is that clinical research is conducted solely on patients by physicians. This was generally correct before the 19th century, but today not all clinical research is conducted on patients, and individuals with many backgrounds are also involved. *Clinical research* is defined as research conducted on either an entire human or on any part (e.g., blood, isolated organ), whether or not that part is viable. This broad definition allows a wide variety of people to claim that they are conducting clinical research. The broad definition does *not* include research on medical devices or medical equipment unless they are *directly* in contact with patients or their biological samples. Thus, research on human blood and its constituents comes under the heading of clinical research, but research on equipment used in blood research does not. A narrower definition that restricts the concept of clinical research to studies on a whole person also raises many objections to the use of the term by research professionals who study such areas as organ transplants, biological fluids (e.g., blood, urine), and pathological tissues.

TYPES OF CLINICAL RESEARCH

Within the broad definition presented above, it is useful to consider two basic types of clinical research. The first type is patient-oriented research: the whole viable patient is the subject of the study. The second type includes all other studies in which a live human is not involved (e.g., on urine, blood, tissues, organs, and cadavers).

The terms *clinical studies* and *clinical trials* (i.e., those studies conducted during Phases I to III) refer to patient-oriented studies. Clinical trials may be primarily designed to evaluate therapeutic, preventive, or diagnostic characteristics of a medicine or nonmedicine regimen. Studies on urine, blood, and cultured specimens are often referred to as clinical laboratory studies. Pathological studies include gross, histological, and other microscopic evaluations on tissues, organs, or cadavers. Other types of clinical research include evaluations of (1) X-rays, (2) outputs of physiological testing, and (3) in vitro study of human tissues.

BASIC MODELS OF HOW CLINICAL RESEARCH IS CONDUCTED

Although the following nine models are described as if they are independent, many researchers follow two (or more) models simultaneously and others use different models during the course of their careers. Models are initially described in terms of their practitioners and outputs. They are also described as patient-oriented or in terms of other clinical research.

Model 1. Investigators with various professional degrees who personally conduct clinical research in academia, government, industry, private medical practice, or contract organizations. This model involves direct patient contact (i.e., patient-oriented research). It includes practitioners of many clinical disciplines including psychology, psychiatry, surgery, acupuncture, and less accepted (or validated) fields of medicine (e.g., chiropractors). Clinical studies and clinical trials are the initial output. A final output may be a publication, talk, or other presentation.

Model 2. Investigators who do not *directly* participate in research on patients. Their roles in patient-oriented research may be as supervisor, advisor, reviewer, or consultant. The output is the clinical study or trial itself and also may involve a publication.

Model 3. Investigators who directly participate in other types of clinical research (e.g., clinical laboratory studies, pathological studies, physiological studies).

Model 4. Staff of the investigator who participate in a patient-oriented or other type of clinical study or trial. This group includes individuals with different backgrounds whose roles vary from those that are essential to those that involve progressively less responsibility or involvement in the study. The clinical study or trial itself is usually the only output, but some staff may participate in publications or other presentations.

Model 5. Readers of the literature who are primarily concerned with reviewing clinical research (of either type) that has already been conducted. The usual outputs of this model are reviews that are published in the literature.

Model 6. Scholars who use clinical research already completed to generate new ideas and hypotheses. There may be either a fine line or a wide gulf separating this model from model 5. Outputs include talks, articles, books, and other presentations that contain a highly creative component. There are relatively few practitioners of this model.

Model 7. Medical personnel at a sponsoring organization who plan, initiate, and monitor clinical studies or trials, and then analyze and interpret the results. Individuals who follow this model have extremely wide variation in their training, experience, skills, and creativity. The group, which includes most professionals within medical departments of a pharmaceutical company, is not solely limited to physicians. Some professionals at government agencies [e.g., National Institutes of Health (NIH)] would also fit this model. Outputs include clinical trial protocols, final medical reports, publications, regulatory submissions, and clinical development plans. Patient-oriented clinical research is the primary type of research affected, but many laboratory and other nonviable patient studies are also sponsored.

Model 8. Medical and other scientific personnel at regulatory agencies who guide clinical trials and medicine development via their influence on sponsors or investigators. A common output is a clinical trial or part of a trial that is modified according to their suggestions. In some instances an entire clinical development plan may be modified by a sponsor based on views of a regulator. Patient-oriented clinical research is the major type of research affected.

Model 9. Contract organizations who place studies with investigators. Many of the individuals in these organizations relate both to sponsors and to investigators. Individuals within the medical department of such contractors are analogous to those described in model 7. Outputs are the same as model 7. Investigators at contracting companies that conduct clinical research themselves are best considered as members of models one or two. Although both types of clinical research may be undertaken, most studies are patient oriented.

CHARACTERISTICS OF CLINICAL RESEARCH PERSONNEL

Marked differences occur among clinical research personnel in regard to their professional degrees, training and experience, perspectives (e.g., scientific, clinical), activities followed in conducting research, and environmental settings.

Professional Degrees

There is, in theory, no minimum professional degree necessary to conduct or assist in at least some non-invasive forms of clinical research (e.g., interviews). Medical interventions on patients require professional degrees, and each country has legal requirements relating to this issue. The important point is that excellent clinical research may be and is being conducted by individuals who are nonphysicians. This is discussed in the section describing activities conducted in each of the nine models above.

Training and Experience

The degree of clinical training or experience necessary to conduct clinical research depends entirely on the particular situation and varies over a wide spectrum.

PERSPECTIVES OF CLINICIANS VERSUS SCIENTISTS

Ideally, there should be no difference between clinicians and scientists in the approach they take to clinical research. In some cases, however, their background and training lead them in different directions. This difference is based primarily on a need for clinicians to treat a patient even though much (or most) data needed are not available at the time a decision must be made. A scientist is taught to withhold judgment until most (or all) data are available. This topic is discussed elsewhere in more detail (Spilker, 1989a). This difference sometimes has practical consequences.

A few examples in which a nonphysician scientist's zeal for logic and rigorously designed studies generally leads to problems in clinical trials are:

1. A scientist requests more blood samples in a protocol than is clinically reasonable or appropriate in volunteers or patients.
2. A scientist requests too many clinic visits, too frequent tests, or too arduous a schedule for clinical trial patients.

These problems and other related ones may be avoided by ensuring that all protocols are reviewed at the appropriate stage by an experienced physician.

ACTIVITIES OF PERSONNEL ENGAGED IN CLINICAL RESEARCH

The nine models are used as the basis for describing the activities of the groups described below.

Investigators Who Directly Interact with Patients in Clinical Research. Investigators who interact with patients are either involved with patient care as part of their day-to-day activities or interact directly with volunteers or patients, primarily in the conduct of clinical research. Professional relationships in this model may therefore be limited to a clinical trial or may be part of an ongoing longer-term relationship. In addition to physicians, investigators include doctoral level psychologists, pharmacokineticists, and doctoral level scientists.

Investigators Who Do Not Directly Interact with Patients in Clinical Research. Investigators who do not interact with patients delegate the actual conduct of a clinical trial to assistants or residents. The investigator's name may be on the protocol merely to have a physician involved for legal, ethical, and regulatory reasons. This type of investigator may provide advice and supervision to the staff, and may occasionally interact directly with patients (i.e., model 1). A second group of investigators works with patient data that it did not collect. This includes economists conducting cost-effectiveness studies using data furnished by others, and epidemiologists who analyze data collected in the field.

Laboratory Investigators. Investigators may study biological samples and not be directly involved with patients. This group includes biochemists, histologists, pharmacologists, and hematologists conducting laboratory studies.

Staff of the Investigator or Those Related to a Clinical Trial. The staff is a heterogeneous group including nurses, nurse practitioners, physician assistants, study coordinators, research assistants, other physicians, plus support staff. Their activities cover a broad range and include administrative or managerial roles in addition to helping with the actual conduct of a clinical trial.

Reviewers. An individual from one of the seven other groups may also act as a reviewer. This individual assimilates published literature on a clinical topic and prepares review articles (see last section of this chapter) or meta-analyses (see Chapter 104).

Scholars. Scholars differ primarily from reviewers in the amount of creativity in their work. They approach the literature or other sources of information with important questions and help advance medical science by generating new approaches, new ways of viewing information, and novel ideas. As opposed to the literature reviewer, they tend not to participate in the other models.

Medical Personnel at a Sponsor's Site. The sponsor's medical personnel includes a heterogeneous group of physicians, scientists with doctoral degrees, and many others with different training and experience (e.g., PharmD, MS, BA). Activities include writing protocols, monitoring studies, analyzing data, interpreting data, and planning clinical development. People who prepare data collection forms, enter raw data into computers, or perform other related types of support services are not included in this model because of their limited involvement in clinical research.

Medical Personnel at a Regulatory Authority. Selected reviewers participate in clinical research by interacting with sponsors who develop medicines. Regulatory input may be made into a clinical development plan or into design aspects of a single clinical trial. Their input often involves clinical research.

Contract Organization Personnel. Those who place and monitor studies at other organizations generally span the range of personnel and activities at sponsoring companies. The degree to which these personnel may be said to participate in clinical research is usually less than those at their client's organization. This is because the client (i.e., sponsor) has usually made most or even all of the creative decisions prior to contracting the work.

ENVIRONMENTAL SETTINGS IN WHICH CLINICAL RESEARCH IS CONDUCTED

Most people immediately think of clinics and hospitals when this question is raised. Specific settings at which clinical research is conducted include:

1. Hospitals (e.g., general wards, operating rooms, intensive care units).

2. Outpatient clinics (e.g., in hospitals, Health Maintenance Organizations, various institutions).
3. Outpatient medical practices (e.g., private medical practice).
4. Laboratories in any of the above settings where blood, microbiological, or biological samples are assayed or evaluated. These are found in hospitals, clinics, and institutes of all types, as well as in independent facilities.
5. Physiological measurements (e.g., electroencephalograms, respiratory functions, echocardiograms, sonograms) are conducted in laboratories or elsewhere in each of the first three types of settings listed above.
6. Libraries. Research is often conducted entirely within a library setting when literature reviews or meta-analyses are prepared. In addition, libraries are important for literature searches or reviewing other published material when planning a study, writing a study for publication, or addressing a specific question. This category includes archives of raw and other data.
7. Regulatory authorities. Some groups have their own scientific laboratories and some personnel work at other sites part-time (e.g., hospitals). The type of research referred to however, is primarily that conducted on the discipline in which they are working (e.g., clinical trial methods, regulatory issues).
8. Sponsor's offices, clinics, and laboratories.
9. Contractor's offices, clinics, and laboratories.

Research settings 1 through 6 above may be located in an academic institution, government agency, government laboratory or hospital, private corporation, Health Maintenance Organization, community hospital, contract organization, or other source.

CLINICAL REVIEWS AND REANALYSES OF PUBLISHED DATA

It is a truism that one need not conduct clinical trials in order to make a significant contribution to medicine. Case reports on individual patients sometimes provide important information that advances patient diagnosis, care, or treatment. Another method that may have a major impact in medicine is the careful review of published clinical trials conducted by other groups of investigators. A third method is to reanalyze published data. Reviews may concentrate on a narrow topic or cover a broad area. The type of review described in this chapter is one that concentrates on a specific question or topic of medical interest.

Levels of Interpretation

The interpretation of data by an investigator who has conducted the clinical trial and generated the data may be viewed as a "primary level" of interpretation. A reinterpretation of someone else's data in a published article may be defined as a "secondary level" of interpretation. Secondary-level interpretations are often found in the letters to the editor or discussion sections of various publications. An example occurs when a reviewer either challenges or provides an alternative interpretation of someone else's data. When two or more trials are evaluated and a reinterpretation or reanalysis of the data is performed, it is defined as a "tertiary level" of interpretation. This section considers tertiary levels of interpretation.

Reasons to Reanalyze the Literature

There are several compelling reasons why a review and reanalysis of the existing clinical literature offer valuable opportunities for interpretations or reinterpretations of data. Some of these reasons are:

1. Multiple clinical trials may be reviewed.
2. Data from multiple trials may be pooled to obtain a more comprehensive interpretation of the overall results than may be obtained in any single trial.
3. More appropriate or newly devised statistical techniques may be used to reanalyze previously published data.
4. A greater degree of objectivity and a more balanced perspective may be utilized in analyzing the data. This improved objectivity would be expected to yield more definitive and convincing interpretations.
5. Data from clinical trials with relatively few patients and low power may be included in the review rather than being discarded because of their small quantity of data and low power.
6. Important influences on the data may be discerned that were not apparent or were not clear in the individual trials.
7. Extrapolations to different patient populations, physicians, settings, times, or levels of organization may be made with stronger evidence than is available in a single trial.
8. The value of certain clinical approaches may better be evaluated.

A number of possible objectives are listed in Table 109.1.

TABLE 109.1 *Possible objectives of writing and publishing a clinical review article*

1. To determine the current state of the art in a given area
2. To assess the clinical value of a specific treatment
3. To assess the role and use of a particular factor in clinical trials
4. To address a specific clinical or nonclinical question
5. To compare two (or more) types of controls, blinds, randomizations, endpoints, or other trial-related characteristics
6. To assess the quality of clinical trials being conducted and published in a specific (or general) area of therapy
7. To assess the quality of clinical trials being published in a specific journal(s)
8. To evaluate trends in diagnosis, treatment, or prevention of disease
9. To assess the validity of a particular test, measure, or parameter
10. To assess the clinical importance of anecdotal reports of suspected adverse reactions[a]
11. To assess the quality of adverse reaction or other safety data reporting[b]

[a] Venning (1982).
[b] Venulet et al. (1982).

Methods of Conducting a Clinical Review

The techniques used to conduct this type of data review vary but begin with a clear determination and expression of the question to be addressed (i.e., the objective of the review). Next, it is necessary to collect all clinical trials in the literature that meet the criteria established [e.g., year(s) of publication, language(s) of publication, minimum number of patients, type(s) of trial design, type(s) of control groups].

After the clinical trials are collected, pertinent data from each are often listed in a tabular format. If there are a large number of trials, then subheadings by type of trials, by result, or by another factor (e.g., doses used, duration of treatment, definition of patient response, patient or disease characteristic) may be used to create multiple categories for facilitating the listing and analysis. A statistician should be consulted to determine the appropriate approach(es) that can be used. At that stage, the results, approaches, interpretations, or other aspects of the trials being evaluated are compared. Unless the original authors of the articles reviewed have provided sufficient information on the statistical methods used to analyze their data, it may not be possible for reviewers to reanalyze their data adequately.

Summaries and comparisons of the clinical trials reviewed may be based on tabular approaches of either efficacy or safety data. One approach to summarizing a review is to state that X of Z total trials showed . . . , whereas Y of Z trials showed. . . . Another approach is to tabulate the number of patients (e.g., A of B total patients showed . . .). Numerous types of comparisons may be made, each of which could be the basis of separate interpretations and conclusions. Data may sometimes be pooled and reanalyzed to arrive at a global consensus of all trials considered.

PART XI

Planning and Conducting Multiple Clinical Trials

6 Phases of a Project
1. Enthusiasm
2. Disillusionment
3. Panic
4. Search for the guilty
5. Punishment of the innocent
6. Praise and honors for the nonparticipants

—Author unknown

There must be no barriers to freedom of inquiry. There is no place for dogma in science. The scientist is free, and must be free to ask any question, to doubt any assertion, to seek for any evidence, to correct any errors.

—J. Robert Oppenheimer

CHAPTER 110

Golden Rules of Clinical Development of Pharmaceuticals

DEFINITIONS

Golden rules are universal principles that are not specific to a particular company or set of companies. They are credos that companies should adhere to if they wish to follow state-of-the-art principles. In addition to these *golden rules* or guiding principles, each company's research and development group or department has general *objectives* to attain over the long term and more specific *goals* to achieve over a 1- to 3-year period. These goals may often be quantitated. In addition, a research and development group must develop *strategies* of how to attain these objectives and goals: strategies describe how the group will proceed from its current state to achieve its desired goal(s). Strategies are therefore general plans that describe the path to follow. Specific mechanics and detailed plans followed by groups to accomplish strategies are called *tactics*. By keeping the distinction between these terms in mind, medicine discovery and development plans may be developed and progress monitored with greater clarity. One final term that is often used in this context is *mission*. This describes the overall purpose of the group and is often a succinct statement that may or may not be prepared in a written form. Each of these terms has been described in more detail (see Chapter 112).

In assessing the most important principles, (i.e., golden rules) of clinical medicine development, it is worthwhile placing these in the context of medicine development. To do this the overall principles of medicine development should be identified. Eighteen general principles of medicine development were described (see below), as were golden rules for discovering medicines (Spilker, 1989b).

GOLDEN RULES OF MEDICINE DEVELOPMENT

The overall principles identified are:

1. Focus development activities in a relatively limited number of therapeutic areas.
2. Formulate an overall concept and strategy of how each medicine, indication, and formulation will be developed.
3. Create an international development plan that minimizes duplication and stresses efficiency.
4. Avoid tangents that depart from the chosen path of development, except under conditions described.
5. Hire the best people possible for all positions in a company.
6. Assign personnel and other resources according to both the value and importance of each indication and formulation being developed.
7. Encourage openness, honesty, cooperation, teamwork, and shared goals among research and de-

velopment, marketing, production and other groups.

8. Adhere to the highest standards of ethics in scientific, medical, marketing, and other activities.
9. Create and use systems that assist medicine development.
10. Develop a portfolio of investigational medicines that balances high- and low-risk projects.
11. Reevaluate each project and the overall portfolio on a regular basis.
12. Identify the rate-limiting steps of each medicine's development and ensure that appropriate and adequate resources and attention are focused on these areas.
13. Develop a clear licensing policy.
14. Attempt to create and maintain a cooperative relationship with all regulatory authorities.
15. Prepare logical and straightforward regulatory submissions.
16. Protect and extend the medicine's indications and formulations after initial marketing.
17. Attempt to learn everything of importance about a medicine, even what may be considered as bad news.
18. Ensure that activities to implement and carry out these principles follow an appropriate pace.

A number of other principles could be added to this list that may be applied to many areas of medicine development. Their omission does not signify that they are of lesser importance.

SELECTED TYPES OF STANDARDS USED IN CLINICAL TRIALS

Availability of Valid Clinical Methods

Standards relate to the quality of the methods available and how well they measure what they are attempting to measure. Concepts of sensitivity and selectivity are important to assess.

Utilization of Clinical Methods

In several areas (e.g., pharmacoeconomics) there are well-defined, well-validated, and useful clinical methods. Nonetheless, there are no agreed-on standards as to how or when these clinical methods should be used (i.e., in which situations a specific method should be used).

Computer Processing and Quality-Assuring Clinical Data Obtained in Trials

The quality-assurance techniques used to confirm clinical data entered into computers are well established and widely used.

Statistical Analyses of Data

The standards used to analyze data vary greatly depending on the amount and types of data obtained. In some situations the approaches used by statisticians are well established (i.e., clear standards exist). However, with many data bases the most appropriate statistical approaches to use are not well agreed upon, and different groups (e.g., regulatory authorities, pharmaceutical companies) often have widely divergent approaches (e.g., intention-to-treat analysis versus using another statistical approach) to analyzing the same set of data.

Interpretation of Clinical Data

Standards exist in regard to the quality of the interpretation made of clinical data. Relevant issues include consideration of the following questions. Is the interpretation a complete review of all data? Does the interpretation consider all possible factors that could have influenced the data? Does the interpretation consider alternative treatments and compare all relevant groups of data? Is it consistent with and supported by statistical analyses of the data?

Standards also may be described for specific discipline areas or technical departments. Each department has its own standards that should be adhered to for their operations.

GOLDEN RULES OF CLINICAL MEDICINE DEVELOPMENT

At a more specific level than the rules listed above, it is possible to describe principles that focus on a particular function or department (e.g., medical, toxicology, chemical scale-up, pharmaceutical formulation, patents, regulatory affairs).

The following principles include many of the most important ones that underlie modern clinical medicine development, and are discussed in this book and elsewhere in more detail (Spilker, 1989a). They are divided for convenience into a few broad categories.

Personnel and General Issues

1. *Adhere to high standards of ethics, medicine, and science.* In this manner it is less likely that a development program and the data obtained will be challenged or criticized by a regulatory authority, the medical community, or the press. Although a program adhering to high standards will require more time, effort, and money than a program using lower standards, the benefits of the former approach far outweigh the additional time and money spent. For example, it will almost always lead to a more rapid regulatory review, which leads to a greater commercial return.

2. *Establish and maintain a positive and close working relationship between statisticians and clinicians.* Statisticians should be involved in most aspects of a clinical trial, including trial design, protocol review, trial conduct, data collection, data processing, data analysis, and report writing. If this is not done, then data may be collected that are not analyzable, or an excessive amount of data may be collected and processed. Other problems may be created by inappropriate interim or other analyses. Standard operating procedures and sound management techniques should encourage this principle.

3. *Do not readily give medicines to physicians for use in compassionate plea protocols until well-designed protocols are established and data collection procedures are assured.* Freely giving out medicines requires significant company resources and may lead to many problems requiring even more resources. Carefully designed programs adhere to ethical standards, benefit patients, and do not jeopardize a medicine's development.

Clinical Plans

1. *Design a clinical program that develops the medicine from its initial evaluation to its initial registration in the fewest number of trials consistent with good scientific, medical, and marketing standards.* Anticipated or desired clinical advantages of a medicine over available therapy should be evaluated. If demonstrating the advantage is crucial to a medicine's development, that aspect should be assessed early. If the advantage is less critical it may be assessed at a later stage. Advantages may be sought in terms of efficacy, safety, quality of life, compliance, cost effectiveness, or other factors. Conduct as many clinical trials simultaneously as practical and realistic during those periods of medicine development when it is possible to do so.

2. *Ensure that every clinical trial planned is necessary to conduct and is designed to address a specific issue or question on the path to a medicine's marketing.* Do not pose too many or too few questions to address during a medicine's clinical development. Clinical trials that are merely desirable or would provide information that is nice to know should either be eliminated from the plan or conducted after the go/no-go decision point. Do not initiate clinical trials in new therapeutic areas, diseases, or patient populations until it is established that the medicine is active in the primary indication. While there are some exceptions to this principle it is usually not appropriate to expand greatly the efforts on a medicine's development until reasonable efficacy and safety are established.

3. *Develop clear principles relating to the appropriate timing of each type of clinical trial in a medicine's overall development.* A number of examples follow.

A. *Breakthrough drugs for serious diseases.* Placebo-controlled trials should be conducted, if possible, early in Phase II, because after the medicine's benefits are demonstrated it will no longer be possible to conduct such a trial. Otherwise, case studies or crude pilot trials may strongly suggest activity, but it is no longer ethical to conduct a placebo-controlled trial. It may then be impossible to conduct a placebo-controlled trial and obtain definitive data to convince skeptics who challenge the pilot trial results.

B. *Pharmacokinetic trials.* These should be incorporated into all early (i.e., Phase I) trials. A number of separate pharmacokinetic trials are usually conducted after the medicine passes the go/no-go decision point late in Phase II.

C. *Quality of life trials.* These trials are usually conducted late in Phase III, after the initial regulatory application has been submitted, or during Phase IV.

D. *Academic type trials.* These are generally conducted in Phase III after a definitive go/no-go decision has been reached, in Phase IV, or not at all. These mechanism-of-action or "nice to know" trials should only rarely be conducted during Phase I or II.

E. *Market-oriented studies.* Studies of this type are generally conducted late in Phase III or in Phase IV.

4. *Plan clinical trials in which the degree of extrapolation is acceptable.* The conditions of at least some of the trials must resemble those of the broad patient population in terms of dosage recommended, type of disease, age and sex distribution of patients, concomitant medicines, concurrent diseases, severity of disease, and various other factors. For example, trials carried out by tertiary care investigators may help get

the medicine approved for marketing, but may not be suitable for publications directed at primary care investigators who see a different mix of patients and utilize different types of treatments in their patients.

5. *Consider a feasibility trial if the clinical trial is a major one that will require significant resources.* While this is rarely a requirement it often helps government-sponsored or other large multicenter trials develop the best possible protocol and methods for conducting a trial.

6. *Develop a plan for postmarketing Phase IV trials before the medicine is initially marketed.* This plan will usually include observational trials, specifically desired clinical trials, and marketing-oriented studies. Clinical trials seeking additional regulatory licenses for other indications, formulations, and routes of administration are not included in this plan. These types of trials are conducted as parts of Phases I, II, and III for newly marketed medicines.

Clinical Trial Design, Initiation, and Conduct

1. *Conduct virtually all trials in Phases I and II of medicine development using double-blind designs.* To prevent being misled about a medicine's safety or efficacy, it is necessary in all but a few situations (e.g., cancer) to blind both investigators and patients. Monitors who interact with investigators should also be blind to patient randomization. This is sometimes referred to as a triple-blind trial. Pilot trials are particularly important to keep blind, because open-label trials have an exceedingly high likelihood of yielding false-positive results that are not confirmed in more carefully controlled trials. Initial false-positive results could cause a company to spend additional money and additional years of study unnecessarily, before it is learned that the initial efficacy observed cannot be confirmed. These problems may often be avoided or minimized through conducting double-blind pilot trials that provide more definitive data at an earlier time.

2. *Use validated instruments (e.g., questionnaires, scales, tests) in a clinical trial.* Data obtained with non-validated scales will be less convincing to all knowledgeable people who read about the trial. This includes regulatory authorities who must approve the medicine for sale and physicians who must prescribe the medicine. The most convincing data are usually those that are obtained with clinical, biochemical, and other endpoints that are accepted by most physicians as appropriate or state of the art. Positive data obtained by elaborate transformations, or when elaborate statistical tests have been used to show significance, are more likely to be questioned or rejected.

3. *Do not pose too many questions in a clinical trial (i.e., minimize the number of objectives).* The pitfall of posing too many questions is one of the most appealing lures in clinical medicine development, especially to neophytes or to scientists who are used to controlling many parameters in animal studies. Marketing staff often encourage clinicians to conduct trials that are too ambitious. The chances of a trial yielding clear results are usually enhanced if the objectives are not too complex and few questions are posed. Trial objectives must be specified as precisely as possible.

4. *Do not collect more data than needed to answer the questions posed.* There is a great temptation, especially among neophytes, to collect more data than necessary. This often creates a huge amount of excess work to process and analyze the data.

5. *Design each clinical trial at a high standard, unless there are sound reasons not to do so.* Use adequate sample size and appropriate randomization methods, minimize the number of interim analyses, and discuss the major contingencies that may arise, and how each is to be handled.

6. *Choose the best investigators to conduct each clinical trial.* It was common in the past to utilize investigators who had important reputations and political connections. The quality of the trial they conducted was often less important to the sponsor than what their opinion was about the medicine. There are still thought leaders and opinion setters today in medicine, although their importance depends to a large degree on the specific country and therapeutic area involved. For example, in Germany and France the opinion of "The Professor" is still highly important and particularly in these countries it is usually necessary to have them conduct a pivotal trial (i.e., generally the most well-controlled trial) on a new medicine. It may be undesirable from the sponsor's perspective to have these people participate in critical trials for solely political reasons, unless they also have the resources and interest to conduct the trial at the required standards. If pivotal trials are not carefully conducted they may create problems that could take years for the sponsor to undo. Important or well-known clinicians may be asked for political reasons to assist in a medicine's development by performing an ancillary trial to provide supportive data or to help marketing. This approach allows them to be involved in an "important" way while protecting the company's interests. If it is imperative to have them conduct a pivotal trial, it may be possible for the sponsor to pay for additional staff to help ensure that the trial is conducted in an appropriate manner.

7. *Utilize common-design data collection forms across trials conducted on one medicine and multiple medicines.* Develop a library of data collection forms that are used in as many trials as possible. This will

simplify data processing and analysis. This goal should also be in place for an international medicine development program.

8. *Monitor trials in a modern and not old-fashioned way.* This subject is discussed in detail in Chapter 62. Lasagna's law must be considered in monitoring trials as well as in choosing and educating investigators.

9. *Develop checklists, computer programs, and other forms to help initiate and track clinical trial progress, data editing, data processing, data analysis, and medical report writing.* Remote data entry should be considered when both the investigator and sponsor desire to use this option.

10. *Use a Data Monitoring Committee of independent, well-respected scientists and clinicians if the trial has significant political, medical, or ethical implication.* See Chapter 17.

11. *Establish the magnitude of response in efficacy trials that is clinically significant and incorporate this in the trial design.* The difference between statistical significance and clinical significance must be considered during the trial's design as well as during the interpretation of data. If the magnitude of a clinically significant response is not obvious, then assemble a group of clinicians to address this question in terms of how large a change in the key efficacy parameter(s) would lead them to use a new medicine.

12. *Review and approval of protocols should be performed by people with a great deal of experience, including a statistician.* Any protocol that includes pharmacokinetics should be reviewed by one or more of the company's senior scientists in this area. Clinical aspects should be reviewed by at least two people who are not directly involved in the trial. At least one physician must review every protocol to ensure it makes "clinical sense," is not too difficult for patients, and adheres to appropriate clinical and ethical standards.

13. *Pay close attention to all details in each trial protocol.* It is important to process patients through a trial mentally, imagining as many problems as possible. Approaches to all common problems should be described in the protocol. For example, measure electrocardiograms at the approximate time of peak medicine levels in Phase I trials and not solely before the trial and at its conclusion, when medicine levels are low or absent. Do not dose outpatients who arrive at a clinic without ensuring that their blood values (e.g., SMA-12, CBC) are within the expected range. Otherwise, unanticipated abnormalities may be made worse by the medicine, and its development, as well as the patient, may be placed in jeopardy.

14. *Utilize appropriate resources to conduct each clinical trial.* It is important for both practical and ethical reasons to have sufficient resources available to conduct a clinical trial.

INTERNATIONAL MEDICINE DEVELOPMENT

1. *Create an appropriate size core package of clinical trials.* There is a balance between creating a large core package that is cumbersome and too inefficient for use in most regulatory applications and one that is so small that the benefits of a core package are not obtained.

2. *Senior managers should resolve different philosophies of medicine development that affect an international development plan prior to its approval.* Differences between two pharmaceutical companies or two development sites of a single company are described elsewhere (Spilker, 1989a). Cooperation between sponsor sites involved in developing a medicine should be stressed.

3. *Stress utilization of agreed-on protocols between two or more sites of a multinational pharmaceutical company that are developing a medicine, and avoid unnecessary duplication of efforts.* Prior agreement is important for identifying the types of protocols that should be utilized. Joint review of specific protocols will foster cooperation and should enable a unified interpretation of the data to be made. A single international data base across all clinical trials on a medicine will facilitate its development as well as creation of regulatory dossiers.

4. *Do not conduct multinational medicine trials (as opposed to multicenter trials) unless they are sufficiently large in scope and financial support to have a good chance of success.* Differences in medical cultures and practices lead to many problems in most multinational trials. These may be possible to conduct if the countries are generally similar (e.g., some Scandinavian countries, United States and Canada). See Chapter 40.

5. *Develop a strategy for regulatory dossier preparation and submission.* Consider which countries should be targeted and in which order. Consider the Dual Pyramid Concept (see Chapter 127) when developing multiple regulatory packages for submission.

6. *Reach agreement on a single format and approach to data analysis and final medical report preparation for each clinical trial.* Statistical analyses and clinical interpretation of trials should not be repeated by other parts of the same company. International agreement on approaches and formats should be reached, either prior to each clinical trial or prior to data processing and analysis. This concept will prevent disputes, reanalysis, and reinterpretations by different statistical or medical groups. That possibility could raise significant problems for a company.

7. *All patients should be discussed under patient accountability and the safety analysis must include all*

patients entered in a clinical trial. Efficacy analysis should usually include all patients entered, but may occasionally delete those patients who did not achieve certain milestones. This group of excluded patients should be indicated in the protocol.

Perhaps the most important principle underlying most, if not all, of these golden rules is that *good data in a few patients are far better than mediocre or poor data in many patients.*

Other golden rules of comparable importance could be added to this list. Their exclusion must not be in-terpreted as any suggestion that they are not as critical to consider, especially in specific situations that arise. One of the author's personal views, which cannot be promulgated as a golden rule, is that interpretations and conclusions based on statistical analyses and methods that do not make clinical sense should be distrusted. When complex or sophisticated statistical methods that cannot be easily explained to a clinician are required to show an effect, it generally indicates that more meaningful analyses were not positive. Statistics must never be allowed to overwhelm nor undermine clinical judgment.

CHAPTER 111

Choosing a Project or Medicine for Evaluation

GENERAL PROCEDURES

This chapter is written from the perspective of individuals within an industrial, academic, or government organization who have choices to make about which projects to develop. The projects would usually be oriented toward developing an investigational medicine, medical device, or diagnostic test. The same approaches may be used by scientific and clinical investigators in academia who are also choosing a project to develop that will require multiple clinical trials. A few considerations that specifically apply to academicians will be mentioned. Chapter 56 presents a dis-

cussion on how physicians in private practice may choose a project or medicine for evaluation.

Limiting Factors

The projects that a company is willing to undertake depend on which other projects the company is pursuing. If there are many other projects under development and limited resources are available, then standards for accepting a new project will be higher than if there are only a few interesting projects or if resources are "unlimited." Projects that fall outside the company's usual "comfort zone" usually have a more

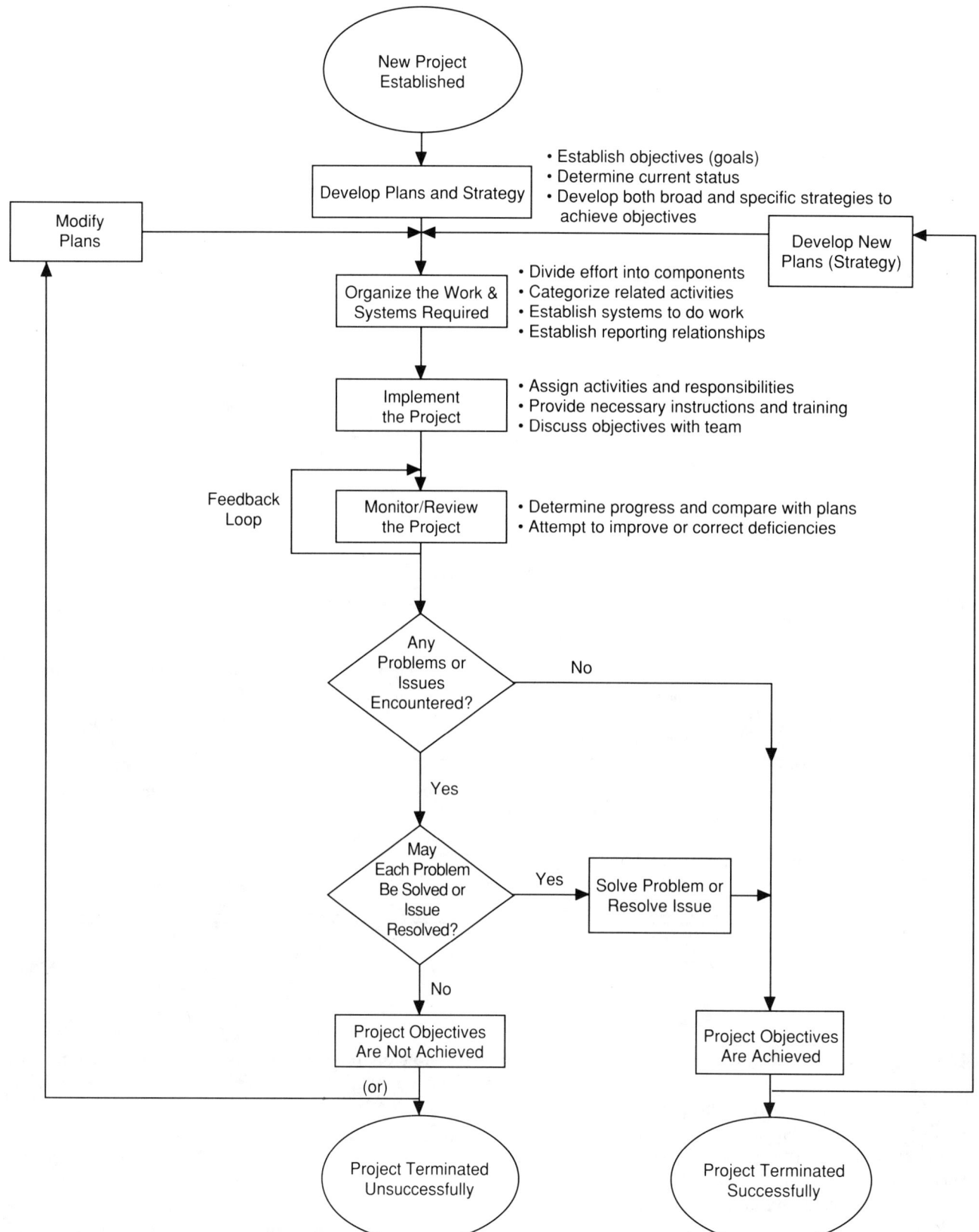

FIG. 111.1 Flow diagram model for establishing and monitoring a project.

difficult time gaining resources, unless a strong commitment is made for their development.

Steps to Reach a Decision

In reaching a decision about whether to initiate a new project, the following few steps will usually ensure that a reasonable sequence has been followed. These processes may be used to judge each specific criterion as well as the overall project proposed.

1. Specify the objectives to be achieved in making the decision. Do all the relevant people agree on these objectives?
2. Determine and examine each of the available alternatives. Various techniques such as algorithms, flow charts, or decision trees may be useful in creating or looking for additional alternatives.
3. Obtain the necessary information on each alternative.
4. Analyze the uncertainties inherent in each alternative. This may be done qualitatively or quantitatively.
5. Evaluate the alternatives and discuss each with relevant people.
6. Based on all of the above information and inputs,

reach a decision. The general methods by which a project is established and monitored are shown in Fig. 111.1, and the types of reviews conducted within a company are illustrated in Fig. 111.2.

Evaluating Projects Based on a Score

A number of years ago some companies used systems that gave scores to potential projects to determine if they had enough points to enter the project system. The points were based on the types of criteria discussed above and various other considerations. A number of systems that have been used are discussed by Faust (1982). This approach is rarely followed today in the pharmaceutical industry because the elaborate models were found to have numerous shortcomings that were critical factors to consider in selecting projects, but were difficult to include in the models. These factors include (1) personal biases, (2) intuition, (3) assessing long-term risks at the time the decision is made, (4) status of other projects, and (5) corporate financial health. More emphasis is now placed on how the proposed project is perceived to fit into the overall project portfolio, which in turn is defined in terms of medical and commercial objectives plus long-term and short-term goals.

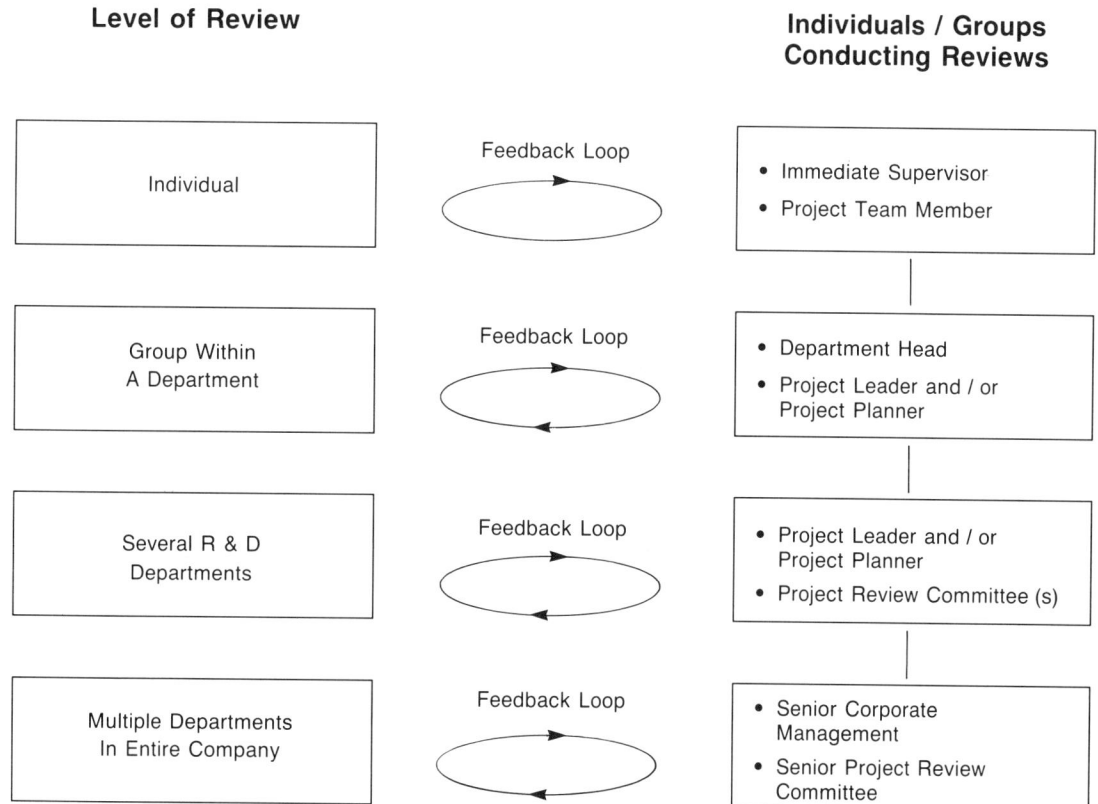

Level of Review

Individuals / Groups Conducting Reviews

Level of Review		Individuals / Groups Conducting Reviews
Individual	Feedback Loop	• Immediate Supervisor • Project Team Member
Group Within A Department	Feedback Loop	• Department Head • Project Leader and / or Project Planner
Several R & D Departments	Feedback Loop	• Project Leader and / or Project Planner • Project Review Committee (s)
Multiple Departments In Entire Company	Feedback Loop	• Senior Corporate Management • Senior Project Review Committee

FIG. 111.2 Levels of project reviews within a company.

CRITERIA TO APPLY

Categories

There are many criteria to use in selecting a project or medicine for evaluation; although some are highly specific, many are general. The primary categories of criteria to be discussed are (1) scientific merit, (2) medical utility and uniqueness, (3) commercial value, (4) practical considerations, and (5) organizational factors.

Scientific Merit

Scientific merit includes consideration of how scientifically interesting the project or medicine's preclinical, biological, and chemical profile is assessed to be. Scientific interest, in turn, is often based on the differences and similarities between the new medicine and known agents, how well the medicine's profile meets the minimal and ideal goals set for the medicine, and how the medicine works. In addition, the project may have special attributes of interest to the developers or scientists.

Medical Utility

Medical utility and uniqueness are often clearer for major breakthroughs than for medicines that may play a more minor role in patient therapy, prevention, or diagnosis. One gauge of assessing medical uniqueness is to determine the number of patients who would be expected to be treated per year if the medicine is shown to have the expected clinical profile. If this criterion is used to make a choice among multiple medicines it will favor that medicine (or medicines that will be used most often).

A more humanistic approach to choosing among multiple medicines with different indications is to consider the percent of patients with the disease who will be treated and helped with each medicine, and not solely the numbers of patients treated. Thus, a novel medicine for a rare disease that has no current therapy should acquire 100% of that small market (e.g., 1,000 patients) and may represent a more important project to develop (in terms of medical interest and humanitarian concerns) than one that will only attain a 10% share of a larger market (e.g., 1,000,000 patients) in which adequate therapy already exists. It is also possible to consider both aspects (i.e., number of probable patients to be treated and market share) when determining which project to develop.

Commercial Value

Commercial value is usually an important factor for pharmaceutical companies to consider in choosing a project and may be assessed in many ways. Marketing considerations include (1) projections of sales and profits, (2) fit of the potential project with marketed products and other projects, (3) commercial need for a new medicine with the characteristics anticipated in the potential project, and (4) status of the competition in terms of existing and investigational medicines.

For academicians who do not envision a commercial product resulting from their project, the commercial aspects usually relate to relative costs in terms of staff, equipment, and time required to pursue a particular project and also the likelihood that a given project will be funded through competitive grants or other mechanisms.

Practical Considerations

The fourth and fifth major types of criteria used to choose projects are practical considerations and organizational factors. The term "practical considerations" refers to how easily and conveniently the project fits into the particular investigator's plans or sponsor's organization. Timing is an important consideration since the ability to pursue a project depends to a large degree on which other projects are ongoing and what potential each of those projects has in medical and commercial terms. The situation is actually more complex for many companies that wish to maintain a balance of short-, medium-, and long-term projects, in terms of the anticipated duration of their premarketing clinical studies. In addition, companies often have short-, medium-, and long-term objectives in terms of therapeutic areas or types of products they wish to emphasize.

Resource Implications

The impact of the proposed project and ability to pursue it expeditiously in terms of resource requirements and availability (e.g., number of staff, expertise, equipment, facilities, money) must be considered, as well as the likelihood of success. A resource-intensive project that will have a major impact on other projects in terms of staff requirements for a protracted period must be considered differently than a project that has only a negligible or temporary effect on the others. Another resource issue is whether the appropriate expertise is available to carry out and complete the project.

One particular aspect of the resource issue that is often relevant relates to short-, medium-, and long-term financial commitments in taking on a new project. Some companies consider this issue through brief informal conversations among research managers using as a theme the questions "Can we afford to take this project on?" and "Can we afford not to take this project on?" Other companies resort to detailed business analyses of what the market for the therapeutic class is expected to be like in 10 or another number of years and the expected market share for the proposed medicine, based on established and projected new competitive products. Common analyses and estimates include consideration of specific advantages of the new medicine, date of launch, and strength of the patent(s). These companies then determine anticipated sales and profits considering the above factors plus manufacturing, marketing, promotion, and other costs.

Alternative Development Approaches

If new compounds that may become breakthrough medicines are not being developed because of financial limitations, then the potential medicine may be licensed to another developer such as the federal government, independent foundation, institute, or another company. Another possibility is to establish a collaborative approach or joint venture to pursue the new medicine's development. Joint development may make consideration of selected orphan medicines more attractive.

Public Exposure

Another criterion to consider in choosing which medicines to develop is the public exposure one receives by deciding to develop a given project or medicine. There are clearly diseases for which medicine development will enhance the image of the sponsor, either because the development may be viewed as an altruistic effort (such as for rare diseases, when the sponsor may actually lose money) or as a valuable service in an area of great societal need (e.g., a major advance in chemotherapy for lung or colon cancer).

Applying the Criteria

The manner by which the criteria used to choose a project are applied depend in large measure on the nature of the group that must choose a project to develop. If there is a preponderance of either medical, scientific, or marketing personnel involved in the final decision, then that particular aspect will likely have a major influence on the decision reached.

Some groups apply these criteria in an overall subjective approach, whereas others resort to sophisticated scales that delve into many details (Mazzoni, 1972). There is a wide spectrum between simple and complex approaches to this discussion and the pharmaceutical industry appears to be moving away from complex approaches.

ROLE OF MARKETING INPUT IN CHOOSING RESEARCH DIRECTIONS AND PROJECTS

Short-term versus Long-term Outlooks

Many pharmaceutical corporations attempt to avoid placing a heavy emphasis on short-term marketing considerations in choosing corporate goals. One danger of this marketing approach is that the organization may focus too closely on what appears to be profitable in the short term (e.g., line extensions of marketed products) at the expense of important medical opportunities and long-term commercial success.

Traditional Marketing Approaches and a Newer Concept

A traditional marketing approach to choosing future areas for new medicine discoveries and innovations is based on examining the past performance of medicines in various therapeutic areas. A previously successful therapeutic field from the perspective of medicine sales is usually viewed as having great potential to be taken over by a more therapeutically valuable medicine. Therapeutic areas in which current sales are small or are actually declining are often viewed with skepticism. On the other hand, a creative individual will view a number of these "unpromising" therapeutic areas as providing great opportunities to make important medical breakthroughs, while also reaping large commercial success. For example, prior to the introduction of cimetidine (Tagamet), medicine therapy of ulcers was a small market primarily limited to the use of antacids, but cimetidine markedly enhanced total medicine sales in the entire therapeutic area. Cimetidine paved the way for other antiulcer medicines to become both scientifically acceptable on a rational basis and commercially attractive. Unless unexpected adverse effects are reported, or other toxicities develop, cimetidine and other histamine 2-antagonists will continue to be both commercially and medically successful for many years. Similar situations have occurred in other therapeutic fields influenced by breakthrough medicines. If a new safe and effective medicine were discovered for weight reduction or dementia it would stimulate an enormous demand and a huge new commercial market would be created overnight.

Developing novel approaches to patient treatment in important therapeutic areas in which some therapy already exists is a worthwhile concept to explore, especially when there are significant limitations in the safety or efficacy of current therapy. This situation can be illustrated through the use of propranolol in hypertension. At the time of its development there were many medicines for hypertension, but none were ideal. Propranolol was not ideal either, but it offered greater benefit to many patients with hypertension than previous therapy and spawned the discovery and development of a large number of other β-receptor blocking medicines. Propranolol was not the ultimate antihypertensive medicine; both calcium channel blockers and angiotensin-I-converting enzyme (ACE) inhibitors have made further advances in this field.

When Should Marketing Input Be Sought?

There are many appropriate stages of medicine development at which to consider commercial information. The first such time is during the early stages of research when targets are sought for new chemical compounds. Many compounds, however, are often found to affect targets other than those for which they were originally intended. This is discovered either early in the research process during screening and testing in animal models, or later during the clinical development or marketing phases. Nonetheless, commercial input is relevant when decisions are made about the original targets chosen by scientists and scientific management.

Marketing Forecasts

As a medicine moves through a variety of tests, hurdles, and problems, its profile becomes progressively better defined, especially in terms of relative benefits and risks. The estimates of the medicine's potential commercial return becomes more accurate, especially toward the end of Phase II clinical trials. Usually the best marketing estimates may be made of the medicine's commercial value at the time of launch, after many years and many millions of dollars have been spent. Even these estimates are based on many unknown factors and may prove to be highly inaccurate.

Attrition of Compounds and Potential Medicines

It is generally well accepted that approximately 1 in 3,000 to 10,000 newly synthesized compounds becomes a marketed medicine, so the rate of attrition is extremely high for newly synthesized compounds.

Most compounds are synthesized with hopes for their success, whereas others are made for improved patent protection or for different reasons. The ratio of medicines that become marketed to those compounds tested in humans varies from approximately 1 in 4 to 1 in 10, depending on the source of information and also what standards are used to choose those medicines that are tested clinically.

As the costs of taking new compounds into clinical trials increases in developed countries, fewer sponsors are willing or able simultaneously to progress two or more compounds from the same chemical series to initial clinical tests in humans. Instead, they select the best compound from a single chemical series for clinical evaluation based on animal and other data. This has meant that the fraction of medicines marketed to those tested in humans has increased over the last two decades and a greater percentage of apparent success in medicine development has been achieved. The increased cost of the entire medicine development process has also put pressure on sponsors to increase the standards used for choosing medicines to test in humans.

LICENSING OF MEDICINES OR PRODUCTS

There are few major pharmaceutical companies that rely entirely on discovering new medicines within their own research and development departments and that are not proactively seeking to license medicines from other companies. Other companies have adopted a reactive posture and respond to offers received. When sponsors are considering either licensing in compounds from other companies or licensing out compounds to other sponsors to develop or market, the importance and influence of commercial input is often paramount to the decisions made. In licensing medicines the company must strongly consider commercial potential for the compound, medicine, or product being discussed, as well as commercial aspects of the proposed business arrangements (e.g., royalties, fees, countries involved).

Although licensing medicines from other sponsors that have been tested in (or are approaching) Phase I human trials may seem to be a means of avoiding the high costs of research, many of the major clinical, toxicological, and technical development costs usually remain. These latter costs are almost always much more than those spent on the discovery and early animal studies of the compound that is being developed.

Sources of Medicines to License

In addition to the licensing of medicines from other companies, medicines may be licensed from the academic community, which often has the chemical and biochemical means to synthesize medicines, but lacks adequate resources for testing or developing them through formulation development, toxicology, and clinical trials. There are also instances of commercial or research groups outside academic centers or corporations who synthesize medicines that eventually are tested by companies.

At What Stage of Development are Medicines Licensed?

Medicines may be licensed in (or out) at any stage of development. The further along the development track the product is at the time of licensing, the more accurately its potential value may be estimated. A newly synthesized compound that is found to have activity in an initial screen may have enormous long-term commercial potential but relatively little value for licensing. As the compound survives additional rounds of biological testing, its real value steadily increases. Each stage in the medicine development process usually represents a difficult hurdle and culls out many candidate medicines, usually for reasons of toxicity or insufficient therapeutic activity.

Medicines may also be licensed (in or out) after they have been approved for marketing. A major reason why a sponsor might license a medicine to another company *after* it has been approved for marketing would be because the original sponsor could not market the medicine as effectively as the company to which it was licensed. For example, a relatively small company with a limited number of marketing representatives usually cannot generate as much revenue with a specific medicine as a sponsor with a much larger number of sales representatives. A company may also wish to expand its sales in regions of the world where its presence is currently small or non-existent.

Cross-Licensing

If two companies develop medicines that are outside their usual zones of marketing, then swapping products (with appropriate financial, legal, and other safeguards) may be a sound business arrangement for both. For example, if one company's products are primarily concentrated in the cardiovascular area and those of another company are concentrated in the surgical area, then each of their sales forces will normally direct their promotional campaigns and efforts toward different types of specialists and practitioners. A new product in a different therapeutic area might be difficult for them to promote and a cross-licensing agreement could be a mutually beneficial solution. Two companies that

sell medicines in different regions of the world could also benefit in some cases from a cross-licensing arrangement.

Joint Development or Marketing

The original developer of a medicine might wish to retain the rights to sell it as well as license it or obtain expertise or funds for its development. Thus, there could be an agreement between two sponsors to develop or market a medicine jointly.

The types of arrangements for joint development vary enormously. Sometimes one company does all the technical and clinical work and the other company provides financial support. In other situations, the two companies either divide the work equally or work jointly on all tasks.

Under confidentiality agreements many companies are willing to discuss openly most of their ongoing efforts on hot leads and new medicines with a competitor if a cross-licensing or joint-marketing arrangement is considered likely or merely possible. By initially discussing results in general terms there is little chance of divulging information that is unprotected.

Licensing Agreements

The licensing patterns and product "mix" of large and medium-size pharmaceutical companies reveal an amazing variety of business arrangements. Many research-based companies have a few products that they have licensed out to other companies, whereas other products may have been licensed in, and certain other medicines are being jointly developed.

This discussion has so far omitted one of the most important factors—that each agreement covers certain countries but not others. Therefore a company may license a single medicine to several different companies, but each company will get the rights to sell the medicine in a different country. Another complicating factor occurs when a medicine is available in multiple dosage forms such as an oral capsule, intravenous solution, and eye drops. Each of these dosage forms may be licensed-out separately to different companies for development or marketing in the same country.

BIOTECHNOLOGY

Medicines produced by biotechnology techniques have been part of the physician's armamentarium since bread made with yeast was used to treat hunger and alcohol drunk for a wide variety of reasons. Recent advances have dramatically increased the potential for biotechnology to help produce some medicines more efficiently and develop others for the first time.

For many proteins, polypeptides, and other chemicals that could not be made without biotechnological methods, design considerations are similar to those for chemically simple compounds in clinical trials to evaluate safety, efficacy, and pharmacokinetics. Ethical considerations require that great caution be exercised before some of these products are evaluated in the environment (e.g., as agricultural modifiers) or in humans (e.g., for genetic manipulation). This is a complex and rapidly changing area, and is not covered in this book.

Biotechnology has led to medicines that replace low-level or absent hormones (e.g., growth hormone, insulin) or other chemicals (e.g., factor 8), or that cause direct biological effects (e.g., tissue plasminogen activator to dissolve intravascular clots, or interferon to treat hairy cell leukemia, juvenile laryngeal papillomotosis, and other diseases). All of these medicines are evaluated through techniques described elsewhere in this book, even though the routes of administration may be different (e.g., intralesional). Regulations and patent issues are also different for biotechnology products.

Future advances using biotechnology include gene therapy. This therapy is still in its infancy, but should utilize the same features of clinical trial design that are described in this book. Products used as diagnostics have their own set of requirements. Technical and manufacturing issues are usually far greater for biotechnology products. Animal testing requirements must be clarified with various regulatory agencies.

Efficacy of Biologicals

When a biological product derived from humans is given to a patient who is deficient in that product (e.g., thyroid hormone, growth hormone, corticosteroids) it can be assumed that efficacy should be observed. Unless the product is outdated, not absorbed, or subject to another problem, replacement doses (i.e., physiological doses) are effective. On the other hand, when a biological product derived from humans is given to patients at high multiples of the normal level (i.e., pharmacological doses), neither the efficacy nor safety of the biological can be assumed. Any biological product at high doses may have a wide range of effects and interactions that may lead to major safety problems. These have been observed with probably every natural biological product.

PREPARING FEASIBILITY REPORTS

Before making a firm commitment to conduct clinical or preclinical research in a therapeutic area, initiate a new biological project, or develop an interesting chemical lead as a new medicine, it is usually important to prepare a feasibility report. In the academic community, a feasibility evaluation or report may assist in the preparation of a grant application, whereas in the pharmaceutical industry a feasibility report is usually related to the development or licensing of a new medicine. Feasibility reports vary in scope and magnitude, ranging from a superficial review of the proposed project, medicine, or area for investigation to a thorough evaluation and analysis of the project requiring a major commitment of time, effort, and money.

Purposes

The feasibility report usually presents a global view of the proposed strategy that has been designed to achieve the project's objectives. For the purposes of this discussion it is considered that the feasibility report is prepared either shortly prior to or shortly after the decision is made to initiate a project. In the former case the document is created to assist in the decision-making process, whereas in the latter case it is used as one of the initial steps to assist in the planning of a project's development. Other possible uses of a feasibility report are to (1) define the goals and objectives of the project, (2) identify the most efficient and rapid route(s) for reaching the goals, and (3) show that the steps in this route are possible to conduct.

The major purpose of a feasibility report is to examine the factors that may affect whether the project or clinical development can be conducted successfully. If certain factors are uncovered that will probably or definitely play a critical role and affect the success of the project, then additional attention can be given to those factors as the strategy for the project is developed. A detailed strategy to achieve or fulfill the goals of the project should not be developed until after it has been determined that an overall strategy is feasible. There is usually some overlap in discussing feasibility and strategy. For the purpose of this discussion, however, these two processes will be separated, and the development of strategies is discussed in Chapters 112 and 113.

One of the most important reasons for preparing a feasibility report is to identify both actual and potential problems that may be encountered in pursuing a project. If significant problems are uncovered it may be necessary to (1) terminate the project, (2) establish a new goal that will avoid the anticipated problem(s), or (3) develop a strategy that will overcome the anticipated problem(s). The unstated axiom in this situation is that the better one is able to anticipate problems, the better one is able to deal with them. Although this is not always correct it is usually in the interests of the leaders of a project to have a clear view of the path they are traveling and the obstacles that may block their route.

Another objective of the feasibility report is to convince others of the project's value. For instance, in preparing a grant application in the area of clinical research, one attempts to convince the group that is deciding how to dispense funds that the goals indicated within the grant are both worthwhile and attainable. Thus, the feasibility report will help the investigator define the objectives or goals, describe the path to follow, to reach, or to approach the goals; and identify potential problems that are likely to arise.

Styles

There are many different styles for preparing a feasibility report. Three styles are shown in Tables 111.1 to 111.3. The first is intended as a more informal approach that addresses the basic questions about most projects. The second is a more structured and detailed approach, better suited for situations in which a formal review of the report will be conducted. The third emphasizes strategies and international development of a project. These tables indicate major areas that should be included (or at least considered) in most feasibility reports.

TABLE 111.1 *Sample table of contents for a clinical feasibility report—I*

Section headings	Section contents
1. What?	What is proposed?
2. Why?	Why is it proposed? How does the clinical trial fit the overall strategy?
3. Where?	Where are the proposed trials to take place?
4. How?	How will the project be organized, monitored, and reviewed?
5. Who?	Who will run the project, manage the project, design the protocols, conduct the trials, monitor the trials, analyze the data, and interpret the analyses?
6. When?	When will the trials be started, reach various milestones, and be computed?
7. How much?	How much will the trials cost individually and for the entire project? What are the other costs?
8. Verification?	Has it been verified (insofar as possible) that the trials can be conducted as planned within estimated times and budgets? What steps were conducted to verify these factors?
9. Success?	What are the chances of success (i.e., achieving the objectives)?
10. Recommendation?	What are the recommendations for the project?

TABLE 111.2 *Sample table of contents for a clinical feasibility report—II*

A. Abstract
B. Background
C. Summary information on the medicine
  1. Chemical structures of pertinent compounds or medicines
  2. Pharmacological synopsis of the primary compound or medicine
  3. Clinical pharmacology synopsis on the project medicine and standard medicines
D. Pharmacology and other preclinical data (e.g., biochemical, physiological)
  1. Summary of pharmacological and other tests related to primary activity
  2. Summary of any other biological tests
  3. Suspected or known mechanism of action
  4. Additional nonclinical studies that will be (or may be) performed
  5. Toxicological results
E. Clinical data available
  1. Activity of the project medicine and of standard medicines
  2. Clinical conditions that cause, result from, or are associated with the target disease
  3. Physiological and biochemical mechanisms underlying or associated with the target disease
  4. Currently available medicine and nonmedicine therapy for treating the target disease—advantages and disadvantages
  5. Interactions among medicines
  6. Other available data
F. Patent status
G. Regulatory considerations
H. Formulation and other aspects of technical development considerations
I. Marketing considerations
  1. Present market size
  2. Future trends in market growth
  3. Present medicines available
  4. Limitations of currently available medicines
  5. Competitive medicines currently under investigation (e.g., indications, pros and cons, pharmacological characteristics, current status)
  6. Estimated ranges of future sales plus caveats
J. Financial considerations (e.g., development costs, payback time, projected profit)
K. Rationale for human investigation
  1. Summary of primary clinical objectives
  2. Clinical data available
  3. Animal data and extrapolatability of those data to humans
  4. Potential advantages of the project medicine versus currently available medicines and other therapies
  5. Potential disadvantages of the project medicine versus currently available medicines and other therapies
  6. Overall strategies for clinical development
L. Clinical trials to be considered
  1. Overview of clinical trials proposed[a]
  2. Protocol for initial trial (or trials)
  3. Estimated costs and time of initial clinical trial and for entire program
  4. Clinical personnel required
    a. At pharmaceutical company (sponsor)
    b. At academic institutions
    c. At private clinics or other facilities
M. Summary
N. Recommendations
O. Bibliography
P. Appendixes
  1. Details of medicines currently marketed for the proposed indication
  2. Details of medicines chemically related to the trial medicine
  3. Additional chemical, pharmacological, clinical, or other information

[a] This list may not be complete and may only cover Phases I or Phases I and II.

TABLE 111.3 *Sample table of contents for a clinical feasibility report—III*

1. Rationale for clinical development
2. Comparison of the proposed medicine with an ideal medicine
3. Comparison of the proposed medicine with presently available medicines and those under development
4. Current clinical data available (if any)
5. Proposed strategy for clinical development
6. Proposed clinical trials to be conducted
7. Proposed development of a core package of clinical trials
8. Coordination with medicine development in other countries
9. Timetable of regulatory submissions
10. Work-force requirements
11. Financial costs
12. Summary
13. Recommendations

Review and Evaluation

After a feasibility report has been prepared it may be used in many different ways. One common use is for the supervisors or managers who control the decision making to evaluate the report and to reach a decision as to whether the author(s) have demonstrated that the project is feasible. It should be mentioned that a feasibility report does not necessarily have to be a positive report in favor of conducting a project. There are many situations in which a negative report is far more valuable. For instance, a well thought out and logically developed feasibility report that strongly criticizes the proposal may save the sponsor many millions of dollars on a project with flawed logic or undesirable goals, or on one that has an extremely small chance of meeting its objectives.

ASSESSING THE FEASIBILITY OF AN OVERALL PROJECT

In an ideal medicine development scenario, the individual who is planning the clinical program of a new medicine will develop a list of the types of clinical trials that should be conducted in all four phases of development. Questions relating to postmarketing surveillance (what will need to be known about a new medicine in 10 or more years) will often influence the direction that is taken at the outset of the initial clinical trials. If the general planning and strategy of a clinical trial program is haphazard and random, then errors in the project's direction will undoubtedly occur. These errors may become part of that medicine's history and reputation and may affect the entire medical and commercial life of the medicine, even years after it is eventually marketed. For example, if an inappropriate indication is initially chosen to be pursued and the medicine performs badly, then a stigma will probably be created, which may take a long time to overcome

even after the medicine is developed for a more appropriate indication. Moreover, valuable time will be lost in the medicine's development when such tangents are pursued.

Factors to Consider

Various types of projects that usually require multiple clinical trials are listed in Table 111.4, and factors to consider in determining whether to initiate a new project are shown in Table 111.5. With any of the types of projects shown in Table 111.4, one must assess or consider all information available before deciding to undertake the project. This information should be examined for hints of potential problems to avoid at different stages [e.g., avoid including patients in Phase II trials who are receiving concomitant medicines (if possible) or who have renal disease with compromised renal function]. Also examine preclinical and clinical data available for potential toxicities that should be carefully monitored in future trials with special tests (e.g., ophthalmological examinations) and determine whether more frequent use of commonly used tests (e.g., electrocardiograms, blood tests) is advisable to monitor patients. In some situations it is useful to evaluate data available on close chemical analogs of the trial medicine for hints of potential value. Careful review of the data will minimize the chance of obtaining either false-positive or false-negative results with the medicine being evaluated.

TABLE 111.4 *Multiple clinical trials are generally required for the projects listed*

1. Phase I, II, III, or IV clinical evaluation of a new medicine
2. Postmarketing surveillance studies of a newly approved or marketed medicine
3. Pharmacokinetic profile of an investigational or marketed medicine
4. Comparison of a test medicine, treatment, or procedure with a standard medicine, treatment, or procedure
5. Evaluation of a theory, hypothesis, or mathematical model of a biological effect
6. Evaluation of a new or modified medical device
7. Evaluation of a new indication of a marketed or investigational medicine
8. Evaluation of a new formulation, dosage form, or dosing schedule
9. Evaluation of a new therapy in a specific patient population (e.g., geriatrics, infants)
10. Evaluation of a medicine's general safety profile or a specific question about a medicine's toxicity
11. Marketing-oriented studies designed to compare a test medicine and a competitor's medicine. Evaluations may focus on the medicine, formulation, indication, dosage form, dosing regimen, route of administration, or other factor
12. Evaluation of a new methodology for assessing safety or efficacy of a medicine or other modality
13. Evaluation of known or potential medicine interactions

TABLE 111.5 *Selected factors to consider in determining whether to initiate a new project*

1. Determine how worthwhile the project is from scientific, medical, and commercial viewpoints
2. Determine whether adequately trained personnel are available for all aspects of the project. If not, estimate the probability that they can be recruited and hired by the time they are needed or may be recruited as consultants
3. Determine whether adequate financial resources are available to conduct the entire program. If not, estimate the likelihood that they will be obtained
4. Determine whether some or all of the financial and other resources necessary for the project have to be taken from other projects. If so, determine which projects have a greater priority
5. Determine the adequacy of the facilities and equipment that are presently available
6. Determine how much time the project will require to complete. Estimate the probability that the project will be completed by a given date if the medicine or treatment has the desired properties
7. Estimate the likelihood that most (or all) technical, ethical, patent, legal, and regulatory problems that will be encountered during the project are presently known and can be effectively addressed and solved
8. Determine the activities that are currently being conducted at other academic centers, institutes, and pharmaceutical companies that might influence the project (e.g., compete for a limited patient population, compete for a limited number of investigators, solve the same medical problem, evaluate the same issue, reach the market sooner) and decrease its value or affect the overall objectives
9. Determine the potential impact that the project will have on publicity

Formulating the Initial Approach to Developing a New Medicine

Four questions one usually desires to answer in formulating an approach to developing a new medicine in the most rapid and efficient manner are:

1. Which appears to be the best or most nearly optimal dosage form, formulation, patient population, indication, and dosage regimen to utilize *initially* in clinical trials?
2. What is (or are) the *ultimate* dosage form(s), formulation(s), patient population(s), indication(s), and dosage regimen(s) desired?
3. At what phase of development will other dosage forms, formulations, patient populations, indications, and dosage regimens be added or evaluated in the clinical program as a transition is made from the initial to hopefully final goals?
4. What claims does one want to make and at what time points after eventual launch? These must be prioritized and appropriate clinical trials designed and scheduled.

Determinants of Success

Once these questions have been considered and a decision reached to proceed with a medicine's devel-

opment, then additional strategies and plans may be developed that will assist progress in reaching the goals identified.

Whether a medicine is developed successfully primarily depends on the nature of the medicine and the individual people who are collectively developing it. The type of organization and systems used by the company or sponsor are usually secondary considerations. Well-developed plans are important, but they can only cover a limited number of possibilities and often have limited usefulness when problems arise. It may only be possible to design a Phase I program at the outset of a project, and to design Phase II clinical trials after all data are reviewed and assessed. The individuals running and managing the development must have "prepared minds" as well as a sense of readiness to deal effectively with any uncertainty and unanticipated problems that arise.

CHOOSING A PROJECT FROM AMONG SEVERAL CANDIDATES

A series of steps is described to assist in choosing a single potential medicine candidate when several or many compounds are available for consideration.

1. Determine the relevant criteria to be used in evaluating the compound. Include criteria (objectives) of activities the compound should both possess and not possess. Limit the number of criteria to about six if possible.
2. Establish minimum standards that a compound must meet to be selected for development.
3. Rank order the objectives. Assign approximate weights to each objective (if possible), depending on its relative importance.
4. Rank order the potential candidates according to how well they achieve each objective.
5. List important caveats about each compound that may affect the decision.
6. Determine if additional tests should be conducted on the lead compound(s) before a decision can be made.
7. Determine which compounds, if any, meet the minimum criteria needed to choose a compound for development.
8. Determine which non-compound-related factors (e.g., financial resources, other projects underway, work force) will affect the decision, and list how they will affect it.
9. Consider all of the above factors and choose the best compound.
10. If the best compound to choose is not obvious, consider and critique each compound in turn. Then compare the evaluations.

Avoiding Red Herrings (Poor Choices)

Everyone would like to work for an organization in which each medicine or medical device chosen for development has an excellent chance for success and offers important medical and commercial opportunities. Unfortunately, this scenario does not always occur. When multiple compounds (or sometimes even a single compound) are being considered, the quality of the proposal presentation may influence or even determine which medicine is chosen. The people who serve as backers of a compound are usually a critically important influence in the choice. One means of controlling for these factors is to arrange for an independent person or group to review the decision. This group could consist of consultants or scientists who do not report to the group that made the decision. This independent person (or group) should be able to reach a decision based on scientific and business criteria only.

CHAPTER 112

Missions, Objectives, Goals, Strategies, and Tactics

A few years ago, each of the terms in this chapter's title were invariably used with different meanings by various authors, and there was no consensus about their separate definitions. The word objectives was used so broadly that a 1964 Harvard Business Review article (Granger, 1964) titled "The Hierarchy of Objectives" discussed 11 levels. This is no longer true. Each term has important distinctions that differentiate it from the others. This chapter seeks to define each term, show how these concepts relate to each other, indicate how these concepts may be applied to different levels within any organization, and show how these concepts may be applied to various functions. Additional discussions on several of these topics are found in Chapter 113. These concepts apply equally well (in most situations) to academic, government, industry, or other organizations.

DEFINITIONS

Mission. The mission is the overall purpose of the group and is usually expressed succinctly in no more than four sentences. It is a reflection of the group's values and needs. It usually reflects the drives of the primary individual(s) who establishes policy for the group.

Objectives. Objectives are nonquantifiable goals, usually with a long-term (i.e., multiple-year) horizon.

These are general statements about the future direction of the group or organization. Objectives explain how a mission will be achieved, but are not tied to specific completion dates. Objectives are often related to values and philosophies and may describe a desired state of being. It is not essential for an organization to have clearly established objectives.

Goals. Goals are quantifiable endpoints, often with a time limit (e.g., 1- to 3-year horizons are common). It is possible to divide this category into short-term and intermediate-term goals. Goals are developed to explain how each objective will be achieved, and they address the question of what a group wants to get or

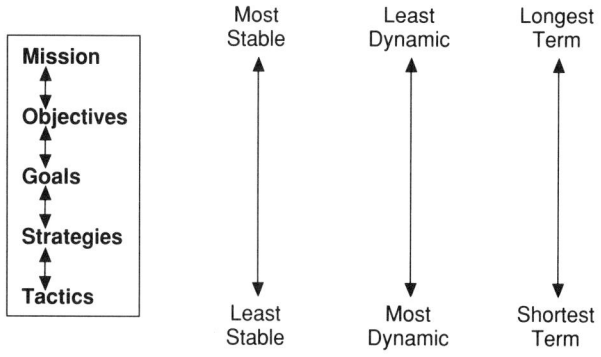

FIG. 112.1 Interrelationships and selected characteristics of the five concepts listed on the left side of the figure.

849

State University System

Overall Group of Universities (e.g., The State of North Carolina System)

$\updownarrow$

University-Wide (One University Campus-University of North Carolina at Chapel Hill)

$\updownarrow$

School (e.g., Medicine)

$\updownarrow$

Department (e.g., Pharmacology)

$\updownarrow$

Section or Group (e.g., Cardiovascular)

$\updownarrow$

Individual Professional (e.g., Dr.J.A.B.)

Pharmaceutical Industry

Overall Multinational Co.

$\updownarrow$

Company Based in One Country

$\updownarrow$

Division (e.g., Research and Development)

$\updownarrow$

Department (e.g., Pharmacology)

$\updownarrow$

Section (e.g., Cardiovascular)

$\updownarrow$

Individual Professional (e.g., Dr.J.A.B.)

Government Regulatory Agency

Overall Agency (e.g., Department of Health and Human Sciences)

$\updownarrow$

Specific Agency (e.g., Food and Drug Administration)

$\updownarrow$

Major Activity (e.g., New Drug Evaluation)

$\updownarrow$

Division (e.g., Cardio-Renal)

$\updownarrow$

Section or Group (e.g., Pharmacology)

$\updownarrow$

Individual Professional (e.g., Dr.J.A.B.)

FIG. 112.2 Line management levels at which the five concepts operate in a state university system, pharmaceutical industry, and government regulatory agency.

MATRIX FUNCTIONS IN WHICH THE FIVE CONCEPTS APPLY

- Overall Project System
- Individual Projects
- Project Champion/Leader
- Project Manager/Administrator
- Project Planners/Coordinators

FIG. 112.3 Matrix functions in which the five concepts apply.

be. One or more goals should be identified for each objective. Goals may be combined with objectives in some situations, especially at lower levels in an organization. In that situation, they may be referred to either as objectives or goals.

Strategies. Strategies are plans, concepts, and principles of how goals will be achieved. Strategies describe the means or approaches that are to be followed to achieve goals. Each goal should have one or more strategies indicating how the goal will be obtained. More specific strategies may also be created to focus on means of attaining short-term goals or milestones that are established. The three major elements to describe a strategy fully are (1) the current position, (2) the goals, and (3) the means of moving from the current position to the goals.

Tactics. Tactics are detailed methods and plans used to initiate, implement, and complete each strategy. They usually deal with the shortest term for which plans are created. There may be two or more levels of tactics (e.g., tactics for the next week and others for the next 2 months). Tactics are the most specific, detailed, dynamic, and shortest-term of the five concepts.

The interrelationships between the five concepts is simplistically illustrated in Fig. 112.1. This figure emphasizes their hierarchical nature, and how they compare in terms of stability, dynamic nature, and permanence. The various levels at which these concepts operate within an academic institution, a pharmaceutical company, or a government agency are shown in Fig. 112.2. These concepts are also important within the matrix function of project development. Five aspects of a matrix that may be involved in projects are listed in Fig. 112.3. Usually either a project champion/leader or a project manager/administrator is involved with a particular project. A single organization generally manages projects with only one of these groups, although both types could be present to lead different types of projects (e.g., prescription versus over-the-counter medicines). These topics are discussed further in Chapter 124.

Although missions, objectives, goals, strategies, and tactics may be created or determined independently for different levels, departments, divisions, matrix individuals, or projects within a company, there are also important interrelationships among different levels, in-

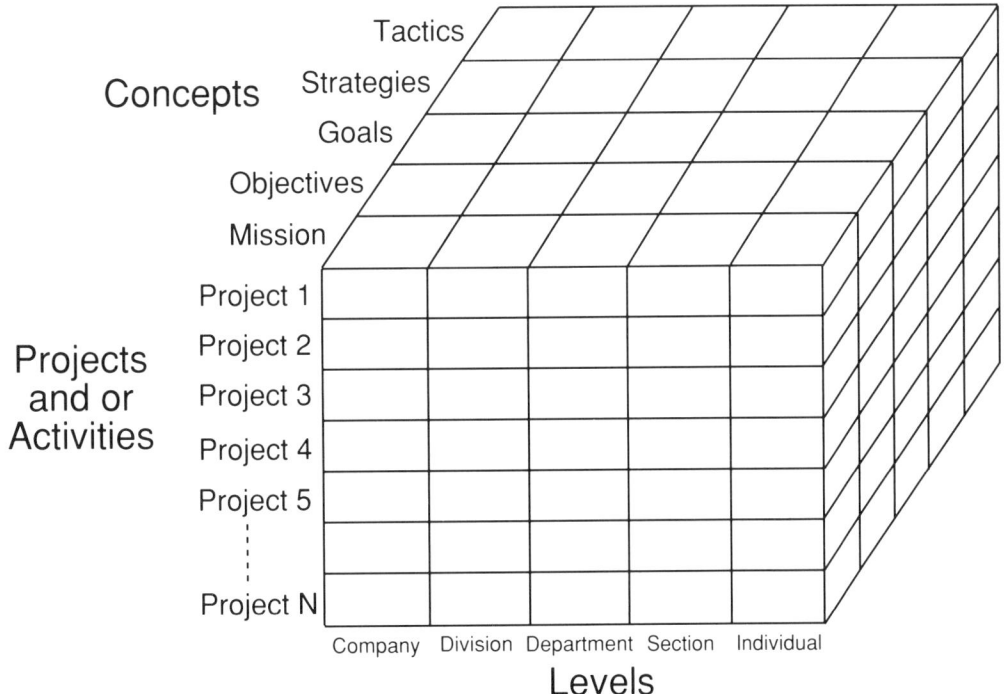

FIG. 112.4 Matrix of company levels, projects, and concepts.

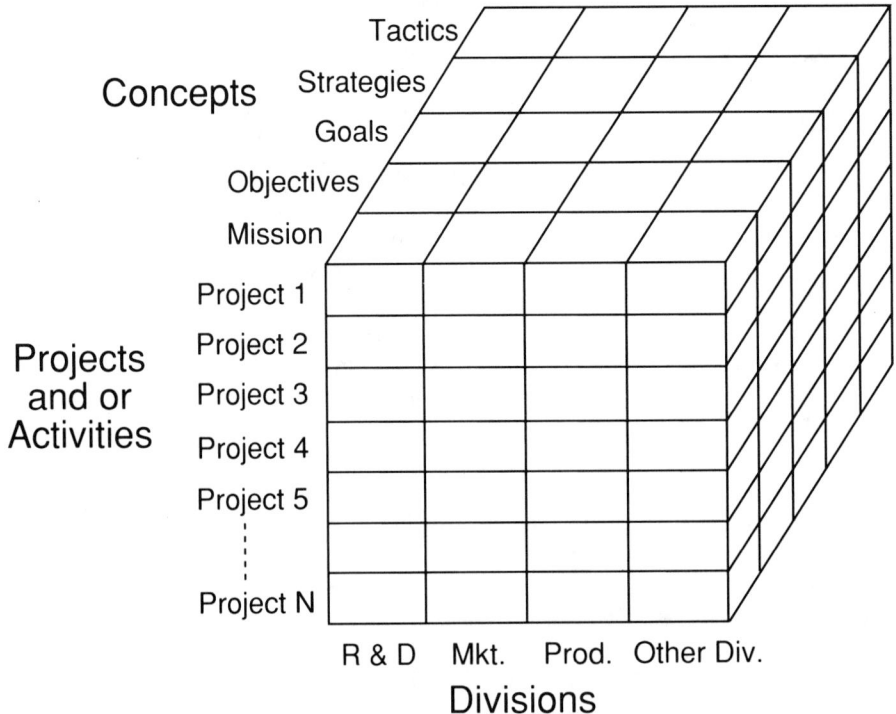

FIG. 112.5 Matrix of divisions, projects, and concepts. Mkt., marketing; Prod., Production; R & D, Research and Development; Div., Division.

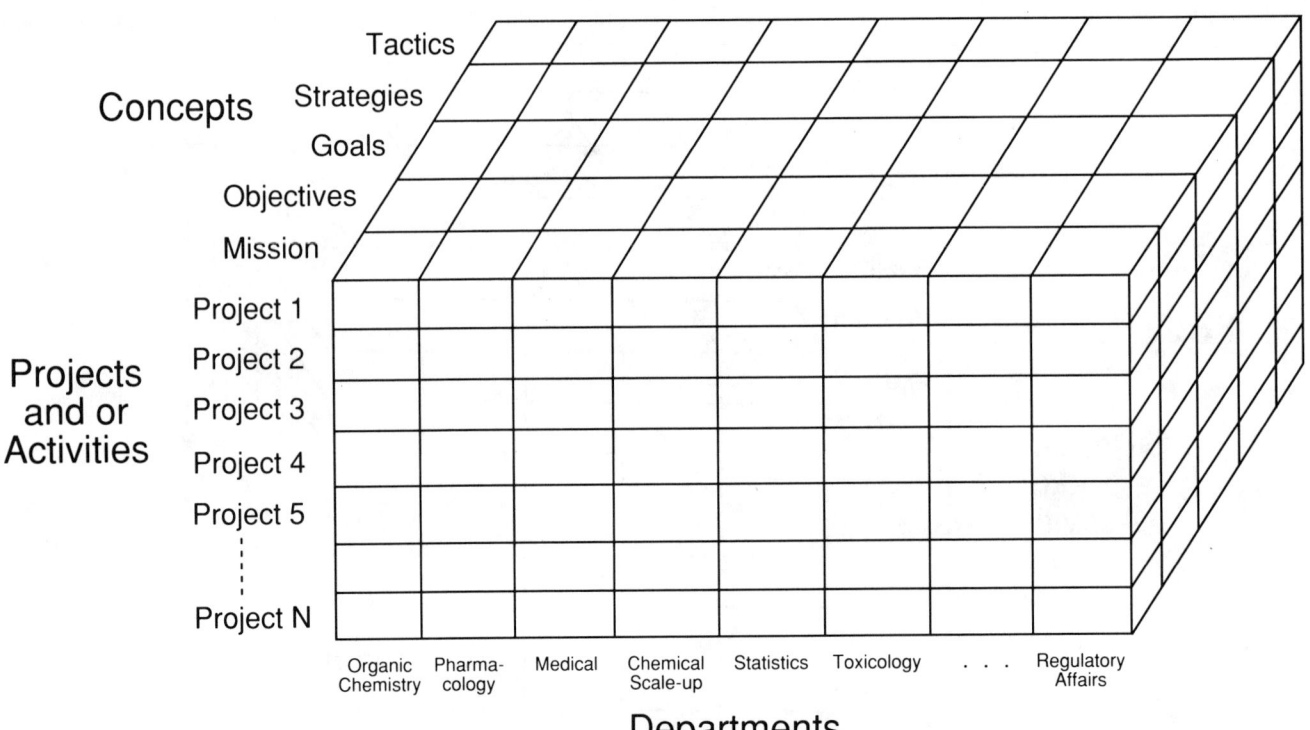

FIG. 112.6 Matrix of departments, projects, and concepts.

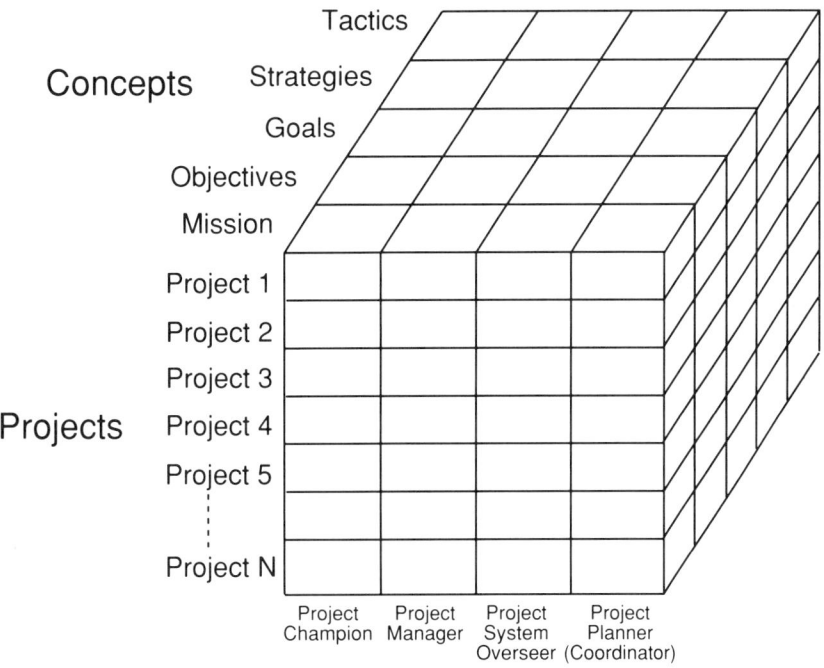

Individuals in Matrix Functions

FIG. 112.7 Matrix of individuals who function predominantly within the matrix function, projects, and concepts.

dividuals, projects, or groups. Some of the relationships are illustrated in three-dimensional block diagrams (Figs. 112.4 through 112.7). Each of the smaller cubes that together form a large cube shown in these four figures may be nearly 100% different from or identical to the small cube next to it. Even these diagrams are too simplistic, because each of the minicubes inside the larger cube changes over time. Time is a fourth dimension that could be illustrated by showing a series of identical large cubes at specific (or general) time points.

DEVELOPMENT OF THE FIVE CONCEPTS

It is theoretically possible to develop the five concepts stepwise starting with desirable tactics and building strategies, etc., until the overall mission is created. Nonetheless, this would be a backward and inefficient process. The natural order of creating these concepts is to develop the mission first and then systematically proceed in a stepwise manner to describe objectives, goals, strategies, and finally, tactics. This enables each concept to be tied to those both above and below it in the hierarchy. When the exercise is completed, it should be possible to move both upward and downward between the concepts to show how certain specific strategies will lead to desired goals and how each

of the goals will be achieved by following the strategies described.

The plan described above can be utilized for any level (e.g., section, department, company) within an organization. Nonetheless, it is most efficient if the overall organization conducts this exercise first. This will allow the lower organizational levels to create individual concepts that also integrate with the overall organization's concepts (Fig. 112.4). While a conglomerate of distinct companies may allow each subsidiary a great deal of independence in developing these concepts, a single pharmaceutical company discovering and developing medicines at two or more sites cannot allow the same degree of autonomy to exist at each site. It is easy to predict the outcome if each major part and level of an organization creates these five concepts independently.

The ground rules for creating these concepts at any level should be clarified. Ground rules relate to the creative freedom or latitude of the group developing the concepts, the time allocated for the exercise, the level of quality desired in the product, the degree to which the group adopting the concepts should be forced to stretch to achieve the desired ends, and an indication of what level of resources may realistically be expected to be applied after the exercise is complete. In some situations a number of alternatives may be created for each stage. Overall, the exercise should almost always be realistic, and not idealistic, if any benefit is to be gained.

ASSUMPTIONS AND CAVEATS PRIOR TO DEVELOPING THE FIVE CONCEPTS

Important assumptions and caveats about each concept must be discussed before the process of developing them is initiated. This is colloquially described as ensuring that everyone is on the same wavelength. These basic concepts are understood differently even by people with similar backgrounds, training, and experience. It is particularly important to ensure that those whose backgrounds, training, and experience differ have the same understanding of what they are doing before the actual process is begun. Adoption of all concepts should be by consensus rather than by a vote or dictatorial decree. Separate points should not be mixed in a single concept item but presented separately. The most important assumptions may be described or listed in writing for any concept developed. This will enhance its understanding by all individuals.

THE IMPLEMENTATION STAGE—AFTER THE FIVE CONCEPTS ARE DEVELOPED

These five concepts should enable people at all levels and positions within the organization to make decisions on a daily basis that are steps toward achieving the realization of the concepts. Adopting contradictory concepts will clearly lead to conflicting actions and inefficiency within the group.

Creating a perfect set of five concepts throughout an organization only establishes ideas and plans that represent the best views of various levels of managers and workers. These may be arrived at through democratic procedures and represent a consensus or shared view. Alternatively, one or more senior managers may literally dictate what each of the concepts will be and force each level within the organization to support their views. Whichever path is followed to derive these concepts, their existence and nature should be widely promulgated throughout the organization.

Plans are implemented and carried out by managers who assign resources to agreed-on activities according to set priorities. The processes of priority setting and resource allocation are discussed in Chapter 123. Implementation of the objectives, goals, and strategies will be enhanced if each is assigned to relevant people as a primary responsibility. Solely making them the group's responsibility may not be sufficient to achieve successful implementation. It is ideal if the people responsible were involved in the concepts' development. The number of objectives and goals delegated to a single individual should be limited, and responsibilities should be shared within the group.

Priority setting has a great influence on which strategies are adopted to achieve the goals. If every project or major activity is awarded the highest priority, there will be few (if any) companies that could effectively assign adequate resources to achieve these strategies. The point is that priority setting plays a major role in the degree to which specific objectives, goals, strategies, and tactics are adopted and enacted.

PERIODIC REVIEW

Once the system is running and initial fine tuning has most people agreeing with (or accepting) the overall direction of each part of the organization, a few options exist for future review. The first is for the group to keep the plans in view, but not to review them until they go out of date and a strong need is felt for a new exercise to bring the organization or group in step with current events. Alternatively, the concepts can be reviewed by each group on an ongoing basis. This generally makes much more sense than the former approach. Continually reviewing these concepts means that a periodic review, usually on an annual, semiannual, or biannual basis is conducted to update the concepts. A periodic review that solicits input from all relevant people ensures that the concepts are meaningful, current, and have become part of the ethos of the organization. The results of the review must be effectively communicated both upwards and downwards through the organization.

Brief examples of the five concepts are given for a pharmaceutical company, a cardiovascular section within that company, and an individual physician within that section.

EXAMPLES OF THE FIVE CONCEPTS

Three of the various levels in a pharmaceutical company are used to create examples of the five concepts discussed. The largest and smallest levels, plus one in the middle, have been chosen. Three concepts are illustrated for a cardiovascular section and all five concepts are illustrated for an individual physician.

Pharmaceutical Company: Overall

Mission

The mission is to be a health care company whose core business is in pharmaceuticals.

Objectives

1. Achieve the status of being one of the top ten pharmaceutical companies in terms of sales and profits

2. Attract the most creative staff
3. Discover or license important new medicines with both commercial and medical values
4. Develop new medicines with increasing efficiency
5. Market all new medicines to attain the maximum market share possible

A maximum of 16 to 25 objectives should be sufficient for a group at any level of an organization. Each major part of the organization should have at least one objective.

Goals

1. Increase sales by X% per year and achieve before tax (or after tax) profits of Y%.
2. Hold staff turnover to Z% annually
3. Identify creative individuals outside the company who may be hired
4. License in medicines each year with estimated third-year sales of XX million dollars

Pharmaceutical Company: Cardiovascular Section in a Medical Department

Goals

1. Submit an NDA on medicine A within 2.5 years
2. Reach Phase III for medicine B within 2.0 years
3. Initiate all studies on medicine C within 1.5 years, complete them in 2.5 years after they start, and submit an NDA in 3.0 years from initiation

Additional goals should be listed on the document created by the cardiovascular section.

Strategies (General)

1. For medicine A, use a "broad front" approach (see Chapter 115) and evaluate the medicine in four specific indications using three dosage forms in all three of the company's development sites.
2. For medicine B, use a "laser" approach and only develop an intravenous form of the medicine. All development will be conducted in country 1.

Additional general strategies should be listed on the document created by the cardiovascular section.

Strategies (Specific)

An overall clinical development plan is created for each medicine. This plan considers each country in which the medicine will be developed and registered, identifies the trials to be conducted, and represents the specific strategy to be followed for each medicine.

Tactics

Specific plans are developed that allocate resources to achieve each step in the strategy. These plans indicate the number of sites per clinical trial, names of investigators to be contacted or hired, monitoring approaches, data-processing plans, and various other aspects of the clinical trials (e.g., frequency of site visits).

Pharmaceutical Company: Individual Physician in the Cardiovascular Section of a Medical Department

Mission

The physician's mission is to contribute to the section, unit, and company's goals and objectives for developing cardiovascular medicines.

Objectives

1. Oversee the development of medicine A and the Product License Application (PLA) submission
2. Provide management functions within the section

Goals

1. Plan and implement five clinical trials, including two pivotal trials, to evaluate medicine A over the next 2 years
2. Direct three junior staff in monitoring these trials

Strategies

1. Develop clinical development plans for medicine A and review these plans quarterly
2. Assign two junior staff to the pivotal trials and the other staff member to the other trials; after the pivotal trials are completed, evaluate the medicine's status and reassign the staff to other medicine A trials or to medicine B trials

Tactics

Specific tactics to achieve each of the goals would be developed.

CHAPTER 113

Establishing Project Strategies and Goals

DEFINITION AND DESCRIPTION OF STRATEGIES

There are many uses of the word "strategy" and many types of strategies that may be developed. Strategies were operationally defined in the preceding chapter as dynamic concepts, plans, or principles (written or unwritten) that describe the means or approach to be used to move a project from its present or current position to achieve the goals that have been established. Strategy is a dynamic term that describes how a project (or other well-defined entity) will move from its current status to achieve its goals. The three major elements of a strategy are (1) the current position, (2) the goals, and (3) the means of moving from the current position to the goals. The term "tactics" denotes the specific details and methods that are used to initiate, implement, and complete the strategy.

In developing strategies for specific projects or activities it is necessary to consider six major factors:

1. *Duration* of time that the strategy will cover (e.g., 1 week, 1–3 years, indefinite).
2. *Level* at which the strategy will operate (e.g., within a specific department, corporation, medicine or nonmedicine project, single-medicine trial, or single activity within the clinical trial).

3. Whether the strategy will emphasize *general or specific details*. A research and development strategy may be created along general or specific lines. A general research strategy may describe how a specific therapeutic area will be explored to search for new medicines. A less general strategy may describe how both targeted (e.g., disease-oriented) and nontargeted research within that therapeutic area will be pursued to achieve specified goals. Specific aspects of a research strategy used for each target might include: (1) the nature of activities to be followed, methods to be used, and how resources will be allocated for targeted and nontargeted research; (2) how the balance of research efforts in targeted and nontargeted areas will be monitored and reviewed; and (3) how short-, mid-, and long-term research programs for each target fit into the general strategy. At a certain level of detail one ceases to describe strategies and enters the area of tactics (specific mechanisms and details followed to implement a strategy).

4,5. *Description of the present position and the goal.* In formulating a strategy it is possible to consider either one aspect of the present position and goals or else to consider the total complexity of each. Each of these two focal points may be considered in general terms and attention may be concentrated on the methods of completing the in-be-tween area (i.e., the strategy for achieving the goals). It is also possible to define and describe the present position or one's goals in too much detail. Detailed documents or reports that focus too strongly on either current status or goals are not describing strategies. At the other extreme it is not always necessary to define current status or final objectives if only general strategies are derived, although not to do so may lead to serious problems.

6. *Degree of risk you are willing to take.* The degree of risk that an organization takes is based on the opinion of its most senior managers as well as the culture and traditions of the groups involved. The risk is manifested by (1) the clinical indication(s) chosen for study, (2) the therapeutic areas in which one chooses to compete, (3) the type of patient population chosen for study, (4) the standards of clinical research adopted, and (5) whether a conservative approach is taken, whereby small steps are taken in the development process, or large steps are taken to reach the submission stage more rapidly.

TYPES OF OBJECTIVES AND GOALS

Goals are more specific targets than objectives. Goals may be quantified and time limits may be associated with them. Organization-wide goals are usually developed after objectives and are intended to help achieve the objectives. Goals usually are established to include measures of performance. Goals usually answer the question of "What" a group wants to get or be.

At lower levels in an organization the distinction between objectives and goals tends at first to blur and then to disappear altogether. One reason is that a general business philosophy and values, which are criti-

TABLE 113.1 *Example of general project goals*[a]

1. Submission of an IND, NDA, PLA, or other regulatory application[b]
2. Solve a current issue or problem
3. Support (or challenge) a current view, theory, hypothesis, or scientific model
4. Develop the characteristics and profile of a new medicine, medical device, or surgical procedure either in various populations or under various conditions
5. Evaluate the mechanism of action of a medicine
6. Evaluate the incidence of adverse reactions in a large patient population
7. Compare a new or established medicine with other standard medicines or other treatment modalities

[a] Two or more of these goals may exist for any project.
[b] IND, Investigational New Drug Application; NDA, New Drug Application; PLA, Product License Application.

TABLE 113.2 *Establishing specific scientific and clinical goals of a project*[a]

Goals may be to:

1. Improve patient compliance
2. Decrease dosing frequency
3. Increase duration of the therapeutic effect, especially with medicines having short half-lives
4. Avoid plasma peak concentrations and hopefully decrease toxicity
5. Avoid plasma trough levels that may lie below minimal therapeutic concentrations
6. Avoid first-pass effects

[a] The example used is that of a medicine delivery system that provides constant blood levels.

cally essential at the overall organizational level, are not necessarily important for each individual department. The department's overall mission tends to be seen in this context as a manifestation of their contribution toward the organization's objectives. Department goals that may be quantitated may be viewed as indistinguishable from their objectives.

In the rest of this chapter and book no distinction is made between objectives and goals. It is clear that such distinctions may be made, but they are not generally considered useful except as they relate to an overall organization.

Types of Project Goals

In the broadest context, development of a new medicine involves several types of goals. These include humanitarian (including medical), scientific, and commercial goals. In addition, goals may include discovery of a medicine, conduct of preclinical studies, and development of a medicine to the market. Within each of those general goals of the medicine discovery and development process, other goals are established [e.g., develop a clinical plan, prepare a New Drug Application (NDA) in an efficient manner and with a minimal amount of time]. Examples of general project goals are listed in Table 113.1, and a few specific goals that could be sought for a medicine that would provide delivery of a constant dose are listed in Table 113.2.

TYPES OF STRATEGIES

Deriving a useful strategy to achieve a goal requires knowledge of both the current status of the project and its therapeutic area, as well as the goal. Goals are generally more ambiguous and speculative than one's current position. If only the current status is considered, then the strategy created may lead in numerous directions, many of which would be tangents and not lead to the desired goals. If one focuses on only the past and the present status of a project, a direction may be created that will lead forward. However, without establishing a clear goal, the place one is headed toward may be uncertain or unknown.

Types of Overall Research and Development Strategies

Three examples of the type of information included in a research and development unit's general strategy are presented to illustrate the wide diversity possible in establishing even a single type of strategy:

1. Principles, philosophy, and values with which the unit operates to achieve its goals.
2. General and specific scientific and clinical approaches to develop medicines that result from the principles, philosophy, and values of the group. These approaches will theoretically be the same in future years as they are today. This definition does not depend heavily on the specific characteristics of current products and activities, but is a reflection of underlying approaches and methods to be followed.
3. Discussion of therapeutic areas of interest. To achieve corporate and research and development goals it may have been decided to concentrate efforts in certain therapeutic areas. There are other therapeutic areas that may be considered for development if certain circumstances (e.g., chemical leads) are present. There is a third group of therapeutic areas that are not to be considered as targets for various reasons (e.g., they lie outside the corporate "comfort zone"). Research efforts and projects must be targeted to the first two groups of therapeutic areas, and the identity of the third group should be discussed.

Examples of Overall Strategies for Specific Projects

It is important to have an overall strategy for each individual project. Agreement on an overall strategy for pursuing each individual project usually precedes discussion and agreement on the specific project strategies and tactics that enable the overall strategy to be achieved. Individual projects have a variety of overall strategies associated with them. Some specific examples of overall strategies for individual projects of new chemical entities (NCEs) include (1) focusing all efforts on the single indication and dosage form for which an NDA may be achieved most rapidly, (2) conducting Phase I and early Phase II clinical trials only and then licensing the medicine to another company, (3) choosing the most commercially rewarding indication as the initial target for the medicine's first NDA, (4) developing a combination product prior to the single entity, (5) initially developing the medicine for a specific patient population, and (6) screening many potential indications in early Phase II before targeting one (or more) for further development. The initial overall goal for these projects would generally be similar, namely, to reach the market in the shortest possible time with the best labeling possible and in the most cost-effective manner.

TABLE 113.3 *General purposes, durations, and levels of various types of strategies*

A. Purpose
 1. Global strategies[a] may be used to:
   Establish general types of mechanisms and procedures to be used
   Develop the values, philosophy, and approaches to be used
   Determine the specific projects to be pursued
 2. Operational strategies[b] may be used to:
   Solve a specific problem
   Address a specific issue
   Guide a specific project or multiple projects
   Conduct a single activity or multiple activities
B. Duration of an established strategy[c]
 1. Definite
   No revisions are anticipated
   Revisions required at fixed time intervals (e.g., monthly, yearly)
   Revisions required at variable times[d]
 2. Indefinite
   No revisions are anticipated
   Revisions required at fixed time intervals (e.g., monthly, yearly)
   Revisions required at variable times[d]
C. Line management level within the organization at which the strategy will operate
 1. Top managerial level (e.g., corporate-wide, university-wide)
 2. Multidepartmental within the same division or unit
 3. Single department
 4. Group or section within a department
 5. Single individual
D. Matrix level within the organization at which the strategy will operate
 1. Across different functional groups at the top of the corporation or university
 2. Across different departments within one or multiple divisions
 3. Across different groups or sections within a department or departments
 4. Among different individuals from different groups but working as a team
E. Level of activity[e]
 1. Activity within a department on one part of a medicine's development
 2. Activity within a department on an entire medicine's development
 3. Activity within multiple departments on a single medicine
 4. Activity within multiple departments on multiple medicines

[a] Global strategies provide a general approach that will be used to achieve the goals.
[b] Operational strategies provide the specific details required to achieve the goals.
[c] For both operational and global strategies.
[d] Criteria may or may not be established for determining when revisions are required.
[e] Selected examples only.

To carry out development of a new medicine that is to enter Phase I clinical trials and to adhere to an overall strategy, an entire series of other strategies must be created. Many of these will be oriented toward enabling the individual departments or groups to complete their part of the effort. A number of types of strategies are shown in Table 113.3.

Overall NDA or PLA Strategy

The overall NDA or Product License Application (PLA) is often initially articulated in a clinical feasibility report prepared by medical personnel, which is reviewed and accepted by senior managers. This report may indicate, for instance, (1) that the most rapid way to achieve an NDA is to develop indication A before indications B or C and to not explore indications D and E until after an NDA for indication A is submitted, (2) that patients who have certain disease characteristics (e.g., anatomical locations, severity, or classification) would be easier to enroll in clinical trials than other patients with the same disease, (3) that a specific formulation or dosage form might be preferable to develop first, or (4) that certain investigators should (or should not) be contacted for any of a variety of reasons. Numerous other factors could be explored that would be part of the detailed strategy to reach a successful NDA in the shortest possible time and still obtain acceptable medicine labeling.

Specific Strategy To Develop Each Indication and Dosage Form

A specific strategy could be prepared either for the entire period from initial testing in humans through

TABLE 113.4 *Factors to consider in choosing and prioritizing indications to pursue*

1. Scientific merit of the medicine
2. Medical value of the medicine
3. Commercial value of the medicine
4. Chance of regulatory success
5. Animal pharmacology
6. Indications of structurally similar medicines
7. Indications of medicines with similar animal pharmacology data
8. Time required to conduct the development program
9. Probability of success
10. Political and social risks
11. Costs of development
12. Availability of patients
13. Availability of investigators
14. Availability of people to develop the medicine in terms of their background, experience, number
15. Ease of measuring the clinical or other pertinent endpoints
16. Availability of alternative therapy (e.g., medicine, nonmedicine)
17. Special factors (e.g., orphan medicine designation)

TABLE 113.5 *Factors to consider in choosing and prioritizing dosage forms to pursue[a]*

1. Chronic versus acute treatment of a disease
2. Pharmacokinetics in animals
3. Stability of the various dosage forms
4. Availability and utilization of dosage forms on the market
5. Characteristics of the disease
6. Manufacturing issues
7. Commercial value
8. Cultural value

[a] The first dosage form(s) evaluated may only serve the purpose of ensuring efficacy (or absorption) and may not be put on the market.

NDA approval, or could be limited to the period between two project milestones. Alternatively, this type of strategy could focus on a specific time period, such as a few months, a year, or some other fixed period. Short-term strategies must be periodically updated, because they rapidly become outdated and obsolete. General purposes, durations, and levels of various types of strategies that may be used for projects are presented in Table 113.3. Factors to consider in choosing and prioritizing indications, dosage forms, claims to pursue, and patient populations to pursue are listed in Tables 113.4 to 113.6. Do not initiate clinical trials until all essential strategies are established.

Production and Marketing Strategies on a Project

Specific production and marketing strategies may be developed for relevant projects. Although production considerations usually become relevant only when a medicine reaches Phase III there may be specific production issues that should be discussed when a compound is first considered for project status, or even before this time, so that optimal input into a medicine's development may be achieved. This is particularly critical for biotechnology-derived products. Relevant production issues might relate to the lack of equipment or technology, the hazardous nature of the chemical synthesis, or problems associated with certain types of production. In practice, many medicine companies only seek production input during late Phase II or dur-

TABLE 113.6 *Factors to consider in choosing and prioritizing patient populations to pursue*

1. High-risk versus low-risk patients for having clinically significant sequelae
2. Patients with mild forms of a disease versus more severe forms
3. Age groups available and those targeted for marketing
4. Patients with concurrent diseases
5. Patients requiring treatment with concomitant medicines
6. Availability of patients for enrollment
7. Regulatory considerations for special populations (e.g., geriatrics, pediatrics)

ing Phase III after efficacy has been demonstrated, and an NDA is being planned or assembled.

The research-and-development-oriented strategies described in this chapter are generally intended for a project on an investigational medicine. Analogous overall and specific marketing and production strategies will also be developed for each investigational medicine. There are (or should be) clearly delineated marketing and production strategies for each marketed medicine. Marketing strategies may also be developed for early preclinical research programs or projects. A discussion of marketing strategies is presented in Chapter 129.

DEVELOPING A STRATEGY

Once the feasibility report is reviewed and accepted by management, the information included may generally be converted into a global operating strategy. The feasibility report usually includes information on the current status of knowledge in a field or on a known chemical compound and describes goals of the project. The means (i.e., strategy) of achieving these goals may be presented in general or specific terms. A number of formats that may be used to delineate and present strategies are shown in Table 113.7.

Overall Approach

The traditional means of developing a strategy starts with goals and then develops one or more alternative ways (i.e., strategies) to achieve those goals. If the goals relate to an entire corporation or large organization, rather than to a specific project or activity, then it may be relevant to start with the resources available and develop a strategy before establishing the goals. This approach was advocated by Hayes (1985). The author believes that this approach may be relevant for a large organization but is inappropriate for developing the strategy for a particular project.

TABLE 113.7 *Potential formats to delineate and present strategies*[a]

1. Algorithms
2. Flow charts
3. PERT[b] network, critical path method, precedence charts
4. Activity schedules of descriptions by department or group
5. Preset forms of questions to complete
6. Tables of activities to conduct
7. Grid charts
8. Prose—from short terse statements to expanded discussions
9. Gantt charts
10. Milestone charts
11. Critical path method

[a] See Chapter 124 for a discussion of most of these formats.
[b] PERT, Program Evaluation and Review Technique.

How Many Strategies Must Be Developed?

It is usually impossible to develop a single strategy to meet all of a project's needs. This is partly because of the great differences that exist in approaching short-term and long-term goals within a project. For example, one cannot develop a global strategy using the long-term ultimate goals to be achieved in several years and incorporate all short-term specific goals one hopes to achieve on a month-to-month (or other) basis. Multiple strategies are also necessary because many types of workers and managers at various hierarchical and functional levels will need different strategies to plan their work and to judge completed efforts.

When multiple goals exist it is important to determine whether they will be approached simultaneously through one strategy or whether each will require a separate strategy. It is usually possible to establish and clarify goals that can be pursued simultaneously. When there are also a series of goals to be approached sequentially, it may only initially be possible to develop a strategy that addresses the first or first few goals to be pursued.

Strategies exist at many hierarchical levels in an organization, and in many projects multiple strategies are operating at the same time. Some are general strategies, whereas others are extremely specific. Some relate to complex coordinating activities among many departments or groups, and others refer to activities conducted by a small cadre of people. Some strategies require a few days or weeks to complete, whereas others require years or are indefinite in length. Therefore, there are many "current positions" and "goals" to consider within any given project and these differ greatly from each other, depending on the nature of the particular strategy that is being developed.

How to Develop an Overall Strategy for Many Projects

Bottom-Up Approach

If an overall strategy is to be developed for all projects, it may evolve through "bottom-up" or "top-down" techniques. In the bottom-up approach, consideration is given to combining the desirable aspects and principles of individual project strategies. An attempt is made to discern what is common to most or all projects and to bring those aspects together.

Top-Down Approach

The top-down approach starts from an overall view of research and development goals and seeks to identify the specific project strategies that would best fit that overall approach. This overall strategy concept is then used as a model from which the individual strategies are derived. Certain elements of this overall strategy might be (1) to concentrate activities on a few (e.g., three to six) selected projects to reach the NDA or PLA submission stage most rapidly, (2) to spread resources thinly across many projects to increase the chances that some will reach an NDA or PLA stage, or (3) to focus attention on a single indication for each project so that an NDA or PLA for each project may be attained most rapidly.

Specific Approaches to Developing Strategies

The person or group responsible for developing strategies must initially determine:

1. The level(s) in the organization to be included in the activities or plans created
2. The duration of the strategy or strategies
3. The number and purpose of each of the strategies to be developed
4. The degree of specific details to be used

The next step in developing a strategy is to produce a clear statement and description of both current status and goals for the project or activity. It is sometimes impossible to define goals clearly. A general description of the area in which the goals exist or a clear direction to be followed may be used in such cases, and specific goals may be identified later. There may also be occasions when the current status of a project is not clear and cannot be well defined. In such situations a broad description of this area may suffice.

After these aspects are established the following approaches may be considered from the perspective of identifying specific strategies that will best address their objectives. Five types of approaches to developing strategies are briefly described (in no particular order):

1. *Backward approach.* In this approach it is necessary to focus initially on the goals and then develop strategies on the basis of their likelihood of achieving these goals. Activities may combine both intergroup (i.e., matrix) and intragroup (i.e., line management) aspects.
2. *Forward approach.* This approach focuses on the resources, current status, and interests of the group and creates strategies that allow those factors to be developed in the manner determined by the decision makers. This approach is more suited for some large companies than it is for a research department or other group that usually has clearcut goals.
3. *Line-function approach.* This approach limits strategies to those that lie within the purview of a specific function, department, or other group. It avoids considerations of matrix strategies.
4. *Matrix approach.* Developing a matrix strategy (or strategies) cuts across multiple units or groups within a company or research and development group.
5. *Key question approach.* Strategies are developed on the basis of how they fit key questions that are identified as focus points. A person or group assigned to each question could develop the specific strategies to answer or pursue that question. Examples of relevant questions could be:
   a. What therapeutic areas should be emphasized?
   b. What types of projects should the portfolio contain?
   c. How may projects be developed more efficiently?

A series of questions to address in developing a strategy on publications is shown in Table 113.8.

Different types of project, department, or even institutional strategies will require different approaches. These approaches are not mutually exclusive, as either the forward or backward approaches may be combined with either line-function or matrix approaches. After the strategies are created they must be tied in with other strategies that already exist. Selected elements that may be used to summarize a project's strategies are listed in Table 113.9.

A Few Pitfalls

One potential danger in developing strategies occurs when a single strategy document attempts to accom-

TABLE 113.8 *Questions to address in developing a strategy on publications*

1. How many publications are desired for each indication?
2. How many publications should have comparisons with specific medicines (e.g., market leaders, future market leaders, standard medicines)?
3. Which type of journals should be targeted (e.g., specialty, general)?
4. Which specific journals should be targeted?
5. Which articles have priority to prepare?
6. Should the sponsor's representatives or monitors be authors in addition to investigators?
7. Which investigators should be authors and in what order should their names appear?
8. Who should write the articles (e.g., sponsor, investigator, commissioned consultant)?
9. Which topics should be covered in publications (e.g., safety or efficacy in specific populations, mechanism of action, cost-effectiveness, quality of life)?
10. Which patient populations should be covered (e.g., pediatric, debilitated, renal-compromised, geriatric)?
11. Which advantages should be stressed to tie in with marketing plans? This question also relates to several of the choices made on preceding questions (e.g., to focus on renal-compromised patients).

TABLE 113.9 *Selected elements that may be included in a brief document summarizing a project's strategy*

A. Identification material
   1. Project name and medicine name
   2. Date of report
   3. Project code number
   4. Project leader or manager
B. Clinical synopsis[a]
   1. Specific indication or disease studied or to be studied
   2. Dosage form
   3. Status of each indication and dosage form (e.g., 1, U, P, F)[b]
   4. Next decision point for each type of clinical trial (e.g., efficacy, safety pharmacokinetic)[c]
   5. Date next decision point is expected for each trial being conducted. Identify protocol numbers and nature of the decision
   6. Other present or future activities of importance and estimated dates of completion
C. Operational strategies for each clinical indication[c]
D. Technical development issues and activities
   1. Present activities
      Analytical development
      Chemical development
      Pharmaceutical development
      Final formulation
      Stability studies
   2. Issues or problems
      Analytical development
      Chemical development
      Pharmaceutical development
      Final formulation
      Stability studies
   3. Comments
E. Toxicology
   1. Studies in progress
   2. Studies planned to start within 1 year
   3. Issues and problems
   4. Comments
F. Other relevant activities and issues

[a] The first five points may be used as headings for a table, to present the data.
[b] 1, Primary indications or dosage form studied; U, trial (or trials) underway; P, trial (or trials) planned to start within 1 year; F, future trial (or trials) planned to start after 1 year.
[c] A one- to three-sentence synopsis is given for each indication listed.

plish too many different functions, which could create confusion in the minds of those who must use these documents to plan their activities. Consideration of multiple levels or multiple time frames within a single document may lead to confusion. Mixing principles, values, current status, and goals with strategies is common and often hinders, rather than facilitates, communications. Another common problem is to identify a goal that is not the most appropriate one and thus to initiate activities in pursuit of secondary or inappropriate goals. Examples of poorly conceived strategies are shown in Table 113.10.

Evaluating the Initial Strategies Proposed

While strategies are being developed (or after a draft is completed) it is necessary to ensure that they make sense. This is achieved through various analyses. The analyses should demonstrate that the proposed strategies are both realistic and have a reasonable probability of achieving the intended goals. Either before or after the strategies and analyses are accepted by managers, methods of implementation must be established. The proposed means may include simple or highly complex methods whereby everyone necessary is informed about the strategies and understands their roles in the implementation process.

In critiquing a proposed strategy the first step is to ensure that both the current status and the goals are clearly defined and appropriate for the basic purposes. Then the strategy must be evaluated as to how effectively and efficiently it will allow and facilitate progress toward the goals. Next, evaluate whether any relevant problems or issues have been overlooked and determine if there are unanswered questions. Several different strategies should usually be developed on any one project to (1) expedite decision making by project leaders, (2) allow for delegation of responsibilities, (3) facilitate management review, and (4) achieve an overall uniformity in approach.

Monitoring and Periodically Reviewing a Strategy

It is important to have a mechanism for periodically reviewing and updating strategies. This process may be conducted at fixed intervals or on an as-needed basis. Although neither approach is *a priori* preferable, it is useful to consider the question of periodic reviews and revisions at the outset of a project. It is also im-

TABLE 113.10 *Examples of poorly conceived clinical strategies*

1. Evaluating three or four indications in a mediocre way rather than one indication well
2. Evaluating three or four indications in a slower way because of limited resources rather than the most important indication more rapidly
3. Choosing a dose for testing a medicine in Phase II clinical trials based on animal data rather than on dose-ranging trials in humans that establish the top of the dose–response relationship
4. Collecting small amounts of data at many doses hoping to attain regulatory approval for a dose range, rather than focusing on two or three doses
5. Developing a sustained release form without specifically identifying which patients are being targeted and why
6. Developing a large capsule or tablet for young children that will pose problems in swallowing
7. Choosing between two highly different chemical compounds for the same important disease, based on animal data, rather than studying both compounds in humans
8. If a medicine has an extremely long half-life, waiting 4 to 8 weeks between subsequent doses in the first Phase I clinical trial rather than dosing different groups of volunteers or patients at more frequent intervals

portant to determine the number and nature of different strategies that will be helpful to use in a project. These strategies should be developed in the early stages of a project's life to facilitate their acceptance and increase their usefulness.

One of the major purposes of a strategy is as a monitoring tool to assist an individual, group, department, or larger unit to adhere to a preset course. When the person or group deviates from the agreed-on course, the strategy should serve to raise a warning flag. Alternatively, the deviation may indicate that the strategy itself has to be modified to incorporate the implications of the new information that has made the departure necessary.

CHAPTER 114

Elements of a Clinical Strategy

One of the major determinants for developing a medicine successfully involves the quality of the clinical strategy created. After identifying a compound or medicine to be developed and marketed, it is important to determine the clinical strategy that will be followed. This strategy may be as simple as deciding that "we will develop an oral form of the medicine for indication X." With a simple clinical strategy, the sponsor may plan and initiate clinical trials on a one-by-one basis and hope that the trials will eventually lead to a regulatory submission. A more modern approach, however, is for sponsors to prepare a carefully conceived and detailed clinical strategy and development plan at the outset of a project, and to review and update it at periodic intervals. Nonclinical strategies (e.g., marketing, production, technical development) are eventually developed and hopefully integrated with the clinical approach.

CLINICAL DEVELOPMENT PLAN

A clinical development plan is the blueprint by which the overall clinical strategy is to be implemented and achieved. A poorly conceived or simplistic development plan is similar to using an incomplete and illogical blueprint to help create a large and complex building. Many people will provide conflicting advice and suggestions to the builders and the structure created may not suit anyone. It is far better for the builder to have a detailed plan, even if it only takes him or her to the first milestone, at which time an additional plan can be created.

This chapter describes specific factors that make up a general clinical strategy and enable one to create a clinical development plan. The following chapter describes the methods to follow in designing a clinical development plan.

CLINICAL STRATEGIES

Examples of a general clinical strategy include the following:

1. Develop the medicine for indications A and B, rather than C, D, or E. If clinical activity cannot be demonstrated for indications A or B, then evaluate (or do not evaluate) indications C, D, or E.
2. Develop the medicine in country A first, and in countries B and C at a later date, after efficacy has been established in well-controlled clinical trials.
3. Develop medicine A at a slower rate than medicines B and C until efficacy is established. At that point raise the priority of medicine A within the company and accelerate its development.
4. Develop the medicine only at site A until efficacy is established. Then have another development site of the same company begin development activities.
5. Develop the medicine to Phase I completion in country A and compare data with a similar medicine developed to that stage by another site of the company in country B. Then choose one of the medicines for further development by both sites.
6. Develop the medicine through Phase I (or Phases II or III) and then license it to another company.
7. Develop the medicine slowly until a patent infringement suit is settled. If the outcome is favorable, then accelerate development.
8. Utilize regulations that allow breakthrough medicines to condense Phase II clinical trials and avoid Phase III trials altogether.

Two or more of the factors identified in these examples could be combined into a more detailed clinical strategy. Nonetheless, a single factor is sometimes of paramount importance in determining the overall strategy conceived. Each factor's importance in the general strategy differs.

It is often desirable to develop a clinical strategy for each group of clinical trials with a common indication, common target population (e.g., pediatrics), or other common goal.

PHASES AND SUBPHASES OF MEDICINE DEVELOPMENT

The elements of a clinical strategy described in Table 114.1 subdivide Phases II and III clinical trials into a and b categories. All phases of medicine development are briefly defined in the terminology section at the front of this book. Definitions are based both on the function of trials conducted, as well as their relative timing, although the former is more important.

With the exception of the very first Phase I clinical trial on a new medicine, all other trials conducted in Phases I to IIIb may evaluate a marketed or unmarketed medicine (Table 114.1). A single medicine is often studied in multiple development phases at the

TABLE 114.1 *Phases when various elements of a clinical strategy are evaluated[a]*

Specific element of a clinical strategy to evaluate or identify	Phase(s) when usually evaluated
1. Dose that has an adequate safety profile	I, IIa, b, IIIa
2. Dose that elicits a sufficient magnitude and quality of efficacy	IIa, b
3. Dosage regimen (e.g., b.i.d., q.i.d., q.h.s., q.o.d.)	I, IIa
4. Dosage schedule (e.g., for anticancer agents)	IIa, b, IIIa
5. Loading and maintenance doses	IIa, b, IIIa
6. Duration of treatment necessary for short episodes or to obtain adequate labeling for chronic therapy	IIa, b, IIIa
7. Dose ascension schedule that is slow enough to avoid excessive adverse reactions and rapid enough to yield a therapeutic effect as soon as possible	IIa, b, IIIa
8. Schedule to wean patients off medicine (e.g., preventing a sharp rebound of disease symptoms, preventing withdrawal symptoms)	IIb, IIIa, b
9. Overall medicine safety and the therapeutic ratio; consider all safety and efficacy data	I through IV
10. Goals for long-term data required for regulatory submissions (e.g., 100 patients treated for 1 year)	IIa, b, IIIa
11. Appropriate efficacy parameters to measure	I, IIa
12. Definition of a responder (i.e., identify the difference between clinical significance and statistical significance)	I, IIa
13. Should quality of life studies be conducted? If so what factors should be evaluated and at what phase?	IIIa, b, IV
14. Disease type or subtype for which the medicine is particularly effective or ineffective	IIa to IIIb
15. Medicine interactions (e.g., with other medicines, food, environmental factors, other treatments)	IIa, b
16. Controlled trial(s) (e.g., use of placebo, active medicine, no treatment, or dose response)	IIa, b, IIIa
17. Number of patients necessary for an NDA (PLA)[b]	IIa, b
18. Various other studies conducted to answer safety, efficacy, or other questions raised by any of the above studies	I to IV
19. Comparisons with standard medicines	IIb to IV
20. Evaluation in special populations (e.g., elderly, renal impaired)	IIIa
21. Absorption of the medicine	I
22. Metabolism of the medicine	I
23. Elimination of the medicine	I
24. Pharmacokinetic comparison of two or more formulations of one or more dosage forms	IIIa
26. Cost-effectiveness and other economic studies	IIIb, IV

[a] Points 1 to 8 relate to dosing issues. Points 21 to 24 are conducted throughout Phases I, IIa, b, and IIIa, although they are considered as part of Phase I.

[b] NDA, New Drug Application; PLA, Product License Application.

same time. This may occur when a phase is initiated before a prior one concludes or because several types of trials are being conducted simultaneously.

May a Single Clinical Trial Be Part of Two Phases of Development?

Finally, some clinical trials are really part of both Phases I and II, or Phases II and III (Table 114.1). An example of a Phase I and II trial would be the very first trial of a new dermatological medicine that was being tested topically on patients with the disease to be treated. Both safety and efficacy parameters would be studied. An example of a combined Phase II and III trial would be an extremely large trial that provided more patients than needed to demonstrate efficacy in a well-controlled trial. The large number of patients would be enrolled at the request of the sponsor to acquire data needed for Phase III.

ELEMENTS OF A CLINICAL STRATEGY CREATED PRIOR TO INITIATION OF CLINICAL TRIALS

A clinical strategy is generally developed from 6 to 18 months prior to initiation of clinical trials. The identity of the person or group that has responsibility for creating or proposing the clinical strategy should be clear. Likewise, each of the reviewers and groups who must approve the strategy should be known. Specific steps used to review the strategy relate to a sponsor's standard operating procedures and are not discussed. Nonetheless, prior to developing a detailed clinical strategy, senior research and development managers should discuss and agree on general elements of the strategy with appropriate medical staff. This process would prevent staff from developing a strategy and development plan that were not consistent with views of senior managers. These elements of a clinical strategy include the following.

Indications To Be Pursued

Determination of the initial indication or all indications to be pursued is included in this category. The simultaneous or sequential order in which each indication of interest will be studied is proposed. One indication is usually identified as primary (or major) and the others as secondary (or minor). The milestone or stage of the primary indication's development (e.g., end of Phase IIb, end of Phase IIIa) is identified when the evaluation of secondary indications is initiated. Even if the identities of secondary indications are initially unknown or uncertain, the earliest stage at which their

development may be considered should be determined. The guiding principle is that it is always better to evaluate one indication well than several indications in a mediocre way.

Dosage Forms To Be Developed

Specific dosage forms to be developed should be identified. This includes choices among numerous dosage forms such as solutions for intravenous use, capsules for oral use, and ointments for topical use. As above, the order and timing should be established (if possible) for evaluating each dosage form. Two or even more dosage forms may be developed simultaneously from the outset of the project.

Patient Population To Be Studied

The choice of patient population(s) to be studied is heavily influenced by the indication(s) pursued. Other factors that must also be considered include severity of patient illness, patient availability, and the ability to measure validated and appropriate efficacy endpoints. A medicine may be targeted for initial evaluation in patients with severe, mild, or a broad range of disease severity. A company that desires to study their medicine's efficacy in responsive patients may have problems with investigators who wish to enter and treat their most resistant patients in the sponsor's trial. Regulatory pressure may force the sponsor to use a specific population of patients (e.g., for disease modifying antiarthritis medicines, a regulatory agency may require that only patients with severe disease who have failed previous treatment with two disease-modifying medicines be studied in the initial clinical trials). Regulatory authorities, investigators' sponsors, and ethics committees often have differing views on this and many related issues.

International Plan To Be Followed

The international plan should be discussed even if no firm decisions are reached at this early point in the medicine's development. The discussion may be as simple as stating that country A will conduct all clinical trials and that country B will eventually use some or all data from country A (along with marketing studies to be conducted later) to submit regulatory submissions. See Chapter 121.

Regulatory Strategy To Be Pursued

This includes the order in which regulatory submissions are to be submitted and the contents of each submission. A decision should be reached on whether a core package of clinical trials will be used and, if so, what its contents will include. The extent to which local medical studies prior to medicine registration will be permitted in each country is another factor to consider.

Companies differ in the extent to which they want to anticipate and address regulatory questions about their applications prior to submission. Although some companies attempt to anticipate and address *all* regulatory concerns, this goal may never be achieved. There are always large numbers of new tests and additional details that may be requested *or* required by regulatory authorities. It is unreasonable for a sponsor to try and anticipate all regulatory questions. A few companies may try and cut many corners and do substantially less work than they believe may be required or requested for marketing authorization. This strategy often backfires and leads to regulatory delays that may be longer than the time initially required to do the work. Finally, regulatory dossiers should be submitted to most (if not all) registration authorities at about the same time, to avoid the necessity for time-consuming updates.

Magnitude of the Plan To Be Implemented

Both the number and size of trials to be conducted should be considered. Although the overall magnitude is illustrated in the clinical development plan, a general strategic approach should initially be discussed and adopted. This is usually influenced by the company's traditions, degree of competition, regulatory experiences, and risk-taking or risk-aversion behavior of senior managers. Specific characteristics and issues revolving around a fat versus a lean plan are discussed later.

Practical Issues To Be Considered

Practical issues include organizing a project team to carry out the medicine's development, organizing an efficient system of coordinating efforts of many different groups, and ensuring adequate medicine synthesis and supplies. Resources required to complete the strategy successfully must be determined. These are important factors to deal with and although they are not literally part of a clinical strategy they may exert a great influence on which specific strategy is chosen, and whether it is successful. Finally, the key people for major roles should be identified if they have not been previously named.

Other elements of a clinical strategy—the ones usually created or modified during the conduct of a trial—are described in the next section. Nonetheless, those

elements may also be discussed prior to the initiation of clinical trials.

The overall clinical strategy created may be described in terms of the various visual models of medicine development as shown in Fig. 115.4. An advantage of using a visual model is that it helps ensure that relevant people view the project in the same way. This helps prevent individuals from pursuing unauthorized tangents, improves efficiency, and expedites the review process. Using one of these models also facilitates creation of the clinical development plan.

ELEMENTS OF A CLINICAL STRATEGY CREATED OR MODIFIED DURING THE CONDUCT OF CLINICAL TRIALS

Each of the general elements described in the preceding section must be reviewed and updated throughout the course of a medicine's development. The project leader and review committees must pay particular attention to ensure that unauthorized tangents are not pursued.

Most specific elements mentioned below may be evaluated during any phase of development, but it is usually most appropriate and convenient to evaluate them during particular phases. Trying to force an exception (e.g., conducting efficacy evaluations in Phase I) is often inappropriate and likely to cause problems. The timing for evaluating these elements for most medicines fits the pattern shown, although exceptions exist. Whether the timing slides forward or backward for evaluating any one element depends on the nature and priority of the medicine plus the company's policies and circumstances.

FACTORS THAT INFLUENCE CLINICAL STRATEGIES AND DEVELOPMENT PLANS

Degree of Risk the Sponsor Is Willing To Take

The degree of risk taken with a medicine varies widely and is predominately a reflection of the personality of the most senior research and development manager, as influenced by advisors, supervisors, and company traditions. Risk refers specifically to whether all possible and logical clinical trials are conducted (a highly conservative style), some trials are skipped to gain a more rapid appraisal of a medicine's profile, or most possible trials are omitted. The latter approach takes the risk that all of the essential questions may not be answered and that it will be necessary to redo some trials or conduct others.

Another type of risk refers to medicines that have a small probability of being effective (or safe). Companies that develop those medicines usually believe that the commercial potential justifies the small chance for success.

Degree of Speed Required

The degree of speed that is *possible* to achieve in a medicine's development is quite different from the degree of speed *required,* because of competition, patent expiration, financial problems, or other issues. The most critical point to stress is that an emphasis on speed must never be allowed to affect sound judgment about which steps must be taken in a medicine's development, their appropriate rate, and which clinical trials or activities cannot be abbreviated.

Overall Medicine Development Strategy

Overall strategy is often the most important factor that influences the choice of specific elements of the clinical strategy. The overall clinical development strategy may be similar to or quite different from the overall medicine development strategy. For example, a clinical strategy might be to use only case reports to achieve an NDA or to follow a laser approach to attain the medicine's registration. The overall strategy for this same medicine might be to develop a bioengineered product that would utilize available production facilities.

Magnitude of the Clinical Development Plan (i.e., Fat versus Lean)

Characteristics that make a clinical development plan fat or lean are the number of (1) indications, (2) patient populations, (3) dosage forms, (4) routes of administration, (5) dosing schedules, (6) medicine interaction trials, (7) pharmacokinetic trials, (8) mechanism-of-action trials, (9) marketing trials, and (10) other trials conducted. The number of patients in each specific trial also influences whether a clinical development plan is fat or lean.

Some sponsors attempt to obtain regulatory approval for a Product License Application (PLA) with a minimum amount of clinical data (i.e., a lean plan), whereas others go to the opposite extreme (i.e., a fat plan). This factor should be reviewed and controlled prior to initiating clinical trials. Data obtained as a result of a fat plan take much longer to process, analyze, interpret, and write up. This may be a major problem if a competitor uses a lean plan and submits a PLA earlier. A plan that is too lean, however, may backfire and not achieve PLA approval. Additional trials may be required.

A clinical development plan may also be fat or lean in another sense than the number and scope of trials included. This refers to the amount of data collected on each patient entered in a clinical trial. Quantities of data obtained in similar trials may vary widely, depending on the experience and goals of those who prepare the protocols and data collection forms. Therefore, a fat clinical development plan may collect a lean amount of data from each trial and vice versa.

Amount of Forethought, Consensus Building, and Discussion Required Prior to Proceeding with a Development Plan

The amount of previous planning depends on the judgment and style of the group that is determining which clinical strategy and medicine development choices to make. The need for consensus building when undertaking development of a new medicine can vary widely. This aspect must be considered by senior research and development executives prior to launching a new project that may engender resistance and be counterproductive to the company's interests.

Degree of Insistence That Each Step in a Clinical Plan Be 100% Complete Before Proceeding to the Next Step

The degree of completion of each step is related to the amount of speed needed for a particular project, the amount of risk a sponsor is willing to take with a specific project, and the personalities of key managers. Virtually all managers believe that they personally reach the appropriate balance in this regard, but it is apparent that there is a wide range of possible decisions about when to proceed to the next step. It is almost never appropriate, nor desirable, to study all aspects of each element. It is also necessary to make decisions about which aspects are not to be evaluated. For example, it may be possible to study a medicine regimen or schedule in which a medicine is given at X, Y, or Z dose q.i.d., b.i.d., q.d., by infusion, by bolus, once a week, twice a week, up to daily, for a certain number of cycles and then stopped for a period. Because of practical constraints only a few of the possible schedules may be tested in the clinic.

The Scientific and Clinical Standards Required by the Sponsor for Their Medicine Trials, Especially the Most Well-Controlled Ones

Although some readers may raise their eyebrows at the suggestion that different scientific (or clinical) standards exist for different sponsors, important differences do exist among clinicians and among sponsors in the standards they follow. Even a single sponsor or clinician applies different standards to the design and conduct of different protocols. For example, both the degree to which a clinical trial is controlled and the blind is ensured reflect the standards chosen. Standards for clinical trials are presented and discussed in Chapter 110.

Amount of Resources Required and Available

The amount of resources required by the sponsor to plan, initiate, and analyze studies should be determined. This is primarily expressed in terms of numbers of people at different levels necessary to develop the medicine, the duration of their participation, and external costs (i.e., grants) required to conduct the trials in the clinical development plan.

Trials That Compete for Resources at the Sponsor's and Investigator's Sites

Competition represents the "real world" factor. An ideal development strategy often may not be followed because of resource constraints, and the group must adopt a more realistic strategy. No matter how strongly one believes in and proposes a particular development plan, providing resources to a new project usually requires that they be taken away from other projects. The financial status of a company is one influence on the sponsor's ability to expand its current staffing level in response to pursuing new projects.

CHAPTER 115

Designing a Clinical Development Plan

A man was driving in rural Vermont to a town called Valdemeer. He came to a crossroads and the signs pointed in two directions to Valdemeer. At that moment he saw a house to the side of the road where an old man sat rocking on the front porch. The driver stopped, got out, walked up to the old man and asked "Does it make any difference which road I take to Valdemeer?" The old man turned to look at the driver, stopped his rocking, and slowly said, "Not to me it don't."

There are many paths of medicine development that a single medicine may follow. No one directing this effort should be in the position of this driver, who has to ask an unknown person with unknown expertise which road to take to reach his destination. The route should be charted in advance, at least to the next major milestone, at which time the next part of the route may be established. If the crossroads in the above story represents a major milestone, then a clear map to the town should be available or knowledgeable experts should be consulted to help plan the route. Even though it is often necessary to take detours, the same principles apply to revising the map and continuing toward the regulatory goal(s).

TYPES OF PROJECTS

In designing an overall project the initial step is to establish the type of project to be created. Common types of new projects include:

1. Development of a new chemical entity (NCE) from discovery of its biological activity, or from the time of licensing, to its marketing as a new medicine.
2. Development of a line extension for an already marketed medicine.
3. Development of a new indication for a marketed prescription medicine.
4. Conversion of a marketed medicine from prescription to nonprescription [i.e., over-the-counter (OTC)] status.
5. Development of a combination medicine.
6. Development of marketing-oriented evaluations (e.g., comparisons with standard therapies for efficacy, safety, quality of life, cost effectiveness).

There are many similarities among these six types of projects in the approaches followed to design, monitor, and manage the clinical trials. The similarities will be discussed in this chapter rather than concentrating on the many differences that also exist. Some considerations that apply to the different phases of medicine development will also be discussed. Combination medicines are specifically discussed in Chapter 50.

INITIAL STEPS

Choosing the Indication and Dosage Form

For projects involving medicines it is usually mandatory to identify the clinical indication and dosage form that will be the initial focus of activity. Once this goal is agreed on, a detailed clinical plan may often be drawn. If the project involves a therapeutic area in which the natures of most Phase I, II, and III clinical trials are well worked out and accepted, developing a clinical plan will be a relatively straightforward exercise. Even in this situation, however, various modifications will be required throughout the medicine's development. If the medicine is intended for use in a new therapeutic field or in a field that does not have clear guidelines and well-established clinical endpoints for medicine development (e.g., irritable bowel syndrome, senile dementia), it may be impossible to develop a detailed clinical plan for the entire develop-

ment process. Nonetheless, plans for a few initial studies and a general direction must be established.

Illustrating the Order of Steps/Tasks/Clinical Trials

There is no single best order of the many steps necessary for initiating and designing a project. A selected list is given in Table 115.1. Establishing a project plan generally follows the order shown in Fig. 115.1. Individual tasks may be illustrated with the type of bar chart shown in Fig. 115.2 or with the charts that show the interactions between various activities (see Chapter 124). Individual studies planned may also be illustrated with bar charts (Fig. 115.3). Concomitantly with the development of the project's plans it will be necessary to hold meetings at which the choice of specific steps and tasks are discussed. It is also possible to divide the clinical trials shown on this type of chart according to their phase of development. The hatched marks could also represent ongoing versus completed trials. Another possibility is to use shading of the bars

TABLE 115.1 *Initial activities conducted to establish a new project*

A. Establish an overview for the project
  1. Determine overall objectives
  2. Determine how strategies to accomplish overall objectives will be established, reviewed, and reestablished
  3. Develop an overall plan using networks and charts to document how the overall objectives will be accomplished
B. Activities related to project management
  1. Assess the relative priority of the project
  2. Assess the resources needed to accomplish the project's objectives
  3. Assess the resources available to the project
  4. Determine the major milestones and decision points
  5. Determine how progress will be monitored and status reported
C. Activities related to project personnel
  1. Choose the leader or manager of the project
  2. Determine which disciplines and departments should be involved
  3. Choose the members of the project team
  4. Determine workloads and responsibilities for each member
  5. Establish reporting methods to be followed
D. Activities related to progressing the medicine toward human trials
  1. Determine the preclinical studies that must be conducted
  2. Determine all reports that must be prepared prior to testing the medicine in humans
  3. Identify and evaluate actual or potential problems
  4. Determine quantities of medicine needed for the initial phases of development
E. Activities related to testing the medicine in humans
  1. Choose the indication(s) to pursue
  2. Choose the initial route(s) of administration to be developed
  3. Choose the initial dosage form to be developed
  4. Identify the initial clinical trials to be conducted
  5. Determine the type(s) of patients to include in the initial trials
  6. Choose the most relevant endpoints and parameters to measure

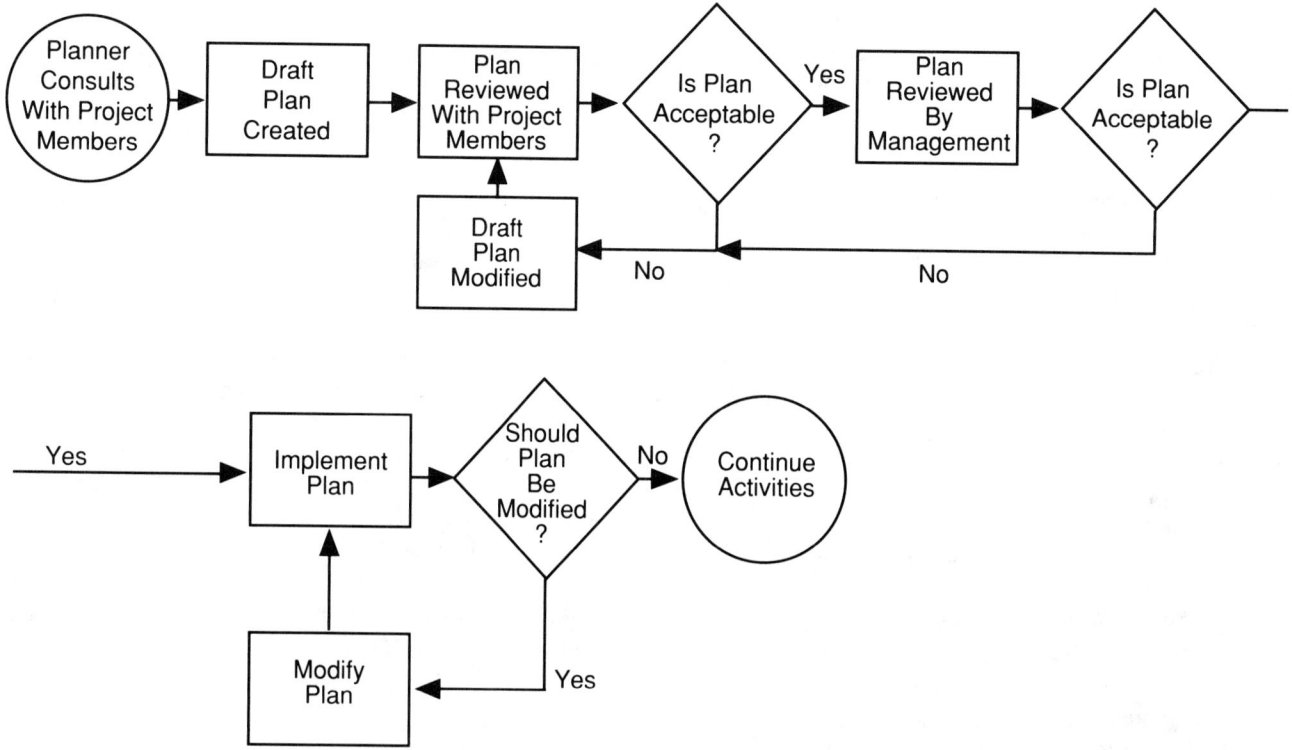

FIG. 115.1 Establishing a project plan to achieve certain objectives. General procedures for reviewing and approving a project plan. The modified plan may have to be reviewed by management prior to implementation.

Events in the Project (Task Description)	Months (Weeks) After Project Initiation												
	0[a]	2	4	6	8	10	12	14	16	18	20	22	24
Identify Relevant Literature		▭											
Acquire Relevant Literature			▭										
Review Existing Methodologies				▭									
Prepare Working Hypothesis				▭									
Prepare Monthly Reports	•	•	•	•	•	•	•	•	•	•	•	•	•
Hold Bimonthly Meetings		•		•		•		•		•		•	
Management Meetings			•			•			•			•	
Prepare Feasibility Report				▭									
Prepare Strategy Document					▭								

[a]0 date is set at the initiation of the project (e.g., January 15, 198 __).

FIG. 115.2 Selected tasks in a hypothetical project illustrated by a Gantt chart.

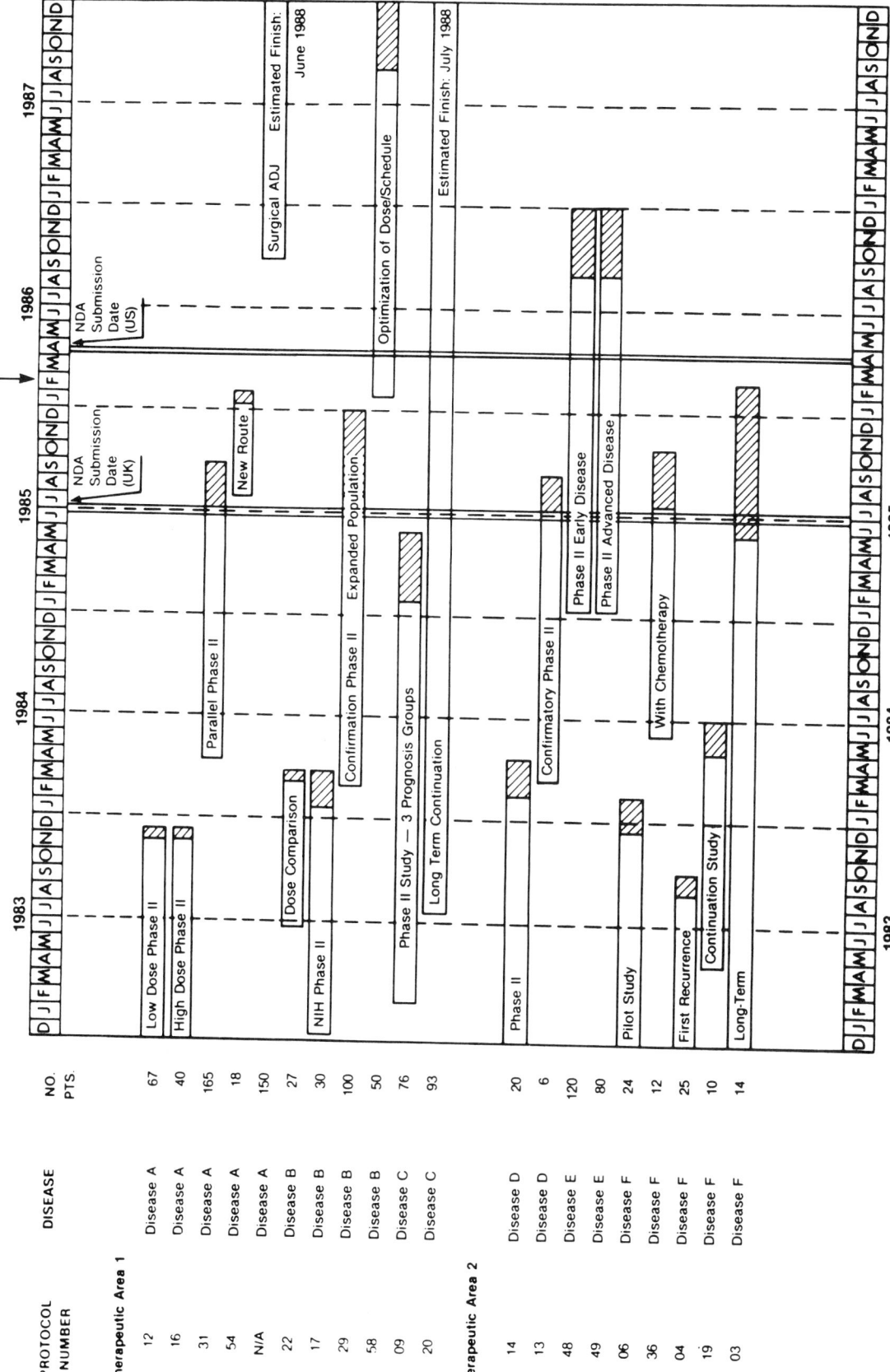

FIG. 115.3 A hypothetical bar chart illustrating the initiation and completion dates for numerous clinical trials on a single medicine. The hatched lines indicate the time required to process the data on the trial. Times required to prepare statistical and medical reports could also be illustrated with other types of hatches or marks. N/A, trial number not yet assigned; NDA, New Drug Application; NIH, National Institutes of Health. The letters at the top and bottom represent the months of the year. ADJ, adjuvant trial.

to indicate which are on the critical path of development.

Approaches

Establishing the overall goals of a project is essential at the start. The nature of the initial steps will be determined by the general framework of the organization sponsoring the project's development. There will be numerous organizational constraints within which the project leader or manager must operate to initiate and develop activities. Depending on the nature of the organization, more or less flexibility in approach or style may be permitted. Individual approaches to project activities are not permitted in some organizations and would probably not flourish, whereas in other institutions, individual solutions to designing and conducting project activities are actively sought and encouraged.

Technical Development

After the clinical direction of a project is established, certain aspects of technical development may be determined. The most basic aspect of technical development concerns the choice of dosage form(s) to be developed (e.g., parenteral, enteral). If the medicine is to be given orally, then the amount of medicine in each capsule (or other dosage form) must be determined. This determination is usually based on anticipated human doses to be used in the initial clinical trials. The fewest number of separate dosage strengths should be prepared because of the large amount of work and quantity of medicine required for each size. Based on the numbers of volunteers and patients in the first few trials, plus medicine requirements for toxicology and other preclinical trials, one or more orders for additional chemical synthesis will probably be necessary. Formulation development and stability testing will be initiated. Analytical development work to develop assays will be initiated based on known compounds, analogs, early chemical studies, and other data. Additional activities required to file an Investigational New Drug Application (IND) or to achieve the initial milestone in the project are similarly planned and scheduled.

Investigator's Brochure

One important activity involves the creation of an investigator's brochure. A sample table of contents is shown in Table 115.2. This brochure should be updated periodically with new data. Between revisions the new data may be indicated in the clinical protocol so that

TABLE 115.2 *Sample table of contents for an investigator's brochure*

1. Summary
2. Introduction (e.g., proprietary name, generic name, chemical name, salt, empirical formula, structural formula, type of medicine)
3. Chemistry (e.g., physical characteristics, PK_a, solubility in different solvents, stability under different conditions, assay method)
4. Pharmacology
   Primary activities (e.g., animal tests used, results)
   Secondary activities (e.g., animal tests used, results)
   Mechanism of action studies
   Effective dose range and duration of action
   Biochemical effects
   In vitro effects
   Other studies
5. Toxicology and experimental pathology[a]
   Acute studies (e.g., species, routes, results)
   Subacute studies (e.g., species, routes, doses, duration, results)
   Chronic studies (e.g., species, routes, doses, duration, results)
   Special studies (e.g., teratology, mutagenicity, reproduction)
6. Metabolism and pharmacokinetic studies[a]
   Animal data (e.g., absorption, distribution, metabolism, excretion)
   Human data (e.g., absorption, distribution, metabolism, excretion)
7. Clinical data[a]
   Diseases in which the medicine is being studied
   Rationale
   Safety profile
   Efficacy profile
8. Pharmaceutical results (e.g., pH, physicochemical compatibilities, stability, expiration date, packaging and storage requirements, dissolution data)
9. Regulatory history and status
10. Marketing status of other dosage forms
11. Basic information for clinical investigators[b]
12. Published literature and unpublished references

[a] Each section may be subdivided depending on type and amount of data available.
[b] May be written in the form of a package insert. This should include information on manifestations and treatment of overdosage.

it may be reviewed by the investigator and his or her Ethics Committee/Institutional Review Board (IRB).

Assembling Data for an Initial Regulatory Submission

Various activities required to assemble an IND are scheduled in a way that prioritizes certain steps which take place before others. If an individual is assigned the role of planner for the project, he or she helps organize and coordinate various activities with the project leader or manager. These activities are described further in Chapter 124. As one progresses from trial to trial there are numerous clinical aspects to modify. Some of these are shown in Table 115.3. A number of selected pitfalls to avoid in conducting clinical trials are listed in Table 115.4.

TABLE 115.3 *Selected aspects to modify or consider as one progresses from trial to trial within the same project*

1. Patient inclusion criteria
2. Duration of medicine exposure
3. Dosing regimens
4. Indications
5. Formulations
6. Initiation of continuation protocols
7. Compassionate plea protocols
8. New types of patient populations
9. Revision of estimates of patient entry rates

Golden Rule of Clinical Development

Possibly the single most important point to consider in designing the clinical development of a medicine is that it is better to have fewer clinical trials of higher quality than many trials of lesser quality.

Go/No-Go Decision Points

There are three different answers to the question of: How many go/no-go decision points exist in the process of developing a medicine?

The first answer is one. Toward the end of Phase II, when it is known that the medicine has sufficient activity to be developed for the market, a commitment to pursue development is usually made.

TABLE 115.4 *Selected pitfalls to avoid in conducting clinical trials*

1. Overestimating the number of suitable patients that are currently available or will in future be available to enter the clinical trial
2. Overestimating the rapidity with which patients can be entered
3. Underestimating the demands of the trial in terms of time requirements for (1) evaluating patients, (2) discussing patient's clinical status and requirements with staff, (3) completing data collection forms, or (4) performing other necessary administrative activities
4. Applying the inclusion criteria inappropriately and entering unsuitable patients, or entering patients before all of their laboratory data are returned
5. Failing to notify the sponsor or the Ethics Committee/Institutional Review Board (IRB) within 24 hours after a serious adverse reaction has occurred
6. Failing to notify the sponsor or the Ethics Committee/IRB about serious clinical events that are not believed by the investigator to be medicine related, but that could be trial related (e.g., suicide of a patient who was receiving placebo)
7. Paying inadequate attention to important details in the protocol for conducting the trial (e.g., how to modify doses after adverse reactions occur)
8. Failing to complete data collection forms adequately
9. Handing out bottles of medication or assigning patient numbers haphazardly, instead of following the randomization code. Patients are therefore not entered and randomized to treatment in the appropriate predetermined sequence
10. Underestimating time to prepare a clean data base

It is also possible to say that there are about seven such decision points, corresponding to each of the major milestones in a medicine's development. These include (1) establishment (or not) of a project, (2) submission of the IND, (3) completion of Phase I, (4) completion of Phase II, (5) data cutoff during Phase III, (6) submission of the NDA or Product License Application (PLA), and (7) regulatory approval of the medicine.

The last answer admits that issues can arise every day that influence a medicine's development and future. Each of these issues represents potential go/no-go situations. The most commonly used definition of go/no-go decisions is the second one.

CHOOSING THE APPROACH

In choosing an approach to be used in developing a medicine there are two major influences that are not discussed in this section. They are the nature of the medicine and the specific situation of the institution that will develop the drug.

Spectrum of Endpoints

The nature of the medicine has to do with whether objective clinical criteria or endpoints may be used to evaluate the medicine and reach a go/no-go decision during Phase II. Medicines such as diuretics or weight-reducing agents have clear clinical endpoints. If this type of endpoint is present then a highly focused approach may be initially followed. If the medicine is an anticancer agent or in a therapeutic area in which many disease targets may be affected, then it will often be advisable to evaluate the medicine in several different areas during Phase II clinical trials. Even during Phase I trials numerous approaches may be used to identify the maximally tolerated dose using various dosing regimens and schedules. If the endpoints are generally nonobjective, such as for antipsychotic medicines, then a different type of approach must be used, which emphasizes well-controlled trials.

Establishing the Basis of a Go/No-Go Decision

If criteria on which to base a go/no-go decision with regard to developing the medicine to a NDA status are not established before clinical trials begin, then there is more of a chance for personalities and nonscientific influences to affect this decision.

Types of Sites at Which to Conduct Trials

Pharmaceutical companies pursue Phases I to III evaluations of medicines at various types of sites and in a variety of ways. These can be generally summarized as utilizing a mixture of the following types of options:

1. Clinical facilities, owned and operated by the sponsor, that conduct clinical trials. These facilities are primarily, but not exclusively, used for Phase I trials.
2. Clinical facilities established by the sponsor in a hospital that may be part of a medical school. The hospital is often located near the sponsor, but some notable exceptions exist.
3. Some academic institutions have established clinical facilities that are used to conduct clinical trials. These trial sites are sometimes physically separated from the hospital wards. They may be reserved for faculty members and may be primarily oriented toward sponsored clinical trials.
4. Some departments within a medical school have established facilities that solicit sponsored trials as a source of training for the staff and students; these facilities also act as a source of revenue for the department, staff, and institution. These funds are sometimes directly applied to support other clinical trials that are of particular interest to the unit's staff or recipients of the funds.
5. Some contract organizations have established independent clinical facilities that pursue clinical trials as a business enterprise. The physicians who are part of these groups may or may not be associated with a nearby hospital to which patients may be brought if an emergency develops.
6. Some contract organizations have organized a network of hospitals in which clinical trials are conducted.
7. Some contract organizations have organized a network of private practitioners or group practices who are able to conduct clinical trials. The physicians may be located in one city, a particular region, or throughout the country.
8. Some contract organizations do not conduct any clinical trials themselves, but act as intermediaries to find a solution for the sponsor's needs, and attempt to place each trial where it may be successfully conducted.

Choosing the Sites at Which to Conduct Clinical Trials

In choosing among these options (and others), sponsors usually balance (1) consideration of expected quality of the trial, (2) control of the trial retained by the sponsor, (3) turnaround time to initiate and complete the trial, (4) costs, (5) reputation of the site(s), and (6) numerous other factors.

It is important that the priority assigned a given project at each development site be sufficient to com-

plete the work assigned. If that does not occur, then the international development will be seriously affected. Moreover, there may be stress within a group when one site expects the other to be doing much more than they are in fact doing. This may lead to conflicts of various types. A number of models that may be used to develop multiple medicines for a single indication are described in Table 115.5 along with a potential drawback of each.

Should a Sponsor Establish an Independent Phase I Unit?

It is a significant step for a company to establish an independent Phase I unit. This unit must have excellent staff and should be close to a population of potential volunteers. In Phase I clinical trials the major factors in most sponsors' deliberations on whether to establish an independent facility are control, cost, and anticipated turnaround time. When Phase I trials are conducted by physicians who are employees of the company the sponsor has more control on the timing of the trial and ordering of priority than for trials conducted by outside investigators. The costs and maintenance of the physical facilities, plus salaries of the staff and anticipated degree of use must be balanced against the expected convenience, added control, ease of utilizing other Phase I facilities, and costs of those trials.

TABLE 115.5 *Models for developing multiple medicines for a single indication*[a]

Name of Model	Approach	Potential problem
1. Separate site	Each medicine is studied at a different group of investigational sites	May have huge intersite differences
2. Simultaneous, with intrasite randomization	All medicines are studied at all sites. Patients are randomized within investigational sites	May have an insufficient number of patients at some sites
3. Simultaneous, with randomization among investigational sites	Medicines are randomized to different investigational sites for each clinical trial	May not test all medicines at all sites
4. Sequential	All medicines are studied at all investigational sites, but medicine A is studied before medicine B, etc. Some overlap is possible	Takes too long to complete the evaluation of all medicines

[a] These models are based on the premise that each medicine is being evaluated individually. When medicines are being studied in combination (e.g., in oncology) or by comparison with one another, various other permutations of these models may be described.

Potential Problems in Enrolling Students in Phase I Trials

A local college or university will not necessarily provide a reliable source of volunteers, because (1) the school may have rules that prohibit certain types of activities, (2) the unit may not be able to advertise in the school paper or post notices on bulletin boards, (3) there may be difficulty gaining access to students, or (4) students may have religious or philosophical views that do not allow them to volunteer for medicine trials. Moreover, students usually take long summer and mid-semester breaks that may adversely affect scheduling student participation of some important trials.

Phase II and III Trials

Phase II and III clinical trials are generally conducted through a variety of mechanisms (e.g., contractor organizations) at various types of institutions and with both narrow and broad patient populations. Although the majority of trials on most new medicines are conducted at teaching institutions, Phase III trials are often conducted at community hospitals (Begg et al., 1982) and at other facilities (e.g., nursing homes, private clinics).

Clinical Facilities Established by Sponsors

Clinical facilities that are established or financially supported by companies at hospitals have certain advantages over an independent unit that is entirely owned and operated by the sponsor. A unit at a hospital would be especially useful to a sponsor who did not have the volume of clinical trials to keep an independent company-owned unit operating at or near full capacity. Arrangements with the hospital could be established to allow trials by other sponsors or the hospital faculty to be conducted during slack periods. This unit could be located in a private community hospital or in a hospital that is part of a medical school.

VISUAL MODELS OF MEDICINE DEVELOPMENT

What Do These Models Describe?

A few simple models are described as a means of establishing a frame of reference for considering how medicine development changes within a project during the years it takes to proceed to an NDA. These approaches do not illustrate the quantity of work involved in moving from the project's initiation to an NDA. The magnitude of work required is almost always believed to multiply manyfold as a compound progresses toward an NDA. In some cases there appears to be more of a logarithmic, rather than an arithmetic, increase in the amount of work. Some people have described the increasing quantity of work as an inverted pyramid or a mushrooming effect.

The models refer primarily to the number of (1) different dosage forms (e.g., solution, capsule, tablet) that are studied, (2) different indications pursued, (3) different routes of administration being tested, and, to a lesser degree, (4) different formulations, (5) different claims for each indication, (6) patient populations, and (7) dosing regimens. These models are illustrated in Fig. 115.4 and refer primarily to Phases II and III of clinical development. These models may be used to include or to focus on technical development, toxicological, and other nonclinical activities. Consideration of Phase I clinical activities may sometimes be included in these figures. Hybrid and other models may also be described.

Choosing a Model

Some companies generally adopt one or more of these approaches. No company will be entirely representative of a single approach. Ideally, the model should be chosen to fit the medicine. Two of the major influences on the model chosen relate to the nature of the medicine being developed and the personality of the individual who has the major "say" or makes the final decision regarding the approach taken. At most pharmaceutical companies, this individual is usually the head of research and development.

Laser Approach

The laser approach targets a single dosage form and single disease indication at the initiation of the project. This target is pursued without expanding the clinical trials to other indications, formulations, or dosage forms until after the NDA is filed (or approved). In the purest form of the laser approach, a variety of dose schedules and patient populations are not necessary to evaluate. This type of project moves along a highly focused path. An intravenous neuromuscular blocking medicine is one type that could be developed using this approach.

Cone Approach

In the cone approach, a single dosage form, formulation, and target disease are initially evaluated. Gradually, as the compound progresses toward an NDA or PLA, more and more dosage forms, formulations, routes of administration, or indications are pursued.

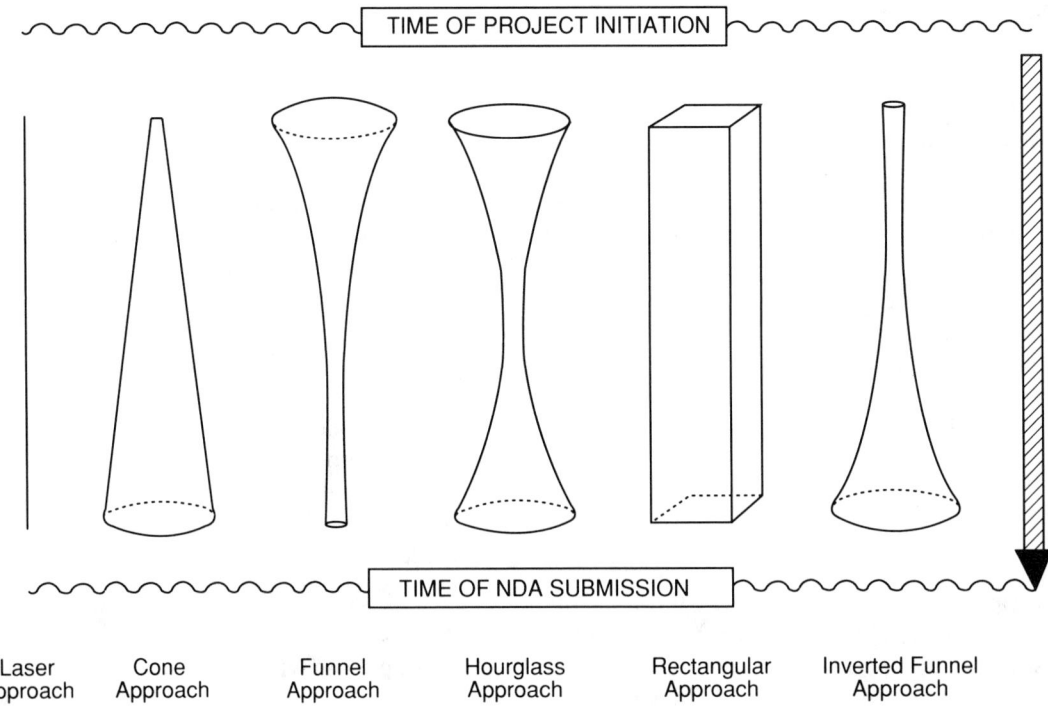

TIME OF PROJECT INITIATION

TIME OF NDA SUBMISSION

| Laser Approach | Cone Approach | Funnel Approach | Hourglass Approach | Rectangular Approach | Inverted Funnel Approach |

FIG. 115.4 Visual models of medicine development illustrating different types of approaches followed. See text for details. NDA, New Drug Application. The arrow represents time.

This is the most common approach followed in new medicine development. The pertinent question is whether this is the intended development plan or not.

Funnel Approach

After initial Phase I trials demonstrate that a medicine should enter Phase II, multiple indications are evaluated in the funnel approach. From the results of numerous trials, a single or small number of the more promising indications are chosen to be pursued. These are followed in well-controlled Phase II trials and Phase III evaluations. The size of the funnel's stem will vary, depending on how focused the activities are during later Phase II and Phase III.

Hourglass Approach

As in the situation above, multiple indications are focused to a small number in the hourglass approach. The number of activities are then gradually expanded in terms of additional dosage forms, formulations, dosage regimens, and patient populations as the project nears the NDA. The top part of the hourglass usually illustrates a focusing of indications, and the expanding lower part illustrates an increase of other aspects of the project (e.g., multiple dosing regimens, multiple dosage forms). Some anticancer medicines are devel-

oped using this approach. For such medicines the upper part of the hourglass usually represents types of cancers evaluated and the lower part represents different dosing schedules evaluated.

Rectangular Approach

The rectangular approach is a "broad-front" approach, whereby multiple dosage forms, indications, and routes of administration are followed throughout the life of a project. Whereas some of these will probably drop out, others may be added. A comparable image would be that of a cylinder. This approach is often used by companies that want to go "all out" on developing a particular medicine.

Inverted Funnel Approach

The inverted funnel approach gives a narrow focus for most of a project's life. Shortly before (or after) the NDA or PLA is submitted, the number of activities greatly increase. Other possible indications are pursued and other dosage forms or routes of administration may be studied. This approach is used to conserve resources until it is known that the NDA is going to be submitted within a short period. This represents a conservative use of resources.

A. Focused Approach (Ideal Plan)

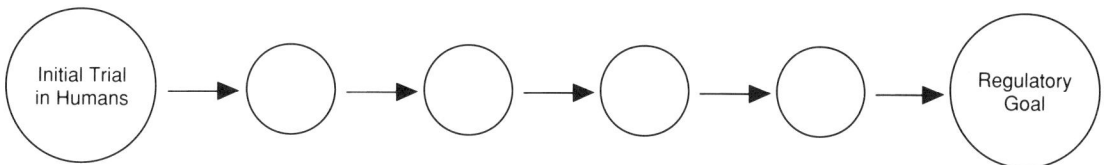

B. Focused Approach With Change of Goals (Usual Plan)

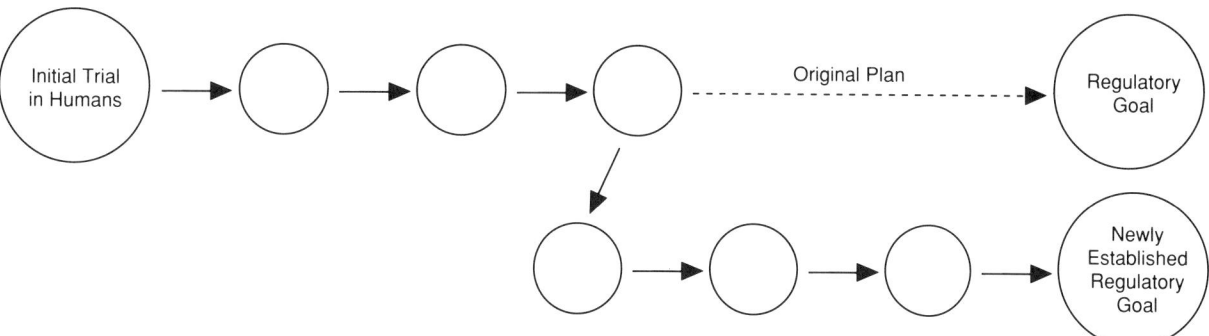

C. Nonsystematic Approach (Foolish Plan)

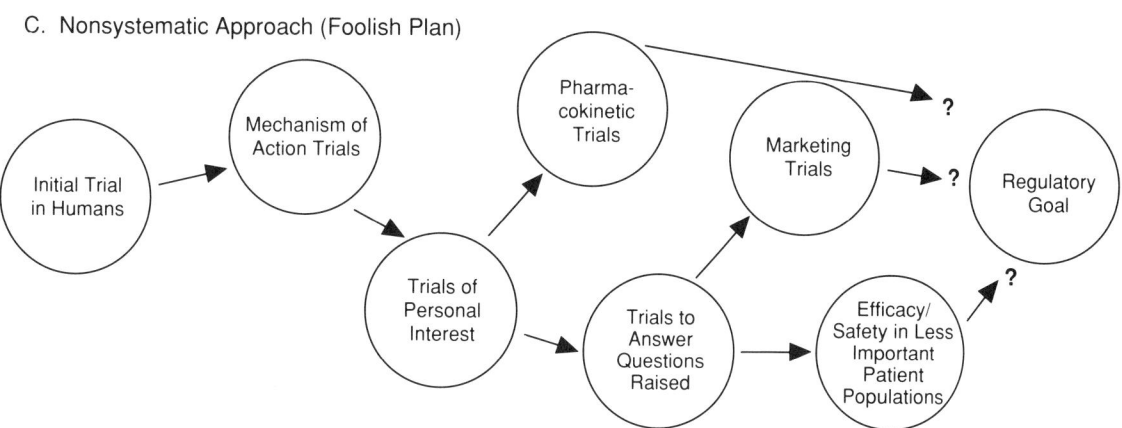

D. Nonfocused, Broad-Front Approach (Scattergun Plan)

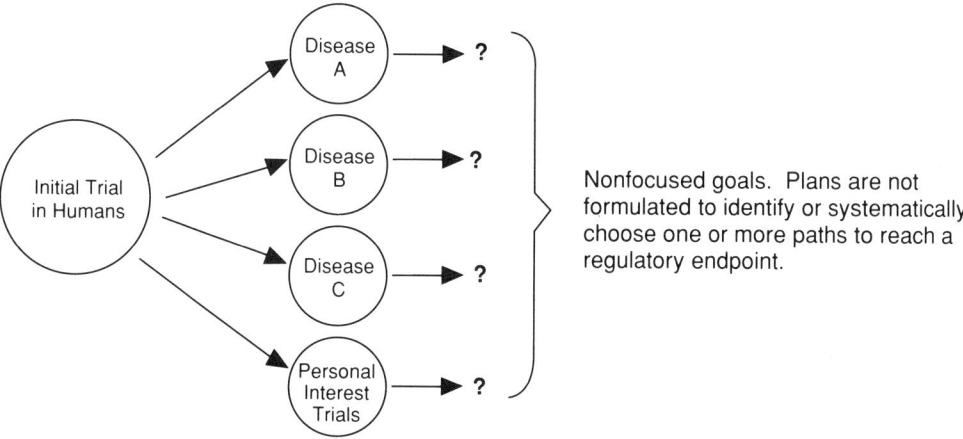

FIG. 115.5 Selected approaches to clinical medicine development. Goals are defined in terms of indications, formulations, patient populations, and other factors. (Reprinted from Spilker, 1989a, with permission of Raven Press.)

Shotgun Approach

To proceed from project initiation to an NDA or PLA requires planning, vision, persistence, and many other desirable attributes. When some of these characteristics are missing from a project team or management, the project may proceed in different directions either simultaneously or sequentially. When this occurs the project rarely succeeds. The difference between the shotgun approach and the funnel, hourglass, and rectangular approaches is that the latter three represent an organized approach to pursuing a project that builds continually in an effort to reach a goal. If the project's efforts are not constantly directed toward the goal, it is easy for a project's direction to wander.

It is often only in hindsight that a shotgun approach may be diagnosed. At the time that clinical trials are in progress the project may be presented to others on the team, or to management, in the guise of funnel, hourglass, or rectangular approaches.

Schematics

A few selected approaches to medicine development are illustrated in Fig. 115.5.

TANGENTS

Tangents are activities on a project that do not adhere to the general agreed-on approach. These activities may be purposely initiated to explore specific issues, questions, or therapeutic areas. As such, they may rep-

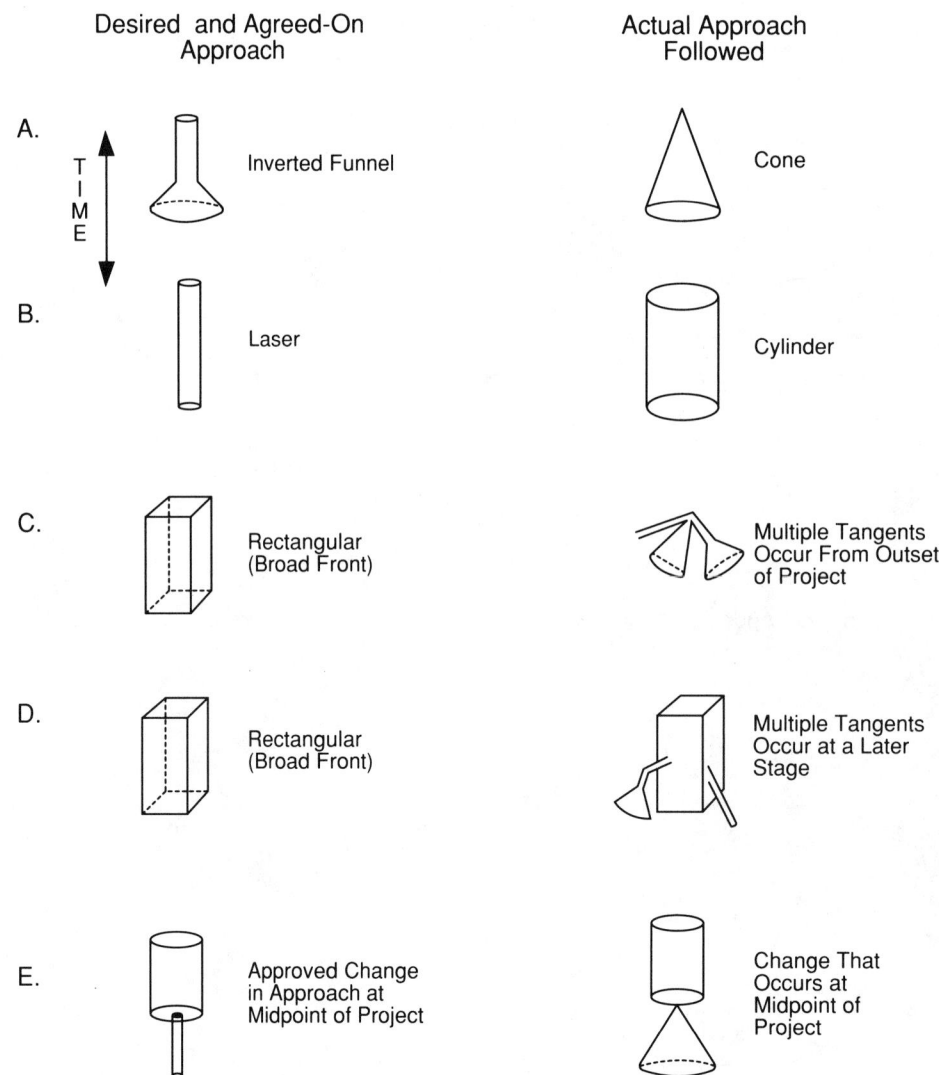

FIG. 115.6 Examples of negative tangents in a medicine's development. (Reprinted from Spilker, 1989a, with permission of Raven Press.)

A. Tangents occur one at a time. The direction and focus of the project keep changing.

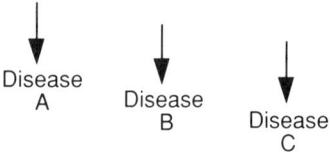

B. Multiple diseases targeted at the outset of a project to learn which approach is best.

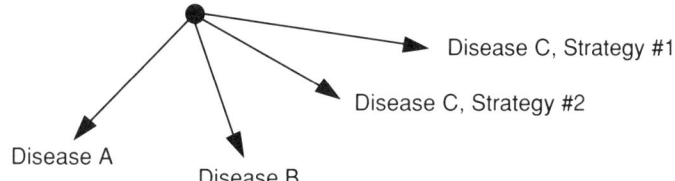

C. A combination of the above approaches is followed.

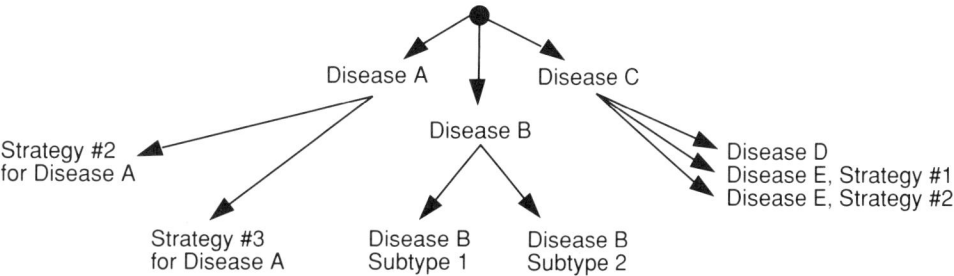

FIG. 115.7 Medicines in search of a disease. Each arrow differs in the amount of time, effort, and resources expended. Strategies may differ in terms of route of administration, dosage form, dosing schedule, or other factors. (Reprinted from Spilker, 1989a, with permission of Raven Press.)

resent or lead to modifications. Thus, a project that starts out following one of the diagrams shown in Fig. 115.4 may change and become one of the other approaches, or a hybrid approach may result (Figs. 115.6 and 115.7).

Avoiding Tangents

Tangents may also develop inadvertently or purposely, but without appropriate sanction. In either case it is the responsibility and one of the major roles of management to prevent or minimize the number and extent of tangents. Many individuals associated with a project will present "good reasons" for exploring an area or a question that is later diagnosed as going off on a tangent. The most effective means of preventing tangents is to question how the proposed clinical trial or activity will help achieve the project's goals. Hopefully, this question will be asked at the stage when the work is proposed and not after it has been initiated or completed.

Potential Danger of Tangents

It is rare for most projects to reach their goals without having explored a number of unplanned tangents. Many tangents offer the potential of valuable benefits that may improve the project. Nonetheless, if tangents become too commonplace in number or too extensive in size they may threaten progress on a project. Tangents require company resources and will diminish productive work that will help move a project toward its goals. Clearly a balance must be achieved among the interest, excitement, and creativity often associated with exploring tangents and work on the main thrust of a project. Management must determine which tangents to allow because most will not be successful and there are usually insufficient time and resources to try all possible tangents. Tangents that occur within a single clinical trial often represent protocol violations and are not discussed in this section. A more detailed discussion of tangents is presented in *Multinational Drug Companies: Issues in Drug Discovery and Development* (Spilker, 1989a).

CONSIDERATIONS FOR A CLINICAL PROGRAM IN PHASES I, II, AND III

Various factors that may decrease the time to proceed from the Investigational New Drug Application (IND) to the NDA are listed in Table 115.6. A number of suggested approaches to increasing the efficiency of clinical trials are presented in Table 115.7, and typical types of trials conducted in each phase of development are in Table 115.8. Finally, sources of scientific information to help in planning projects are given in Table 115.9. The definitions of the four phases of clinical development are given in the terminology section.

Different individuals or groups sometimes use other definitions, such as ones based entirely on the chronological order in which clinical trials are conducted. Using that approach, Phase I trials are the first clinical trials conducted on a new medicine. This is often an unsatisfactory definition, because later in a medicine's development program during Phases II or III it may be necessary to conduct additional Phase-I-type trials (e.g., to explore a higher medicine dose in normal volunteers), which should be referred to as Phase I. Another reason against using a chronological definition is that pharmacokinetic trials are often referred to as

TABLE 115.6 *Factors relating to clinical trials to consider in minimizing the interval between submitting an IND and NDA*[a]

1. Adopting a feasible clinical strategy
2. Developing a regulatory strategy and core clinical package by which each clinical trial serves an important purpose for the indication(s) that will be requested
3. Reviewing each strategy periodically and revising them appropriately
4. Utilizing appropriate staff and resources to carry out the clinical strategy
5. Utilizing appropriate trial designs to achieve trial objectives and overall objectives
6. Utilizing well-developed protocols that have a high likelihood of being successfully completed
7. Utilizing efficient investigators and staff who are highly motivated and have demonstrated their abilities
8. Ensuring rapid patient entry—insofar as possible
9. Utilizing a sufficient number of trial sites to achieve objectives
10. Conducting trials with adherence to high standards
11. Monitoring studies both at the trial site and sponsoring institution on an appropriate periodic basis, paying close attention to effective monitoring
12. Utilizing reasonable and effective project management systems to ensure efficient allocation and use of resources
13. Processing and analyzing data according to a plan developed prior to trial initiation
14. Conducting meetings with regulatory authorities to present data and plans and to solicit feedback on their responses to the clinical plan for medicine development
15. Developing a realistic and efficient plan to write and assemble the various parts of the NDA

[a] IND, Investigational New Drug Application; NDA, New Drug Application.

TABLE 115.7 *Means to increase efficient conduct of medicine trials*

1. Incorporate elements of proven value from earlier protocols
2. Eliminate problem areas encountered in conducting earlier protocols
3. Choose collaborators (or investigators) who have proved their reliability, dependability, cooperativeness, and overall ability
4. Include a research coordinator at the clinical trial site, especially for complex trials, whose primary or sole responsibility is to help conduct the trial
5. Establish both formal and informal systems that have been proved to be useful in initiating, conducting, and monitoring trials
6. Periodically review how different aspects of conducting a trial can be improved (e.g., follow-up of missed appointments can be handled with telephone calls and reminder cards)
7. Discuss problem areas with staff and colleagues to reach acceptable solutions
8. Discuss issues or problems with a consultant or panel of consultants
9. Determine which individuals have specific responsibilities

Phase I trials, although they are conducted throughout a project's three phases.

Phase I Trials

The types of clinical trials conducted during Phase I are listed in Table 115.8. These trials usually progress from single-dose trials to multiple-dose trials and include as much pharmacokinetic evaluation as appropriate.

Choosing an Upper Dosing Limit

The philosophy of attempting to identify a maximum tolerated dose is stressed, because it provides an upper limit to use in planning Phase II and III trials. Some individuals have questioned the ethics of this approach because it doses normal volunteers until at least moderately severe adverse reactions occur, and this may be at doses higher than those considered necessary to test for efficacy in Phase II trials. The counterargument is that an adequate degree of efficacy may not be observed at the expected doses in Phase II trials and it may be necessary to evaluate higher doses, which will not have been tested in normal volunteers. If that has to be done, then additional Phase I trials in normal volunteers must be considered. Moreover, Phase I testing is relatively safe and few volunteers who provided an honest medical history have ever been seriously injured (see Chapter 33 for references).

Pharmacokinetics

The pharmacokinetic program should be developed by experts in the area, but most specialized clinical trials

TABLE 115.8 *Typical types of clinical trials conducted on investigational medicines*[a]

A. Phase I
1. Single-dose tolerance trial in volunteers or patients who are exposed to a single dose of the medicine[b]
2. Multiple-dose trial in volunteers or patients. This typically lasts for 3 to 28 days. The subjects usually receive a fixed dose of medicine, although dose titration is sometimes permitted
3. Increasing the dose range of a new investigational medicine to define the upper limit of safety or to ensure safety when lower doses have failed to demonstrate activity in Phase II trials
4. Initial pharmacokinetic evaluations. These are often combined with, and conducted as part of, the above trials
5. Interactions of the medicine with food or other interventions in normal volunteers
6. Pharmacokinetic trials in normal or various patient populations (e.g., elderly, hepatic impaired) using unlabeled or radiolabeled medicine
7. Infusion trial to determine the maximally tolerated dose with different dosing regimens (e.g., varying the concentration or duration of the infusion)
8. Concentrations followed after the first oral dose to measure absorption and other pharmacokinetic parameters
9. Concentrations followed after a single intravenous dose to measure pharmacokinetic parameters
10. Evaluation of pharmacokinetic parameters after multiple doses (e.g., follow the disappearance of concentrations of the medicine in plasma after the Nth oral dose)
11. Evaluation of distribution, metabolism, and elimination in normal volunteers using radioactive or cold methods of analysis. An example of a specific elimination trial would be to evaluate biliary excretion
12. Bioequivalence trials to compare two or more formulations

B. Phase IIA[c]
1. Pilot trial (or trials) of a medicine in patients. These trials may be conducted in either an open-label or a single- or double-blind manner
2. Pilot trial (or trials) of a medicine in normal volunteers challenged to determine the efficacy of a medicine (e.g., castor oil may be used to cause diarrhea, citric acid may be used to produce cough, syrup of ipecac may be used to produce emesis)
3. Dose–response trial in patients to identify the range of active doses
4. Trials evaluating variations in dose level or dosing schedule
5. Initial pharmacokinetic trials in patients as opposed to volunteers, who are enrolled in most Phase I trials[d]
6. Dose ascension (or withdrawal) trial evaluating how rapidly doses may be escalated (or withdrawn) safely
7. Duration of dosing required to achieve a sufficient magnitude of efficacy
8. Dose-interval trial evaluating the time between doses

C. Phase IIB
1. Placebo-controlled double-blind trial (or trials) conducted at one or at multiple sites
2. Placebo-controlled and active-medicine controlled, double-blind trial (or trials) conducted at one or at multiple sites
3. Active-medicine controlled, double-blind trial (or trials) conducted at one or at multiple sites
4. Dose–response-controlled, double-blind trial (or trials) conducted at one or at multiple sites

5. Trials to focus on one or more aspects of Phase IIa
6. Trials to focus on issues raised in previous trials or on potential issues identified

D. Phase III
1. Open-label and both single- and double-blind trials of larger numbers of patients with fewer protocol exclusions than in Phase II
2. Humanitarian studies conducted in severely ill patients
3. Evaluation of potential new indications
4. Evaluation of new dosage forms
5. Evaluation of new formulations
6. Evaluation of new dosing regimens
7. Pharmacokinetic trials required for characterizing a medicine's activity
8. Large-scale open-label trials to obtain broad exposure in a wide variety of patients
9. Medicine interaction trials (e.g., with other medicines, food, alcohol)
10. Premarket surveillance studies to characterize the safety profile better
11. Marketing-oriented studies (e.g., comparisons with standard therapies)
12. Long-term trials to evaluate efficacy or safety
13. Quality of life trials
14. Cost-benefit, cost-effectiveness, and other pharmacoeconomic studies
15. Special efficacy trials (e.g., using different endpoints)
16. Clinical trials in special populations (e.g., geriatric, pediatric, liver failure, renal failure, heart disease, outpatients, inpatients)
17. Clinical trials in patients on concomitant medicines or with concomitant diseases
18. Different routes of administration
19. Mechanism-of-action trials
20. Special types of safety trials (e.g., hemodynamics, respiratory function)
21. Evaluation of a well-known toxicity of standard medicines and comparison with a new medicine
22. Clinical trials to evaluate how long patients remain symptom free after a medicine is withdrawn
23. Evaluate other subpopulations of patients with the major indication

E. Phase IV
1. Observational post-marketing surveillance studies of a medicine's use under usual conditions
2. Same as above using a case-control study design
3. Same as the first example for a special cohort of patients
4. Evaluation of a hypothesis (e.g., a medicine may cause a specific adverse reaction) using a large automated multipurpose data base
5. Clinical well-controlled randomized (or with other characteristics) prospective studies to evaluate one or more aspects of the medicine
6. Marketing-oriented studies
7. Quality of life trials
8. Cost-benefit, cost-effectiveness, and other pharmacoeconomic studies
9. Field trials
10. Community intervention studies
11. Monitoring of possible adverse events and reports received by companies and regulatory agencies and reported in the literature
12. Comparison of a brand name medicine with its generic "equivalents"

[a] The actual trials utilized to evaluate an investigational medicine depend on many factors, including the pharmacological nature and characteristics of the medicine, disease, and patients, plus ethical and commercial considerations.
[b] In some trials a second (or third, etc.) dose is given to the same volunteer a number of days or weeks later. A period of at least five half-lives is used between doses.
[c] Studies in Phases II and III may evaluate the medicine either as monotherapy or as add-on therapy.
[d] Pharmacokinetic trials are considered as Phase I trials by most individuals.

TABLE 115.9 *Sources of scientific information available to clinicians, scientists, and the public*

1. Computerized data bases of clinical and scientific data (e.g., Medlars, Medline, Toxline)
2. Computerized data bases of clinical and scientific reports
3. Computerized collections of data bases (e.g., Dialog)
4. Medicine information services (e.g., hospital based)
5. Poison control centers
6. Pharmaceutical companies
7. Trade associations (e.g., Pharmaceutical Manufacturer's Association, Association of the British Pharmaceutical Industry)
8. Professional associations
9. Disease-oriented societies (e.g., American Cancer Society, American Heart Association)
10. Medical societies (e.g., State Medical Society)
11. Under the Freedom of Information Act (e.g., companies such as FOI in Rockville, MD)
12. Foundations[a]
13. Professional colleagues, friends, and peers
14. Well-known experts in the area
15. Medical libraries at universities, institutions, and the National Library of Medicine
16. Various government agencies [e.g., National Institutes of Health (NIH), Food and Drug Administration (FDA), and the United States Department of Agriculture]

[a] See the *Foundation Directory* (10th edition, Foundation Center, New York, 1985) for an extensive listing of foundations.

are generally not conducted until after a medicine has demonstrated sufficient activity to warrant full clinical development. Many pharmacokinetic trials are thus conducted during the period when the medicine is being evaluated in late Phase II and throughout Phase III.

Patients versus Volunteers

Patients are evaluated instead of volunteers in Phase I clinical trials when:

1. The medicine is too toxic to test ethically in volunteers (e.g., many anticancer agents)
2. The expected therapeutic ratio is too narrow to test the medicine ethically in volunteers (e.g., antiarrhythmics)
3. It is believed that the therapeutic dose in patients will be greater than normal volunteers can tolerate (e.g., a neuroleptic)

Phase I clinical trials may enroll patients in addition to volunteers (although in separate trials if it is believed that patients may metabolize the medicine differently than normal volunteers. This is often the case in epileptic patient populations, because these patients are often receiving medicines that affect hepatic microsomal enzymes.

Two other possibilities are (1) to study patients with a serious disease who are in remission, or (2) to study those patients who do not have the specific concom-

itant illness that the new medicine is designed to treat. A good example of the latter situation occurred recently. The Food and Drug Administration (FDA) required a company to test a new chemical entity in acquired immunodeficiency syndrome (AIDS) patients without *Pneumocystis carinii* pneumonia (PCP), even though the medicine was intended to treat PCP in AIDS patients.

Phase II Trials

Pilot Efficacy Trials

Pilot efficacy trials should almost always be double blind, because open-label trials in all therapeutic areas studied yield far more false-positive results than do double-blind trials. This topic is discussed in Chapter 4.

Dose Range Evaluated: A Key Issue

A medicine's entire dose–response range should be evaluated. This issue refers back to the discussion about identifying the maximum tolerated dose in Phase I. Unless this is done, it often creates problems in deciding about the maximum dose that may be used in Phase II clinical trials. If this maximum tolerated dose is known, then Phase II dose-ranging trials may titrate patients up to this level, while evaluating both safety and efficacy. Because the maximum dose is known it is easier to identify the dose that achieves maximum efficacy with minimum adverse reactions. If Phase I dosing has only explored the range of doses predicted to be effective in Phase II, it is generally only possible in Phase II to evaluate those doses that were studied in Phase I. The major drawback of this approach is that an effective dose may be found and subsequently evaluated in many new trials, but that dose may be substantially lower than one that yields a greater degree of efficacy with minimal or no loss of safety. Thus, using a limited approach to exploring doses in Phase I may not lead to evaluating an important part of the dose–response relationship in Phase II. It is important in Phase II trials to evaluate the entire range of doses that may be used to treat patients. If a company has two research locations that approach this medicine development issue from different perspectives, then a different dosing regimen may eventually be recommended for marketing in different countries. This will not arise because of relevant differences (e.g., weights of patients, cultures, genetic differences), but because the two research groups each explored different parts of the dose–response relationship.

Patient Population

In choosing the patient population to evaluate it is essential to consider whether the risks of treatment are justifiable on the basis of the benefit-to-risk ratio, for all patients with the disease. It may be necessary to limit medicine exposure to those patients with either mild or severe forms of the disease.

Phase III Trials

Issues to Address

Major issues include (1) identifying the specific patient populations to evaluate, (2) whether to expand clinical trials to new indications, formulations, and routes of administration, (3) the numbers of patients to be included in a regulatory submission, (4) whether to initiate marketing studies and when they may be initiated, and (5) when to decrease the number of trials and increase the efforts spent on preparing a regulatory submission(s).

At some point during clinical development of a new medicine (or of a marketed medicine for a new indication), whether the medicine affects the natural history of the disease should be considered. If this has not been considered or evaluated in Phase II clinical trials, then it should be explored during Phase III. Unfortunately, little is known about the natural history of many diseases.

Where to Conduct Phase III Clinical Trials

There has been a general trend away from conducting many Phase III clinical trials in the offices of private practitioners over the last 20 or so years. Nonetheless, many Phase III trials are still performed by practitioners working in solo or group practices. Some contract companies have established networks of private offices/clinics to conduct medicine trials.

Phase IV studies are discussed in chapters on postmarketing surveillance studies.

"CATCH-22" AND OTHER ISSUES

"Catch-22" (Circular, Paradoxical, or No-Win) Issues in Planning Multiple Trials

"Catch-22" situations often arise when many activities of medicine development are attempted simultaneously. It is not advisable to conduct all development on a medicine sequentially nor is it possible to do it simultaneously. Neither approach on its own is sat-

isfactory, and judgment should be applied in each separate case in arriving at a reasonable balance. This balance will vary during the stages of medicine development.

Development of a Promedicine

If the metabolism of a medicine is studied in animals before human trials are initiated and a number of metabolites are identified, then it is easier to look for active metabolites in humans. If a parent medicine is found to be acting as a promedicine, then there might be advantages in developing the active metabolite instead of the parent medicine (e.g., to minimize adverse reactions, to reduce dosing variability). To develop this degree of knowledge at an early stage of medicine development, however, usually requires additional time to conduct metabolism trials, which would be obtained at the expense (in part) of conducting clinical trials (as rapidly as possible) to learn whether the medicine possesses efficacy. If efficacy is not found, then the medicine will be dropped and there is usually no reason to evaluate or consider the development of a metabolite. Resources spent on identifying metabolites could have been used to develop metabolic profiles on other medicines that had demonstrated efficacy. This is clearly a circular argument.

Use of the Final Formulation in Clinical Trials

Another example of a "Catch-22" situation is that the most important well-controlled Phase II clinical trial should ideally be conducted with the final medicine formulation, but it often takes significant time and experience to identify and produce the final formulation, shape, and color of a solid (or liquid) dosage form. If a company waits to finalize each of these (and other) characteristics before the major Phase II trials are initiated, too much lost time will occur. The alternative that is usually followed is to use a temporary dosage form (e.g., capsule) and to conduct a bioequivalence trial at a later time with the final dosage form (e.g., tablet). It is assumed that the data for the temporary and final dosage forms will be comparable. If not, then additional clinical data with the final dosage form will be required. For biotechnology-derived medicines it is essential to conduct pivotal clinical trials with the final formulation.

Ceiling Effect

In a model of mild pain (e.g., dental pain from tooth extraction) the degree of patients' pain may be adequate to allow a statistically significant separation between pain relief from a standard analgesic medicine and placebo to be observed. There may not, however, be adequate residual pain (below the ceiling effect) to show that a new medicine relieves more pain than the standard medicine. Therefore, it would be necessary to study a new versus old analgesic using a different pain model, which could be used to evaluate medicine responses to more severe pain. In this model there would be adequate residual pain to demonstrate a significant pain-relieving effect of the test medicine if it were more active than the standard medicine. However, mild analgesics are not expected to be active in models of severe pain, and therefore the clinical trial would not be worthwhile to perform.

Project Champions

Another example of a "Catch-22" situation concerns the aggressiveness and enthusiasm of project champions. If they are too cautious or even negative about their project in reports and verbal presentations, then management will be reluctant to commit significant resources to their project. It is also possible, of course, that management will replace the project champion with a more forceful and dynamic individual. Champions who are enthusiastic beyond what the data justify may acquire large quantities of resources too early in the projects' life, before it is even known whether the medicine has demonstrated activity. If a company encourages and rewards this type of overoptimistic reporting of a medicine's progress, then it has a negative effect on the other champions who attempt to present a balanced view of their projects and who do not seek resources before it is appropriate. In addition, resources inappropriately allocated to one project are unavailable to others.

Conducting All Studies and Trials at an Earlier Time

Listening to speakers at national meetings, one often hears that the secret to efficient medicine development is to "conduct clinical trials in parallel rather than in series; prepare final trial reports earlier, so that regulatory submissions may be prepared and submitted earlier; do toxicology studies earlier so that longer duration clinical trials may be conducted; do metabolism studies earlier so that metabolites may be identified that could be developed as medicines instead of the current one."

These statements seem reasonable on the surface, but they usually are not. Everything cannot be done earlier or in parallel. First Phase I clinical trials must generally proceed in series, and sometimes this is true during part of Phase II or even Phase III. Second, supplies of medicines (i.e., as a chemical) are usually limited at early stages of a project, which is the time when many activities are competing for these supplies. Third, if many metabolism and toxicology studies are done earlier and clinical trials are delayed, by the time Phase II clinical trials show that the medicine is either ineffective or unsafe in patients, significant resources will have been expended that did not have to be spent or expended. Fourth, these statements are often hollow clichés, because a good plan considers the balancing of many factors and many demands to arrive at the most reasonable balance. Moreover, there are numerous other projects and activities competing for resources that greatly affect whatever plans are created for a single project.

CREATING THE ACTUAL CLINICAL MEDICINE DEVELOPMENT PLAN: NINE STEPS TO FOLLOW

After a clinical strategy is chosen it is necessary to move it toward reality by creating a clinical development plan that implements the strategy. A series of steps to follow in creating a clinical development plan are listed below. This plan should begin with the clinical strategy and be consistent with the overall medicine development plan. Is the strategy to have a fat, lean, or in-between-sized plan? This should influence which studies are included in the plan.

1. Identify the major indication and dosage form to be pursued.
2. List each of the clinical trials expected to be required for each development phase (i.e., Phases I, IIa, IIb, IIIa, IIIb) prior to marketing. Estimate the number of patients in each. Ensure that clinical trials to address all relevant elements of the clinical strategy are included. Phase IV studies should also be considered and identified, if possible. Identify whether each clinical trial is essential, highly desirable, or nice to have if possible.
3. Delete those clinical trials that are outside the comfort zone of the sponsor. Alternatively, these (or other) trials could be contracted to other groups (see step 7).
4. Based on the information to be obtained from each clinical trial, determine which ones can be conducted simultaneously and which must be conducted sequentially.
5. Estimate the amount of time and resources required for each clinical trial's (1) planning and initiation, (2) conduct, (3) data editing and processing, (4) statistical analysis, and (5) final medical report preparation.
6. Plot the above data on a Gantt or other type chart.

Identify the time and resources required for each of the five parts listed above for each clinical trial.

7. In view of projected resource requirements and resource availability, identify which clinical trials should be conducted by other groups (e.g., foreign sites of the sponsor, contract organizations, government agencies).

8. Determine whether a second indication or dosage form will be studied. If so, determine if clinical trials will be initiated before or after the time when the first indication (or dosage form) is firmly established (i.e., well-controlled clinical trials have demonstrated efficacy).

9. Incorporate other clinical trials that fit the visual model of medicine development chosen or are required for other countries' regulatory packages.

The overall plan should be reviewed with knowledgeable consultants and investigators before being submitted to senior managers. If insufficient information is available to create this plan, then a 1-, 2-, or even 3-day meeting should be held with knowledgeable professionals who can debate the separate elements of a plan and determine reasonable and realistic alternatives.

REVIEWING AND UPDATING THE CLINICAL DEVELOPMENT PLAN AFTER ITS ADOPTION

As internal and external environments change, the clinical development plan must remain appropriate to achieve desired goals. This requires using some measurements to assess the plan. Measurements should assess the quality of data obtained (as well as its quantity) to ensure that the original strategies remain appropriate. Other measures include personnel and other resources available and needed to fulfill the strategies, and assessment of the external climate (e.g., state of the art of practicing medicine in the disease area of interest, regulatory views and reactions). In addition, progress should be monitored as the clinical development plan is implemented and progressive milestones are achieved. This step ensures that the rate of progress is appropriate for the specific medicine being developed. Any changes in the rate of progress may lead to a review of options available or to a review of the strategies adopted.

It is not always possible to describe fully the clinical trials to be conducted beyond Phase I or the first Phase IIa trial. This limitation occurs because major uncertainty exists about one or more aspects of the clinical program. Under these circumstances the clinical development plan should only be created, reviewed, and approved up to an appropriate stage (i.e., milestone). In addition, the clinical plan should describe the specific events that will occur at that time to determine

the project's future course. These may be such events as (1) assembling a group of consultants to review the data and determine the next steps, (2) presenting the data to a regulatory agency and discussing next steps, (3) reviewing the alternative options in-house, or (4) reviewing the plan with other sites or groups participating in the medicine's development. If two or more of these (or other) options will be followed, then the order that will be used is important to discuss and to determine.

QUESTIONS AND ISSUES TO CONSIDER IN DEVELOPING, REVIEWING, AND UPDATING A CLINICAL DEVELOPMENT PLAN

1. Does the plan fit the visual model of drug development chosen?

2. May the medicine's efficacy be evaluated using a marker (i.e., a surrogate endpoint of the disease)?

3. Under what conditions is the medicine cost effective when compared with standard therapy? Should this be evaluated in Phases IIIa or IIIb trials?

4. Is the benefit-to-risk ratio believed to be better than that of standard therapy? If so, how may this be demonstrated most convincingly?

5. What is the likelihood that a competitor will get its medicine to market first? If so, will this impact on one's clinical plans and what countermeasures may be taken?

6. What are the risks to a sponsor that could arise from conducting each clinical trial in the development plan? Are any of these risks much greater than the others, or are any unacceptable?

7. Is everyone who has been consulted in agreement that each of the clinical trials in the development plan is appropriate? If not, what are the pros and cons of their reasons?

8. What options are available to the sponsor for sharing the costs and risks of developing the medicine (e.g., codeveloping with another sponsor, asking the government to codevelop the medicine, licensing or cross-licensing the medicine)? Are any of these options realistic and also commercially attractive?

9. Is it ethical to conduct a placebo-controlled trial with the medicine? If not, what alternative clinical trial designs are available that would maintain a controlled double-blind trial?

10. If one plans to conduct placebo-controlled trials in Phase IIb after a medicine is shown to be active in pilot trials, will it still be ethically acceptable to conduct the trial or will it become unethical? If the medicine is a new life-saving medicine, it will probably become unethical to conduct the clinical trial in Phase IIb after its therapeutic value has been

demonstrated in Phase IIa. It is important under these circumstances to conduct a well-controlled double-blind placebo trial in Phase IIa.

11. What comparison medicine(s) should be used in the clinical trials? Would regulatory authorities agree with this choice? If not, this issue should be discussed with them. For example, if the active medicine to be used as a control is not on the market in a commercially important country, those data may not be acceptable to the regulatory authority as a pivotal trial.

12. How will resources used for a medicine's development impact on the development of other medicines? What steps can be taken to minimize any negative impact? For example, some of the work may be contracted to other organizations, or a foreign development site of the same company may be able to conduct more of the clinical trials.

13. Has the clinical development plan been integrated with current and future plans at other development sites within the company? Is the medicine's development viewed as an international effort, or merely as one of "their" medicines?

14. What type of clinical development model(s) will be used for the second and third indications? The use of one visual model for the first indication may have little bearing on the model chosen to evaluate subsequent indications.

15. Has the temptation been resisted to address too many questions in a single clinical trial? Inexperienced professionals "always" want to design a few clinical trials that address many questions. The opposite problem also occurs (i.e., designing a separate trial to address every question). Elements 7 and 8, for example, may easily be evaluated in conjunction with other elements.

CHAPTER 116

Combining Efficacy Data from Multiple Trials

THE SPECTRUM OF APPROACHES

Data from multiple clinical trials on a single medicine may be combined in several ways. The least integrated manner is merely to arrange sets of data obtained from each trial alongside each other and to combine the data solely through discussion of the conclusions reached for each set of data. At the opposite extreme, the data from all trials may be combined (i.e., pooled) into a global (i.e., single) data set so that a single unified interpretation may be developed, as well as separate interpretations of each subset.

Various other possibilities for combining data lie between these two extremes of the spectrum. For instance, only similar data of identical parameters may be combined. This is commonly done with laboratory parameters on samples collected at comparable times after medicine initiation, administration, or termination. It may also be done for data obtained using standard tests of efficacy.

Combining Dissimilar Data

Dissimilar data may be combined if they were obtained for similar parameters. One means of accomplishing this is to convert or transform some or all of the variables so that all data have a common basis. For example, data collected on the same efficacy test derived with different equipment in different clinical trials

could be converted to a three-part qualitative scale to indicate whether the patient improved, remained unchanged, or deteriorated. Alternatively, a five-point (or larger) scale could be created and all data could be converted to fit this scale and then combined. This particular example is often undesirable or unsatisfactory because much of the potential value obtainable from quantitative data is lost when they are converted to qualitative data.

A more satisfactory approach is to create ranges that may be used to combine dissimilar data. For instance, if patients have been able to tolerate a medicine for different lengths of time (e.g., 3 days to 3 months) then broad categories may be utilized to create an appropriate number of categories in which all patients' responses may be entered, with only minimal loss (in most cases) of the quantitative value in the data. In this case, data may be presented from patients who received a trial medicine for 0 to 2 weeks, 2 to 4 weeks, 4 to 8 weeks and 8 to 12 weeks, rather than using a specific number of days or weeks that could, in theory, place each patient in a separate category.

It is obviously easier to integrate data from clinical trials that utilize identical or similar protocols and methods of obtaining and measuring efficacy data than from trials using different protocols. It is important to design both protocols and data collection forms with an eye toward eventual integration of efficacy (and safety) data. If that has only been done to a limited degree (or not at all) and many trials have been conducted, then the integration of data will be more difficult.

A Practical Approach

One of the first steps to consider in integrating efficacy data is to evaluate the general results and relevant aspects of all clinical trials to be combined. A useful approach is to list all trials by name or number on the left column and to list all of the important elements about each trial that are of interest along the top of a spreadsheet format. These elements may include the number of patients treated, the doses of medicine tested, the frequency of dosing, the duration of the trial, whether a placebo group was included, plus any other pertinent features of the trial design. On the same or different table indicate overall results in terms of efficacy. Table headings could include measurements made, equipment used, tests conducted, plus synopsis of the data resulting from the evaluations.

From these tables a number of combinations of clinical trials may suggest themselves, such as combining trials in newly diagnosed patients, in patients receiving no concomitant medications, pediatric (or geriatric) trials, mild or severe disease, inpatient or outpatient, oral or parenteral therapy, and so forth. A further breakdown of these trials by key elements or data may be made, whereby similar data within each trial would be combined. Examples of efficacy data that may be combined across trials are given in Table 116.1. Examples of sample tables used to combine data across trials were published by Guy (1979). Selected uses of clinical data are listed in Table 116.2.

Tables may be used to present general overviews of data across many clinical trials or specific subgroup analyses within individual trials. Group means for baseline and overall or final treatment periods may be presented in addition to group means for each dosage level and each time treatment effects were measured. Multicenter trials should usually have results presented for each separate investigator to evaluate whether site-related differences occurred.

Forward versus Backward Approaches

The above approach may be defined as a "forward approach," i.e., starting out with a large amount of apparently dissimilar data and seeing the ways one can extract pertinent parts to combine together.

Another approach to combining various types of efficacy data is to use the "backward approach." In this system one determines at the outset where one desires to end up. This may take the form of a specific format of a conclusion, figure, or table of data one wishes to generate, or alternatively an entire series of blank ta-

TABLE 116.1 *Examples of efficacy data that may be combined across clinical trials[a]*

1. Specific values or scores obtained in standardized tests or any tests that are used in a standard way. These tests measure physical performance, laboratory measures, or other objective parameters. Data combined across clinical trials may be chosen as either one or more values for each test. If one value per patient per test is used, it may be the first value obtained, last value obtained, mean value, median value, or modal value of all applications of the test. Other choices may be made but should be defined in advance. If multiple values from a single patient's test are combined across trials, consultation with a statistician is strongly advised to ensure that appropriate methods and approaches are followed
2. Data from patient diaries (e.g., number of events, maximum or mean intensity of events, maximum or mean duration of events, scores of events using an arbitrary scale, number of entries)
3. Data from efficacy scales obtained and measured by written tests or verbal interviews (patient or investigator completed)[b]
4. Clinical global impression scores (patient or investigator completed)
5. Scores of disease severity
6. Percentages of patients improved or cured at different time points
7. Medicine formulations, dosing regimens, and combinations of medicines used by patients for which maximum efficacy was observed
8. Dosages found to elicit a maximum therapeutic effect

[a] Raw data should be combined whenever possible, before converting it to percent response or by another data transformation whereby the nature of the effects measured become less clear. Normalization of data is one statistical method of transforming data that usually causes little distortion of raw data. Patient populations should be similar for defined characteristics in the trials being combined.
[b] If different scales were used in different trials to measure efficacy, then broad categories (e.g., improved, unchanged, deteriorated) are a possible (though often undesirable) means of transforming data so that dissimilar data may be combined.

TABLE 116.2 *Selected uses of clinical data that are collected[a]*

1. For preparation of regulatory submissions (e.g., IND, NDA)[b]
2. For preparation of reports (e.g., review of the clinical trials or project)
3. For preparation of an article for publication
4. For assistance in monitoring future trials
5. For providing clinical guidance or decisions for future trials or patient treatment (e.g., what dose should be used)
6. For comparison of results with those from other trials (a) for general interest, (b) to address specific questions, (c) to support a theory or belief, (d) to challenge a theory or belief
7. For providing information for advertising or other marketing activities
8. For exploring new indications, formulations, or product line extensions
9. For providing an enlarged data base to assess safety and to have the information available for dissemination
10. For addressing a specific question about efficacy, safety, or pharmacokinetics
11. For generating a new hypothesis for additional trials

[a] A set of clinical data may be useful for two or more of these objectives.
[b] IND, Investigational New Drug Application; NDA, New Drug Application.

bles and figures may be created. With these specific endpoints in mind it is possible to go through available reports and data on clinical trials to cull out those parts that may be pieced or combined into the final tables or figures.

If all trials provide the necessary pieces to create final tables and figures, then the "forward approach" works well. The choice of a system to combine data usually depends on the nature of the individual conducting this effort as well as the specific type of available data. However, if small or large portions of the tables or figures are found to be missing when everything is put together, the options to consider should be discussed with a statistician.

Are Identical Parameters Always Identical?

When combining certain parameters across clinical trials it is important to confirm that they are measuring, or refer to, the same thing. For example, investigators may look for different attributes or rate the same attributes differently in assessing their clinical global impressions (CGI). The best means to help standardize this parameter is to create operational definitions and examples for the investigators to use. This will hopefully prevent or at least minimize the problem whereby multiple investigators in the same trial (or different trials) apply different criteria. Review the definition(s) of CGI and other relevant parameters at both individual and group pretrial meetings with investigators.

Weighting the Components of Efficacy

Figure 71.2 illustrates the individual components of efficacy that may be measured in clinical trials. These are the (1) natural progression of the disease, (2) nonmedicine personal factors, (3) concomitant medicines, (4) nonmedicine treatments, (5) placebo response, and finally (6) clinical effects of the medicine being tested. Not all of these factors are always present and if they are, not all will lead toward a patient's improvement over a defined period. Few investigators attempt to

measure all of these factors in a single patient because it would be difficult (if not impossible) to measure or assess their influence accurately.

The overall summation of these components includes some or many interactions among these factors. Assessing interactions among these factors is usually an extremely complex activity. Relative importance (i.e., weight) of each factor varies, and statistical analyses traditionally subtract the average placebo response from the medicine group's average response. This subtraction simplifies the analysis but minimizes the true complexity of the relationship between placebo and medicine-induced effects. Unfortunately this subtraction approach is the best one can presently do to assess a medicine's effect. The assumption that all other relevant factors are evenly distributed between treatment groups is a major one that cannot be proved. The other assumptions often made (e.g., placebo response is constant over time, placebo response is the same in patients receiving medicine as in those receiving placebo) are also unproved.

DOSE–RESPONSE RELATIONSHIPS

One goal of integrating data from multiple clinical trials may be to construct a dose–response relationship of the trial medicine. Various types of trials and data that may each be used to generate the same dose–response relationship are illustrated in Fig. 116.1. Characteristics of these figures are described in Table 116.3.

Approaches

It is possible to conduct dose–response evaluations in a single patient, single clinical trial, or multiple trials. The choice of approach to follow depends on the characteristics of the trial medicine, the disease or problem being treated, and the availability of patients. It is undesirable statistically (and often clinically) to construct a dose–response relationship when each dose was tested in a different trial or trials. Doses studied must be carefully chosen to be within an appropriate range.

TABLE 116.3 Types of characteristics of dose–response relationships

Type of dose–response relationship[a]	Number of groups of patients	Number of doses per patient	Washout between doses[b] (*)	Order of presenting doses
A	1	≥2	No	Cumulative
B	1	≥2	No	Random
C	1	≥2	Yes	In order of ascending dose
D	1	≥2	Yes	Random
E	Multiple (one trial)	1	No	Single dose or fixed range per group
F	Multiple trials	1	No	Single dose or fixed range per group

[a] The letters refer to dose–response relationships illustrated in Fig. 116.1
[b] The "*" in Fig. 116.1 indicates that time was allowed for a washout period between doses.

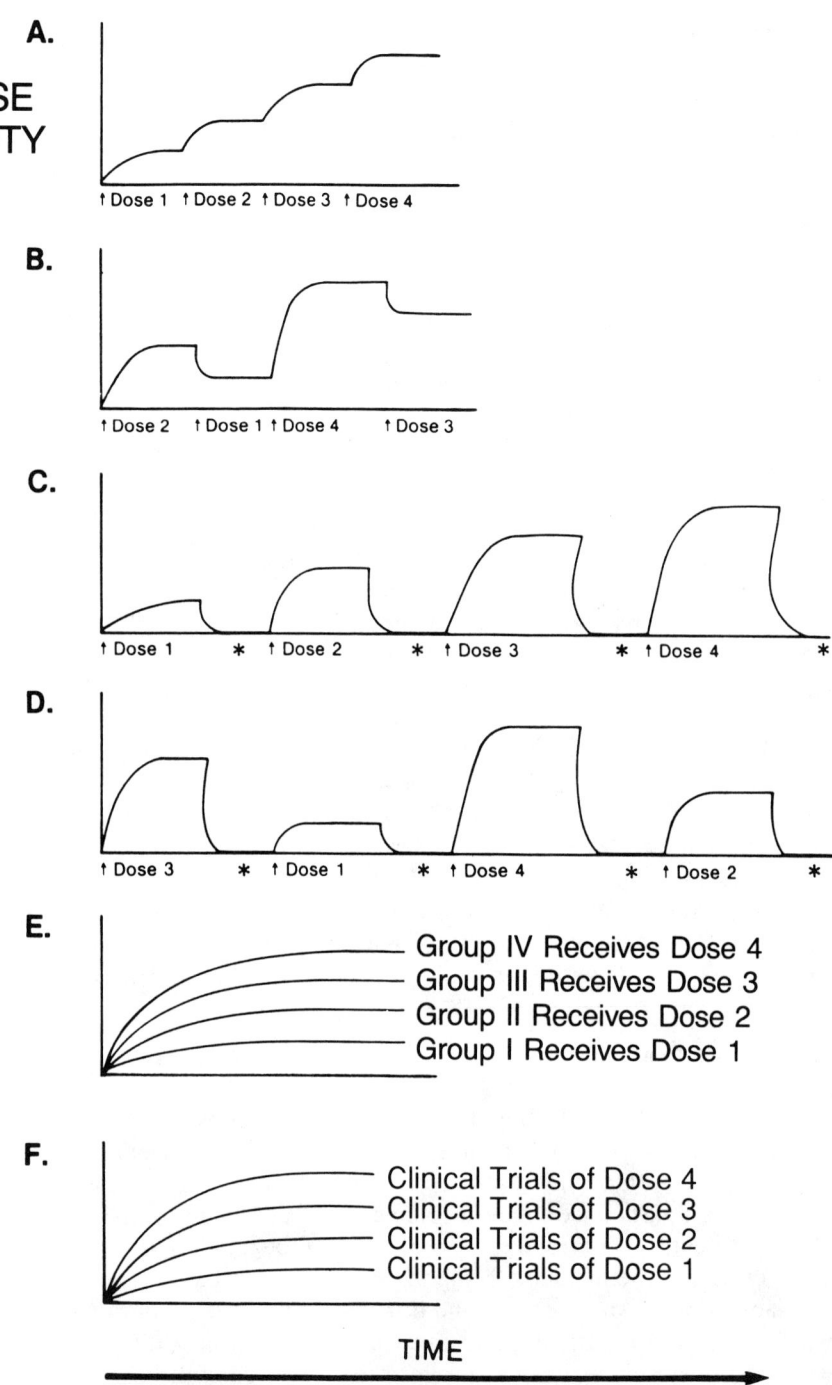

FIG. 116.1 Types of clinical trials that may generate data for creating dose–response relationships. The same dose–response curve may be created from any of these six graphs (graphs not drawn precisely to scale). *Asterisks* denote periods of washout. **A:** Cumulative doses administered to a group of patients in a stepwise manner without washout (in one or multiple trials). **B:** Doses administered in a random order to patients, without washout (in one or multiple trials). **C:** Progressively increasing doses administered in a stepwise manner with washout periods between each dose (in one or multiple trials). **D:** Doses administered in a random order to patients with washout periods between each dose (in one or multiple trials). **E:** Each patient in a group receives a single dose, and several groups in one trial each receive different doses. **F:** Each patient in a group (or trial) receives a single dose and several groups in different trials each receive different doses.

If they are too low they may be below or at the threshold of the dose–response curve; likewise, if the doses are too high they may be at (or beyond) the peak or plateau phase of the dose–response curve. In addition, they must cover an appropriate range so that a dose–response relationship may be observed.

Dose-Escalation Trials

In dose-escalation trials that are conducted to develop a dose–response relationship, only those patients who do not respond to a given dose are given a higher dose. This is a highly ethical design because all data may be used and each patient contributes to the dose–response evaluation, even if they drop out of the clinical trial. This approach is also similar to the way patients are often treated in a clinical practice. In addition, inter- and intraindividual variability are distinguishable and one can obtain a population dose–response curve. On the other hand, there are some potential problems with this method, primarily because simple pooling of data may produce biased results. A statistician should be consulted for techniques to minimize or eliminate such biases.

Approaches A through D in Fig. 116.1 may be utilized in a single patient, a single group, a single clinical trial, or in multiple trials. The choice between these approaches depends on several factors, such as how rapidly a medicine's effect wears off and whether it is practical to give cumulative doses.

Panels B and D show approaches to studying the dose–response relationship that are strong tests for whether a true dose–response exists. These approaches minimize the chances of a false-positive result, as compared to the approaches in panels A and C, in which a stepwise progression of doses is used.

If a patient is responding positively to treatment the protocol should specify whether he should be given still higher doses. Forced escalation is not usually done because physicians rarely would increase the dose further in clinical practice unless the patient's response was inadequate, and one of the major goals of Phase III clinical trials is to approximate usual clinical practice. In addition, it could be considered below ethical standards to raise the dose of a patient already benefiting from therapy to a point at which new adverse reactions or more intense ones could occur.

Two additional cautions about using the dose-escalation techniques are that (1) the natural history of the disease may change over time and (2) effects may be attributed to medicine when, in fact, these effects are not medicine related. Also, it is possible to increase the dose when no effect is observed, but the patient may not yet be at a steady state pharmacokinetically or clinically at that particular dose. Therefore, it is advisable to have a minimum period required before a patient's dose may be raised to the next higher dose or dose range.

Absence of a Dose–Response Relationship

If no dose–response relationship is observed with a medicine it may be a true effect or it may mean that (1) inappropriate efficacy parameters were used, (2) the efficacy parameters were inappropriately measured, (3) the data demonstrate great variability, (4) the doses chosen to study were all at the plateau part of the dose–response relationship, (5) the doses were too close together to illustrate the shape of the curve, or (6) human homeostatic mechanisms compensated and blunted dose-related effects.

Are Dose–Response Relationships Always Possible?

Dose–response relationships are sometimes difficult to demonstrate in humans. Outside of all-or-none effects, this is particularly true when a large placebo effect occurs and efficacy itself is difficult to establish. This is particularly true for psychiatric diseases, in which a large subjective component is present. In many (if not most) of these diseases it has not been possible to demonstrate dose–response relationships to a medicine. Nonetheless, individual patients with those same diseases have shown dose responses to specific medications. When their data are combined or when groups of patients are given different doses, however, the combined data fail to show a dose response. Given the small increments over most of the active dose range, it should be possible to show a dose response by either enrolling very large numbers of patients or just exploring threshold responses. Neither of these approaches is realistic either in the context of developing new medicines efficiently or conducting academically oriented clinical trials.

The most realistic approach to this issue is to titrate patients individually and to illustrate individual dose–response relationships. Another approach is to examine a secondary measure of efficacy. In depression, for example, the onset of therapeutic benefit is delayed, and it may be possible to demonstrate a faster onset of activity with a higher dose than with a lower one, even though the amount of activity observed (i.e., the response) may be the same with each dose.

Dose-Responses for Safety Parameters

In addition to dose–response relationships to illustrate and evaluate a medicine's efficacy, dose–response relationships may be used to illustrate safety parameters.

A dose–response curve may be constructed for each adverse reaction, using each of the following as a parameter on the ordinate: percent of patients affected, median effect observed, maximum effect observed, or another measure of the intensity of the response. A different approach is to present all significant or frequently observed adverse reactions on a single dose–response curve by indicating the dose at which each of the effects is known to occur. This approach would be useful to illustrate that different adverse reactions usually occur at different doses. A recent book edited by Lasagna et al. (1989) focuses on dose–response relationships.

Threshold Effect of Dose–Response Relationships in Toxicology Studies

The issue of the shape of the dose–response relationship at low doses of carcinogens or teratogens is actively debated in the fields of toxicology and oncology. Indications of the true shape are quite significant at very low doses of medicines. If the true shape of the dose–response curve was linear and without a threshold dose (i.e., the curve passed through the origin), it would mean that there is always some risk of that medicine causing cancer, even at relatively low doses. A supralinear dose–response curve (i.e., curved above a

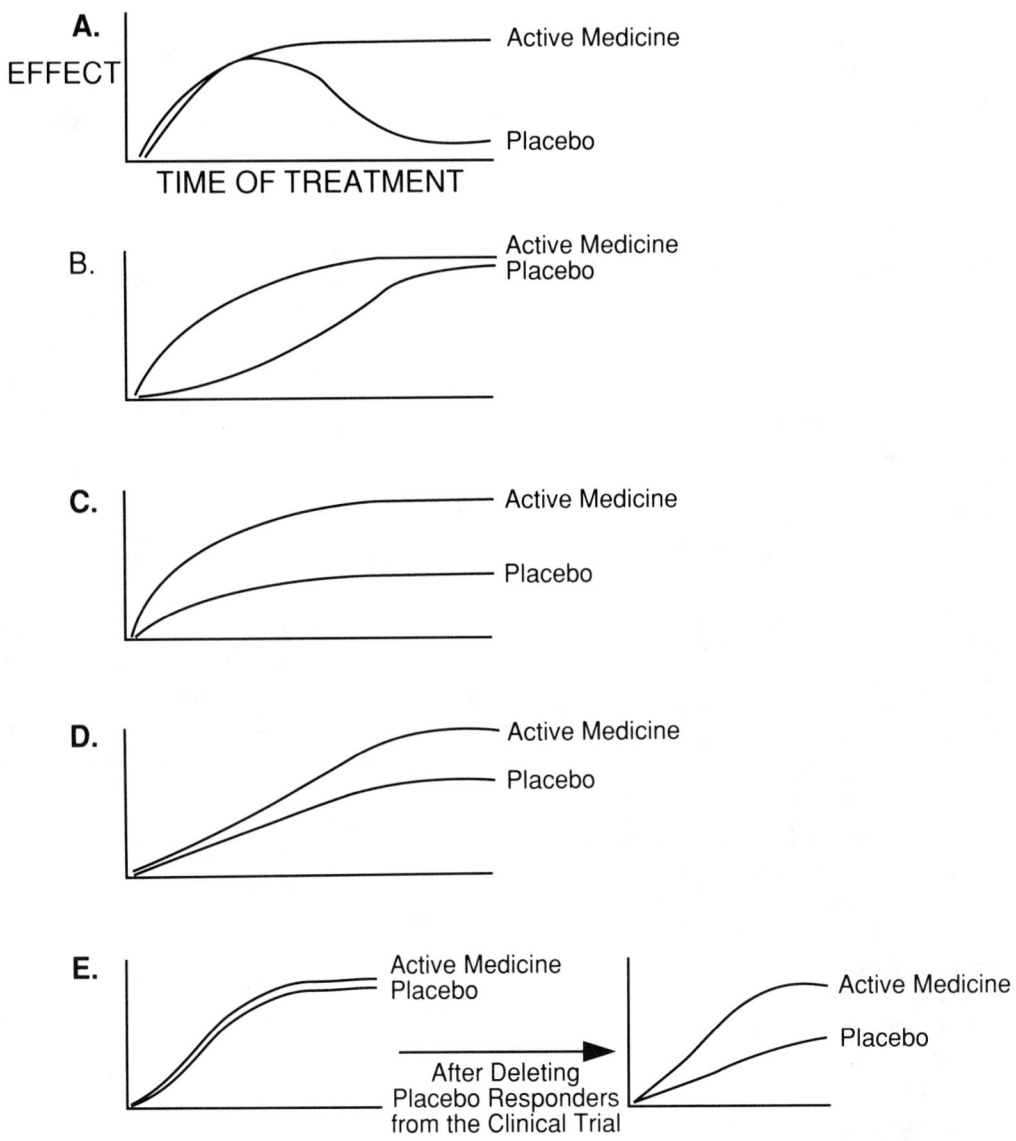

FIG. 116.2 Time course of placebo response. Five patterns illustrate selected means to separate placebo and medicine effects. This information, if known historically, may help determine the appropriate design and duration of a clinical trial. When the situation in the left of part E is expected, all patients may be placed (single blind) on placebo and evaluated at a predetermined time. All responders are then discontinued. Remaining patients are then placed double blind on either trial medicine or placebo to give the curves on the right.

straight line, but meeting the line at its two endpoints), starting at the origin, would have the same interpretation. A linear dose–response curve with a threshold dose would mean that there is a dose below which there is no risk of the medicine causing cancer. A sublinear dose–response curve (i.e., curved below a straight line, but meeting the line at its two endpoints) with a threshold dose would have the same interpretation (see Chapter 88).

PLACEBO EFFECT

Another goal of combining data from multiple clinical trials is to evaluate the nature of the placebo effect. The magnitude and time course of this effect is important to evaluate but may not be apparent in a single trial. Various types of time courses of a placebo response are illustrated in Fig. 116.2. If this information is known or estimated prior to a trial, it can help determine the optimal duration of a trial that is necessary to separate medicine and placebo effects. There are obviously several other factors that influence the du-

ration chosen for a trial. More extensive discussions of the placebo effect are included in Chapters 12 and 93.

DETERMINING WHY PATIENTS FAIL THERAPY

A potential means of improving efficacy may result from careful analysis of why patients fail therapy. It is therefore important not only to determine the number and percent of patients who fail therapy but also to determine why they fail and the amount of time it takes for them to fail after the medicine is initiated. Reasons given may relate to the rigors of the protocol and not to the medicine. Reasons may also relate to factors that may be modified (e.g., taste of the medicine, frequency of dosing, adverse reactions from rapid peak concentrations), which will allow the clinical trials to be completed successfully. In an extreme case, a suitable means of evaluating a medicine may be elucidated. It is important to explore this issue for clues to successful conduct of both current and future trials and to better data interpretation from completed patients and trials.

CHAPTER 117

Combining Safety Data from Multiple Trials

HOW MUCH SAFETY DATA SHOULD BE COLLECTED?

It is important to determine how much safety data are adequate and necessary to collect in each clinical trial in terms of both scope (i.e., the number of different parameters and tests to evaluate) and depth (i.e., the amount of data required for each parameter). The answer to this question depends on the (1) characteristics of the medicine, (2) previous clinical experience and data available on the medicine, (3) disease being treated, (4) regulatory considerations, (5) safety of alternative therapy, and (6) the time in history that is being discussed.

Requirements in the quantity and quality of data necessary to demonstrate safety of a new medicine have steadily increased over recent decades, and the requirements of many national regulatory authorities differ. One may address the question of how much data to collect by establishing the scope and magnitude of the safety data that a prudent physician in the relevant country would desire to know prior to prescribing a new medicine for a patient. It is also possible to address this question by attempting to second guess the relevant regulatory authorities on the amount of data required for approval.

Collecting Laboratory Data

Detailed laboratory data from normal volunteers and patients should be relatively extensive. These examinations include evaluation of clinical chemistry and hematology analytes in blood (even for topically applied medicines) and routine urine analytes. Specialized tests suggested by the specific actions of a medicine or by its chemical relationship to other known medicines should also be evaluated. Except in unusual circumstances, a minimum of approximately 100 patients should be evaluated with broad screening tests, in addition to the normal volunteers who are evaluated in Phase I clinical trials. There are exceptions to this generalization. For example, some orphan medicines for a rare disease will never be able to enroll 100 patients, and if over-the-counter status is sought for a marketed medicine then many more than 100 patients will be required to establish a reasonable level of safety.

If the above data suggest that abnormalities may occur as a result of a medicine, then those parameters should continue to be closely monitored, until the reason for the abnormality is determined (e.g., a concomitant medicine) and evaluated. If the reason is not found, a sufficient characterization of the abnormality and its clinical importance should be achieved. Issues regarding benefit-to-risk considerations are discussed in Chapter 99.

It is important during Phase I clinical trials of most new medicines to evaluate normal individuals who do not abuse drugs or alcohol. These groups of abusers generally have a higher rate of abnormal laboratory results and are usually less reliable in complying with a protocol. Nonetheless, it is common for normal individuals to have one or more laboratory parameters fall outside the reference range and for this event to be clinically unimportant. The abnormality observed is often not reproducible.

CATEGORIZING ABNORMAL DATA

In comparing laboratory data from several clinical trials it is possible and usually meaningful to categorize the data by degree of abnormality, in addition to the generally all-or-none question of whether the data are defined as abnormal. One means of categorizing abnormalities is by the percentage deviation both above the top of the normal range and below the bottom of the normal range. Various categories that classify degrees of abnormality may be created. One such example is to choose ranges of 20 to 40% above normal values, 41 to 60% above normal values, and so on. Alternatively the actual laboratory units of measure may be used (e.g., 201–400 mg/deciliter, 401–600 mg/deciliter, and 601 mg/deciliter and above). Similar categories would be created for percents or values below normal values for most laboratory analytes. For a few biochemical parameters, abnormalities are not considered to exist when a value is below the reference range (e.g., serum cholesterol).

Apart from establishing broad categories as described above, there are numerous other ways to classify laboratory results. These are described by Spilker and Schoenfelder (1990) and include categorizing:

1. Values that extend beyond an expanded normal range, so as to include only those values that are clinically significant abnormalities
2. Differences of before and after medicine values that are greater than a fixed percentage of the normal range
3. Differences of before and after medicine values that are greater than a fixed percentage of the baseline value
4. Values greater or less than a fixed number (e.g., platelets >500,000, platelets <100,000)
5. Patients with a specified group of laboratory abnormalities indicative of a specific organ dysfunction (e.g., renal analytes, hepatic enzymes)
6. Patients whose laboratory abnormalities are char-

acterized by the investigator as probably or definitely medicine related
7. Abnormalities that have been confirmed by repeating duplicate samples or have been reported as abnormal on at least two separate occasions. Any of the above categories may be used with this additional criterion
8. Duration of abnormality after medicine treatment is discontinued. The time for the return of an abnormal value to the normal range (or to baseline) may be used as a parameter
9. Association of the degree of abnormality with (1) dose of medicine given, (2) duration of treatment, (3) total quantity of medicine given, or (4) another parameter

Clinical Significance

Another approach to the categorization of abnormal data is to concentrate on the patients whose abnormalities are defined as clinically significant by the investigator. An important positive aspect of this approach is that this evaluation brings clinical judgment into the assessment and presents a measure of the clinical significance of the abnormality, which allows a better perspective of the laboratory value(s) than merely stating the fact that a value is abnormal. This later statement often has no clinical importance. There may be several problems, however, with using this approach. First, using clinical judgment introduces a subjective evaluation that often differs among different physicians. Second, the physician may not have sufficient information on which to arrive at a well-based conclusion as to whether the abnormality has clinical significance. Third, another physician evaluating the patient and abnormality at a subsequent visit may arrive at a different conclusion.

PRESENTING DATA ON LABORATORY ABNORMALITIES

If both objective and descriptive judgmental approaches are used to present abnormalities it will increase the likelihood that an accurate clinical impression will be created. It is important to categorize laboratory abnormalities by magnitude (i.e., degree of abnormality) and according to other parameters (e.g., duration of abnormality) and according to other parameters (e.g., duration of abnormality), as well as incorporating an investigator's clinical judgment as to the clinical significance of an abnormality. The degree of association between the medicine and the abnormal event is often best assessed by the sponsor, because much more information on the medicine is available to them than to a single investigator.

Some of the basic approaches to presenting laboratory data are to illustrate statistically significant (1) within-group changes, (2) changes within prespecified categories, (3) detailed within- and between-group changes, and (4) specific data on individual analytes. Various tables may take the reader or reviewer progressively from tables, figures, and descriptions of (a) general cross-study presentations of data to (b) overall clinical trial data, to (c) specific within (and combined)-trial analyses, and finally to (d) specific patient data.

Other crucial issues to consider in presenting data relate to (1) whether or not the abnormality is reversible, (2) the time required from discontinuation of the medicine until the effect is reversed, and (3) whether rechallenge with the medicine leads to reoccurrence of the abnormality. These considerations have a resemblance to Koch's postulates for confirming that a specific disease results from a specific type of bacteria. A description of several commonly used methods to present laboratory data in publications or regulatory submissions are shown in Table 117.1. Specific examples are illustrated in *Presentation of Clinical Data* (Spilker and Schoenfelder, 1990).

TABLE 117.1 *Methods of presenting abnormal laboratory data in publications or regulatory submissions*[a]

1. Plot or tabulate the overall number of abnormalities for each parameter in each clinical trial and cumulatively for all trials
2. Conduct subgroup analyses to determine the influence and associations of age, sex, race, and other relevant patient factors
3. Tabulate (or plot with histograms) the number and severity of abnormalities observed with different medicines treatments. Compare number and percent of patients on each treatment with different degrees of significant increases above normal (and those with decreases below normal)
4. Define categories of mild, moderately, and severely intense abnormalities and plot or tabulate number of abnormalities in each category
5. Tabulate data based on whether the baseline was normal or abnormally high (or low) with laboratory values obtained during treatment (normal, abnormally high, or abnormally low)
6. If multiple values were obtained, tabulate the number of patients with all values normal, those with no two successive values abnormal, or those with two or more successive abnormalities. Further describe data in the latter group
7. Transform data to standardized scales[b]
8. Describe noteworthy abnormalities in the text, presenting sufficient details

[a] Approaches to developing and presenting summary statistics of overall and abnormal results are provided in the appendix of *Guide to Clinical Studies and Developing Protocols* (Spilker, 1984). The term abnormality must be carefully defined. It is sometimes used to denote all values outside the normal range or only those values that are outside the normal range by a prespecified amount.
[b] If this technique is used it should be followed for the same data from all clinical trials on a medicine.

PRESENTING LABORATORY DATA USING TRANSFORMATIONS

One means of clinically interpreting laboratory data is to categorize the degree of abnormality. This may be done in many ways from a simple scale (e.g., mild, moderate, severe) to a highly sophisticated scale developed by Dr. Joann Data and colleagues (*personal communication*). Their method utilizes a grading system with transformed data on a five-point scale of −1 to −5 for values below the lower limit of the reference range or with a +1 to +5 scale for values above the upper limit of the reference range. The range of laboratory values associated with each grade on the scale is determined by a consensus of expert clinicians. Each positive or negative number further from zero represents a more severe state.

Types of Data Transformations

A few types of data transformations are described below.

Type I. Raw data are changed by a single process. The data either maintain the same units or are changed to different units.
Type II. Data that have been transformed (i.e., type I) are subjected to an additional transformation.
Type III. Transformation of data that have already been transformed at least twice.

A schematic description of these types is shown in Fig. 117.1, which also illustrates how each type of transformation may be used to determine derived parameters.

Examples of Type I Transformations

1. SGOT values have a reference range at site 1 that equals 6–42 units/ml and the reference range at site 2 equals 4–39 units/ml. It is decided that all SGOT data are to be transformed to a reference range of 5–40 units/ml. Patient B from site 1 has raw values of 41, 76, and 95, and his transformed values are now 40, 75, and 93.
2. Values may be transformed from an arithmetic scale to a logarithmic scale.
3. Data are changed to percent of control values.
4. Data are changed to percent of maximal observed response.
5. Data are changed to percent of maximal possible response.
6. Data are normalized.

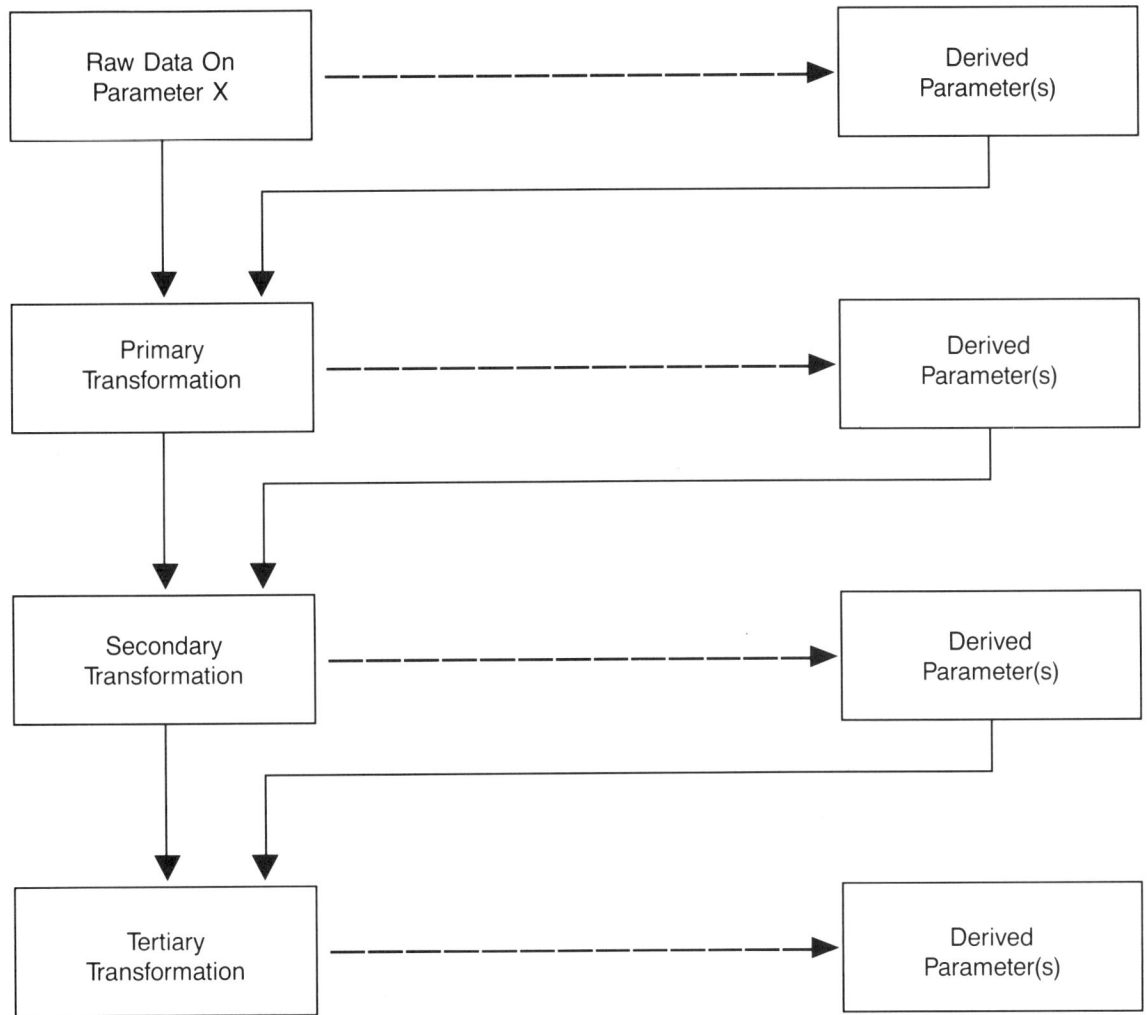

FIG. 117.1 Relationship between transformed data and between transformed data that may be used to create derived parameters. Some of these relationships are only hypothetical. Dashed lines represent determination of derived parameters and solid lines represent transformations of the data.

Examples of Type II Transformations

1. All SGOT data in the first example above are transformed to a fraction, where 40 is defined as unity (1.0). All normal values are therefore less than 1.0.
2. Patient B has raw values of 41, 76, and 95. His type I transformed values are 40, 75, and 93 and his type II transformed values are 1.0, 1.8, and 2.33.
3. Another example is to transform data that have already been transformed to percent change from control, to percent of maximal observed response.

Examples of Type III Transformations

From the initial example using SGOT, the percent changes from baseline of the secondary transformed values are 88% and 133%.

Examples of All Three Types of Data Transformations with the Same Data

Example 1. Blood pressure values:

$$\text{value of blood pressure measured} = \text{raw number (mmHg)}$$

$$\text{type I transformed value} = \text{a number converted to a standard scale (mmHg)}$$

$$\text{type II transformed value} = \text{percent decrease from control}$$

$$\text{type III transformed value} = \text{percent of patients with 50\% or greater decrease from control}$$

Example 2. Transformation of left ventricular function values:

$$\text{values of pressure in left ventricle} = \text{raw number (mmHg)}$$

$$\text{type I transformation} = \text{differentiated value, i.e., } dp/dt$$

$$\text{type II transformation} = \frac{\text{percent increase in}}{dp/dt \text{ observed with medicine}}$$

$$\text{type III transformation} = \begin{array}{l}\text{percent of patients with a 50\% increase in } dp/dt \text{ with medicine}\end{array}$$

Example 3. Values for a laboratory analyte (raw numbers):

$$\text{type I transformation} = \begin{array}{l}\text{number of patients with an abnormality}\end{array}$$

$$\text{type II transformation} = \begin{array}{l}\text{percent of patients with an abnormality above a certain level}\end{array}$$

$$\text{type III transformation} = \begin{array}{l}\text{trend of the secondary transformation in ten different studies}\end{array}$$

Transformations of Laboratory Data: Proposals in the Literature

There are various proponents of different methods of data transformation as a technique to combine laboratory data across patients and across clinical trials more easily. Transformations of data are intended to eliminate any influence of different normal ranges or different analytical techniques at different laboratories. Sogliero-Gilbert et al. (1986) and Abt and Krupp (1986) each present their own version of data transformations of laboratory data. Sogliero-Gilbert et al. (1986) propose two concepts for "simplification of lab data monitoring and interpretation." First, they propose normalizing data by dividing each value by the upper limit of the normal range for the particular laboratory in which the data were obtained. This means that all analytes have an upper limit of 1.0 for normals, a lower limit of 0, and all transformed values are positive. Their second concept is a multivariate scoring system that determines a number from normalized values for a functionally related group of analytes (e.g., liver function group). This number is called a "Genie Score" and the authors of this article state "Just as the Genie in Aladdin's lamp made Aladdin's work easier, so the Genie Score introduced here will simplify the management and assessment of the lab parameters." Abt and Krupp (1986) propose that laboratory data obtained in multicenter trials be combined by transforming data from each center into percent-scaled values from 0% to 100% for the upper range of normal at each site.

The Case Against the Above Types of Laboratory Transformations

The author strongly disagrees with the concept of transforming laboratory data for reasons given below. These methods and other transformation techniques often allow data to be combined more easily, but the process of interpreting the data becomes more complex and difficult. Depending on the specific transformation used, the data themselves usually have little or no meaning to clinicians who are trained and experienced in interpreting data presented in actual units. Clinicians develop a "feel" for the data based on the specific analyte measured, its degree of variability within (and between) most normals and patients, and their knowledge and experience with accepted interpretations. For example, potassium is tightly regulated by the body, laboratory measurements are highly accurate if the blood is not hemolyzed, and small increases or decreases in mEq/L (milliequivalents per liter) often have a marked clinical significance. Glucose values, on the other hand, vary widely during the course of a day and depending on when a sample was taken and under which circumstances, there would be less clinical significance if values changed to the same degree as for potassium.

It is not reasonable at the present time to expect clinicians in practice or at a regulatory authority to develop a "feel" for how to interpret data transformed in each of the various ways proposed. The interpretation of a change of 10% or a doubling of the value in one system would obviously differ from the same percent change in another system. Clinicians at regulatory agencies would have an extremely difficult job if many companies submitted laboratory data transformed with different techniques. If one transformation does become popular and accepted over time, then that particular method would certainly be a useful approach for standardizing the combination of laboratory data in a study as well as across studies.

International Units

The conversion of the American medical community to the international system (SI) units for laboratory values required over a decade of planning (Lundberg, 1988). This goal has still been incompletely realized, despite the fact that many values are unchanged between systems and many others are modified by a simple multiple such as 10, 0.1, or 0.001. Other analytes have conversion factors provided in easily available handouts or nomograms. Considering the near impossibility of converting the American medical community to a single logical system with international acceptance, it is difficult to imagine how any one system of data transformation could be accepted by a sufficient number of either companies or medical practitioners so that it would become a standard. Moreover, it is difficult to imagine that a large national regulatory authority would accept a system of data transformation when their reviewers are trained to interpret data using currently accepted standards, and there are numerous systems of data transformation, each vying for attention in the literature.

ADVERSE REACTIONS

Safety data include much more than just laboratory data. Probably the most well-known area of safety relates to physical and psychological adverse reactions to medicines. These effects are often particularly difficult to combine and integrate from multiple clinical trials or even in some cases from within a single trial. A few representative approaches to this issue will be described.

Obtaining Adverse Reaction Data

In the simplest case, several clinical trials may have been conducted on relatively few patients, as in certain orphan medicine applications. In this situation a tabular presentation of adverse reactions may be prepared with a relatively complete description of each moderate or severe adverse reaction that occurred.

It is extremely important that adverse reactions, especially serious ones, be diagnosed accurately throughout the world. This is not only so that patients may be promptly and appropriately treated but also to ensure that, when data on the cases are combined and incidence figures are created, all cases of a certain adverse reaction really did have the same problem. Another reason why adverse reactions must be diagnosed accurately is that the benefit-to-risk ratio of a medicine may change when a serious adverse reaction is reported. This could affect the medicine's use or may even cause it to be withdrawn from the market. Criteria to use in identifying some adverse reactions such as seizures are generally well understood. However, when no direct observations of a patient have been made, it may be difficult or impossible to know if, for example, a seizure has actually occurred. In addition, certain adverse reactions (e.g., various type of rashes) are labeled differently by different physicians, depending on their knowledge of the medical area, the state of knowledge in the particular field of medicine,

and other factors. It is thus important to define the criteria carefully for any serious adverse reactions that may be anticipated to occur and to have a specialist consulted on all serious or potentially serious adverse reactions that lie outside the investigator's area of expertise.

In combining data on adverse reactions from different clinical trials, it is usually important that the means of obtaining the adverse reactions was similar. If unsolicited comments were collected in one trial, a general probe used in a second trial, and a specific list of symptoms read to patients in a third trial, then simply adding the results to determine incidence figures would probably be highly misleading. In Phase IV postmarketing studies data are often obtained in many different ways and by many different physicians, but in trials conducted during Phases I to III, attempts should be made to standardize methods of collecting data on adverse reactions.

Categorizing Adverse Reactions

In most New Drug Applications (NDA) submitted to regulatory authorities, 500 to 3,000 patients are evaluated. Within each NDA, different types of clinical trials have usually been conducted and highly diverse adverse reaction data accumulated. These adverse reactions may be categorized in numerous ways, including (1) type (e.g., behavioral, cardiovascular, topical, neurological), (2) severity (e.g., mild, moderate, severe), (3) counteractive treatment provided (e.g., discontinued medicine, increased surveillance, prescribed an antidote), (4) duration of effect (e.g., weeks, months, number of occurrences), and (5) degree of association with the medicine (e.g., possible, probable, definite, unknown). Adverse reactions present at baseline that did not worsen during the clinical trial should be separated from those that emerged or worsened during the trial. Steps to follow when patients report adverse reactions are given in Table 117.2. COSTART and other systems to categorize adverse reactions are described in Chapter 67.

Presenting Data on Adverse Reactions

In several types of clinical trials adverse reaction data are not appropriate to combine. An obvious example is when some trials were conducted in children and others were conducted in adults. Also, if one (or more) trial was conducted in severely ill patients and the other trials were all conducted in mildly ill patients (for whom the medicine was intended) then it might be preferable to present the data separately from the severely ill patients. Many adverse reactions observed in severely ill patients may not be directly attributable to

TABLE 117.2 *Steps to follow when patients report adverse reactions*[a]

1. Quantify the rate (incidence), intensity (severity), duration, and total number of episodes
2. Obtain information on related events and determine possible causes[b]
3. Consider countermeasures to deal with adverse reactions
4. Establish a reminder system to contact the patient for a follow-up visit. Suggest that the patient contact the clinic or investigator if the problem persists, recurs, or worsens
5. Consider additional follow-up by telephone, letter, or by scheduling another visit
6. If the adverse reaction is severe or serious, complete a Food and Drug Administration (FDA) 1639 form or UK "yellow card"[c]
7. Contact the sponsor for severe or unexpected adverse reactions if the clinical trial is sponsored
8. Contact the Ethics Committee/Institutional Review Board (IRB) if the adverse reaction is severe[c]

[a] The flow of information for reporting serious adverse reactions is shown in Chapter 126.
[b] As part of determining the cause of the adverse reaction, it may be relevant to ask the patient for his/her opinion.
[c] See Chapter 126.

the medicine, and those that were attributable to the medicine might have occurred because of the nature of the patient population studied.

Many of the tables shown in *Presentation of Clinical Data* (Spilker and Schoenfelder, 1990) for presenting data are extremely laborious to compile and evaluate. The highly detailed manner described is usually not followed for most multicenter trials initiated in academic centers. Rarely does one encounter this level of detail in clinical publications. A detailed style is adhered to, however, for the majority of regulatory submissions on new medicines in the United States.

Creation of a single large data base in a computer is usually essential in order to combine data easily on adverse reactions from multiple clinical trials. A single data base allows future reanalyses of the data should that become necessary, and also allows new adverse reaction data to be easily integrated with existing data.

Another style for presenting adverse reactions is referred to as the "summary style." In this scenario, it is assumed that a great deal of data has been collected on adverse reactions. These data could be presented in the exhaustive manner described above, but for various reasons a general overview is desired.

In the "summary style" of presenting adverse reactions, tabulations are made of the incidence of all observed adverse reactions. This can be either on paper or with the aid of a computer program (e.g., Lotus 1,2,3). The left-hand vertical column could list all of the observed adverse reactions and the horizontal headings could list each of the clinical trials. The number of patients entered in each trial could be entered in parentheses under the trial titles. After data are entered in this table, a column could provide both total

numerator (i.e., cases) and denominator (i.e., exposed patients) figures for each adverse reaction. These totals could also be converted to a percent incidence. Separate tabulations could also be made of all serious adverse reactions attributed to the medicine. These two tables would provide a broad view of adverse reaction types, incidence, and severity that could be interpreted in the text of a report. Separate summary tables of adverse reaction durations and also patient outcomes (e.g., died, nonreversed, reversed) could be prepared.

Calculating the Incidence of Adverse Reactions

The incidence of a specific adverse reaction always relates to the rate of its occurrence. In its simplest form, it is the number of patients with the adverse reaction divided by the number of patients treated with the medicine. This ratio may be converted to a percent by multiplying by 100, but most commonly both the numerator and denominator are presented.

There are many other ways of presenting incidence figures of adverse reactions. The most appropriate way depends on the particular therapeutic area and situation (e.g., duration of treatment, severity of the adverse reaction, whether patients have one or multiple episodes). The value of these ratios will often differ for a medicine evaluated in Phase II or III versus a medicine evaluated in Phase IV. Moreover, the quality of data used to establish the ratio also differs markedly between these two categories of studies (see Chapter 121 for additional discussion of this point).

Some of the possible means of presenting incidence figures are listed below:

1. $$\frac{\text{Number of patients with the specific adverse reaction who received medicine for at least X days (or weeks)}}{\text{Total number of patients who received medicine for at least X days (or weeks)}}$$

2. $$\frac{\text{Number of episodes (events) of the specific adverse reaction reported in a clinical trial}}{\text{Total number of possible episodes (events) of the specific adverse reaction that could have been reported}}$$

3. $$\frac{\text{Number of patients with severe adverse reactions of a specific type}}{\text{Total number of patients treated with the medicine for at least X weeks}}$$

4. $$\frac{\text{Number of patients with severe adverse reactions of any type}}{\text{Number of patients with mild, moderate, or severe adverse reactions}}$$

5. $\dfrac{\text{Number of patients with a specific adverse reaction that is severe}}{\text{Total number of patients in the clinical trial treated with the medicine}}$

6. $\dfrac{\text{Number of patients treated in the clinical practice who had the adverse reaction to the medicine}}{\text{Total number of patients treated in the practice with the medicine}}$

7. $\dfrac{\text{Number of patients with the specific adverse reaction}}{\text{Total number of patient years of treatment with the medicine}}$

8. $\dfrac{\text{Number of episodes of the adverse reaction lasting over X hours}}{\text{Total number of episodes possible}}$

For ratio number 7 the total number of patients treated is also important to present, so that this ratio may be adequately understood. Without this information the reader could not determine whether one patient year represented 365 patients treated for 1 day each or one patient treated for the entire year. For ratio number 8 (and 2) the total number of possible episodes equals the total number of patients in a clinical trial multiplied by the number of clinic visits or times when adverse reaction reports are collected.

Note that some of these ratios are more appropriate to a clinical trial and others to clinical practice. In any report of adverse reactions the most appropriate ratios must be determined. It may be relevant to present several different ratios in a report, in order to convey a more accurate impression of the data. The ratio may also be based on the patient's age, sex, race, type of disease, or dose of medicine given. Other approaches to either calculating the incidence rates of adverse reactions or to illustrating their characteristics are possible (e.g., denominators may be expressed as number of units sold or number of people exposed). There is no best ratio to use, since only some can be applied to any clinical situation. For example, (1) some adverse reactions (e.g., agranulocytosis) are graded as all-or-none and not as mild, moderate, or severe; (2) acutely administered medicines are not described in terms of patient years; (3) the number of episodes possible to record are only applicable to clinical trials and not to clinical practice.

Potential Confusion of Incidence and Prevalence

When an interaction of a new, seldom, or moderately used medicine with a widely used medicine has a low incidence, there will still be so many people taking the common medicine that the prevalence of the interaction will be high. The medical impression is likely to be that the interaction has a high incidence. The opposite also is true. A new, seldom, or moderately used medicine that interacts with a seldom used medicine with a high incidence will have a low prevalence. The medical impression is likely to be that the interaction has a low incidence.

Data from other evaluations of safety (e.g., physical examinations, electrocardiograms, microbiology, immunology) may be combined from multiple trials using methods described above.

CHAPTER 118

Specific Therapeutic and Disease Areas: Methodological Considerations

DIFFERENT LEVELS FOR CONCEPTUALIZING CLINICAL TRIAL METHODOLOGIES

This chapter is based on the premise that there are four distinct levels on which one may consider and discuss clinical trial methodologies (Fig. 118.1), as described below.

First Level: Concepts, Principles, and Considerations of All Clinical Trials

The first level is the most general, and concerns the overall concepts, principles, and considerations of methodology that apply to almost all clinical trials. These include considerations of clinical trial size, blind, duration, treatment groups, design, randomization, and other factors that could be applied to clinical trials in virtually all therapeutic areas and with virtually all therapeutic modalities. A distinction may be made (if desired) in this level between medicine and nonmedicine clinical trials. Almost all clinical methodology chapters in this book describe this level.

Second Level: Clinical Trials of a Specific Therapeutic Area

The second level of clinical trial methodologies concerns that of a single therapeutic area or field. Examples include psychiatric disorders, cardiovascular

diseases, oncology, pulmonary diseases, dermatology, and nephrology. There is a general consensus within medicine about the identity of most therapeutic areas, although controversies exist about the placement of some specific diseases into one or another therapeutic area.

Third Level: Clinical Trials of a Specific Disease, Syndrome, or Condition

The third level concerns the specific concepts, principles, and considerations that apply to trials of a specific disease, syndrome, or condition. For example, within the therapeutic area of neurology many different diseases require different methodological considerations when evaluating new treatments in clinical trials. Designing a clinical trial to evaluate patients with Parkinson's disease, for example, requires measurement of the three major hallmarks of the disease (i.e., rigidity, tremor, and bradykinesia) as well as measurement of the ability of patients to deal with physical requirements of daily living. Clinical trials may last from 2 to 4 weeks to determine a medicine's efficacy. In epilepsy, the number of seizures, as well as their intensity, and other seizure characteristics are the focal points for evaluations of efficacy of a new (or old) treatment or medicine. Clinical trials often last from 6 to 12 weeks to determine a medicine's efficacy. Crossover trial designs may be used to study patients with epilepsy, but

Level 1:

All Clinical Trials

Level 2:

Clinical Trials in a Single Therapeutic Area or Field (e.g., Cardiology)

Level 3:

Clinical Trials in a Specific Disease, Syndrome, or Condition

Level 4:

Individual Clinical Trials

FIG. 118.1 Four levels at which various concepts and principles of clinical trials may be considered.

are rarely used to study patients with Parkinson's disease.

One variation of level three refers to a critique or review of methodological approaches to a particular issue. The issue may be related to a diagnosis, therapy, or preventive approach. For example, Tunnessen and Feinstein (1980) conducted a methodological critique of papers that focused on the steroid/croup controversy.

Fourth Level: Specific Clinical Trials

The fourth level of clinical trial methodologies is the most detailed and specific level. It is the level of the individual clinical trial. Considerations at this level are rarely the same for any two different clinical trials, even if they are carefully designed to mimic other trials. Specific conditions, patients, and many other factors vary from trial to trial. The reputation of a medicine and its medical use also changes over time. The protocol of the clinical trial is the document that best expresses the plan for the fourth level. Each of the factors that may affect the specific objectives and other aspects of a clinical trial should be considered when creating the protocol. Information and considerations from the first three levels are important when creating a specific protocol.

The final medical report or a published paper of a clinical trial is the document that describes the results of level four. In addition to the protocol and report of a clinical trial, a number of publications have described experiences with one or more aspects of the methodology (e.g., recruitment, compliance) for a specific clinical trial.

PUBLISHED INFORMATION ON CLINICAL TRIAL METHODOLOGIES THAT DESCRIBE EACH OF THE FOUR LEVELS

No single source describes each of the four clinical levels described. This book and a few others (see Appendix of *Multinational Drug Companies: Issues in Drug Discovery and Development*, Spilker, 1989a, for a list) primarily discuss the first level. Numerous articles discuss one or more aspects of the first level. The second level (therapeutic areas) has the least amount written about it. References to methodological aspects about this level are presented in Table 118.1.

TABLE 118.1 *Specific references to methodological articles or books concerning a therapeutic area (i.e., level 2)*[a]

Therapeutic area and references

Cardiovascular diseases: Cohn (1985); Friedewald and Schoenberger (1982)
Central nervous system: Spilker (1987b)
Chronic obstructive pulmonary disease: Sexton (1983)
Fertility: Olive (1986)
Oncology: Sedransk and Carter (1980); Buyse et al. (1984); Muggia (1978); Muggia et al. (1980); Scheurlen et al. (1988); Gehan (1988); Rotmensz (1989)
Ophthalmology: Seigel (1984)
Orthopedics: Laupacis et al. (1989)[b]
Parasitic diseases: Botero (1976)
Rheumatology: Brewer and Giannini (1982); Tugwell and Bombardier (1982)
Psychosocial oncology: Morrow (1980)
Maternal–infant behavior: Thomson and Kramer (1984)

[a] Many papers purportedly describe methodological information in a specific therapeutic area, but are quite general and contain little information specific to the therapeutic area.
[b] Primarily contains information on level one.

TABLE 118.2 *Selected references to methodologies for specific diseases or types of medicines (i.e., level 3)[a]*

Disease and reference(s)

Acute musculoskeletal injuries: Honig (1988)
Affective disorders: Pietzcher and Muller-Oerlinghausen (1984)
Alcoholism: Nace (1989)
Analgesics: Sriwatanakul et al. (1983)
Antidepressants: Little et al. (1977); Angst et al. (1989)
Antiemetics: Pater and Willan (1984); Olver et al. (1986); Krasnow (1989)
Anxiolytics: Wang et al. (1977)
Acquired immunodeficiency syndrome (AIDS): Broder (1989); Green et al. (1990)
Arrhythmias: Keefe et al. (1986); Bigger (1987)
Arthritis—using biological response modifiers: Pinsky (1985); Herberman (1985); Bates (1987)
Back pain: Bloch (1987); Waddell et al. (1982)
Biotechnology: Lasagna (1986a)
Brain tumors: Allen (1985)
Breast cancer: Baum et al. (1982); Carter (1979)
Caries prophylactic agents: Worthington (1984)
Congestive heart failure: Packer (1988); Guyatt (1985)
Contrast media in radiology: Belloni et al. (1986)
Dementia: McConnachie (1978)
Dyspepsia: Nyren et al. (1985)
Epilepsy: Morselli (1986); Cramer et al. (1983); Mattson et al. (1983); Commission on Antiepileptic Drugs of the International League Against Epilepsy (1989)
Hip joint arthroplasty: Gross (1988)
Irritable bowel syndrome: Cann (1987)
Leukemia: Carter (1973)
Lung cancer: Miller (1980)
Memory disorders: Alperovitch (1989)
Migraine: Tfelt-Hansen and Nielsen (1986); Couch (1987); Diamond (1987); Hedman et al. (1987); Kunkel (1987); Lewis (1987); Solomon (1987)
Multiple sclerosis: Weiss et al. (1988); Bates (1987); Robinson (1987); Compston (1987)
Myelomatosis: Birgens et al. (1985)
Perioperative chemotherapy: Gelber (1985)
Rheumatoid arthritis: Gotzsche (1989)
Schizophrenia: Pietzcker and Muller-Oerlinghausen (1984); Curson et al. (1986)

[a] Many of these and other related publications only discuss a limited number of methodological issues.

More is written about the third level (individual diseases) than any other level. Numerous books, chapters, and articles discuss methodological considerations that are applicable to specific diseases or to a related group of diseases. Selected references to published information at this level are listed in Table 118.2. Readers who are interested in obtaining additional information about level three should consult librarians, information specialists, experts in the area, professional associations, or others.

Writings about the fourth level are primarily included in papers that discuss methodological considerations and experiences of the specific clinical trials. Most of this literature focuses on large multicenter trials whose actual results are usually published independently of the papers on methodology. Methodological considerations and experiences are usually published because they are deemed of interest to help interpret the clinical trial's data or to provide lessons that could be applied to other trials. Selected examples of articles describing specific reports at level four are listed in Table 118.3. Many articles that present results of clinical trials also make one or more points about methodological aspects of the specific trial discussed.

CLINICAL TRIAL DESIGNS IN A SELECTED THERAPEUTIC AREA: ONCOLOGY

Because medicines available in oncology are relatively poorly effective and highly toxic, the standards by which new medicines are judged are quite different than in most other therapeutic areas. Thus, concepts of partial response, combination therapy, multiple-stage clinical trials to gain the most out of patients enrolled, and maximal tolerated doses were developed.

TABLE 118.3 *Selected references to methodologies about specific clinical trials (i.e., level 4)*

Name or description of clinical trial	Major aspects described	Reference
β-Blocker Heart Study	Design features	β-Blocker Heart Attack Study Group (1981)
Coronary Drug Project plus brief discussions of 13 additional specific cardiovascular or diabetes trials[a]	General experiences and results	Canner (1983)
The Hypertension Prevention Trial	Multiple aspects	Meinert et al. (1989)
Macular Photocoagulation Study	Changing the protocol	Macular Photocoagulation Study Group (1984)
National Cooperative Gallstone Study	Design, organization, and implementation	Lachin et al. (1981); Marks et al. (1984)
National Cooperative Crohn's Disease Study	Design and conduct	Winship et al. (1979)
Lipid Research Clinic's Coronary Prevention Trial	Recruitment	Benedict (1979); Agras and Bradford (1982)
Schizophrenia	Interrater reliability	Busch et al. (1981)
Systolic Hypertension in the Elderly	Various issues	Furberg and Black (1988)

[a] A list of numerous references to other papers with methodological discussions is included.

Simon (1987a) reviewed several Phase II trial designs used in oncology and proposed a new model. His proposed two-stage design uses a target of 35 to 50 patients per clinical trial. Active medicines would require two or even three such clinical trials for Phase II evaluation. In this field it is generally important to explore various dose schedules prior to conducting the pivotal trial(s).

Ellenberg and Eisenberger (1985) suggested a two-stage design for Phase III combination chemotherapy trials. In the first stage an equal number of patients are treated in each arm of the clinical trial. Only if more responses are observed with the experimental combination than with the standard combination is the clinical trial continued to stage two. Stage two enrolls the remaining patients according to the sample size consideration determined in advance of the clinical trial. This method has the advantage of terminating a clinical trial at an early point if it cannot demonstrate an important advantage of the experimental treatment. Thus, fewer patients will be evaluated in those trials and results will be obtained more rapidly.

Placebo treatment may be considered in some trials, particularly if it is given as an add-on. But, it is difficult to do this if the response rate to active treatment is small (i.e., few patients respond).

Surrogate endpoints are extensively discussed (see Wittes, 1987) and chapters in this book.

CHAPTER 119

Safety Data Required for a New Medicine at the Time of Initial Marketing

Research-and-development-based pharmaceutical companies frequently address the question of how much clinical safety data, efficacy data, and other types of data (e.g., pharmacokinetic, quality of life) should be included in the initial regulatory submission [i.e., Product License Application (PLA) or New Drug Application (NDA)] for each new medicine under development. This chapter discusses how a company may identify the amount of safety data required when a new medicine is marketed. Both general and specific factors that influence this decision are discussed. The perspective used is primarily that of a pharmaceutical company developing the medicine, but perspectives of

a regulatory agency and a practicing physician are also mentioned.

LIMITATIONS OF SAFETY DATA AT THE TIME OF A MEDICINE'S LAUNCH

Before describing the factors that influence the decision of how much data to collect, it is important to understand the limitations of safety data that are usually present at the time a medicine is initially marketed. The reasons for those limitations should also be understood. It would be ideal if the full profile of a medicine's adverse reactions, as well the incidence of each of these adverse reactions, were known at the time of marketing. This is impossible for several reasons.

Numbers of Patients Evaluated

First, only several hundred to a few thousand patients are usually evaluated at the time a new medicine is initially marketed. This number is insufficient to identify the nature and clinical importance of rare adverse reactions, although most common and unusual ones will be known. It was estimated that zomepirac sodium was administered to 15 million patients before it was withdrawn as a result of a rare but severe anaphylactic reaction. An incidence of 0.007% resulted in five deaths (0.00003% of all users) (Reines and Fong, 1987). Generally, the number of patients that must be studied to be reasonably sure of having observed any specific adverse reaction is three times the adverse reaction incidence. Thus, to identify a medicine-related adverse reaction with an incidence of 1 in 5,000 patients, 15,000 patients must be studied. Algorithms, global introspection, and other techniques are used to identify whether any specific adverse event is medicine related.

The problem of having safety data on too few patients to understand which uncommon adverse reactions are medicine related at the time of initial marketing is even more severe when a medicine is developed to treat a rare disease. Data on fewer than 100 patients may be all that can be included in a regulatory application; therefore, relatively little safety data will be available at the time of marketing. In the 1980s, pimozide was approved for Tourette's syndrome using data from approximately 60 patients, although it did not have an orphan drug designation (Abbey Meyers, personal communication). Since the Orphan Drug Act in 1983, several drugs have been approved for marketing with data on fewer than 100 patients [e.g., hemin, 1-carnitine, sodium benzoate, sodium phenylacetate; personal communication from Aleta Sindelar, Office of Orphan Products Development, Food and Drug Administration (FDA)]. Benefit-to-risk considerations often suggest that orphan medicines should rapidly be made available to patients, despite what may be obvious shortcomings in its safety profile.

Observation of Uncommon and Rare Adverse Reactions

The second reason why limited safety information is usually available at the time a new medicine is first marketed is that some severe adverse reactions may not be recognized for many years after the medicine

is marketed. Diethylstilbestrol (DES) is an example of this situation. The potential for precancerous and cancerous genital lesions that sometimes occur with this agent many years after maternal exposure is difficult, if not impossible, to recognize in the early years of a medicine's development and marketing. Major improvements in toxicological methods and standards used to evaluate medicines since DES was first marketed should minimize and hopefully prevent future occurrences of this type of problem. These changes include the necessity of conducting teratology studies and more elaborate reproduction studies in animals to evaluate fertility, reproductive function, perinatal, and postnatal aspects.

Predicting Areas in Which Safety Problems May Arise

Third, it is impossible to study fully or even to predict all areas in which safety problems may arise. There is an almost infinite combination of concurrent diseases, potential medicine interactions, patient ages, genetic predispositions, and other factors that may affect the safety of a new medicine. Few of these possible factors can or should be specifically studied during Phase III, unless there are particular reasons to do so.

Use of Medicines for Nonapproved Indications

Fourth, medicines are often used for nonapproved indications in patients who differ significantly from those entered in clinical trials. These patients may have quite different profiles of adverse reactions.

Making Breakthrough Medicines Available to Patients Earlier in Their Development

Fifth, there are increasing pressures in society to make important new efficacious medicines (i.e., breakthrough medicines) available for medical treatment at an earlier time than ever before. This means that some of the human safety studies traditionally conducted during Phases II and III are now delayed until Phase IV. This is appropriate when the benefit-to-risk ratio favors the new treatment over existing therapy. Examples of types of medicines targeted for abbreviated Phase III development and for rapid regulatory review include important anti-acquired immunodeficiency syndrome (AIDS) and anticancer medicines.

Including Relevant Patient Populations

Sixth, certain patient populations are either excluded from all clinical trials or so few patients are studied that their adverse reaction profile is virtually unknown.

This includes both pediatric patients and pregnant women. Recent attention is also focusing on different races.

Methods to Treat Patient Overdose

Seventh, the optimal method of treating patient overdose is often not established at the time of initial medicine marketing. The profile of clinical effects observed after an accidental or purposeful overdosage may be incomplete or even unknown, because few cases of overdose may have occurred. As a result, determining the method to treat those patients would be mere speculation.

TOTAL SAFETY PACKAGE REQUIRED FOR NEW MEDICINES

Golden Rules

There is no simple formula to define an acceptable size of a safety package for new medicines. The algebraic sum of interactions, pressures, and opinions of groups shown in Fig. 119.1 will determine the appropriate size. Not all groups shown in Fig. 119.1 are always involved, and additional groups may express opinions on this issue, particularly for controversial medicines. *Although a single precise formula cannot be established, an important principle is that the greater the benefit-to-risk ratio of a new medicine over existing* *treatments, the smaller the safety package may be at the time of the medicine's initial approval.* When the benefit-to-risk ratio of a new medicine represents a clinically significant improvement over current therapy, there should be a shifting of some (or all) Phase III trials to Phase IV. This last point has not been generally accepted by regulatory agencies, except for a limited number of clinically important breakthrough medicines.

Groups That Influence the Size of the Safety Package

The two most important groups that influence the size of the safety package are usually the sponsor and regulatory agency. Other groups generally play little, if any, role. For novel and newsworthy medicines such as tissue plasminogen activator (tPA), most of the groups shown in Fig. 119.1 became heavily involved in attempting to influence the size and nature of the efficacy package required.

Types of Safety Trials Conducted

Three types of safety trials are conducted on new medicines. These are (1) basic package of safety trials, which is generally similar in nature, and often size, for most new medicines; (2) specialized safety trials that depend on the particular medicine (e.g., ophthalmological, gonadal, sleep studies); and (3) additional safety trials that explore abnormalities observed or possible safety issues raised during clinical trials.

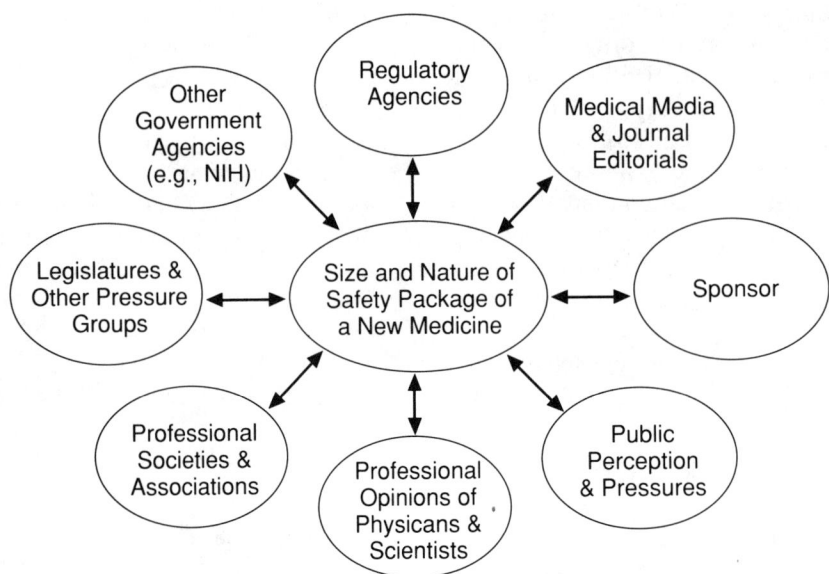

FIG. 119.1 Groups that influence the relative size of a new medicine's safety package. The arrows are double headed to illustrate the potential for a two-way interaction. NIH, National Institutes of Health.

Basic Package of Safety Trials

The basic package of safety trials required on all new medicines includes evaluations of laboratory parameters (e.g., electrolytes, basic chemistry analytes, basic hematology analytes), complete physical examinations with vital signs and body weights, electrocardiograms, and ophthalmological examinations, plus assessment of adverse reactions observed. The number of patients who should have a complete battery of assessments is generally at least 100 for almost any new medicine. Virtually all patients exposed to a medicine during the investigational period should have at least a minimal safety profile obtained. This number usually varies from 1,000 to 3,000 patients, but numerous exceptions occur that may make the safety package required for marketing either greater or lesser than this range. There must be some balance in the number of patients studied in each of the separate tests of the basic safety package. This means that it makes little sense to have data on only 25 patients with complete hematological profiles to demonstrate a lack of medicine effect, and totally negative data on 500 patients with multiple 12-lead electrocardiograms on a new medicine to treat a noncardiac disease. Any abnormal safety findings or unexpected signals of potential safety issues will require a sufficient number of additional trials to convince the sponsor, regulatory authorities, and physicians that there is either no problem or that the problem has been adequately explored and described.

How To Count the Number of Patients Exposed to a New Medicine

Clinical safety evaluations must be determined at therapeutic dose levels of a medicine. If a medicine studied for several years at 50 mg/day is found to be ineffective and a dose of 250 mg/day is necessary to provide clinical benefits, then the basic safety package must be reassembled for the higher dose.

The number of patients required to be evaluated with a new medicine does not refer to the total number of patients entered in a clinical trial, but to those exposed to therapeutic levels of the new medicine. The total number of patients treated with a therapeutic dose for the full treatment period is usually far fewer than the number who receive the medicine under various other conditions. Numerous reports state, for example, that the safety profile of medicine X is based on data from 3,000 patients. However, closer examination of the data often reveals that this number includes patients given placebo, subtherapeutic doses, therapeutic doses for inadequate treatment periods, doses for patients with other indications in pilot trials, or patients receiving active medicines who were used as controls.

Specialized Package of Safety Trials

Based on data from the basic package of safety and efficacy trials, as well as knowledge of the chemical class of a medicine, a number of specialized safety trials are almost always conducted prior to a medicine's approval. These trials may focus on a particular target organ (e.g., eyes, heart, liver, lungs) or a particular physiological function (e.g., digestion, metabolism, absorption), or certain interactions (e.g., with other medicines, with food). The exact nature of these specialized trials varies from medicine to medicine, but the most important principle in determining how much data are required to obtain is: *Enough data must be gathered so that a physician who prescribes the medicine can understand the relative risks of the medicine from the package insert, and can assess the benefit-to-risk ratio for the particular patient being treated.*

The specialized package of safety trials overlaps the third category of safety trials, i.e., studies to explore abnormal results observed. The principles for guiding both types of trials are similar, so that a separate discussion of this type of trial is not presented.

Major Influences on Assessing the Quantity of Safety Data to Collect

Three major factors affect the decision of how much clinical safety data to include in the initial submission of a new medicine for marketing approval. These are the (1) regulatory strategy adopted, (2) type of medicine being developed, and (3) nature of the disease being treated. Each of these is discussed below.

REGULATORY STRATEGIES

Is It Best to Submit a Dossier Initially to a Less Demanding Regulatory Authority?

Regulatory authorities vary widely in the type and amount of clinical safety data they require before they are willing to approve a new medicine for marketing. A company that attempts to attain regulatory approval first in a less demanding country may take either of two views. It may decide to seek more rapid approval by submitting a minimal safety data package, or it may wait until a relatively complete safety package of data has been assembled. The strategy of submitting a minimal amount of safety data may easily backfire if the regulatory authority requests more data, and this delays the medicine's approval. If a company desires to minimize the total amount of work in rewriting reports, assembling and reassembling documents, and submitting regulatory applications, it makes sense to obtain a relatively complete amount of data before submitting the initial application.

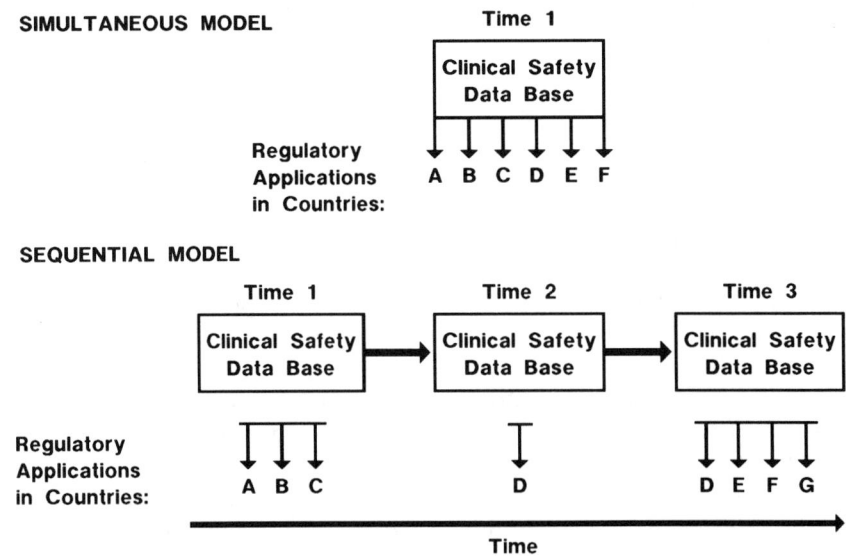

FIG. 119.2 Models (**A**, upper and **B**, lower) of clinical safety package assembly for multiple regulatory submissions.

Submitting Dossiers Simultaneously or Sequentially

The actual quantity of safety data included in regulatory applications on a single medicine submitted to different national authorities often varies widely. This depends on the time (i.e., year) of submission, rather than on an attempt to withhold data. Figure 119.2 illustrates two models of how clinical safety packages are assembled for multiple regulatory submissions. Model A minimizes the difference in time between regulatory submissions as compared with potential differences that arise if a company follows model B. In model B, it is possible that safety reports in regulatory applications sent to agencies A, D, and G, not only contain different quantities of safety data, but may also contain conflicting information, interpretations, and conclusions. This could readily lead to multiple regulatory problems for a company if different safety results or interpretations were present, although the company would not be guilty of any wrongdoing. In fact, pending PLA and NDA regulatory submissions in multiple countries may (and in some sense should) be periodically updated to minimize any substantial differences between them. The practice of frequent updating, however, is frowned upon by regulatory authorities, although they generally are interested in a final updating of safety data shortly prior to the medicine's approval.

Companies may be unable to utilize model A for a variety of practical reasons. When the sequential model B is used, the duration of time between submissions to major agencies should be kept to a minimum. The longer this time becomes, the greater is the chance that conflicting information, interpretations, or conclusions will arise. In addition, the longer the time that elapses between submissions, the greater are the

number of new personnel at the company and at regulatory authorities. These new people will have to familiarize themselves with the data and are more likely to challenge the conclusions reached than are those individuals who previously worked with the data.

A company may initially submit an application to a less demanding regulatory agency but intend to follow up rapidly with applications to more demanding authorities. Model A still makes the most sense to use in that situation. One of the difficulties in using model A is that it requires more time and effort to acquire necessary data than if a company desired to market their medicine as rapidly as possible. The counterargument is that acquiring postmarketing data in one or more countries often helps speed regulatory approval elsewhere. A corollary of this view is that a medicine should be marketed first in a major market in which postmarketing data may be obtained and not in a minor market with little scientific or commercial significance.

Factors Influencing the Regulatory Strategy

The preceding discussion demonstrates that the regulatory strategy established for a particular medicine depends on more than just the nature of the medicine and its therapeutic usefulness. Other critical factors that influence regulatory strategies are the nature and traditions of the company, its leaders' personalities, and the degree of risk they are comfortable taking.

Fat versus Lean Clinical Development Plan

The clinical development plan indicates which trials will be conducted for a regulatory submission. At some stage during a medicine's development, each of the trials that will be conducted is identified. The number of trials and number of patients targeted for enrollment in each study for any specific medicine would vary at different companies. At one extreme, these clinical development plans are designed to be lean or skimpy; the company decides to accumulate the least amount of safety and efficacy data possible to achieve marketing authorization. At the other extreme, a company adopts a fat plan and accumulates much more data than necessary for market approval. Of course, it is possible to propose a development plan in which a fat plan is chosen for efficacy data and a lean plan for safety data (or vice versa).

Expert Reports

The contents of regulatory applications in model A vary in the amount of data presented, but the data base from which the information is drawn does not. *Expert reports are critical evaluations and not merely summaries (up to 25 pages in length) that describe one type of data (e.g., clinical, preclinical safety).* These reports are required for PLA regulatory submissions in many countries and are usually prepared by experts either in academia or within the pharmaceutical company. It is clear that the in-house expert may have a conflict of interest in discussing some less than desirable information, particularly if more senior management wishes to have the critical evaluation presented differently. External consultants who serve as experts also have potential conflicts of interest if they wish to continue their professional relationships with the company. It becomes more problematical to prepare multiple versions of expert reports when they are based on a changing data base. The question of what types of changes in the data base require a new expert report to be written must then be addressed.

TYPE OF MEDICINE BEING DEVELOPED

A company that uses model A for regulatory submissions must determine the standards to be used in acquiring clinical data. These standards depend to a large degree on the type of medicine being developed. An acceptable safety package is discussed for the following types of drugs: (1) breakthrough medicines; (2) "me-too" medicines; (3) "average" new medicines with substantial medical value; (4) lifesaving medicines; and (5) orphan medicines that are not lifesaving. A single medicine may fit two of these categories. In describing these categories the primary question to discuss is what safety questions should be addressed, if not answered, at the time of initial marketing. A related

question is what safety questions or information may be reasonably delayed to Phase IV?

Breakthrough Medicines

The amount of safety data necessary at the time of initial marketing for a breakthrough medicine has traditionally been viewed as approximately the same as an average new medicine with substantial medical value. One of the arguments for requiring a smaller safety package for marketing this category of medicines would be the desire of companies, physicians, and the public to reach the market more rapidly with an acknowledged medically superior medicine. Whether regulatory authorities agree with this premise and would approve a medicine for earlier marketing under these circumstances is uncertain. However, there is not always agreement on whether a specific medicine represents a breakthrough.

Most regulatory authorities accept the logic of deferring some safety assurances for breakthrough medicines to the postmarketing period. Nonetheless, two successive medicines of this type could be treated entirely differently by a single regulatory authority. Discussions with regulatory authorities to achieve an agreement and commitment to defer some safety trials to Phase IV would be an ideal solution to reach at the end of Phase II. The FDA welcomes these discussions. Unfortunately, such types of discussions and commitments are the exception worldwide rather than the rule, and companies must use their own judgment about whether or not to submit a PLA without Phase III data. Examples of breakthrough medicines that were not lifesaving treatments of previously untreatable diseases include propranolol and cimetidine. The sponsors of these medicines had to conduct substantial Phase III trials prior to their approval for marketing in the United States and other countries.

"Me-Too" Medicines

"Me-too" medicines represent agents that are relatively equivalent to one or more medicines already on the market. The exact number is arbitrary and depends on the type of medicine, the differences between them, and the views of the person referring to them as "me-too." Another term for this type of product is "follow-on medicines."

Medical Reasons for Developing "Me-Too" Medicines

"Me-too" medicines are often developed because some or many patients are not adequately treated with their current therapy or have developed tolerance or adverse reactions. The medical rationale for developing and marketing "me-too" medicines is that some of the patients who are inadequately treated might be helped with a related, but different medicine. This occurred commonly with nonsteroidal antiinflammatory medicines. Another reason for their development is that some of these medicines were major breakthroughs at the time of their discovery and early development, but were beaten to the market by a number of competitors. Yesterday's breakthrough medicines may become today's "me-too" medicines.

Commercial Reasons for Developing "Me-Too" Medicines

A commercial reason for developing "me-too" medicines is that attaining even a small share of a very large market often justifies the development effort. Market research may suggest that there is a chance the total market will expand, the medicine will become widely used, or that other medicines will lose market share and that development should therefore continue.

Safety Packages for "Me-Too" Medicines: Opposite Perspectives

Two points of view are often expressed about safety packages for "me-too" medicines. The first states that since there are several (or many) similar medicines on the market (e.g., beta-receptor blockers, thiazide diuretics, calcium channel blockers), their safety has been firmly established and potential problems are well understood. The proponents of this view state that companies and regulatory authorities should not require as substantial a total safety package as for the average new medicine that is chemically and medically unique.

The opposite perspective states that because there are other similar medicines available, it is mandatory to acquire as much, if not more, safety data on a "me-too" medicine to get its application approved. Companies that develop "me-too" medicines with the philosophy of acquiring a limited safety package prior to regulatory submission risk the chance that their medicine will not be expeditiously approved in a major market. They also risk the possibility that regulatory authorities will raise safety questions that will brand the medicine with a negative stigma. Most stigmas are difficult to erase. The company may also be branded with the negative stigma within the regulatory authority.

Regulatory Pressure to Approve "Me-Too" Medicines

Little, if any, pressure is ever placed on a regulatory authority to approve "me-too" medicines, and in numerous cases these applications sit for many years on regulators' desks. If these applications were eventually to be picked up and reviewed, the safety data might be found lacking by new, higher standards used at that time. Regulators can then easily justify their denial of marketing approval, or request additional safety data. The latter response places companies in a difficult position because of the possibility that this cycle will continue. Similar problems may also occur for efficacy data.

This negative approach to "me-too" medicines usually is found at important regulatory authorities, and must be considered if a decision is made to develop a "me-too" medicine. Nonetheless, there are often sound medical and commercial reasons for developing "me-too" medicines, and no medium or large pharmaceutical company should eschew this practice. Additional discussions about "me-too" medicines are presented by Spilker and Cuatrecasas (1990).

Average New Medicines with Substantial Medical Value

Average new medicines with medical value are those medicines that do not have special labels such as breakthrough, lifesaving, orphan, or "me-too." The safety package of medicines in this group is judged on an individual basis as described in other sections.

Lifesaving Medicines

There is universal agreement that the safety package of a new lifesaving medicine may be smaller than that for most other new medicines. Despite this agreement, there is no consensus on exactly what are lifesaving medicines and exactly how much smaller the safety package may be.

The difficulty of defining lifesaving medicines arises because most clinical situations and diseases cannot be described easily. Some of the issues that complicate this definition are:

1. If alternative therapies currently used to treat the disease are adequate or almost adequate, should the new medicine be considered as lifesaving?
2. Must a new medicine be more effective than existing therapy to be considered lifesaving?
3. If a medicine is agreed to be lifesaving, but the quality of a patient's life is severely compromised, should the size of a safety package be smaller than for other medicines at the time of initial approval?

4. What percent of patients with a disease must find the medicine to be lifesaving before that label is appropriate?

After these and other issues are settled, there still remains the issue of how much smaller the safety package may be for the new medicine. This should be addressed in the same manner as for breakthrough medicines.

Orphan Medicines That Are Not Lifesaving

The safety package for orphan medicines that are not lifesaving must be determined case by case. Each of the factors that influences the safety package must be considered. Various myths abound about orphan medicines and rare diseases. Regardless of which general definition of orphan medicines is accepted, there are many types or categories of orphan medicines. They represent a heterogeneous group of investigational and marketed medicines. The vast majority do not represent breakthrough or lifesaving treatments. In fact, many are developed for diseases that already have treatments, albeit inadequate ones. A well-known example is Wilson's disease, which may be treated with penicillamine, dimaval (2,3,dimercaptopropane 1-sulfonate), trientine, or zinc sulfate. The need for new therapies varies widely among orphan diseases, and the appropriate safety package for a new orphan med-

icine will depend on the need for the medicine in terms of its medical value and safety.

NATURE OF THE DISEASE BEING TREATED

The third major element in the equation for determining the amount of safety data to obtain on a new medicine relates to the disease being treated. If the disease is one with high mortality or morbidity and is not adequately treated, then a smaller safety package may be acceptable at the time of initial marketing. The less the mortality and morbidity of a disease, (e.g., allergic rhinitis, nausea, hiatal hernia) the greater must be the safety package of a medicine used to treat it. Medicines given on a chronic basis to prevent a disease (e.g., by decreasing a risk factor such as hypertension) must have a relatively complete safety package at the time of marketing.

CONCLUSIONS

There has been a change in recent years to delay some safety trials on new medicines from Phase III to Phase IV, but this primarily affects major breakthrough medicines that are also lifesaving and does not represent a trend that will affect the development of most new medicines.

CHAPTER 120

Standards of Postmarketing Surveillance: Past, Present, and Future

Few fields of medicine have evolved as rapidly over the last 15 years as postmarketing surveillance. This evolution is evident in the methods, standards, and results of this scientific discipline. It is informative to examine and compare the status of postmarketing surveillance as it existed at the dawn of the last decade, as it exists today (at the dawn of the 1990s), and also as it will most likely look in ten years, at the dawn of the next century. Standards of postmarketing surveillance are briefly defined and discussed in terms of their

development, after which the following selected issues are discussed:

1. Principles governing relationships between regulatory authorities and pharmaceutical companies
2. Reporting adverse reaction data to regulatory authorities
3. Organizing postmarketing surveillance activities within companies

4. Standards for establishing adverse reaction causality
5. Standards of methodology for postmarketing surveillance studies
6. Establishment of standards and guidelines for conduct of postmarketing surveillance activities
7. Standards for regulatory agency conduct regarding postmarketing surveillance

DEFINITION OF STANDARDS AND HOW THEY ARE DEVELOPED

Standards are operationally defined in this chapter as the scientific principles that underlie commonly accepted practice. Standards are not immutable but evolve over time, as scientific practices and professional behavior change. Pharmacoepidemiologic standards are established and influenced by a variety of groups involved in conducting studies, reporting adverse events, writing about this area, and developing the practice of the field in other ways. Standards are probably most strongly influenced by regulatory authorities when they pass regulations or promote guidelines to influence current conduct and practice. Government task forces and committees outside the aegis of regulatory authorities have also played a role in this field, as described later in this chapter. Pharmaceutical companies influence standards, particularly when they determine that obtaining the best data possible makes good business sense and this goal is encouraged. Academicians who are active in this field also influence standards. Another group that affects the form standards take are professional societies. The recently formed International Society of Pharmacoepidemiology has members from academia, industry, regulatory authorities, and various other institutions and plays an important role in the development of postmarketing surveillance standards. Professional trade associations (e.g., the Pharmaceutical Manufacturers Association) have also played a major role in influencing both direction and growth of this field. Finally, there are many individuals associated with pharmacoepidemiology who influence standards through their writings, speeches, and peer pressure.

PRINCIPLES GOVERNING RELATIONSHIPS BETWEEN REGULATORY AUTHORITIES AND PHARMACEUTICAL COMPANIES

It is difficult to generalize about relationships in this area, but a few basic principles are evident. The most important one is that cooperation between regulatory authorities and pharmaceutical companies is in everyone's interests. This principle existed in the past and will persist into the future. What does change over time

is how well this principle is fulfilled through the standards of postmarketing surveillance practice and through the spirit of cooperation. Fortunately, positive interactions are occurring in this field.

A marked degree of cooperation has existed between several of the larger regulatory authorities (e.g., in the United States and France) and corporate sponsors. While some disagreements previously existed, currently exist, and probably will continue to exist, both groups approach most issues with a positive attitude toward seeking agreement and improving standards.

Most regulatory authorities have begun to allow earlier marketing of important new breakthrough medicines in exchange for sponsor guarantees to conduct adequate postmarketing surveillance studies. The most well-known example to date is zidovudine (Retrovir) of the Burroughs Wellcome Co. The early marketing of zidovudine is an important event for future breakthrough medicines. All companies would like to see this approach expanded to include most new medicines. Given current trends, however, the author believes it is doubtful that this will occur to any significant degree by the year 2000. Some skeptics state that the more rapid approval of breakthrough medicines has occurred at the expense of all other medicines. The data to prove or disprove this assertion are not yet available.

REPORTING ADVERSE REACTION DATA TO REGULATORY AUTHORITIES

Ten years ago, few regulatory authorities in industrialized countries had requirements about what types of adverse reactions they wanted reported and at what frequency the reports should be made. Practice was governed by impressions and inferences of regulators and the regulated, but was not widely codified in regulations outside of the United States and the United Kingdom. Practices such as whether or not labeled (i.e., included in the package insert) or only unlabeled adverse reactions were reported within a short specified period often differed within a country, as well as from country to country. The allowable time for reporting adverse reactions after they occurred also differed among countries, but most large regulatory agencies were primarily concerned with adverse reactions that occurred within their borders.

The situation today is quite different and some regulatory authorities (e.g., Sweden, West Germany) want to learn about all serious adverse reactions of medicines marketed in their country, regardless of where in the world the adverse reactions occur. This change has been relatively rapid and, even within a short span of 10 years has gone through several phases. Ten or more years ago, each interested regulatory authority began to evolve its own rules for types of adverse reactions to report and how frequently to report them. Each authority designed its own forms and created its own definitions. This increasingly complex situation was becoming a nightmare for pharmaceutical companies. Some described postmarketing surveillance as building a Tower of Babel. It was rapidly seen that cooperation between regulatory authorities and companies could resolve many unnecessary complexities and benefit both groups as well as physicians and, ultimately, patients.

The Council for International Organizations on Medical Sciences (CIOMS) is an informal coalition of medical associations (e.g., American Medical Association), trade associations (e.g., International Federation of Pharmaceutical Manufacturers Associations, or IFPMA), and regulatory authorities. It is a neutral forum where form, format, and content of adverse reactions reports are discussed. A working group of regulators and industry representatives initially convened in 1987 under the auspices of CIOMS and made several recommendations. A pilot test of these recommendations for alert reporting has been judged successful. This effort originally involved regulatory authorities from six countries and manufacturers from seven. Uniform forms in English were designed to promote rapid and efficient submission of relevant adverse reaction data from manufacturers to regulators. The primary goal of this program is to facilitate postmarketing reporting using common definitions and uniform reporting forms, categories, and frequencies. The final report of the CIOMS Working Group has recently been issued (CIOMS Working Group, 1990). A second phase is focusing on the content, format, and timing of reports for important adverse reactions that are labeled and not serious. This program is another example of extraordinary cooperation in the postmarketing surveillance field that has benefited all groups.

Future needs for collaborative efforts include steps to minimize, if not eliminate, variances between the forms, format, frequency, and content of all types of periodic adverse reaction reports. This is part of European Economic Community harmonization that will hopefully occur over the next decade and may be based, in part, on the CIOMS model. A more distant goal relates to the formalization and harmonization of epidemiologic studies on a worldwide basis.

ORGANIZING POSTMARKETING SURVEILLANCE ACTIVITIES WITHIN COMPANIES

Establishing Departments Within Companies

To gather, assemble, and report on adverse reactions, most research and development-based companies

have established postmarketing surveillance departments over the last decade. In 1980 there were extremely few departments in the industry, although many, if not most companies, had specific professionals to correspond with physicians who reported adverse reactions to the company. This early precursor of the modern postmarketing surveillance department is as different from the large computer-assisted postmarketing surveillance groups of today as are the accounting scribes sitting on high stools, carefully writing numbers in a ledger book in a Dickensonian novel from computer-assisted financial departments today. The modern postmarketing surveillance group designs a specific postmarketing surveillance program for each investigational medicine during Phase III. This package of studies is designed to obtain important medical data as early during the postmarketing period as possible. The postmarketing period may be considered to begin during Phase IIIb (i.e., after the regulatory submission has been made, but prior to the medicine's initial approval). The current state of postmarketing surveillance organizations within companies should be interpreted as representing important progress, and not as being an ideal state.

Data Bases Within Companies

Numerous problems remain to be resolved in the area of postmarketing surveillance. One of these is how to determine whether a pharmaceutical company with two (or more) adverse reaction surveillance sites should use a single worldwide data base or whether they should have separate data bases in each site and share information on an open and periodic basis. The pros and cons of each approach are not presented here.

It is predicted that in 10 years almost all pharmaceutical companies will have centralized their adverse reaction data reporting facilities for ease of operations. Most companies will use a single worldwide data base despite a number of important limitations and potential problems with this approach (e.g., combining adverse reaction data of different qualities). Subsetting the data within the data base according to its quality and validity will undoubtedly occur. Data may also be partitioned based on country of origin, or according to any other factor that can be flagged as the data are entered into the computer.

STANDARDS FOR ESTABLISHING ADVERSE REACTION CAUSALITY

Relevance of Causality Assessments in Clinical Trials

Causality is the assessment of a cause-and-effect relationship between two associated events. The likelihood of the cause-and-effect relationship is usually expressed in such terms as definite, probable, possible, unlikely, and definitely not. Causality assessments may be viewed on several levels. For individual patients it is often critically important to determine whether a medicine is the cause of the patient's adverse event. The specific causality assessment helps determine whether or not the medicine should be discontinued for that patient. For individual clinical trials, the causality assessment often determines whether the trial itself must be prematurely terminated. For individual companies, it is usually critically important to be aware of causal relationships between their medicines and serious adverse events that are reported. This assessment often plays a major role in the company's decision to continue or terminate the medicine's development.

Relevance of Causality Assessments in Postmarketing Surveillance Studies

For large postmarketing surveillance studies, and adverse event evaluations, the assessment of causality usually is not relevant for interpreting the data. This is because it is usually not possible to obtain sufficient information on reported adverse events to determine if they are caused by the medicine. Information obtained is often fragmentary, unverified, and of variable quality. It is often impossible to obtain sufficient additional data to answer important questions. The interpretation of such data, even from many large, well-known data bases is subject to substantial error if the data are analyzed too finely (i.e., to assess causality). Although causality has been found to be an important, and even critical, tool for Phase I and other clinical trials, it is less valuable, and sometimes even counterproductive, to evaluate causality in postmarketing studies.

Tools Used to Assess Causality

The tools to assess causality have evolved over 20 years from an emphasis on global introspection (i.e., assessment by an expert using clinical judgment, experience, and data on the specific case), to the use of algorithms (i.e., simple or complex preestablished questions that lead to an answer), to formal Bayesian logic, and finally, to the use of natural history registries to establish background rates.

Global Introspection

Up to the mid-1970s, global introspection was the method most widely used to establish causality be-

tween a medicine and an adverse event. This approach was criticized by various professionals who were able to demonstrate a lack of agreement among experts who used these methods (Kramer, 1986). Global introspection approaches also have been criticized by proponents of algorithms as being a less scientific and less valid method for establishing causality.

Algorithms

Ten years ago, we were at the height of the "algorithm phase" for establishing the causality of purported medicine-induced adverse reactions. At least 15 separate algorithms were developed and published. A highly logical approach was apparent in many of the algorithms created. It is no accident that many of them were developed by individuals trained as scientists and not by practicing clinicians.

During the decade of the 1980s a sense of frustration developed with algorithms, particularly when insufficient clinical data were available to utilize the algorithm as designed. This was particularly common with complex (i.e., elaborate) algorithms that posed many questions. Algorithms are utilized retrospectively, often when some important information either is unavailable or was never obtained. Algorithms are not patient specific and are not necessarily correlated with medical decision making. The simpler algorithms proved easiest to use.

Bayesian Approaches

A group of active professionals in this area developed a Bayesian approach to the causality issue during the mid-1980s using concepts of formal logic. This methodology is probably as able as any other method to yield a definitive answer to the cause and effect issue. The method is well suited for assessing causality for individual patients and therefore could assist clinical treatment. This approach is unsuitable, however, for medicines for which a great deal of data are unavailable, because the method requires a substantial amount of prior knowledge. Therefore, the method is only useful for medicines in Phases III and IV. This method is also extremely time consuming and is not appropriate to use except when the importance of the clinical question justifies the use of a relatively large amount of resources (see Jones, 1985).

Present and Future Approaches

At present the need to assess causality during clinical trials differs from the need to assess it during postmarketing surveillance. Clinical trials must consider it.

In the future, as well as today, when serious unlabeled adverse reactions arise in clinical trials, a sponsor might want to use *both* global introspection and a moderately simple/complex algorithm. If results differ, the author would place more reliance on the former method to establish the strength of the association of the event with the medicine.

Natural History Epidemiology

For postmarketing surveillance studies there will be an increased demand for natural history epidemiology. This means that registries of the natural history of diseases will be used more in the future to establish the background rate(s) of adverse events in patients with that disease. This information will be compared with medicine-induced rates. Comparing the rates for medicine-related adverse events with rates obtained in natural history registries will be more important for postmarketing surveillance evaluations than for focusing on the attribution of individual adverse events with the medicine.

Registries of Adverse Event Data

Several registries that gathered adverse event data in selected therapeutic areas were founded prior to the 1980s. In the United States this includes National Registry of Drug-Induced Ocular Side Effects, Registry of Tissue Reactions to Drugs, and Hepatic Events Registry. The Dermatological Adverse Drug Reaction Reporting System was begun in 1980.

STANDARDS OF METHODOLOGY FOR POSTMARKETING SURVEILLANCE STUDIES

Several large and costly postmarketing surveillance cohort studies (e.g., prazocin, cimetidine) had been mounted by 1980 with a goal of enrolling approximately 10,000 patients each. This number had a somewhat mystical connotation and was often described as representing a balance between the minimum size necessary to observe most rare adverse events (i.e., those with an incidence of less than 1 in 3,000) and the maximum size that could be practically managed by a single company. Standard methods of assembling large cohorts of patients (e.g., conducting multicenter studies) were used for these postmarketing surveillance studies. These methods were usually applied to all medicines for which prospective postmarketing surveillance was considered, rather than custom designing different approaches for particular medicines. Postmarketing surveillance studies sometimes involved retrospective analyses of data already collected, to look for increased incidence rates of adverse reactions in specific groups of patients.

The balance between conducting retrospective and prospective studies has switched over the last decade from a preponderance of large, prospective, cohort studies to a preponderance of studies involving a retrospective or mixed examination of data in large multipurpose, automated, linked data bases. The pendulum has also swung from most information and signals about possible adverse reactions coming from passive intelligence gathering to a greater proportion of signals coming from active searching of published literature and more active solicitation and evaluation of spontaneously generated reports.

Cardinal Rule for Large Automated Multipurpose Data Bases

The most important single change in postmarketing surveillance over the last decade has been the development and use of large, automated, multipurpose data bases to evaluate purported medicine-induced adverse reactions. *The cardinal rule today for using these multipurpose data bases for record linkage studies is that patient diagnoses must be confirmed.* Without this essential step, erroneous interpretations and conclusions based on misclassifications of patients are possible.

Clusters of Adverse Events

The same principle of validation also applies to other types of studies, such as those of clusters of adverse events. This situation is well known to public health investigators. For example, a report that 50 people who had emesis at a dinner party all ate the chicken salad, or that 50 people who lived in a polluted environment developed cancer, must be checked carefully. It may turn out in the former case that there was a contact psychological reaction that began when someone was overheated and felt nauseous; and in the latter case, many of the people involved may have had unassociated types of cancers or may have only recently moved to the area.

RAD-AR

The discipline of postmarketing surveillance is currently in the midst of a substantial effort to develop additional and broader large automated, linked, multipurpose data bases. Without sufficient linkages within each data base and without a sufficient number of data bases, it is impossible to address relevant postmarketing surveillance questions and important issues adequately. Risk Assessment of Drugs—Analysis and

Response (RAD-AR) is an important industry-wide group (initiated by Ciba-Geigy) that helps build sufficient data base capacity for pharmacoepidemiology, and helps clarify the relationship between medicine benefits and risks. This group has four major functions or goals:

1. To explore and support the appropriate role of epidemiology in the pharmaceutical industry
2. To serve as a forum for exchanging epidemiology and related information
3. To serve as a coordinating group for intercompany activities relating to epidemiology
4. To act as a liaison between the pharmaceutical industry and other organizations (e.g., regulatory agencies, universities) for epidemiology-related activities.

One of RAD-AR's first projects was to assemble and issue a four-volume series titled *International Drug Benefit/Risk Assessment Data Resource Handbook* (Pharma Corporation and the Degge Group, 1988). The four volumes cover North America, United Kingdom, Japan, and West Germany/The Netherlands/Switzerland. These volumes are the most complete list of sources of data bases and available information. RAD-AR has achieved success at both the national and international levels. At the national level, numerous groups have evaluated pharmacoepidemiologic methods, standards, and capacity within their own country. At the international level, RAD-AR has achieved a network of many national groups and has helped foster the formation of the International Society of Pharmacoepidemiology.

Large Automated Data Bases: Present and Future

Major pharmaceutical industry resources are currently being spent to evaluate current data bases in terms of validity of diagnoses and data, as well as completeness and linkability. Numerous large automated data bases with record linkage currently exist, primarily in the United States, and are described elsewhere in the text. By the year 2000 many more will probably have been established in most other countries where new medicines are developed. One of the keys to developing more large linked data bases outside the United States is their endorsement by large international health organizations (e.g., the World Health Organization). That would encourage some countries to overcome their current reluctance to build such data bases. This reluctance is often based on the perceived need to protect the privacy of individuals.

These large data bases will become more efficient in the future as they are used to address important postmarketing surveillance questions. Most of the existing data bases are available to companies on a contractual basis. They include data bases of health maintenance organizations, states, Medicaid, consortiums of hospitals, and selected registries. It should be noted that these data bases were not designed with pharmacoepidemiology studies in mind, and they differ significantly from each other in the data they collect and their ability for linking different types of data. As a result, there are numerous pros and cons of using each data base from a pharmacoepidemiologic viewpoint.

Prescription Event Monitoring

Current major experiments in postmarketing surveillance methodology include Prescription Event Monitoring (PEM) by the Drug Safety Research Unit (DSRU) in England. This technique involves systematic sampling of up to a million prescriptions per year, chosen (from 350 million written) because of the medicine prescribed. Each of the prescribing physicians of these million prescriptions is sent a green form requesting information on whether the prescription involved a new diagnosis, referral, unexpected improvement, or change of treatment, and on whether any adverse event occurred. The goal of the DSRU is to conduct PEM on all new major chemical entity medicines used within the National Health Service. Eventually, PEM may also be used to test specific hypotheses in England (Wales, Scotland, and Ireland are not included in this survey).

Caveats and Cautions in Interpreting Prescription Event Data

Data obtained through PEM must be interpreted with a great deal of caution because (1) patient diagnoses are not confirmed and validated, (2) a causal relationship of an adverse event with a medicine cannot actually be established, and (3) a high reporting rate of adverse reactions may falsely suggest that the medicine is less safe to use than others. For example, if a new medicine is promoted as being *less* liable than others to cause a certain adverse reaction, physicians will tend to place more of their high-risk patients (for getting that adverse event) on the medicine. Thus, a higher rate of that adverse experience may be noted with the medicine, but may not reflect a true incidence figure for that adverse reaction.

Results of PEM and other population-based methods are expected to differ from data obtained in medicine development studies sponsored by pharmaceutical companies. This is because the adverse reaction profile of a relatively healthy or select group of patients receiving a medicine, in a study conducted in a limited patient population (e.g., in clinical trials), will differ from the adverse reaction profile obtained in *all* patients in a large population who receive the medicine. However, many physicians do not return *any* data on their patients to the DSRU, and the data returned may not represent a true cross section of what is occurring. Even if physicians return data to the DSRU, the validity of the data is uncertain. Moreover, the background incidence of most adverse events measured is unknown. Thus, without population controls, excesses in frequency are difficult to interpret. The type(s) of patients who are prescribed new medicines is also unknown. One final drawback of PEM is that it requires a minimum of several months to gather sufficient data, whereas a multipurpose automated data base may take only 1 hour or even less to obtain suggestive postmarketing surveillance results.

Epidemiologic Intelligence

Epidemiologic intelligence from sentinel sources such as physician observations in letters sent to pharmaceutical companies, regulatory agencies, and the literature will remain an important source of information for identifying the adverse reactions that should be further evaluated. Allegations from the media of important medical risks from marketed medicines will also remain a mechanism to trigger responses in both companies and regulatory agencies.

ESTABLISHMENT OF STANDARDS AND GUIDELINES FOR CONDUCT OF POSTMARKETING SURVEILLANCE ACTIVITIES

Joint Commission on Prescription Drug Use

Prior to the Joint Commission on Prescription Drug Use, there were no guidelines or standards for postmarketing surveillance studies. The United States Congress established a commission (Joint Commission on Prescription Drug Use) in 1976 "to describe a postmarketing surveillance system that could be used to detect, quantitate, and describe the anticipated and unanticipated effects of marketed drugs, and to recommend a means by which information on the epidemiology of prescription drug use in the U.S. could be distributed regularly to interested parties in the United States." The commission's final report was issued on January 23, 1980 (Melmon, 1980) and contained five major recommendations, as follows:

1. A systematic and comprehensive system of postmarketing drug surveillance should be developed in the United States.
2. Such a system should be able to detect important adverse drug reactions that occur more frequently than once per thousand uses of a drug, to develop methods to detect less frequent reactions and to evaluate the beneficial effects of drugs as used in ordinary practice. New methods will have to be developed for the study of delayed drug effects, including both therapeutic and adverse effects.
3. An integral function of the postmarketing surveillance system should be to report the uses and effects of new and old prescription drugs.
4. Recognizing the progress that the Food and Drug Administration (FDA) has made in the area of postmarketing drug surveillance in the last 3 years, the Commission recommends that postmarketing surveillance should be a priority program of the FDA and that the FDA should continue to strengthen its program in this area.
5. A private, nonprofit Center for Drug Surveillance should be established to further the development of a postmarketing surveillance system in the United States. This center should foster cooperation among existing postmarketing surveillance programs, develop new methods for carrying out surveillance, train scientists in the disciplines needed for doing postmarketing surveillance, and educate both providers and recipients of prescription drugs about the effects of these drugs.

The first four recommendations have been initiated to a large degree by the FDA and the pharmaceutical industry in the United States, working jointly as well as independently. The last recommendation has not been implemented, but the need for a national center could certainly be debated.

Grahame–Smith Working Party

In the United Kingdom, a group analogous to the Joint Commission on Prescription Drug Use was the Grahame-Smith Working Party. There are currently no formal requirements, however, that serve as standards for postmarketing surveillance studies in either country.

Is There a Need for Standards and Guidelines?

Many regulatory agencies believe that there should be formal criteria or decisional standards to determine what medicines require tests, what types of studies are needed, and how postmarketing surveillance studies should be established, monitored, and reported. In other words, many groups believe that the postmarketing period of a medicine's life should be evaluated as systematically and carefully as the premarketing period. There are generally well-designed standards for the premarketing period of new chemical entities and these are being reviewed in a search for appropriate postmarketing surveillance standards.

No guidelines existed for postmarketing surveillance in 1980. Ten years ago, the data used and combined in postmarketing surveillance often contained contaminants (inaccurate or incomplete data), and data were not validated for accuracy. The few studies conducted were mainly designed by clinical groups without training in epidemiologic methods. There were no guidelines at regulatory agencies to decide which medicines should be subject to postmarketing surveillance studies.

Proposed Guidelines

A set of 19 guidelines for postmarketing surveillance was proposed (Joint Committee of ABPI, BMA, CSM, and RCGP, 1988) by a joint committee of the Association of the British Pharmaceutical Industry (ABPI), the British Medical Association (BMA), the Committee on Safety of Medicines (CSM), and the Royal College of General Practitioners (RCGP). These guidelines were particularly developed for observational cohort studies sponsored by pharmaceutical companies.

These 19 points are primarily principles and managerial guidelines rather than scientific guidelines or standards useful for the design and conduct of postmarketing surveillance studies. The British guidelines include a definition of postmarketing surveillance and describe basic principles underlying most studies (e.g., there should be a valid medical reason for undertaking the study). The guidelines state that studies should not be designed solely for promotional purposes, and that any breaches of this guideline are to be reported to the Code of Practice Committee of the ABPI. Another guideline is that appropriate fees may be paid to physicians for completing data forms, but no other financial inducements may be offered. These guidelines might best be viewed as starting points for the development of scientific guidelines.

Investigational New Drug Application (IND) and New Drug Application (NDA) rewrites, plus regulatory commentary and additional guidelines written by the FDA during the 1980s indicate gradually increasing and clarified regulatory requirements on what adverse event data to report. This pertains to adverse events that occur in clinical trials as well as after the medicine is marketed. The frequency and timing of these reports are also more precisely specified, both for short-term serious, unexpected, and unlabeled adverse events, and for those included in quarterly or annual reports.

Current Activities at the Pharmaceutical Manufacturers Association

In the United States, the Emerging Epidemiological Monitoring Techniques Committee of the Pharma-

ceutical Manufacturers Association (PMA) is actively and aggressively exploring the development of standards for the field of postmarketing surveillance equivalent to Good Laboratory Practices. Forty companies are participating in discussions on this topic. In sharing their problems and perspectives, they have followed the public health approach that encourages multiple groups to work together to help protect the well-being of patients using pharmaceutical products. Many practices that were standard 5 years ago are no longer acceptable today.

Pharmaceutical Companies' Views on Postmarketing Surveillance Guidelines

Most research-and-development-based pharmaceutical companies are opposed to the establishment of regulatory guidelines for the postmarketing period. They do not believe that the FDA has the regulatory authority or mandate to put forth these guidelines. Thus, no guidelines currently determine which medicines require postmarketing surveillance studies in the United States and what types of studies to perform. These decisions are handled on an individual basis between the sponsor and regulatory agency. The European Economic Community is looking for concordance with the United States and it is hoped that a general consensus between these groups can be reached. As a general principle, any guidelines enacted should consider the ability of sponsors to conduct postmarketing surveillance studies with available methods and data bases, and should not force sponsors to adopt standards and methods that are beyond current capabilities.

More formal postmarketing surveillance guidelines will undoubtedly exist in the future. It is hoped that these scientific guidelines will be put together as a consensus of all interested parties and will represent state-of-the-art scientific principles that are realistic to achieve. Setting standards that are unrealistic in terms of methodologies or resources required to meet those standards will be counterproductive and not in the best interests of patients, the ultimate group for whom standards are created.

STANDARDS FOR REGULATORY AGENCY CONDUCT REGARDING POSTMARKETING SURVEILLANCE STUDIES

"Fishing Expeditions"

An undesirable pseudoscientific practice of the past has been termed the "fishing expedition." In this nonscientific method, someone at a regulatory agency or academic center with access to a large data base would punch into his or her keyboard the name of a medicine and a number of adverse medical events to determine whether any association existed. If an academician, in his or her initial evaluation, found a higher rate of adverse events associated with a medicine than anticipated, then an academic paper or a letter to the editor often resulted. The report could be picked up by the media or by a regulatory authority and pursued further. If a regulatory person conducted this fishing expedition, then they would ask the relevant company how they intended to respond to any associations found. This letter might require the company to conduct a survey or study, but at the minimum would require that the company respond. Because of the ease of deriving possible associations by looking at one adverse event across multiple medicines or by examining various patient populations and multiple adverse events for a single medicine, a single individual could potentially keep the entire pharmaceutical industry busy investigating such associations. This could occur despite the fact that most, or almost all, of these associations were not meaningful and could not be confirmed.

Obviously, the actual situation never deteriorated to this extent, and it is currently scientifically unacceptable for causality assessments to be derived in this nonscientific manner. Associations that should (or must) be analyzed usually arise from case studies, in the literature, or from reports received by a company or regulatory authority from physicians, sales representatives, or other sources.

Regulatory Authority Publications of Purported Associations of Medicines and Adverse Events

Both the FDA in the United States and the Department of Health (DoH) in the United Kingdom periodically publish reports of purported associations. For example, if either agency receives an increased frequency of blood dyscrasia reports occurring with a particular medicine, they will often include those data in the newsletter that all physicians receive. Their intention is quite worthwhile, i.e., to alert physicians about a potential problem and to seek additional data to define better the numerator and denominator of its incidence. Unfortunately, this method may have the effect of eliciting many additional reports that complicate rather than simplify the assessment of a medicine's benefits and risks.

Recommended Approaches for Regulatory Authorities Regarding Adverse Events

In the future, perhaps all regulatory agencies will adopt a more logical and scientifically sound approach to in-creased frequencies of reports of known adverse reactions or to reports of serious new adverse reactions. The first step should be to contact the medicine's sponsor, manufacturer, or distributor and to notify them of the purported medicine-induced adverse reaction. One company's response may be to dispatch trained monitors to visit the sites where the reported cases occurred and to evaluate all available data. At the same time, both the company and regulatory agency would review their existing data bases to determine what cases were previously reported and the details of those cases. Potentially, these assessments could better establish the importance of the signal, evaluate whether specific risk factors were involved in the cases, and describe any characteristics common to two or more of the cases. Benefit-to-risk assessments would be determined and a meeting would be arranged (if necessary) to plan the next stage of follow-up.

Any one or more of the following additional steps could be taken. A group of experts from academia and/or government could be brought together to review the data and make recommendations. The regulatory authority or sponsor could issue a notification to all physicians in the country, in order to seek further information (i.e., examples). At this point, it would have to be determined if the name of the specific drug or just the chemical or therapeutic class of the medicine should be identified. The latter approach would prevent biasing physicians against a single medicine, and would also minimize the chance of a "fishing expedition." This approach would determine more fairly whether the adverse reaction was characteristic of an entire class of medicines. Large, automated, multipurpose data bases could be used to evaluate the hypothesis. Other types of epidemiologic studies could also be conducted. Additional prospective epidemiologic studies could be undertaken to evaluate the adverse reaction. Finally, if specific risk factors were identified and the benefit-to-risk consideration dictated that specific patients should not receive the medicine, then package labeling changes could be negotiated and the new data disseminated using a variety of techniques.

CONCLUSIONS

This brief discussion illustrates some of the vast changes in postmarketing surveillance that have evolved over the last 15 years and indicates a number of potential future trends. The field has moved from its own Dark Ages of the 1970s, when little consensus and no standards existed, into the light of the 1990s. Pharmacoepidemiology needs to continue to move forward and further develop and refine the scientific standards and guiding principles that represent signs of a more mature discipline. It is for the practitioners of pharmacoepidemiology individually or through appropriate organizations to accept this challenge. Let us hope that the scientific growth of the field of postmarketing surveillance and the development of standards for its conduct continue, and that the once fledgling and fragmented field reaches adulthood by the turn of the next century.

CHAPTER 121

Developing Medicines Worldwide

OBJECTIVE OF AN INTERNATIONAL DEVELOPMENT PROGRAM

Multinational companies with discovery and development activities in two or more countries are increasingly stressing the value and importance of coordinated activities (Reich and Hilleman, 1985). The objectives of this approach are generally straightforward and similar for most companies to (1) increase the efficiency and speed of each medicine's international development, (2) increase the commitment of all parts of the company to the international objectives, (3) increase the efficiency and speed of the overall development, and (4) increase the ability to pursue a more sophisticated and proactive licensing policy.

ORGANIZATION OF A MULTINATIONAL COMPANY: FIVE MODELS

A simplified view of large multinational companies is described. These models view companies as primarily utilizing a centralized, decentralized, or balanced approach to conducting their business. Nonetheless, each model is part of a continuum.

Model A: Centralized—Dictatorial Style

In the centralized model (Fig. 121.1), the real power and decisions within the company are made at the company's headquarters. Most important decisions are made by a single leader, a committee, or a combination of the two. The subsidiary sites that conduct research, production, marketing, and other functions are primarily directed from the central site. Modifications of the centralized directives to the subsidiaries requested by local representatives must be approved at the central location.

Local physicians must submit protocols (or at least summaries) to the central headquarters for approval before they may initiate and sponsor a clinical trial.

Model B: Centralized—Collaborative Style

This model differs from the above in that the central headquarters solicits input from subsidiaries before making decisions (Fig. 121.1 with arrows in both directions). The decisions are made, nonetheless, by the central headquarters.

Model C: Equality of Major Sites—Collaborative Style

Two or more development sites are considered as equals in developing and managing clinical development (Fig. 121.2). This model contains both centralized and decentralized elements. The two major sites collaborate and attempt to function as a single central authority. The areas in which each of the other peripheral groups (i.e., subsidiary sites) retains autonomy and in which the joint central authority predominates should be clearly specified.

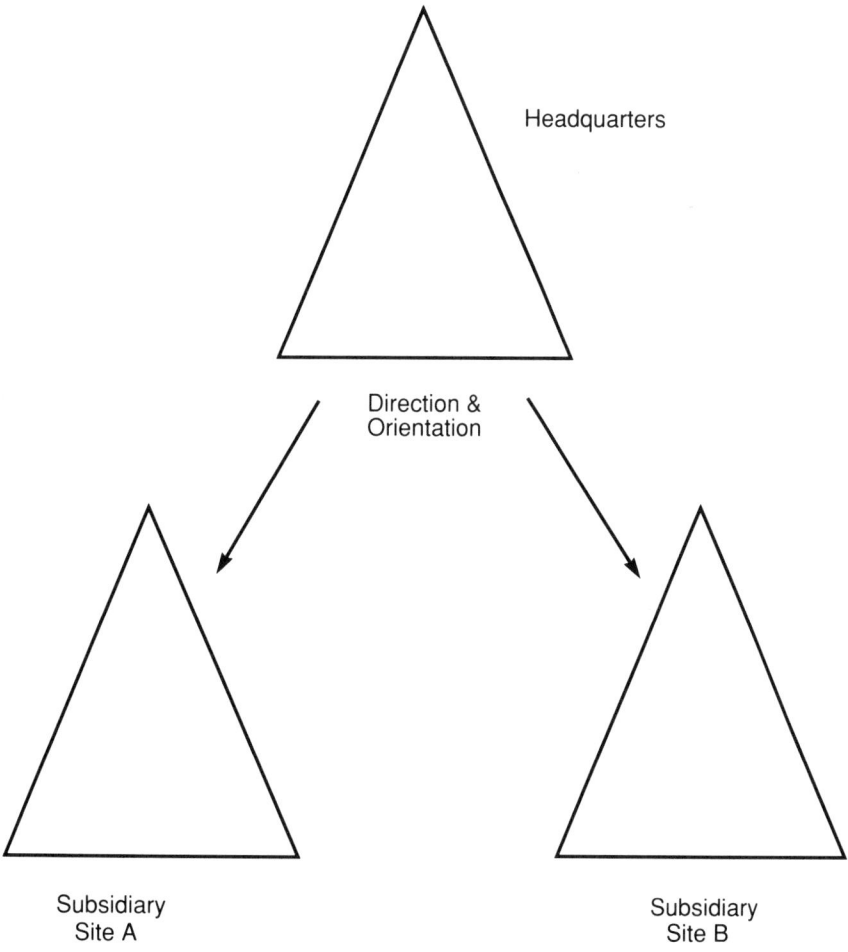

FIG. 121.1 Centralized model of internationally organizing two (or more) subsidiaries that conduct development activities on new medicines. Direction and orientation emanate from the centralized headquarters.

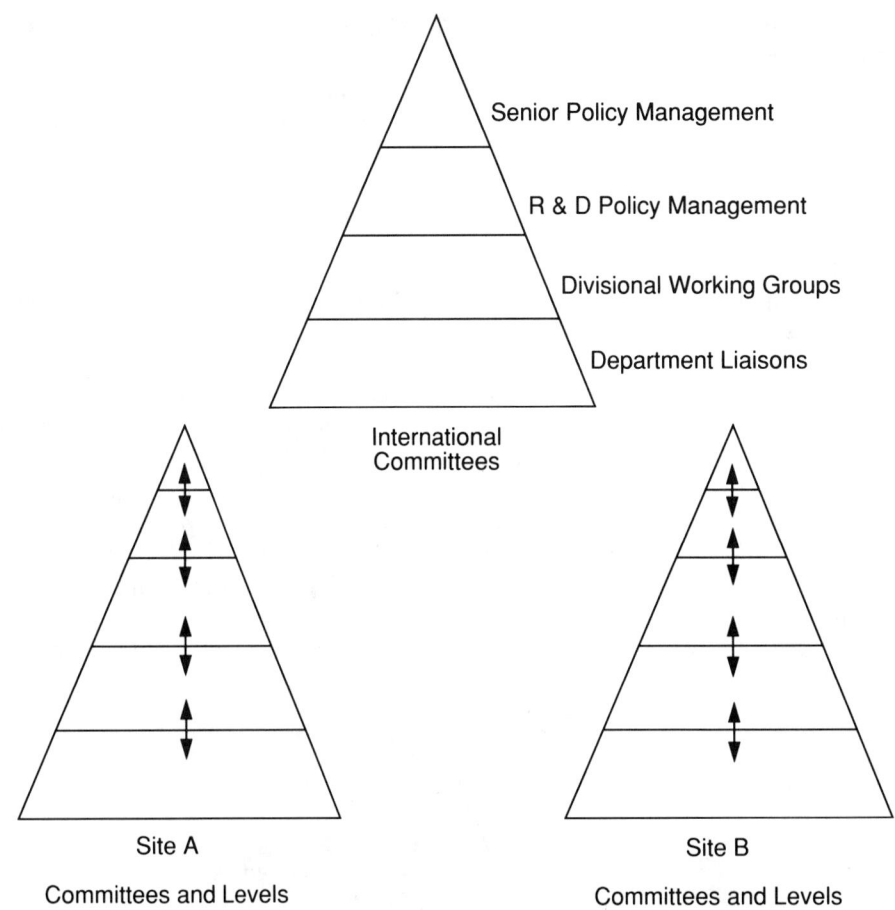

FIG. 121.2 A separate series of international committees may be established to manage and coordinate international development activities on new medicines. Communications flow both up and down within each site both prior to and after the meetings of international committees. This approach may operate for a centralized, equal-partner, or decentralized model. R & D, research and development.

Model D: Decentralized Sites—Semiautonomous-Coordinated Style

In the decentralized model (Figs. 121.2 or 121.3), the relative independence and decision making of subsidiary sites is substantial in some or all operating areas. One extreme occurs when each of the peripheral sites or regions retains autonomy over most of their actions and decides which of the parent company's medicines each wishes to develop and market. The central site may or may not have a core package of data available to obtain regulatory approval, which is supplemented by clinical trials conducted in the local countries or regions. Financially, the subsidiary may be relatively dependent or independent of the central site. Local laws govern many aspects of company behavior that affect the degree of autonomy possible. Some of the advantages and disadvantages of the centralized and decentralized models are listed in Table 121.1.

Model E: Decentralized Sites—Totally Autonomous Style

The sites are not coordinated in any formal way (Fig. 121.3). Each site retains its autonomy to develop medicines independently. Companies may change along this scale over time. Also, part of a company may operate using one model and another part of the same company may use a different model. This is particularly possible for decentralized companies or for those in which one or more parts are run independently (e.g., agricultural business, pesticide business).

A Different Type of Model

Another model of multinational pharmaceutical organizations is of a conglomerate consisting of several independent companies. Each of these companies is au-

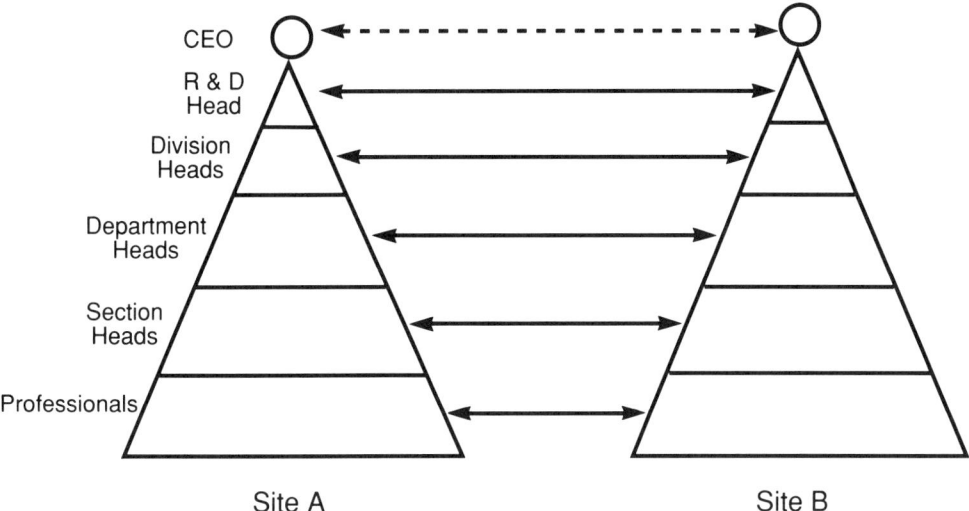

FIG. 121.3 The independent development site model. This model could also be used to show the equal-partner development site model with joint collaborative decisions flowing up and down throughout each pyramid as well as between similar levels at each site conducting development activities on new medicines. The decentralized development site model would have dotted lines between the comparable levels of each site conducting development activities on new medicines. R & D, research and development.

tonomous and may have its own approach to medicine development. Each company within the conglomerate may emphasize a centralized, decentralized, or balanced approach to management.

Meetings of regional directors or general managers with the overall board of directors or chairman of the board may be a forum at which the appropriate balance is established and maintained. The central board of

TABLE 121.1 *Pros and cons of centralized versus decentralized forms of corporate management*

A. Centralized management advantages
  1. Clearer understanding by all employees in terms of who is setting the corporate course, making decisions, and giving directions
  2. Allows integration of overall strategies
  3. Enables the entire corporation to change direction most easily
B. Centralized management disadvantages
  1. Local territories may lose their identity, image, and control of studies, regulatory submissions, marketing strategies, and other business decisions
  2. Centralized management may not be sufficiently sensitive to ideas coming from subsidiary companies or satellites
C. Decentralized management advantages
  1. Sensitive to local needs in each territory
  2. Allows many units to have some autonomy and to be differentially treated
  3. Permits more rapid decision making and action in response to local issues
D. Decentralized management disadvantages
  1. More duplication of effort occurs, at least some of which is unnecessary and unproductive
  2. More difficulties are present in communications between territories and headquarters and between one territory and another

directors may establish policies within which regional and local directors may operate according to clearly established guidelines. Needs of local directors also flow up through the organization in this system.

WORLDWIDE STRATEGIES AND SYSTEMS

Clinical strategies and development plans are discussed extensively in Chapters 112 to 115 and will not be repeated here. The major issue is for the international group to choose the best possible strategy and to then assign work to the various sites involved in development activities.

Three models of approaches to developing international systems that can be developed are shown in Fig. 121.4. These systems primarily involve computer links to transfer information. One modification of approach B is to have a satellite of site A at site B and a satellite of site B at site A to enable communications to occur. This approach may be used when sites A and B are unable to communicate directly because of differences in hardware or software. Another approach to viewing this international system at a more detailed level is shown in Fig. 121.5.

International Steering Group

Even with the best of intentions, work on international projects at two or more sites tends to move away from

Model A: Common System

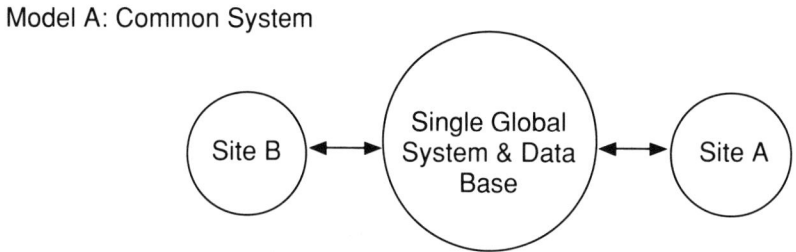

Model B: Compatible Systems: Varies from Identical Systems to Totally Different Systems at Each Site

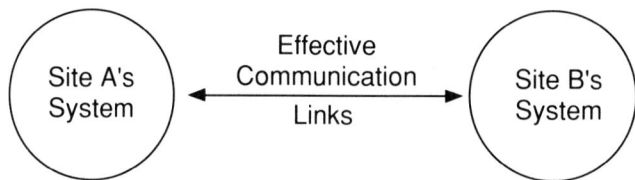

Model C: Incompatible Systems

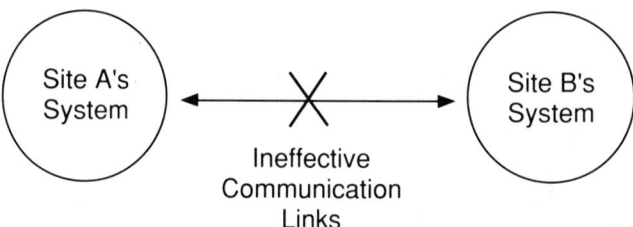

FIG. 121.4 Models of international systems for medicine development, relating to communications between hardware and software.

the agreed-upon plans over time. The potential reasons for this are many: (1) key individuals leave the company or are transferred, (2) new employees cannot be hired and trained as rapidly as anticipated, (3) priorities shift on other projects and affect the project in question, (4) new regulatory events arise that affect the project more at one site, or (5) new medical findings occur that affect progress or direction of the project at one site. It is thus essential for a committee to meet at regular intervals to ensure that different groups are following the agreed-upon strategies. This steering group oversees all international projects to "steer" them in the appropriate direction, both individually and collectively. In summary, an international steering group should decide which indications, dosage forms, and clinical trials *should* be studied and which *can* be studied with available resources. They may constitute a subgroup of experts to review quality of life and pharmacoeconomic trials. The group should also determine which trials can be contracted out. This group must also prevent the Himalaya Syndrome.

Himalaya Syndrome

Some people who establish certain clinical trials do so simply "because they are there." Even though the need to conduct certain clinical trials may appear to be obvious, such trials could represent tangents of scientific interest and could be either delayed until Phase IV or omitted entirely from the development program. Professionals in the academic community are always seeking to conduct meaningful clinical trials and might appreciate an opportunity to conduct trials with great scientific merit.

International Meetings within a Single Pharmaceutical Company

When two separate development sites are involved as equals, meetings may often:

1. Rotate venue between the two sites
2. Rotate the chair between each site

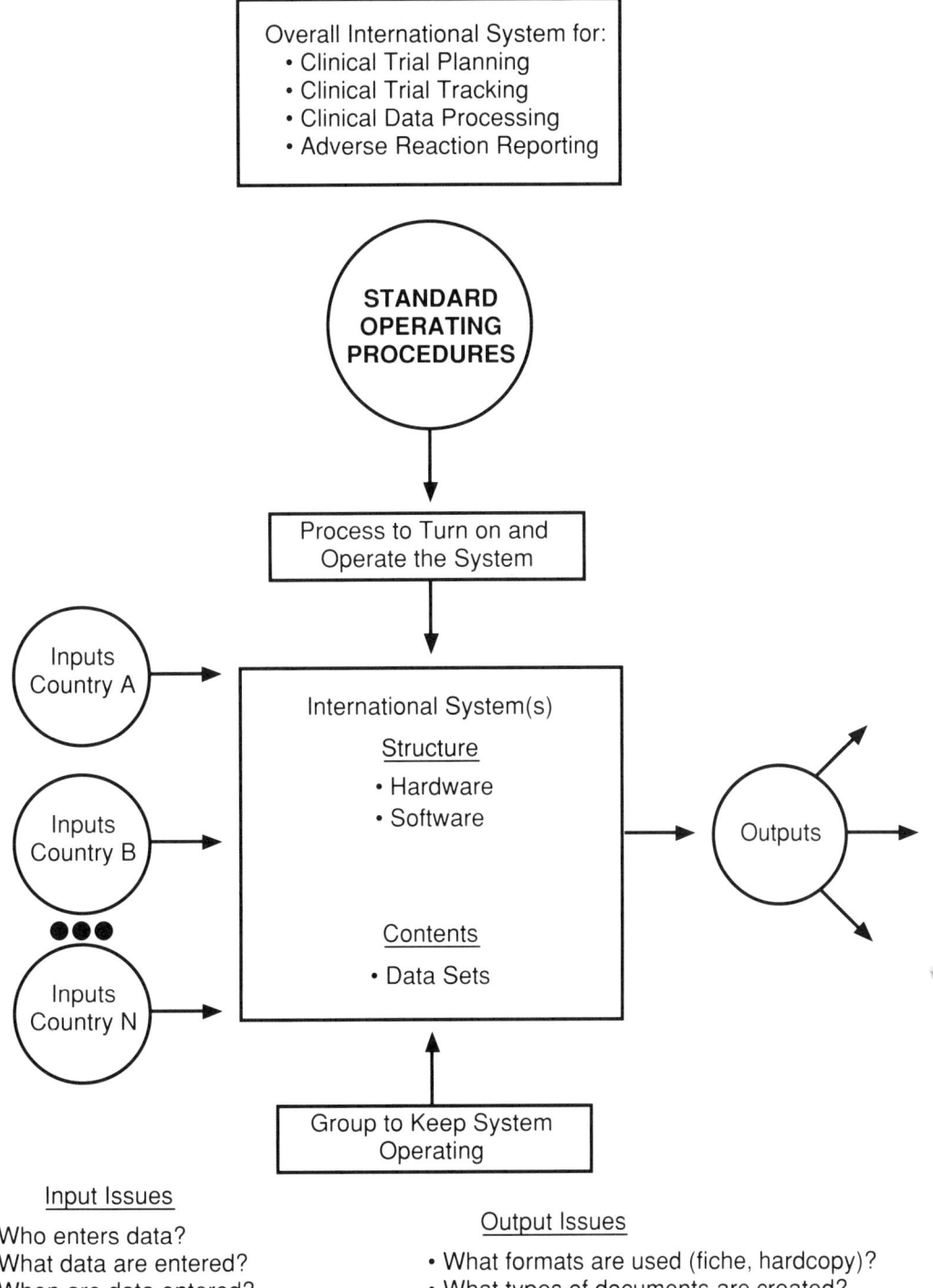

FIG. 121.5 How standard operating procedures, inputs, and outputs relate to international systems used to develop new medicines.

3. Have an equal number of representatives from each site who are at equal managerial positions
4. Have each site present their views on an issue and then get a consensus view if possible—or identify each site's views on points where they differ

WORLDWIDE PROJECT TEAMS

The worldwide project team is a group of individuals who plan and execute the activities needed to achieve the goals of worldwide development. Membership on

A. Centralized (Controlled/Shared) Model

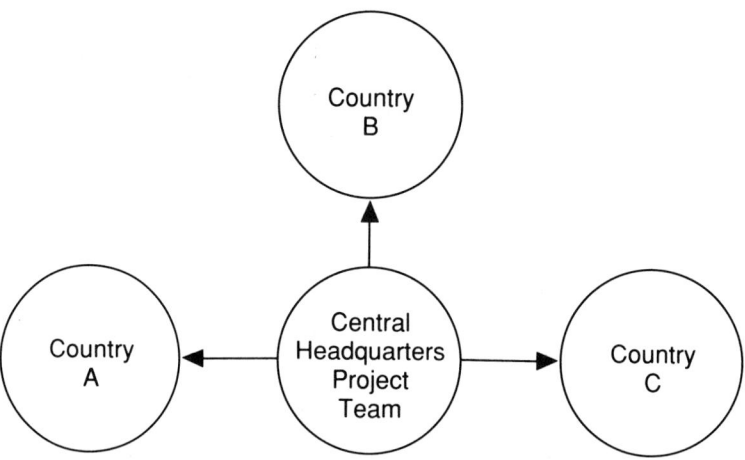

B. Decentralized (Independent) Model

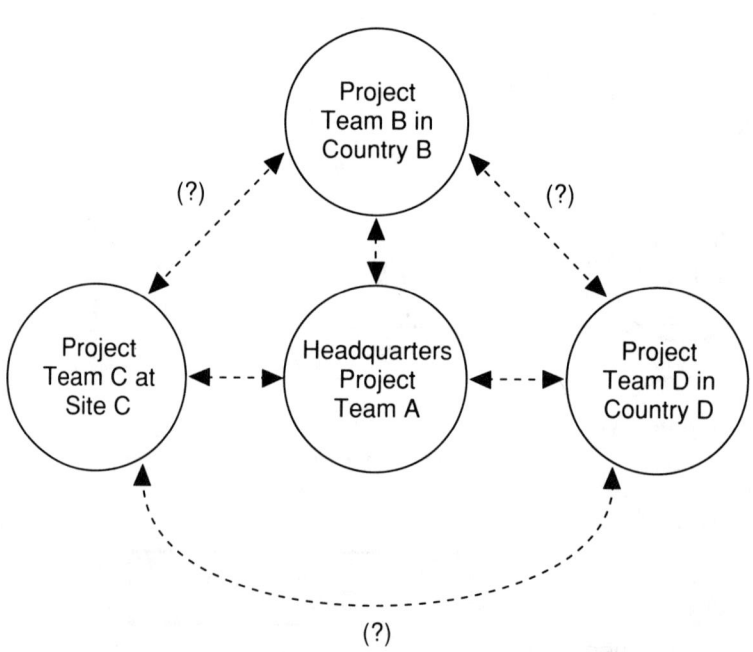

FIG. 121.6 Models of project teams that may be created for international medicine development. (Reprinted from Spilker 1989a, with permission of Raven Press.)

the team will probably include at some point during the life of the project (or perhaps for its duration) representatives of research and development (e.g., preclinical sciences, clinical, toxicology, regulatory, chemical development, technical development, metabolism, statistics), marketing, production, and coordination departments.

Although some companies develop a new medicine by utilizing a single international project team, many others operate with separate teams at each independent research and development site in addition to or instead of a worldwide team. Each site may have a project team leader and their own team. The teams may coordinate their activities through various mech-

C. Network (Integrated) Model

D. Combination Model of Panels B and C

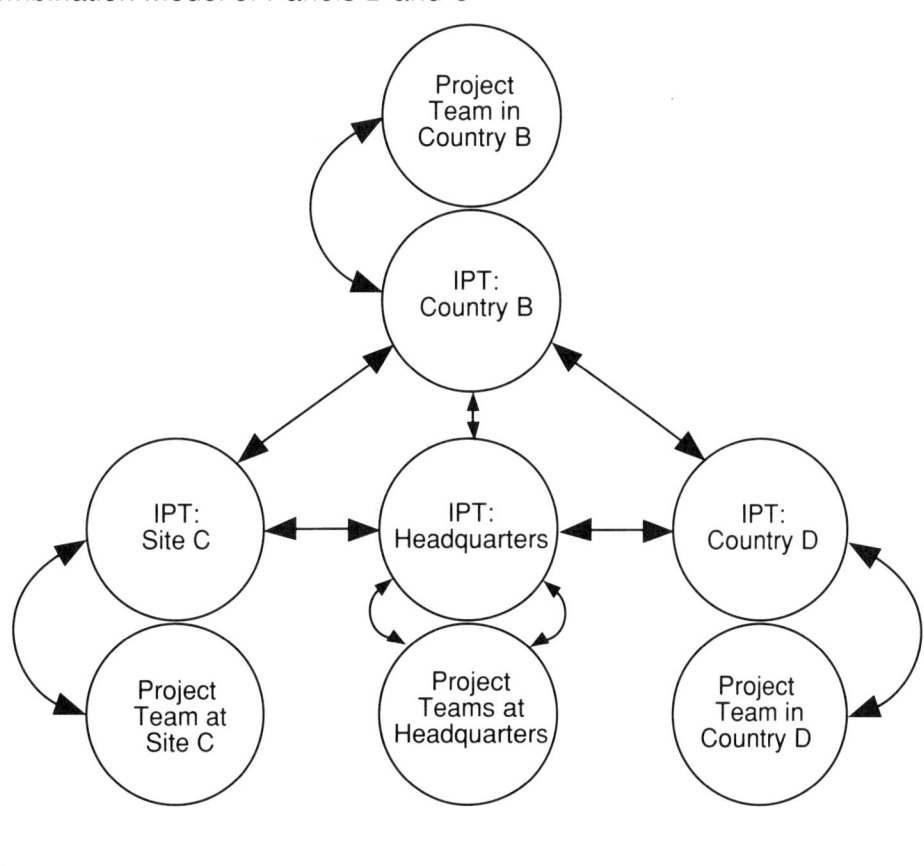

◀------ =Primarily informal relationships and influences
◀——— =Primarily formal relationships and influences (i.e., control)

FIG. 121.6 (*Continued*)

anisms (e.g., memoranda, telephone calls, visits) or they may each report to a central management group or individual who coordinates their efforts. This individual would generally be part of a matrix system or senior management. An international group composed of some of the members from each site could also function in the role of coordinating the overall activities of the various independent project teams, which are developing all of the company's investigational medicines. Models of project teams are shown in Fig. 121.6.

Model of Interactions Between Project Leaders and Members in Different Sites

Unless a company developing medicines at two (or more) sites has specific policies governing interactions of clinical and other staff between sites, many people will be uncertain about the appropriate procedures to use in many situations. Figure 121.7 shows a model intended to provide a communications framework that could be modified as necessary. The model illustrates a means of conceptualizing interactions within the matrix system. It does not relate to the traditional line management organization.

The following points may be made based on the model:

1. Requests for specific information, material, data, or work from the project team should be funnelled through the project member of the relevant department at site I to his or her counterpart at site II after appropriate approvals at site I. Copies of requests and correspondence should be sent to project leaders and appropriate management.

2. Project leaders at the two sites should communicate directly on project-related matters, but should not directly request help or services that would be appropriately dealt with by specific departments at either site. Those requests should flow via the other pathways shown.

3. Interactions between the two sites related to requests (as opposed to general conversations or vis-

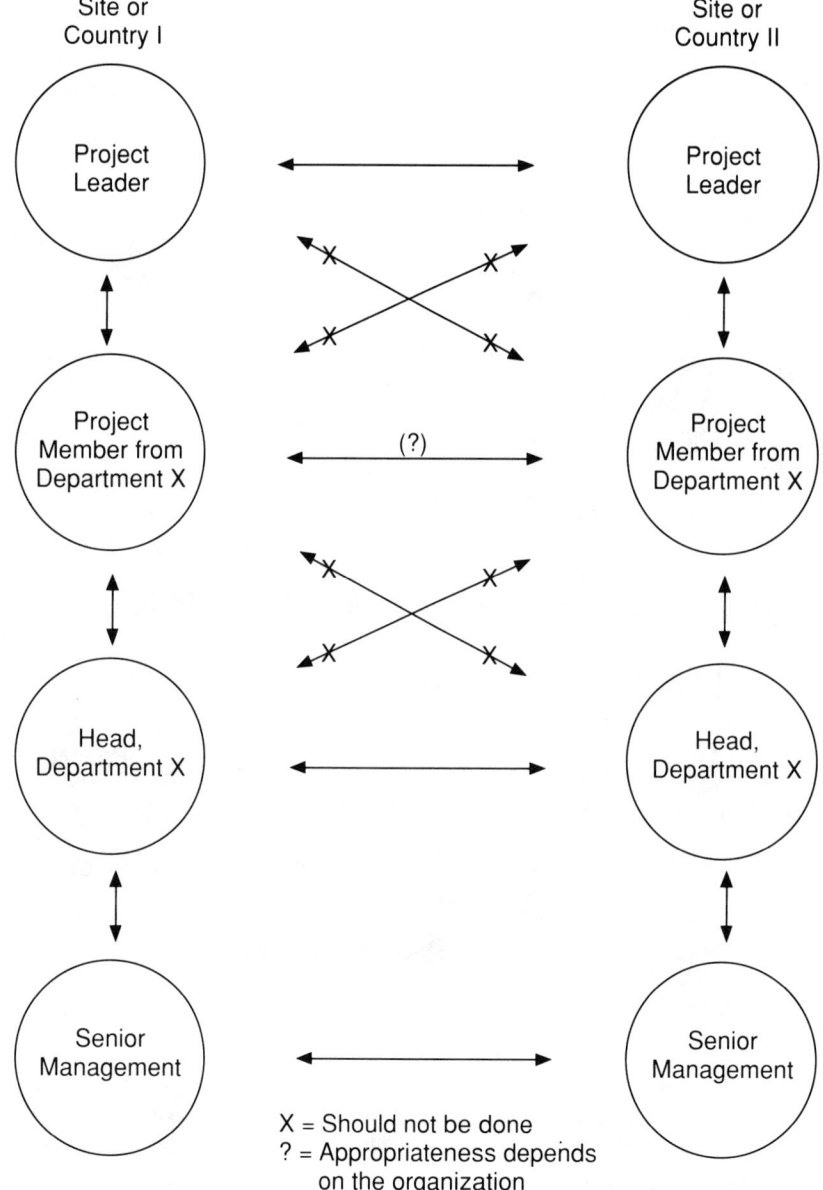

FIG. 121.7 Model for communications of various individuals and groups within and between two sites developing new medicines.

its) should not proceed from project leaders in either site directly to project members (or their department heads) in the opposite site. Similarly, interactions related to requests from project members at either site should not go directly to project leaders at the opposite site.

4. A department head may wish to have all intersite interactions proceed between department heads. A policy within a department should be adhered to by the project representative from that department and the project team.

5. For projects that only operate at one site the same general system of communication should operate. For example, if a project exists at site I, then the project liaison or correspondent at site II should take the place (in the model) of the project leader. This means that the site I project leader would use the top pathway in the same manner as when there is an official project in both sites. Project members at site I would act through their department head or via the project leader, because there would not be any project members at site II.

6. Although this model illustrates lines of direct letter or phone communication, copies of documents should be disseminated to all relevant individuals.

7. This model does not address the question of which individuals may make firm commitments, but if all levels of management are consulted in this decision process, then that issue should not become a problem in most situations. Scientists should consult their department heads if they are unsure about the types of commitments that they may make.

8. Projects should have all relevant departments represented on the project committee or team. There could be a problem when site II personnel are requested to provide documents, materials, or other work and there is no site I representative of a comparable department on the project committee. If a member of the relevant site I department were named to the project committee in order to interact with the site II member of the comparable department, this person would also act to keep the site I department informed of ongoing activities. This in turn would provide better scheduling of resources within the department's structure and organization.

9. If communications outside the recommended pattern are undertaken in a particular situation, then the person or people concerned should notify those who would be expected to be involved if the guidelines were followed.

10. All official documents and reports from sites I or II that are to be included in a regulatory submission in the other site *must* flow between the two regulatory departments.

Assigning Work on Individual Projects to Various Development Sites

1. The project is only of interest to one site and the other(s) will not become involved.
2. The project is only of interest to one site, but the other(s) will conduct one or more clinical trials during a specific phase of development.
3. The project is of interest to both (or all) sites, but one site will initiate and conduct all of the clinical trials and the other(s) will register the medicine wherever appropriate.
4. The project is of interest to both sites, but one of the sites will initiate work only after Phases I, IIa, or IIb clinical trials are completed.
5. The project is of joint interest and each site will conduct clinical trials on different indications.
6. The project is of joint interest and each site will collaborate, but with different intensities of resource commitment.

Once one of these (or another) strategies is adopted, a detailed clinical plan may be developed. Depending on the nature of the medicine and disease area, the plan may only be created up to a certain milestone.

DESIGNING CORE STUDIES AND A CORE PACKAGE

What Is a Core Package?

Many multinational pharmaceutical companies are trying to integrate their international activities and function as a single worldwide company. One of the issues they are grappling with is the question of whether a core package of studies will increase the efficiency of their medicine development on an international scale. A "core package" refers to a group of clinical and nonclinical trials that require only minor revisions to be suitable for submission to multiple regulatory agencies in different countries. The core package contains data from preclinical and clinical trials necessary to answer most or all safety and efficacy questions of major interest (Table 121.2) to a regulatory authority. Locally conducted trials of interest to each specific regulatory agency are generally submitted with the core package.

Size of a Core Package

This issue of core packages may be discussed in several contexts, but one of the most important relates to the magnitude or size. The greater the number of clinical trials included in the core package and the more

TABLE 121.2 *Example of a core dossier of clinical trials and data*

A. Phase I clinical trials
1. Single- and multiple-dose tolerance trials
2. Pharmacokinetics (e.g., effects of single dose, multiple doses, dose–response, medicine interactions, bioequivalence; effects in children, elderly, renal-compromised patients; effects of food)
3. Special pharmacology or physiology studies (e.g., mechanism-of-action studies)

B. Phase II clinical trials
1. Efficacy trials: dose-ranging trials, active medicine control with placebo (if possible), and placebo-controlled[a]
2. Special patient populations (e.g., those with decreased cardiac function, elderly)
3. Efficacy trials: dose–response trials if ethics prevent use of a placebo[b]

C. Phase III clinical trials
1. Long-term Phase III trials of up to 1 year (or longer—if appropriate)
2. Short-term Phase III efficacy clinical trials

D. Trials conducted in all phases
1. Special safety trials
2. All adverse medicine reactions obtained, with particular reference to incidence data

[a] Two pivotal trials per indication, including data on the dose–response relationship.
[b] Use of placebo treatment is restricted in certain countries.

completely they are described, the less likely it is that only minor revisions will be required in order to submit the core package to many regulatory authorities. The smaller the number of clinical trials in the core package, the easier it will be to modify the core package to make it suitable for meeting requirements of multiple regulatory authorities. A smaller core package has greater flexibility than does a larger core package. However, the smaller core package will require a greater number of additional trials, conducted either locally or in another country, to complete each dossier.

Theoretically, it initially appears that a small core package would save less time than would be saved with a larger core package. If the core package is too large it will be impractical and inefficient to use, and if the core package is too small it will not yield the benefits desired. Thus, there is a need for balance in determining an appropriate size of the core package that will decrease time required for multiple submissions and reduce the total work and costs. Finding the ideal magnitude of a core package is complicated by the fact that all medicine development programs at a single corporation differ from each other, and the optimal core package size for two medicines will vary widely. The nature and number of the trials in the core package also will vary depending on the particular regulatory agencies to which the dossiers will eventually be sent.

Regulatory Input

Both direct and indirect regulatory input affect the design of a core package of studies. Indirect input results

from current regulations in the countries for which the core package of clinical trials is being prepared. Regulations have enormous influence in shaping almost every trial on investigational medicines. Regulations are probably the most important single factor responsible for the improved standards in design, conduct, and analysis of clinical trials over the last several decades. Regulatory input will affect both the type and number of trials to be done.

Direct regulatory input refers to statements, suggestions, and directives from regulatory agencies. These may occur at any or all stages of a medicine's life. Initial planning and development meetings may be held with regulatory agencies to help plan clinical trials that would be a part of the core package. During the conduct of the trials there will often be regulatory input, especially when an agency has specific questions or concerns to be addressed. While the registration dossier is being prepared, regulatory considerations directly affect the format and manner of data presentation. The type and nature of the direct interactions between regulatory agencies and pharmaceutical corporations during the planning, conduct, review, and approval stages is discussed in Chapter 126. The nature of these interactions varies greatly between different countries. For example, there are traditionally more interactions between a sponsor and the Food and Drug Administration (FDA) in the United States than there are between a sponsor and the Department of Health (DoH) in the United Kingdom, or regulatory authorities in most other countries.

Making a Core Package System Work

Innumerable difficulties are associated with creating a practical system for developing and using core packages of data. There are also innumerable difficulties for a multinational pharmaceutical company if a core package system is not used. Once the decision has been reached to utilize a core package system there are a number of principles that will facilitate its implementation and successful outcome.

If a company is initiating or experimenting with a core package system, it may be desirable to choose one or two projects that have a high likelihood of success and are at an early stage of development as test cases. The sponsor will gain invaluable experience using such medicines as models. Initial questions for the project group to consider are listed in Table 121.3.

1. Whenever possible, have a multinational group develop the plan for a medicine's development prior to initiating clinical trials. If clinical trials are already in Phase II it may be exceedingly difficult to develop and implement a successful core package system. This is because (1) some appropriate trials may not have

TABLE 121.3 *Selected questions for an international project group to consider initially*

1. Which dosage form(s) of the compound are to be developed?
2. Which countries will develop the medicine and in which order?
3. How will the project team be constituted and who will be in charge?
4. How will the project team operate?
5. How will the overall strategy be developed, reviewed, and revised (when necessary)?
6. How will the plans be developed both nationally and internationally for:
   preclinical studies?
   clinical trials?
   data management?
   coordination of efforts?
7. How will standards be maintained at an acceptable level in each country? Will standardized international monitoring practices be developed?
8. How will this matrix approach be coordinated with ongoing work conducted using line management systems and control?

been conducted, (2) some appropriate trials may not have been properly designed, (3) some inappropriate trials may have been conducted that have raised new issues to be addressed, and (4) the individuals involved may not have the experience, skills, and authority needed to develop and implement a core package for a complex project.

2. It is more efficient in developing a core approach for most medicines to wait until a medicine has demonstrated initial efficacy in Phase II trials before implementing many activities requiring detailed coordination between two or more company sites that are each directing the medicine's development. This approach will preserve the company's resources and efforts for those medicines that are most likely to reach the market, since most new medicines that are tested in humans are terminated during Phases I and II.

3. The project team should develop criteria and implement procedures to identify which countries will receive the core package and to determine all of the relevant regulatory considerations from those countries that may influence the design of toxicological, preclinical, clinical, technical development, and marketing studies. The criteria and procedures used for this purpose with other medicines will generally require little or no modification. The team must also be able to incorporate modifications into the core package so that it will meet any special requirements of the regulatory agencies for which it is intended. Table 121.4 describes roles of the regulatory representatives on the project team in planning worldwide regulatory strategies.

4. The medical representatives on the international project team may jointly plan the clinical trials to be included in the core package. This includes planning

of the following information for specific trials: (1) indication(s), (2) dosage form(s), (3) trial designs, (4) resources and equipment required, (5) locales to conduct trials, (6) specific or general types of investigators to use, (7) number of patients needed per trial and per phase, (8) monitoring strategy, and (9) various other factors. Specific considerations for a core clinical protocol have been presented (de Maar, 1986).

5. The relevant representatives from various company sites who are members of the international project team may plan the technical development and toxicological development for the core package. One aspect of the plan is to determine which parts of the company will have responsibility for which parts of the core package.

6. The amount of documentation relating to a clinical trial is a major issue in determining whether the core package system will work. Since the FDA requires more documentation than almost all other countries, the core package system is generally agreed to work best for medicine companies that are most familiar with conducting trials that meet FDA regulations. Most of these companies are either based in the United States or have major subsidiaries here.

7. Company representatives in each country to receive the core package must discuss and agree on various issues with the parent organization. These include dosage forms to be developed, indications to be pursued, and technical specifications of the formulation (e.g., dyes, duration of stability, size of capsule or tab-

TABLE 121.4 *Roles of the regulatory representives on the project team in planning worldwide regulatory strategies*

1. Identify each country's requirements for registration and pricing studies
2. Develop an international dossier to assist local groups in registering the medicine
3. Discuss pertinent issues with regulatory authorities
4. Discuss pertinent issues with national opinion makers and local experts
5. Reply to questions on regulatory dossiers from subsidiaries
6. Confirm that dossiers are submitted to local regulatory authorities
7. Reply to questions on dossiers from local regulatory authorities
8. Confirm that each subsidiary understands the role of the project team in providing the dossier, in communicating with the local company
9. Determine comparative agents to use in Phase III clinical trials (e.g., in some countries the price a company may charge for a medicine is heavily dependent on the medicine(s) used as an active control in Phase III trials)
10. Identify appropriate countries in which to conduct Phase III trials
11. Develop or utilize a method of keeping up with changing requirements and situations in relevant regulatory authorities
12. Determine responsibilities of each group that will contribute to the international regulatory submission and to each local dossier

TABLE 121.5 *Roles of the marketing representative(s) on the project team in planning worldwide marketing strategies[a]*

1. Determine marketing interest in each territory where the medicine could be sold
2. Participate in choosing dosage forms, formulations, and colors for all forms of the medicine to be marketed
3. Propose and discuss which clinical trials would meet common marketing needs in all or most territories
4. Participate in focus groups[b] and roundtable discussions on marketing issues
5. Design a flexible approach that may be used for worldwide promotion of a new medicine
6. Consider capabilities of the marketing organization in each territory when designing the strategy and setting goals
7. Assist marketing representatives in each territory to plan the best launch possible

[a] Other roles of marketing representatives on the project team are discussed in Chapter 129 (Table 129.10).
[b] Focus groups conduct interviews with a specific group of potential users (generally physicians) to determine their views and reactions to statements or questions about a product. The questions may relate to a real or hypothetical product.

let). If disagreements or problems arise and modifications of the development program are requested or required, then these modifications must be factored into decisions regarding the type of product to be made and tested, the target indications, and which countries will be able to benefit from the results obtained (Table 121.5).

8. Most companies believe in tailoring the core package to meet the requirements of the most demanding major regulatory authority. This is generally agreed to be the FDA in the United States, although there are certainly exceptions. In certain situations, standards of the European Economic Community (EEC) should be used as a guideline for organizing the

TABLE 121.6 *Selected questions for clinical representatives on an international project group to consider*

1. Which clinical trials should be conducted to demonstrate medicine safety, efficacy, and pharmacokinetics?
2. How will dose-ranging trials be conducted to evaluate the maximally tolerated dose and also the optimal dose(s) to demonstrate efficacy?
3. Which trials should (hopefully) be the pivotol trials and where should they be performed?
4. Who will prepare the clinical protocols and data collection forms?
5. How will these be reviewed to maximize their usefulness?
6. How will differences in ideas and viewpoints be arbitrated and decided?
7. What standards will be used for the clinical protocols?
8. How can data from trials be rapidly shared among all relevant individuals?
9. How can each relevant group have appropriate input into decision making on expected issues and unexpected problems?
10. Which group will have responsibility for preparing statistical analyses of the results? How will differences of opinion be resolved and at what stage of analysis?

TABLE 121.7 *Levels of detail in reports of a single clinical trial[a]*

1. Synopsis of one paragraph to one page
2. Manuscript that may be published as an article in the medical literature
3. Comprehensive medical and statistical reports—prepared separately or combined
4. Supportive information (e.g., protocol, listings of adverse reactions, abnormal laboratory data, patient discontinuations, reasons for exclusion of patients from a trial, pharmacy records, statistical analyses)
5. Raw data and data collection forms

[a] These are listed in order from the most general to the most detailed and specific. Not all of these data are required by a regulatory agency for all clinical trials. The appropriate amount of data submitted must be determined for each application submitted. See Fig. 121.8 for additional details.

nature of clinical trials to be conducted. If this is done, then separate well-controlled major Phase II efficacy (i.e., pivotal) trials may be planned for the United States if a New Drug Application (NDA) is to be submitted to the FDA.

9. It is likely that any core package of clinical trials will be inadequate to meet regulatory requirements in all targeted countries. Depending on regulatory requirements, ethics, culture, and other factors of the targeted countries, it may be necessary to exclude one or more countries from receiving the entire core package. It is nonetheless likely that different parts of the core package will be included in the regulatory dossier submitted in each country. Some of the questions for the clinical representatives on the international project group to consider are listed in Table 121.6. The basic levels of detail in clinical reports that may be submitted to regulatory authorities are listed in Table 121.7. Additional levels are illustrated in Fig. 121.8. This figure shows multiple levels of clinical data and summaries in a single clinical trial and in a single regulatory submission. The term *pyramid* has been used to describe this concept of multiple levels of detail in a single trial (Snoddy et al., 1985), but the term also is appropriate for a regulatory submission.

TABLE 121.8 *Administrative roles of the project team*

1. Recommend proceeding to full-scale development
2. Inform subsidiaries about new projects and the status of ongoing activities
3. Prioritize regulatory submissions based on available information (e.g., market forecasts, regulatory requirements, anticipated availability of data)
4. Develop a plan that addresses medical, regulatory, and marketing considerations
5. Determine the target countries in which the medicine will be investigated
6. Recommend discontinuing development in one or more countries
7. Recommend terminating the project
8. Agree on a plan, methods to monitor progress, and methods to facilitate disputes
9. Review deviations from the plan
10. Refer disputes or disagreements to more senior managers

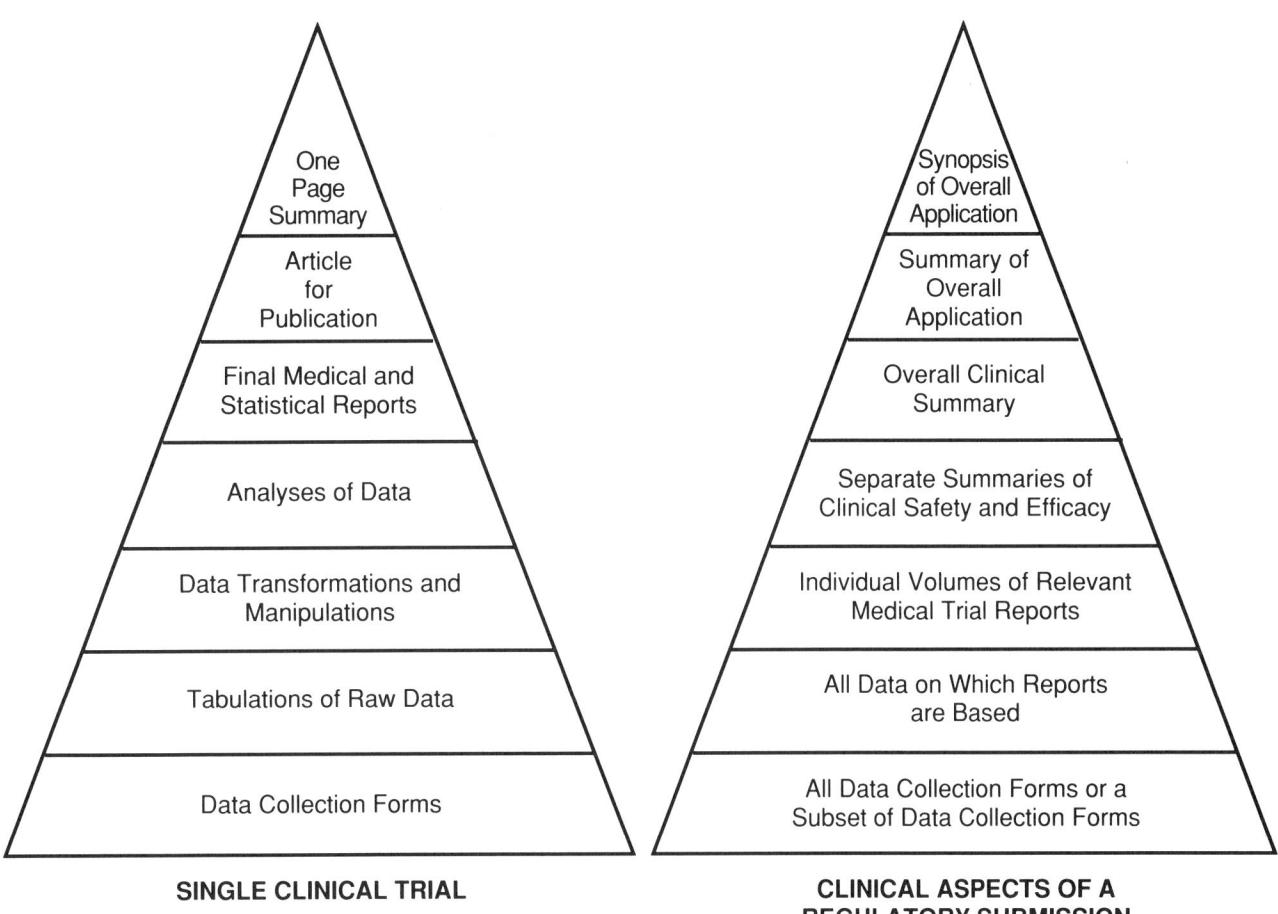

FIG. 121.8 The pyramid concept. Progressive summaries of clinical data in a single clinical trial and in a regulatory submission. The synopsis of the overall application is approximately 1 to 5 pages, whereas the one-volume summary is generally 50 to 500 pages. Not all components are necessarily required for a regulatory submission.

10. Various administrative roles of a project team must be considered, discussed, and determined (Table 121.8) to develop a medicine effectively.

Major Types of Foreign Trials from a United States Perspective

In many clinical trials conducted by a single company, parts of the trial are performed in another country. Five of the many possible variations are presented (Table 121.9). The activities performed, plus the management and coordination functions differ for each. In the following examples it is assumed that the company in the United States is a subsidiary of a foreign company. If not, then more of the management decisions will probably be made in the United States, unless the foreign subsidiary is given autonomy to make decisions on these issues. A core submission may include several types of these trials (see Table 121.2).

Type 1 Trial. The entire management and coordination of type I clinical trials are performed in the same manner as trials that are initiated and conducted domestically. One of the few differences is to keep informed the relevant medical, regulatory, marketing, and other representatives who are in the country in which the trial is being conducted. It is assumed that all regulatory and company permissions have been obtained to do the trial in the specific country.

Type 2 Trial. The major difference in type 2 clinical trials compared with type 1 is that the initiation and monitoring is jointly organized and run. This requires coordination among the monitors and project leaders. The management is the same as for type 1 trials.

Type 3 Trial. In type 3 models all activities are jointly established and conducted. The balance of activities will vary on a given clinical trial for each aspect. The trial is viewed as a joint venture, although one site usually has more of a leadership role. If the United States has the leadership role, then the major

TABLE 121.9 *Major types of foreign (i.e., non-United States) clinical trials conducted by a single company*[a]

Protocol prepared by	Trial initiated by	Trial monitored from	Final statistical and medical reports[b] prepared by	Data intended for regulatory submission primarily in
1. United States	United States	United States	United States then foreign country	United States
2. United States	United States and foreign country	United States and foreign country	United States and possibly foreign country	United States
3. United States and foreign country	United States and foreign country	United States and foreign country	United States and foreign country	United States and foreign country
4. United States and foreign country	Foreign country	Foreign country	Foreign country then United States	United States and foreign country
5. Foreign country	Foreign country	Foreign country	Foreign country then United States	Foreign country

[a] Numerous variations occur on these types. For foreign-based companies, an additional country (i.e., that of the parent company) may be involved. Other variations would include joint development by two companies, use of a contract organization, and collaboration with a government organization.
[b] Reports and data prepared by one site will be reviewed and may be reanalyzed or reinterpreted by the other site (or other sponsor).

management decisions are usually made here. If the foreign (i.e., parent) country has the leadership role, then management decisions are made there. The coordination functions would be operated semi-independently at each site, but with frequent communication to keep individuals informed and plans up to date.

Type 4 Trial. In type 4 trials the balance of activities has clearly shifted to the foreign country, which is now the group playing the greatest role. The original impetus for the trial may have come from either the United States or the foreign country. Both groups will be involved with management issues, but most decisions will be made by the specific group that "owns" the trial, usually after consultation with the other group.

Type 5 Trial. In the "all-foreign" trial, the comparable United States project leader (if the project exists in the United States) or project correspondent (if there is no project in the United States) passively monitors activities on the clinical trials. No coordination or management activities are routinely conducted, except for review of reports generated by the project leader or correspondent to keep management informed.

Overall Coordination and Management Review

Regardless of the type of clinical trial, reports prepared for management committees at one site are sent to and reviewed by senior managers at the other site. Thus, important issues relating to clinical trials are usually discussed at both sites, although there is often a time lag before the other site hears about the issue. The magnitude of the time lag depends on the importance of the trial and on the importance of the issue.

Coordination occurs at multiple levels between people at both sites, including project leaders, project planners, heads of research, heads of the matrix function, heads of development, plus department heads of all functions involved (e.g., regulatory, medical, statistics, chemical development, pharmaceutics, toxicology).

How Are Core Packages Perceived?

Perception by FDA

It is possible for a pharmaceutical company outside the United States to assemble a core package of data for a medicine and to license that medicine to a company in the United States. Although the company in the United States has the option, in theory, of submitting the package as is, without conducting any clinical trials in the United States, this approach is not generally viewed favorably by the FDA. Although the FDA has become more willing in recent years to accept foreign data, they apparently prefer that some studies be conducted within the United States. One reason for this viewpoint is that the FDA is less able to conduct an audit of trial sites to assure themselves that the trials have been conducted in an adequate and acceptable manner. Other reasons are discussed by Lasagna (1986b).

When the FDA views foreign data they prefer to examine a published article by a recognized authority (when available) rather than solely having data reentered in computers and reanalyzed by a sponsor in the United States. The former technique allows them to understand and assess the interpretation of the trial from the investigator's perspective, whereas this is not usually possible when the latter technique is used.

Perception by Multinational Companies

The way that pharmaceutical companies view the core package system depends in part on the size of the company and whether the company's headquarters is based in the United States. Large multinational companies either based in the United States or with a large subsidiary here are more likely to favor the core package system than are large multinational companies based outside the United States if they do not have a large subsidiary here. This occurs because it is generally easier to use data from clinical trials conducted in the United States for regulatory submissions in other countries than to use data from studies conducted in other countries for regulatory submissions in the United States. Moreover, companies with a large group in the United States generally have a better understanding than do other companies of how to conduct trials that meet FDA standards.

Each country that is a major market for pharmaceuticals has different regulations. It is uncertain whether the time necessary to complete and submit regulatory submissions, plus the time for regulatory approval, will be significantly diminished by utilizing a core package of data. Differences in dossier format and often content require significant amounts of time to modify appropriately for each new country. Clinical trials conducted in one country may not be acceptable as major or pivotal studies in another.

The Case Against Multinational Project Teams and a Core Clinical Package

A worldwide project team is an important mechanism to help turn a multinational company that is operating inefficiently into a more efficient single international company. However, there are also some reasons against using worldwide project teams (Table 121.10). These considerations should be evaluated each time a new project is adopted, even though there may be

TABLE 121.10 *Synopsis of arguments against using worldwide project teams*[a]

1. There is a shortage of suitable leaders for these teams in many companies
2. Errors made in strategy by the team may be major ones
3. Committees in general tend to be conservative
4. There is a potential loss of input from advisors from local countries who can often provide valuable information on submitting a dossier and on expediting its approval
5. Trying to develop and complete a worldwide plan may take more time than if a number of subsidiaries developed their own plans that are loosely coordinated with other subsidiaries and the parent organization
6. Many projects are of local interest or are concentrated in only a few territories and do not require a worldwide project team
7. Many projects are too small in commercial potential to justify the effort and expense of a worldwide project team

[a] There are numerous counterarguments to these reasons. The soundness of the counterarguments must be judged by senior research managers.

worldwide project teams in the same company for other projects.

Despite the obvious appeal and apparent value of a core package of clinical data, several reasons suggest that it is not a panacea and has significant drawbacks. Most of the following points may be overcome with a carefully developed core package, but consideration of these issues is often necessary.

Variation in Regulations. Regulations differ widely in most countries and the core package may require so much adjustment from country to country that its value may be severely compromised. Some countries require specific trial designs to be used for clinical trials conducted in their country and possibly may not accept some of the trials that are included in the core package.

Differences in Medicine Characteristics. Most medicines are developed using different dosage strengths, dosages, formulations, colors, and other specifications for different countries. There are often sound reasons for many of these differences and despite vigorous attempts to standardize most aspects of a medicine's development, there are usually certain limitations. For example, the choice of colors for a capsule or tablet may create problems in certain countries because few dyes used to create colors are universally acceptable. There may be sound reasons related to local customs or culture as to why certain colors are undesirable or even unacceptable in some countries. Many excipients are not universally acceptable. Preferred dosage forms often differ between countries (e.g., capsules, tablets, suppositories, liquids). For some products there may be strong desires in some countries to market certain specialized forms (e.g., aerosols, powders, shampoos, lotions, ointments, talcs) and not others.

Statistical Reanalyses of Data and Reports. A statistical group in one country may desire to reanalyze and reinterpret data from a clinical trial originally performed and analyzed by another subsidiary or the parent company located in a different country. In that situation, the final medical report may differ substantially from the original document. If the trial was performed outside the United States, the detailed documentation required by the FDA may not be available, especially if the sponsor is a foreign pharmaceutical company that is not extremely familiar with FDA requirements or if it has not adhered to those requirements in the trial. This may create problems in terms of a core package, especially if different interpretations are reached. Currently, this is less of a problem since the trials may be easily downgraded from pivotal to supportive, or in some cases not even described in detail. In some companies, statistical and medical reports are only written once. This is done by the group that ran the trials, although input is accepted on the methods to use and results to include from other national groups of the same company.

Pressures to Increase Quantity and Quality. The quantity of data that must be submitted with a regulatory dossier varies between countries. In general, the core package will have to contain both the maximum quantity and quality of data obtained in all clinical trials included. In addition, some countries require more pharmacokinetic data than do others. Some countries require more pharmacy or geriatric data. If each of these supplementary pieces is added to all core packages it may raise problems in the future because of (1) "too much" data in the application increasing the standards expected of all applications, (2) additional preparation time, and (3) longer time for regulatory review.

Differences in Philosophy Within a Company. Dose-ranging trials to evaluate safety in humans must be performed so that doses appropriate for efficacy may be chosen. These data also permit an understanding of the therapeutic window that is eventually determined. However, dose-ranging studies performed in some countries are based on a different philosophy or goal than in others. For example, dose-ranging trials in normal volunteers in the United Kingdom usually stop at the dose expected to yield efficacy in patients, whereas dose escalation trials in the United States usually continue in volunteers to the point at which toxicity is observed. This may lead to differences in doses studied in Phase II trials and eventually to (1) different recommended dosing regimens between different countries and (2) use of different trials to support the recommendations.

Issue of Active Controls. It is sometimes necessary to use different active controls in different countries. The price that may be charged for a new medicine depends, in some countries, on the active medicine chosen to compare with the test medicine in Phase III clinical trials. Some medicine trials may therefore be conducted in one country when they are not suitable for use as part of a core package for other countries. Moreover, some standard medicines included for comparison purposes may be chosen because they are widely used by specialists in one country, but may not be used by the same group of specialists in another country. Some comparison medicines may not be marketed in some of the countries where data are submitted. Another issue arises when general practitioners use a standard medicine that is different from that used by specialists for the same disease.

Ethical Standards. Ethical standards vary widely in clinical trials conducted between different countries. It may be impractical to conduct trials that will meet standards in all countries in terms of placebo, informed consent, Ethics Committees/Institutional Review Boards, and other issues.

Use by Thought Leaders. National thought leaders who use a medicine in one country may use it differently than in another country, based on differences in experience or opinion. It may not be easy for a core package of clinical trials to accommodate these differences by designing multiple trials that explore different types of medicine use in different countries.

Standards of Monitoring Used. If clinical trials are performed at foreign locations that have less stringent monitoring than in the United States, serious issues that were either unknown by the monitors or inadequately addressed may arise. Since most investigators are (rightfully) more oriented toward clinical results and helping their patients than they are to adhering to protocols, there may be a greater tendency to stray from the protocol in some foreign trials, unless monitoring is rigorous.

Differences in the Language of Medicine. The language of medicine is not used the same way in different countries. This may lead to problems in combining data on patient diagnosis, measurement of effects, or adverse reactions from different countries.

Each of these situations may create pressures to use different clinical trials for each major dossier. The group of efficacy trials that support one dosing regimen may not generally be used to support others. Trials using one dosing regimen in one country may not be useful in another country where the dosing regimen differs. Trials performed with the formulation to be marketed in one country could not be used in countries where the final formulation differs, unless appropriate bioequivalence trials were conducted and yielded acceptable data. Additional considerations of these issues are listed in Table 121.11.

As part of the planning activities it may be prudent and possible to develop an international team of individuals who will ensure intelligent, realistic, and imaginative plans to develop the medicine efficiently. This step may occur without using any but a minimal core package of trials.

Mini-Core Package

In a large core package each local (i.e., national) affiliate of a pharmaceutical company removes the parts it does not want in its regulatory submission and adds any pieces necessary. One alternative to a relatively complete core package of clinical trials is to develop a small nucleus of trials, such as those for safety, pharmacokinetics, and supportive Phase III efficacy trials that could be utilized as a mini-core package in most countries. Each country would add the major efficacy or other trials deemed necessary for registration. Nonetheless, even this alternative or a different type

TABLE 121.11 *Synopsis of arguments against the core package system[a]*

1. The core system may act to increase time and costs of medicine development[b]
2. The core system is not useful for all countries (e.g., Japan)
3. The worldwide project team concept that is necessary to develop the core package system has various drawbacks[c]
4. If the company is foreign based it may be difficult for it to plan a development program that adequately meets U.S. standards
5. The absence of a systematic approach that leads to more apparent (or real) disorder may work to the advantage of larger companies. A highly organized and simplified system permits more competition to develop from smaller companies
6. When trials from one country are reanalyzed and reinterpreted in another, different interpretations may be drawn that tend to diminish or compromise the usefulness of the core package
7. Different philosophies of medicine development in different countries may make it extremely difficult to reach consensus on (1) the trials to include in a core package, (2) how to design those trials, or (3) the order in which trials should be conducted

[a] See footnote to Table 121.10.
[b] The core system adds to pressures to increase the time and costs of medicine development by raising standards all over the world. Many countries have a particular area in which their requirements tend to be more stringent than in other countries (e.g., pharmacokinetic data in Scandinavia, geriatric data in England, pharmacy data in Belgium). If the core package attempts to meet all of these standards in all submissions there will probably be a major increase in both costs and time of medicine development.
[c] See Table 121.10 for several examples.

of mini-core package will require that dossiers be rewritten for most major countries in which the medicines will be registered. By the time the core group of trials for each country are rewritten and reformatted, it may not have saved time over the traditional method of planning each country's submission independently, using as many studies from other locales as possible.

Potential Problems With a Fully Integrated Clinical Development Plan

The major problems that may arise during the conduct of a fully integrated international clinical plan are clinical, regulatory, and commercial in nature. Clinical problems include differences in diagnostic criteria of certain diseases, different parameters used to assess the outcomes, different endpoints measured in various countries to assess disease improvement, different magnitudes of change to determine a clinically significant effect, and different approaches to treating patients.

Regulatory differences are mentioned elsewhere in this chapter. Each investigational medicine requires a fully developed regulatory strategy. That strategy must tie in with worldwide marketing needs and assess-

ments. The marketing plan must be based on data obtained in the integrated plan. This may be difficult if different markets worldwide have different needs in terms of types of claims desired, types of patients treated, types of treatments used, and numerous other factors. These points all indicate that an integrated international plan is not necessarily an ideal approach for developing a new medicine.

Conclusions

Careful planning of medicine development to (1) obtain consensus on the strategy and approach, (2) seek input from marketing, (3) minimize duplication of efforts, (4) conduct trials at as high a standard as possible, (5) monitor all activities frequently, (6) maintain open communications, and (7) adjust the development program as necessary are among the most important factors in expediting registration of a new medicine in multiple countries. The core package system should be developed to the extent that it expedites regulatory submissions worldwide. The appropriate size of the core package must be determined for each medicine, but an extensive core package should be avoided in most situations.

There will probably never be complete congruence between the specific trials that must be conducted in the United States to obtain an NDA on a particular medicine and those trials conducted outside the United States. Nonetheless there is some overlap, and certain trials conducted in foreign countries will meet the FDA's requirements.

ISSUES IN INTERNATIONAL MEDICINE DEVELOPMENT

How Should a Company Choose the Countries in Which to Conduct Clinical Trials?

Although there are some logical approaches to addressing this question, many companies answer it on the basis of the most senior medical manager's opinion. Criteria used include (1) largest commercial markets, (2) countries where development sites are located, (3) countries where expert investigators are located, (4) broadly spreading the clinical trials, and others. The ability to have high quality monitoring is also important. Another approach is to consider at least two important parameters in order to create four quadrants (Fig. 121.9). Table 121.12 lists additional criteria.

Each country being considered may be designated by a single mark (not shown) on the grid and then the four quadrants are created to assist in the choice. An-

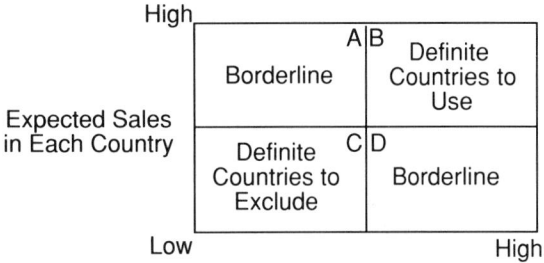

FIG. 121.9 Grid to illustrate one means of choosing countries in which to conduct clinical trials.

other approach is to classify each country by quadrant (i.e., A, B, C, and D) and then to focus attention on those marked with a B. Regardless of the approach used, other factors often markedly affect whether the outcome is accepted. For example, the company may have a large amount of available resources in a country marked as ''borderline.'' A country in the ''definite'' quadrant may not accept good clinical practice standards or it may be impossible to conduct an acceptable clinical audit there.

A few reasons to focus development activities in a few countries include (1) to simplify logistics of planning and conduct of the trials, (2) to simplify regulatory activities, (3) to maximize efficiency, (4) to minimize the number of protocols, and (5) to decrease cost. Not all of these reasons will always hold for all countries or for all medicines. Priority countries should also be identified for manufacturing and for marketing.

Conducting Clinical Trials in Developing Countries

If patients do not want to remain in a hospital for a clinical trial or if there are too few or inadequate hospital facilities, then it may be possible to:

TABLE 121.12 *Criteria to use in choosing a country for a clinical trial*

1. Availability of suitable investigator(s)
2. Availability of an adequate number of suitable patients
3. Ability to conduct a clinical trial according to acceptable standards
4. Ability to monitor the trial in the manner desired
5. Physical accessibility and convenience of the trial site(s)
6. Cooperation, resources, expertise, and quality of local staff
7. Speed with which the trial can be initiated and completed
8. Acceptability of previous trials conducted in that country by regulatory authorities in other countries
9. Manner in which the trial fits worldwide medicine development and registration plans
10. Projected impact on company's profitability in conducting the trial in a specific country

1. Have patients leave the hospital during the day and return at night.
2. Have physicians travel to the patient's location to test patients and ensure adequate compliance.
3. Enlist family members to give medicines, take measurements, or maintain a diary.
4. Schedule fewer patient visits, while lengthening the period between visits.
5. Shorten the duration of trial treatment.

Other considerations relating to the planning and conduct of clinical trials in underdeveloped countries include:

1. Definitions of diseases sometimes vary between countries. This is especially true of syndromes and conditions that are ill defined.
2. Criteria of efficacy may vary greatly. Investigators in some countries may emphasize different endpoints that relate to pharmacological, clinical, or quality of life measurements.
3. Definitions of what is considered an adverse reaction, as well as judgments of its severity, may differ.
4. Collecting data on adverse reactions is often difficult (Table 121.13). Specialists may not be available to evaluate patients, provide consults, or use sophisticated testing methods.

Two other considerations that relate to the sponsoring company are: (1) resources may not be efficiently used if clinical trials are duplicated unnecessarily in less developed countries; (2) the needs and goals of a company's local subsidiary may not match those of the central headquarters or those of an integrated international development program.

TABLE 121.13 *Problems of collecting data on adverse reactions in developing countries*

1. Many patients are illiterate and unaware of the identity of medicines they are receiving
2. Many medicines that are available over-the-counter are only sold by prescription in other countries
3. Difficulties are involved in maintaining adequate patient care, especially in rural and overcrowded areas
4. Many physicians are overworked and do not have sufficient opportunities to report or study adverse reactions
5. Patients are often treated by multiple physicians with little or no continuity of patient care
6. Many patients have concurrent illnesses that complicate detection and evaluation of adverse reactions
7. People may have in their homes many potent and potentially dangerous medicines that they are willing to use, which decreases compliance with the prescribed regimen
8. Patients may be following local medical ''folk'' practices at the same time they are taking medicines developed in industrial countries
9. There may be difficulties in hiring and maintaining an adequately trained staff

Should International Development Work for a Single Activity Be Done at a Single Site?

The most efficient international medicine development often occurs when a single site conducts all activities of one type. Involving too many workers or leaders from multiple development sites may slow progress considerably. Developing a dosage form, developing an assay, conducting Phase I clinical trials on an anticancer medicine, and conducting early stage toxicology studies are a few situations in which one site should be doing all the work on a new medicine, at least initially. Considerations for coordinating multinational trials are mentioned in Table 121.14.

Each site should have 10 to 14 days, however, to review protocols generated by the other site, to ensure that the trials will not create problems for one or more sites at a later date.

Will a Single Regulatory Application Be Possible Worldwide?

There are strong signs and indications that the number of unique regulatory applications that a company must submit worldwide is decreasing. This is most apparent in the European Economic Community, which is standardizing the application process. The standardization of adverse reaction reporting to regulatory authorities is another area in which unification of multiple regulatory forms is occurring (see Chapter 120). A single form, even if it is submitted to multiple regulatory authorities will make the development process for new and modified medicines more efficient and more rapid. Fewer duplicative clinical trials will be conducted and fewer trials should have to be repeated to obtain additional endpoints or data required by local authorities.

On the other hand, the world is quite far from a single regulatory dossier and different countries currently have vastly different requirements in terms of studies for most areas, including mutagenicity, reproduction, stability, formulation development, chemical synthesis, and pharmacokinetics.

Should One or More Countries Be Targeted for the Initial Registration?

Initial marketing of a new medicine in countries with less stringent regulatory requirements serves to generate patient exposures while additional clinical trials are conducted elsewhere. It also tends to provide some comfort to most regulatory authorities to know that a new medicine they are evaluating is already marketed and patients are receiving the same medicine elsewhere. Another positive aspect is that significant adverse reactions have a greater chance of being discov-

TABLE 121.14 *Coordinating multinational clinical trials*[a]

1. Establish the specific requirements of each country in terms of regulatory, patent, legal, ethical, political, social, marketing, and other perspectives
2. Determine if a multinational trial is necessary or important and feasible to conduct, based on regulatory requirements and potential benefits of each prospective country that will participate
3. Develop a detailed integrated strategic plan that addresses these national considerations
4. Identify key personnel and assignment of responsibilities that minimizes duplication of effort. Many similar trials are often performed in multiple countries
5. Establish standards that protocols, data collection procedures, and statistical analyses must meet if the data are to be used in multiple countries. These are usually determined to be the standards of the strictest regulatory agency, provided that the efforts of achieving these standards are found to be cost effective
6. Provide reports of medical and other trials in a format from which local submission packages (dossiers) may be easily compiled
7. Plan Phase IV and marketing studies with the same thoroughness used to plan investigational studies
8. Consider using a central group to monitor clinical activities at each separate trial site to help ensure uniformity of data
9. Consider any changes in scientific, regulatory, financial, political, medical, ethical, and social aspects throughout the trial (or trials) that may influence the trial in any way
10. Meet on a periodic basis with the project manager and others to review and update the overall development plan
11. Communicate the revised plan, dates, and responsibilities to all relevant individuals

[a] These factors relate to a single trial as well as to a series of multinational trials on one or more medicines. Almost all factors also relate to coordinating efforts of an international project group that does not have any multinational trials in their clinical plan. A multinational trial refers to a single clinical trial conducted in two or more countries. All multinational trials are multicentered, but not all multicentered trials are multinational. See Chapter 40 for additional discussions on multinational trials.

ered at an earlier date. The probability of discovering new serious adverse reactions with a moderate frequency progressively diminishes as a medicine is used more widely. This is a beneficial aspect of increasing patient exposures under monitored conditions.

What Role Should Marketing Play in Establishing Research and Development Goals?

Marketing should provide input (but not decision making) into research and development goals. At some companies the marketing division identifies marketing needs and creates a business opportunity list of desirable research objectives. The question is whether marketing objectives control the areas in which research is conducted or whether research innovations provide marketing with medicines to sell and therapeutic opportunities to develop.

Ideally, marketing provides information to the research and development division at all stages of a project. That information assists in the decisions on management and direction of research, but without controlling the direction of that research. A prototype package insert is used by some marketing groups at the initiation of a project to establish and link communications with clinicians inside the company. This technique may (in theory) allow a project to be terminated relatively painlessly if the insert contains the minimally acceptable clinical profile and it is not supported by data obtained.

Which Formulations Should Be Developed?

Each company attempts to balance the savings generated by having the least number of formulations developed with the needs, desires, and requirements of different countries and marketing groups. This is a highly complex issue. It is usually necessary and prac-

tical to develop several formulations of a single medicine that is to be sold in several different countries. Technical and clinical development of multiple formulations may be conducted simultaneously, sequentially, or in an overlapping manner. Both cost and benefit should be evaluated for each dosage form and formulation that is considered for development.

Should Manufacturing Be Centralized or Diversified?

Despite numerous benefits that accrue as a result of centralizing the manufacture of a medicine there are various reasons why this procedure is often impractical or impossible. For instance, (1) some countries require production to take place within their borders before a medicine is allowed to be sold, (2) production facilities may be fully committed at one location and available at one or several other locations, (3) multiple formu-

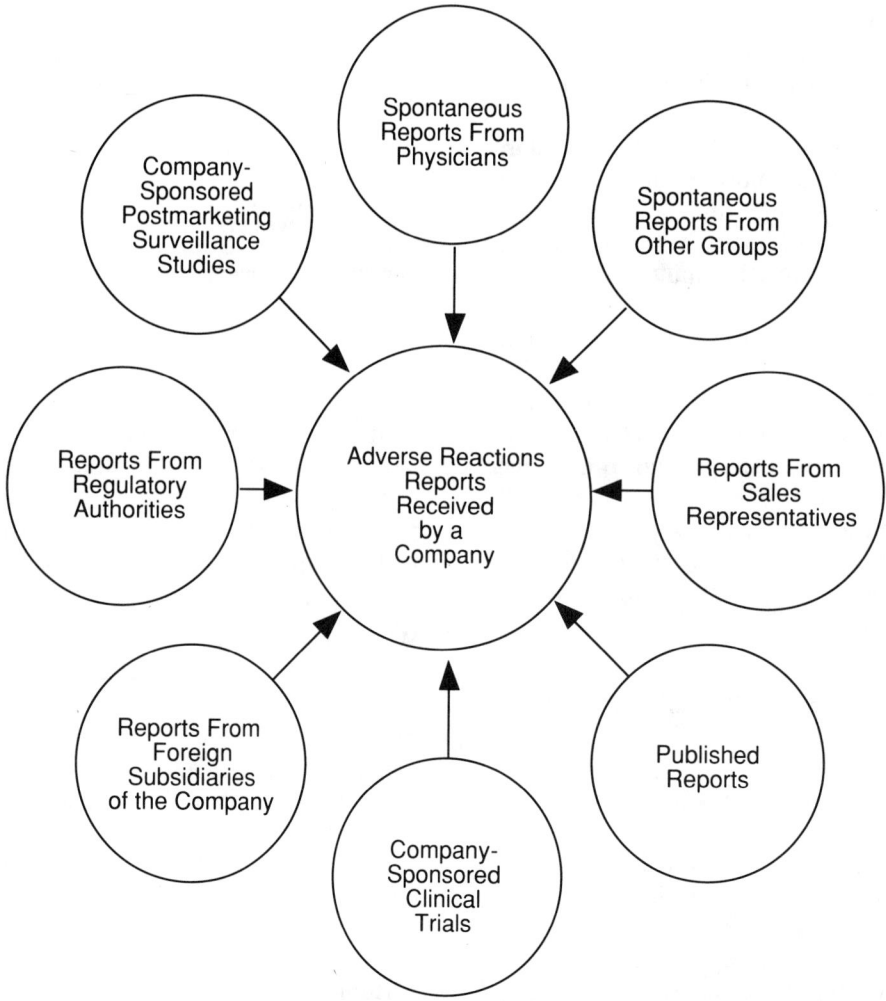

FIG. 121.10 Source of adverse event reports received by a pharmaceutical company. Consumers or attorneys may be a source of adverse events in some countries, but not in others.

lations may make it impractical to produce all varieties of a medicine at a single site, (4) cost savings or tax benefits may make local production attractive, (5) a final step in a synthesis may be the only part of the synthesis performed locally, (6) in event of a fire or other disaster at one site there will be another facility that can increase production to supply the affected markets, (7) special equipment (e.g., for manufacturing sterile products) may only be available at certain locations, and (8) there may be regulations preventing export of a finished product for sale in another country when the medicine is not approved for sale in the country of manufacture. A related issue is whether all stability tests should be conducted in each of the multiple locales where a medicine is made or whether they should be performed at a central site.

Are Statistical Approaches Applied Identically to All Trials Worldwide?

Just as standards of conducting clinical trials vary from country to country, so too do statistical techniques and standards. A worldwide consensus of approaches and methods to use can be developed by each company. A potential problem may arise when statisticians in two or more countries analyze and view data differently. This is a relatively common occurrence and may lead to different clinical interpretations of the same data.

One approach to minimize or prevent problems is to have the group that conducted the trial derive the company-wide interpretation. This can only work if all relevant groups have an opportunity to review the data

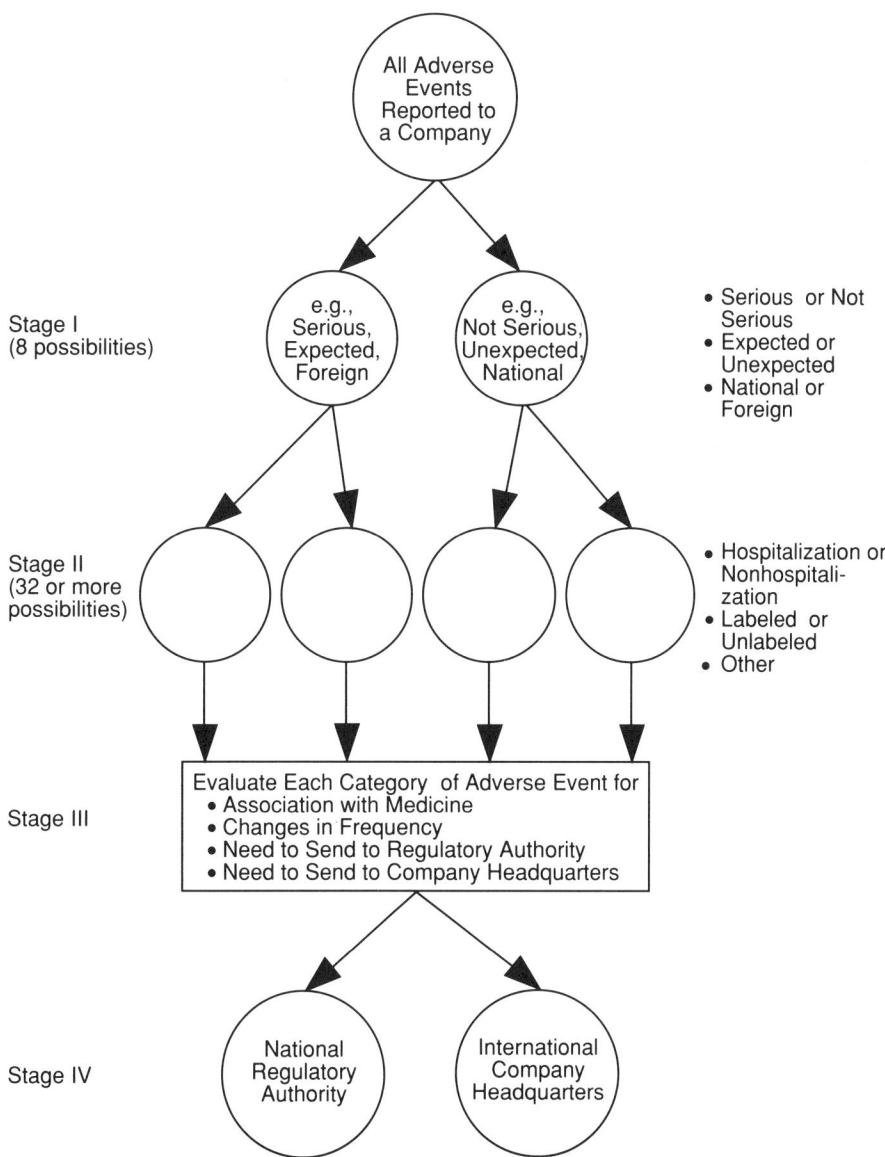

FIG. 121.11 Progressive classification of adverse events to marketed medicines received by a pharmaceutical company.

and results, as well as having input into the methods chosen to analyze the data. This approach will sometimes fail, however, when different people are not able to reach agreement, or some regulatory authorities require new methods to be used or challenge interpretations presented. Thus, even a unanimous consensus by all company statisticians and academic statisticians on how to perform data analyses may not prevent regulatory authorities (with or without statistical training) from challenging the methods used.

Adverse Reactions

1. More than ten countries currently require reporting of adverse reactions that have occurred in other countries. There are various definitions of adverse reactions used, various forms to use, and various timetables for filing reports in different countries. It is easy to imagine the administrative complexity for many pharmaceutical companies. Recent efforts by regulatory agencies, pharmaceutical companies, and trade associations are attempting to standardize reporting of adverse reactions between countries (see Chapter 120).

2. A number of national regulatory agencies (e.g., in Australia, Canada, England, Norway, Sweden, New Zealand) issue reports on adverse reactions caused by various medicines. The issue of causality assessment becomes more complex when a parent pharmaceutical company receives these reports plus those of its subsidiaries in these and other countries (see Figs. 121.9 to 121.12). Assessments are not made using uniform criteria or applied in a uniform manner in all countries (or even within one country). For example, the assessment of the probability of causation may be made by the treating physician, manufacturer, or regulatory agency. Patients may be taking multiple medicines and the medicine responsible for the adverse reaction may not be known or may not be identified on the report.

3. The issue of distortion of adverse reaction data is a major one. A company may attempt to minimize distortion between its subsidiaries and the central office, but assuring the quality of data at an earlier point (i.e., between physician and patient, or between physician and local company) is extremely difficult, if not impossible. Another problem is that of obtaining all information needed to understand adequately and interpret the clinical significance of the adverse reaction report.

4. The incidence of adverse reactions reported by physicians on a new medicine (as opposed to the true incidence) goes through different periods. Most new medicines generate medical interest and attention to most of its adverse reactions. After an unusual type or frequency of an adverse reaction is reported, there is often a flurry of other reports on the same event. There may be overreporting during this period because physicians are alerted to the possible occurrence of the unusual or un-

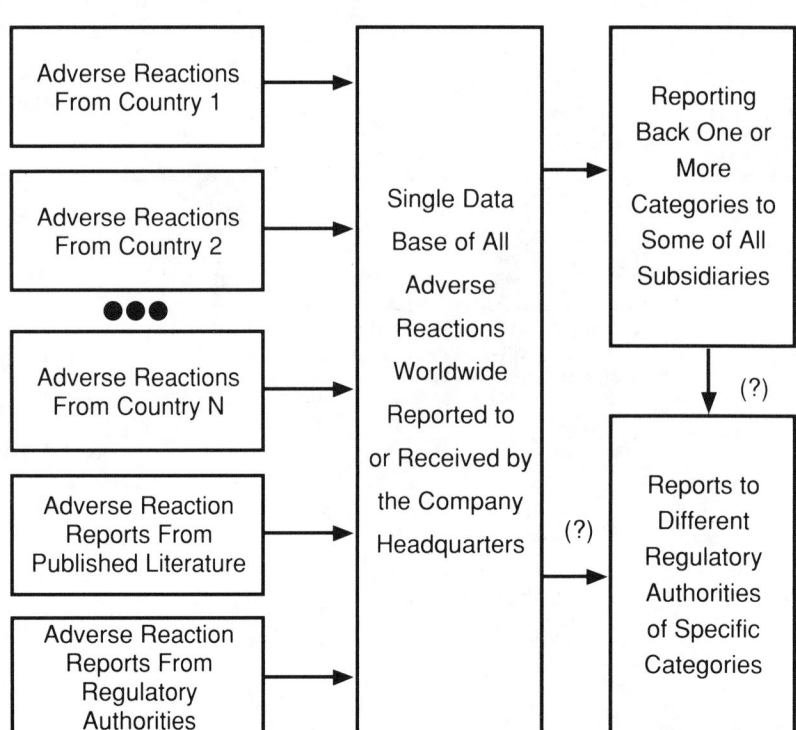

FIG. 121.12 Processing adverse event reports to marketed medicines received by a pharmaceutical company from worldwide sites.

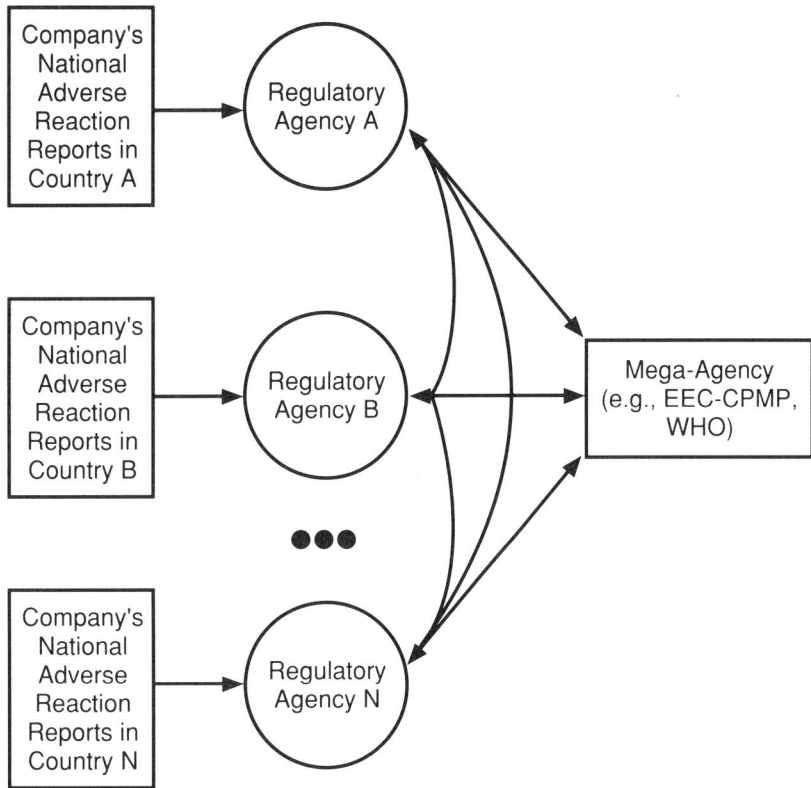

FIG. 121.13 Sharing of a pharmaceutical company's adverse reaction reports among regulatory agencies in different countries. EEC-CPMP, European Economic Community–Committee for Proprietary Medicinal Products; WHO, World Health Organization.

expected adverse reaction and may diagnose possible or questionable cases as definite examples of the adverse reaction. Physicians may also attribute these adverse reactions more readily to the medicine than would otherwise have occurred. After a number of years, however, the incidence of almost all adverse reaction reports (except for possibly the most serious) generally fall below the expected rate. This occurs because many physicians have little or no interest in reporting well-established adverse reactions and leads to a period of underreporting adverse reactions.

Multinational companies should instruct all of their staff involved with adverse reactions to report any unexpected and serious adverse reactions to the central company within 48 hours of learning about them (Fig. 121.10). The processing of adverse reactions received is illustrated in Figs. 121.11 to 121.13.

Information on adverse reactions reported in package inserts is available in the *Physicians' Desk Reference* in the United States. Comparable sources of information from other countries may be identified in *Drug Information Sources* (Revill, 1978). Additional issues on international adverse reaction surveillance were presented at a Drug Information Association Workshop (Jones, 1985) and in a recent monograph (Inman, 1986). A review of international voluntary systems for reporting adverse reactions was presented by Griffin and Weber (1985, 1986).

Selected Inconsistencies in Adverse Reaction Reporting Worldwide

1. Most regulatory authorities do not inform companies of adverse reaction reports they receive, but insist on companies providing their own data to the regulatory authority (i.e., there is no true sharing of information with most regulatory authorities).
2. The rates of adverse reaction reporting for any one medicine may be extremely different between countries. This could be either a real or spurious difference, and determining this distinction may be difficult (Griffin and Weber, 1989).
3. Dates of occurrences of adverse reactions are often quite different from the dates they are reported to a company, yet regulatory authorities sometimes expect reports from a company within a few days after occurrence. On the positive side, most regulatory authorities are quite familiar with this issue and do not place unreasonable demands on pharmaceutical companies. This is, therefore, a potential issue.

PART XII

Management of Multiple Clinical Trials

We trained hard—but it seemed that every time we were beginning to form into teams, we would be reorganised. I was to learn later in life that we tend to meet any new situation by reorganising—and a wonderful method it can be for creating the illusion of progress while producing confusion, inefficiency and demoralisation.

—*Gaius Petronius, Roman, 1st Century A.D.*

How seldom a fact is accurately stated; how almost invariably when a story has passed through the mind of a third person it becomes . . . little better than a falsehood; and this, too, though the narrator be the most truth-seeking person in existence.

—*Nathaniel Hawthorne*

Man's chief purpose . . . is the creation and preservation of values: that is what gives meaning to our civilization, and the participation in this is what gives significance, ultimately, to the individual human life.

—*Lewis Mumford*

Management Styles, Staff, and Systems

The innumerable issues and complexities that arise during the conduct of a single clinical trial become exponentially more complex when multiple clinical trials must be managed. The term "multiple clinical trials" is used in the context of two or more separate and independent trials on one specific medicine, or of several independent trials on each of two or more different medicines. In either of these situations it is important to develop systems and procedures that will assist in the orderly and efficient management of the myriad activities involved.

The chapters in this section present little information on the standard management techniques that are discussed in numerous textbooks and business or management courses and may be applied to almost any industry. The information included differs from most available material in two major ways. First, it minimizes theoretical discussions and emphasizes a practical, straightforward approach to management. Second, it is directed primarily at pharmaceutical companies and medicine development, and only secondarily at academicians or medical device manufacturers, or others who conduct multiple clinical trials.

MANAGEMENT STYLES

Spectra

Styles of management vary along several different spectra, and no single style is universally best or most appropriate in each situation. The spectra range from (1) authoritarian to democratic, (2) loose control to tight (rigid) control, (3) centralized to peripheralized, (4) matrix to line management, (5) ends oriented to means oriented, and (6) willingness to try the latest new management idea or fad to grudging acceptance of ideas only after they have been accepted by most other people. Appropriate management styles for an individual are based on the specific work environment, tradition of the institution, personality of the individual, and other factors. The most rapid movement of a project toward a goal usually occurs when a single authoritarian figure determines the goal and controls the resources allocated and the vigor with which the goal is pursued. On the other hand, a more conservative approach, which is usually adopted by most committees and institutions, is less likely to make a major error in going in a wrong direction for a long period without recognizing the error.

Styles at Individual Companies

Individual companies often go through periods during which they shift from one style to another. This may be a result of change in leadership or a desire to try something new. Different parts of an organization often utilize different and possibly even conflicting styles at the same time. Selected management styles are summarized in Table 122.1.

Styles of Individuals

Different management styles emphasize a variety of approaches. Some individuals believe in emphasizing analytical tools and techniques in helping to make complex decisions. These techniques include quantitative methods described in management systems [e.g., Program Evaluation and Review Technique (PERT), critical path method]. Another group approaches management through consideration of the general functions conducted by most managers. These functions include planning, organizing, directing, reviewing, and controlling. Finally, some managers emphasize interpersonal relationships, since managers must complete a work assignment through the efforts of other people. Knowledge of group behavior, motivation, and other personal characteristics allow some managers to direct projects efficiently and effectively. Although multiple

management styles may be used by the same person, each individual balances the use of these styles in different ways. One useful frame of reference for evaluating personal styles of behavior and management is presented by G. D. Bell in his book, *The Achievers* (1973).

Another perspective focuses on styles of communication. Individuals usually develop preferences in the techniques they use for communication. These more or less include use of (1) personal notes sent to others, (2) telephone discussions, (3) short informal meetings generated as the manager walks around an area, (4) meetings of small informal groups, (5) more formal meetings, and (6) memoranda, as well as other methods of communication. When individuals are promoted or are given a new assignment they usually do not greatly alter their personal habits or style in the methods they use to communicate.

MANAGEMENT STAFF

Management staff is composed of numerous individuals whose responsibilities vary greatly and include:

1. Investigator(s)
2. Coinvestigators and assistant investigators
3. Members of Ethics Committees/Institutional Review Boards (IRBs)
4. Professional consultants
5. Regulatory agency reviewers
6. Trial coordinators
7. Trial monitors
8. Monitoring committees, data review committees, and other staff
9. Project champions
10. Project managers
11. Supervisors of data processors and data entry operators
12. Statistical reviewers
13. Executives at the sponsoring institution
14. Contract organization staff and executives
15. Data analysis committees
16. Independent auditors of diagnoses, laboratory data, trial conduct, or other aspects of a trial
17. Independent review committee of trial results and interpretation

Trial personnel requirements vary from a single individual who performs every role from investigator to appointment clerk, to situations where large numbers of people with specific responsibilities are involved. This section describes several of the major management functions that are usually performed by different individuals. A subset of the staff positions listed above will be individually discussed. Their roles are summarized in Table 122.2.

TABLE 122.1 *Styles of management*[a]

1. The style is rigid and authoritative: one individual controls a group, determines most of the rules to be followed, and usually does not delegate real power or decision-making responsibility. This individual does not seek nor accept opinions from individuals willing to disagree or act independently
2. One individual runs a group, but delegates power and decision making appropriately (participative leadership)
3. One individual makes decisions, but only after consulting with others (consultative leadership)
4. A committee is established to make important decisions, as well as to monitor and review projects and issues. The committee follows highly formal monitoring and reporting procedures
5. A committee is established as above, but follows a loosely structured and flexible system for monitoring and reporting activities and for arriving at decisions
6. No formal systems are created. Managers depend on ad hoc meetings and discussions to solve problems and to provide a review of activities

[a] These styles are not mutually exclusive within a large organization, and several approaches are often observed to be used simultaneously. Most managers or small committees of about three to 12 people also exhibit different approaches in different situations.

TABLE 122.2 *Possible management roles within a clinical trial*

Position or responsibility in a clinical trial	Aspects of their managerial role
1. Receptionist	Schedules clinic visits and sends out (or telephones) reminders
2. Nurse	May be assigned duties of receptionist, nursing assistant, research coordinator, or assistant investigator
3. Research coordinator	Usually supervises data collection forms, schedules activities, dispenses medicines and may assist or conduct other functions at the investigator's discretion
4. Assistant investigator[a]	Assists the principal investigator in managing the trial, or may solely supervise the trial. Usually conducts patient examinations and may sign data collection forms
5. Principal investigator[b]	Overall manager of trial. Details of specific activities vary greatly between investigators. Often delegates many responsibilities to others
6. Clinical monitor[c]	Helps to plan and implement the trial. Reviews conduct of the trial, plus completeness and accuracy of data collection forms. Often monitors data processing, analysis, and report writing
7. Sponsor's medical representative	In charge of the particular trial for the sponsor. May also act as trial monitor
8. Project leader or manager	In charge of managing the development of the medicine, medical device, or project for the sponsor
9. Medical department head	Academic (or sponsor's) department head, who has a formal or informal review function over the trial
10. Executives of the sponsoring institution	Individuals who must approve and review the overall strategy and allocation of funds given the project trials or an individual trial
11. Institutional Review Board members[d]	Approve initiation of the trial conducted at their institution and review its progress on a periodic basis. They must ensure that appropriate ethical standards are maintained and may intervene in the management of a trial
12. National regulatory agency	Usually reviews each protocol. Must approve the initiation of each trial in some countries. Reacts to issues that arise and may intervene in the management of a trial

[a] May be resident or fellow.

[b] Usually a physician. Coprincipal investigators may share this responsibility.

[c] For sponsored trials, one or more people from the sponsor or contract organization share this responsibility, or it may be conducted by a committee. This is performed by an individual at the trial site for nonsponsored trials and for some sponsored trials as well.

[d] Known as an Ethics Committee in many countries.

Investigator(s)

From an organizational perspective the investigator is the central figure in a clinical trial. He or she is the focal point for contact with the patients, staff, Ethics Committee/IRB, professional advisors, assistants, and sponsor. Many investigators direct the conduct of the trial through contact with each of these individuals or groups. Other investigators, however, deputize assistants or other staff (e.g., residents, fellows, study coordinator) to conduct the trial. These investigators often limit their involvement to the use of their name on a protocol and the eventual publication. Between these two extremes are investigators who participate to varying degrees in the conduct of a trial.

Degree of Involvement

It is important for sponsors to identify the type and degree of personal involvement that an investigator is able and willing to accept in a clinical trial. Confirming the degree of the investigator's involvement is in the sponsor's interest, since an investigator may have been chosen for his or her special skills or talents. This often occurs in complex surgical trials in which the investigator's assistants may not yet have mastered various techniques. The quality of a trial may be seriously com-

promised if the investigator does not participate at a previously agreed on level.

In nonsponsored clinical trials, an investigator may wish to minimize his or her own involvement and to delegate most or all parts of the trial to assistants, residents, fellows, or others. In sponsored trials, a well-known investigator may not have the time (and possibly interest) to become involved personally with a trial, yet has the facilities, staff, and patient population to conduct an excellent trial. The degree to which the investigator is able to participate in a clinical trial must be viewed individually, and an understanding must be reached as to the nature and necessary extent of the investigator's personal involvement.

Coinvestigator or Assistant Investigator

Two (or more) coinvestigators equally share overall responsibility for a clinical trial, although each may have their own spheres of responsibility and activity. Depending on the arrangements made for a trial, a single coinvestigator may have authority over the financial arrangements and allocation of funds. Reasons for utilizing coinvestigators include (1) recognizing an already existing partnership, (2) recognizing an already existing collaboration, or (3) indicating that two or more individuals initiating a trial are to be considered as equals in the venture.

Assistant investigators differ from coinvestigators in that they are at least nominally directed by the investigator. An assistant investigator is empowered to sign data collection forms and to act for the investigator regarding administrative matters, if required.

Members of Ethics Committees/Institutional Review Boards

The functions of this group are briefly summarized in Chapter 27.

Professional Consultants

Several types of consultants may be used in a clinical trial, including:

1. Consultant physicians who are requested on an ad hoc basis to evaluate or treat patients in a trial for unforeseen events (usually specialists in a specific discipline).
2. Consultant physicians or medical specialists who are requested to treat patients as part of the established clinical protocol.
3. Consultant specialists who are requested to assist in the diagnosis or evaluation of patients as part of the protocol (e.g., pathologists, electroencephalographers, individuals who conduct and interpret pulmonary function tests).
4. Consultants who review data or problems occurring in a trial and make suggestions as to means of solving or addressing these issues.
5. Consultants who are asked to help plan a specific trial, or the broad development of a single medicine or nonmedicine project.
6. Consultant contract organizations that either act as intermediaries to place a sponsor's trial at an appropriate site for its conduct or perform the trial themselves.
7. Lastly, there is a saying that anyone who calls himself (or herself) a consultant is one.

This topic is discussed in more detail in *Multinational Drug Companies: Issues in Drug Development and Discovery* (Spilker, 1989a).

Regulatory Agency Reviewers

The roles of regulatory agency reviewers are discussed in Chapters 126 to 128.

Trial Coordinator

The trial coordinator may also be termed the research coordinator, site planner, clinical coordinator, administrative director, and so forth. The trial coordinator handles most of the administrative responsibilities. Some of the tasks, such as scheduling appointments and sending out reminder cards to patients, may be delegated to another individual, if the size of the trial and workload at the trial site warrant. The trial coordinator may also assist in conducting the trial. The specific responsibilities assigned, plus the types of assignments made by the investigator, depend on the abilities and training of the coordinator. The trial coordinator may either devote 100% of his or her efforts to a single trial or may be involved with many trials.

The clinical trial coordinator is usually the contact person for the sponsor in most situations, both expected and unexpected. Data are usually reviewed for completeness and accuracy (i.e., to ensure that they are quality assured) by the coordinator before the trial monitor reviews them. Data may be entered on the data collection forms by the coordinator, who usually plays a pivotal role in ensuring that the trial is conducted as efficiently as possible.

Monitoring or Data Review Committees

In large multicenter studies a separate committee is sometimes established to oversee the monitoring of the clinical trial. In some cases the monitoring function is subdivided and assigned to several committees. See Chapters 39 and 62.

Other Staff

Numerous other individuals may be involved in planning, conducting, and analyzing clinical trials, particularly sponsored trials. Many of these individuals are located at the sponsoring institution and include statisticians, pharmacokinetic specialists, data entry operators, data editors, medical writers, report editors, and regulatory personnel.

Project Champion

An old adage is that jobs do not get done on their own and projects die when they are not pushed. A champion of a project is considered particularly important by those who emphasize this viewpoint. Strong proponents of a project champion believe that this concept is essential to optimize a project's overall progress.

In a management system with a project leader, this individual usually (although not always) acts as the project champion. The true project champion could be a senior executive, department chairman, or dean who is not even on the project team, but who encourages progress from "behind the scene." Numerous articles and books detail the ideal characteristics of project champions (e.g., entrepreneurial spirit, compulsiveness, workaholic nature, creativity) and indicate means through which potential champions may be identified and cultivated. Some of the major factors used to evaluate project champions/managers/leaders are presented in Table 122.3, and advantages of having projects led by champions are discussed in Chapter 124.

Multiple Champions for a Project

It is also possible for a project to have more than one champion, sometimes a primary and a secondary one(s). The primary champion is not necessarily the more senior person in the organization. Each champion will probably play different roles. Sometimes a champion of a project in its early phases turns it over to another individual later.

Pet Projects

When a senior individual has a "pet" idea (i.e., an idea of great personal importance) that is not widely shared by individuals less senior in the organization, the senior person is often forced, willingly or unwillingly, to become the champion. It behooves the senior executive to be relatively certain about the importance and likely outcome of the project, since significant company resources are often expended with few of the checks and balances that are usually applied. For staff morale and sometimes even for the sponsor's economic vitality, it is generally important to apply the same standards to the boss's pet projects as to other projects.

Project Manager

One alternative to the project champion is a project manager. This individual's primary professional objective is to guide a project through a maze of processes to a successful outcome. He or she usually controls (or manages) several projects at the same time. Proponents of this system claim that many of the emotional factors that often complicate the approach of the project champion do not concern the professional manager, since the project manager is not usually as emotionally involved. Also, the project manager is often described as a professional administrator who is experienced in managing a project or projects and does not have to also contend with the specific discipline-related tasks that confront most champions. Proponents of the project manager approach also claim that a project champion is often a professional scientist, clinician, or other individual who is usually relatively unskilled in the administrative requirements for leading a project. Advantages of having teams led by professional project managers are discussed in Chapter 124. Some of the functions that a project manager must track (monitor) are listed in Table 122.4.

TABLE 122.3 *Selected factors used to evaluate project leaders/managers*

1. Interpersonal and communication skills, which facilitate interactions with many different people who have widely different backgrounds
2. Effective leadership of the project team as evidenced through motivation of others
3. Ability to concentrate on details and an overall perspective of the project being managed
4. Adequate self-confidence to seek help elsewhere when required, while still functioning independently and avoiding dependence on others
5. Organizational abilities to establish an effective monitoring system that observes each important area of the project for early signs of potential problems or other matters that require attention
6. Initiative and self-motivation to start activities without prompting, and perseverence to continue them to completion
7. Ability to plan, organize, and coordinate activities in a project. Ability to move the project toward its objectives in the most direct and efficient means practical
8. Taking necessary steps to keep activities as close to schedule as possible
9. Adjusting strategies and goals as appropriate and in a timely manner
10. Technical skills in area(s) of expertise
11. Ability to be imaginative in selecting the approaches taken
12. Using resources appropriately and only requesting resources necessary to meet objectives
13. Ability to write clearly and communicate effectively in reports
14. Ability to use sound judgment to make decisions and adjust priorities and plans as required
15. Ability to determine, in a timely manner, when the project should be terminated

TABLE 122.4 *Administrative functions to consider monitoring during a project's life[a]*

1. Tracking the status of the clinical data
2. Tracking the status of ongoing and completed nonclinical studies conducted by the sponsor, contractors, and others
3. Tracking both published and unpublished articles and reports
4. Tracking bulk chemicals and formulated medicine supplies
5. Tracking funds that are committed and spent for both internal and external costs
6. Tracking the time and effort expended by various departments
7. Tracking the fate of all medicine supplies sent to various sites
8. Tracking the status of competitive medicines under investigation
9. Tracking the market for which the medicine is being targeted
10. Tracking trends in FDA reviews of similar medicines

[a] Forms may be created for each of these activities that are monitored.

STAFF MOTIVATION AND MORALE

Changes in Motivation over Time

The amount of time that each investigator and his or her staff devote to any one clinical trial varies widely. This aspect often depends on, and in turn influences, their degree of interest, involvement, and motivation to conduct a trial at the highest level. Unless some unexpected positive results occur, the high point of most people's interest in a trial they are conducting usually occurs at or near the outset. This implies that if the investigator or staff members are lukewarm about conducting a trial at the outset, the chances are great that their interest will rapidly decline after the trial is initiated.

An investigator and staff members who spend relatively little time on a clinical trial (e.g., below 10–20% of their work week) often do not invest the effort, enthusiasm, and emotional commitment necessary to complete it in a timely manner. If a trial is extremely long in duration (i.e., a number of years) or extends beyond the original plans (usually due to slower patient enrollment than anticipated), then the interest of the investigator and staff may be expected to wane. Improving the efficiency with which a project is managed also served to improve morale. A number of areas in which efficiencies are often obtained are listed in Table 122.5.

Maintaining Motivation

To maintain motivation at a high level there are a number of techniques that a monitor (as well as the investigator) should consider. The most important is to discern at the outset what motivates the staff, primarily the investigator(s), and then to address their desires.

TABLE 122.5 *Selected project management areas in which great efficiencies may often be achieved*

A. Meetings
1. Conduct well-organized and targeted meetings
2. Terminate meetings when they are not productive
3. Eliminate periodic or ad hoc meetings that are not necessary
B. Documents
1. Eliminate unnecessary paperwork
2. Eliminate unimportant periodic reports
C. Travel
1. Cancel periodic business trips unless essential or expected to be productive
2. Replace trips with telephone calls plus letters whenever possible
D. Allocation of time
1. Evaluate whether one's time is spent on the most important issues and tasks that are pending
2. Delegate matters that may be handled by others

Common sources of motivation include (1) professional recognition, (2) career advancement, (3) financial reward, (4) advancement of science, and (5) ability to treat a certain patient group more effectively. Motives often overlap, and several of these (plus others) may be present in any one individual.

Professional recognition may be stimulated by publications and by encouragement and travel funds to present data at professional meetings. Some sponsors assist investigators in preparing their posters, slides, or other materials. Career advancement may be stimulated through (1) publication, (2) public speaking at various meetings about important results, and (3) informing (directly or indirectly) the investigator's institution about the financial contribution that certain clinical trials make to that institution. Financial considerations may be stimulated by providing bonuses for meeting target enrollments and by sponsoring trips to scientific meetings for the investigator and appropriate staff. Advancement of science is dependent on the importance of the trial and the quality of the data. Treating one's patients in a trial leads to its own rewards. Care must be used in offering financial bonuses to prevent any conflicts of interest or undesired influences on the trial conduct (e.g., entering of inappropriate patients, excessive discontinuation of patients, sloppy study conduct).

CONSIDERATIONS IN ESTABLISHING AND MAINTAINING MANAGEMENT SYSTEMS

The choice of a suitable system of forms, reports, and meetings to review and manage multiple clinical trials and the personnel assigned to them depends on whether the clinical trials are to (1) be conducted on one medicine by a single person or group, (2) involve one type of trial (e.g., pharmacokinetic, Phase I, population survey) on many medicines, or (3) involve a variety of different types of trials on many different medicines. In many management situations all three of these types are followed, but by different individuals or groups within an institution. Questions to consider in implementing a management system are listed in Table 122.6, and issues relating to meetings and reports are discussed in Chapter 125.

Organizational Factors

In choosing the most appropriate management system(s) to oversee the planning, conduct, and analysis of multiple clinical trials there are several considerations that relate to the nature of the managing organization. Academic managers and clinical investiga-

TABLE 122.6 *Questions to consider in implementing a management system*

1. Are most people in agreement with the nature of the proposed system?
2. Do most people support the individual managers who will operate the system?
3. Have adequate descriptions of the system been written and distributed to relevant individuals?
4. Have adequate meetings been held with the staff to explain the system?
5. Has everyone had ample opportunity to raise questions and point out potential problems with the proposed system?
6. Has a pilot program of the system been tested in a group smaller than the entire group to be affected?
7. Should outside consultants review the system for possible flaws or potential problems?
8. Has the system been endorsed and approved by all of the relevant senior managers?
9. Have countermeasures and other mechanisms been developed for all the possible major exceptions and problems that have been anticipated?

tors often have different reporting relationships and pressures than do the government agencies that sometimes manage clinical trials (e.g., National Institute of Neurological Disorders in their Antiepileptic Drug Development Program). Both of these groups differ markedly in organizational structure and objectives compared with those of the pharmaceutical industry, which sponsors many clinical trials. Research-based companies within the pharmaceutical industry that are developing medicines also differ from (1) contract companies that conduct trials or act as intermediaries to place and monitor trials and (2) other companies in the health area, such as manufacturers of equipment or medical devices.

Individual management systems used in academia, government, and industry may differ because of both general and specific variables. Each department, committee, or group of people in these three types of general organizations have different reporting responsibilities and groups with whom they interact. Some of these interactions necessitate the creation and use of certain types of management systems and preclude others. Secondly, each specific institution within each type of organization (i.e., academia, government, pharmaceutical company, independent company) differs in size, goals, historical tradition, personnel, and resources, so that there will be major differences in the optimal systems that each institution develops. These factors have a major influence on the management system chosen, but in a few instances the type of institution will have a greater influence.

Individuals in management in academia, government, and industry all have to deal with questions of prioritization and allocation of resources (see Chapter 123). Other management issues at all institutions involve the coordination of multiple projects (see Chapter 124).

Size of the Organization

Several other factors, which are independent of whether the institution is academic, governmental, or industrial, also influence management systems. For instance, some management systems are more appropriate to large institutions, and other systems are more appropriate to smaller ones. Personalities of senior managers and traditional methods of management at some institutions often have the greatest influence on the choice of systems and the degree of formality.

Although more formal methods are usually associated with large institutions and more informal methods are associated with smaller groups or institutions, there are numerous exceptions to this principle. An informal system can work well in a larger institution when people are trusted to be conscientious about performing their job well. This requires that the most senior managers have a great deal of trust in subordinates. When this method works well, the most senior scientific manager is usually able to remain aware of most activities and is able to react quickly as decisions have to be made. There are not many strong, self-confident scientists who possess both the scientific and managerial skills necessary to make this approach work in a large company, government agency, or university. In small institutions with relatively few scientists it is much easier to make this style of management work effectively.

It is more common for large institutions to follow formal systems for managing projects and multiple clinical trials. These systems usually involve forming various committees and periodic reports to provide checks and balances to ensure that each project is progressing at an appropriate pace and in the correct direction. The systems are intended to provide increasingly general summaries of the work, problems, and progress of the project as they are directed to progressively higher levels in the institution.

KEEPING SENIOR MANAGEMENT ADEQUATELY INFORMED

One means for senior managers to remain current with project status is to receive brief reports on a periodic basis. These reports should contain essential information on the project such as that listed in Table 122.7. The other major mechanism is for senior managers to receive briefings from the relevant senior manager, project manager, or another individual. Most institutions use both the techniques of reports and meetings to keep management informed. Every institution, department, and other group should periodically reassess whether their balance of meetings and reports is satisfactory for their needs and whether it may be im-

TABLE 122.7 *Issues that may be covered in a project summary for senior management*

1. Project name, number, therapeutic category
2. Medicine generic name and trade name
3. Project leader or manager
4. Proposed initial indication(s)
5. Phase of current development
6. Background material and summary of the project's history
7. Milestone dates (e.g., project formation; IND submission; Phase I, II, III; NDA submission; product launch)[a]
8. Project costs (e.g., actual to-date, estimated total costs)
9. Major technical issues
10. Major clinical issues
11. General market background (e.g., market size in sales and prescriptions, growth trend, competitive environment and intensity, disease demographics, need for improved therapy)
12. Major marketing issues
13. Marketing considerations (e.g., final formulation, names of competitive products plus their sales and market share)
14. Patent status
15. Potential therapeutic and competitive advantages
16. Major production and manufacturing issues
17. Projected sales for first 3 years
18. Major uncertainties and questions to address
19. Potential indications
20. Significant changes since the previous report
21. Date of report

[a] IND, Investigational New Drug Application; NDA, New Drug Application.

proved. The quality and speed of senior managers' decision making and workers' productivity both suffer when there is an excessive amount or total lack of reports and meetings. Both formal and informal reviews by management should be used to facilitate progress on projects rather than impede it. It is clearly impossible to describe the appropriate blend of reviews, since this varies enormously between situations and institutions. The best management decisions can usually be reached when all information is available, all relevant people have given their opinions, all possible alternatives are known, and a thorough discussion has occurred among the relevant people.

CONCLUSIONS

A management style that emphasizes a strong leader is usually most effective when the environment of the organization is weak. The strong leader is best able to stimulate career growth, communications, and efficient work habits in this type of environment. In organizations with a positive climate, a team-oriented management style is the more productive. It is unfortunate that as institution's environments change, the styles of the leaders do not often follow. Thus, many strong organizations become weakened, in time, by the very skills and management techniques that once made them strong. A related aspect is that when top managers retire they usually choose successors who most clearly resemble themselves, without adequate consideration of what style would best suit the institution in the years ahead.

CHAPTER 123

Prioritization of Activities and Allocation of both Resources and Supplies

PRIORITIZATION

Why Have Priorities?

Prioritization of activities, projects, or clinical trials is not required unless two or more activities are competing for the same resources. On the other hand, it is virtually impossible to plan, conduct, and analyze data from even a single clinical trial without frequent need to prioritize various activities to help guide most people involved with the trial. This necessity becomes much more critical when multiple clinical trials are considered. If no priorities are set within and between trials or projects one must deal individually with every issue and conflict of resources as they arise, and often one must reanalyze the same or similar decisions on several occasions. Even without establishing formal priorities in every trial, *de facto* priorities exist. Finally, prioritization assists the process of allocating resources.

Types of Prioritization

Prioritization in its simplest form does not require documentation or special planning. It is performed by applying common sense to determine what activities should be done in which order. This simple approach to prioritization is usually not sufficient to handle large numbers of activities or potential activities that require resources and attention. A more formal approach to prioritization is to create lists to keep track and organize various activities. These lists may assign an order of priority to all items from 1 to n, or assign general classes of priorities, such as A, B, or C. Alternative techniques are to establish a "high" and "low" system or to describe functions that take priority over other functions (e.g., clinical activities take priority over technical development, which in turn takes priority over basic research), or to state that activities on marketed medicines have priority over activities on Phase III medicines, which in turn have priority over medicines in Phase II, and so on. The numerous priorities for the activities within each trial may be identified with the same or different type of prioritizing system.

Hierarchies of Priorities

In addition to assigning priorities to different investigational or marketed medicines, there is an entire hierarchy of priorities. Above the level of individual medicines, certain groups of medicines, such as those in a specific therapeutic area, may be given a high or low priority. Below the level of individual medicines, priorities may be assigned to certain trials, indications, dosage forms, routes of administration, etc. Within any of these categories certain activities will be given higher or lower priorities. It is important to prioritize separately the indications of a medicine that are being (or will be) pursued from the specific claims that the sponsor wants to make for all indications together, or for each one individually.

Criteria Used to Establish Priorities

Criteria used to establish priorities often emphasize the potential medical and/or commercial value of the projects. Other criteria include (1) the availability of resources and expertise both within and outside the institution, (2) scientific value, (3) quantity and type of resources required to develop the medicine, and (4) public health/political/regulatory issues surrounding the particular medicine (or type of medicine) being developed. For example, a new medicine to treat a problem of importance to national health such as acquired immunodeficiency syndrome (AIDS) will generally be given a higher priority by its sponsor than most other medicines.

Establishing Priorities Based on Assigning Scores and Using Elaborate Systems

Elaborate systems of prioritization may be developed that involve establishment of criteria and scores by which to judge the major competing elements (e.g., projects, clinical trials) for resources. A range of possible scores is usually established for each criterion; the scores may be equal (e.g., a maximum of 5 points is assigned for each criterion) or weighted to reflect importance. Criteria that are scored should be those that impact on the decision of how best to allocate resources (e.g., time, efforts, money). Interrelationships between two or more criteria may or may not be considered. The goal of this type of exercise is to determine a numerical ranking of competing projects so

that one may allocate resources either proportionally to their importance (assuming that this was the basis for the ranking) or to a project or projects at the top of the ranking. This approach is rarely useful for prioritizing investigational medicines because their status often changes rapidly. A summary of systems used to prioritize projects or activities is given in Table 123.1.

Who Establishes Priorities?

In most instances there will not be one individual, or even one group of individuals, that establishes each of these priorities. The broad type of medicine development program described requires integration of many types of departments, individuals, and skills. Therefore, assigning priorities among different medicines when conflicts arise must be made by senior managers. It would be ideal if each individual could establish his or her own priorities for achieving objectives assigned by his or her immediate superior and fit these together with priorities of other individuals with a minimum of conflict. Unfortunately this does not usually occur, and conflicts frequently have to be resolved by others.

Can a Formal System of Priorities Be Avoided?

If there is a general agreement on medicine development goals and the methods of operation to achieve those goals, then avoidance of a formal priority system is possible. The most important elements of a successful system for developing medicines are (1) a de-

---

TABLE 123.1 *Systems to prioritize projects or activities[a]*

1. Do not establish any formal system for assigning priorities; instead, allow decisions on priorities to be made as they are required
2. Establish a priority sequence of 1 to n (for n activities)
3. Establish a classification of "A" (high priority), "B" (moderate priority), and "C" (low priority). Divide all projects or activities into one of these three (or other number) classes
4. Establish a two-tiered informal system of having "high" and "low" priority projects, possibly with a single project designated as a "top" priority
5. The priority system used may not be based on specific whole projects but on subparts (e.g., chemical development, analytical assays) of all or certain projects
6. Differentiate between marketed and investigational projects and establish separate systems of priorities for each group
7. Establish a two-tiered system. In the first tier, prioritize marketed medicines ahead of medicines with a pending NDA, which in turn come before Phase III medicines which precede Phase II medicines, etc. The second tier refers to priorities made within each of these broad classes

[a] More flexible systems appear to work best in most situations within the pharmaceutical industry because of the frequent changes of medicine status and the frequent modifications required in prioritizations.

sire of the relevant people for it to work, (2) a clear statement and understanding of the objectives for each medicine's development, and (3) periodic reviews to ensure that activities are progressing appropriately and in the correct direction. Reviews are performed both by the individuals who supervise the system and by a person or group (e.g., matrix group) who is (are) different from the people who are responsible for conducting the work (e.g., line-function departments). Reevaluating relevant priority issues, either formally or informally on a periodic basis is an important part of this review, as well as reviewing the strategies for the medicine's development.

Why Priorities Differ in Different Departments

Achieving harmony in a large organization often requires apparently conflicting priorities within various parts of the organization. As an example, assume that a corporation has informally placed its highest priority on developing and marketing three investigational medicines (medicines A, B, and C) and has assigned a low priority to three other medicines (medicines E, F, and G). Further, assume that medicines A, C, and E are close to having a New Drug Application (NDA) submitted, whereas medicines B, F, and G are in an early stage of development. Some departments are primarily active during the early part of a medicine's development (e.g., pharmacology, organic chemistry, analytical chemistry) whereas other departments are primarily involved as the medicine gets closer to the market (e.g., postmarketing surveillance, production, data processing). Thus, the priorities within those departments whose activity is greatest during the early phases of a medicine's development will be different (medicine B will have the highest priority and medicines F and G will have high priority) than in those departments with responsibilities at the later points of development, where medicines A and C will have the highest priority and medicine E will have high priority. The actual situation would have to include consideration of other factors as well, as such as the technical ease of conducting the work, the skills of the staff, costs of development, availability of raw materials, or medicine to work with, and possibilities of contracting the work to others. In addition, some departments operate best with continuous input or flow of work, whereas others prefer job work (each job is actually a discrete bolus of work that may come every X months or weeks).

Use of Priorities in Actual Practice

An actual case of medicine development is usually more complex. Priorities at all levels are frequently changing because of (1) unexpected toxicities, (2) delays, (3) problems, (4) regulatory requests, (5) movements of personnel, (6) opportunities, or (7) other factors. It is partly for these reasons that formal systems of priorities are usually impractical except as a general guide. An elaborate or formal system that changes frequently requires meetings, documents, and resources to confirm each change and rapid communication of changes throughout the relevant parts of the organization. Changes in an informal prioritization system are usually more easily communicated because they do not require several steps to formalize and disseminate information. Low-priority activities tend to never be completed.

ALLOCATION OF RESOURCES

Approaches

In allocating resources one may use any one, or combination, of various systems. The simplest approach is to give all required resources to the project that has top priority. Any remaining resources are then applied to the second priority project, and so forth, until all resources have been allocated. This approach may make sense in some situations, such as when a financially troubled company has one project that stands out above the others in terms of its commercial potential coupled with ease of development. In most situations, however, a company has many viable projects and focusing resources on a single project makes little sense.

Resources of time, effort, and money in terms of people, equipment, and other factors (e.g., prestige, image) must often be apportioned to different projects. The intensity, duration, and quantity of resources are often allocated according to priorities. In an ideal world there would be a perfect correlation between allocations and priorities. In the real world, however, people do not often establish clear priorities because priorities are not all-or-none, but vary by degree and may change frequently. In addition, often people do not reevaluate priorities as conditions change. People may also not pursue their most important priorities because of many reasons, including judgment errors or psychologically denying the correct priorities.

Who Allocates Resources?

Resources may be allocated by senior management with little input by department and section managers, or may result from joint discussions and decisions. The systems established by a group to allocate resources may be broadly based, narrowly based, formal, informal, or nonexistent. In nonexistent systems, resources

TABLE 123.2 *Methods to expand capabilities of fixed resources temporarily*

1. Contract a facility to serve as a core laboratory to assay samples off site
2. Use outside contract groups to (1) obtain investigators, (2) monitor clinical trials, (3) process data, (4) analyze results, or (5) prepare regulatory dossiers
3. Collaborate with government agencies interested in developing medicines (e.g., National Cancer Institute, National Institute of Neurological Disorders)
4. Collaborate with United Nations organizations (e.g., World Health Organization) on development of medicines intended for Third World countries
5. Contract synthesis or evaluation of compounds to outside scientists or to contract laboratories
6. Conduct only a partial analysis of data to expedite decisions. Complete data analyses at a later date only for viable projects
7. Hire temporary employees to assist in handling a short-term excess of work
8. Reassign permanent employees to handle a specific issue or task for a limited period
9. Delay work on less important activities to free additional staff

may be allocated to those champions and projects who make the loudest din or to those areas in which crises occur, or may be based on a manager's whim, personal preference, or various nonrational bases.

Expanding Fixed Resources

It is sometimes necessary to increase resources for a short period to satisfactorily deal with a temporary need. Selected methods that may temporarily expand the capabilities of fixed resources are listed in Table 123.2.

How Many Projects Should Each Person Work On?

Individuals may be assigned to work on only one project so that each project has a certain number of unique individuals assigned to it. Alternatively, each individual may be assigned to various projects and his or her time must then be allocated according to priorities established either for or by that individual. Com-

bination approaches are often used in industry and academia, whereby some individuals work only on one project and others work on several. The reasons for choosing between these approaches may be based on the specific department involved or on the methods used to allocate resources. Sample headings of tables used to summarize work-force allocations are given in Table 123.3.

Reviewing the Allocation of Resources

The portion of total resources allocated to each project and to each clinical trial within individual projects should be periodically reviewed. This review can be done at several levels within an organization or by the individual or group responsible for the allocation of resources. Reviews may occur on either a fixed or variable time basis, or only when forced by a "crisis." If reviews occur on a fixed interval, that interval may either be tied to time (e.g., monthly, quarterly) or to the stage in a project's life [e.g., Investigational New Drug Application (IND) submission, Phase I, Phase II].

ALLOCATING SUPPLIES OF A MEDICINE OR COMPOUND

How to Distribute Medicine for Clinical Testing When There Are More Demands than Supply

The first principle in medicine distribution is to determine the total quantity of a medicine required, the amount needed by each group or individual, and exactly when it is needed. Groups that are requesting the medicine are often from numerous areas of a company outside the medical function. If there are requests for more medicine than is available, then supplies to some preclinical or clinical departments or for some clinical trials will have to be delayed.

Important considerations in allocating the available supply of a medicine include: (1) if additional medicine

TABLE 123.3 *Sample table headings to summarize work-force allocations to specific clinical trials or activities*

A

Project number and protocol number	Title of trial	Investigator name(s)	No. of patients	Current status	Name or initials of personnel	Percentage of time allocated for the period (*X* months)

B

Project activity	Current status	Name or initials of personnel	Percentage of time allocated for the period	Maximum total work force needed during the period

C

Project activity	Total work force allocated for the period (worker months/month)	Total worker months for the period	Senior level headcount assigned	Junior level headcount assigned

TABLE 123.4 *Suggested procedure to allocate a limited supply of a medicine or compound[a]*

1. Identify every group that wants or needs the medicine
2. Determine how much medicine each group needs
3. Identify the critical path for the medicine's development
4. Identify the schedule for future syntheses (at all manufacturing sites) and the amounts scheduled to be made at each time
5. Determine the relative certainty that these dates and quantities will be met
6. Identify the commitments made for present and future medicine supplies
7. Determine which allocation of medicine would minimize delays on the critical path of pharmaceutical development
8. Allocate small amounts of medicine to those departments that only requested small amounts or can begin (or conduct) all their work with small amounts
9. Ensure that any group beginning work with less than their total needs will not lose the value of their work if future medicine supplies cannot be met. Explore this issue in depth

[a] The term "compound" is also assumed in the table when the word medicine is used.

TABLE 123.5. *Goals in preparing medicines and placebos for use in double-blind clinical trials*

1. Error-proof procedures
2. Procedures that are easy to implement
3. Placebos that are similar to active medicine in all characteristics[a]
4. Documentation of all procedures that uses simple language and is easily understood by staff
5. Documentation of how to use medicines that is easy for investigators to understand and implement
6. A method of medicine use that is easy for patients to understand
7. Readily available method to break the blind, if needed
8. Procedures that adhere to required regulations and guidelines

[a] See Table 25.1.

is available elsewhere in the company (e.g., at another site, in other laboratories), (2) which groups require the medicine for ongoing studies that should not (or must not) be readily stopped (e.g., toxicology, clinical trials), (3) what are the absolute quantities needed by each group, (4) which groups requesting medicine are on the critical path to creating the regulatory application, and (5) where delays would be most disruptive if they occurred.

Another point to consider is that a toxicology study may be begun with a fraction of the total dose required for the study, if the supply of the remaining compound required can be assured at appropriate times, while the study is underway. Providing medicine from different batches or lots, however, may cause problems for a company if a different impurity profile is found.

A group that requires only a very small amount of compound can usually be given this amount despite the fact that its need is not as great as groups needing large amounts. Procedures for allocating a limited supply of medicine and goals in preparing medicines are listed in Tables 123.4 and 123.5.

Monitoring the Use of Available Compound Supply

The internal stock of a company's compounds and investigational medicines must be carefully monitored to

prevent unexpected drains that would deplete stocks of important compounds/medicines. A system may be readily developed so that the individual responsible for a research program or medicine project is notified each time some of the compound or medicine is removed (or alternatively, is requested) from a central stock. This could be done by having the stock controller complete a preprinted form. The balance of stock remaining should be indicated so that reorders could be placed at appropriate times.

Alternatively, the key individual involved in activities on a particular compound or medicine could be required to give permission for all withdrawals made from the central stock. Although this process allows greater control of available supplies, such tight control may not be necessary for all compounds and could inhibit innovation in research. Both systems could be used in a sequential order: an informal system (or no system) could be used until compound or medicine stock fell to a level that was prespecified for each compound or medicine, at which time a mandatory system for approving further withdrawals would be invoked. Various methods and aspects of tracking medicines are shown in Tables 123.6 to 123.8.

Can Unused Medicine Supplies Be Transferred to a Different Clinical Site?

Whether unused medicines may be sent to another site depends on the particular policies and regulations of the country and sponsor. In general, unopened sealed

TABLE 123.6 *Sample table headings to determine clinical supply needs*

Clinical trial number[a]	Total number of patients	Anticipated daily dosage per patient (average no. of mg)	Duration of trial per patient (days, weeks, months)	Total medicine supply needed per patient (mg)	Total medicine needed per year (month) for the trial
A					
B					
C					

[a] Each site of a multicenter trial could be listed separately or as a combined total.

TABLE 123.7 *Sample table headings to track requested supplies of a medicine*

Date of current update _____

Code number of the request for the compound	Date and quantity of the request for chemical synthesis	Date raw materials ordered and received	Status of the chemical synthesis (planned, in progress, completed)	Chemical passed by the analytical department (yes, no, date)	Amount of bulk chemical currently available for use	Formulated chemical prepared as the medicine	Number of tablets and other dosage forms prepared (per strength)	Amount of packaged medicine available for use (per strength)	Date medicine shipped to sites

bottles may be sent to another site in the same clinical trial when identical packaging is used. Appropriate medicine disposition forms must be completed, and all documents must be transferred to the new site. Anticancer medicines, however, are not sent to other sites. The pros and cons of sending unused noncancer medicine supplies to a new site must be assessed separately for each case and a decision made based on weighing costs and benefits involved.

It is almost never practical to take unused medicines from a clinical trial and return them to bulk stock. This practice raises the possibility of numerous types of potentially serious errors arising, such as putting the tablets or capsules in the wrong large containers (e.g., in placebo versus active medicine bins), or combining them with the wrong dosage strengths (e.g., placing tablets in the 100-mg versus 200-mg bins).

What Happens When an Investigational Medicine's Shelf Life Is About to Expire?

During the investigational period a long shelf life is rare for a new medicine. Developing new formulations, dosage forms, dosing strengths, and shapes means that the clock on measuring stability and shelf life of samples starts anew each time a change in made.

Medicine samples from the batch used in a clinical trial are periodically retested and "repassed" to extend the shelf life of existing supplies and continue the trial. There is no limit to the number of times that medicines may be repassed during the investigational period. The information on a medicine's repass is sent to the investigators.

How May a Company Convert a Medicine's Development from Capsules to Tablets?

Conversion from capsules to tablets is a common event during a medicine's development program. It ideally

occurs at the start of a new phase of clinical trial study. A less ideal, but acceptable approach is to make this conversion at the start of a new trial. Another less desirable approach is to convert dosage forms during a long-term trial. It is undesirable and ill advised to make this change during a relatively short (e.g., 6-week) clinical trial, even if that trial lasts for a total of 1 or 2 years. It will definitely raise regulatory questions in the future and places the regulatory acceptance of the entire clinical trial in jeopardy. This change must never be made during a well-controlled pivotal trial.

To avoid this last possibility it is necessary to ensure that adequate supplies of an old dosage form exist at the start of a clinical trial. If the medicine is poorly absorbed then there is a greater risk that bioavailability between a capsule and tablet will differ. Film coating tablets may delay a medicine's absorption; such tablets must never been introduced during a clinical trial. It is strongly desirable (some would say mandatory) to confirm that the film-coating process has not affected the pharmacokinetics of the medicine, before it is introduced in any efficacy trial.

TABLE 123.8 *Various aspects of pharmaceutical supplies that must be tracked*

1. Amounts requested by each department and individual
2. Dates that each requestor needs the material requested
3. May amounts requested be delivered in parts? If so, how much must be delivered by which dates
4. Schedule of batches to be made
5. Status of each batch
6. Potential or actual delays and what is being done to address these problems
7. Amounts prepared and a comparison with amounts requested
8. Analytical profile, identity, and quantity of impurities present in each batch
9. Priorities of all requests
10. Location of material remaining from each batch
11. Code numbers of clinical trials that received medicine of each batch prepared for clinical use
12. Twelve- and 18-month forecasts of future medicine and placebo requirements

CHAPTER 124

Coordination and Management of Multiple Projects

DESCRIPTION OF PROJECTS

Within the pharmaceutical industry and a number of other health-care-related industries, (e.g., medical device or equipment manufacturers), innovation and technology are primarily directed toward development of new products that will eventually be launched on the market. Conducting the myriad steps necessary to develop a new medicine or product requires coordination of the input and substantial activities occurring in numerous departments.

Projects are defined differently in different pharmaceutical companies. In some companies, a project represents one potential medicine no matter how many formulations, dosage forms, or indications are evaluated. In other companies, each dosage form, formulation, and indication studied is considered as a separate project. A second aspect of defining projects relates to the stage of development at which a project is formed. A project may be formed at any stage, from an early chemical lead to a medicine that has demonstrated activity in Phase II evaluations. A third consideration relates to whether one or more than one chemical compound may be considered to be part of a single project. Thus, it is apparent that the number of projects existing at different companies can only be compared when each of the above factors is considered. The quality of a compound in terms of its potential medical and commercial value are probably the most important criteria in creating new projects. Companies use different standards in determining whether a compound should be developed as a medicine with regard to these two criteria. The implementation of these standards also has a great influence on the number of projects that are present in a company at any one time.

PROJECT TEAMS

To develop medicines efficiently, it is useful to bring together at least one member of each of the various departments that will be involved in the development. This usually occurs before a compound has been tested in humans. These members may be referred to as a team, project group, project team, project committee, or by another term. This group is usually given a certain level of autonomy plus limited authority by senior management to pursue the development of their project. The team meets to determine goals, set strategies, develop and revise plans, set priorities within their project, and solve problems. Their efforts are reviewed formally and informally by other groups or individuals at periodic intervals or on an ad hoc basis.

Structure of Project Teams

The number of members of each project group varies enormously between (and even within) companies. There is no ideal number of members on the project group. For most projects there will probably be anywhere from 5 to 20 members on the committee, although the precise number is highly dependent on various factors, including (1) tradition and practice of the corporation, (2) type of project involved, (3) current phase of development, (4) plans and goals of the project, and (5) constraints on resources due to the presence of other projects. A summary of the various alternative organizational structures that constitute a project team is given in Table 124.1.

Seniority and Authority of Project Team Members

The seniority and authority of the members of the project team vary between companies. Team members at many companies are those who lead the work within their own departments, but individuals may be appointed to the project team for other reasons. Some administratively oriented individuals (e.g., department heads) may also be members of a project team to act as a bridge between line management and the matrix management concept (see next section) or for other reasons. Service and support departments (e.g., statistics, data entry processors, metabolism, toxicology) may also be represented on the team at relevant

TABLE 124.1 *Alternative organizations and characteristics of a project team[a]*

Alternative	Approach to completing work on project	Approach to developing a team	Responsibility for work	Project leadership	Coordination with limited authority	Coordination with full authority	Periodic and ad hoc review and control
A	Divide work into subprojects for functional departments	No team exists (pure functional organization)	Each functional manager or department head	None	Generally none	Department heads or functional leaders	Upper levels of management
B	Divide work into subprojects for functional departments	Functional managers appoint representative (pseudomatrix)	Each functional manager or department head	None, committee, or other	A member within each department	Department heads or functional leaders	Upper levels of management
C	Divide work into subprojects for functional departments	Functional managers appoint representative (matrix)	Each functional manager or department head	Project manager[b]	Project manager or individual from outside the departments	Department heads and project manager	Upper levels of management
D	Divide work into subprojects for functional departments	Functional managers appoint representative (matrix)	Department heads and project manager	Project manager[b]	Individual jointly appointed by functional and project managers	Project manager	Upper levels of management
E	Divide work into subprojects for functional departments	Functional managers assign personnel to join a team full time (task force)	Project manager	Project manager[b]	Individual on team	Project manager	Upper levels of management
F	Core group exists to handle multiple disciplinary functions	Core group functions as a team (pure project)	Project manager	Project manager[b]	Individual on team	Project manager	Upper levels of management

[a] Many variations on these six alternatives are possible.
[b] Project managers may be champions or full-time professional managers.

stage(s) during the life of a project. At some companies the project team is composed entirely or almost entirely of more-senior staff (e.g., department heads). A description and models of international project teams are given in Chapter 121.

Roles of Project Leaders, Managers, and Members

The roles of the project head depend on whether he or she is viewed or instructed to act as a true leader and champion or as an administrator and manager. Both types of individuals conduct many activities and typically run meetings in a similar way. Outside meetings, however, the project leader acts as an enthusiastic and dedicated troubleshooter, cheerleader (i.e., morale booster), and politician, supporting the project team in its effort to accomplish the project's goals. The champion usually has other line function responsibilities (e.g., running a section, department, or division, directing the clinical trials on the project).

The project manager is more administratively oriented and does more coordinating of the various elements than working hard to shape them. This person often spends more time than the project leader champion on the daily "nuts and bolts" because he or she is working full time on the project. Some project managers act as bureaucrats and administer projects by adhering to all details of standard operating procedures, whereas other project managers are more creative administrators.

Roles of project members are described in Table 124.2.

TABLE 124.2 Roles of project team members[a]

1. Represent their department on the team
2. Share technical expertise with the team on issues that arise
3. Maintain expertise within their discipline and specific areas of the project
4. Consult other members of their department
5. Maintain awareness of evolving regulations and guidelines
6. Develop and maintain contacts with outside experts and consultants
7. Learn about aspects of one's field that are changing or might provide a competitive advantage
8. Develop an ability to predict accurately how long it takes to accomplish various activities and learn how to consider all major influences (e.g., priority, amount of resources needed and available) that affect time
9. Inform department managers about the status of the project and any requests for changes in the level of resources needed
10. Inform the project leader of any events that will affect (e.g., delay) the project (i.e., adhere to the golden rule of "no surprises" at meetings)
11. Coordinate activities with counterparts in other sites of the organization
12. Arrive at all project meetings prepared to present or discuss topics on the agenda

[a] Roles of several types of specific project team members (e.g., regulatory affairs, marketing) are listed in Tables 121.4, 121.5, and 129.10.

Another variation is for a company to have therapeutic area teams for development. Each team leader is usually a vice-president for a functional area. This makes the team quite powerful and the leader able to make important decisions. These teams usually meet on a periodic (e.g., monthly) basis and deal with all projects within that therapeutic area. Team chairpersons may meet as a separate group with the head of the company on a scheduled basis.

MATRIX ORGANIZATIONAL STRUCTURE

Vertical and Horizontal Management

In the traditional system of management, generally referred to as "line-function" or vertical management, individuals report through the chain of command to the top of the organization. This type of management is usually described as having a pyramid structure, because there are progressively fewer managers as one ascends the corporate or institutional ranks. A newer system of management that has become more widespread in recent years is called a "matrix organizational structure." This is usually described as a horizontal system.

In most instances the matrix system does not replace the more traditional hierarchical-oriented line management system, but is superimposed on it. All individuals continue to report through the line-function organization, but many (possibly most) employees also have a second reporting responsibility. Those individuals report to a member of the project team or group. Each member of the project team reports to the leader of the project, and all project leaders report to a central coordinator of all projects who then reports up the pyramid (or directly) to the head of research and development.

The reporting relationships in the matrix system may be as formal as those of the line-function system or they may be quite informal. The optimal system for each organization probably varies to some degree depending on the (1) historical traditions of the organization, (2) personalities of the people doing the work, (3) nature of their projects, and (4) styles of management used in the line-function system. Other considerations (e.g., personalities of the senior managers) are also of importance in determining the optimal manner in which to establish the matrix system.

Advantages of the Matrix Structure

A matrix system is often adopted for managing projects because it allows the organization to (1) conduct a larger number of complex projects efficiently, (2) better allocate resources, (3) coordinate activities more

TABLE 124.3 *Generally perceived benefits of the matrix system*

1. Improves management control. Provides an alternative to line management and is an easier means to monitor progress and current status on multiple projects. Helps resolve conflicts between project requirements and the functional roles of various departments
2. Improves flexibility of the system used to achieve New Drug Applications (NDAs)
3. Improves visibility of more individuals to senior management
4. Improves the visibility of a project's objectives, status, and problems
5. Improves cross-functional communication and dissemination of information between different departments and groups working on a project
6. Provides a simple mechanism to solicit, receive, and use input from all relevant departments, groups, and functions
7. Applies expertise and resources flexibly and efficiently to multiple projects
8. Achieves project objectives more efficiently than without the matrix, since the entire project team usually operates as a group
9. Allows skilled professionals to work on multiple projects while working within their area of expertise
10. Allows the entire project portfolio to be easily viewed as a whole and may be more readily reviewed, modified, or directed
11. Provides more leadership positions within an organization
12. Provides more training of staff for leadership roles
13. Tends to improve staff morale

easily between various groups, (4) facilitate communications between separate departments, (5) assist individuals (or a group) who have difficulty identifying important tasks of high priority, (6) provide intellectual stimulation to team members, and (7) remove some degree of the high emotional stakes in the outcome of studies supervised by line managers. Other benefits of this system are listed in Table 124.3. This approach requires management support to all levels in an organization for it to operate effectively. If the managers do not want the matrix system to be successful it will not work.

Disadvantages of the Matrix System

The case against the matrix system is that it dilutes authority and creates dual loyalties, especially when a formal reporting system is established on the same administrative level as line managers. This may lead to an undesirable competition between line managers and matrix managers. The matrix system requires greater interpersonal skills to operate effectively and is more time consuming to operate. Also, it is often difficult for project managers to assess accurately the contribution of each member of the team, since most of their work is performed within their line-function responsibilities. See Table 124.4.

Resolving Conflicts in a Matrix Environment

When problems arise within any section or department, the individuals involved must decide whether to pursue its resolution through line management or through the matrix system. Ideally, both avenues are open and there should be little or no friction or difficulties between the two when one system is used rather than the other.

This idealized view of two systems working in complete harmony is difficult to achieve in practice. An important consideration for some individuals in determining the system that should have priority in solving a problem relates to the system that is tied to promotions, salary adjustments, and other administrative matters. If each system's representative has equal input into these administrative matters, then a strong conflict is more likely to result as they each attempt to gain a superior position. If, however, one system is defined or created as having dominance then there is a better chance of achieving harmonious relationships in operations and facilitating solutions to problems. Within each of these spheres, certain problems and administrative matters will tend to become centered. Making these distinctions as clear as possible to all employees included in or concerned with both systems is an important goal to pursue.

Conflicts Between Matrix and Line Management

Conflicts that occur between line and matrix managers are often over clearly defining the types of decisions that lie within each's purview. One approach toward resolution of complex situations when many people are involved is to clarify the major roles of the individuals involved in decision making. These roles include those of individuals who (1) have final approval, (2) should be consulted but who are without veto power, (3) may develop alternatives and provide analyses, (4) should be informed about decisions made, and (5) have responsibility for implementing a decision once it is made.

TABLE 124.4 *Disadvantages of the matrix system[a]*

1. Project members and leaders report to two separate bosses
2. An additional organizational structure must be monitored and controlled
3. Allocation of resources may be more difficult
4. Additional administrators must be hired and trained
5. Potential is significant for disagreements and power conflicts between line and matrix managers, particularly over priorities and competition for resources
6. Policies and standard operating procedures may require excessive amounts of time to create and operate

[a] Most of these may be avoided by making either the line management or matrix system dominant.

Strong versus Weak Matrices

In a perfectly balanced matrix the power and authority of line managers are on an equal basis with that of matrix managers and project leaders. This situation is, ironically, the most unstable type of matrix because there are forces within both groups that are constantly seeking to tip the balance in their favor. If the matrix managers and project leaders (or project managers) win, then a strong matrix results. If line managers win, then a weak matrix results. Strong matrices emphasize speed of performing work and coordination of activities. Strong line managements emphasize expertise within that discipline.

The balance of power is usually determined by the most senior manager(s) in a company or other organization. One way to affect the balance is to modify the level in the organization at which matrix managers and project leaders (or project managers) report. Another important mechanism that affects this balance of power is the nature and strength of the matrix managers' and project leaders' support from the most senior managers. Bringing project members physically together to work as a group (i.e., team) tends to strengthen the matrix, just as keeping them within areas assigned to their functional department tends to weaken it.

The amount of decision-making ability and responsibilities of line managers and project leaders on project activities is the major factor that indicates whether the matrix is strong or weak. The main areas to review are (1) budget responsibilities, (2) assignment of staff to projects, (3) reviewing performance of staff, (4) hiring and firing staff, (5) promoting staff, (6) counseling staff for errors, (7) assigning activities to staff, and (8) maintaining scientific oversight of the project.

SCHEDULING PROJECT ACTIVITIES

Some of the most popular approaches currently used to schedule project activities are (1) milestones, (2) Gantt, and (3) Program Evaluation and Review Technique (PERT). Each of these is briefly discussed. The spectrum of project management approaches are shown in Table 124.5.

Milestone Schedules

Milestones are the major time points and stages in a project's life. For projects involving medicines, these milestones usually include the time of (1) project formation, (2) Investigational New Drug Application (IND) filing, (3) Phase I (start, end), (4) Phase II (start, end), (5) Phase III (start), (6) New Drug Application

TABLE 124.5 *Selected approaches to managing projects*

Approach	Potential problems
1. Totally informal (i.e., no system)	Complex projects are difficult to manage
2. Periodic review	May be inadequate as a method on its own
3. Gantt charts	Too many details or insufficient number of details may be present
4. Milestone projections	Too few milestones exist to use without additional methods
5. Work schedules	Not suitable for all departments, particularly research-oriented ones
6. Scheduled meetings	Purposes of all meetings should be clear to participants
7. PERT[a] charts	Most people do not understand or relate well to these charts

[a] PERT, Program Evaluation and Review Technique.

(NDA) filing, (7) NDA approvable letter, (8) NDA approval letter, and (9) project launch. Table 124.6 lists a similar series of milestones.

Milestone schedules are rarely sufficient on their own to serve as an adequate project schedule. The milestone listings may summarize a great deal of information, avoid complexity, and present "the bottom line" for individuals to use as a measure to gauge progress. Both start and completion dates for a variety of activities may be listed. Although milestone schedules are easy to prepare and review, they do not indicate interrelationships between activities or any details of the project plan.

Gantt Chart

A Gantt chart is a bar or line chart along an axis of time, usually expressed in weeks, months, or years. Figure 115.2 illustrates one example. This type of chart is easily understood and is therefore widely used. It may be modified in many ways, such as illustrating the

TABLE 124.6 *Major milestones in the development of a new medicine[a]*

1. Project formation
2. IND[b] or CTX[b] or other initial regulatory submission
3. Phase I completed
4. Phase II completed (or) go/no-go decision point reached
5. Clinical data cutoff
6. Submission of NDA[c], PLA[c], or other marketing authorization document to regulatory authority
7. Marketing authorization received, i.e., NDA or PLA approved
8. New medicine introduced

[a] Any number of minor milestones may be created by the project to measure its progress. Each department represented on the project team may create its own series of milestones.
[b] IND, Investigational New Drug Application; CTX, Clinical Trial Exemption.
[c] NDA, New Drug Application; PLA, Product License Application.

time necessary to complete various parts of the overall task represented by one bar, through subdividing it with hatched lines, open spaces, or other markings. One of the drawbacks of this approach is that it is not suitable for most large and complex projects and it does not illustrate interactions between activities. As with the milestone chart, the Gantt chart may be used in conjunction with more complex schedules. In that situation, the Gantt chart may illustrate one or a few aspects of a large project. Activities that lie on the critical path may be identified (e.g., with specific symbols such as hatch marks).

Program Evaluation and Review Technique (PERT)

PERT is more complex than the preceding two methods and illustrates the interdependence of many activities. The IND and NDA models shown in Figs. 124.1 and 124.2 are illustrations of the PERT technique. This network chart is usually accompanied by a listing of all of the separate activities shown. It is usually desirable to list activities for each individual group or department responsible for those activities. Those lists may then be used as a planning tool by those groups.

PERT, along with the closely related methodologies of Critical Path Method and Precedence Scheduling are often referred to as network methods because they illustrate and document how multiple processes may be followed in a project. This approach may document the critical path whereby those activities are indicated that are rate limiting. If activities noted as critical are delayed then the time for project completion will be delayed. Each event on a PERT chart may be viewed as a milestone, albeit a minor one in most instances.

Whereas the Critical Path Method provides a single estimate of time required to complete an activity, the strict definition of PERT requires three time estimates for each activity. These estimates are for the best case, worst case, and most likely case. These three estimates are then used to create a single time estimate, using a standard formula.

To use the PERT system it is necessary to have:

1. A well-defined set of activities that constitute a project (usually 20 to several hundred events are listed).
2. Activities that are interrelated with other activities and conducted in a predetermined order.
3. The ability to designate which activities may be initiated and stopped independently of each other.
4. An indication of the time required to complete each activity or the probability that each activity will be successful.

Comparisons of the various techniques may be found in texts or reviews on project management (e.g., Cleland and King, 1983; Graham, 1985; Cori, 1985). It is usually most relevant to create PERT charts for medicine projects for the IND, NDA, and launch milestones, if the method is used at all. These charts are not generally as useful at other times of a project's life, unless the sponsoring organization has implemented an ambitious overall cost and resource tracking and management system.

PROJECT MANAGEMENT

Project management represents a rational basis for allocating resources to project activities and provides a means to focus attention on plans to achieve the institution's goals for the future. It identifies rate-limiting steps in current and planned work and improves the efficiency with which work is accomplished. In companies with numerous projects simultaneously under development, the matrix approach is usually viewed as the most efficient approach to manage those projects.

Choosing an Approach to Project Management

Possible approaches and a major (potential) drawback for each are listed in Table 124.5. Ideally, in a large organization, several, if not all, of these approaches will be used. Some approaches are more effective in different departments, others work best at an early (or late) stage of a project, and some work best for complex projects. The author does not believe that PERT charts are a valuable tool for planning a medicine's development, and believes few people find them useful.

Predictors of a Project's Success

Success is usually defined as the attainment of the project's objectives as soon as possible. This means that the termination of an unsuccessful project is also judged as a success, if it is achieved rapidly and efficiently. The best predictors of project success are (1) attitude of the project team, (2) ability of the project leader to act as a champion, (3) quality of the development plan, (4) medical and commercial value of the medicine, (5) support of senior management, and (6) traditions of the organization.

Breadth versus Depth in Project Management

To calculate the number of people and amount of resources needed for a project it is important to consider both the breadth and depth of the project system. Breadth primarily refers to the number of projects in

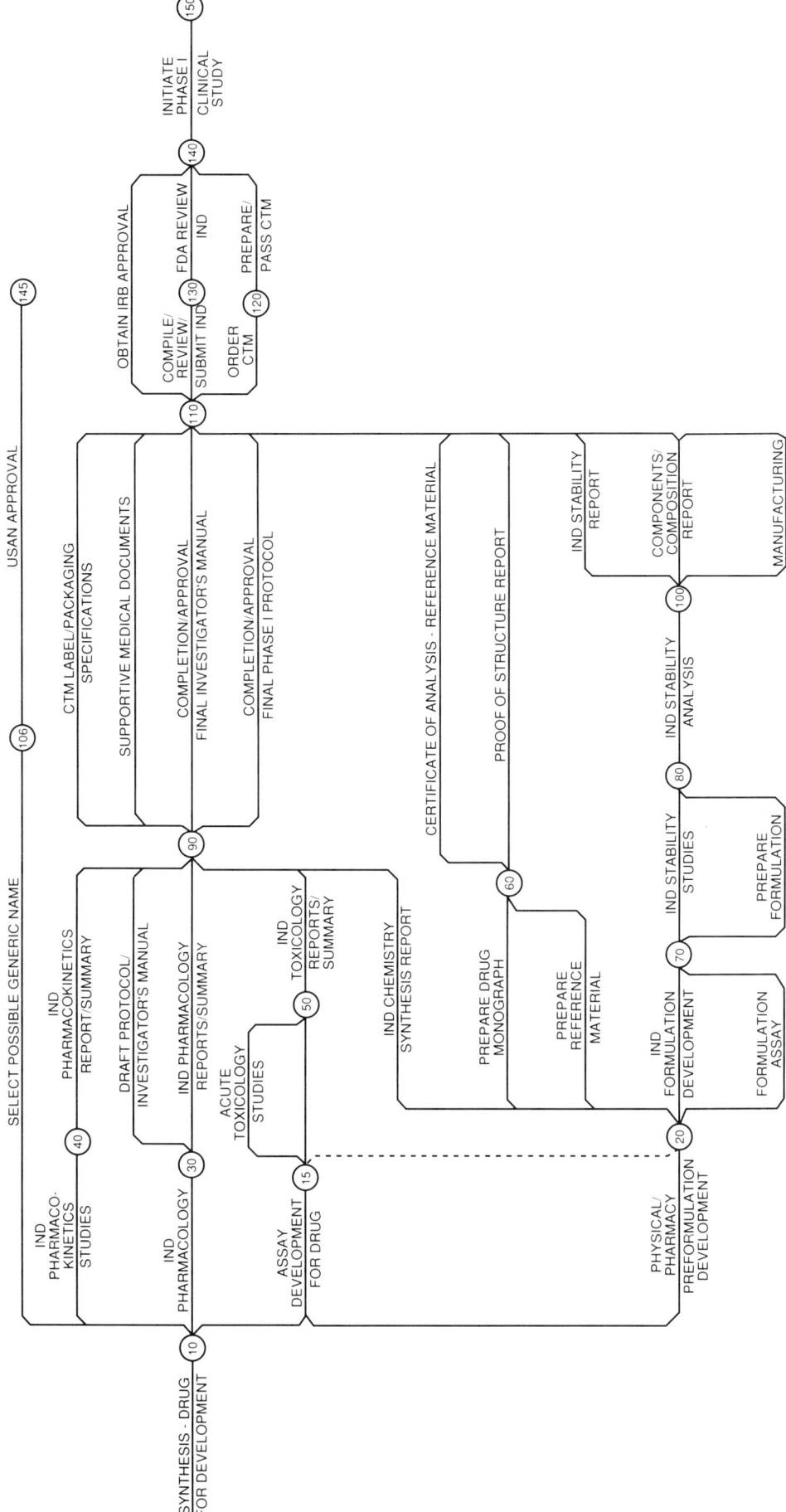

FIG. 124.1 Model of activities needed to submit an Investigational New Drug Application (IND). [Program Evaluation and Review Technique (PERT)]. IRB, Institutional Review Board. For other abbreviations, see Fig. 124.2 legend.

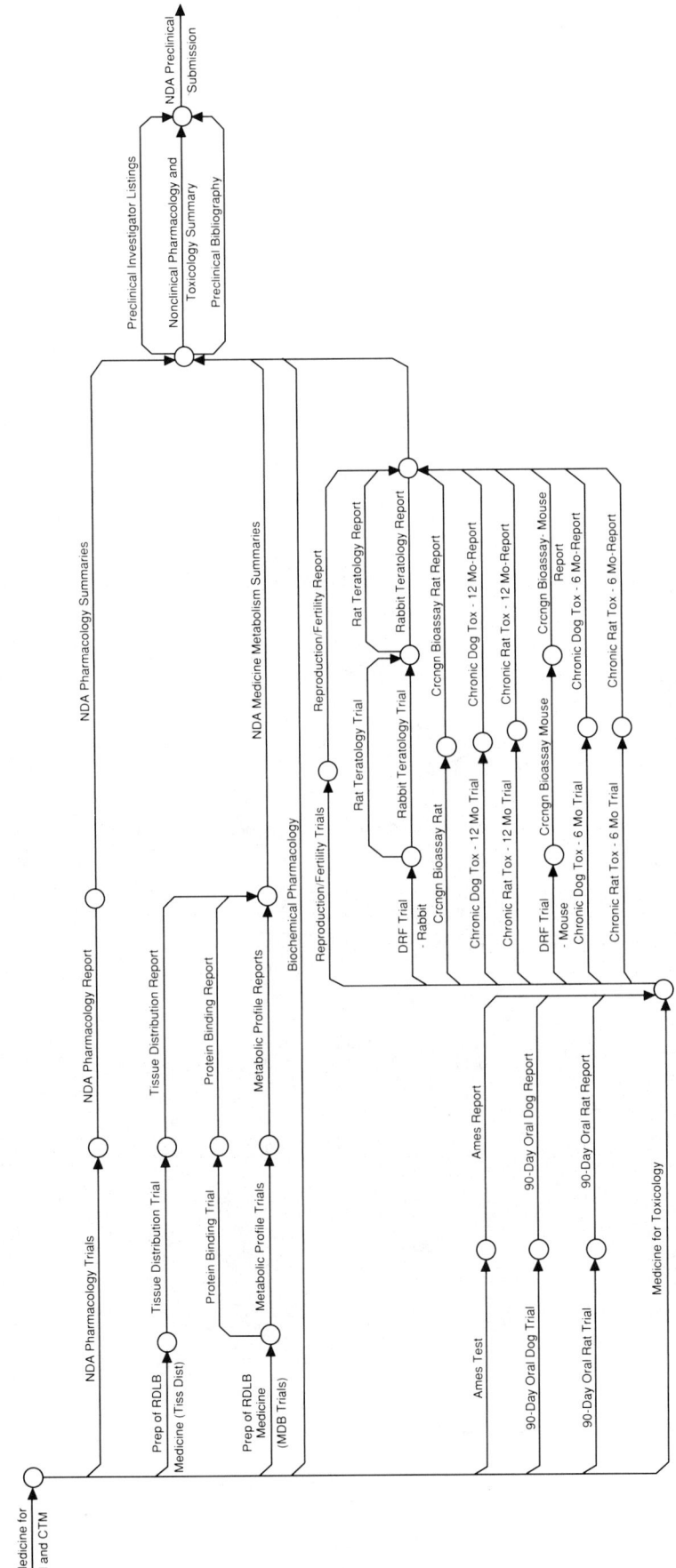

FIG. 124.2 Model of activities needed to submit an NDA (PERT chart). **A:** Preclinical activities. **B:** Clinical activities. **C:** Technical development activities. Abbreviations in A: CTM, clinical trial material; RDLB, radiolabeled; Tiss Dist, tissue distribution; Crncngn, carcinogen; Mo, month; DRF, dose range finding: Tox, toxicology; MDB, Metabolism, distribution, binding; NDA, New Drug Application. In B, new abbreviations: USAN, United States adopted names; PO, oral; IV, intravenously, FDA, Food and Drug Administration.

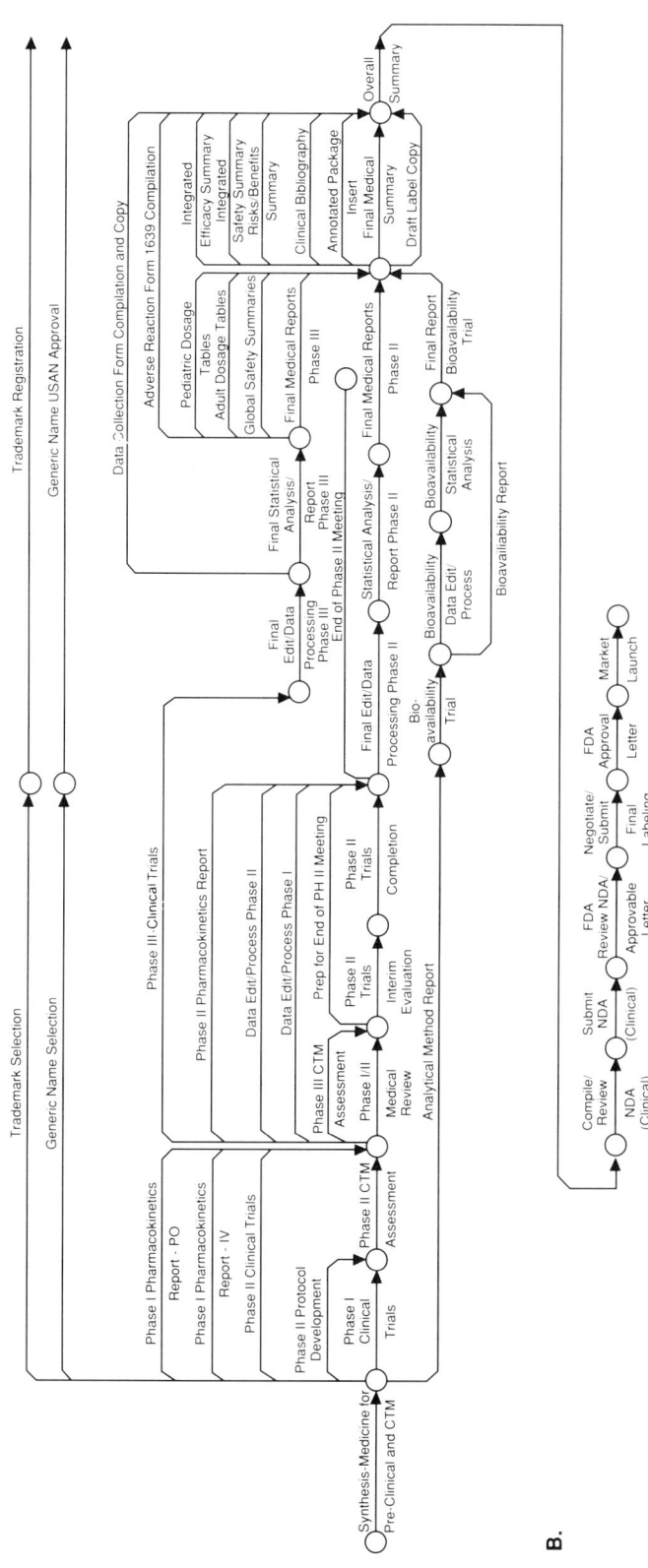

FIG. 124.2 (*Continued*)

975

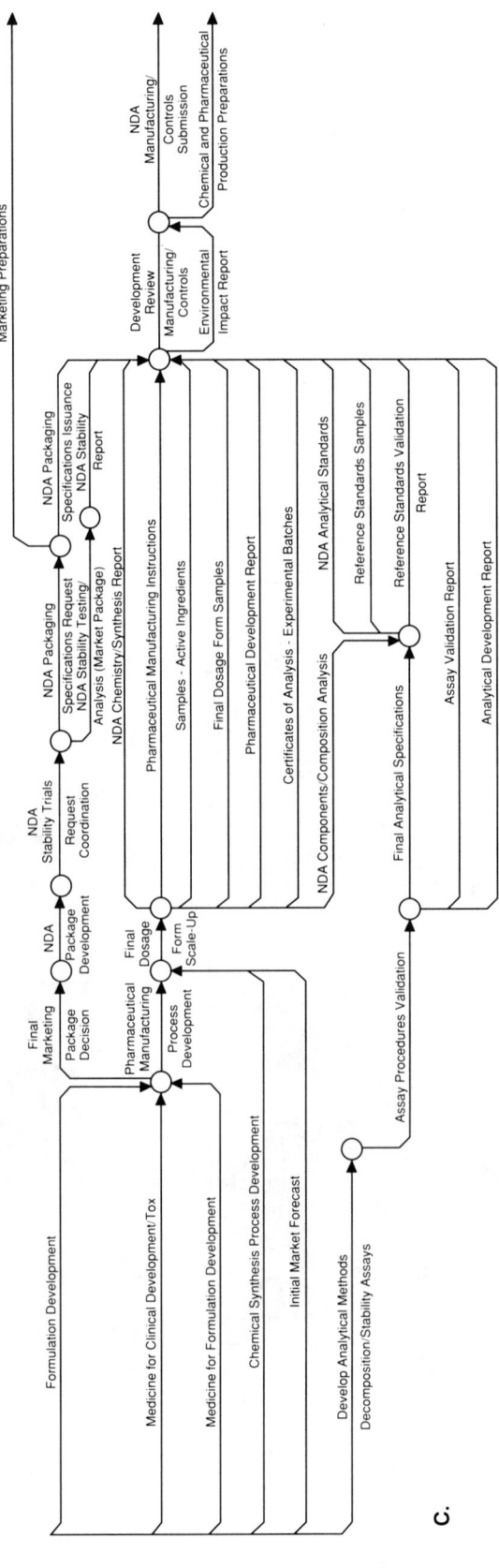

FIG. 124.2 (*Continued*)

C.

976

TABLE 124.7 *Representative example of a planning matrix*

Level within the organization	Time frame		
	Short-term (0 to 12 Months)	Mid-term (1 to 3 Years)	Long-term (3 to 10 Years)
Chairman			
Unit (e.g., R & D)[a]			
Division (e.g., Medical)			
Department			
Section			
Individual			

[a] R & D, research and development.

the system; depth refers to the number of activities conducted on each project.

Expansion in either breadth or depth must be frequently evaluated by every organization that has some control over the balance between these two. One objective of this evaluation is to ensure that the project team is not expanding beyond its original charge, is not embarking on tangents, and is meeting its objectives. Breadth and depth must also be assessed for the overall project system.

Types of Matrices

The organization of medical projects within the pharmaceutical industry is a well-known matrix used to develop medicines and is described in this chapter. A comparable matrix organization may exist in the discovery phase of new medicines, focusing on individual research projects or topics.

Either of these matrices may be viewed from various levels within the organization. The perspective of the person viewing either matrix will differ greatly, depending on their level. The chief executive officer will be more concerned about overall costs and the likelihood (and magnitude) of commercial success as compared with an individual scientist or clinician.

Another type of matrix may be called a planning matrix (Table 124.7). This matrix actually has three axes: the time frame (e.g., short, medium, and long term), the level of the individual or group creating the plan, and the type of plan created. This last category could focus on one or more of the following: strategic plan, headcount changes, equipment and capital expenditures, and priority issues.

CENTRAL COORDINATING FUNCTION

Need and Size

It is generally useful to establish a central coordinating function to assist in tracking and monitoring various activities within multiple projects. This is especially relevant if the multiple projects impinge on each other in terms of their need for resources and require central overall monitoring and administration. Some companies that have established this function utilize a single individual, but most larger companies have created a smaller group or department to fulfill this role. The size of the department varies between pharmaceutical companies, but is usually kept to a relatively small size of approximately 3 to 15 people. Larger groups do exist.

Functions

The role of this group in any company varies from simply consulting on planning to having a strong central management role in budgeting, expenditure review, global status reporting, or central control of investigational medicine usage. A summary is shown in Table 124.8. Selected procedures to follow in project management are shown in Table 124.9.

Planning and Creating Models

Coordination involves both planning activities that occur simultaneously in one or more departments and identifying those activities that occur sequentially. In a complex project such as developing a medicine, both simultaneous and sequential processes must be planned. All of the activities within departments may be considered by creating a model that prepares a plan for each individual medicine under development. The plans shown in Figs. 124.1 and 124.2 are generic ones and must be modified to include specific characteristics, requirements, and available resources for the particular investigational medicine.

Road Map

In theory, the plan developed for each particular project (e.g., Fig. 124.1) may be used as a road map.

TABLE 124.8 *Selected functions of a central coordinating group within a matrix organization*

1. Plan the integrated development of a medicine
2. Monitor progress toward that plan and advise members of their commitments to the plan
3. Inform members of the project team and the project leader of potential or actual problems or issues
4. Modify the development plan as needed
5. Assist the project leader or manager in scheduling meetings and writing reports
6. Store project records
7. Analyze financial aspects of the project
8. Facilitate discussions or meetings to resolve issues
9. Maintain morale and enthusiasm on the project
10. Assist the project leader or manager in all aspects possible

TABLE 124.9 *Selected procedures to follow in project management[a]*

1. Define project objectives in terms of final tangible outputs
2. Develop a progressive breakdown of the project until manageable units of work (activities) are established
3. Establish a list of all activities required to achieve the project objectives
4. Establish a network, using all of the activities in a time sequence
5. Evaluate the network to establish early and late start and completion dates, plus the amount of slack time. Establish which activities constitute the critical path
6. Create a schedule that utilizes the network, availability of resources, priorities, and the calendar
7. Estimate the times to complete each activity. In some situations (e.g., with PERT[b] techniques) an optimistic, pessimistic, and most likely estimate may be made
8. Assign responsibility for completing activities to appropriate individuals
9. Establish a method to monitor progress
10. Establish a method for management review and dealing with problems
11. Use milestones and other systems as needed to gauge progress and review activities
12. Revise network and schedule as necessary

[a] This list excludes financial aspects (e.g., costs, budgets), which must often be included.
[b] PERT, Program Evaluation and Review Technique.

The plan outlines the route that each involved department will follow to reach the final goal. A medicine rarely follows the original route without numerous modifications to the plan. There are two major types of reasons why the original plan is only an ideal route. The first reason is related to modifications that occur in the development plans of medicine X itself. The second reason is that in most instances, the development project on a single medicine is not the only major ongoing project, and demands for resources, priority, or other factors related to different projects often influence the development of medicine X.

Modifications to a Plan

Plans for a medicine's development are modified throughout the course of implementing and conducting the various activities. This occurs because only incomplete information for planning the entire development program is known at the outset of the project. As more and more technical and clinical information becomes available the plans for the regulatory submission usually become clearer. In addition, problems or significant issues invariably arise during the development of any medicine that require modifications of the plans. Serious problems may cause the entire plan to be scraped, revised, or placed on hold. Numerous causes of a delay are possible. Many delays do not require major modification of the plan's logic and activities as much as they prolong the time necessary to carry out the activities in the plan.

Functions of the Central Coordinating Group

Personnel within the central coordination unit may act as planning consultants or as leaders or managers of the project teams. In certain instances these project managers are fully accountable for their projects, prepare regulatory (e.g., IND and NDA) summaries, and monitor details of their projects' activities. Most individuals who have this magnitude of responsibility can only manage a small number of projects (e.g., two or three).

Leading the Project Team

The project team may also be led by a scientist or clinician. The choice of one or the other usually depends on the specific stage of a medicine's development. This individual may or may not act as a project champion. He or she will have other (i.e., departmental) responsibilities in addition to managing the project. In this situation, personnel from the central coordination unit may act as assistants to the project team leader or they may be restricted to a planning and coordination function. The project planner may then handle more projects. This number varies, but is often in the range of approximately 6 to 12 projects. Advantages of having project teams led by professional managers or by project champions are summarized in Table 124.10, and methods of assigning work among project planners are listed in Table 124.11.

When choosing one of the approaches in Table 124.10, consider number of available staff, number of projects, interests of people involved, traditions of the organization, and opinion of the department head.

Head of the Coordination Department

The training and background of leaders of coordination departments vary to a great degree, as does the training of the individuals within the departments. The department leaders usually, but not always, have a substantial background in science, but individuals with business, production, or other backgrounds have also been appointed to these positions. Orientation, attitudes, interpersonal skills, and managerial abilities appear to be more critical determinants of success than area(s) of previous training. The academic degrees achieved by these coordination heads also vary. If this individual has additional responsibilities in the organization, then the nature of these other tasks will greatly influence the background, training, and experience necessary for the coordinating position.

TABLE 124.10 *Advantages of having project teams led by professional managers or by project champions*

A. Advantages of professional project managers
1. Usually have a more even-handed and objective approach to all projects
2. Usually are more experienced with the methodologies used to develop medicines than project champions
3. Usually are more experienced with management methods
4. Less training is usually required in administrative methods and procedures
5. Can usually facilitate agreements between projects more easily
6. Improves the chance of choosing the most suitable individual to lead the project
7. They may be better leaders of a project than the champion(s)
8. Less chance of enthusiastic champions draining resources to a project prematurely (e.g., before efficacy is demonstrated) or to a less promising or less important project
9. Avoids problems that may develop when project leadership is given as a reward to an individual instead of giving it to the most appropriate person
B. Advantages of project champions
1. Usually have more enthusiasm for their particular project. This generates a sense of excitement and a commitment to push the project forward
2. The process of utilizing project champions trains more individuals in managerial techniques
3. Provides more challenges to the most exceptional staff
4. Provides a goal for many potential champions to aspire to
5. Diversifies responsibilities within a company or organization
6. Usually have better political positions within the organization
7. Often have people reporting to them and can get work done
8. Have more technical understanding and scientific credibility when dealing with internal or external experts
9. Usually are greater risk takers; willing to take calculated career risks to move the project forward
10. Usually will find a way around problems (if possible) or else develop alternatives to solve a problem, rather than merely accept a delay

Members of the Coordination Department

Members of coordination departments who perform various planning activities and monitor progress of these plans usually interact with all members of the project team. These planners also have a wide range of training and experience. A scientific background is highly desirable, and in some companies it is essential. Probably their most important attributes are interpersonal skills and attention to detail. If either of these skills is absent the abilities of these individuals to function effectively will be diminished. Experience with computers is becoming a more important part of success in these positions. Potential functions and issues to address for project planners are listed in Tables 124.12 and 124.13. Mechanisms for deciding how to allocate their time are shown in Fig. 124.3.

TABLE 124.11. *Assigning work among project planners*

1. Assign different therapeutic categories to each planner, who then becomes involved with all projects in that area
2. Rotate projects periodically among planners
3. Balance quantity of work independent of therapeutic area
4. Assign planners to specific departments or sections within departments
5. Assign different phases of clinical development to different planners
6. Assign different specialities (e.g., NDA[a] preparation, IND[a] preparation) to different planners

[a] IND, Investigational New Drug Application; NDA, New Drug Application.

Career Advancement in Coordination Departments

The field of project planning and coordination is a relatively young one in the pharmaceutical industry. Current activities within the Project Management Institute and the Pharmaceutical Manufacturer's Association demonstrate that the group of project planners is searching for a professional identity and also for an

TABLE 124.12 *Potential functions of project planners*

1. Develop a network chart(s) (e.g., PERT,[a] Gantt) and schedule(s) for each project to help organize all activities necessary to complete the IND[a], NDA[a], or other goal
2. Monitor progress of all activities listed in the schedule to determine whether they remain "on time" and "on course"
3. Modify or expand the network or schedule as required to keep it current
4. Develop a network and schedule for the launch of either (1) a new medicine or (2) an old medicine with expanded indications, new dosage form, new formulation, or other modifications
5. Develop a network and schedule to plan and monitor Phase IV studies, toxicology, or studies within a specific department. Develop other plans as needed
6. Develop procedures and forms to monitor the flow of clinical, toxicological, or other data. Implement use of forms and monitor progress
7. Assist in the coordination between the group(s) representing the research and development function and marketing, production, financial, or foreign groups
8. Assist in interdepartmental communications to clarify and resolve issues
9. Follow the financial status of the project. If the company allots a certain sum to be used by each project, assist in the plans for its disbursement and monitor funds spent
10. Accompany project leaders to relevant meetings with regulatory personnel, senior managers, or other groups
11. Act as a secretary for the project at both official and unofficial meetings
12. Provide other assistance to the project leader as requested on an ad hoc basis (e.g., provide specific analyses, documentation, graphics, or other information on a project)
13. Facilitate meetings or actions that attempt to solve problems
14. Derive estimated times for completing disparate activities using a criterion of either optimistic, pessimistic, or realistic appraisals of time required[b]

[a] IND, Investigational New Drug Application; NDA, New Drug Application; PERT, Program Evaluation and Review Technique.
[b] Estimates may include or exclude consideration of other currently active projects that may possibly (or definitely will) affect the schedule.

TABLE 124.13 *Selected issues for project planners to address*

1. Should planners passively accept dates that project members provide to devise a project schedule and network, or critically evaluate and question those dates to increase the speed of completing the project?
2. Should all departments submit work schedules and resource allocations to a central person or group? This might allow more rapid recognition of either underutilization or overcommitment of resources
3. Should planners closely monitor adherence to the schedules by all relevant groups?
4. Should estimated times to complete activities be based on the best possible, worst possible, or average times? Should other approaches be used to estimate time requirements?
5. How much effort should be expended in each project on strategies, PERT[a] charts, and other planning activities? Is the amount of time and effort spent on these activities cost effective?
6. If activities are falling behind schedule who should evaluate whether the reasons for the delay are legitimate and, more importantly, determine whether priorities must be adjusted?
7. Who has the responsibility for enforcing scheduled dates?

[a] PERT, Program Evaluation and Review Technique.

accepted role that allows professional career opportunities for growth and advancement. Preliminary efforts into certification, and acceptance as a profession within the pharmaceutical industry by outside groups, have not been totally satisfactory to date, but efforts are continuing that will hopefully improve the professional image and career opportunities for project planners in the future.

One of the difficulties in developing this area as a profession is that people almost always enter the profession from another one; they become expert at their new roles and then they are promoted or transferred to a different area. Another difficulty is that there are relatively few people working in this area.

Project Coordinators Within Each Major Function

It is possible to organize a matrix so that individual project coordinators are located within medical, mar-

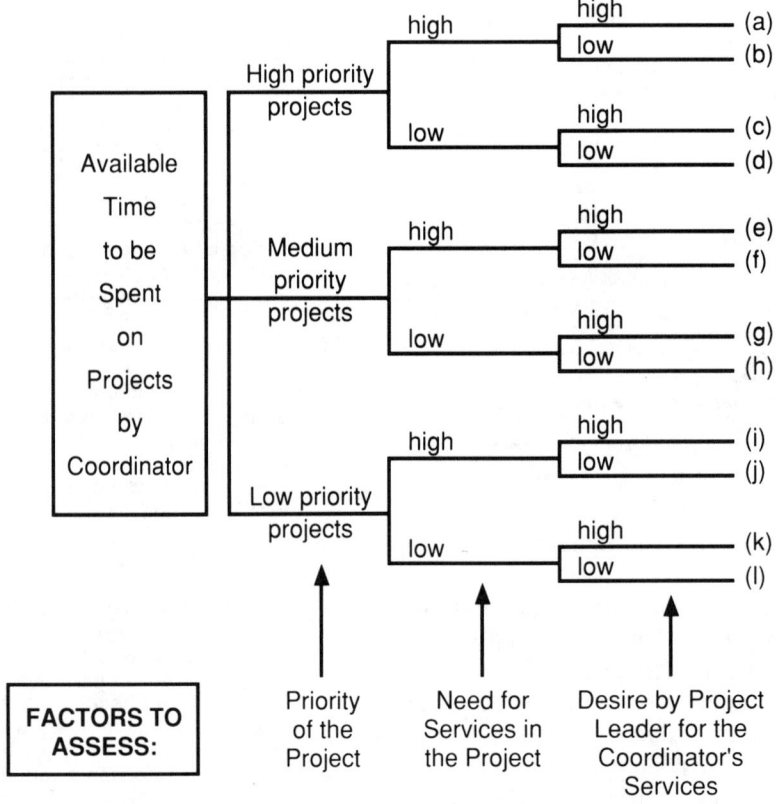

Assessment of where to allocate time

Project a = Top priority for the coordinator
Project b = Create a desire for services
Project c = Services not needed
Project d = Cyclical need and may increase in future
Project e, i = High priority because input will have a major impact

FIG. 124.3 Mechanisms to decide the most efficient allocation of a project coordinator's time to multiple projects.

keting, and technical development functions, instead of within a centrally organized group. Alternatively, or in addition, each of these functions could have a centralized coordinator for all projects to help the overall functioning of project activities (Fig. 124.4).

Amount of Work on a Project Performed by a Coordinator

The amount of work performed on a project usually shows a biphasic relationship (Fig. 124.5). Work

reaches its first peak shortly prior to IND submission and then reaches a second, higher peak at the time of the major regulatory submission.

Types of Project Teams

Although most people think of project teams in terms of a multidepartmental group of professionals, there are also project teams within some departments (Fig. 124.6). For example, a group within a medical department working together on the clinical development

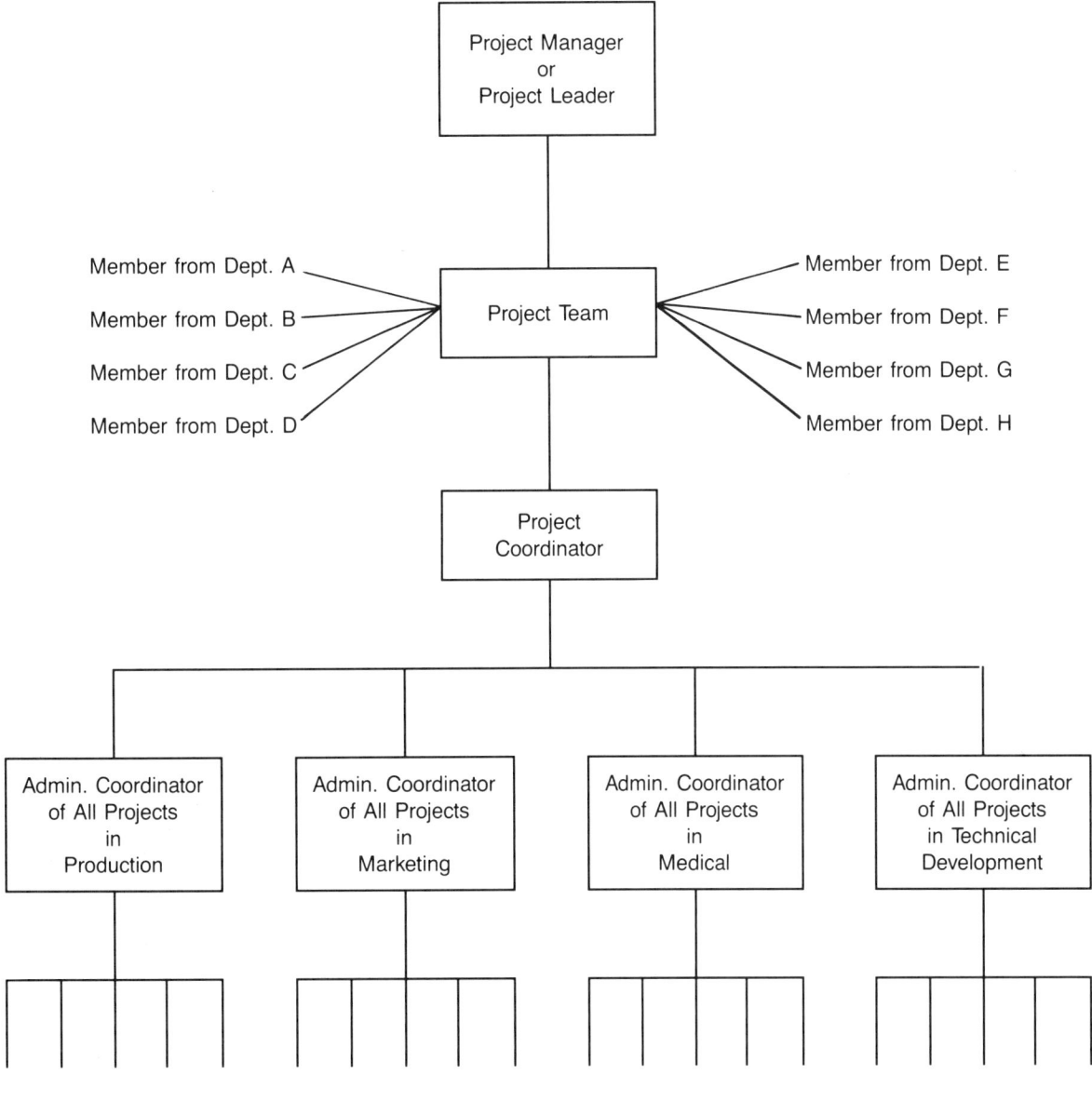

FIG. 124.4 Various organizational aspects of coordination within a single project. The major coordinators are part of the project team.

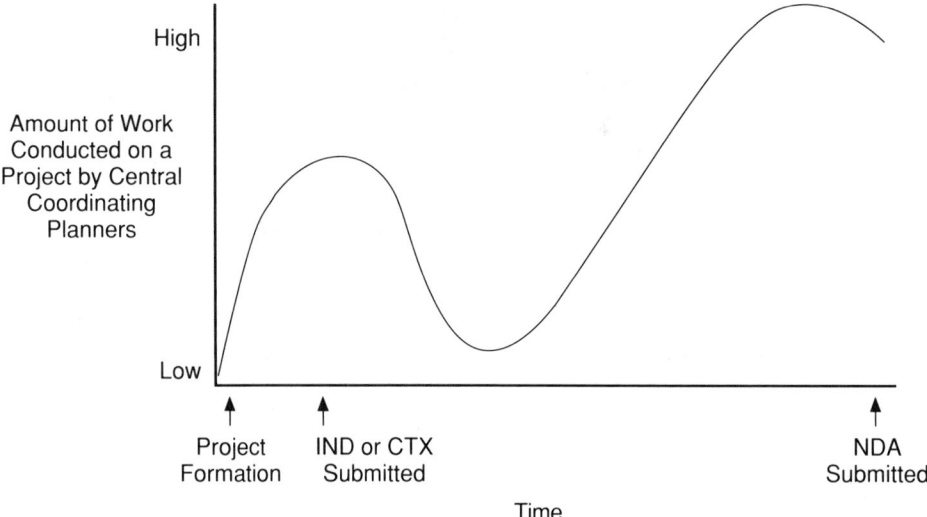

FIG. 124.5 Biphasic nature of work conducted by coordinators on a single medicine development project. Work is also often conducted by coordinators prior to the project's formation and after the New Drug Application (NDA) has been submitted. CTX, Clinical Trial Exemption; IND, Investigational New Drug Application.

of a specific medicine constitutes a department or line-management team. Departmental teams coexist with matrix project teams in many departments, but only one type of team or the other may exist. It is important to identify which type of team is being referred to in discussion or documents where ambiguity may arise. Figure 124.6 illustrates other variations on teams (e.g., subproject teams, joint department teams) that work on a single project.

GOLDEN RULES FOR PROJECT MANAGEMENT AND PLANNING

Some of the essential principles that should usually be followed are listed below.

Project Management

1. Provide at least one development plan for each project.
2. Identify the critical path on the project's development plan.
3. Analyze various aspects of the overall project system on an ongoing basis to provide trends and information needed in order to consider modifications to the project plan.
4. Offer a menu of services to various groups within the organization.
5. Become involved in *inter*department issues, but not *intra*department issues, unless invited to do so.

Project Planning

1. Consider the entire process and final step(s) or outcome(s), even if one only plans a portion of it.
2. Illustrate the plans in multiple ways and evaluate each to determine which one(s) is most clear.
3. Review all plans with relevant people affected prior to officially promulgating the plans.
4. Run through "what if" exercise (i.e., problems are imagined to occur at every step of the plan).
5. Conduct dry runs to test the feasibility of the plan, insofar as possible.
6. Decide whether one or more consultants are necessary to review the plans.
7. Divide the plans into those for shorter periods and those dealing with longer periods.

TYPES OF ESTIMATES MADE OF COMPLETION DATES

Dates are usually estimated when planned activities are to be completed. This practice is important because it enables resources to be better allocated, i.e., plans for reserving equipment use and people's efforts may be prepared.

Estimates may be entirely *idealistic*, i.e., made without reference to other projects competing for the same resources. Estimates may be *pessimistic*, made by skeptics who have had many bad experiences or who prefer to be conservative and think that if they forecast a date with a large cushion of time, they will seem more like a hero if the dates are met. Neither of these ap-

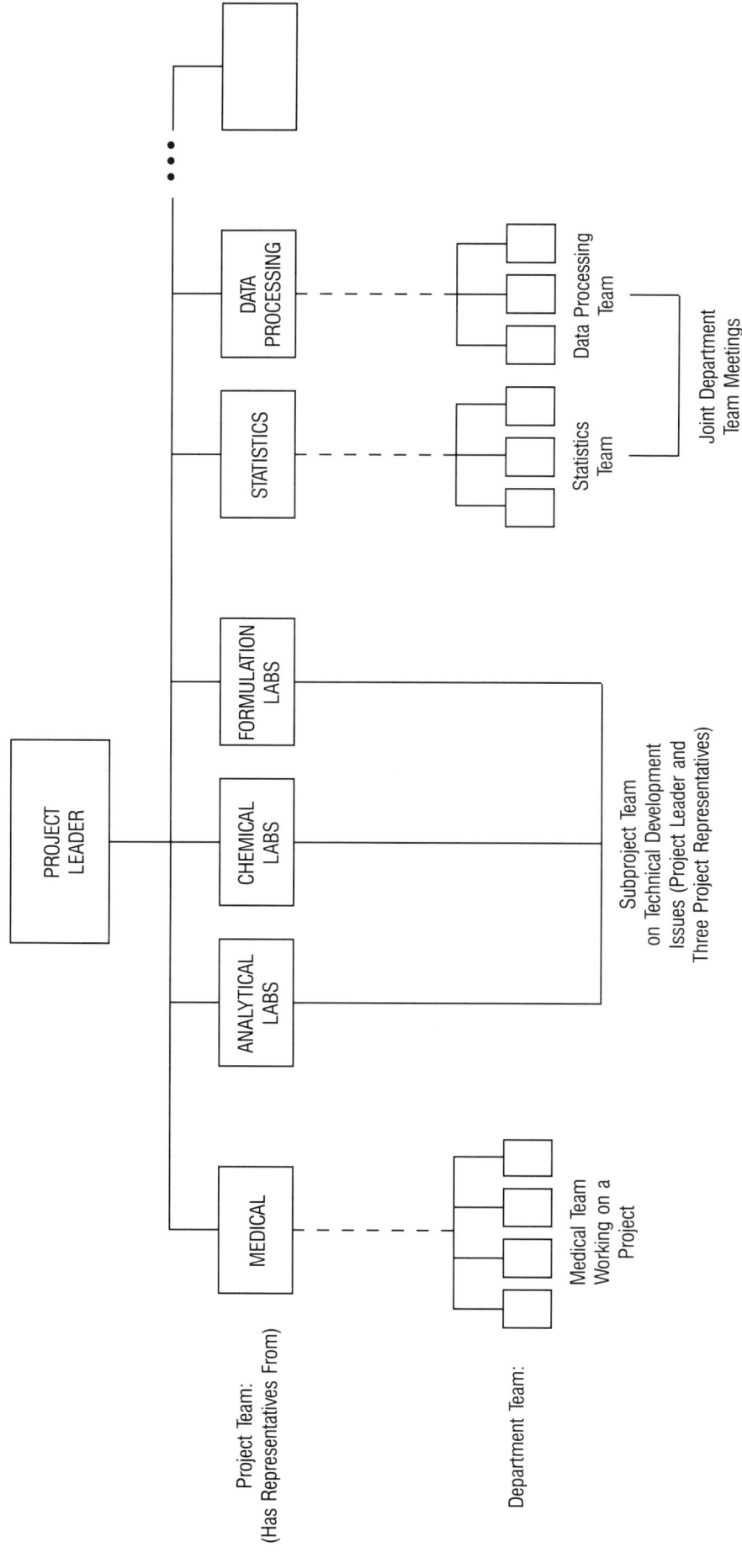

FIG. 124.6 Types of project teams.

proaches is correct. A *realistic* estimate of the date for completing any activity is the best way for a company to develop its new medicines efficiently.

Estimates of the date when specific activities are to be completed may be inaccurate for two types of reasons. The first type is under the control of the person who made the estimate; this includes using incomplete or inappropriate information to generate the dates. The other category of reasons includes those that are not under the direct control of the person who made the estimate. A delay by any internal or external group (e.g., regulatory agency) that represents a rate-limiting step is an example of this second category.

Resource Allocation and Utilization

Headcounts assigned to each project and subproject (e.g., specific indications, dosage forms, routes of administration) may be tracked on their own as well as in comparison to the resources utilized. Most nonacademic organizations have their employees report time spent on projects on a periodic basis (e.g., weekly, biweekly, monthly, quarterly). These data, in terms of hours, percent of total effort, costs, or percent of total costs may be listed and plotted according to (1) a numbering system of projects, (2) therapeutic area, (3) marketing forecast, (4) level of effort spent, or (5) amount of money spent. Other tables and graphs are prepared based on the section (e.g., angina), department (e.g., cardiovascular), division (e.g., medical), and unit (e.g., research and development) level.

In all of the above cases it is useful to evaluate the last period measured (e.g., 3 months), on its own as well as its changes in relation to one or more previous periods. It is generally most helpful if at least a 2- or 3-year period is shown in some graphs so that a sense of trend is achieved. A large number of presentations may be made if they are of interest to the senior managers who are evaluating the results.

If an organization assigns priorities to certain projects then it may wish to monitor and compare activities within each separate priority category. One of the problems with this approach is that while the overall priorities may be established for an organization, those for any one department or other subgroup may differ significantly. This is usually appropriate because some departments are mainly involved at early stages of a project (e.g., organic chemistry, pharmacology), whereas others become more involved at later stages (e.g., data processing, pharmacoepidemiology). A scattergram graph of the overall costs within research and development versus those of the group involved will illustrate how closely the two are in harmony. Project code numbers inside circles may be placed on the graph and a separate key to the project's identification provided. A separate scattergram of each category of priority (e.g., A, B, C) for any group versus

the level of effort or percent of costs, and so on, would indicate how closely the priorities within that group are reflected in efforts.

TRAINING OF PROJECT LEADERS/MANAGERS

Traditionally, project leaders receive most of their basic training while "on the job." Recently, some companies have created more formal systems to improve the quality of training. There is no single approach to training that meets everyone's needs, and a variety of programs are important to establish. Some of the specific approaches that are used to train project leaders/managers are:

1. An experienced individual may be assigned to act as a *tutor* in an initial period and to act as a resource person in later stages. This experienced person may be another project leader, a project planner, or another type of individual.
2. An *orientation program* may be established for new project leaders. This may be organized such that interactive sessions are scheduled throughout a day, or it may be divided into separate sessions occurring over a period of weeks. The instructors are generally department heads and other senior individuals whose departments or functions will interact with project leaders. Experienced project leaders may also instruct the group on various issues that may arise during one's tenure as a project leader. It is usually best if these orientation sessions are limited to small groups, to facilitate discussion.
3. A *periodic meeting* of all project leaders may be conducted with (or without) senior management to provide an opportunity for discussing issues of mutual interest. Problems that exist in the project system may be discussed. The opportunity for interaction and problem solving is an essential part of this meeting. The format of the meeting should be chosen to allow this interaction to occur, and new formats may be tried from year to year. Retreats, work-dinner sessions, and small workshops are a few possible formats. Meetings between project leaders in research and development with product managers in marketing or production may also be useful.
4. A *written guide* or manual provides valuable information for project leaders to use as a reference. The guide may contain information along the lines of standard operating procedures, but should also contain background information on departments, their organization, and general means of performing functions that are of interest to the project leader. This type of guide rapidly goes out of date because many procedures change significantly or are replaced entirely. Thus, providing this guide

in a loose-leaf binder with sectional tabs that serve as an index has advantages over creating a permanently bound version. The loose-leaf album allows new parts to be added or substituted for out-of-date material. The guide will then have a longer period of useful life. A separate guide presenting information on regulatory issues may also be useful to prepare. The purpose of this guide must be established in advance, or it can readily turn into one that never achieves its goals and that, furthermore, is complex to produce. The purpose of such a guide could be (1) to educate the staff with general information appropriate to any company or organization, (2) to provide a reference to standard operating procedures, (3) to provide a guide to the company's culture, values, traditions, philosophy, or (4) to provide a working guide of recommendations on practical issues.

5. A *mentor* approach may be followed formally or informally, either as a substitute for point 1 above or as an additional technique. Most individuals are able to learn from the experience and wisdom of a mentor. This system usually achieves best results when it is implemented by project leaders informally on their own volition. It is uncertain whether formally establishing a mentor approach will achieve the same degree of success as providing encouragement to those interested in this approach.

6. *Outside courses* are being heavily promoted to the government, academicians, and the pharmaceutical industry. Some emphasize technical skills that the project leader may lack, whereas others focus on management and interpersonal skills. These courses are offering to fill a need that is usually not met in the training of scientists and professional managers who become project leaders.

7. A *roundtable meeting* of project leaders or managers may be conducted to discuss useful points and techniques they have learned that might be helpful for others to learn. Although every project teaches innumerable lessons about better ways to avoid and deal with problems, many of these relate to the highly specific nature and conditions of that project and the people involved. Nonetheless, many lessons are more generic and may be used by others.

8. *Ad hoc seminars and meetings* designed to train managers or improve their managerial knowledge have a role in improving skills, but are best viewed as supplemental material to the other parts of the training program.

Other educational opportunities for project leaders are to (1) tour manufacturing facilities, (2) spend a day with a sales representative to obtain a better understanding of their role, (3) listen to prepared cassette programs, (4) spend time with each project member and (5) solve

TABLE 124.14. *Techniques to use in training new investigators or staff*

1. Utilize lecture courses, seminars, and other types of formal verbal instruction
2. Provide video tapes of other investigators who are either interacting with, or examining patients. These tapes should illustrate points about patient diagnosis, treatment, identification of adverse reactions, or other aspects of the clinical trial
3. Make video tapes of the investigator-in-training with patients. Use these as a learning tool to help new investigators improve their techniques
4. Hold a roundtable discussion with the sponsor and other investigators, consultants, and staff. Review the protocol and other aspects of the trial
5. Have the new investigator or staff work with an experienced investigator or trial coordinator for a specified period
6. Have the new investigator or staff practice specific techniques or procedures with their colleagues
7. Monitor the site frequently to assess progress of the new staff

problem situations in a written or oral format that are based on previous company experiences. A number of qualities that are usually valuable for an effective project leader to possess are listed in Table 122.3 Additional information on staff training is presented in Chapter 54. Techniques to use in training new investigators or staff are listed in Table 124.14.

Evaluating the Performance of Project Leaders

In a weak matrix, the performance of project leaders is evaluated completely by their line managers. This means that if a line manager is unhappy about the amount of time and energy the project leader is spending on his or her project [as opposed to functional responsibilities (e.g., as a scientist, as a clinician)], the project leader will be pressured to spend less time working on project activities. This situation is more likely to arise in a preclinical department, because responsibilities are likely to be almost entirely non-project related (e.g., service oriented, basic research oriented, or oriented toward targeted medicine discovery). Clinical project leaders spend most, if not all, of their efforts on project-related activities, so that this issue should rarely arise.

Project leaders who operate in a weak matrix are not evaluated for their project-related accomplishments. This evaluation should be viewed as a means of recognition for and strengthening of the matrix system. The ideal individual to provide an evaluation of each project leader would be the head of the project system. This review could be provided to the line manager to assist in completing official performance appraisals. A simple evaluation system is probably best. An annual rating (excellent, good, needs improvement) could be made of any number of categories desired, but evidence of leadership, creativity, and success in reaching objectives are the major aspects to evaluate.

CHAPTER 125

Use of Meetings and Documents to Assist in Planning and Managing Clinical Trials

MEETINGS

The types of meetings held to plan and manage projects vary, depending on the nature of the project, its needs, the personalities of the people involved, and the historical traditions and systems of the institution. A few general comments and principles are pertinent to mention.

Meetings are required at each relevant level within an organization to handle project-related matters effectively. These levels include section, department, interdepartment, and corporate (or institution) groups. The major factors in considering the nature of meetings relate to their (1) level within the organization, (2) time of scheduling, (3) objectives or goals, (4) degree of formality, and (5) size. After these points are considered, the relevant people who should attend that meeting are chosen.

Scheduling

Scheduling of meetings may be viewed in the context of (1) those scheduled at periodic intervals (e.g., once a month, three times a year), (2) those scheduled at variable intervals to coincide with project milestones or other events, or (3) ad hoc meetings called for specific reasons.

Purposes

General goals of meetings are to (1) establish objectives and plans, (2) deal effectively with and solve problems, (3) communicate information, (4) coordinate activities, (5) advise an individual or group, (6) discuss, review, or evaluate various aspects of a project, (7) formulate policy, (8) brainstorm, and (9) make decisions. Meetings may also deal with issues in a highly detailed technical manner and/or general issues when appropriate.

The purpose of a meeting should be made known to all participants in advance. This will assist their preparation, both in terms of presentations and of effective participation.

Golden Rules

One of the most important principles of meetings (a golden rule) is that the leader should encounter "no surprises.'' Previously unknown and unexpected information should be communicated to the leader as far ahead of the meeting as possible. The flow is often disrupted and meetings are sometimes unable to accomplish their purpose(s) when unexpected information is presented that significantly affects the topic or project. Shock value is counterproductive to efficient project management. The practice of surprising people should be *strongly* discouraged by all project leaders and line managers. There should also be no surprises in who shows up at meetings.

Meetings called to solve a problem should initially define its nature and character, preferably prior to the meeting, but at the meeting itself if necessary. A clear description of the problem may be simply stated or may require a great deal of time, discussion, and energy. It is often helpful if background material is prepared and distributed prior to the meeting to help expedite the discussion. Wise leaders will have previously lobbied attendees. They will attempt to achieve commitment to their point of view by persuading others to assist in planning or decision making. Involving others in a new idea or solution prior to a meeting will increase commitment and help ensure its adoption and eventual success.

Types

Two basic types of meetings are held to review and evaluate progress, current status, future plans, and other aspects of a clinical trial or project. First, the group that formulated the plan (or other information being considered) reviews or evaluates information that it has either directly generated or has had clear responsibility for generating. Second, the group reviews or evaluates various aspects of a project that it did not either create or directly request. The second type is often conducted by a senior management review group. A mixed type often exist: one or more of those who helped formulate the plans are also members of a higher reviewing body, or the more senior reviewing group has had some direct input into the plans.

Formality and Agendas

The degree of formality of a meeting may not always be established in advance. Sometimes plans for one type of meeting are not carried through (for any of a number of possible reasons) and the meeting is treated either more or less formally than was anticipated or planned. In hindsight, the reasons for this disparity are often clear and should help in planning future meetings of a similar type.

TABLE 125.1 *Three types of sample agendas for project meetings*[a]

A. For a routine meeting held to share information
  1. Department status reports
  2. Issues and questions to discuss
  3. Requests for information (e.g., requirements for compound) from members
  4. Future plans and action[b]
B. For a meeting held to solve a problem, develop a plan, or make a decision
  1. Presentation of the problem and purpose of the meeting
  2. Reports of relevant departments
  3. Development of alternatives to pursue
  4. Discussion of further steps
  5. Summary of points of agreement[b]
  6. Summary of action items (to be taken after the meeting) and responsibility assignments[b]
C. For any meeting
  1. Presentation of specific topics to discuss or goals to achieve
  2. List of relevant questions for each topic (e.g., who, what, when, why, where, how, and how much)
  3. Summary for each conclusion and action point[b]

[a] These agendas may contain much more detail if desired, including names of those responsible for each point on the agenda, and possibly the time allotted for discussion.
[b] To do this effectively, the person leading the meeting or someone else must take appropriate notes during the meeting. Taking notes to identify action items is completely different from taking notes for the meeting's minutes.

Meaningful agendas should be prepared for most meetings and distributed in advance (Table 125.1).

Size

Various studies of a meeting's size show that the type of interpersonal interactions changes as the size of the group increases. Meetings tend to become more formal as their size increases. Meetings may be broadly categorized as small (5 or fewer people), medium (5–20 people), or large (20–75 people). A meeting of more than 75 people is generally a lecture, and discussion becomes difficult. These numbers are not precise and sometimes may be much larger or smaller. The number of people invited to attend a meeting should be considered in the context of what types of discussions are desired.

Technical Details

Technical details that must be planned for conducting a meeting also change markedly as the size of the meeting increases. Factors must be considered such as (1) voice enhancement with microphones, (2) suitable audiovisual displays, (3) introductions of people present, (4) ability to have informal interactions, and (5) a smooth flow and control of the meeting itself. Characteristics of poor meetings are listed in Table 125.2

TABLE 125.2 *Characteristics of poor meetings*[a]

1. Participants are too guarded and do not participate adequately
2. Participants do not prepare adequately
3. Participants have hidden agendas
4. Participants do not listen to the discussion
5. The leader or facilitator is inadequate
6. Participants do not cover all topics
7. Participants are not focused
8. Participants go off on tangents or discuss inappropriate topics
9. Participants talk too long and engage more in monologue than dialogue
10. Participants do not develop specific recommendations
11. Participants do not attempt to reach a consensus
12. No one summarizes decisions reached

[a] By implication, characteristics of a good meeting are the opposite of these points.

and a few factors that may improve the conduct of meetings are listed in Table 125.3.

Danger of Superficial Agreement at Meetings

Many individuals attempt to avoid disagreements at a meeting, using whatever efforts they must. Thus, they will nod their heads in agreement, state "I hear you," "I understand," "I see," "That is a fine point," or even agree directly with the speaker. When such people leave the meeting, however, they either refuse to

TABLE 125.3 *Questions to consider prior to a meeting that may improve its conduct and productivity*

A. Objectives
  1. Is there a real need for the meeting?
  2. Who should attend the meeting?
  3. What outcomes of the meeting are desired?
  4. What outcomes of the meeting are specifically not desired?
B. Decision making
  1. Who should lead this meeting and control its flow?
  2. What items will be on the agenda and in which order?
  3. What methods will the group use to deal with each agenda item?
  4. What processes will be used to reach decisions?
  5. Who will make the final decision?
  6. Will the meeting be allowed to continue past its scheduled conclusion? If so, by how much time?
C. Administrative matters
  1. What type of meeting will be held?
  2. When should the meeting be held?
  3. Where would the best place be to hold the meeting?
  4. What will be the length of the meeting and will there be breaks?
  5. How should the chairs and tables be set up?
  6. Who will keep notes/minutes of the meeting and how will these be reviewed and issued?
  7. What equipment will be needed (e.g., flip chart, slide projector)?
  8. What food/beverages will be available or served and at what times?
  9. What documents should be distributed prior to and at the meeting?
  10. What materials (e.g., pens, paper) should be available for participants?

follow through on what they agreed to, state that it has to be looked into further, state that they are working on it, or use another delaying tactic (i.e., excuse). In a culture or company that does not tolerate this kind of behavior, they will be forced to discard it, or they will be transferred or fired. (There are cultures in which superficial agreement is openly tolerated, if not encouraged.)

People who leave meetings and do not implement agreements, ignore them, or actively work against them should not be tolerated in a pharmaceutical (or any other) company. This behavior cannot be justified by claims of diplomacy or politeness. It is, simply stated, counterproductive to the entire organization and makes the goal of efficient development of medicines extremely difficult to achieve. It is one major reason why certain cultures are relatively poor in developing medicines or conducting clinical trials efficiently.

Increasing Efficiency

To increase the efficiency of meetings it is often possible to (1) decrease their number by eliminating unnecessary ones or by combining two or more meetings, (2) use agendas, (3) use a time schedule, (4) decrease the number of participants, (5) limit discussion on each agenda item, and (6) assign activities for individuals to complete after the meeting. It is necessary to keep track of these latter assignments so that those people will report back to the group at a subsequent meeting or via a different mechanism. A highly readable account of how to run a meeting is presented by Jay (1976).

The arrangement of tables and chairs sometimes may encourage participation and discussion of the group or may serve as a barrier. For example, if everybody sits around a single table there appears to be better involvement and more active participation than when several sit in chairs behind or away from a table where the main focus of discussion takes place.

It is sometimes valuable to have an individual at the meeting who (1) summarizes discussions on a subject after it is clear that additional constructive comments have ceased, (2) brings the discussion back to the relevant topic if it wanders on a tangent for too long a period, (3) recommends taking up the next subject if too much time is spent on one topic, and (4) recommends that highly detailed issues be handled by a small group outside the larger meeting. This type of individual is often self-appointed, but a leader may easily encourage or discourage this type of behavior.

Concluding a Meeting

The final event of a meeting should be a summary by the leader that ensures that everyone leaves the meeting on the same "wavelength." Points to be pursued outside the meeting should be reviewed and can also be put in the minutes as action points. Specific assignments may be made. Communications of committee members after a meeting may take numerous forms (Fig. 125.1).

Consultants' Meetings

Two types of meetings are discussed in more detail because of their special nature. A meeting with consultants is discussed below, and a pretrial roundtable meeting is discussed in Chapter 60.

There are often occasions in the life of a project when it is valuable to bring a group of consultants together to discuss an important issue or problem. The two major occasions are: (1) the outset of a project, when a general direction or emphasis is being charted and the strategies are being developed; (2) when an important problem has developed that will benefit from expert input into the decision that senior management has to make.

Purposes

The general purpose(s) of a consultants meeting is to:

1. Review available data and recommend or propose part or all of a clinical strategy and clinical development plan.
2. Compare results from various clinical trials and rank two or more medicines based on their safety or efficacy.
3. Acquaint potentially new clinical investigators with a medicine, learn more about their knowledge, and judge their interest in participating in a clinical development program.
4. Familiarize the sponsor's management (in research and development and in marketing) and support groups (e.g., statistics, data processing, project management) with views of experts in the field.

Choosing Consultants to Attend

The group of consultants will be chosen because they are (1) already acting as consultants to the sponsor, (2)

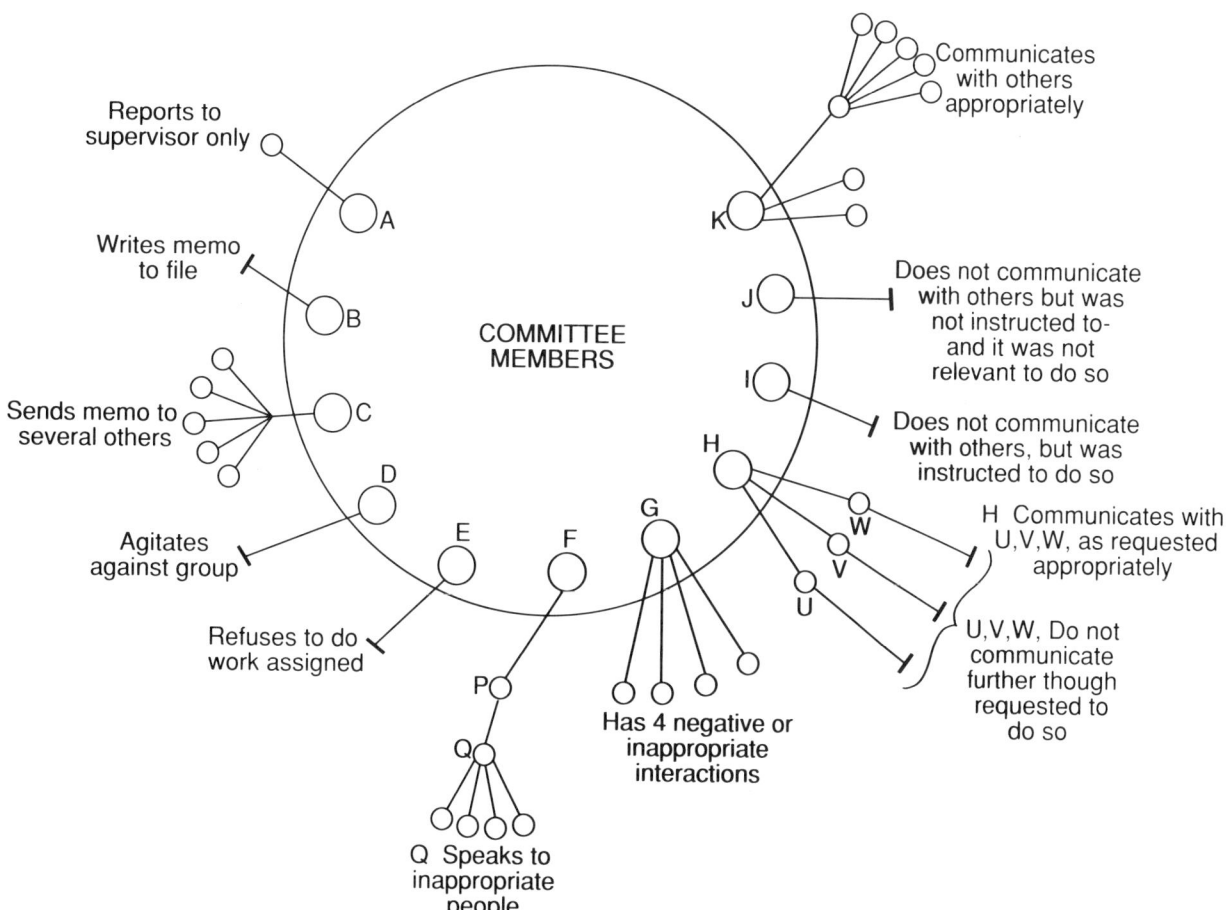

FIG. 125.1 Possible types of postmeeting communications by committee members.

other experts in the field, (3) thought leaders in the field, or (4) other individuals who may have a special contribution to offer, such as general practitioners. Consultants will provide suggestions and recommendations based on their own experiences and patients. The choice of specific consultants and their backgrounds will have a great influence on the type of advice they will offer. Consultants who understand the complexities of medicine development have a marked advantage in many cases over other experts who do not. If only tertiary care experts from academic institutions are assembled, the sophisticated opinions and advice they offer may be totally inappropriate for a medicine that will be almost totally used in primary care medicine. Another criterion for choosing consultants is based on identifying potential investigators to conduct future clinical studies. In addition to the type of consultants invited to a meeting, the advice they offer will be highly dependent on the specific questions posed and also how the questions are posed. Careful consideration should be given to this issue and to communications with the consultants prior to the meeting.

Other Attendees

A group of four to eight consultants is often assembled, plus members of the project team, senior managers, and individuals who are in charge of the project at a foreign subsidiary or parent company. This latter group (or individual) is extremely important to include in the discussions and decision making process to facilitate international cooperation and acceptance of decisions reached.

Technical Details

The agenda for the meeting should allow time for (1) presentation of background, (2) statement of the issues, (3) discussion, and (4) recommendations. It may be useful to allot separate times for panel (i.e., consultant) discussion and discussion with the audience. Although the duration of the meeting may last from 1 hour to several days, it is usually impractical to have a meeting that lasts more than a single day. Almost all consultants are extremely busy and, with few exceptions, would prefer not to spend more time. A meeting that discusses an entire therapeutic area, however, may require several days. Selected types of questions for expert consultants to consider are listed in Table 125.4.

Teleconference Meetings

Use of satellites to conduct meetings of groups located in different regions or continents is now a common

TABLE 125.4 *Selected types of questions for expert consultants to consider regarding a clinical project*

1. Dosage forms to develop
2. Efficacy parameters to measure
3. Methods to measure efficacy parameters
4. Choice of patient population(s)[a]
5. Methods to recruit patients
6. Estimated rate of patient enrollment
7. Methods to identify an appropriate dosing regimen
8. Approaches to establish a safety profile
9. Choice of criteria to stop a clinical trial prematurely
10. Role of continuation trials
11. Priority of different indications and routes of administration
12. Choice of trials for Phases I, II, and III
13. Choice of criteria and measures to determine the benefit-to-risk ratio
14. Methods to diagnose patients
15. Choice of an active control medicine

[a] This may include consideration of whether a placebo control group is ethically possible.

occurrence. Discussions with several participants in such meetings and personal experience suggests several tentative conclusions.

1. The technology appears to be generally operational, although major snafus (i.e., technical problems) do occur periodically.
2. The conferences allow relatively small groups (i.e., up to 8 or 12 at each site) to meet without the expense of international travel and often (more important) without the exhaustion and jet lag that accompanies the travel.
3. The abilities to simultaneously transmit documents and send facsimiles enhance the productivity of the meeting.
4. The need for television screens and separate groups in each location enhances the we–they effect of having separate groups.

These meetings should not be used to replace all-important face-to-face meetings. Teleconferences are a reasonable means of conducting selected meetings in a cost-effective manner, particularly for those meetings (1) that are short, (2) that focus on a single straightforward topic, (3) that require an urgent decision, or (4) for which major staff travel is undesirable.

DOCUMENTS

Functions of Records

Although many people prefer to run projects without producing formal reports, there is always a need for documentation. Many of the reasons why documentation is important relate to the functions that it serves. These functions include a need to:

1. Communicate and disseminate information among relevant individuals, some of whom may be many miles away.

2. Serve as a basis to discuss various issues or problems: everyone concerned may read the same background material and statement of the issues.
3. Serve as a means for speculation about a point for which input is requested.
4. Provide a blueprint of current and proposed plans and operational strategies to help allocate resources and assign priorities and work responsibilities.
5. Seek response to a request or proposal.
6. Provide an archival document for future use, as an "institutional memory."
7. Provide a formal source of agreements, statements, commitments, and decisions made by individuals and by groups.

Types of Reports and Issues in Record Keeping

Various types of reports are generated. Almost any type of meeting may generate minutes, consensus agreements, points for action, or other information that may need to be documented. In addition, numerous reports are written independently of meetings. These reports include feasibility reports, project plans, project strategies, current status on one or more issues, issues to be resolved, plus many others. Outlines of final medical reports are shown in Tables 125.5 to 125.7. Information deleted from these reports in a publication is listed in Table 125.8.

In addition to reports that are many forms, lists, and schedules that will assist in the management of multiple clinical trials. Some are shown or described later in this chapter. A number of types of records that an investigator may adopt are listed in Table 125.9, and selected issues in record keeping are listed in Tables 125.10 to 125.12.

An Integrated Statistical and Medical Report

Creating an integrated statistical and medical report with two different groups of authors (i.e., statisticians and clinicians) may involve difficulties, including use

TABLE 125.5 *Contents of a final medical report*[a]

1. Title page[b]	5. Clinical trial design	9. Conclusions
2. Abstract	6. Methods[c]	10. References
3. Introduction	7. Results[d]	11. Tables and figures
4. Objectives	8. Discussion	12. Appendices

[a] Each of these sections may contain all of the items described in Chapter 102. Two or more sections could be combined.
[b] May contain a sign-off sheet.
[c] Methods may be broken down into separate sections on medicines, dosages, measures, evaluations, project management, and analysis.
[d] Results may be broken down into separate sections on demographics, patient and trial accountability, and prognostic variables, as well as clinical trial results.

TABLE 125.6 *Table of contents for a final medical report*[a]

0. Synopsis
1. Introduction
2. Objectives
3. Trial design
4. Materials and methods
  A. Formulation of medicine
  B. Dosage
  C. Methods
    i. Investigators participating in the clinical trial
    ii. Ethical approval procedures
    iii. Inclusion criteria
    iv. Exclusion criteria
    v. Timing of events
    vi. Patient self-assessment
    vii. Visual analog scales
    viii. Clinician's assessment
    ix. Additional treatment period
    x. Hematology, clinical chemistry, urinalysis
    xi. Adverse events
5. Data processing
6. Results
  A. Patient and trial accountability
    i. Patient details
    ii. Protocol adherence
    iii. Concomitant medication
    iv. Patient compliance
  B. Demographics
  C. Clinical assessments
    1. First treatment period
      i. Patient self-assessment
      ii. Visual analog scales
      iii. Clinician's final assessment
    2. Additional treatment period
      i. Patient self-assessment
      ii. Visual analog scales
  D. Hematology, clinical chemistry, and urinalysis
  E. Adverse events
7. Discussion
8. Conclusions
9. References
10. Appendices plus relevant data listings

[a] Page numbers would be listed. A simpler outline could merely consist of (1) demographics and background, (2) dosing and compliance, (3) efficacy, and (4) safety.

of different jargon, differences in emphasis, and the need for the statistical part to be completed first. Many problems may be avoided if an agreement on procedures to be followed is established or a standard format is utilized (e.g., the first part of the report could be a statistical evaluation and the second part a medical evaluation). If desired, most statistical tables plus data listings could be placed in an appendix.

Standard Operating Procedures

The typical hierarchy beings with (1) national laws and, at subsequently more specialized levels, includes (2) regulations, (3) regulatory guidelines, (4) department guidelines, and (5) standard operating procedures. The first three levels refer to a regulatory agency and the last two to a specific organization. The hierarchy of these five categories is generally established chronologically in the order of laws, regulations, regulatory guidelines, organizational guidelines, and standard op-

TABLE 125.7 *Outline of a combined medical and statistical report of a clinical trial*

A. Title page
1. Title of report
2. Protocol number and title
3. Investigator(s) names and institution(s)
4. Dates clinical trial performed (i.e., from enrollment of the first patient to the final evaluations of the last patient)
5. Date of report
6. Summary of results or abstract
B. Table of contents
C. Introduction
1. General objectives
2. Design of the clinical trial
3. Special considerations or features of the clinical trial
D. Clinical trial objectives
1. Primary objective(s)
2. Secondary objective(s)
3. Subgroup hypotheses
E. Clinical trial design
1. Overall design
2. Specific characteristics (e.g., blinding, randomization, treatments compared, patient populations) and reasons why each was chosen
F. Materials and methods
1. Medicines
2. Dosages
3. Efficacy parameters
4. Safety parameters
5. Biological samples
6. Other tests
7. Patient well-being and management (e.g., Ethics Committee/Institutional Review Board (IRB) approval, informed consent)
8. Criteria for patient discontinuation
G. Statistical tests
1. General tests planned and any deviations in any tests used
2. Planned patient exclusions
3. Interim analyses conducted
4. Data-processing methods
5. Quality-assurance methods
6. Statistical software
7. Statistical models and methods
8. Statistical assumptions
9. Test statistics
10. Determination of sample size and power calculation
H. Patient and trial accountability
1. Accounting of all patients contacted (if available) and enrolled
2. List of patient dropouts and discontinuers, plus reasons for their failure to complete
3. Demographic data on each group of patients
4. Exposure to clinical trial medicines
5. Data Review Committees and other committees used to monitor the clinical trial
I. Efficacy data
1. Intention-to-treat results
2. Other analyses used, plus definition of valid patients included in each analysis
3. Analysis of each efficacy measure and tabulation of individual patient data (overall and by site)
4. Listings of any patients excluded plus reasons for exclusion
5. Listing of all pertinent data (e.g., concomitant medicines)
6. Statistical issues (e.g., adjustment for covariates, handling of dropouts, interim analyses, ability to pool data across centers, multiple endpoints)
7. Examination of subgroups and testing of subgroup hypotheses
8. Dose–response relationships tested or demonstrated
9. Interactions among medicines or between the test medicine and other factors
J. Safety data
1. Overall adverse events and adverse reaction data (e.g., incidence, severity, treatments used, relationship with efficacy or other adverse reactions)
2. List of all important adverse reactions and characteristics on an individual patient basis (e.g., demographics, dose, time of onset and duration, intensity, action taken, rechallenge, outcome, relationship to medicine)
3. Laboratory evaluations
4. Other safety tests
K. Discussion of results
1. Statement of results of the clinical trial
2. Comparison with other data on the medicine
3. Comparison with other medicines
4. Extrapolations
L. Conclusions
M. References
N. Appendices
1. Tables
2. Figures
3. Protocol
4. Protocol amendments
5. Sample set of data collection forms
6. Publications resulting from the clinical trial
7. Names and affiliations of all investigators
8. Randomization code used
9. Descriptions of statistical tests used and data
10. Individual patient data
11. Reports of clinical audits conducted

erating procedures. Standard operating procedures should be considered the servant that assists in achieving the goals of a group. When the standard operating procedures are too old or no longer useful they should be changed and revitalized.

Standard operating procedures are intended to provide guidance for many of the activities needed to plan, conduct, and manage single or multiple clinical trials. This guidance reflects the policy of the institution in which the activities are conducted. Standard operating procedures are a useful guide in numerous activities, and a few selected areas are listed in Table 125.13. They are an important part of quality assurance activities necessary to ensure that Good Laboratory Practices (GLPs), Good Manufacturing Practices (GMPs), and Good Clinical Practices (GCPs) are followed in developing a medicine or medical device.

Standard operating procedures should only be established if they are going to be followed. A balance must be established between the ideal, practical, and actual case in using standard procedures in many situations. There should not be a discrepancy between the official procedures and actual practice, because legal complications may ensue. For instance, if established guidelines suggest one code of corporate behavior for adverse reactions reported to the company, but a different code is followed, then ethical and possibly legal problems may arise.

TABLE 125.8 *Information sometimes included in a final medical report (or its appendix) that is usually deleted from a publication*

A. Statistical processes and methods
 1. Details of data processing
 2. Quality-assurance procedures
 3. Software packages used
 4. Statistical models and details of analyses used
 5. Statistical assumptions
 6. Interim analysis results and any modifications made
 7. Raw patient data
 8. Data tabulations
 9. Data listings
B. Administrative information
 1. All relevant personnel connected with the clinical trial, including their roles, addresses, and qualifications
 2. Résumé of all investigators and coinvestigators
 3. Protocol plus any amendments
 4. Blank copy of the data collection forms
 5. Instructions given to patients
 6. Informed consent form
 7. Details about the Ethics Committee/Institutional Review Board (IRB) and its members
 8. History of the protocol approval by the Ethics Committee/IRB and a copy of the approval form
 9. Randomization schedule used
 10. Source of clinical trial materials
 11. Table of dosing schedule
 12. Lot numbers of all clinical trial materials
 13. Diagnostic criteria
 14. Assay procedures to measure test medicine in biological samples
 15. Any other guidelines or procedures used
C. Clinical trial results detailed and summarized in terms of tables, listings, and/or graphs
 1. Patient demographics
 2. Patient accountability
 3. Medicine exposure
 4. Laboratory data
 5. Adverse reactions
 6. Other safety measures
 7. Pharmacokinetics
 8. Efficacy

Standard operating procedures differ widely from company to company, and within a company they will change over time. This book does not attempt to provide specific procedures. It does contain, however, many factors to be discussed or considered when such procedures are developed.

Preparing Standard Operating Procedures

The most senior managers who have direct responsibility for establishing standard operating procedures and for a specific topic meet and discuss the overall major and minor goals they wish to achieve. They must decide how the standard operating procedures will be developed. Four possible approaches to developing standard operating procedures are (1) the same group of managers do all the work, (2) the work is delegated to a task force, (3) a consultant is hired to complete the task, or (4) a task force and the managers agree to meet in order to determine the approach.

The people developing the actual procedures often start by creating flow charts and identifying activities of all relevant groups. Subcharts and other more detailed plots and descriptions are also developed. Flow charts of activities are reviewed and after approval has been obtained, they are used to develop standard operating procedures. These procedures may be developed by a single group or divided into multiple sections, each of which is assigned to a different person or group. The final stages involve discussion, revision, review, and acceptance by the creators, and then review, revision, and approval by relevant managers. The final step is dissemination to all involved individuals, possibly accompanied by meetings to discuss the implications or conduct of the new standard operating procedures.

Standardized Forms

Forms are often used to expedite dissemination of information about clinical trials and serve numerous

TABLE 125.9 *Types of record keeping that an investigator may adopt*[a]

A. Individual patient records for patients who are also part of a physician's clinical practice
 1. Maintain separate files of a patient's medical records and records for each medicine trial in which they participate. Place these files together under the patient's name
 2. Maintain separate files of a patient's medical records and records for each medicine trial in which they participate. Write "progress notes" for each clinical visit conducted as part of a medicine trial on the patient's permanent medical records. Place the two sets of records in separate files, one devoted to practice patients and the other to medicine trials
 3. Cross-index all hospital records in a patient's medical record, with hospital number, dates of each admission, reasons for admission, and other pertinent data
 4. Cross-index all laboratory reports maintained in a medicine trial if the reports are not photocopies in the patient's permanent medical records
B. Individual patient records for patients who are not part of a physician's clinical practice
 1. Duplicate basic information from the medicine trial record to a new file that is kept in the practice's permanent medical records
 2. Insert a form (or file) only with the patient's name in the clinical practice medical records. This serves as a cross-index to the data collection forms and medicine trial records
 3. Do not maintain any medical records for patients who are not part of an investigator's clinical practice, apart from the data collection forms and medicine trial files
C. Maintain one master set of all files, whether or not patients in a medicine trial are part of a physician's private practice[b]
 1. Order files by patient's last name, social security number, date of first visit, or using another system
 2. Files or file tabs may be color coded using a variety of methods to facilitate retrieval of information

[a] Some or all of the information collected may also be placed in a computer data base.
[b] Data collection forms will have to be maintained separately.

TABLE 125.10 *Selected issues to consider in record keeping*

A. Design and nature of the record
  1. Physical form of the record (e.g., hard copy, computer disk)
  2. Design of the forms used should be suitable to record data from the investigator's private practice and clinical trials
  3. Content of each form and changes in the format of the record form that may occur over time or be required to collect a different type or amount of data
B. Completing the form or record
  1. If different physicians treat the same patient include the physician's name on each relevant record
  2. If different technicians test the same patient include their name on each relevant record
  3. Determine who will be responsible for filling in and maintaining the records
  4. Ensure legibility of the records
  5. Ensure that an adequate amount of data is recorded
  6. Utilize black pens for all data recorded if a typewriter or computer is not used
C. Other issues
  1. Measuring quality of recorded observations and devising a means to indicate this in the records
  2. Procedures to allow for patient follow-up
  3. Confidentiality of the data (e.g., sponsors should only receive pages with patient initials)
  4. Similarity of records in different institutions conducting a multicenter clinical trial (e.g., retrospective, prospective)
  5. Changes in trials' tests and laboratory reference ranges over time (e.g., specific efficacy tests, equipment) may affect data placed in the same record
  6. Changes in patient diagnoses or severity of illness over time

TABLE 125.11 *Administrative matters for a sponsor to track in a clinical trial for each site*[a,b]

1. Important milestone dates [e.g., trial initiation, medicine shipment, Ethics Committee/Institutional Review Board (IRB) approval]
2. Sites enrolled in a clinical trial, plus names, addresses, telephone and FAX numbers of all relevant staff and ancillary sites
3. Contracts and budgets agreed, payment schedules, and how checks are to be made out and mailed
4. Orders for manufacture of medicine(s) and placebo (i.e., a list of dates and weights)
5. Orders for shipment of medicine(s) and placebo
6. Regulatory and other documents sent to each site
7. Ethics Committee/IRB approvals requested and received for the protocol and any amendments
8. Periodic trial reports sent to Ethics Committees/IRBs
9. Telephone log reports
10. Site visit log reports
11. Requests for payment received and processed
12. Receipt of data collection forms and their processing
13. Current status of patient enrollment per site, versus projected enrollment goals
14. Current status of serious adverse events and reporting of those events to regulatory authorities
15. Sites terminated and in process of being terminated
16. Unused medicine returned to sponsor
17. Periodic reports to generate for various groups
18. Expiration date of medicine and the process required to have it extended
19. Overall financial accounting of the clinical trial
20. Overall use of medicine in the clinical trial

[a] For each item, list original projected date or number, any revisions to the estimate, and the final actual date or data.
[b] For each appropriate item that is ongoing, list the current status and the projected current status to assess where future problems may develop (e.g., will patients run out of medicine at certain sites).

other functions. Although forms may be created *de novo* for each clinical trial or project of multiple trials, it is generally useful to have a number of standardized forms available for many projects. This also saves the time and effort that would otherwise be required to develop forms each time they are desired or needed.

Modular Forms

In some situations it may be possible to devise a modular approach to reports, using a series of standardized forms. Reports for many different purposes would be created by completing and combining a number of standardized forms. The purpose of this approach is to simplify report writing and the reviewing of multiple reports. There are numerous pros and cons to using multiple standardized forms for creating reports. In general, this approach is not recommended because it does not easily permit variations to allow for differences between medicines, exceptions, and special cases that frequently arise and do not fit the general pattern. If these variations were met by including additional prose, then an entire prose report would often be preferable to using modular forms.

Basic Forms

This section describes some types of forms that have been developed and illustrates a few examples. Selected forms used for manufacturing clinical supplies were published by Bettis (1985). A basic library of various schedules and forms used in managing previous clinical trials will simplify the creation of new forms.

TABLE 125.12 *Selected records that may be maintained by investigators for a clinical trial*[a]

1. Patient appointment book
2. Patient sign-in book
3. Log of sponsor (if any) visits
4. Log of medicine(s) dispensed
5. Log of laboratory samples sent
6. Log of laboratory results received
7. Log of payments made to patients
8. Log of payments received from sponsor
9. Log of appointments for patients at specialized clinics (e.g., ophthalmology) or laboratories (e.g., pulmonary function tests)

[a] For each log it is relevant to identify the date, name of patient or visitor, name of staff person involved, plus details of the medicine, sample, or other item discussed. Items mentioned in the preceeding table may also be relevant to track.

TABLE 125.13 *Representative types of standard operating procedures*[a]

A. Related trial medicine(s). How to:
1. Request that medicine be synthesized
2. Request that medicine be formulated into a specific dosage form
3. Request that a finished dosage form of a medicine be packaged for a clinical trial and shipped to a trial site
4. Request points 1, 2, or 3 above from a facility in a different country, subsidiary, or parent company
5. Return medicine to the sponsor from a trial site and have it destroyed
6. Transport and store compounds
7. Request that specific compounds be tested in specific (or general) tests
8. Acquire clinical trial medicines from other companies or from other parts of the same company
9. Request for biological screening or advanced testing on a specific compound/medicine
10. Request that a new formulation of a medicine be developed and placed on stability
11. Complete laboratory notebooks as well as arrange for their storage, duplication, and safeguarding
B. Related to the clinical trial. How to:
1. Choose a trial site
2. Report on pretrial and periodic visits to a trial site
3. Report on a telephone conversation
4. Request that money be sent to the investigator
5. Request that data from a clinical trial be entered in a computer and be quality assured
6. Transmit data from the investigator's site to the sponsoring institution
7. Correct data collection forms after they have been received by the sponsor
C. Related to the sponsor's institution. How to:
1. Prepare a feasibility report and have it approved
2. Prepare an investigator's brochure and have it approved
3. Prepare a final statistical report and have it approved[b]
4. Prepare a final medical report and have it approved[b]
5. Prepare an annual report on a medicine for the FDA[c] and have it submitted
6. Request changes in membership on a project team
7. Request that reports be prepared for an IND or NDA[c]
8. Change labeling on a marketed medicine
9. Report adverse reactions to the FDA
10. Communicate with the FDA or other regulatory agencies
11. Set up a meeting with the FDA
12. Register compound numbers for both internal and external use
13. Review and approve protocols and amendments to protocols
14. Request that plasma, urine, or other samples be assayed for medicine levels or concentrations
15. Request that data on a clinical trial be analyzed statistically
16. Request that a new indication be considered for a medicine's development
17. Develop a new or modified standard operating procedure
D. Related to investigator. How to:
1. Identify duties of each staff person
2. Assign responsibilities in the investigator's absence

[a] Some organizations would divide several of these topics into multiple standard operating procedures.
[b] It may be desirable to prepare a joint statistical and medical report.
[c] IND, Investigational New Drug Application; NDA, New Drug Application; FDA, Food and Drug Administration.

Forms should have prepunched holes if they are to be placed in loose-leaf binders. Computer forms are becoming popular, not only for remote data entry, but for use and communication within offices. A problem with this trend is that many people become too enthusiastic and want to develop one or more forms for every possible use; these people also tend to create forms that are too detailed. Such dangers must be avoided. A description of a few basic forms follows.

Tracking Patients, Trials, Grants, and Data

Tables 125.14 to 125.16 and Figs. 125.2 to 125.6 illustrate some forms that may be used to keep track of patients, trials, grants, and the flow of data obtained in most trials. Other forms were published by Frelick and Kyle (1984). Many of the forms used for these purposes may be entered in a computer and easily updated by the monitor or other staff.

Schedules for Staff

Schedules may be developed for each staff member (e.g., physician, nurse, coordinator, receptionist, specialist). These schedules present a list of activities that must be performed on each patient at each visit or *in toto*. These lists may include dates or times when the scheduled activities are to be performed. Other staff activities in a clinical trial may also be scheduled (e.g., completion of data collection forms, discussion of results and issues, contacts with the sponsor).

Telephone Conversation Sheet

This form basically consists of a blank page with lines. A few lines at the top may be preprinted with headings such as date, time, medicine, and clinical trial involved, as well as individual(s) on the telephone (see Fig. 125.5). If all forms used by one individual are for a single trial or project, then some of the information on this form may be preprinted or stamped on the form.

The person completing the form should indicate the reason for the call as well as a synopsis of advice or information given. Any decisions reached or comments made that affect the clinical trial should be recorded. Forms of all conversations should be copied (if carbonless paper was not used to create copies) and placed in both permanent and trial record files. Some companies send a copy of all telephone reports to the investigator as well.

Patient Screening Forms

Many clinical trials have data collection forms that are used as soon as a patient has been enrolled in a clinical

TABLE 125.14 *Sample table headings to monitor status of individual patients enrolled in long-term clinical trial protocols*

Site code or name	Patient no.	Pt starts medicine (date)	Pt ends medicine (date)	Duration on medicine to date	Current dose of medicine	Length of time since last dose changed	No. of dose changes	Completed treatment (C) or dropped out (D)	Date when Pt will complete X months on medicine	Comments

[a] Pt, patient.

trial. If it often useful to have a special form that can be used for patients who are undergoing various procedures in the screening phase of a trial. If a patient either does not "pass" the screen or passes but does not agree to sign the informed consent and enter the trial, a set of data collection forms will not have had to be used and the patient will not have been assigned a trial patient number. Unless there is a specific reason to retain these forms on patients who are not entered in a trial, they may be discarded after the trial is completed.

These forms may be used to process patients through inclusion criteria. While some inclusion criteria may be answered rapidly by patients, others require tests and take additional time to complete. During this phase of the clinical trial it is useful to use screening forms, particularly if the percent of patients screened who eventually qualify and enter the trial is below 80% (or any other percent that seems more appropriate to the monitor or investigator). These screening forms are, therefore, practical, although their use *may* require recopying information onto data collection forms. On the other hand, these forms could be the first part of data collection forms and could be placed in an appropriate

notebook when a patient passed the screen and signed the informed consent.

The patient screening form should indicate the patient's name, address, telephone number at work and home, source of referral, and a checklist of the inclusion and exclusion criteria. The disposition of the patient must be indicated (i.e., the patient either entered or did not enter the clinical trial). A form to be used for telephone interviews should be a condensed version of the inclusion criteria. Telephone interviews are usually used as a preliminary screen to decrease the number of potential enrollees to those most likely to be suitable for enrollment.

Patients entering a clinic or place where screening occurs usually go through a carefully planned series of steps culminating in their agreement to participate in a study. It is usually unwise and unnecessary to have anyone undergo an expensive test (e.g., electroencephalogram, CAT scan) prior to ensuring that they meet other parts of the entrance criteria. The reasons why patients fail the inclusion criteria are usually important to record so that trends or important factors may be determined. A form for this record is shown in Figure 79.2. The reasons and number of patients

TABLE 125.15 *Sample table headings to track clinical trials in Phases II and III*

A

Type of trial[a]	Protocol no.	Purpose of trial[b]	Number of patients	Start date	Actual end date	Data processing (due date)	Statistical report (due date)	Medical report (due date)	Manuscript[c]

B

Product	Trial objective	Dose, route, frequency	Investigator and site	Monitors and staff	Start data	Target end date	Progress and comment about priorities and reasons for objective		

C

Protocol no.	Number of patients	Number of treatments	Date of data cutoff for NDA[d]	Date of last DCF[d] entered	Date data base available	Date stat. report due	Stat. author	Date medical report due	Medial author	Date report to regulatory affairs

[a] This column may list the indication, general type of patients enrolled, or whether the clinical trial is evaluating pharmacokinetics or efficacy, or is being conducted for a specific purpose.
[b] To evaluate a specific indication, formulation, dose, or to provide support to marketing.
[c] The status may be either planned, in preparation, in press, or already published.
[d] NDA, New Drug Application; DCF, data collection form.

TABLE 125.16 *Status of requests for medicine supplies to be sent to an investigator's site*

Request number	Project number	Name of medicine	Study number	Priority code	Medical requestor	Date of request	Proposed date of shipping	Comments
1								
2								
3								
—								
N								

who pass the screen but decline to enter the clinical trial because of the information in the informed consent or for other reasons may also be collected (Fig. 79.3). Prognostic characteristics plus demographic data of these patients should be collected if possible.

Reviewing Data Collection Forms by Investigators and Staff

At some point prior to a patient's visit it is usually valuable if one member of the clinical trial team is assigned to review the patient's data collection forms for completeness and accuracy. A separate single-page form could be completed and attached to the front of each chart; it would indicate the points that had to be completed or answered by relevant people prior to, or at the time of, the patient's next visit. These points include: (1) adding any missing data that are now available, (2) noting any abnormal laboratory, adverse reactions, or other data that have to be followed up at the upcoming visit, (3) having signatures put in all relevant places, (4) raising questions that should be asked at the upcoming visit, or (5) providing information that will enable the next visit to run more efficiently and be more productive. Some of these points may be handled by the monitor if the investigator and staff do not complete this function.

Other standard forms may be prepared at the clinical trial site that will complement those prepared by the sponsor. These forms will provide the investigator and staff with a straightforward means of implementing the trial with the least number of difficulties.

Name of Medicine _____

Project No. _____

Date of Update _____

Page _____

Protocol No.	Clinical Trial Code	Site No.	Investigator(s) Name(s)	Clinical Trial Status	First Patient Enrolled (Date)	Total No. Patients Actual (A) Planned (P)	No. of Patients Enrolled (%)	No. of Patients Completed (%)	Estimated Completion Date of Trial
1									
2									
3									
•••									
N									

FIG. 125.2 Form to track clinical trials status: planned, in progress, or completed.

Project: No.: _____   Prepared By: _____   Current Status for 1. Planned Trials _____

Date: _____   Approved By: _____   2. Ongoing Trials _____

Previous Update: _____   3. Completed Trials _____

(Check 1 or more)

Type of Trial (Indication, Route)	Blind (DB, SB, Open)	Purpose/ Objective	Phase No.	Trial No.	Investigator Name(s)	City, Country	Monitors	Total Cost ($)	Start Date	Original End Date	Current End Date	Total No. of Patients To Be Enrolled	No. of Patients Enrolled	No. of Patients Completed
Atrial Fib.	DB	Efficacy	II	2125	Jones	Munich FRG	Smith, Taylor	16.525	Jan '86	Jan '87	Feb '87	45	24	12

Comments: _____
_____
_____
_____
_____

FIG. 125.3 Tracking current status of clinical trials on a specific medicine. DB, double-blind; SB, single blind. A separate form may be employed for planned, ongoing or completed trials, or all three may be combined on one form.

Company Location: _____

Medicine Name: _____

Protocol Number: _____

Grant Number: _____

Total Amount of Grant ($): _____

Checks Are Made Payable To: _____

Agreed On Payment Schedule: _____

Address To Which Payments Are Sent: _____

(If different than investigator's address) _____

Investigator's Name: _____

Investigator's Address: _____
_____
_____

Payment Number	Date Check Requested	Date Check Received	Person Requesting Check	Work Being Paid For	Check Number	Type of Currency	Amount of Payment (US $)	Exchange Rate	Date of Check	Amount of Check	Total (US $)	Balance (US $)

FIG. 125.4 Tracking grant payments on a clinical trial.

Telephone Conversation Report

Project: _____

Study No: _____

Investigator: _____

Spoke To: _____

Date & Time: _____

Reason(s) for Call: _____

_____

Important Points: _____

_____

_____

_____

_____

_____

_____

_____

Who originated call? _____

Place top copy in the study file and the other copy in the telephone log.

Send copies to: _____

Signature: _____

FIG. 125.5 Telephone conversation report form.

Organizing Clinical Trial Files

There are numerous ways to organize files on multiple clinical trials. It is important for investigators as well as sponsors to adopt a single or primary method for organizational consistency within their project of multiple trials. This practice will help in the rapid retrieval of information as well as in case of an audit from a regulatory agency. A workable hierarchy should be used. Two examples are:

1. Project name and number/specific indication/protocol number/trial site number/patient number
2. IND number/site number/trial number/patient number

A more complete type of file organization for investigators is shown in Table 125.17.

Creating a Clinical Trial Visit Log and Report

At each clinical trial and sponsor's location it is generally important to maintain a log for documenting each visit by (1) representatives from the sponsor, (2) FDA personnel, (3) consultants, (4) contract group representatives, or (5) other individuals regarding the trial. This log should contain (1) name, (2) date, (3) purpose of visit, and (4) comments. Reports of periodic visits by trial monitors for their own records and the

Periodic Site Visit Report

Project: _____

Product or medicine: _____

Trial no: _____

Investigator: _____

Date of visit: _____

Conducted by: _____

Personnel with whom visit was conducted: _____

Purpose of visit: _____

Number of data collection forms edited: _____

Data collection forms returned to sponsor: _____

DCF errors found that were not corrected by the staff during the visit: _____

_____

_____

Protocol violations (if any): _____

_____

Items to receive from site: _____

_____

Items to send to site: _____

_____

Other follow-up: _____

_____

Is a more detailed report of this visit available? _____ Yes _____ No. If yes, doc. no. _____

Comments:

Signature and date: _____

Copies to: _____

FIG. 125.6 Periodic scheduled site visit report form for trial monitor to complete. DCF, data collection form.

TABLE 125.17 *Possible organization of an investigator's files on a clinical trial*

A. Regulatory documents
  1. Curriculum vitae of investigator (or coinvestigators)
  2. Signed copy of the clinical trial protocol
  3. Ethics Committee/IRB[a] approval to conduct the trial
  4. Copy of informed consent and pregnancy waiver
  5. Copy of data collection forms
  6. Copy of laboratory certification and reference range of values
  7. Copy of all correspondence with regulatory groups
  8. Copy of protocol amendments
B. Study documents
  1. Financial records and correspondence
  2. Forms regarding medicine shipments to and from the site and disposition of medicine to patients
  3. Visits by monitors (e.g., reports, correspondence, trial log)
  4. General correspondence
  5. Trial reports (e.g., statistical, medical)
  6. Publication(s)
C. Patient records
  1. Signed informed consents
  2. Completed or current data collection forms
  3. Medical records relating to the trial
  4. Laboratory and other reports
D. Correspondence with Ethics Committee/IRB
  1. Information submitted for approval
  2. Approval letters from all relevant groups
  3. All correspondence and reports submitted (e.g., annual, final, unexpected events)
  4. Any amendments to protocol submitted
E. General information
  1. Elements of the informed consent
  2. Investigator's manual
  3. Background material about the medicine
  4. Obligations of clinical investigators

[a] IRB, Institutional Review Board.

sponsor's official files are generally prepared as separate documents. Figure 125.6 shows one typical form that may be used for this purpose.

Contents and Monitor's Review of Data Collection Forms

A short table of contents for all pages of the data collection form can be prepared. Either insert one copy in front of each patient's "book" of data collection forms or prepare a single copy for the investigator and staff to use for all patients. Monitors may also use a different form (Fig. 125.7), that lists the general contents of data collection forms to point out items that the investigator has to complete, modify, or change.

Physician's Medical Chart on Patients in a Trial

In addition to the data collection form, the physician must also maintain independent medical records on each patient in the clinical trial who is also in his or her private practice. Some physicians maintain separate patient charts on all patients in a trial in addition to data collection forms. This patient chart record should include the following:

  1. A list of each patient visit that was part of the clinical trial, including the date.

Data Collection Form Checklist

Trial No. _____ Patient No. _____ Monitor Initials _____ Date _____

Part of Data Collection Form	Page No.	Specific Questions
Admission Criteria		
Medical History		
Physical Exam		
Electrocardiogram		
Blood Chemistry		
Hematology		
Dosage Record		
Pill Count		
Adverse Reactions		
Clinical Global Impression		
Etc.		

FIG. 125.7 Data collection form checklist for the investigator and/or coordinator to use in monitoring. A copy of this form may be attached to the front of data collection forms containing unanswered questions. A new form (per patient) is used for each visit.

Form for Evaluation of Potential Investigator

Name of Potential Investigator _____

Address and Telephone No. _____

Protocol Name and Number _____

Medicine Name and Phase (I to IV) _____

Reviewer Who Made the Visit _____

Date of This Report _____ Date of Visit _____

People Visited and Title _____

Final Recommendation

        Definitely Use Site   _____

        Use Site if Necessary   _____

        Definitely Do Not Use Site _____

        Consider Only If _____

Specific Rating and Comments:

  (Rate from 1 [Unacceptable] to 10 [Top in Field or Acceptable]; NA = Not Applicable)

Comments

1. Investigator's qualifications and previous experience   _____ _____
2. Investigator's interest in the clinical trial   _____ _____
3. Investigator's time availability for the trial   _____ _____
4. Adequacy of support staff (list names and positions)   _____ _____
5. Adequacy of physical facilities and security   _____ _____
6. Adequacy of laboratories and pharmacy   _____ _____
7. Patient population — numbers (how was it determined?)   _____ _____
8. Patient population — quality for trial (same as above)   _____ _____
9. Cost of the trial (proposed budget)   _____ _____
10. Additional comments _____

_____

_____

Prepared by _____
                 (Signature)

FIG. 125.8 Form for evaluation of potential investigators.

1004 / MANAGEMENT OF MULTIPLE CLINICAL TRIALS

Shipment of Trial Materials to Site

Medicine Name and Protocol Number: _____

Investigator's Name and Location: _____

Name of Contact at Site and Telephone Number: _____

Item	Sent (Date)	Received (Date)	Comment
Final Protocol			
Medicine			
Medicine (Second Shipment)			
Medicine (Third Shipment)			
Data Collection Forms (DCFs)			
DCFs (Second Shipment)			
Plasma Sample Tubes			
Plasma Tube Labels			
Plasma Forms to Accompany Samples			
Box for Shipping Plasma Samples			
Pharmacist's Book			
Investigator's Log			
Other _____			
Other _____			
Other _____			
Other _____			

FIG. 125.9 Form for shipment of trial materials to a trial site. It may also be desirable to identify the batch and lot numbers of medicine sent.

2. A typical office visit note may be written.
3. A rubber stamp may be used to refer to the trial record for additional details.
4. A statement could be added that the patient's trial record is part of this medical chart.

Other Forms

Many other forms are used in most clinical trials, including forms for monitors to choose investigators (Fig. 125.8), transmit medicines to sites (Fig. 125.9), return medicines from sites, plus forms used for various other purposes.

COMPUTER USE IN MEDICINE DEVELOPMENT

The rapid and enormous expansion of computer applications over the past decade has made them an integral part of many, if not most, clinical trials. Their role will undoubtedly continue to grow, although the exact pace and nature of future uses are not certain.

Areas of Use

Selected areas in which computers may assist in the conduct of clinical trials are given in Table 125.18. This table illustrates many applications related to the ac-

TABLE 125.18 *Selected areas in which computers may assist in the conduct and management of clinical trials*

A. Pretrial
1. To develop PERT[a] charts and schedule of activities for planning the conduct of a project and monitoring its progress
2. To provide randomization codes
3. To assist in preparing information labels that are applied to containers
4. To weigh capsules automatically after their manufacture and ensure correct weight
B. During trial
1. To develop various graphs illustrating progress of individual projects or of an entire program
2. To enter data from data collection forms
3. To obtain data online or direct from distant sites of clinical investigation
4. To obtain data online or direct from distant laboratories
5. To develop data bases and monitor trial progress
6. To communicate between sites using electronic mail
7. To monitor current status of some or all patients
8. To track and plan medicine supplies, patient enrollment, and other aspects of the trial
C. Posttrial
1. To compile data and compare doubly entered data
2. To analyze data from clinical trials
3. To analyze plasma and other biological samples with analytical equipment connected to a computer
4. To track completion and receipt of data collection forms
D. Throughout trial program
1. As word processors in preparing protocols and other documentation
2. Maintain current status of ongoing and completed clinical trials
3. Follow grants, payment records, travel records, expense items, contract laboratories, and publications
4. Data storage and retrieval

• [a] PERT, Program Evaluation and Review Technique.

quisition and processing of data. Functions that are not listed in this table related to the involvement of computers in many efficacy tests that are conducted, plus areas of administration such as making appointments and billing patients for services rendered. Although relatively few clinical trials *require* the use of computers for their conduct, it is clear that computers possess an incredible potential to expand the abilities of the people who are involved in all parts of a clinical trial. Improvements in data collection through use of a computer system in oncology studies are described by Kent et al. (1985). Computers are an integral part of artificial intelligence (see Table 72.5).

Measuring Clinical Parameters

Some efficacy parameters may only be measured with the use of computers. For example, the computer is essential to obtain evoked responses, and thus this efficacy parameter is impossible to measure or obtain without computers. Various types of radiological imaging (e.g., computerized tomography, positron emission tomography) also require computers.

Handling Data

The computer has expanded the abilities of individuals to handle data and to conduct analyses that previously were impossible or extremely arduous. Nonetheless, the essential core of most clinical trials continues to be the interaction of physician and patient. Computers should be viewed as important aids to assist the investigator or others involved with the trial, rather than being an integral part of the trial's conduct.

Integration of Computers

The integration of numerous types of computers is being carried on today to create wider networks and increased functions, including the use of computers in remote data entry (Chapter 28) and retrieval (Yu, 1986), which will undoubtedly become even more common practice in the future. Numerous uses of an integrated computer system are described by Bleich et al. (1985) for a teaching hospital (Boston's Beth Israel Hospital). Although this system is not specifically designed to conduct clinical trials it is clear that this system may be used to assist such trials in many ways.

Electronic Searches of Data Bases

A final use of computers that has become indispensable to many clinicians and scientists is in the search of electronic data bases for information regarding medical literature, patient treatment, and many other areas. This enormously diverse area has been summarized by Williams (1985), and is discussed widely.

CHAPTER 126

Interactions of Regulatory Departments, Regulatory Authorities, and Medical Departments

Regulatory submissions (and approvals) play a major role in the livelihood and survival of a company. This chapter briefly describes the major types of regulatory submissions and how they are generally planned and compiled. It also discusses the types of interactions that occur between regulatory affairs departments in pharmaceutical companies, regulatory agencies, and medical departments. Many activities conducted within a pharmaceutical corporation are either directly or indirectly targeted toward an eventual filing of a regulatory submission.

Academicians who conduct unsponsored clinical trials (with or without active participation of a pharmaceutical company) usually have few interactions with a regulatory agency or department. In some situations, however, academicians may interact with a regulatory group either at their own institution, at the national level, or with a pharmaceutical company. Common interactions of these types will be described.

ORGANIZATION OF THE FOOD AND DRUG ADMINISTRATION

Figure 126.1 gives us (1) a perspective of the Food and Drug Administration (FDA) organization in the Department of Health and Human Services, one of the major cabinets in the United States government, and (2) a description of the various offices of the FDA. A more detailed organization of the Center for Drug Evaluation and Research (CDER) and the Center for Biologics Evaluation and Research (CBER) are shown in Figs. 126.2 and 126.3.

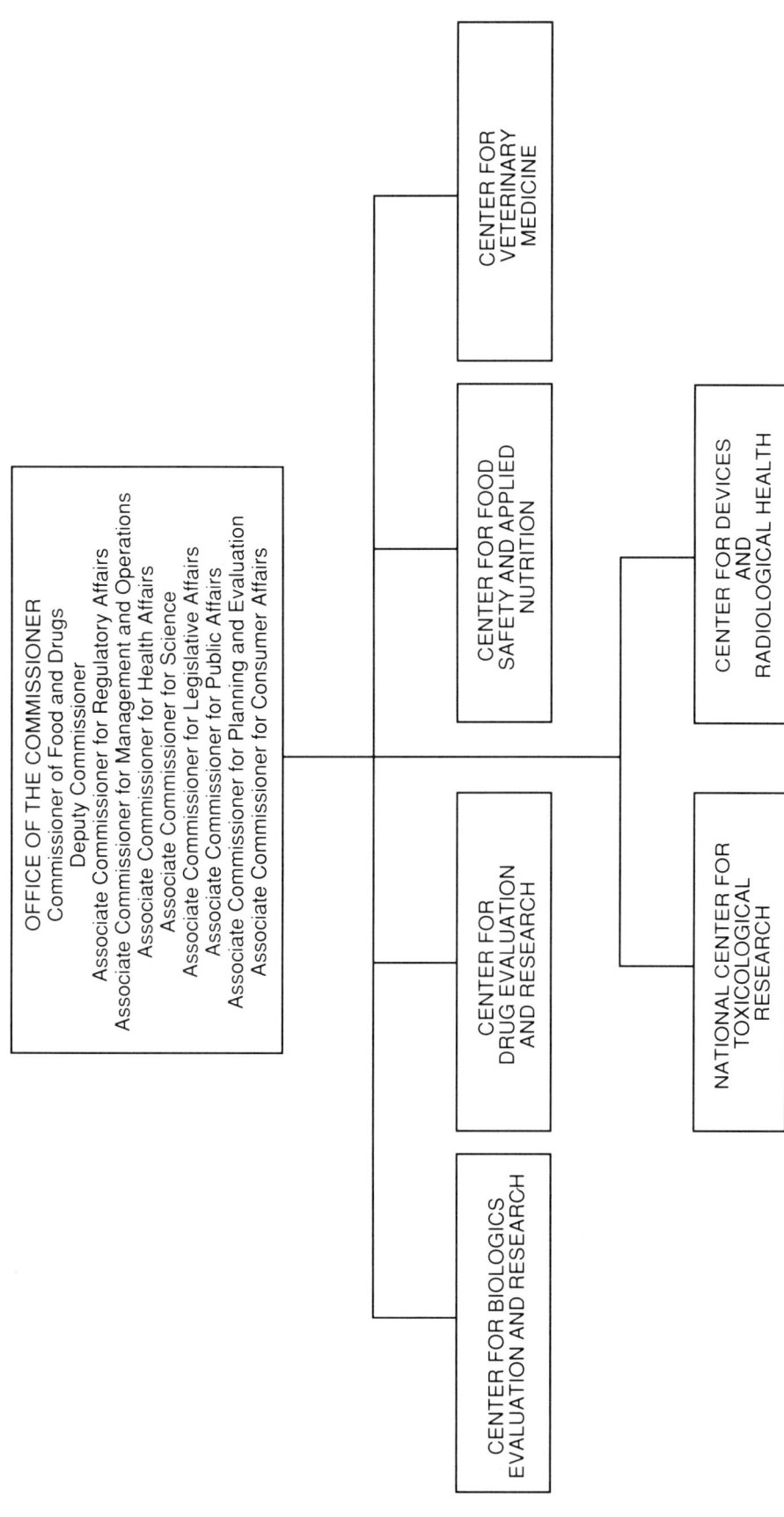

FIG. 126.1 Organization of the FDA.

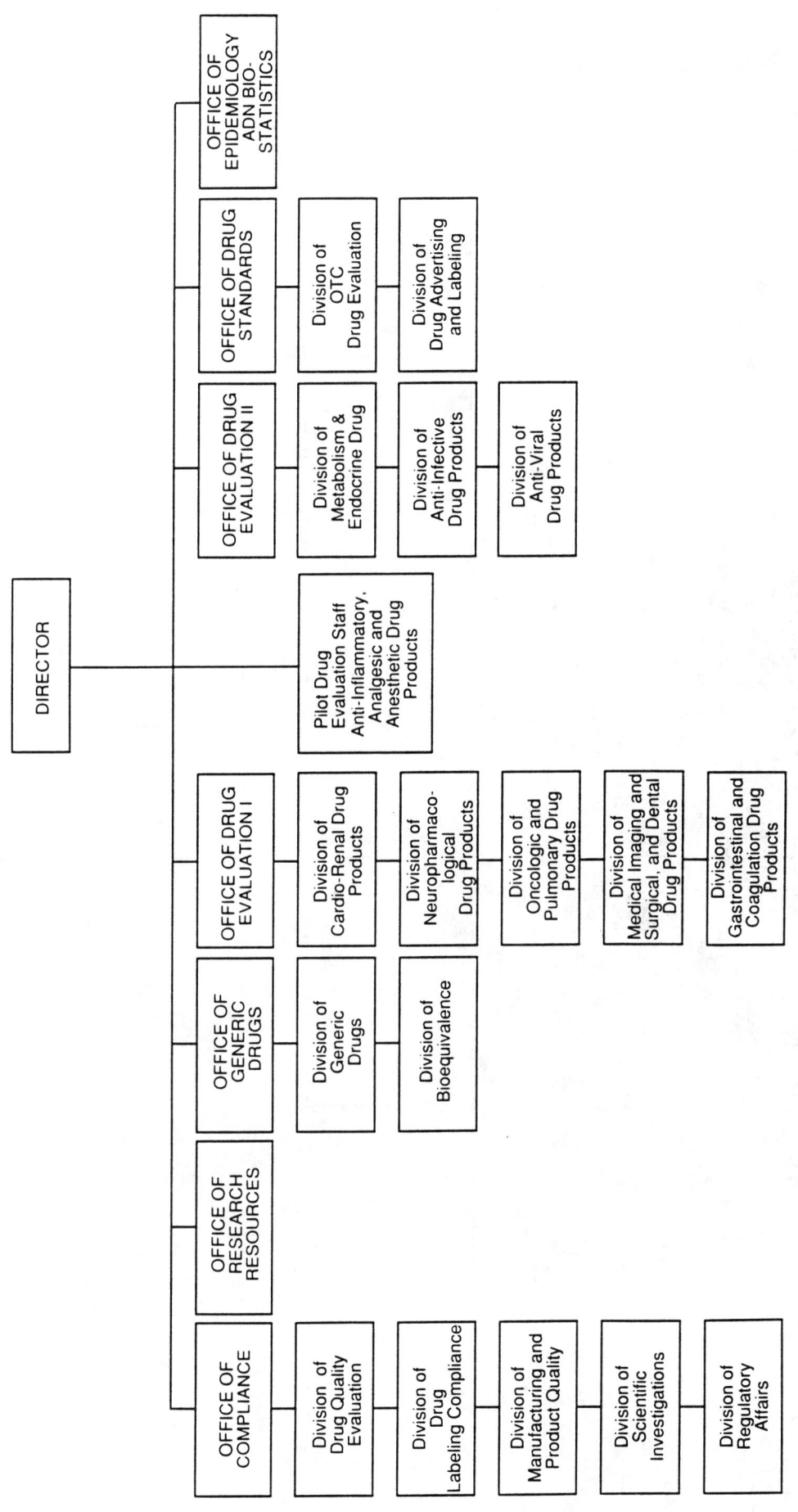

FIG. 126.2 Organization of the Center for Drug Evaluation and Research within the FDA. IND, Investigational New Drug Application.

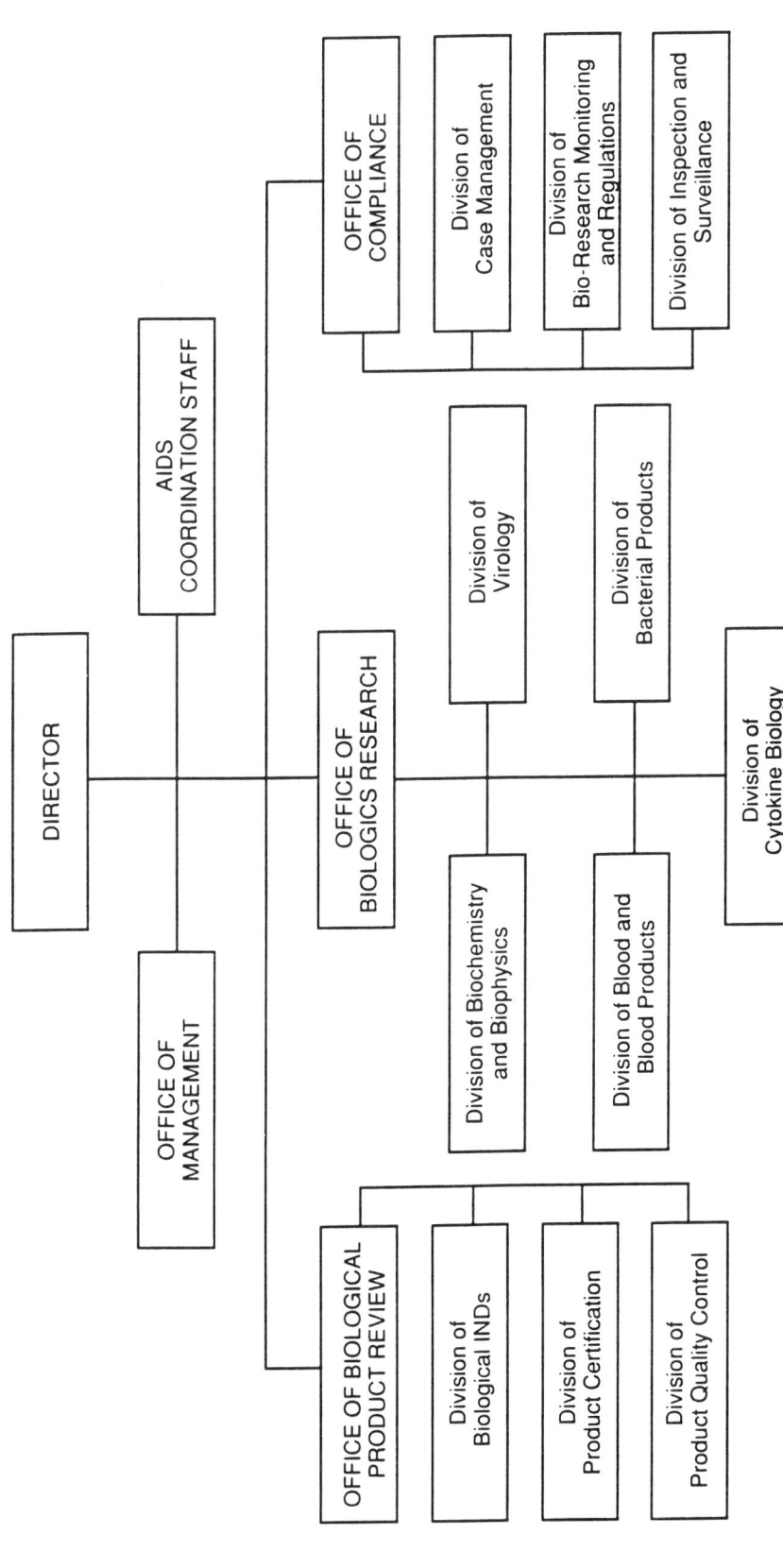

FIG. 126.3 Organization of the Center for Biologics Evaluation and Research within the FDA. OTC, over the counter.

1009

MAJOR TYPES OF REGULATORY SUBMISSIONS

There are many different types of regulatory submissions made by multinational companies to regulatory authorities throughout the world. A few of the most important submissions in the United States and the United Kingdom are indicated.

United States

IND. An Investigational New Drug Application (form FDA 1571) is the documentation that allows initial clinical testing of a new medicine or a new dosage form of an already marketed or investigational medicine. INDs are not approved, but may be disapproved for good cause. Clinical testing may begin 30 days after filing the IND, unless the FDA places the IND on hold or raises questions that must be answered prior to initiation of trials. The 30-day delay requirement may be waived by the FDA if the sponsor demonstrates a good reason for a waiver. Preclinical testing of the investigational compound usually takes from 2 to 4 years prior to submission of the IND. The contents of an IND are outlined in the form required, as shown later in this chapter in Table 126.15 and in Figs. A1 to A3 in the appendix to *Guide to Planning and Managing Multiple Clinical Studies* (Spilker, 1987). The section in the Code of Federal Regulations (CFR) that provides regulatory guidance is 21 CFR 312.

IND Amendment. This is filed for any change in protocol, medicine strength, investigator, or other aspects of a trial or medicine development program.

NDA. New Drug Application (form FDA 356h) requests approval by the FDA to market a medicine for the indications specified in the application. It is usually submitted to the FDA at the end of Phase III trials after most major investigational trials have been completed and the sponsor is satisfied that all requirements for safety and efficacy have been met. In some circumstances, such as when a medicine will be used to treat a rare disease, or a serious disease for which no satisfactory treatment is available, the NDA may be submitted at the end of Phase II clinical trials. The contents of the NDA summary according to the 1985 "NDA rewrite" are shown in Table 126.1, and the general contents are shown at the end of this chapter in Table 126.13. Form FDA-356h is shown in Fig. A4 of Spilker (1987). The section in the CFR that provides regulatory guidance is 21 CFR 314.

The FDA rates New Chemical Entities (NCEs) as A, B, or C. Type A represents important therapeutic gains, Type B represents modest therapeutic gains, and Type C represents those with little or no therapeutic gain. These categories are described in more detail later in this chapter.

TABLE 126.1 *Contents of the overall summary of a New Drug Application (NDA)[a]*

1. Proposed text of product labeling, with annotations to the information in the summary and technical sections
2. The medicine's pharmacologic class, scientific rationale, intended use, and potential clinical benefits
3. The medicine's marketing history, if any, outside the United States
4. A summary of the chemistry, manufacturing, and controls section
5. A summary of the nonclinical pharmacology and toxicology section
6. A summary of the human pharmacokinetics and bioavailability section
7. A summary of the microbiology section (required only for antiinfective medicines)
8. A summary of the clinical data section including statistical analyses
9. A concluding discussion of benefit-to-risk considerations, proposed additional studies, and postmarketing surveillance plans

[a] Based on the 1985 "NDA rewrite."

NDA Amendment. An applicant may submit an amendment to an application that has been filed but not yet approved. An amendment may contain either significant new data from a previously unreported clinical trial or detailed new analysis of previously submitted data. A major amendment may extend the review period of the NDA (see 21 CFR 314.60 for more details).

NDA Supplement. A supplement to an approved application is required for any significant changes in the conditions described in the NDA. It is usually required for substantive modifications. (e.g., in labeling, packaging, manufacturing methods, chemical synthesis). Certain minor changes are permitted without submitting a Supplement to an NDA (SNDA) (see 21 CFR 314.70 for more details). Supplements may only be filed by the holder(s) of the original NDA.

Abbreviated NDA. Approval of this application is required prior to the sale of medicine products that already meet the statutory standards for safety and effectiveness. It is usually reserved for duplicates and medicine products previously approved under a full NDA and has become the standard for requesting approval of generic medicine products (see 21 CFR 314.55 for more details).

Annual Report. Pharmaceutical companies must submit an annual report on every investigational and marketed medicine to the FDA. The contents of the annual report for marketed products are listed in Table 126.2 (see 21 CFR 314.81 for more information). Other records and reports to be submitted to the FDA are detailed in 21 CFR 310.300, 310.302, and 310.303.

Premarket Notification (510k). This is a notice to the FDA, Center for Devices and Radiological Health, of the intent to market a medical device of Classes I [those subject to only the general controls of the Food,

TABLE 126.2 *Contents of annual reports of marketed products submitted to the Food and Drug Administration*[a]

1. Summary of data affecting safety, effectiveness, or labeling
2. Amount of medicine distributed during the preceding year
3. Samples of labeling
4. Changes in chemistry, manufacturing, and controls, including reports of experiences, investigations, clinical trials, or tests involving chemical, physical, or other properties of the medicine. Changes made during the year that did not require prior FDA approval
5. Nonclinical study reports of unpublished data and summaries of published reports of toxicological and in vitro studies
6. Current status of postmarketing studies conducted by the sponsor or on their behalf
7. Published clinical trials of the medicine[b]
8. Summaries of unpublished clinical trials that have been completed

---

[a] Annual reports are submitted within 60 days of the anniversary date of approval of the application using form FDA 2252.
[b] See Trombitas and Simpson (1986).

Drug, and Cosmetic (FD&C) Act] or II (those that are or will be subject to a performance standard in accordance with the FD&C Act).

Investigational Device Exemption (IDE). An IDE is a research permit to allow an unapproved medical device to be tested on humans to evaluate safety and efficacy.

Premarket Approval Application (PMA). A PMA is a permit to allow the sale of a Class III medical device. This application is usually filed after completion of clinical trials that assure safety and effectiveness of the device or that establish an acceptable performance standard.

United Kingdom

There are several major differences between medicine regulations and regulatory agencies in the United States and the United Kingdom. One important difference is that clinical trials conducted in normal volunteers do not require government approval in the United Kingdom, whereas the FDA requires submissions of a full IND. Some other differences in the medicine review process for the FDA and the Department of Health (DoH) in the United Kingdom are listed in Table 126.3.

CTX (Clinical Trial Exemption) Certificate. This application is usually submitted to the regulatory authorities after initial clinical trials have been performed in normal volunteers. (There is no official requirement for volunteer trials to have been carried out beforehand, and indeed it would not always be ethical to conduct volunteer trials with a new medicine.) The Secretariat of the Medicines Division (within the DoH) evaluates the CTX, but does not actively approve it.

TABLE 126.3 *Selected differences between regulatory agencies for medicines in the United States and United Kingdom*

United States	United Kingdom
1. Companies have some access to decision makers during the review period	1. Companies have less access to decision makers during the review period
2. The same reviewer(s) will review all or most applications on one type of medicine	2. Reviewers are assigned applications to review in sequence. It is uncertain who will be the reviewer of a specific application
3. A public advisory committee usually meets to provide a recommendation to the FDA for Class A or B medicine[a]	3. Nothing comparable
4. Appeal process is possible by a sponsor for a rejected application	4. Either a written or oral appeal is possible by a sponsor
5. A fishbowl atmosphere is sometimes present with many observers, which slows speed of approval	5. A more closed environment is present

---

[a] See text for definitions.

After a specified period of approximately 1 month clinical trials may be conducted in patients with the disease or problem for which the medicine is intended. This application is approximately equivalent to pilot Phase II trials in the United States, but could be extended to cover Phase III trials. A summary of the regulatory dossier currently submitted to the European Economic Community countries is shown below in Table 126.14. If initial clinical trials are to be performed in patients with the disease or condition for which the product is to be indicated, the DoH requires a Clinical Trial Certificate (CTC), unless a CTX is obtained.

CTC (Clinical Trial Certificate). This application to conduct clinical trials (in patients) that are usually more extensive than those conducted under a CTX is approximately equivalent to regulatory approval to conduct late Phase II and all of Phase III trials in the United States. The CTC contains more data than a CTX. The licensing authority might request a CTC for a new medicine if they had initially considered a CTX and did not wish to approve it without more complete data and without a second opinion from the Committee on Safety of Medicines (CSM). CTX applications are not reviewed by the CSM but are judged solely by the full-time professional Secretariat of the Medicines Division. The Secretariat can only get the opinion of the CSM by asking a sponsor for a full CTC application.

PLA (Product License Application). A PLA is an application to obtain approval to market a new medicine. There are three major sections: clinical, preclinical, and pharmaceutical. A CTC is not required prior to a PLA.

Comparing Medicines and Biologicals

Medicine approvals are governed by the FD&C Act of 1938 plus amendments passed since that time. Biological products are governed by a different law, the Public Health Service Act of 1944 (58 Stat 682).

Separate registration documents are submitted to the FDA for each of these two types of product. NDAs are submitted for medicines to the CDER, and PLAs are submitted for biological products to the CBER. Anyone, whether sponsor, distributor, or manufacturer of a medicine, may submit an NDA, but only a manufacturer of a biological product may submit the PLA. A PLA in the United States thus differs from a PLA in most other countries, because in other countries a PLA is submitted for either a medicine or biological product.

Estimating the Date When a Regulatory Application Will Be Submitted

Stage One: Guessing Dates

There are various ways that a sponsor may estimate the date of Phase III completion (and consequent submission of an NDA or other dossier). In the early life of a project, before the compound has been tested in humans and also during Phase I clinical trials, most medicines are in a "guess stage." At this time, approximate estimates are made based on past events (approval of medicines in the same therapeutic class), resources devoted to study the medicine, and future expectations of a project's progress.

Stage Two: The Forward Model for Predicting Dates

In late Phase II and early Phase III a medicine enters a period that may be labeled as the "forward stage" for estimating dates. During this period the remaining clinical and development program is planned and dates are estimated at which each step will be completed. Based on an optimistic, but realistic, plan of which clinical trials may be conducted simultaneously and which must be conducted sequentially, plus estimating resources available and potential conflicts with other projects, an estimated date for submission of the regulatory application is determined. This means that all steps are identified, their time requirements are estimated, and a total time is derived from adding up the critical paths or control points.

Stage Three: The Backward Model for Predicting Dates

During Phase III a medicine enters a different period of study, which may be labeled as the "backward stage" for estimating dates. This means that a realistic target date is established for regulatory submission based on many factors, including those listed above. This date is used as a starting point, and plans are established by working backwards from that date to set all of the other dates for required activities to be completed. This process is meant to apply more pressure to complete activities than usually exists in the forward stage. A reasonable time to set a backward-oriented date is when the regulatory submission is expected to occur about 1½ to 2 years in the future.

Overly Ambitious Predictions of Dates

Personnel participating in a project generally realize if a date given for completion of a regulatory submission is too ambitious. Instead of serving to spur activities and enthusiasm of the staff with a large amount of resources moving in a common direction, it will generally lead to (1) sloppy and incomplete work that was rushed to meet the deadline or (2) setting an unrealistic target date that will backfire and cause people to build resentment or ignore the dates completely. In the first case, the submission's flaws will eventually be uncovered and will probably require more time and effort to undo, whereas in the second case, people may lose faith in the plan and any value it has for the project.

The above techniques for estimating dates are not used by all sponsors and probably are not useful for all projects.

STRATEGIES AND PLANS OF REGULATORY SUBMISSIONS

Developing Activities and Plans for Regulatory Submissions

IND Plans

Once a decision has been reached to advance the compound toward an IND, a plan should be developed listing all of the activities needed to meet the requirements of the IND. A generic model of the identity and flow of activities required for an IND is shown in Fig. 124.1. This model or chart must be modified for each specific medicine since the characteristics of each product differ and special requirements may be necessary for inclusion. Modifications of the original plan must be made periodically to allow for time delays, new routes that must be followed to prepare the IND, or additional steps that must be added.

NDA Plans

The NDA model plan (Fig. 124.2) is much more complex than the IND model plan. This plan may be established at any point after the IND is filed (or even before), but many of the necessary steps will not be identified until sometime during Phase II. At that point a fairly accurate understanding of the medicine's clinical activity is usually achieved and the clinical program required for the NDA may be assembled with a reasonable chance of knowing which clinical trials must be conducted prior to submitting the NDA. Phase II determines which indication(s) may be included in the NDA. The technical development of most medicines also cannot be planned with great certainty prior to Phase II. Technical development issues include identifying items such as route of synthesis and manufacturing, final formulation, dosage strength(s), packaging, and so forth.

Quality of Regulatory Submissions

There are a number of general strategies that most pharmaceutical companies follow in attempting to improve the rate at which their submissions are processed by regulatory agencies. Probably the single most important factor relates to the overall quality of the submission. Documents that are well organized, well written, read easily, and internally consistent, and that do not contain major omissions tend to be processed more rapidly than carelessly assembled submissions. Reviewers are understandably exasperated when pages are missing or misnumbered, the text or tables are illegible or difficult to understand, or important descriptions are incomplete. The overall quality of a submission also refers to the standards with which clinical trials are conducted. This is evidenced by the trial design, completeness of data, and other characteristics. Poorly conducted trials will probably initiate a more thorough review of all data, more inspections of participating investigators, and thus, greater delays in processing a submission.

Regulatory Strategies

Some sponsors routinely attempt to obtain regulatory approval through submission of what they believe to be the minimal amount of data necessary to demonstrate safety and efficacy of a new medicine. Other sponsors utilize as much data as they can muster to support their application. One major difference between these two approaches lies in the amount of foreign data submitted. If a medicine is marketed in at least one foreign country, then data should be available to support its use in the United States. Even if pivotal well-controlled data are not obtained outside the United States (generally a positive point in an American application), data from clinical trials or postmarketing surveillance efforts in foreign countries provide additional information, which may influence the reg-

ulatory review, especially if the foreign data are of a high quality.

If multiple submissions are anticipated on a single medicine for different dosage forms and indications, then a strategy is needed to obtain approval on the most important applications in the most timely matter. This may entail temporarily delaying submission of an application for a relatively minor dosage form until favorable regulatory action has occurred on a more medically and commercially important submission, even if the former application was prepared first. If both applications are submitted simultaneously there is a possibility that regulatory reviewers will process the less important one first, or that they will process both together and not issue a regulatory decision until both can be approved or rejected. Also, if the medicine represents a major therapeutic breakthrough and a minor dosage form is approved, it will probably decrease pressure to approve the medicine that might be exerted on the regulatory agency from sources outside the sponsor (e.g., investigators, medical community, patients, Congress). It is important to hold a pre-NDA meeting(s) with the FDA reviewer(s) and to learn (insofar as possible) whether a simultaneous or sequential review of the applications will occur.

TYPES OF INTERACTIONS BETWEEN CLINICAL DEPARTMENTS, REGULATORY DEPARTMENTS, AND REGULATORY AGENCIES

Contact With a Regulatory Agency

Some sponsors believe that maintaining close contact with regulatory agencies (whenever possible) assists in a rapid and efficient review, whereas other companies follow the opposite approach. The author has not noticed evidence where one general approach yields uniformly better results for a sponsor. It is probably preferable to use both approaches. The choice of the appropriate response should depend on the particular individuals the sponsor is dealing with at the regulatory agency and on the nature and importance of the regulatory submissions involved. Contact with many national regulatory authorities is not permitted.

It is uncommon for most clinical departments and regulatory agencies to interact without representatives of a regulatory department present, or without their initial input. Individuals in most regulatory agencies prefer to deal with each major submission through a single company representative for more formal actions. Regulatory reviewers will occasionally contact their counterparts in industry to discuss various issues or questions that may be easily resolved.

A number of common types of interactions that occur between clinical and regulatory departments within a pharmaceutical company are listed in Table 126.4. This table is organized to illustrate those inter-

TABLE 126.4 *Types of interactions between clinical and regulatory departments in the pharmaceutical industry*

A. Interactions initiated by the clinical department
 1. Request for information or clarification about regulatory requirements, laws, practices, or company procedures
 2. Submission of data and reports as part of a regulatory application
 3. Request to schedule a meeting with a regulatory agency
 4. Submission of data and reports as part of a request for a meeting with a regulatory agency
 5. Request to obtain information, guidance, or an advisory opinion from a regulatory agency
 6. Request for an interpretation of a regulation, guideline, or legal action
B. Interactions initiated by the regulatory department
 1. Request for information solicited by the regulatory department or government regulatory agency
 2. Provide information obtained from a regulatory agency
 3. Provide information or advice about regulatory issues, opinions, problems, or commentary
C. Interactions initiated by either department
 1. Discussions of regulatory strategies and procedures to be followed either in response to a regulatory agency request or independent of a regulatory agency
 2. Regulatory assistance in planning or compiling a regulatory submission

TABLE 126.5 *Types of interactions between regulatory departments in the pharmaceutical industry and government regulatory agencies*[a]

A. Formal meetings[b]
B. Informal meetings may be held on occasion, to discuss problems or issues
C. Information transmittal from a pharmaceutical company to a regulatory agency
 1. Company submits and requests approval of regulatory submissions of various types (e.g., NDA)
 2. Company submits regulatory documents (e.g., IND)
 3. Company informs a regulatory agency about modifications covered by an existing regulatory submission (e.g., additional protocols to be conducted under an IND)
 4. Company provides data on adverse reactions according to statute, provides annual reports on open INDs, and provides other required documentation
 5. Company provides data and other information in response to regulatory requests
 6. Company requests clarifications and responses to specific questions
 7. Company provides responses pertaining to proposed new regulations or changes in existing regulations
D. Information transmittal from a regulatory agency to a pharmaceutical company
 1. Responses are provided to company requests for (1) approval of various submissions, (2) formal meetings, (3) information on specific questions
 2. Statements are made to companies about (1) violations of the FD&C Act,[c] (2) minor problems, or (3) potential problems
 3. Responses are made about actual or potential issues or problems relating to one of the company's medicines
 4. Questions are posed about one of the company's medicines

[a] These interactions are primarily those concerned with new medicine development.
[b] See examples listed in Table 126.6.
[c] FD&C Act, Food, Drug, and Cosmetic Act.

actions that are usually initiated by the clinical department, by the regulatory department, or by either department.

Table 126.5 illustrates various types of interactions that occur between regulatory departments in a pharmaceutical corporation and a government regulatory agency. Many other types of interactions are not described, because they have less relevance for investigational medicines.

Meetings: General Considerations

Meetings with regulatory authorities to discuss clinical plans, problems, contents of submissions, and other issues provide a valuable basis for developing a submission of the quality and format that will be most acceptable to the individuals who will have to review and approve the application. It is important for both the sponsor and regulatory agency to strive for agreement in the approach to be used for regulatory submissions. Effective use of these meetings to define an appropriate development path is an important strategy for many sponsors. Unfortunately, there is a relatively high turnover of staff at the FDA and new reviewers are not bound by any agreements reached by their predecessors about a particular medicine. Moreover, reviewers may change their own minds.

Some sponsors prefer informal meetings at the FDA to identify preferable approaches to follow in medicine development. At meetings with the FDA, company representatives usually make proposals or ask for FDA responses to specific questions. Open-ended questions

(e.g., What do you suggest we should do?) should almost never be posed, because answers given may place a company in an extremely difficult position.

Meetings: Specific Considerations

There are many reasons why requesting meetings with the FDA to discuss development plans and issues is beneficial to a medicine's sponsor. Various types of meetings are listed in Table 126.6. A few circumstances in which it is desirable to have a pre-IND meeting with the FDA are listed in Table 126.7. In setting up meetings between the FDA and a sponsor it is important to agree on which individuals should be present and the major points on the agenda, which improves the possibility of agreement. Table 126.8 lists additional considerations for initiating and preparing for a formal meeting with FDA personnel. Some of the points that may be discussed at an end-of-Phase II conference are in Table 126.9. Following meetings of company representatives with the FDA (Table 126.5) a summary of the meeting may be sent to the FDA by the company. A reply is requested if their understand-

TABLE 126.6 *Types of meetings held with regulatory authorities*

1. Prior to submittal of application to evaluate an investigational medicine in humans. The purpose of this meeting is to discuss the nature of the application and possibly the clinical approach and plan to be followed ("pre-IND[a] meeting")
2. Any time that a problem or situation arises when regulatory input would be useful
3. At the conclusion of Phase II clinical trials ("end-of-Phase II meeting")[b]
4. To discuss overall or specific aspects of the medicine development strategy, plans, or protocols at any time during the medicine's investigation
5. To discuss contents to be included in the NDA and the format for its organization, prior to submittal of the application for medicine approval ("pre-NDA[a] meeting")[b]
6. At the time of NDA submittal to review its contents and organization
7. Between the time of NDA submittal and NDA approval, to address issues that arise[c]
8. To discuss final labeling after an "approvable letter" has been received ("labeling conference")[b]

[a] IND, Investigational New Drug Application; NDA, New Drug Application.
[b] These are the types of meetings that are most frequently held.
[c] Meetings, conference calls, and correspondence between the FDA and the sponsor usually occurs with greatest frequency during this period.

ing of the discussion differed from that presented in the letter, or to confirm that the FDA's minutes of the meeting are in agreement with the company's minutes.

Adverse Reactions

Information on serious adverse reactions reach a sponsor from many sources and trigger responses that often include interactions between various departments of the sponsor and regulatory agencies. Figure 126.4 illustrates some of the activities and interactions that often occur as various groups become involved in the implications and flow of information about serious adverse reactions. This chart does not consider the various processes involved in diagnosing and treating the

TABLE 126.7 *Selected circumstances in which it is desirable to have a pre-IND meeting with the FDA[a]*

1. When the IND will consist mainly of foreign data
2. When an unorthodox approach will be followed in the initial clinical trial (or trials)
3. When there is an unusual aspect of the IND application which should be discussed or explained (e.g., amount of data of a certain type, unusual metabolism, toxicology profile, mechanism of action)
4. When apparently conflicting data are presented on an important issue
5. When data are included which are expected to raise serious questions
6. When input from the FDA is desired relative to proposed clinical trials
7. To discuss a waiver of the 30-day review period

[a] FDA, Food and Drug Administration; IND, Investigational New Drug Application.

TABLE 126.8 *Considerations for initiating and preparing for a formal meeting with Food and Drug Administration (FDA) personnel*

1. Contact the FDA's Consumer Safety Officer (CSO) by letter or telephone to propose a meeting and outline the purpose as clearly as possible
2. Discuss the attendees but do not attempt to determine who the government should have at the meeting
3. Submit a proposed agenda and any other information requested by the CSO
4. Provide sufficient background material to the FDA prior to the meeting
5. Bring only those individuals who will contribute to the meeting
6. Rehearse relevant portions of the company's presentation
7. Consider questions that the FDA or others at the meeting might pose
8. Be totally clear about relevant FDA procedures and regulations
9. Remain courteous at all times, even if provoked. Do not embarrass FDA staff
10. Refer to FDA Bureau of Drug's Guide BD 4800.3-81-11, issued May 29, 1981, for additional information on meetings with the FDA

adverse reaction, evaluating its severity, or assessing its relation to medicine intake. This chart includes consideration of adverse reactions that reach the pharmaceutical company via clinical trials, postmarketing surveillance, or voluntary reporting systems. Numerous variations of this scheme are possible and depend on the particular circumstances of the adverse reaction, company, and country (or countries) involved. Some of the major categories of adverse reactions and reporting requirements are shown in Table 126.10. The FDA's interpretation of postmarketing adverse reaction requirements is presented by Sills et al. (1986).

The form used to report an adverse medicine or biologic reaction to the FDA is the 1639 form (Fig. 126.5). The "yellow card" form (Fig. 126.6) is used

TABLE 126.9 *Points that may be discussed at an end-of-Phase II conference with the Food and Drug Administration (FDA)*

1. Adequacy of safety and efficacy data from Phases I and II clinical trials for the desired indications
2. Reasonableness of proceeding with Phase III trials from a safety perspective. This includes consideration of animal toxicology data
3. Adequacy of Phase III trial designs and possible specific protocols
4. Completeness of preclinical studies
5. Relative completeness of the manufacturing and controls data for the current stage of the medicines
6. Discussion about the adequacy of current data and proposed trials for the NDA
7. Discussion about Phase III plans
8. Discussion on specific topics of interest or particular problems
9. Discussion on the medicine's pharmacokinetic profile
10. Discussion about the intended dosage of the new medicine
11. Discussion of the proposed format and organization for the NDA

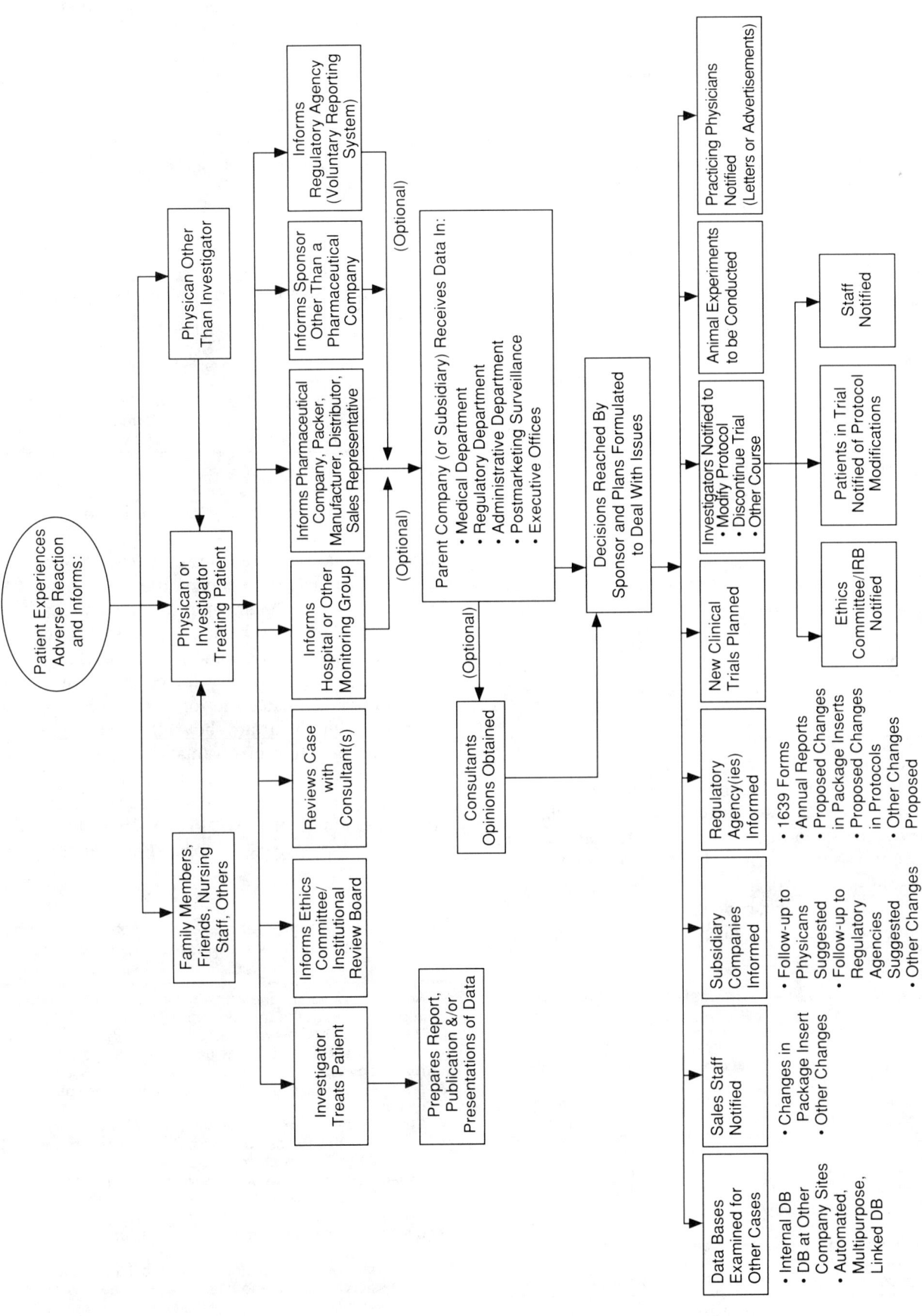

FIG. 126.4 Flow of information resulting from serious adverse reactions. DB, data base. IRB, Institutional Review Board.

TABLE 126.10 *Reporting of spontaneous adverse reactions by sponsors to the Food and Drug Administration (FDA)*

Nature of adverse reaction	Action to be taken	Mechanism to use	Time frame
Serious and unlabeled[b]	Submit 15-day report and follow-up	FDA 1639 form	15 days
Serious and labeled	Submit data periodically	FDA 1639 form and tabulation	Periodically
Serious and labeled	Detect if there is an increased frequency	Narrative	15 days
Nonserious	Submit data periodically	FDA 1639 form and tabulation	Periodically

[a] This table relates to those adverse reactions that occur in the United States and come to the attention of sponsors. Spontaneous adverse reactions reported by physicians to the FDA are often considered as a measure of concern by the physician about the medicine or adverse reaction observed.

[b] The terms "labeled" and "unlabeled" refer to whether the specific adverse reaction has been identified in the package insert.

for this purpose in the United Kingdom. The speed with which serious adverse reactions must be reported to a regulatory agency varies, depending on the particular situation, but is generally clearly described in the regulations. See 21 CFR 314.80 for details pertaining to FDA requirements.

REGULATORY ISSUES AND PROBLEMS

Different types of deep-seated issues and problems permeate the current regulatory environment. There are usually limited methods available to sponsors for dealing with these issues in a satisfactory way. Such issues are described from a pharmaceutical company perspective, and admittedly do not fully present the viewpoint of the regulatory agency. Most of these issues particularly involve the FDA. Issues involving other agencies are not elaborated, because there are many factors that differ between national agencies (see Table 126.11 for some examples).

Several of these situations arise because of congressional pressures on the FDA and the attitude that has risen at the agency that it is "better to be safe than sorry." For the most part these issues cannot be satisfactorily influenced by the pharmaceutical industry. Nonetheless, dialogue is an important step toward making progress on these issues and improving the relationship between the FDA and the pharmaceutical industry.

Escalation of Regulatory Requirements

There is in general a continued escalation of regulatory demands over the years for increased quality and

amount of data (e.g., number of patients, data tabulations) to be generated by the sponsor for INDs as well as NDAs. One aspect of this issue relates to the tendency by the FDA to require more data at an earlier stage of medicine development. Occasionally, manufacturing or control information is requested prior to the NDA to allow ample time for review of those items that have been troublesome for regulators to review in the past. In some instances these data are now being required with the IND. Also, there has been a tendency over the last several years to require steadily more definitive safety and efficacy data on a medicine, particularly before women of childbearing potential may be entered in clinical trials. This often creates a "Catch-22" situation when NDAs are criticized by regulatory personnel for including too large a proportion of male patients.

The FDA has made an effort to decrease the amount of paperwork necessary to be submitted in an NDA by no longer mandating that all data collection forms (case report forms) be sent with the initial application, except for patients who died during a clinical trial or who did not complete the trial because of an adverse event. This is often a relatively minor point for the sponsor, however, since all of the data have been generated and may be requested at any time by the FDA. In addition, it often requires more time and effort to generate the data tabulations required than it does to supply all data collection forms with the submission.

Hitting a Moving Target

One of the most frustrating of all issues between sponsors and FDA involves the changing criteria by which regulatory submissions are judged. This is often referred to as the sponsor's trying to hit a moving target. Some of the changes may be justified if they relate to major changes in the state of the art within a therapeutic area. Other changes are not justified, especially when they relate to the personal philosophy or views of FDA reviewers and are not a reflection of science, medicine, or regulations. When changes occur as a result of new personnel at the FDA desiring to review an NDA differently than their predecessors, it is difficult to know how to resolve this question best. Most companies merely go along with regulatory requests.

The "moving target" issue concerns virtually all areas of medicine testing, manufacture, technical development, and toxicology. Guidelines are often established, such as for toxicology (see Table 126.12), but their implementation and interpretation often depend on the personal views of individuals within regulatory agencies, and it is generally believed that appeals made by sponsors with a strong scientific basis are often not accepted.

DEPARTMENT OF HEALTH AND HUMAN SERVICES
PUBLIC HEALTH SERVICE
FOOD AND DRUG ADMINISTRATION (HFN-730) — ROCKVILLE, MD 20857

ADVERSE REACTION REPORT
(Drugs and Biologics)

Form Approved: OMB No. 0910–0230.

FDA CONTROL NO.

ACCESSION NO.

I. REACTION INFORMATION

1. PATIENT ID/INITIALS (In Confidence)	2. AGE YRS.	3. SEX	4.-6. REACTION ONSET			8.—12. CHECK ALL APPROPRIATE:
			MO.	DA.	YR.	

7. DESCRIBE REACTION(S)

☐ PATIENT DIED

☐ REACTION TREATED WITH Rx DRUG

☐ RESULTED IN, OR PROLONGED, INPATIENT HOSPITALIZATION

☐ RESULTED IN PERMANENT DISABILITY

☐ NONE OF THE ABOVE

13. RELEVANT TESTS/LABORATORY DATA

II. SUSPECT DRUG(S) INFORMATION

14. SUSPECT DRUG(S) (Give manufacturer and lot no. for vaccines/biologics)

20. DID REACTION ABATE AFTER STOPPING DRUG?

☐ YES ☐ NO ☐ NA

15. DAILY DOSE	16. ROUTE OF ADMINISTRATION

17. INDICATION(S) FOR USE

21. DID REACTION REAPPEAR AFTER REINTRODUCTION?

☐ YES ☐ NO ☐ NA

18. DATES OF ADMINISTRATION (From/To)	19. DURATION OF ADMINISTRATION

III. CONCOMITANT DRUGS AND HISTORY

22. CONCOMITANT DRUGS AND DATES OF ADMINISTRATION (Exclude those used to treat reaction)

23. OTHER RELEVANT HISTORY (e.g. diagnoses, allergies, pregnancy with LMP, etc.)

IV. ONLY FOR REPORTS SUBMITTED BY MANUFACTURER

V. INITIAL REPORTER (In confidence)

24. NAME AND ADDRESS OF MANUFACTURER (Include Zip Code)

26.—26a. NAME AND ADDRESS OF REPORTER (Include Zip Code)

24a. IND/NDA. NO. FOR SUSPECT DRUG	24b. MFR. CONTROL NO.

26b. TELEPHONE NO. (Include area code)

24c. DATE RECEIVED BY MANUFACTURER	24d. REPORT SOURCE (Check all that apply) ☐ FOREIGN ☐ STUDY ☐ LITERATURE ☐ HEALTH PROFESSIONAL ☐ CONSUMER

26c. HAVE YOU ALSO REPORTED THIS REACTION TO THE MANUFACTURER?

☐ YES ☐ NO

25. 15 DAY REPORT? ☐ YES ☐ NO	25a. REPORT TYPE ☐ INITIAL ☐ FOLLOW-UP

26d. ARE YOU A HEALTH PROFESSIONAL? ☐ YES ☐ NO

Submission of a report does not necessarily constitute an admission that the drug caused the adverse reaction.

NOTE: Required of manufacturers by 21 CFR 314.80

FIG. 126.5 A: Copy of FDA 1639 form to collect data on adverse reactions.

INSTRUCTIONS FOR COMPLETING FORM FDA–1639

GENERAL

- Use a separate Form FDA-1639 for each patient.

- Additional pages may be attached if space provided on the Form FDA-1639 is inadequate.

- Non-manufacturers should send forms to the Food and Drug Administration, Division of Epidemiology and Surveillance, HFN-730, 5600 Fishers Lane, Rockville, MD 20857.

- For questions call: 301-443-4580.

- Patient and initial reporter identification is held in confidence by the FDA and is not subject to release under the Freedom of Information Act.

- Reports of serious, suspect reactions are encouraged.

SPECIFIC INSTRUCTIONS

I. Reaction Information

Item 2.
Age—For children under 5 years of age, also write date of birth (DOB) in Item 1. For congenital malformations, give the age and sex of the infant (even though the mother was exposed).

Item 7.
Describe Reaction(s)—Give signs and/or symptoms, diagnoses, course, etc. Underline the single most important descriptive phrase.

II. Suspect Drug Information

Item 14.
Suspect Drug—The trade name is preferred. If a generically produced product is involved, the manufacturer should be identified.

Item 15.
Dose—For pediatric patients, also give body weights.

Item 20 and 21.
NA—is defined as nonapplicable (e.g. when only one dose given or outcome was irreversible).

V. Initial Reporter

Item 26c.
Have you also reported this reaction to the manufacturer? Your answer facilitates identification of duplicates in the central adverse reaction file. FDA encourages direct reporting even if a report has been submitted to the manufacturer.

NOTE TO MANUFACTURERS

(Refer to 21 CFR 314.80) Detailed instructions are contained in the "Guideline for Postmarketing Reporting of Adverse Drug Reactions."

*U.S. GPO: 1986-0-491-338/55173

FIG. 126.5 B: Instructions for completing FDA 1639. FDA 1639 is completed by investigators for known medicines and by sponsors for serious adverse reactions reported to them.

IN CONFIDENCE — REPORT ON SUSPECTED ADVERSE REACTIONS

1. Please report all suspected reactions to recently introduced drugs (identified by a black triangle in the British National Formulary), vaccines, dental or surgical materials, IUCD's, absorbable sutures, contact lenses and associated fluids, and serious or unusual reactions to all agents.

2. Record all other drugs etc, including self-medication, taken in the previous 3 months. With congenital abnormalities, record all drugs taken during pregnancy, and date of last menstrual period.

3. Do not be deterred from reporting because some details are not known.

4. Please report suspected drug interactions.

NAME OF PATIENT (To allow for linkage with other reports for same patient. Please give record number for hospital patients.)	Family name				SEX	AGE or DATE OF BIRTH	WEIGHT (Kg.)
	Forenames						

DRUGS, VACCINES (Inc. Batch No.), DEVICES, MATERIALS etc. (Please give Brand Name if known)	ROUTE	DAILY DOSE	DATE		INDICATION
			STARTED	ENDED	
Suspected drug, etc.					

Other drugs, etc. (Please state if no other drug given.)

SUSPECTED REACTIONS	STARTED	ENDED	OUTCOME (eg. fatal, recovered)

ADDITIONAL NOTES	REPORTING DOCTOR (Block letters please)
	Name:
	Address:
	Tel. No: Specialty:
	Signature: Date:

If you would like information about other reports associated with the suspected drug, please tick box —

AR/20   250,000 2/83 / 52/4286   C.BROS(N/C) Ltd.

FIG. 126.6 Copy of "yellow card" used in the United Kingdom to report adverse reactions.

TABLE 126.11 *Selected regulatory factors that differ between national regulatory agencies*

1. Compulsory licensing of a new medicine to nonpatent holders (e.g., Canada prior to 1987)
2. Fees to process regulatory submissions (user fees)
3. "Needs clause," which indicates the basis of why the country has a need for the medicine (e.g., Norway)
4. Prices established for new medicines are negotiated with most governments.[a] The United States is an exception
5. Limited period for marketing is implemented (e.g., Japan). At the end of the period the medicine may be relicensed and also reevaluated by the regulatory agency
6. Review of promotional material by the regulatory agency prior to complete approval (e.g., Canada)[b]
7. Some countries own manufacturing facilities (e.g., Sweden), which may make a medicine that is not being made by a sponsor
8. Specific clinical studies must be performed within the country (e.g., ADME[c] studies in Japan)
9. Specific preclinical studies must be performed within the country

[a] This may be done either before the medicine is approved (e.g., Nordic countries) or after the medicine is approved (e.g., France).
[b] The "approvable" letter in the United States suggests submission of promotional material to the FDA, but is not a requirement.
[c] ADME, absorption, distribution, metabolism, and excretion.

Sponsors would like to reach agreement with the FDA ahead of time (i.e., prior to the NDA submission), on exactly which statistical analyses and stratifications are desired. This would save time and prevent reviewers from stringing out multiple requests for reanalyses of the same data over a long period.

Adversarial Relationship

An adversarial relationship between regulatory agencies and the pharmaceutical industry has built up over the years. Each side has claimed no fault; however, the relationship between many other industries and agencies of the U.S. Government is often different. There is no *a priori* reason why the relationship cannot be more cooperative, and in some situations this has occurred with mutual benefit (e.g., with Retrovir).

Priority of NDA Reviews

A relatively low priority is usually given by FDA reviewers to evaluating NDAs, even on extremely important NCEs. Procedures require the reviewers to give a higher priority to (1) tasks for Congress, (2) tasks for other government agencies, (3) IND reviews, and (4) other tasks assigned by their supervisors.

Clinical Hold

The FDA sometimes places ongoing clinical trials on hold because of perceived problems of patient safety.

This is sometimes done before contacting the company, to determine whether the questions at the FDA may be satisfactorily answered. Occasionally this practice may be justified if the data submitted are unclear or inadequate to allow determination that continued use of the medicine is safe. This has created many unnecessary difficulties in some cases, however, because of the complex and time-consuming processes necessary to interrupt a series of clinical trials.

SELECTED REGULATIONS AND GUIDELINES

Classification of INDs and NDAs by the FDA

The FDA classifies the clinical type and therapeutic potential of commercially sponsored INDs and NDAs. This system provides a simple means of describing the IND and NDA application. The designation given a specific application may change only until the NDA is approved, at which time it becomes fixed. The classification is used as a basis for priority given to the application's review and also as a factor for determining whether an application should be submitted to an advisory committee for review and whether an end-of-Phase II conference should be held. The end-of-Phase II conference is usually restricted to new medicines that are rated by the FDA as having at least a modest therapeutic gain over current treatments. If a lower rating is given a medicine, the sponsor may request that the FDA elevate its rating.

The classification given below is taken from the FDA's Staff Manual Guide.

Chemical Types

Type 1. New molecular entity, i.e., the active moiety is not yet marketed in the United States by any pharmaceutical manufacturer either as a single entity or as part of a combination product.

Type 2. New salt, i.e., the active moiety is marketed in the United States by the same or another manufacturer, but the particular salt, ester, or derivative is not yet marketed in the United States by any pharmaceutical manufacturer either as a single entity or as part of a combination product.

Type 3. New formulation, i.e., the compound is marketed in the United States by the same or another manufacturer, but the particular dosage form or formulation is not.

Type 4. New combination, i.e., contains two or more compounds that have not previously been marketed together in a product by any manufacturer in the United States.

Type 5. Already marketed medicine product, i.e., the product duplicates a medicine product (the same

TABLE 126.12 *Suggested guidelines for required toxicology studies for various phases of medicine development*[a]

Type of medicine	Phase I		Phase II		Phase III	
	Clinical trial	Toxicology	Clinical trial	Toxicology	Clinical trial	Toxicology
Medicine for oral or parenteral use	Small single dose to few people	Acute toxicology in minimum of two species Subacute in two species, three doses, 14 days Special tests	1. Single dose 2. 1–2 weeks 3. 1–3 months 4. 6 months or more	1. As Phase I 2. Subacute in two species for 4 weeks 3. Chronic in two species for 3 months 4. Chronic in two species for 6 months to 2 years Special tests	1. Single dose 2. 1–2 weeks 3. 1–3 months 4. 6 months or more	1. As Phase I 2. Chronic two species for 1–3 months 3. Chronic two species for minimum 3 months 4. Chronic in two species for 6 months to 2 years Special tests
Inhalation anesthetics	One episode of anesthesia	Acute in four species For subacute, 3-hour exposure for 5 subsequent days	One episode of anesthesia	As Phase I Special tests	One episode of anesthesia	As Phase I Special tests
Medicines for dermal application	Single dose	Acute, oral in two species Dermal exposure for 24 hour and observation for 2 weeks	1. Single dose 2. Short-term (2 weeks)	1. As Phase I 2. Subacute dermal for 3 weeks and observation 2 weeks. Sensitivity testing in guinea pigs	1. Brief period 2. Long-term (unlimited)	1. As Phase II 2. 3–6 months, dermal Special tests
Medicines for local ophthalmic application	Single dose	Acute oral and local in two species Rabbit irritation test	Brief period	Subacute in two species for 3 weeks	1. Brief period 2. Long-term	1. As Phase II 2. Chronic for 3–6 months
Medicines for vaginal or rectal application	Single dose	Acute oral and local in one to two species	Brief period	Chronic local in two species for 3 weeks to 3 months	1. Brief period 2. Long-term	1. As Phase II 2. Chronic local for 3 months or more
Combinations, full assay for each single component	Brief period	Acute	Brief period	In rat and dog for 1–3 months	1. Brief period 2. Long-term	1. As Phase II 2. As Phase II
Hormone contraceptives, estrogens and progestagens	Brief period (1 month)	Acute and subacute in rat, dog, and primate for 90 days	3 months	Chronic in rat, dog, and primate for 1 year	3–12 months	Chronic in rat, dog, and primate for 2 years
Contact lenses and lens fluid	Brief period	Acute and subacute tests, locally Oral acute for fluids	Long-term	Chronic in rabbit for 3 weeks or more	Long-term	As Phase II

[a] From *Nordic Guidelines* (Nordic Council on Medicines, 1983).

active moiety, same salt, same formulation, or same combination) already marketed in the United States by another firm.

Type 6. Already marketed medicine product by the same firm—used primarily for new indications for marketed medicines.

These types are not mutually exclusive, since a new formulation (type 3) or a new combination (type 4) may also contain a new molecular entity (type 1) or a new salt (type 2). In such cases, both numbers should be included in the overall classification number for the medicine. For example, a new molecular entity representing an important therapeutic gain would be classified 1A; if the new entity were also in a new combination it would be classified 1,4A.

Therapeutic Potential

Type A. Important therapeutic gain, i.e., medicine may provide effective therapy or diagnosis (by virtue of greatly increased effectiveness or safety) for a disease not adequately treated or diagnosed by any marketed medicine, or provide improved treatment of a disease through improved effectiveness or safety (including decreased abuse potential).

Type B. Modest gain, i.e., medicine has a modest, but real, potential advantage over other available marketed medicines, e.g., greater patient convenience, elimination of an annoying but not dangerous adverse reaction, potential for large cost reduction, less frequent dosage schedule, useful in specific subpopulation of those with disease (e.g., those allergic to other available medicines), etc.

Type C. Little or no therapeutic gain, i.e., medicine essentially duplicates in medical importance and therapeutic usage one or more already marketed medicines.

These types are mutually exclusive. Only one of these letters may be included in the overall classification number.

Filing Times and Review Clocks

The two review clocks used by the FDA are illustrated in Fig. 126.7. The FDA has 180 days (by statute) to complete their review of an NDA and to determine whether the application is approved, approvable, or rejected. Sixty days after an NDA is received, a second clock (filing clock) is started. The filing date is established if the NDA's format, content, and administrative details are acceptable.

When a sponsor submits significant new data or information to the NDA, the FDA can restart the 180-day review clock. The FDA is not known for strictly adhering to this clock.

The filing clock (Fig. 126.7) is used when an applicant requests a hearing. This is an administrative appeal that is usually made to plead a case if an application is not approved. The FDA issues a notice of hearing advising the public of a scheduled hearing. This notice is published in the *Federal Register*. The hearing is public, except for any part in which discussions involve trade secrets. That part of the meeting may take place in private if a prior request is made by the applicant. See 21CFR.314.200 for more information on this process.

The Drug Master File

A drug master file (DMF) is a submission of information to the FDA by a person (the DMF holder) who intends it to be used for one of the following purposes:

1. To permit the DMF holder to incorporate the information by reference when the holder submits an IND, NDA, or other submission.
2. To permit the DMF holder to authorize other persons or another company to reference the information to support a submission to FDA without the holder having to disclose the specific information to the person or company. For example, a manufacturer of packaging components may submit a DMF and allow all of its customers (companies) to refer to the DMF. Each company that purchases packaging components may have numerous NDAs referring to the same DMF of the packaging company.

The FDA ordinarily neither independently reviews drug master files nor approves or disapproves submissions to a DMF. Instead, the agency customarily reviews the information only in the context of an application.

Much of the information that supports an NDA is similar or identical to that required for multiple regulatory applications. A DMF is submitted once and is then referred to in multiple applications by the sponsor to avoid having to resubmit these data with each application.

Five types of DMFs may be submitted, which relate to:

Type I. Facilities, personnel and general operating procedures

Type II. Specific medicine substances, intermediates, or dosage forms

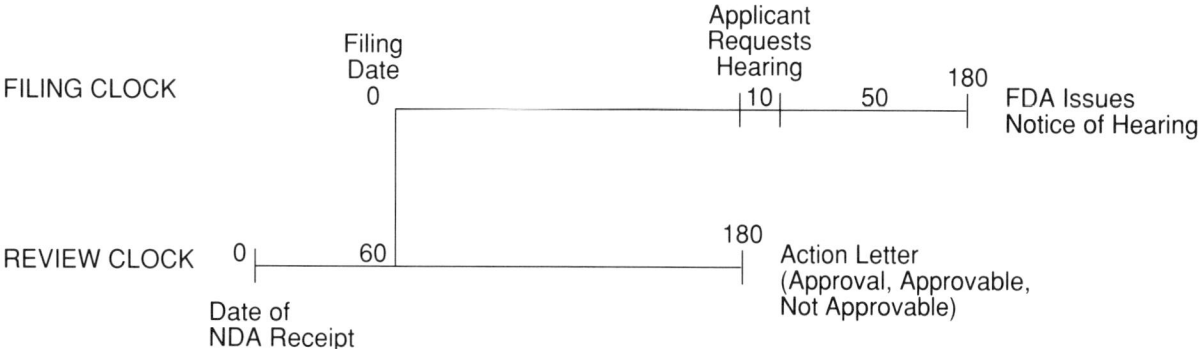

FIG. 126.7 Time frames of the FDA's review clock and filing clock. Numbers refer to days. NDA, New Drug Application.

TABLE 126.13 *Summary of contents of a New Drug Application (NDA)*

I. Overall summary (see Table 126.1 for contents)
II. Technical sections
  A. Chemistry, manufacturing, and controls
    1. Medicine substance
      a. Physical characteristics
      b. Chemical characteristics
      c. Stability
      d. Name/address of manufacturer
      e. Method of synthesis/purification
      f. Process controls in manufacturing and packaging
      g. Specifications and analytical methods as necessary to assure identity, strength, quality, purity, and bioavailability of the medicine substance
      h. Alternate suppliers, process controls, etc.
    2. Medicine product
      a. List of all components used in manufacture
      b. Composition of medicine product
      c. Specifications/analytical methods for each component
      d. Name/address of each manufacturer
      e. Manufacturing/packaging procedure
      f. In-process controls
      g. Specifications/analytical methods
      h. Stability with expiration dating
      i. Alternative components, suppliers, methods, etc.
    3. Environmental impact analysis report
  B. Nonclinical pharmacology and toxicology
    1. Pharmacology studies in relation to
      a. Proposed therapeutic indication
      b. Studies that otherwise define the pharmacologic properties of the medicine
      c. Studies pertinent to adverse effects
    2. Toxicology studies relating to clinical use, including:
      a. Acute studies
      b. Subacute studies
      c. Chronic studies
      d. Carcinogenicity studies
      e. Special studies relating to route of administration or conditions of use
      f. Reproduction studies
      g. Studies on the developing fetus
    e. Studies of the absorption, distribution, metabolism, and excretion of the medicine in animals
    4. For each nonclinical laboratory study, a statement that it complies with Good Laboratory Practices (GLP) regulations or a brief statement of the reason for the noncompliance
  C. Human pharmacokinetics and bioavailability
    1. A description of each bioavailability and pharmacokinetic trial performed in humans, including:
      a. Analytical methods
      b. Statistical methods
      c. Statement that trial was conducted in compliance with Institutional Review Board (IRB) regulations
      d. Statement that trial was conducted in compliance with informed consent regulations
    2. A rationale for establishing a specification or analytical method necessary to assure bioavailability
    3. A summary and analysis of the pharmacokinetics and metabolism of the active ingredients and the bioavailability/bioequivalence of the medicine product
  D. Microbiology section (for antiinfective and antiviral medicines)
    1. Description of the medicine's biochemical basis of action on microbial physiology
    2. Description of the antimicrobial spectra of the medicine (include in vitro preclinical studies demonstrating concentrations of medicine required for effective use)

    3. Descriptions of any known mechanisms of resistance to the medicine
    4. Description of clinical microbiology laboratory methods needed for effective use of the medicine
  E. Clinical data
    1. Clinical pharmacology, including:
      a. Trial description
      b. Trial analysis description
      c. Comparison with animal pharmacology/toxicology
    2. Controlled clinical trials pertinent to a proposed use of the medicine, including:
      a. Protocol
      b. Description of statistical analysis
      c. Include unanalyzed, controlled studies along with a brief description of the results and status of the trial
    3. Uncontrolled clinical trials, including:
      a. Description
      b. Summary of results
      c. Statement explaining why the trial is classified as uncontrolled
    4. Additional information received by applicant from any source, including:
      a. Foreign trials
      b. Clinical trials on additional indications
      c. Commercial marketing experience
      d. Published scientific papers
      e. Unpublished scientific papers
    5. An integrated efficacy summary, including:
      a. Evidence to support dosage and administration in labeling
      b. Evidence to support dosage and dose interval recommended
      c. Evidence to support dosage modifications for specific subgroups:
        i. Pediatrics
        ii. Geriatrics
        iii. Etc.
    6. An integrated summary of all available safety information including:
      a. At initial NDA filing:
        i. Pertinent animal data
        ii. Demonstrated or potential adverse medicine reactions
        iii. Clinically significant medicine–medicine interactions
        iv. Additional information, such as from epidemiological studies
        v. Description of statistical analysis used, unless submitted in II.E.2.b (above)
      b. Periodic updates:
        i. Content and format as in II.E.6.a (above)
        ii. Case report forms for each patient who died or did not complete the trial due to an adverse medicine reaction
        iii. Timing of safety updates
          α. Four (4) months following initial submission
          β. Upon receipt of approvable letter
          γ. At other times, as requested by Food and Drug Administration (FDA)
      c. For controlled substances only: analysis of trials or information related to the abuse of the medicine, proposal for scheduling under the controlled substances act and overdosage information (dialysis, antidotes, etc.)
    7. Risk/benefits summary
      a. Discussion of why the benefits exceed the risks under the conditions stated in the labeling

TABLE 126.13 (*Continued*)

8. Statement that each human trial was conducted in compliance with Part 50 (informed consent regulations) and Part 56 (IRB regulations) of the Code of Federal Regulations (CFR).
F. Statistical section
   1. Describe the statistical evaluation of clinical data, including:
      a. Copy of information submitted in II.E.2 (above) concerning (for controlled clinical trials):
         i. Description
         ii. Analysis
   2. Additionally, for controlled clinical trials, submit:
      a. Documentation
      b. Supporting statistical analysis used in evaluation
   3. Describe statistical evaluation of safety data, including:
      a. Copy of information submitted in II.E.6.a (above)
      b. Documentation and supporting statistical analysis used in evaluating the safety information
III. Samples and labeling
   A. Samples
      1. Four samples of the following (submit upon FDA request):
         a. Medicine product
         b. Medicine substance used in manufacture of medicine product (above)
         c. Reference standards and blanks
      2. Samples of finished market package (if requested)

3. In the archival copy of the application, submit
   a. Three copies of the analytical methods and related descriptive information contained in the manufacturing/controls section (II.A.1 and 2 above)
B. Labeling (in archival copy of application)
   1. Copies of the label and all labeling, as follows:
      a. If draft, four copies
      b. If final, 12 copies
IV. Data collection forms and tabulations
   A. Data collection form tabulations (in archival copy)
      1. Tabulations of all data from:
         a. All clinical pharmacology trials (Phase I)
         b. Each adequate and well-controlled trial (Phases II and III) for indication(s) sought
      2. Tabulations of safety data from:
         a. Uncontrolled clinical trials
         b. Other clinical trials
   B. Data collection forms (in archival copy)
      1. Required for:
         a. Each patient who died during a clinical trial
         b. Each patient who did not complete a clinical trial because of an adverse reaction, whether medicine-related or not, including patients receiving reference medicines or placebo
   C. Additional data
      1. Submit additional data collection forms/tabulations as requested by FDA

TABLE 126.14 *Summary of contents of a registration dossier for the European Economic Community (EEC)*

A. Flyleaf
   1. Name or business name of applicant for marketing authorization
   2. Full address of applicant
   3. a. Name and address of manufacturer
      b. Name and address of importer
   4. Name of the proprietary medicinal product
   5. Pharmaceutical form
   6. Method and route of administration
   7. Number of annexes supplied in support of the application
B. Annex I: General information
   1. Name of the proprietary medicinal product
   2. Pharmaceutical form
   3. Qualitative and quantitative composition in terms of active principles
   4. Therapeutic indications
   5. Dosage
   6. Contraindications
   7. Warnings and precautions (including during pregnancy)
   8. Side effects
   9. Directions for use (where applicable)
   10. Shelf life and storage precautions
C. Annex II: Information and documents concerning physiochemical, biological, or microbiological tests
D. Annex II.A: Complete qualitative and quantitative composition
   1. Name of product
   2. Composition
   3. Container (brief description)
E. Annex II.B: Method of preparation
   1. Manufacturing formula

2. Manufacturing process including in-process control and the pharmaceutical assembly process
F. Annex II.C: Control of starting materials
   1. Active principles
      a. Active principles described in a pharmacopeia
      b. Active principles not described in a pharmacopeia
   2. Other constituents
      a. Constituents described in a pharmacopeia
      b. Constituents not described in a pharmacopeia
G. Annex II.D: Control tests on intermediate products (if necessary)
H. Annex II.E: Control tests on the finished product
   1. General characteristics; other quality control tests required by the nature of the products (appearance, dimension, shape, color, odor, distinguishing features, etc.)
   2. Identification and quantitative determination of the active principle or principles; other quality control tests, with a description of the methods employed [including (if necessary) and depending on the nature of the product; biological and microbiological methods]
   3. Identification and quantitative determination of the other constituents (if necessary)
I. Annex II.F: Stability tests
   1. Proposed shelf life (depending on the type of container)
   2. Information concerning stability, including physical stability:
      a. Number of batches tested
      b. Storage conditions
      c. Methods employed
      d. Description of containers
   3. Results and interpretations
J. Annex II.G: Conclusions

TABLE 126.14 (*Continued*)

Certificate by the expert analyst on the application of the methods and justification of the control methods to be used by the manufacturer

K. Annex III: Toxicological and pharmacological tests (summary of the tasks performed by the expert pharmacologist)

The following information must be provided in respect of each test:
1. Animals used (species, strain, sex, etc.)
2. Experimental conditions, including diet
3. Results

L. Annex III.A: Acute toxicity
M. Annex III.B: Toxicity with repeated administration
1. Subacute toxicity trials
2. Chronic toxicity trials
N. Annex III.C: Fetal toxicity
1. Tests for teratogenicity (dosing during period of organogenesis)
2. Pre- and postnatal dosing of the mother to demonstrate effects on late pregnancy, parturition, and lactation
O. Annex III.D: Fertility studies
P. Annex III.E: Carcinogenicity and mutagenicity
Q. Annex III.F: Pharmacodynamics
1. Actions relevant to the proposed therapeutic uses
2. Other actions investigated
3. Interactions

R. Annex III.G: Pharmacokinetics
1. Absorption (serum levels of the medicinal product)
2. Distribution of the medicinal product
3. Biotransformation
4. Excretion of the medicinal product and metabolites
S. Annex IV: Clinical trials (summary of the tasks performed by the expert clinician)
T. Annex IV.A: Human pharmacology
U. Annex IV.B: Clinical data
1. Individual data—clinical reports
2. Summary
3. Conclusions
V. Annex IV.C: Side effects and interactions

Information on side effects and interactions observed when used in other countries (the extent of usage in terms of number of prescriptions and duration of use is useful in assessing the frequency of the adverse reaction)

W. Annex V: Special particulars
X. Annex V.A: Dosage forms
1. Packaging
2. Label
3. Package insert
Y. Annex V.B.: Samples
Z. Annex V.C.: Manufacturer's authorization
AA. Annex V.D.: Marketing authorization

TABLE 126.15 *Contents of an Investigational New Drug Application (IND)[a]*

Item 1:	Name, chemical structures, dosage form, and route(s) of administration of the new medicine
Item 2:	List of all components of the medicine entity, reasonable alternates for inactive components
Item 3:	Quantitative composition of the medicine entity, including reasonable variations that may be expected during the investigational stage
Item 4:	Source and preparation of new medicine substances used as components; this includes (1) manufacturing processes for new medicine substances(s) and (2) dosage form
Item 5:	Methods, facilities, and controls used for the manufacturing, processing, and packing of the new medicine; the establishment and maintenance of appropriate standards of identity, strength, quality, and purity
Item 6:	Preclinical pharmacology, toxicology, and medicine metabolism data; available clinical data if medicine was used previously (e.g., in another country) or is a combination of previously investigated or marketed medicines
Item 7:	Informational material to be provided to investigators; this includes (1) a copy of the labels to be on the medicine containers identifying the medicines as investigational and (2) a clinical monograph describing the medicine, possible utility, prior investigations, and known hazards, contraindications, side effects, and precautions
Item 8:	A statement of the training and experience required of investigators
Item 9:	The names and credentials of the monitors and investigators. A statement that the sponsor has received from the investigator a signed form that the investigator understands and accepts his responsibilities regarding record keeping, informed consent, and supervision of subjects
Item 10:	Outline of the clinical investigation, including specification of phase involved: Phases I and II (clinical pharmacology) or Phase III (broad clinical trial)
Item 11:	Agreement to notify Food and Drug Administration (FDA) if investigation is discontinued, with explanation
Item 12:	Agreement to notify investigators if investigation is discontinued or a New Drug Application (NDA) for the investigational medicine is approved
Item 13:	Completed only if sponsor wishes to sell, rather than distribute, test medicine free to investigators; the reason for the need to sell must be explained
Item 14:	Agreement not to ship medicine or use in humans until 30 days after receipt of IND by FDA
Item 15:	An environment impact statement when requested
Item 16:	Statement that all nonclinical laboratory studies comply with Good Laboratory Practices (GLPs)

[a] The forms used to file an IND are shown in Figs. A.1–A.3 of Spilker (1987a). These items refer to a synopsis of requirements listed in form FDA 1571 (Fig. A.1).

Type III. Packaging materials

Type IV. Colorants, flavors, essences, and other additives used in medicine dosage forms

Type V. Animal and clinical studies. These are usually submitted, however, in a regulatory application and not in a DMF.

Toxicological Guidelines

Overall Guidelines

The FDA does not have strict requirements and standards for number and identity of species and duration of studies for all categories of medicines. There are, however, approximate guidelines that are similar to those of the Nordic countries (Table 126.12). Specific requirements are often discussed with the FDA during meetings or on other occasions. Regulatory requirements in a number of countries are summarized by Walker and Lumley (1986).

Reproduction

An important part of the toxicology studies are those involving reproduction. These have become the focus of more attention since the thalidomide disaster and are divided into three segments.

Segment I. Study of fertility and general reproductive performance. The studies provide general data for the effect of the medicine on the entire reproductive process (e.g., teratogenesis, late stages of gestation, parturition, lactation) and evaluate the effects on gonadal function, estrous cycles, mating behavior, and conception rates.

Segment II. Study of teratogenesis. Medicines are administered organogenesis to evaluate whether a medicine has a potential for causing toxicity to the embryo or of causing teratogenic effects.

Segment III. Perinatal and postnatal study. The medicine is given during the last trimester of pregnancy and during lactation to evaluate the effects of the medicine on late fetal development, labor and delivery, lactation, neonatal viability, and growth of the newborn.

Acute Studies

There has been a worldwide movement away from conducting acute toxicological studies. In the past, acute studies have been characterized primarily by formal LD_{50} studies that require large numbers of animals and usually provide little information. One reason that the LD_{50} fell into disrepute is that different strains of the same species often yielded greatly different results (Hunter et al., 1979; Zbinden and Flury-Roversi, 1981). When other methods of assessing acute toxicity are inappropriate, however, the LD_{50} remains an alternative.

One alternative to the LD_{50} test to assess acute toxicity is to conduct pathological studies after a single dose of a compound, with or without using a small number of animals to calculate a median lethal dose. Although various professionals and consumer groups have advocated use of in vitro tests to assess acute toxicity, no satisfactory methods have yet been developed.

Finally, it is worth noting that Federal Guidelines are by definition merely "recommendations." Too often the guidelines are interpreted as legal requirements, both by various companies and by the FDA itself. For more detailed information, see 21CFR 10.90.

CHAPTER 127

Regulatory Issues from a Sponsor's Perspective

INTRODUCTION

Innumerable important regulatory issues (from the perspectives of sponsors, investigators, contracting organizations, the public, legislators, and regulatory authorities) exist today. This chapter focuses on some of these issues from the perspective of sponsors. Many of the most frequently discussed issues are not presented here, including European procedures for submitting and reviewing Product License Applications (PLAs), delays in medicine approvals, appeals processes, patent issues, and so forth. These topics are discussed in numerous other sources (e.g., Walker and Griffin, 1989; Spilker, 1989a; Spilker and Cuatrecasas, 1988, 1990). The process of regulatory review in the United States is summarized by Kessler (1989).

Are Regulatory Standards Increasing to Unrealistic Levels?

That standards have increased unrealistically is frequently heard within the pharmaceutical industry. To investigate this issue in detail or to reach any conclusions would require an extensive review. The most essential point is that standards in all scientific and clinical areas of a New Drug Application (NDA) or

PLA may be titrated up or down along several spectra by regulatory authorities. For instance, may certain requirements be satisfied in the NDA or must they be satisfied at an earlier stage [e.g., when the Investigational New Drug Application (IND) is submitted]? Figure 127.1 summarizes this concept. Another spectrum relates to the amount of detail required in an NDA to prove a point to the regulatory reviewers' satisfaction. A third spectrum is the amount of validation required on various points.

DEVELOPING REGULATORY STRATEGIES

The regulatory affairs group of a company should develop an overall regulatory strategy plus specific strategies that are appropriate for each investigational medicine. This strategy should be subject to both periodic and ad hoc review at the company. Many regulatory strategies may be adopted for each investigational medicine during its development. Most attempt to address questions such as:

1. Should a company submit several indications for one medicine in a single PLA (or NDA) or in several separate PLAs (NDAs)?
2. Should a new formulation be submitted as a PLA (NDA) supplement or as a new PLA (NDA)?

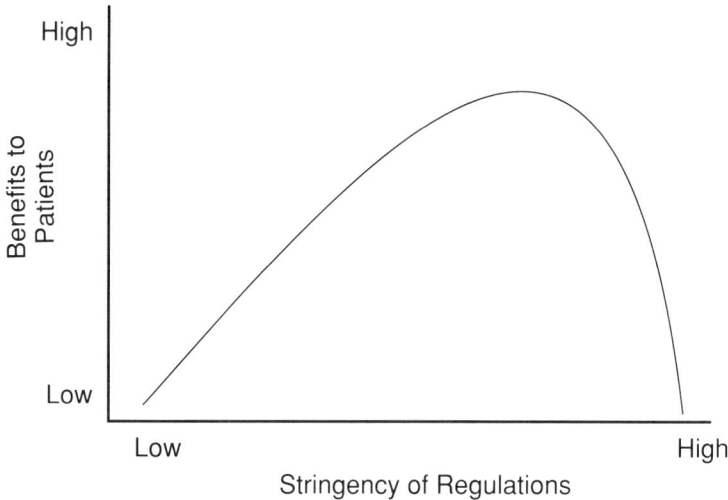

FIG. 127.1 How benefits for patients of strong regulations relate to the intensity of the requirements of regulations.

3. Should a company await approval for a pending PLA (NDA) before submitting a second application for the same medicine (e.g., for a new dosage form, for a new indication)?
4. Should a combination medicine be developed before a single entity?
5. Should the first regulatory submission be made in a relatively less important (commercially) country to obtain more rapid approval, or should more data be collected and analyzed to submit the initial submission in a more important country?

To answer these and other important regulatory questions it is important to understand the regulatory requirements of each country, and the value of having approvals in different countries in terms of ability to generate postmarketing surveillance data and to obtain a significant commercial return.

The factors and groups that impact on the size of the safety package are described in Chapter 119. The pros and cons of submitting many regulatory dossiers on a new medicine simultaneously versus sequentially are also described in that chapter.

Some questions that influence which regulatory strategy is developed are: (1) will any licensing or joint venture partners be included? (2) is a core or modular approach being used? (3) what are the time constraints? (4) what are the marketing considerations? and (5) what pertinent regulatory factors should be considered?

OVERALL APPROACH TO PREPARING AN NDA OR PLA

If the preparation of an NDA or PLA appears to be too formidable a task for a small (or even large) group to handle, each of the separate components and subcomponents should be identified and assignments should be made to complete each. Dividing a single mammoth task into a series of smaller tasks usually allows an individual(s) to cope better with the challenge. When more individuals are assigned to a task, it is usually easier to complete the task when these individuals work together as a team. The team concept helps many people maintain their interest and enthusiasm while working on difficult or tedious tasks. It is extremely important for the individual who organizes the effort either to have had previous experience in assembling an NDA or PLA or to have contact with experienced individuals. A number of suggestions for preparing NDA (or other regulatory) sections of efficacy are listed in Table 127.1.

Classifying Clinical Trials for Efficacy

It is possible to classify clinical trials in a full (or partial) regulatory submission into four categories:

Type I. Efficacy has been demonstrated. These trials may be considered as pivotal trials, i.e., the most well-controlled that have been performed.

Type II. Efficacy has been supported. Partial effects were observed, or alternatively, full effects were observed in a small portion of the population.

Type III. Efficacy was equivocal. It cannot be said that the treatment was effective, or that it was more effective than placebo.

Type IV. Efficacy with placebo was better than with the medicine.

The more subjective the response the more it is likely that type II clinical trials may be accepted by the regulatory authority as valid data to approve the medicine. If objective data are obtained from trials that are expected to be positive with effective medicines almost all the time, then types II and III trials will not be viewed as positively by regulatory authorities.

TABLE 127.1 *Suggestions for preparing New Drug Application (NDA) sections of efficacy data*[a]

A. Relating to statistical analysis and presentation
   1. Present group means for baseline and overall treatment periods for medicine and placebo groups (e.g., number of patients at each week of clinical trial, means at baseline and treatment, difference and categorization of the patient's response as excellent, good, fair, or poor)
   2. Present daily (weekly, monthly) breakdown of the treatment period and possibly stratify patients on basis of their disease severity
   3. Present a list of concomitant medicines taken by all trial patients
   4. Present a list of prior medicine therapy used by patients in the same format as that used directly above
   5. Analyze efficacy parameters by important demographic variables (e.g., age, sex, race) and prognostic characteristics that may be considered to influence the results
   6. Analyze and present data separately for each investigator who participated in a multicenter trial and had a sufficiently large population of patients
B. Relating to document preparation
   1. Present clinical trials on a single medicine in as similar a format as possible
   2. Each final medical report should be preceded by a one-page and a five-or-more-page summary. The one-page summary should include (1) title, (2) investigator(s) name(s) and address(es), (3) a phrase describing the trial design, (4) number and type of patients, (5) test medicine schedule, (6) safety results, (7) efficacy results, and (8) conclusions. The longer summary would expand on each of these points
   3. Use an objective style that does not promote the medicine but judges it fairly and presents it in a reasonable manner
   4. Present data side by side whenever possible for placebo, trial medicine, and active control groups
   5. Have separate individuals track progress on each part of the NDA, write final medical reports, review final medical reports and prepare the expanded summary. The purpose is to prevent delays in NDA preparation
C. Relating to formatting and administration
   1. Group clinical trials of the same type together [e.g., clinical pharmacology, controlled trials for indication(s) pursued, uncontrolled, other]
   2. Provide a list of (1) trial titles, (2) number of investigators, (3) total number of patients, (4) number of patients on each treatment, (5) duration of treatment, (6) NDA volume, and (7) page number
   3. Include information that is believed to be useful to a reviewer, even though it may already be present in another section of the NDA
   4. Delay submission until a relatively complete package of data may be submitted. Additional data in NDA amendments often markedly delay reviews
   5. References to other documents should contain specific date, volume, and page numbers (e.g., to a drug master file). Attach actual copies of documents referenced if they are particularly important. Do not reference documents that the FDA has previously rejected
   6. Ensure that all pages are correctly numbered and that all references to other sections of the NDA and all indexes are correct
D. General comments plus communications with the regulatory agency
   1. A small number of large clinical trials is easier to present and review than a large number of small trials
   2. Indicate whether there were previous discussions with the FDA relating to the study design, conduct, or analysis. If so, provide a synopsis of the situation and agreement (if any). This will help the reviewer understand the background and context of the trial
   3. Indicate which trials support the desired claims of efficacy (or safety)

[a] Several points could be considered in more than one section.

GOLDEN RULES FOR PREPARING REGULATORY SUBMISSIONS

Although the title of this section makes the comments appear as if they are well established and certain, exceptions probably exist to each of these golden rules.

1. Present the application in as simple and straightforward language as possible.
2. Use a logical and straightforward approach to lead the regulatory reviewer through the application. The writers should critique the comprehensibility of their document by imagining that they are also regulatory readers who are unfamiliar with the data presented.
3. Relevant data should be presented in both tables and figures. A regulatory submission is not a publication in which only one format may be chosen. Using both formats avoids criticisms of not showing actual data, because data are shown in tables, and relationships and summaries are presented in figures. Figures are particularly valuable because they present an overview that usually helps people obtain and understand a concept most easily.
4. Present graphs of individual analyses in addition to summary graphs.
5. Ensure that issues or problems raised in one section of the application are adequately considered, addressed, and discussed in all relevant sections of the application. For example, a preclinical issue should often be discussed in the clinical section and vice versa.
6. Attempt to anticipate most of the questions that a reviewer would probably pose, and address each of them in the relevant sections.
7. Do not attempt to anticipate all possible questions that a regulatory reviewer will raise because this is an impossibility, and it is also a foolish objective.
8. Do not hide bad data. This will seriously backfire after the facts are discovered. Present reasons for the data and put them in proper perspective. It is important to present real or potential problems early in the submission in an honest and open manner.
9. Present multiple analyses of data that may be appropriately analyzed in different ways. If a sponsor analyzes data three ways, and likes one analysis best, present all three and state why one is preferred. This approach not only presents other analyses the reviewer might eventually request, but also anticipates this request and saves valuable time. The intention-to-treat analysis is usually one of those done. This approach also demonstrates openness on the part of the company.
10. Do not ask questions of regulatory authorities, unless it is absolutely necessary to do so. Answers received may be unfavorable and may be consid-

ered as immutable. To paraphrase from Ecclesiastes, there is a time to ask questions and a time to refrain from asking questions. It is essential to know which time is which when interacting with a regulatory authority. On the other hand, it is extremely important to describe to regulatory authorities the development plans and strategies being adopted, as early in the process as possible. Their agreement and input may be extremely valuable.

11. Seek to cooperate and even to collaborate with regulatory authorities at those points during a medicine's development process when this is possible. If the authorities have a collegial relationship and have participated in the development plan, their review process should generally be expedited.

12. Do not prepare manufacturing and controls documents too long in advance of the time when the regulatory dossier is to be submitted. Many aspects (e.g., amount of stability data, regulations, methods) may change if there are delays and the entire document may have to be rewritten. This can result in unnecessary duplication of effort.

13. Provide a statement about which clinical trials were audited and certify that they were conducted as reported in the final medical reports. This is reassuring to a regulatory authority even though auditing by the sponsor or an independent group is not required by most authorities.

14. Use two separate data cutoff dates for medicines given on a chronic basis. The first date chosen is based on when data are needed for writing final medical reports. The later date is chosen as the last date to include data from ongoing long-term continuation trials.

16. Labeling for any specific medicine must be consistent from country to country.

17. Develop a document management system to perform the above tasks most efficiently. Contract out those portions that are appropriate, whenever the workload exceeds the staff's capacity.

18. Route the documents to the fewest number of people for reviews, but ensure that their reviews are thorough.

19. Dealing with regulatory authorities should not be a contest of who is right and wrong, or how little do we have to provide, but what information do we have to provide to help them do their job.

20. Pool data separately for controlled and uncontrolled clinical trials. Summarize all clinical experience including trials conducted with volunteers.

Specific Pointers

1. Present the initiation and termination dates for each clinical trial on a single page.

2. Make all indexes that would be useful for a reviewer.

3. Cross-reference all relevant comments within each regulatory submission.

4. Consider making a videotape as an introduction to the entire NDA to identify key points and possibly illustrate patients with specific findings.

5. Establish goals of how much to write each week and month. Do whatever it takes to achieve those goals.

6. If it is impossible to discuss data with a regulatory authority, it may be beneficial in some countries to ask them to interpret the guidelines for a specific situation.

7. Only refer to company documents that are confirmed to have been issued. Regulatory authorities may become quite upset if they request documents that are unavailable.

RESPONDING TO REGULATORY QUESTIONS

Many questions or issues raised by regulatory authorities require significant efforts within a company to formulate a response. This effort may be directed toward conducting new analyses of existing data, new clinical trials, new laboratory tests, or answering some specific (or general) questions.

Range of Responses

The initial step for a company to follow after they receive a regulatory letter is to assess their strategy to respond to regulatory requests, including (1) there are no issues for us to debate, let's just do the work and send it in, (2) let's not do anything until we discuss (debate) their questions in detail with them, or (3) let's have a strategy setting meeting to decide our approach to the authority's questions. At such a meeting it may be decided to meet with regulatory personnel and present the company's view on the subject.

Assigning Responsibility for Generating Responses

One individual within a company may be assigned the overall responsibility for addressing a complex issue or a large number of simple issues raised by a regulatory authority. Others may be assigned responsibility for addressing separate portions of the response. Complex issues are often divided into their component parts to simplify the process of accumulating the necessary responses. Each individual who is assigned responsibility for responding to one or more questions is either assigned a time limit to complete his or her work, or is asked to provide an acceptable period of time to the overall organizer or coordinator.

REGULATORY CATCH 22-ISSUES

Biologicals

Biologicals must be as fully developed as possible from a manufacturing perspective prior to clinical development. If virtually any changes are made during the period of development (e.g., size of column used for purification), then additional clinical trials must be conducted to ensure that the "modified" product retains both the chemical and clinical activity of the original product. The irony of this requirement is that it is almost always impossible to do this at the start of the project, when the goal and efforts of the group are focused on determining whether the biological product is clinically active. Moreover, it would require placing great resources on a project whose future is unknown, again at a time when its eventual outcome is uncertain. The usual compromise is to strive to develop a final formulation and manufacturing process in time to conduct the pivotal clinical trials. These almost always occur after efficacy has been established in pilot trials.

Creating and Using a Common International Data Base

Many companies want to use a common international data base and a common presentation of data in their reports prepared for each regulatory authority to which a PLA or another dossier will be submitted. This is primarily to enhance speed and efficiency, and to decrease costs. Many small points in each dossier, however, must be modified to suit the local authorities both in format and content. An example of an issue relating to content at a national level is that in the United States, "stroke" is a contraindication for patients to receive streptokinase, because of the possibility of an intracerebral bleed. In Japan, streptokinase is indicated and used for treatment of "prestroke" patients, although at a different dose than recommended in the United States. Both regulatory and legal requirements around the world virtually preclude the possibility of having a single worldwide label, but a company must be internally consistent in the labeling of any of its medicines across the countries in which it is marketed.

Dose–Response Relationships

There appears to be increased interest within several regulatory authorities for the full dose–response relationship to be explored at the time a new medicine is approved.

Every academic investigator and company designs a clinical trial to enhance the chances for a positive outcome, regardless of how a "positive outcome" is defined. This is particularly important for companies designing Phase II pivotal (i.e., the most well-controlled) trials. As a result, relatively high doses are often used to demonstrate efficacy. At a later date, there may be a desire to obtain regulatory approval for a lower dose, but the clinical trials conducted at higher doses cannot be used as evidence of efficacy at lower doses. It most cases, the emphasis on speed means that the full dose–response relationship is not established when the pivotal trials are designed. One approach to this potential issue is to include two separate doses of the investigational medicine in most Phase II pivotal trials.

Use of Ultra-Low Doses of Active Medicines

In Phase II pivotal trials the demonstration of efficacy usually depends on showing statistically and clinically significant differences between two treatment groups. Developing medicines for treating cancer and acquired immunodeficiency syndrome (AIDS) are two exceptions to this principle. A company may desire to achieve this goal by having two treatment groups receive the active medicine, one group receiving a standard dose and the other an extremely low dose. The investigator or the Ethics Committee/Institutional Review Board may object to the use of a very low dose (or use of a placebo). Their objection creates a dilemma, which may be difficult to resolve. It should be debated openly by each side. In a limited number of cases, the new medicine may be believed superior to existing therapy and important quality of life endpoints may be used to differentiate it from standard therapy.

FDA Rating System for New Chemical Entities

An A, B, C rating system was initiated in 1978 to expedite NDA review time. No consistent criteria were established to apply these codes, and ratings are based on limited data.

Although the FDA developed this system primarily for internal review, it has become more widely used. The most critical use from a sponsor's perspective is by formulary committees who sometimes decide whether a new medicine is acceptable for placing on the formulary based on the FDA's classification of the medicine as A, B, or C. This raises significant questions for sponsors who want their medicines to have the best chance for commercial success possible.

The FDA's system may be acceptable from an administrative perspective, but it has major flaws from a technical perspective. The flaws include that the classification is usually based on (1) vague criteria, (2) unevenly applied criteria, (3) limited data, and (4) one or a few people's prediction. It is not easy for a sponsor to appeal the FDA's rating of their medicine, because the FDA considers this an internal administrative issue that is not public at an early stage of review.

ELECTRONIC REGULATORY SUBMISSIONS

There is no simple "yes" or "no" as to whether electronic NDAs are a good or bad idea. The spectrum of possible approaches is shown in Fig. 127.2. Various components of an electronic regulatory submission may be discussed as to their advisability.

1. *Optical disk* to present information on actual patient data and reports. This method is advisable because it makes it easier for regulatory authorities to find specific parts of the application. The disk may be considered a hard copy version of the text and is certainly positive for both the sponsor and the regulatory authority.

2. *Word-processing capability.* Regulatory reviewers spend a great deal of time preparing their reports, after having read and assessed the material in the NDA. The optical disk does not allow reviewers to "cut and paste" relevant portions of the application. However, placing the *text* in a word-processing format allows sections to be lifted out. This practice should shorten the time needed by reviewers to prepare their reports.

3. *Raw data.* Providing raw data to regulatory authorities on computer disk or in another electronic format provides benefits in theory to both sponsors and regulatory reviewers. This approach enables regulatory reviewers to use the data to address statistical questions without having to ask sponsors to spend their time generating such data. This approach is not positive for sponsors when it makes it easier for regulatory authorities to reanalyze data without first discussing the request or

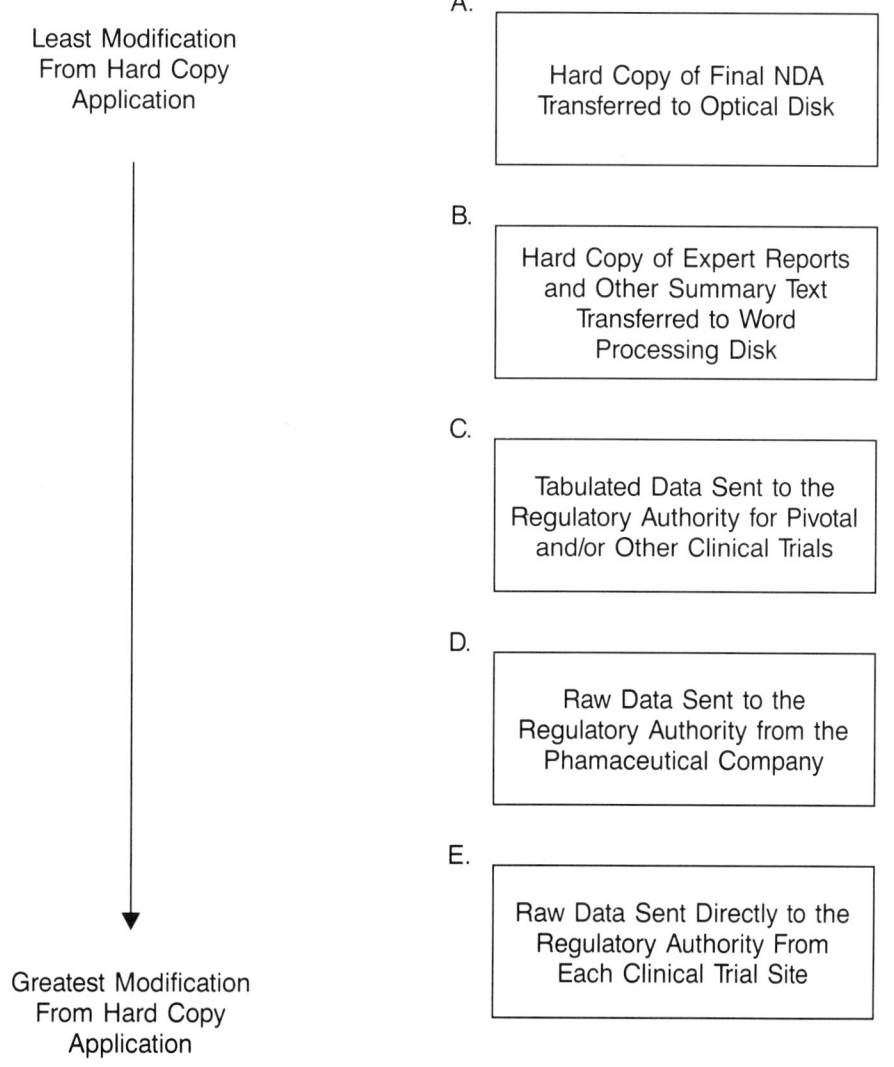

Least Modification
From Hard Copy
Application

Greatest Modification
From Hard Copy
Application

A.
Hard Copy of Final NDA
Transferred to Optical Disk

B.
Hard Copy of Expert Reports
and Other Summary Text
Transferred to Word
Processing Disk

C.
Tabulated Data Sent to the
Regulatory Authority for Pivotal
and/or Other Clinical Trials

D.
Raw Data Sent to the
Regulatory Authority from the
Phamaceutical Company

E.
Raw Data Sent Directly to the
Regulatory Authority From
Each Clinical Trial Site

FIG. 1272. Spectrum of electronic regulatory submissions, NDA, New Drug Application.

concept with the sponsor. Although such a rean-alysis is possible in many countries today, it is rarely practiced by regulatory authorities. Usually a company that is asked to provide further data or analyses may debate the issue with a regulatory authority. The same company, however, will be placed in an undesirable defensive position if a reg-ulatory authority states "We have analyzed your data (using techniques the company believes are inappropriate) and have found the following re-sults."

ADVERSE EVENT DATA

If the review process on an investigational medicine is prolonged (e.g., over 1 year in most countries), it is often appropriate for the regulatory authority to re-quest an update on all adverse event data in the spon-sor's data base. This update should be based on all worldwide data collected by the company.

Companies and regulatory authorities around the world differ on what adverse events or experiences should be considered as adverse reactions with some relationship to a medicine. Minor colds, concomitant diseases, or sequelae of adverse experiences (e.g., sprained neck from falling down some stairs, broken leg from an automobile accident) are sometimes listed as adverse reactions and then explained; at other times they are omitted from data collection forms.

Information on serious adverse reactions reported on marketed medicines is becoming more standard-ized. The categories of information described on a typ-ical one-page form are shown in Table 127.2.

CAUTIONS IN REINVESTIGATING AN OLD MEDICINE

Medicines that are already marketed are often reported to have useful clinical activity in patients who have an unlabeled indication. The question for the sponsor to address is whether to conduct additional clinical trials and to seek regulatory approval for the new indication. It is usually believed that a relatively straightforward issue is being discussed and that the necessary data may be rapidly obtained. Whenever an old medicine is to be studied and a new regulatory submission made, however, it will invariably be found that existing data for technical development, toxicology, clinical trials, or other areas do not meet current regulatory stan-dards.

The amount of effort to prepare a satisfactory reg-ulatory submission will be severely underestimated un-less each of these aspects is thoroughly investigated before committing the resources to develop the med-icine for the new indication. If a company moves blindly ahead to evaluate the medicine, it is likely they will create a complex situation that could possibly jeopardize the medicine's existing market. The cost-to-benefit ratio must be assessed in advance to deter-mine whether the proposed change is truly as valuable as its proponents make it sound.

The same principle and considerations also pertain when there is a request from marketing personnel to introduce a new dosage form, dosing strength, or for-mulation, or to develop another change of an already marketed medicine.

PREPARING STATISTICAL REPORTS FOR AN NDA OR PLA

A few general points are listed that should be consid-ered when preparing statistical reports of clinical trials that will be included in an NDA or PLA:

1. Reports should present a detailed account of all protocol modifications and violations. Reasons for these digressions should be presented.
2. Patients in a clinical trial who do not meet the in-clusion criteria should be identified in the statis-tical report. Explanations should be given in the medical report, although an abbreviated explana-tion may also be given in the statistical report.
3. All relevant baseline variables or combinations of variables should be used to compare treatment groups, even if the data appear to show no differ-ences.
4. It is important to include an accountability section (e.g., the number of patients included at each stage of the study), plus reasons for attrition. It is de-sirable to create a demographic profile at each stage, as well as a table of prognostic criteria.
5. Data should be analyzed separately from each clin-ical trial site, whenever possible.
6. A statistical rationale should be given when data are pooled to use a single statistical analysis.

TABLE 127.2 *Information on a serious adverse reaction placed on a one-page report*

1. Report number
2. Country in which the adverse reaction occurred
3. Medicine(s) involved
4. Adverse reaction being reported
5. Date the sponsor or physician received information about the adverse reaction
6. Type of report (e.g., acute emergency)
7. Date that the CIOMS[a] regulatory form is due in each country on a standard form
8. Date any other form is due, according to regulations
9. Date next action is required
10. Next action proposed
11. Pending dictionary terms

[a] CIOMS, Committee of International Organizations of Medical Societies. See Chapter 120.

7. All patients who do not complete the clinical trial should have relevant data listed [e.g., treatment group, time on medicine, dosage at time of withdrawal, amount of medicine taken, concomitant medicines, adverse reactions if any, reason(s) for dropping out or discontinuation, plus other relevant information].

8. Results of any interim analyses conducted, plus the reasons for conducting an interim analysis should be discussed.

9. It is important for statisticians to avoid making a clinical interpretation of the results, although they may present the interpretation. This issue is discussed in Chapter 100.

CHAPTER 128

Regulatory Issues from a National Regulatory Authority's Perspective

ATTITUDES OF REGULATORY AUTHORITIES TOWARD SPONSORS

There are two basic approaches taken by regulatory authorities in their dealings with sponsors of new medicines. These approaches depend on whether the regulator's national laws, regulations, and guidelines are based on the natural justice system of law (e.g., in the United States) or on the Roman system of law (e.g., in most countries within Europe). In the natural justice system (which grows out of past cases and experience), a company may present data as often as desired (within reason) to the regulatory authority. Data submitted are accepted to be true, although an increasing number of audits are being conducted to confirm these facts. The process of approval of a medicine involves discussions between the two parties trying to reach the best position for both. Some exceptions to this state exist.

Under the Roman system of law, a sponsor may only respond to questions posed by a regulatory authority. It is essentially an inquisitional system because it is based on a legal code that tries to anticipate and to regulate the ways that submissions should be made.

As a result a greater gulf exists between the two parties. Data are viewed skeptically and their truthfulness must be demonstrated.

AUDITING CONDUCTED BY REGULATORY AGENCIES—USING THE FDA AS AN EXAMPLE

Only a few regulatory agencies conduct audits of clinical trials. The Food and Drug Administration (FDA) conducts two major types of audits: for-cause inspections and routine inspections. The audits are conducted as an accounting procedure to verify the data. The major purpose of an audit is to determine whether the records at the investigator's site are complete and agree both with records at the sponsor's site and with data in the NDA. Records at the sponsor's site must also be complete. Further information on this subject is presented by Segal et al. (1985) and Turner et al. (1987). The FDA takes no official position on whether pharmaceutical companies should conduct clinical audits of their own activities.

For-Cause Audits

If there is a specific problem or issue that has initiated the audit, then it may be described as one conducted "for cause." Approximately 30 to 40 of these audits

This chapter is based on many public and private talks by and with regulatory authority personnel, although few specific references are given. The information expressed does not represent the views of any single regulatory authority or regulator. Rather, it is an amalgam of the author's views about the regulator's perspective.

are conducted per year by the FDA. Reasons for conducting for-cause audits are given in Table 128.1. The initial step is to focus attention on clarifying the problem. Once this is done, it should be apparent what type(s) of information are necessary to answer the questions, which can be followed by development of possible solutions. The conduct of a for-cause audit is the same as a routine audit (see below) in terms of what is audited.

Routine Audits

Each routine audit or surveillance type inspection usually follows the same general procedures. Approximately 250 of these audits are conducted each year by the FDA. As with audits by the tax office, however, all audits are not created equal. Some may be total, while others focus solely on specific questions. The purpose(s) of the audit usually influences the decision as to how extensive the audit will be. Even using a single approach (e.g., examining data collection forms for unusual or missing values and then comparing those with original records, following an audit trail of data), an audit may be superficial or thorough.

The FDA routinely audits the information that addresses the following questions:

1. Who did what during the clinical trial (e.g., reported adverse events, obtained consents)?
2. What was the degree of delegation by the investigator?

3. Where were specific aspects of the study performed?
4. How were the data recorded and stored?
5. Was a log documenting contacts (e.g., visits, telephone calls) with monitors maintained?
6. Were records of medicine accountability (e.g., inventory records, site of storage, documenting transactions) maintained at an appropriate level?
7. Were data submitted to the sponsors identical with those on supporting documents?
8. Were the interactions with the Institutional Review Board (IRB) appropriate?

This last item is usually considered by most people to be the most important part of the routine inspection.

Common Problems Found

The most commonly found problem in routine FDA audits is that all elements of the informed consent are not placed on the form (Table 128.2). The severity of all deficiencies is summarized in Table 128.3. The most commonly found problem relating to IRBs is that they are not informed about changes in the protocol. Table 128.4 lists the results of routine data audits at sponsor's sites. It is important to present any problems with a clinical trial submission "up front" and discuss it openly. Trying to bury problems in a submission will only raise the ire and suspicions of a reviewer.

At the conclusion of the inspection the FDA's field investigator prepares a list of his or her observations regarding regulatory violations and discusses it with the clinical investigator. Once the inspector's final report is received by FDA headquarters, a follow-up letter is sent to the investigator that outlines the details of problems found. This list and letter may be obtained under the Freedom of Information Act after the par-

TABLE 128.1 *Reasons why the Food and Drug Administration (FDA) conducts for-cause audits*[a]

1. The investigator is conducting a large number of clinical trials with investigational medicines, particularly if the medicines are in different therapeutic areas
2. The investigator is conducting a clinical trial outside his or her speciality
3. The investigator reports efficacy for a medicine that is much better than that reported in other data for the medicine
4. The investigator reports no adverse reactions or few of a specific type, when other physicians report numerous adverse reactions
5. The investigator appears to have too many patients with a given disease in reference to the practice's setting and location
6. The investigator reports laboratory data that are excessively consistent or are inconsistent with data reported by others
7. The investigator conducts a high media profile clinical trial that may create a demand for the new medicine
8. The investigator conducts a truly important clinical trial. This includes foreign trials that are primary evidence of efficacy
9. The investigator has been complained about by a patient in the clinical trial
10. The investigator has been complained about by the sponsor for a problem of commission or failure to supply data collected

[a] The contents of this table were taken from Turner et al. (1987), with comments by Dr. Alan Lisook of the FDA, and are printed with permission of both.

TABLE 128.2 *Summary of deficiencies found through Food and Drug Administration (FDA) conducted routine inspections of clinical data at investigator's sites*[a]

Most common deficiencies	No. of deficiencies (%)[b]
Inadequate informed consent form	54
Inadequate medicine accountability	25
Nonadherence to protocol	26
Inaccurate or inadequate records	21
Records not available	3
Failure to keep Institutional Review Board (IRB) informed or failure to obtain approval	13
Other deficiencies	5

[a] Sloboda and Currier (1985) plus Lisook (1990). Data obtained from routine audit inspections conducted between June, 1977 and September, 1989. This sample constitutes all of the routine audits conducted, with the exception of a few that were not evaluable.

[b] The percent refers to the number of inspections.

TABLE 128.3 *Summary of severity of deficiencies found through Food and Drug Administration (FDA) conducted routine data audit inspections[a]*

Results of routine data audits	No. of audits (%)
No action required	20
Voluntary action indicated for categories I, II[b]	70
Voluntary action indicated for category III[c]	7
"For cause" audit initiated[d]	3
Total	100

[a] Inspections conducted at the investigator's sites are those described in Table 128.2.
[b] Categories are defined by the FDA. Violations in categories I and II are minor and do not warrant any FDA action.
[c] FDA communicates with the site and requests a response.
[d] An in-depth follow-up inspection is conducted on the clinical trial in question plus other trials conducted by that investigator.

ticular file is closed. Types of letters sent by the FDA as a result of an audit are described in a later section of this chapter.

Audits have become more complex for regulatory authorities to conduct in recent years. This is primarily related to the fact that many different types of software are used to process and handle data in different institutions.

Excuses Reported to the FDA

Excuses from investigators for lack of records or data given to FDA personnel conducting audits range from the credible to the totally incredible. Here are few of the comments collected by Dr. Alan Lisook (personal communication), head of the FDA Clinical Investigations Branch over several years:

1. The records were destroyed in a fire, flood, or hurricane.
2. The records were lost in a boating accident, burglary, robbery, in the mail.
3. The records fell in a sewer and had to be destroyed because of their odor.
4. The hospital closed and the records were lost.
5. The office worker (coinvestigator) is dead or missing, or they were out to get me.
6. The nurse (resident) made the errors, and they were out to get me.
7. The movers threw them out, or my father-in-law threw them out.

Interviews may be conducted with patients who participated in a clinical trial if the FDA headquarters has doubts that (1) a proper and valid informed consent was ever obtained, (2) the patient had the problem they were reported to have, or (3) the patient ever participated in the clinical trial.

Sponsor's Perspective on FDA Audits of Pharmaceutical Company Operations

Although not required by FDA regulations, most pharmaceutical companies have written standard operating procedures to deal with regulatory audits conducted at the company. One of the most important principles is for each company to have trained individuals who accompany the FDA staff during their inspection. Dry runs should be conducted to ensure that inspections are handled appropriately. The company must focus on (1) ensuring appropriate attitudes of their staff, (2) developing and implementing policies for identifying and training staff who accompany the FDA officers, (3) providing information that regulatory officials desire, (4) taking appropriate notes, (5) making corrections to problems identified, (6) participating in an exit interview, and (7) preparing reports. Standard operating procedures should identify documents, records, people, and equipment to which the FDA may have access.

TABLE 128.4 *Summary of Food and Drug Administration (FDA) inspections of sponsors since June 1977[a]*

	No. of sponsors	Percent of sponsors
1. Sponsors with whom no significant deviations from current or proposed regulations were noted	151	67
2. Sponsors with whom significant deviations were noted	74	33
Total	225[b]	100%

	No. of deficiencies	Percent of all inspections
3. Common deficiencies:		
Failure to maintain adequate records of medicine accountability	47	21
Absence of standard monitoring procedures	42	19
Failure to establish adequacy of laboratory facilities used by clinical investigator	37	16
Failure to review patient records	33	15
Failure to assure Institutional Review Board (IRB) approval	29	13
Failure to document monitoring visits	24	11
Failure to visit trial site before and during clinical trial	15	7

[a] This table was provided by the Division of Scientific Investigations of the FDA's Center for Drug Research and Evaluation. It is current as of March 1, 1986.
[b] This number includes some reinspections. Note that percentages have been rounded off to the nearest whole number.

Standard operating procedures should describe the rights of the FDA and the company, plus the company's policies and practices. While these standard operating procedures are particularly important for factory inspections, which lie outside the scope of this book, such guidelines are also relevant for clinical trial audits.

Graded Responses by the FDA to an Inspection

Inspection of a Company

The following are a series of progressively more severe steps that may be taken by the FDA as a result of audits of pharmaceutical companies:

1. List of observations provided to a company by the FDA inspector at the time of inspection. No response is required.
2. Information letter sent to a company; no action is required. (The letter states what the FDA found during their audit.)
3. Notice of adverse findings letter sent to a company; a response is required from the company within 30 days.
4. Regulatory letter is sent to a company; a response is required from the company within 10 days. This letter indicates that the FDA is prepared to proceed with more serious steps.
5. Injunctions.
6. Seizures.
7. Prosecution.

Inspection of an Investigator

Investigators who are disqualified as a result of an FDA audit cannot handle or study investigational medicines. If the investigator signs a consent agreement, it means that he or she agrees not to conduct any more clinical trials or agreement to other restrictions. The FDA may disqualify data, however, and not the investigator. For example, one investigator subcontracted part of a clinical trial to another investigator, and neither one knew what the other was doing, creating so many problems (inadvertently) that the data were judged to be unacceptable. In this case, the two investigators were not judged guilty of any serious misconduct.

Results of Inspections

Data from the FDA's auditing program are published periodically by the FDA staff and others (Lisook, 1990). A recent update by Shapiro and Charrow (1989)

of their earlier study (Shapiro and Charrow, 1985) suggested a decreased rate of serious deficiencies in clinical trials—from 12 to 7%. These authors stated that additional measures should be applied to those found guilty of misconduct. They proposed several methods, which are not discussed further here because they go beyond the scope of this book.

FDA Audits of Foreign Clinical Trials

Foreign clinical trials are more and more likely to be audited by the FDA, particularly if they are pivotal to the approval of a New Drug Application (NDA). The FDA will only audit foreign clinical trials if they can study source documents. Sponsors are always informed by the FDA if a foreign inspection will be conducted. The sponsor may be asked to provide an independent translator on site. Some investigators (both domestic and foreign), however, are not cooperative with FDA inspectors. This may take the form of attempting to place certain records "off-limits" to the inspector or of going on vacation as soon as the inspector arrives. Further information on this topic is presented by Sloboda and Lisook (1987) and Lisook (1990). The most common problems found in foreign audits conducted through October, 1989 are: inadequate or inaccurate records (81%), protocol nonadherence (64%), informed consent issues (45%), and inadequate medicine accountability (40%) (Lisook, personal communication).

COMMON PROBLEMS OBSERVED IN REGULATORY APPLICATIONS

Patterns of NDAs Received

The FDA has described three basic patterns of New Drug Application (NDA) documents received: (1) a single, complete NDA to review (the preferred pattern for new NDAs by the FDA); (2) a few (or many) major amendments to the original NDA are submitted during the review period of the first NDA, (creates innumerable problems during the review process and is frowned on by the FDA); (3) one or more resubmissions of the original NDA are made, with several months or even years between each submission.

Types of NDAs in Terms of Their Quality

The assessment of NDAs from a regulatory authority's perspective may be placed in five broad categories or quality types:

TABLE 128.5 *Selected types of questions posed by regulators who review NDAs and PLAs*[a]

1. What is the minimal effective dose of the medicine?
2. What is the initial dose and how should it be escalated?
3. Are severe adverse reactions results of one or all stereoisomers?
4. How should the medicine be withdrawn from patients?
5. Are all severe adverse reaction reports reported anywhere in the world included in the application?
6. What is the ratio of well-controlled clinical trials that establish or support efficacy to those that do not?
7. Are the expert reports objective scientific critiques of the data, as opposed to mere synopses?
8. Are all major issues and problems with the medicine fully and adequately discussed?

[a] NDA, New Drug Application; PLA, Product License Application.

1. *Good applications.* The term "good" refers both to the quality of the medicine and the quality of the application itself.
2. *Flawed applications.* These NDAs have fatal flaws in the organization or preparation of the NDA and need major additional work if they are ever to be acceptable.
3. *Poor applications.* A clearly beneficial and even important medicine that is poorly developed by the sponsor. The application is unacceptable, in its present form.
4. *Dubious applications.* The medicine is of dubious medical benefit, even if the development was appropriate and the quality of the NDA itself excellent.

TABLE 128.6 *Common problems observed in PLA and NDA regulatory applications*[a]

A. Preclinical problems
  1. Inadequate carcinogenicity studies
B. Clinical problems
  1. Incorrect dose studied
  2. Insufficiently controlled clinical trials
  3. Poorly conceived and written protocols
  4. Foreign clinical trials do not state the primary objectives for all trials and do not discuss whether they were met
C. Manufacturing and controls problems
  1. Incomplete characterization of the medicine
  2. Inclusion of multiple manufacturing sites that have never made the medicine
  3. Incomplete details in the analytical chemistry or other technical areas
D. Overall problems
  1. Some companies believe that exposures of a medicine to 20 million patients worldwide proves that it is safe and effective, and obviates the need for well-controlled clinical trials or a full toxicology program
  2. Although regulations do not generally require clinical data to be obtained in the country in which the medicine is sold, there is a bias toward applications with at least some data collected in each major country in which the medicine is to be licensed

[a] NDA, New Drug Application; PLA, Product License Application.

5. *Premature applications.* This represents a ploy on the part of some companies that attempt to learn what other work is required to have an acceptable NDA. It tends to slow the entire review system at the regulatory authority, and negatively affects all companies submitting regulatory applications.

Regulatory authorities spend a great deal of time validating a sponsor's data, and do not take it on trust. Thus, whatever the sponsor can do to assure the authority that the data are valid should lead to a savings in time. Selected questions often posed by regulatory authority personnel in reviewing NDAs and Product License Applications (PLAs) are listed in Table 128.5, and common problems encountered in these applications are listed in Table 128.6.

CALCULATED TIMES FOR APPROVAL OF A MEDICINE

The time taken for regulatory review of a new medicine is usually calculated by subtracting the date of initial submission from the date of final approval. A certain number of months is determined, but is this an adequate figure to use in judging the speed of an authority's activity? In some countries, this period includes time for a company to respond to an agency's questions; any delays on the company's part are not measured. The time a company takes to address questions raised by an authority includes time taken to solve technical problems and other unavoidable delays, plus (possibly) some avoidable delays.

It would be difficult to measure and then subtract the time that a company is busy preparing its response to a regulatory letter from the total time the submission is "at" the regulatory authority. This is because while the company is busy preparing its response to clinical questions, for example, the regulatory authority may be either awaiting the company's response or continuing its review of other sections of the application (e.g., chemistry, manufacturing).

The length of the review time at the regulatory authority primarily relates to the amount of resources placed on the review. This, in turn, is usually based (to some degree) on the medical value and priority of the submission. The overall time for a review is also dependent on the slowest link in the chain of reviews. On the other hand, the quality of the regulatory submission also has a major effect on the time required to review an application. A well-prepared, complete, easy to read and follow application requires much less time to review than one of lesser organizational quality. It is a golden rule that additional time spent by a sponsor in preparing an easy to read and follow dossier will be more than saved in the speed of the regulatory review.

CHAPTER 129

Interactions of Marketing with Research and Development Departments

ACTIVITIES ORIGINATING IN, AND CONDUCTED BY, RESEARCH AND DEVELOPMENT DEPARTMENTS

This chapter deals with interactions of research and development departments with marketing departments. The word "interactions" refers to both joint activities and joint communications. Activities are usually initiated by a specific marketing *or* research and development department, and are mainly conducted within one of these groups. This section describes the activities of a research and development department.

Conducting clinical studies to support marketing-related activities (see Chapter 51) is an important research and development concern. These studies often involve a direct comparison of an investigational medicine with a known standard medicine. The usual purpose of such studies is to obtain comparative data on safety, efficacy, or pharmacokinetic parameters. These data may eventually be incorporated into promotional materials and publications, and may serve as evidence to support use of the study medicine.

Other marketing-related activities in which research and development's clinical staff may participate include (1) review of advertising and other marketing copy to ensure that it is accurate and not misleading,

(2) participation in the design of scientific exhibits to be used at professional meetings, (3) attendance at scientific exhibits or medicine launches, (4) planning and carrying out symposia or other meetings, and (5) preparation of various monographs, materials for a medicine's launch, and other scientific documents.

Preclinical staff in research departments also assist marketing efforts in many ways. In addition to providing assistance in many of the clinical activities described above, preclinical staff often assay blood or urine samples from ongoing medicine trials in pursuit of new indications, or assist outside laboratories in setting up similar assays. Scientific studies are usually performed to elucidate a medicine's mechanism of action, as well as to investigate reasons for purported medicine–medicine interactions reported in the literature or to the company.

Answering telephone and written requests for routine or emergency information and providing assistance to answer product complaints are additional functions performed by research and development staff. Research staff members also assist in the training programs for sales representatives. Technical departments become involved in the development of new dosage strengths (i.e., size of dose per tablet or unit), dosage forms (e.g., tablet, suppository), and formulations. These products often constitute line extensions for the medicine.

ACTIVITIES ORIGINATING IN, AND CONDUCTED BY, MARKETING DEPARTMENTS

Marketing-Driven versus Research-Driven Companies

Marketing groups provide many important inputs into medicine development. At the early stage of medicine discovery some companies attempt to concentrate their research in the therapeutic areas likely to provide significant commercial returns. If there is a strong influence of marketing views in terms of identifying appropriate therapeutic areas for research and in using marketing criteria to either promote or terminate a project, then the company is said to be "market driven." If marketing influences are not strong at this early stage of medicine development and decisions about choosing research areas to search for new medicines are primarily made by research management, by senior research scientists, or by a combination of the two, the company is said to be "research driven." In this situation the marketing division reacts to new medicines developed by research departments. Some companies experience strong internal conflicts in how the company makes decisions and is oriented.

Areas Where Marketing Input Is Important

Marketing influences and information are important inputs in choosing directions for medicine development once a medicine is tested in humans. Information such as capsule or tablet color, size, shape, and dosage strength are obvious examples for which marketing input is required. In addition, if a choice of indications to pursue is possible or if there is a choice of dosage forms (e.g., liquid or solid), then it is usually important to obtain input from marketing. As the clinical profile of the medicine becomes more clearly established, marketing input is obtained in order to determine which aspects of the profile should be investigated; often, this information is also used to determine which parameters or endpoints should be evaluated. For instance, if a medicine has been administered on a three- or four-times-a-day basis in early clinical trials to demonstrate and confirm its activity, but marketing wishes to sell the medicine on a once-a-day basis, then trials must be planned and initiated to determine if adequate efficacy and safety will be maintained when the medicine is given less frequently. It is often impossible to predict in advance whether a medicine will be active for a sufficiently long period when given on a less fre-

quent basis. One reason is that a medicine's biological activity may persist for a period after the medicine is excreted from the body or is broken down by the body to inactive metabolites.

Toward the end of the clinical program that is followed for an investigational medicine, specialized clinical studies are often initiated specifically for marketing group objectives. These studies usually compare the new medicine directly with a standard medicine presently used for the same indication or they may evaluate interactions of the new medicine with alcohol or other medicines that will be commonly given with the new medicine. The medicine may also be evaluated in a special type of patient population in which results will provide important marketing information.

The time points during an investigational medicine's development when it is important to provide research and development with marketing information are shown in Table 129.1. The type of marketing information of major interest to research and development are listed in Table 129.2.

Marketing Strategies

A marketing strategy may be described as the mix of marketing techniques used by a company to maximize sales and profits. These techniques include variables

TABLE 129.1 *Time points during the development of an investigational medicine when marketing information is desirable or essential to impart to research and development personnel*

1. When a new biological target is being chosen to use in seeking active compounds
2. After a chemical lead is identified that is active in a therapeutic area or for a disease not previously discussed with marketing
3. When a decision is being made to conduct secondary pharmacology and other biological studies on a lead compound that it is hoped will enter project status
4. When a compound is being considered for project status
5. When the clinical plan is being assembled and a decision is being made to file a regulatory submission to test the compound in a specific indication using a specific dosage form
6. At time of the go/no-go decision to continue to Phase III and file a regulatory submission
7. At any time when the clinical profile has changed dramatically
8. If the clinical profile falls below the minimal standards set by both research and development and marketing
9. At any time when a new indication is chosen to develop, or a new dosage form is considered
10. During late Phase II when the Phase III program is being put together and marketing-oriented studies are being considered
11. During late Phase III and after approval when new indications, dosage forms, routes of administration, quality of life, and cost-effectiveness studies are considered
12. After the regulatory submission occurs and marketing trials are being planned

TABLE 129.2 *Selected marketing information of interest to research and development*

1. Statement of the present market size
2. Forecast of the future market size at the time of the new medicine's expected launch
3. Current treatments for the disease of interest and their respective market share
4. Forecast of future market share for each alternative therapy at the time of the new medicine's expected approval
5. Current medicines being developed by other companies and their phase of development
6. Advantages and disadvantages of current medicines under development
7. Changes expected in patient demographics for the disease to be treated
8. Ideal characteristics of a new product in terms of animal and human safety, efficacy, and pharmaceutics
9. Reasonable characteristics to expect in the above categories
10. Minimal product profile that would justify marketing the new medicine
11. Preliminary analysis of sales and return on investment based on alternative clinical scenarios

TABLE 129.3 *Clinical questions that should be considered in developing a marketing strategy*

1. What are the best means to demonstrate superiority of a medicine over its competitors in clinical trials (e.g., use of special patient populations, comparison of specified efficacy parameters, evaluation of their adverse reaction profile)?
2. What are appropriate means to create an awareness in the medical community of important, but as yet unapproved, indications of a medicine (e.g., publications, talks to medical groups, medicine studies)?
3. How may a sponsor/inventor obtain the best patent protection possible for the (1) medicine, (2) medicine uses, (3) dosage forms, and (4) methods of manufacturing?
4. Which clinical trials will provide practitioners with the information needed to treat their patients effectively? This includes the following trials: (1) medicine interactions, (2) special populations, and (3) methods to wean patients off other medicines and place them on the new medicine
5. Which trials must be conducted to obtain data that will enable undesirable medicine labeling to be removed?

such as (1) which established products are chosen to sell, (2) which new products are chosen to introduce, (3) the price of each product, (4) the amount of time for sales representatives to promote the products, and (5) other techniques. Another aspect of strategy relates to the claims made about the medicine that attempt to distinguish it from all other products of its class and other competing products. All of these techniques have a great impact on the percent of a market (i.e., market share) captured by a medicine.

Specific marketing activities conducted on a medicine depend on whether the medicine is established on the market, newly introduced to the market, or investigational. Activities include determining sales strategies primarily based on the medicine's development as a (1) New Chemical Entity (NCE), (2) line extension (e.g., new dosage form, dose size), (3) conversion from prescription to over-the-counter use, or (4) combination medicine. Each of these types of medicines involves specific considerations from a marketing perspective. These considerations plus medicine profile and market needs influence the development of the marketing plan developed for each medicine.

Some relevant questions that may assist in developing a marketing strategy are listed in Table 129.3. Selected types of marketing strategies are listed in Table 129.4. Marketing strategies are described more fully by Slatter (1977) and by Guth (1985). Members of a marketing team are indicated in Table 129.5.

A company's marketing strategy differs for each product. Each medicine is sold in a different therapeutic market, in which doctors' prescribing habits and attitudes differ, the nature and intensity of the competition differs, and many of the other factors that may affect a marketing strategy also differ.

Marketing Research

Marketing research attempts to answer questions that assist in developing a marketing strategy and planning relevant clinical studies. The value of a medicine from a commercial perspective depends on the (1) amount of sales, (2) cost of goods (manufacturing and distribution costs), and (3) costs of promotion, coupled with the company's overall profit objective.

Some of the types of questions that marketing research attempts to answer are described below.

TABLE 129.4 *Selected types of marketing strategies to be addressed through conducting clinical trials*

1. Expansion of available dosage forms (e.g., capsules, tablets, caplets, solutions)
2. Expansion of approved indications (e.g., additional diseases, prophylactic use)
3. Reduction of undesirable aspects of medicine labeling (e.g., removal of a black box around a warning, reduction of a contraindication to a warning)
4. Conversion of a product from prescription to over-the-counter status[a]
5. License-out a specific medicine with a known profile of activity
6. Expansion of number of special patient groups in which the medicine may be prescribed (e.g., children, patients with renal failure)
7. Obtain improved labeling about benefits of a medicine (e.g., state that the risk of cardiovascular adverse reactions is less than with other standard medicines of the same therapeutic class)
8. Expansion of number of packages available (e.g., ampuls, multidose vials, infusion sets)
9. Comparison with a known standard medicine or nonmedicine treatment
10. Demonstration of a particular point for use in advertising
11. Comparison of medicine costs and influence on a patient's quality of life
12. Obtain approval to manufacture a medicine at an additional site or by an additional manufacturer through demonstration of bioequivalence

[a] See reference by Hammes and Ciccone (1985) for details.

TABLE 129.5 *Representative members of a marketing project team for an investigational medicine*

1. Project leader (usually the product manager)
2. Product manager
3. Advertising manager or representative
4. Sales planning manager or representative
5. Professional services manager or representative
6. Physicians who plan marketing-oriented clinical studies
7. Marketing research analyst
8. Copywriter
9. Project leader or representative of the research and development team
10. Project leader or representative of the production team

Before Making New Compounds

1. Which therapeutic areas have a large market size?
2. Which therapeutic areas greatly need medical advances?
3. Which therapeutic areas offer substantial commercial potential for a new medicine?
4. What are the characteristics of a new medicine that would create a major gain in a given therapeutic area?

TABLE 129.6 *Selected types of marketing advantages sought for a new medicine*

A. Improved safety
   1. Less serious adverse reactions (i.e., lower intensity)
   2. Fewer overall adverse reactions (i.e., lower incidence)
   3. Fewer interactions with other medicines
   4. Greater safety in specific populations (e.g., renal compromised, elderly, cardiovascular compromised)
B. Improved efficacy
   1. Faster onset of activity
   2. Longer duration of action
   3. Increased peak effect
   4. Additional clinical or pharmacological activities
   5. More predictable response (i.e., less variability)
   6. Decreased need for concomitant therapy
C. Greater patient convenience or acceptability
   1. Less frequent dosing
   2. Easier to swallow (e.g., film coated, smaller-size capsule)
   3. Easier dosage form to use (e.g., tablet versus aerosol or nasal inhaler)
   4. Easier package to use (e.g., blister pack versus bottle)
   5. Easier storage requirements (e.g., refrigeration no longer necessary)
   6. Improved odor or taste
D. Improved pharmacokinetic profile
   1. More consistent absorption
   2. More predictable metabolism
   3. All patients metabolize the medicine similarly
   4. Preferred distribution pattern (e.g., does not penetrate into the brain)
   5. Preferred route of excretion
E. Greater economic benefits
   1. Decreased direct cost to patient or third-party payers
   2. Decreased length of hospital stay, which saves money for third-party insurers and hospitals
   3. More rapid recovery likely, which allows a more rapid return to work
   4. Decreased costs to institutions for institutionalized patients
   5. Potential savings if traditional concomitant therapies are no longer necessary

TABLE 129.7 *Current sources of published information on pharmaceutical development[a]*

De Haen New Product Survey
Drug Data Report
Inpharma
Investment analyst reports (e.g., Goldman Sacks; Smith, Barney, Harris, Upham, and Co.; Kidder, Peabody, and Co.; Bernstein)
In Vivo
NDA Pipeline
New Drug Commentary
Pharmaprojects
Pharmascope
Pharmaceutical News Capsule
Prospects, Healthcare Forecasting, Inc.
Scrip-World Pharmaceutical News
The Blue Sheet
The Pink Sheet

[a] This is a representative list, not an exhaustive one.

5. What medicines are presently competing in a given therapeutic area? What is their share of that market?
6. What are other potentially competitive companies doing about this therapeutic area? Are there new investigational medicines being evaluated that represent major breakthroughs or advances in this therapeutic area?
7. Is this a new therapeutic area for the company or would it be building on an existing franchise?

The types of marketing advantages sought for a new medicine include those listed in Table 129.6. Some of the sources of published information of investigational medicines under development are listed in Table 129.7.

During the Testing of a New Investigational Medicine

1. What is the desired clinical profile of the medicine (from a marketing perspective) that should be evaluated clinically?
2. How will practitioners use the medicine in actual clinical use?
3. Which of the desired clinical characteristics are essential for the medicine to be successful commercially?
4. If multiple dosage forms or formulations have been prepared and tested, in which order should they be submitted for approval and marketed?
5. What is the range of the anticipated market size for the new medicine? This is based on many factors, including the (1) present market size, (2) market trends, (3) unmet clinical need for an improved medicine, (4) clinical characteristics of the medicine, and (5) technical characteristics of the medicine (e.g., size of pill, taste of medicine).

Prior to, During, and After Launch

1. What tactics and strategies should be adopted to introduce the new medicine?

2. What strategies should be adopted to follow the use and progress of the medicine after it is launched (e.g., use of postmarketing surveillance techniques)?

3. When unanticipated questions arise at any stage of medicine discovery or development, panels of physicians or potential purchasers may be assembled to address the issue (e.g., opinion about a controversial additive; or views about the taste of a syrup among several samples, including those of the competitors).

Sources of Information for Market Research

In order to address these and other questions, the market research staff consults a variety of sources. These include published literature, professional organizations that provide marketing data, surveys and interviews of physicians and consumers, and results of preference tests of flavors or other medicine characteristics. Marketing surveys require consideration of numerous factors (Table 129.8). A number of questions that physicians may be asked are listed in Table 129.9. Research and development personnel should be consulted in the design of marketing surveys and invited to observe the focus groups or other physician interviews to help improve the acceptance of results within the company. Results of these surveys and marketing research are integrated into the overall medicine's development plan through the marketing member on the project team. This member's roles are summarized in Table 129.10.

TABLE 129.8 *Factors to consider in designing a marketing interview*

A. Related to physicians interviewed and their practice
  1. Number of physicians to interview
  2. Choice of physician specialty (or specialties) to interview
  3. Geographical distribution of physicians to be interviewed (e.g., East Coast versus West Coast, city versus rural)
  4. Background of physicians (if desired) in terms of age, training, prescribing habits, and other factors
  5. Number of patients with a specified disease that the physician treats each week, month, or year
  6. Type of practice (e.g., hospital based, solo private practice, group practice)
  7. Selection of physicians interviewed may be made on numerous bases (e.g., with structured or unstructured selection criteria)
B. Related to nature of the interview and data generated
  1. Use of telephone interview versus personal visit or mailed questionnaire
  2. Methods to record data
  3. Methods to analyze data collected
  4. Methods to validate the questionnaire
  5. If interviews are used, what training is necessary for the interviewer?
  6. Determine how the response rate of physicians will be estimated
  7. Determine whether payment will be given to respondents. If so, the amount must be determined

TABLE 129.9 *Selected questions that physicians may be asked in a market research interview[a]*

A. Relating to patients presently in their practice
  1. Type(s) of patients seen
  2. Age range of patients seen
  3. Causes of a specified disease in patients they treat
  4. Frequency of seeing the same patients who have a specified disease
  5. Number of patients seen per day
B. Relating to current methods used for diagnosis and treatment of a specific disease or medical problem
  1. Tests commonly used to diagnose patients
  2. Current treatments used
  3. Rationale for using those treatments
  4. Length of treatment with current therapies
  5. Success rate with current therapies
  6. Usual means of monitoring patients
  7. Degree of dissatisfaction with currently available treatments
  8. Problems with current treatments and changes that would be perceived as improvements
C. Relating to a potential new medicine
  1. Improvements that are desired in a new medicine
  2. Whether a medicine with attributes described by the interviewer would be perceived as an important improvement
  3. Whether a medicine with the attributes described by the interviewer would be used by the physician. If so, in what proportion of his or her patients and in which types of patients?

[a] It is assumed that all questions refer to patients with a specific disease in the physician's practice or clinic.

Market Research versus Venture Research

Market research primarily involves a retrospective analysis of marketing data and information to establish profiles, trends, and characteristics of medicines and therapeutic areas. Market research utilizes historical data when future projections are made. The projections made are often extrapolations of trends and as

TABLE 129.10 *Role of marketing personnel on the project team[a]*

1. Recommend the desired form(s) of the medicine, dose strength (mg), and colors of each dose strength
2. Help determine trade names and provide input into choosing generic names
3. Help determine types of packages (e.g., blister packs, foil samples) and size of packages (i.e., number of tablets per pack or bottle)
4. Coordinate above activities with subsidiaries in other countries or parent company
5. Determine markets to be targeted and in which order
6. Establish needs of physicians through market research
7. Evaluate market sizes; evaluate growth trends of each potential indication
8. Monitor competitive activity
9. Recommend line extensions that are desired
10. Recommend which changes in the package insert would be desirable from a marketing perspective
11. Liaise with other groups in marketing
12. Help instill commercial value in Phase III activities (e.g., recommend quality of life studies, cost-effectiveness studies, and comparisons with standard medicines)

[a] A number of additional roles are listed in Table 121.5.

such have certain limitations, since probable influences of future events are not generally considered.

Venture research is a future-oriented prospective study of evaluating and prognosticating future trends as well as physician needs and desires. Venture research involves physician interviews to establish what information physicians desire in order to make a choice among different medicines of the same therapeutic class. Their responses often differ by specialty, location of their practice, type of practice, age, and numerous other factors. The information from these interviews helps provide answers to several marketing questions that target a new medicine most effectively. Some of these questions are:

1. What information about a new medicine could influence a physician's opinion?
2. How do physicians weigh the various types of information they utilize in choosing a medicine to use?
3. How do physicians obtain information about medicines, and which sources do they use?
4. Do the physicians interviewed prefer to read studies performed by physicians of the same specialty, or is this not an issue?
5. Is the information presented on the characteristics of a hypothetical medicine easily understood by physicians? (The characteristics are those of the investigational medicine.) Would physicians prescribe the new medicine?

Marketing Representatives

An important part of a marketing division is the field staff or marketing representatives. Marketing representatives are the sales force of a pharmaceutical company. They are well trained by their company in the strengths and weaknesses of their products, as well as important selling points. These individuals have become information specialists in recent years and interact with physicians in both private offices and hospitals. Well-trained representatives understand the medical science that underlies their medicine and can help educate physicians about new results relating to one or more areas in medicine, as well as the scientific aspects of the medicines they are promoting. See Table 129.11 for specific functions of sales representatives.

Role of the Product Champion

The product manager in marketing has a role analogous in many ways to the project leader in research and development. The project leader usually shepherds the project from the decision point at which it was decided to study the compound in humans until it is approved for marketing, and possibly longer. In some companies

TABLE 129.11 *Selected functions of pharmaceutical sales representatives*

A. With physicians
  1. Provide information about new products
  2. Provide new information about old products
  3. Provide medical literature and educational materials
  4. Encourage physicians to prescribe certain products
  5. Provide product samples
  6. Help establish and/or monitor clinical studies
  7. Obtain information requested by the physician
  8. Report adverse reactions to the sponsor
B. With pharmacists[a]
  1. Check inventory
  2. Promote over-the-counter medicines
  3. Discuss relevant issues
  4. Encourage pharmacists to dispense the company's products

[a] Most points in part A are also relevant.

a joint research and development plus marketing team is utilized during the transition period. The product manager develops the marketing strategy and approach while the medicine is still undergoing investigation. This includes (1) identifying the target audience that will receive most of the promotion, (2) establishing the position of the product so that it stands apart from the competitors, and (3) determining a promotional platform that remains within the medicine's labeling. He or she also assists in (1) determining the price that will be charged based on a balance of various factors, (2) forecasting the number of units that will be sold during the first year, (3) placing orders with production personnel to make these units, (4) determining the amount of money to spend on promotion and how it will be spent, and (5) planning many other aspects of the medicine's launch and career (see below). This person (or another) represents marketing on the project team. His or her roles include those listed in Table 129.10.

Market Launch of a New Medicine

The market launch of a new medicine is an important milestone in a medicine's life. Planning the various activities involved is important for various reasons, including those listed in Table 129.12. A list of the various activities that may be planned is given in Table 129.13. In addition to all of the activities conducted in

TABLE 129.12 *Selected objectives in planning activities that are part of a market launch*

1. Identify milestone dates
2. Identify decision points
3. Identify activities to be conducted by individual departments or groups
4. Identify the shortest route to a product launch
5. Identify activities in which liaison with production, research and development, and other areas are required
6. Assist in identifying effects of delay

TABLE 129.13 *Factors to schedule and monitor in planning marketing activities to launch a new medicine*[a]

A. Projected milestone events
1. Issue packaging particulars
2. Finalize market plan completed by marketing representative
3. Issue package specifications request
4. Management approves market plan
5. Issue budget schedule
6. Issue production order
7. Develop preliminary launch plan and schedule
8. Review of NDA by FDA and get approvable letter
9. Final pre-NDA approval of market plans
10. Receive FDA approval letter

B. Advertising
1. Determine literature and promotion costs
2. Determine direct-mail costs
3. Contact advertising agency
4. Develop graphic concepts and strategy
5. Prepare preliminary journal costs
6. Submit journal schedule
7. Submit journal advertising proposal
8. Develop and route direct-mail/promotion copy
9. Test and approve journal advertisements
10. Prepare convention panel (mechanicals)
11. Develop promotional layout
12. Prepare advertising film
13. Review and approve journal schedule
14. Route and approve promotional material specifications
15. Prepare and award promotional material bid
16. Print direct-mail and promotional material
17. Have advertising agency send insert order to journal(s)
18. Develop press release
19. Issue press release to trade journal(s)
20. Mail promotional material

C. Management committees, coordinating committees, board of directors
1. Approve market plan
2. Review progress of marketing activities

D. Marketing services
1. Collect and analyze marketing data
2. Prepare initial market plan
3. Conduct focus group interview(s)
4. Request works cost analysis
5. Conduct initial market forecast
6. Request stability studies
7. Issue NDA packaging specifications
8. Determine product and package cost
9. Focus group data analysis
10. Issue product and package pricing
11. Develop final sample package
12. Develop and route package mechanicals
13. Issue packaging particulars
14. Issue packaging specifications request
15. Issue budget
16. Issue production order

E. Marketing product planner
1. Finalize market plan
2. Submit market plan to management
3. Contact wholesale services
4. Contact sales promotion
5. Contact government services
6. Contact hospital services
7. Contact convention department
8. Contact retail services
9. Prepare initial market forecast
10. Prepare preliminary product report
11. Prepare unit forecast
12. Propose budget
13. Request works cost analysis
14. Finalize forecast

F. Production
1. Prepare final packaging specifications
2. Estimate package plan
3. Approve bill of materials
4. Order package components
5. Write manufacturing plan
6. Receive package components
7. Write manufacturing schedule
8. Order printed labels and inserts
9. Receive printed labels and inserts
10. Pass printed labels by quality assurance
11. Manufacture bulk medicine for launch
12. Pass bulk medicine supply by quality assurance
13. Pass package components by quality assurance
14. Schedule and prepare package order
15. Compress tablets or fill capsules
16. Package medicine (e.g., tablets)
17. Pass finished product by quality assurance
18. Ship medicine for launch

G. Medicine regulatory affairs
1. Develop label copy

H. Sales administration
1. Set up market plan
2. Contact medicine distribution data services
3. Develop slide, tape, and video program(s)
4. Develop government promotion
5. Government Service Administration price list addition
6. Develop hospital promotion
7. Track sales information to obtain medicine distribution data
8. Develop medicine distribution report
9. Develop retail promotion
10. Medicine distribution reports to regional sales managers
11. Medicine distribution reports to district sales managers
12. Medicine distribution reports to staff
13. Hospital promotion to sales promotion
14. Medicaid and third-party notification
15. Notification of General Services Administration
16. Set automatic ship quantities
17. Mail launch letter to wholesalers
18. Addition of products to territory planning system
19. Develop territory planning system program

I. Sales promotion
1. Assign detailing positions
2. Develop selling sheet
3. Develop preliminary launch plan and schedule
4. Schedule conventions
5. Develop convention panels for exhibit
6. Develop and produce slide, tape, or video program(s)
7. Draft launch and selling plan
8. Send selling sheet to advertising
9. Route convention panels
10. Review launch and selling plan
11. Produce convention panels
12. Print launch and selling plan
13. Send final insert copy to staff
14. Ship convention panels
15. Send staff launch and selling plan
16. Advise staff of final NDA approval
17. Present slide, tape, or video program to staff

J. Sales training
1. Assessment by training department
2. Prepare disease and product learning unit
3. Issue disease unit to test staff
4. Issue product unit to test staff
5. Send final training unit to staff
6. Revise training unit with approved label

---

[a] Each of these activities requires a start and completion date and an indication of whether it is on the critical path. The *critical path* denotes that (1) other activities cannot be initiated, or (2) the project will be delayed until this activity is completed.

TABLE 129.14 *Preparations in medical and other research and development departments for launch of a new product*

1. Prepare a bibliography of published literature
2. Index the published literature
3. Prepare a list of anticipated questions from physicians and the media
4. Prepare responses to these questions that company personnel may use
5. Train personnel who will provide information to physicians and other health professionals
6. Determine which departments will handle which types of telephone and written questions (e.g., medical questions, marketing questions, orders, complaints)
7. Instruct telephone operators on how to forward calls to the correct departments and individuals

various marketing departments that are planning for, and actually launching, a new medicine, medical departments also participate. Some of their activities are listed in Table 129.14.

Various plans for launching a medicine may be submitted to a decision-making person or group for review and establishment of policy. It is usually important to plan carefully as many launch-oriented events as possible to ensure that they are handled well and take the minimum amount of time. Certain steps (e.g., pharmaceutical manufacturing) may be conducted either before or after the final approval letter is received from the regulatory agency. If the company has received an approvable letter, there may be sufficient assurance that the final approval will be received within a reasonable period and a decision may therefore be made to proceed with full-scale manufacturing.

Medical Groups Within Marketing Departments

Several pharmaceutical companies have allowed their marketing departments to establish and control medical groups that initiate clinical studies. These medical groups are not the company's major medical group or department that investigates new medicines, but are intended to plan, initiate, monitor, analyze, and interpret marketing-oriented clinical studies. These studies include those evaluating (1) a new medicine versus established standard medicines, (2) new formulations, (3) line extensions, and possibly (4) new indications. The primary reason why a company would establish a separate medical group within marketing is that marketing studies have traditionally been given a low priority within medical departments. Thus, medical departments often do not initiate and analyze marketing-oriented studies as rapidly as marketing people would like or expect. This often leads to great frustration within marketing, especially when their top priorities for clin-

ical studies are not accorded adequate priority within the medical department and the studies are not performed, or are greatly delayed.

Conversion of Prescription Medicines to Over-the-Counter Status

When marketing groups have determined that an established prescription product should be converted to over-the-counter (OTC) status, a significant amount of clinical and technical development work must often be conducted within research and development departments. The strategy of converting prescription medicines to OTC status has become more important in recent years and will probably continue to grow, at least for the near future.

Professional OTCs

The group of OTC medicines that were formally prescription medicines has been referred to by some people as "professional OTCs;" such medicines are generally seen by the public as being more sophisticated and contemporary than the long-time traditional OTC products. Professional OTCs are believed by the public to have fewer adverse reactions and to be cheaper than prescription medicines. They are increasingly popular as consumers become more sophisticated and more involved in their own treatment.

TABLE 129.15 *Representative questions sometimes raised about marketing in research and development departments*

1. Are marketing personnel making firm decisions on a medicine's dosage form, color, size, and shape early enough in the medicine's development?
2. Are marketing personnel making too many decisions on a crisis basis?
3. Do marketing personnel understand the implications of their decisions (or of changing their decisions) in terms of hours and months of work by technical professionals?
4. Do marketing personnel communicate their decisions to the right people in research and development?
5. Has the marketing group conducted sufficient market research of the appropriate type to support their decisions?
6. Does the marketplace really change as often as claimed by marketing personnel?
7. When regulatory setbacks occur, why does the marketing forecast always seem to fall so dramatically?
8. Are marketing personnel spending too much time developing marketing forecasts too early in a medicine's development?
9. Are the most appropriate and best-designed market research studies conducted by marketing?
10. Are the above market research studies conducted early enough in a medicine's life, so that the project could be terminated if it was not deemed worthwhile?

SELECTED TYPES OF MISUNDERSTANDINGS BETWEEN RESEARCH AND DEVELOPMENT AND MARKETING PROFESSIONALS

The major reason for the large number of misunderstandings between research and development and marketing staff is that there is usually insufficient professional communication between them. In medium- and large-size companies these departments become quite separated and insulated from each other. In that en-

TABLE 129.16 *Representative questions sometimes raised about research and development in marketing departments*

1. Why do so few research and development personnel understand that the company must make money in order to survive?
2. Why do research and development professionals not involve marketing professionals at the earliest stages of research, in terms of deciding in which therapeutic and disease areas to look for medicines and which compounds to progress?
3. Why do research and development people expect an accurate marketing forecast when they supply so little information about the compound?
4. Why are many research and development people so theoretical and impractical when they talk about medicines?
5. Why do many research and development people go on tangents when they develop new medicines?
6. Why do clinical trials not address and answer more questions?
7. Why are the clinical trials not conducted more efficiently, to save more time?

vironment it is generally easy for rumors and misunderstandings to grow and develop into distrust. Rumors and misunderstandings are danger signs and should be heeded immediately.

A number of comments sometimes heard in research and development offices about marketing are listed in Table 129.15, and those heard in marketing offices are listed in Table 129.16.

Some of the steps that may be taken to diminish these feelings are to (1) encourage more joint activities including retreats, symposia, and social events; (2) appoint a variety of people from both functions to serve on important committees and task forces; and (3) transfer professionals from one of these areas to the other whenever practical.

CONCLUSIONS

In conclusion, each sponsor establishes a marketing strategy for each medicine. In developing this strategy the possible alternatives should be evaluated by comparing them to corporate and marketing objectives, rather than merely comparing the available alternatives with each other. This latter type of comparison is a common trap that may lead a group into choosing a wrong alternative, which may not be consistent with the corporate objectives.

CHAPTER 130

Costs of Clinical Trials, Projects, and Pharmaceutical Development

Although some medicines are highly profitable, many others are not expected to make a profit for the pharmaceutical company that discovers, develops, and launches them. Several studies have reported that only about one-quarter to one-third of marketed medicines ever repay their costs of development (Grabowski and Vernon, 1982; Drews, 1985; Joglekar and Paterson, 1986). Most large and medium-sized pharmaceutical companies receive at least 50% of their sales from one to three medicines (Spilker, 1989a).

TYPES OF COSTS IN MEDICINE DEVELOPMENT

After a medicine is discovered, the costs of new medicine development that are perhaps the most visible are those of clinical trials. In addition to costs of clinical trials conducted during Phases I, II, and III there are numerous other types of costs incurred in medicine development. Most of these are summarized in a few broad categories.

Nonclinical Studies Conducted After Clinical Trials Are Initiated

This category includes most of the toxicology program. If the medicine is to be given chronically, instead of acutely, then there will usually be a need to conduct full 2-year carcinogenicity studies in two species. Advanced studies in pharmacology, biochemistry, metabolism, and other relevant disciplines (e.g., microbiology, immunology) will be conducted during this period, as will most of the technical development activities.

Administrative and Patent Costs

Administrative costs are usually quite substantial in the pursuit of a New Drug Application (NDA) on any new medicine. In many (if not most) cases, these costs do not differ substantially when comparisons are made between medicines intended for rare diseases and those intended for common diseases. This category includes activities of the Regulatory Affairs Department, which has the task of assembling, checking, and submitting Investigational New Drug Application (IND) and NDA documents to the Food and Drug Administration (FDA) and other regulatory authorities. This department remains in contact with the FDA during the review process and even after the medicine is approved and marketed. Adverse reactions and other information on the medicine must be maintained and reports must be submitted to regulatory authorities. There is also significant time spent by managers and other personnel who directly or indirectly supervise and review the progress of the myriad activities necessary to give birth to a new medicine.

Patent Costs

Patent costs may be considered as part of administrative costs. Most patents require periodic fees to maintain their viability. Also, patents must be filed in many countries, even if it is not certain whether the medicine will be eventually registered for sale in any of those countries.

Marketing Costs

Since marketing resources are limited, a suitable amount of promotion and advertising must be determined. Marketing personnel inform physicians about the new medicine, train and educate their own sales force, and provide physicians with promotional materials and information.

Providing Professional Information

Specially trained personnel or regular staff in medical or marketing departments must answer letters and telephone calls from physicians, pharmacists, nurses, and other professionals about the new product. These costs will arise regardless of the market potential of the medicine. A new medicine with limited sales potential that receives a great deal of publicity could generate more requests for information than a medicine with much greater sales potential.

Manufacturing Costs

Activities involved in the synthesis and manufacture of the medicine could raise major issues within a corporation if the manufacturing process required specialized equipment or procedures, or if the needed raw materials are rare or expensive. In some situations it is necessary to build a new plant just to make a single

medicine. A small-volume medicine (small in terms of the number of units sold) may tie up manufacturing equipment and production lines required for other products. For example, the cleaning and preparation of large pieces of equipment, for either (1) the next step in the chemical synthesis or manufacturing process or (2) the next medicine to be made, may represent a time-intensive process. These steps are often complex and costly, and the magnitude (and expense) of the efforts involved are independent of the medicine's eventual use and sales potential.

Other Support Costs

Many other activities must be conducted on an ongoing basis for any marketed medicine, regardless of whether the medicine is for a rare or for a common disease. These activities vary in degree and proportion from medicine to medicine and may also change during the life span of any one medicine. Representative activities include: (1) analyzing blood, urine, or other biological samples for medicine levels; (2) analyzing returned medicine samples to evaluate the amount of medicine present; (3) providing information to pharmaceutical compendia; (4) monitoring the published literature and adverse reaction reports; (5) presenting materials to hospital and state formularies; (6) conducting activities to register the medicine in other countries; (7) providing various types of technical support for the medicine's production; and (8) tracking costs and revenues.

TOTAL COST OF A MEDICINE'S DEVELOPMENT

It is difficult to generalize about the total costs of all efforts and studies necessary to establish safety and efficacy and to bring a new chemical entity to market. There are many factors involved, and at the initiation of the development process there are many known and unknown hurdles for each medicine to overcome. This makes early estimates of total costs for any specific medicine only educated guesses.

Costs Based on Averages of Both Successes and Failures

A number of economists have estimated the costs of developing a new medicine. Rather than averaging a number of actual medicine development costs, these figures are usually derived by taking the entire research and development budgets of a number of companies over a period of years and dividing that total by the number of new medicines launched. Thus, all money spent on medicines that were therapeutic or toxic failures, and all research on the compounds that went nowhere or were the ancestors of new medicines, are allocated to the few eventually successful medicines. This seems to be a fair method for establishing the cost of developing a single new medicine because all of the money attributed to medicine failures was actually spent, and at least some of the costs contributed to the discovery of the new medicine. It would be generally difficult, if not impossible, to differentiate accurately among those costs spent on activities that did or did not contribute to discovering the new medicine.

Using this "fully allocated" technique of summarizing all relevant expenses, the cost of a new medicine in 1976 was calculated to be 54 million dollars. This figure had climbed to nearly 90 million dollars in 1983 (Hansen, 1983), 125 million dollars in 1987, and 231 million dollars in 1990. The determination of this value for any specific company should include consideration of a several-year period because most companies do not introduce new medicines each year. The variation in this figure between companies is probably substantial and is a reflection of their research productivity in discovering new medicines and their ability to develop medicines. Both the numerator (total research and development costs) and denominator (number of medicines discovered) are somewhat complex concepts. A number of considerations that enter into each are listed in Table 130.1. This table illustrates that it is not a simple matter to calculate either the numerator or denominator.

Costs Based on Averages of Only Successful Medicines

The actual ("direct") dollars spent on developing any one specific medicine for the market, after it has been "discovered," are always much less than the large totals given by Professor Hansen and others. Actual amounts spent may vary by orders of magnitude from medicine to medicine and usually range from 2 to 50 million dollars. These costs do not usually include all costs of the research program that might have been spent while searching for many years before a new medicine was discovered.

The money necessary to complete a medicine's development may be estimated (usually excluding factors such as inflation and lost financial interest) at the outset of a medicine's development. The fair market value of outside clinical and nonclinical studies and in-house costs of various aspects of the medicine's development must be established. Knowledge of the number and types of studies required to complete the evaluation of a medicine, plus approximate costs of each, will yield a general total figure. "Fudge factors" are sometimes applied to derive a more realistic estimate that allows for unanticipated problems that invariably develop during a medicine's development. Actual costs of developing a single medicine are often significantly higher than the projected costs established at the initiation of a project. A list of some of the factors to consider in determining costs of a specific medicine are listed in Table 130.2.

TABLE 130.1 *Selected factors to consider when medicine costs are determined by dividing total research costs by number of medicines developed*[a]

A. Total research costs
1. Should all research costs of the subsidiaries of the parent company by included?
2. How many years should be included in the analysis, since too short a period may distort the result?
3. Should some management costs of nonresearch corporate officers be apportioned to research, because of time spent by boards of directors on specific research and medicine development issues?
4. How much computer costs should be allocated to research if they are not part of the research budget?
5. How much of all the other nonresearch costs involved in operating a facility should be considered if they are not included in the research budget?
6. How should inflation be considered in adding costs from different years?

B. Number of medicines developed within a defined period
1. Should only prescription medicines be considered or should over-the-counter medicines be included?
2. Should each separate dosage form marketed be counted separately or combined and counted as only one medicine?
3. Should only new chemical entities be included?
4. Should multiple indications for a medicine be considered the same as one indication?
5. Should a medicine with sales of less than a million dollars per year be considered and counted the same as a highly successful medicine?
6. Should a medicine be counted if it is only introduced into a small country with limited sales and has not yet been approved for sale in an industrialized country?

[a] These questions are intended to illustrate the complexity of the simple ratio and the need to define exactly how the figure is derived. Comparing numbers between companies is fraught with additional difficulties since differences in definitions and accounting practices exist. See Table 130.2 for additional factors.

MONITORING AND BUDGETING PROJECT COSTS

Monitoring Direct Costs of a Project

Costs that are monitored by sponsors include direct costs for clinical trials paid either to investigators or to institutions on their behalf. There are also direct costs of chemical starting materials and various outside grants for toxicology, data processing, or other activities. These expenses are usually captured and reported as a routine matter in most companies.

Capturing Time and Effort Costs

Other costs for projects include the time and effort of the staff at the company developing the medicine. This topic is rather controversial in many companies be-

TABLE 130.2 *Selected factors to consider in answering the question: How much does a specific medicine cost to develop*[a]

1. Should costs of research that lead directly to the medicine be included?
2. Should costs of research on the same therapeutic target that did not lead to the medicine be included?
3. Should costs be included for other research that was not or has not yet been successful but is conducted each year?
4. Should only direct costs be included or should indirect costs of that medicine's development be included?
5. Should relevant overhead costs of management, rent, heat, etc., be included? If not, why?
6. Should costs of all the different dosage forms be included, or only the first one to reach the market?
7. Should costs of developing all line extensions be included regardless of when they were incurred relative to regulatory approval?
8. Should costs of developing line extensions be included if they were being developed while the medicine was investigational?
9. Should costs of trials on new clinical indications be included?
10. Should costs of trials on indications be included if the indications failed? What if trials on other indications were completed before the medicine was successfully marketed for its major indication?
11. Should development costs be included after the medicine was initially launched in the first territory, even though the market size in that territory is extremely small?
12. Should all repetitive costs of medicine development in different countries be included if required by several regulatory agencies? What if the trials are only partly repetitive?
13. Should costs of marketing studies be included if they were conducted prior to launching the medicine? What if the medicine were launched in some countries, but not in all of those where the marketing study results would be used?
14. Should costs of synthesizing additional compounds to protect the patent be included?
15. Should costs of related medicines that were never marketed but assisted in learning about the field and the best investigators, consultants, and other individuals be included?

[a] These questions illustrate the complexity of attempting to determine an accurate figure that simply states the answer to the question. Adding up all the separate costs is not straightforward, even disregarding inflation and other financial questions.

cause of the varying perspectives of different individuals who participate in these exercises. Financial managers are used to, and generally expect, highly detailed reports and itemizations of time and efforts reports, whereas research managers vary enormously in their interest and desire for specific, as opposed to general, information on project costs. Some managers are clearly not interested in evaluating any cost information.

Clinical staff, scientists, and other workers whose time and effort are being monitored often resent the chore of having to complete the necessary forms to capture such data. The more detailed, frequent, and time-consuming the forms, the more the staff can be expected to resent the activity. Shortcuts are frequently used to circumvent or minimize the activity, such as by submitting duplicate or near-duplicate forms for each reporting period.

Clearly a balance is needed between the needs of all of these groups. A different balance is needed in different companies. A system that requires "too much" information demands large amounts of administrative time of both staff and management and will invariably decrease their productivity. On the other hand, management groups that collect little or no information often do not really know what their staff members are working on and how their resources are being allocated to various projects.

Designing Forms to Capture Time and Effort

In designing suitable forms to collect these types of data there are several basic questions to address, including:

1. Whose time and effort will be collected? Is it necessary to collect the time and effort of all clerical and service staff (e.g., data entry operators, librarians), or are those of senior (usually scientific) staff who are directly working in the area of medicine discovery and development sufficient?
2. How frequent is it necessary to collect these data? Most pharmaceutical companies that collect them do so on a monthly or quarterly basis.
3. Who will review these data? Is it strictly for research and development personnel or will it be shared with corporate managers? If so, in what form will it be sent to senior managers?
4. What decisions will be made with these data? They are usually entered in computers and easily summarized and sorted by variables of interest. These include project(s) studied, departmental and divisional effort, periodic and cumulative costs, and other variables of interest. Since the data are available they may be sorted by variables not originally intended or desired by those who established the system.
5. How much data should be collected? Would the proportion of time spent by each individual on each medicine or product be sufficient information? Is it necessary to collect information according to work expended on each major activity on each medicine? The amount of time required to complete such forms accurately increases dramatically as the level of detail increases. The reliability of data may decrease as more are collected, unless adequate measures are instituted to ensure data accuracy. One means of increasing data accuracy is by requiring certain staff to maintain daily diaries of their activities.
6. Should work performed by outside consultants or others who are operating on a contract basis be captured separately? "Contracts" may be utilized within a company for work requested by different

subsidiaries, divisions, or other groups. These data may be collected.

7. What codes could be used to simplify the forms without making them difficult to complete and process?

After these time and effort reports are issued it is possible to conduct various analyses of the results to evaluate changes and trends, or to answer specific questions.

Monitoring Indirect Costs of a Project

The issue of whether the indirect costs of running a research and development organization should be apportioned in some way to the costs of projects will not be discussed here. This is handled differently within each company. These costs include overhead categories such as rent for space, fringe benefits, management costs (corporate as well as research and development), and support services of both a technical and administrative nature. Unless this administrative and technical infrastructure is in place it will be difficult to discover and develop medicines.

Converting Time to Money

Another issue relates to the means by which staff time is to be converted to dollar terms. An average salary of all workers may be used to multiply by the total time expended to determine the total time and effort costs. Alternative approaches are to use classes of workers (e.g., senior and junior, grades 1–4, 5–8, 9–12) with an average salary for each class to compute the value of their separate time totals, or to use each individual's exact salary to calculate their precise time and effort costs spent on each project. The total time and effort spent on a specific project would then be the sum of each individual's total time and effort, plus overhead (if relevant).

Budgeting Costs of a Project

This function should be integrated with the process whereby costs of a project are monitored. There may be a separate individual, group, or department charged with the responsibility for maintaining a harmonious balance among activities monitored. Although medicine development has a long-term horizon, the project manager's budget usually focuses on a 1- to 3-year horizon. Other managers within the corporation may be concerned about a longer time-frame for monitoring costs. In some organizations each project has a budget and the project manager has the responsibility for spending the money in the most efficient way possible.

Part of this manager's performance appraisal is based on how effectively the money was spent. Variations of this approach include having a budget for each project, but assigning the responsibility for its control to an individual other than the project manager.

Many companies have a single sum of money within the research and development function that is allocated to projects according to their requests, priorities, and other considerations. The choice of whether to budget by projects usually depends on the traditions of the company and preferences of the research and development director. The total amount of money available for each project's activities may be specified at the start of each fiscal year. If it is not, then the total research and development budget minus fixed and committed expenses are in general available to be apportioned to projects according to some criteria. In these situations, the company does not create a budget for each project. If the money needed to advance a project's development is generally used up well before each fiscal year is over, however, there may be pressure to institute a project budget. Another choice is to institute more restraints on spending.

COMPETITION FOR INVESTIGATORS

Sometimes a sponsor intentionally does not carefully compare the total cost per patient for a given clinical trial across several potential sites. This may occur if the number of sites that can effectively conduct a particular medicine trial are limited, or when some sponsors enter a bidding war because of limited availability of sophisticated equipment, suitable patients, or qualified and interested investigators. If two or more sponsors are attempting to develop medicines in the same therapeutic area and each requires the services of the few available investigators, most of the "rules" for establishing a fair budget will probably not apply. Some sponsors offer investigators larger budgets than they might offer otherwise in this situation, to delay their competitor's medicine development program.

Some sponsors may conduct a clinical trial that is probably not necessary, merely because they were first to contact the investigator and wish to keep the investigator busy with their trials. Investigators' services may also be acquired through (1) bidding wars, (2) long-term contracts, (3) consultancy arrangements, or (4) other negotiations. "Bidding wars" may also be instigated and perpetrated by investigators. Even if an investigator has a monopoly on conducting trials in a certain therapeutic area because of certain equipment, techniques, expertise, or interest, there may not be any need for these types of undesirable negotiations to occur. For example, the investigator may be able to conduct several long-term trials for different sponsors simultaneously or many short-term trials sequentially (or simultaneously). The investigator would thus not have to "choose" between sponsors. These quasi-unethical practices are not believed to be common.

Sponsors rarely require an academic investigator to work exclusively on their products or new medicines. Indeed, it would not be in keeping with the spirit of academic freedom or integrity to do so. An exception to this principle sometimes occurs in medicine evaluation units established in academic centers or hospitals, which are funded and sometimes staffed by a single sponsor.

COSTS OF A SINGLE CLINICAL TRIAL

Establishing a Fair Market Value for a Single Trial

An investigator or sponsor may estimate the fair market value of a single clinical trial by considering the component parts of the trial. An estimate similar to those shown in Figure 130.1 may be established, although there are many different methods and models for dividing a trial into its components (see Figs. 130.2 and 130.3). A standard form may assist in this exercise but is not a necessity, since there are many ways to develop estimates of a trial's costs. Many companies do not use standardized forms for establishing a clinical budget.

Negotiating the Budget for a Clinical Trial

It has sometimes been said that negotiating the budget for a single clinical trial is similar to buying a used car. The sponsor is not sure of what it is buying, or how honorable the investigator will prove to be in honoring the contract, or what the true value of the product is, or whether a better deal could be had elsewhere. The investigator, too, may feel that he or she is "purchasing the used car" from the sponsor, because it is uncertain how much support will be given, the safety or efficacy of the medicine may be unproven, and the future course of the medicine in clinical development is often an unknown factor.

If a large clinical trial has many centers (e.g., above 50) then it is impractical to negotiate each budget separately. Standards must be established based on fair market considerations that would be applied to each site. If some investigators in hospitals must charge more money for patients because of legitimate costs incurred within their city or hospitals, then an exception can be made to the limit set for those sites, or a lower limit could be placed on the number of patients those sites may enroll.

A letter or formal contract stating each of the points relating to financial matters is desirable. Such a state-

ment should prevent later misunderstandings. Because a sponsor has substantial experience with such matters, these letters or contracts should be relatively complete, including a schedule of when payments will be made, what fractions will be paid each time, and other pertinent details.

A separate letter of the sponsor's principles relating to financial matters may be prepared and given to each potential investigator. This letter would discuss whether the sponsor will compensate the investigator for time spent reviewing the protocol and other documents relevant to the clinical trial and time spent preparing a budget, and it would indicate what information is needed to process the grant and issue a check.

Who Negotiates Budgets?

Pharmaceutical corporations differ in their approaches to the question of who negotiates budgets for clinical trials. Whereas monitors play the leading role in certain companies, others give this authority to regional representatives. Although there is no special prerequisite background necessary to conduct this negotiation, it is important for the individual in charge to have experience or training in the approaches and attitudes of the company toward the various financial issues relating to medicine development.

How Are Funds Dispensed?

After the budget is established, various means of disbursing funds must be considered (Table 130.3). Early payment or receipt of funds may have various consequences vis-à-vis inclusion or exclusion of the money in a particular fiscal year or source of funding, which in turn may have other implications for both payer and payee. Dividing the funds into three or more fractional payments allows the sponsor to encourage continued conduct of the clinical trial, to retain necessary leverage in cases of failure to adhere to protocol requirements, and to collect interest on the balance of the grant during the remaining period. In general, it is important to pay for work completed rather than work promised. One exception is for the initial partial payment, which should be sufficient for the trial to start on a high note, yet not so high as to stunt the investigator's motivation to proceed. In all negotiations, a fair settlement and equitable arrangement should be sought, since no investigator will participate enthusiastically in a trial in which he or she believes the agreement or contract is unfair. Many circumstances change during the course of a trial, and these sometimes present a need to alter a contract during a study to bring it in line with the changed circumstances. Sample

Calculating the Costs of a Clinical Trial

		Cost Per Patient
A. Examinations		
Initial patient history and physical examinations		_____
Abbreviated physical examinations	(No. of exams × cost per exam = $ ___)	_____
Ophthalmological examinations	(No. of exams × cost per exam = $ ___)	_____
Other examinations	(No. of exams × cost per exam = $ ___)	_____
_____		
_____		

B. Laboratory

EKG 12 Lead		_____
EKG Lead II (No. of tests × cost per test)		_____
Clinical chemistry	(No. of tests × cost per test)	_____
Hematology	(No. of tests × cost per test)	_____
Urinalysis	(No. of tests × cost per test)	_____
Other tests	(No. of tests × cost per test)	_____
_____		
_____		

C. Efficacy Examinations

Test 1	(No. of tests × cost per test)	_____
Test 2	(No. of tests × cost per test)	_____
Test 3	(No. of tests × cost per test)	_____

D. Administration

Nurse coordinator	(Percent of fulltime × yearly [monthly or other] salary ÷ n of patients)	_____
Telephone, postage, miscellaneous	(Total cost ÷ n of patients)	_____
	Cost per patient =	_____
University overhead	(X% × cost per patient)	_____

_____
Total cost per patient

Number of patients _____ × Total cost per patient = _____ Total cost of trial.

FIG. 130.1 Calculating costs of a clinical trial.

CALCULATING THE COSTS OF A CLINICAL TRIAL

A

Item	Cost Per Item ($)	Per Patient		Total Cost ($)
		Number Of Tests	Cost ($)	

List Each Point of the Protocol for Which There is a Charge.

B

Item	Cost Per Item ($)	Part A of Trial Per Patient		Part B of Trial				Overall Total Cost
				Screen (n=x)		Trial (n=y)		
		Number Of Tests	Total Cost	Number Of Tests	Total Cost	Number Of Tests	Total Cost	

List Each Point of the Protocol for Which There is a Charge and Total Each Column.

C

Group of Patients	Number of Patients Per Group	Number of Analyses Per Patient	Cost Per Analysis ($)	Total Cost Per Patient ($)	Total Cost Per Group ($)
1	A				
2	B				
3	C				
4	D				
5	E				
TOTAL					

FIG. 130.2 Calculating costs of a clinical trial.

forms that may be used to track financial costs for clinical trials are illustrated in Table 130.4.

Payment of Volunteers

Paying volunteers only if they complete the entire clinical trial places undo coercion on them to remain in the trial even though they may feel too ill to participate. This practice is unethical. Volunteers should be paid based on the amount of the clinical trial they complete, although the money may be withheld until the trial is completed.

If volunteers enrolled in a clinical trial have a highly questionable alcohol or drug history, then there is a greater possibility that they will spend the money they receive for participation in the trial on alcohol or drugs.

Although the manner in which volunteers use their money is not the investigators' concern after the clinical trial is completed, it is a pertinent issue to consider while the clinical trial is underway. The major reason for this concern is that physiological changes resulting from alcohol or drugs could be attributed to the test medicine. Patient status regarding alcohol and drugs may be partially assessed by questioning patients directly, as well as by assessing liver enzymes and other laboratory analytes.

MINIMIZING COSTS OF CLINICAL TRIALS

The major technique for an investigator or sponsor to minimize the costs of a clinical trial is to break down the total financial cost into its components and to ana-

CALCULATING THE COSTS OF A CLINICAL TRIAL

A

Amount

Microbiology Cultures. Number of Cultures Per Patient Per Week
× A Weeks × B $ × C Patients

Pharmacy Fees for Dispensing Medicines and Collecting Returns _____

Salaries

    Research Nurse: A Hours at B $ Per Hour × C Patients _____

    Secretarial Support: _____

    Professional Support: _____

Data Analysis _____

SUBTOTAL _____
OVERHEAD (X %) _____
TOTAL _____
COST PER PATIENT _____

B

Equipment

Individual Patient Costs _____

    Patient Recruitment (Includes Advertising Costs) _____

    Patient Stipend (Includes Meals) _____

    Electrocardiograms _____

    Ophthalmological Examinations _____

    Technical Support (Includes Computer Fees) _____

    Medical Support _____

    Physical Examinations _____

    Clerical Support _____

TOTAL COST PER PATIENT _____
TOTAL TRIAL COST _____

C

	Salary	Benefits	Total Cost
Dr. A. at 25% of Time	_____	_____	_____
Dr. B. at 10% of Time	_____	_____	_____
Office Supplies (Copying, Phone, Typing, etc.)	_____	_____	_____
Professional Travel to One Meeting Each for Drs. A & B			_____
		TOTAL	_____

D

Personnel

    Anesthesiologists (n=A)   X Days at Y $ Per Day

    Recovery Room Nurses (n=B)   X Days at Z $ Per Day _____

    EEG Technician (n=C)   X Days at E $ Per Day _____

    Research Coordinator   H Days at F $ Per Day _____

    Secretarial Assistance   J Days at G $ Per Day _____

    Operating Room Use of Space and Equipment   X Days at K $ Per Day _____

    Operating Room: Supplies and Medicines _____

    Pharmacy Supplies _____

    Laboratory Procedures _____

        Each Listed, Plus Number of Times Performed

        Times Cost, Times Number of Patients _____

TOTAL COST PER TRIAL _____
TOTAL COST PER PATIENT _____

FIG. 130.3 Calculating costs of a clinical trial by multiple methods. A–I represent separate methods that may be used.

E
                                                     Total Cost

Laboratory Assessments
    Itemize — Number Done Per Patient at Cost in $ ———
Clinical Assessments
    Itemize — Cost Per Patient   ———
Personnel Costs
    Research Coordinator Cost Per Patient   ———
    Secretary and Clerical Cost Per Patient   ———
Estimated Costs Per Patient Prematurely Discontinued   ———

                        TOTAL   ———

F

Personnel Costs (% Effort of Each Worker Listed)   ———
Trial Administration Costs (Each Aspect Listed)   ———
Patient Management
    Laboratory Examinations   ———
    ECG Evaluations   ———
    Psychiatric Consultations   ———
    Other Aspects Listed   ———

                        TOTAL   ———
              TOTAL COST PER PATIENT   ———

G
                                  Cost Per Volunteer

Hospitalization
    Beds and Food   ———
Volunteer Payment   ———
Test Procedures (List Each)   ———
Personnel Fees   ———
Overhead (× %)   ———

        TOTAL COST PER VOLUNTEER   ———
            TOTAL COST FOR TRIAL   ———

H

	Cost Per Patient	Total Trial Cost
Screening (X Patients)		
Clinic Visit	———	———
History and Physical Examination	———	———
Laboratory Tests (Specify)	———	———
Special Tests (Specify)	———	———
Baseline Period (Y Patients)		
Clinic Visit	———	———
Laboratory Tests (Specify)	———	———
Special Tests (Specify)	———	———
Treatment Period (Y Patients)		
Clinic Visit	———	———
Physical Examination	———	———
Laboratory Tests (Specify)	———	———
Special Tests (Specify)	———	———
Posttreatment Period (Y Patients)		
Clinic Visit	———	———
Physical Examination	———	———
Special Tests (Specify)	———	———
Personnel		
List Each	———	———
Institution Overhead	———	———
Total Cost Per Patient	———	———
Total Trial Cost		———

FIG. 130.3 (*Continued*)

Cost Per Patient

I (A) Patients Screened But Not Entered:

Initial Visit, Medical History, and Physical Examination _____

Efficacy Assessments _____

Research Coordinator's Fee _____

Laboratory Fees _____

Patient Fees for Meals and Transporation _____

TOTAL _____

(B) Patients Who Complete Screening and Interim Visit:

Initial Visit, Medical History, and Physical Examination _____

Interim Visit Physical Examination _____

Efficacy Assessments (×2) _____

Research Coordinator's Fee (×2) _____

Laboratory Fees (×2) _____

Patient Fees for Meals and Transportation (×2) _____

TOTAL _____

(C) Patients Who Complete the Clinical Trial (Three Visits):

Initial Visit, Medical History, and Physical Examination _____

Interim Visit Physical Examination _____

Final Visit Physical Examination _____

Efficacy Assessments (×3) _____

Research Coordinator's Fee (×3) _____

Laboratory Fee (×2) _____

Patient Fees for Meals and Transportation (×3) _____

TOTAL _____

Estimated Number of (A) Patients _____ × $ _____ = _____

Estimated Number of (B) Patients _____ × $ _____ = _____

Estimated Number of (C) Patients _____ × $ _____ = _____

Estimated Budget Total (A+B+C) _____

FIG. 130.3 (*Continued*)

lyze each component for potential savings. A number of questions to pose for different parts of a trial are described below.

Overall Questions for a Sponsor

1. Would the clinical trial be less expensive if it were conducted in a different country? If the answer is yes, then many other types of costs must be considered to determine whether this is a viable option. This issue is discussed further in Chapter 121 and at the end of this chapter. Also, would the foreign data be accepted by the FDA or other regulatory authorities?

2. Would the clinical trial be less expensive if it were conducted in a small city or less well-known hospital? Expenses in large cities are often greater

TABLE 130.3 *Various means of paying investigators to conduct clinical trials*

1. A lump sum for a clinical trial, regardless of what data are eventually collected
2. Payment only for precisely those tests and procedures actually performed
3. Payment that specifies some or all of the following amounts to be paid for each patient who:
   a. Is screened
   b. Passes the screen
   c. Is enrolled
   d. Completes baseline period
   e. Begins treatment
   f. Completes part of treatment (payments may be prorated based on length of treatment completed)
   g. Completes entire treatment (this period is usually defined as at least a specific proportion of the trial)
   h. Completes follow-up
4. Payment for patients who drop out because of adverse reactions is sometimes given as if they were completed patients
5. Payment for patients who either drop out without reason or are discontinued for lack of cooperation or inadequate compliance is often given on a prorated basis

than in smaller ones. One must be extremely cautious about the approach to this question because of differences in quality of the investigators, conduct of the trial, diagnosis of patients, and many other factors.

Laboratory Evaluations

1. Could the number of different laboratory tests listed in the protocol be decreased without affecting patient safety?
2. Could the number of times each test is requested be reduced without affecting patient safety?
3. Could the tests be conducted at lower cost by an outside laboratory rather than the hospital laboratory, or by a *different* outside laboratory if one is already being used?
4. Could assays for blood or urine levels of the trial medicine be conducted by a central facility rather than at each trial site? If so, is this a less costly

method after including shipping and other costs brought about by this approach?
5. Could a better price be obtained for a trial in which several specialized laboratory studies are to be performed at a single laboratory (e.g., assays of various hormones)? Even if only a single test is being performed, it may be performed on many patients or on many samples of a few patients and negotiations might lead to decreased laboratory costs.
6. Could samples be frozen to analyze for blood levels of the trial medicine at a later date, when specific criteria about the medicine's safety and efficacy are met? If these criteria are not met, then the samples never need to be analyzed.

Safety Evaluations

1. Could an abbreviated electrocardiogram (i.e., lead II) be used rather than a complete 12-lead electrocardiogram for some or all recordings?
2. Could an abbreviated physical examination be conducted at different points in the clinical trial, rather than a complete physical each time a physical is requested? The same question applies for neurological, ophthalmological, and other examinations.
3. Could a trained nurse or other professional conduct certain examinations, rather than the principal investigator or a physician?
4. Could some parts of an examination or test be modified or deleted to save money (e.g., deleting the sleep, photic stimulation, or hyperventilation parts of the electroencephalogram)?

Efficacy Evaluations

Questions similar to those for safety evaluations and laboratory evaluations apply.

TABLE 130.4 *Sample table headings to track financial expenses for clinical trials on a project*[a]

A

Project no. and name	Trial no.	Name of investigator and city	Title of trial	Total no. of patients to be enrolled	Grants budgeted ($)	Grants spent to date ($)	Grants remaining ($)

B

Project and trial no.	Name of investigator	Patient no.	Screen	Baseline	First third of treatment	Second third of treatment	Total treatment	Follow-up	Additional charges	Total cost per patient	Cumulative cost of trial
			Check after completed								

[a] Figure 125.4 contains a form that may be used to monitor grant payments on a single trial.

Trial Design

1. Could the clinical trial be conducted at two or more sites at a lower total cost than at one site (or vice versa)? The decision to use two or more sites for a clinical trial raises many issues, and financial cost is often one of the least important issues. From the point of view of the statistical analyses of data obtained, it is generally preferable to conduct a trial at one site.
2. Could the trial be conducted in outpatients instead of inpatients?
3. Could inpatients be discharged when improved, and continue to receive treatment as outpatients?

Monitoring

1. Could monitors who are based near the clinical site (rather than at a central location) oversee the trial?
2. Could data be transmitted electronically in a cost-effective manner?

Trial Conduct

Would it be cost effective to have the sponsor pay for a full-time research coordinator in terms of (1) having improved rate of patient enrollment because of more efforts expended on this task, (2) increased patient compliance because of greater attention to patient reminders and other details, (3) decreased patient dropouts due to more personal involvement, and (4) more accurate and complete data, because of time to devote to this effort? In certain cases the answer is clearly yes.

Overhead

1. More and more organizations (e.g., hospitals, academic centers, clinics) are including overhead as a separate line item in their budget. The percent used to calculate this value varies enormously and may often be negotiated.
2. Avoid paying overhead on items for which overhead is already built into the price. It is important to determine whether overhead is already included in a charge prior to the application of a general overhead factor.

Other Costs

In addition to financial costs, several other types of costs are associated with many clinical trials. These costs should be considered when the "real" price of a trial is being determined and evaluated.

1. *Lost opportunity costs.* For each trial conducted, there are usually a number of other trials that could have been conducted in its place on the same (or different) medicine. If the medicine actually conducted has little inherent value or fails to answer its objectives, then there is a cost of lost opportunity. Such a cost occurs even though the preferable trial can still be conducted at a later date.
2. *Costs of slow development.* For investigational medicines that are being developed there is a cost associated with the time that the medicine is not available on the market. An actual figure may be determined, based on the time delay and anticipated sales, which in turn is affected by patient need and by competitive advantages of a medicine. If the development process of a medicine is slowed, then costs associated with that medicine will be markedly increased. Another aspect of this issue relates to delays in regulatory reviews.
3. *Costs of additional resources.* There are finite resources available for each project within a sponsoring institution. When these are allocated to one project they are unavailable elsewhere, and if new resources are not obtained the development of other projects would be slowed. To prevent this occurrence, new resources of equipment and staff are sometimes obtained.

CHAPTER 131

Terminating a Project

WHY ARE PROJECTS TERMINATED?

General Reasons for Terminating a Project

Medicine projects are eventually terminated for one of three reasons. The first and best reason is that a project has successfully achieved its objectives [usually New Drug Application (NDA) approval] and the reasons for its existence no longer exist. The second reason is that the medicine may have failed to meet its objectives, usually because of toxicity or lack of efficacy, and the project is terminated. In this case the project itself may be viewed as successful if it efficiently revealed the medicine's negative characteristics in a timely fashion. The third and least frequent reason is that the project itself may have failed to meet its objectives, but the medicine may still be viable and may be taken over by a new project group or it may be licensed to another company for development.

When Is a Project Deemed Successful?

In the case of the pharmaceutical industry, the successful end of a project may be viewed as the time of (1) submission of an NDA to the Food and Drug Administration (FDA), (2) approval of the NDA by the FDA (and subsequent launch), or (3) sales of a medicine that pay back the money invested. There are pros and cons to each of these three definitions and no clear reason why only one definition should be used as a yardstick for measuring success of all medicines. It is the author's view that approval of the NDA or other regulatory application(s) by regulatory authorities and launch of the medicine should usually be considered as the point at which the project may be stated to have attained success. In addition, the timely termination of an unsuccessful project, for whatever reason, is also a successful end to a project.

The Importance of Viewing Projects Objectively

It is important to view projects objectively, because it assists in the process of reaching a dispassionate decision to terminate them at the appropriate time. When one or more senior managers have vested their reputations in a medicine's success, they sometimes exert pressures to keep the project alive past its realistic time of demise. Sponsors are sometimes unwilling to accept the obvious truth about a medicine's likelihood of success, and often resort to progressively less probable scenarios of how the medicine can be shown to be active and worth marketing.

Benefits in Terminating an Unsuccessful Project

Numerous benefits accrue to a sponsor when an unsuccessful project is terminated expeditiously. These include: (1) resources become available to use on other projects, (2) staff morale generally improves as new challenges emerge and problems from what may be an albatross around the corporate neck are shed, and (3) the terminated project is disassembled and future costs are saved. If there is a back-up medicine or medical device candidate to study, then most or all of the experiences plus contacts with investigators and consultants will be useful for investigating and developing the new medicine or device. Lessons learned from the terminated project may often be applied to ongoing or new projects, especially to those in the same therapeutic area.

WHEN TO TERMINATE A PROJECT

Specific Reasons for Terminating a Project

Although the major reasons for project termination usually relate to safety and efficacy, there are numerous other reasons. An unacceptable pharmacokinetic profile may be sufficient grounds for termination (e.g., inadequate medicine absorption, inadequate medicine half-life), as would the inability to solve problems of technical development (e.g., inadequate formulation in terms of dissolution). Patent or regulatory difficulties that cannot be resolved are additional reasons for project termination. Nonetheless, agreements between two or more companies on patent issues may sometimes resolve what would otherwise be difficult or impossible issues to circumvent. Two other reasons for terminating a project include (1) changes in medical practice that make the project medicine or device obsolete and (2) new products on the market that make the project medicine or device noncompetitive.

Safety Reasons

The least controversial reason for terminating a project usually relates to safety considerations. If unexpected (or even expected) toxicological findings of a significant nature occur in animal studies that are not acceptable to patients and physicians from a benefit-to-risk consideration, and there is a reasonable possibility of these occurring in humans, there may be great pressure to terminate the project. Even when no human cases have been reported and the possibility of observing a severe toxic effect in humans is totally unknown, the project is usually terminated.

Projects may also be terminated for occurrence of toxic events (adverse reactions) in humans. Many severe adverse reactions are not acceptable, if observed in humans. The major criteria used to judge the implications of a severe adverse reaction that occurs in humans are: (1) How severe is the reaction? (2) What are the clinical repercussions? (3) What is the incidence of the event? (4) What are the risk factors? (5) Can it be predicted? (6) How safe are alternative treatments? (7) How severe is the disease being treated? (8) What is the therapeutic index (dose at which a toxic effect is noted, divided by the minimal therapeutic dose)? Overall, how is the benefit-to-risk ratio affected by the adverse reaction?

Efficacy Reasons

Another reason for terminating projects involving new medicines is a lack of efficacy determined in well-controlled clinical trials. One difficulty with terminating a project as a result of inadequate efficacy is that there are usually individuals who claim that if the medicine were tested under other conditions there is a likelihood that it would be active. Such situations may rarely be clearly predicted. In addition, some patients may benefit from treatment, but they may represent a small proportion of the total patient population and cannot be readily identified with objective measures prior to treatment.

Actual Reasons for Project Terminations

Prentis and Walker (1986) reported that seven United Kingdom pharmaceutical companies tested 197 New Chemical Entities in humans for the first time during a 17-year period (January 1, 1964 to January 1, 1981). Of these compounds 35 (18%) were marketed by early 1984, and 25 (13%) were still in development. The balance (137 compounds) were terminated. The reasons for termination were adverse reactions (7%), toxicity in animals (6%), lack of efficacy (16%), pharmacokinetic reasons (34%), and miscellaneous reasons (6%). The percents given are calculated based on the total number (197) of compounds studied. Prentis and Walker point out that the high percentage of failures attributable to pharmacokinetic reasons reflects the specific therapeutic areas of the medicines in the sample. Antiinfective medicines accounted for 42% of the data base. When all of the values were recalculated excluding antiinfectives, the category of pharmacokinetic reasons decreased to 25%.

Preventing the Lazarus or Phoenix Project Syndrome

Setting minimal standards in advance for the project to reach will assist the decision to terminate, and avoid the ''what if'' game that is sometimes used to keep projects alive long after their effective demise. These projects are sometimes referred to as ''Lazarus'' or ''Phoenix'' projects, because of the hopes of their champions for the project's eventual resurrection.

Methods to Facilitate Project Termination

Certain techniques facilitate the termination of projects. One of the most important is to establish minimum requirements at the outset of a project to continue development of a project. If these standards are not met then there are grounds for terminating the project. Unfortunately, life is rarely that simple and all of a project's goals are seldom totally met or unmet. Some goals will probably be achieved or at least partially achieved, and others will not be met. As the medical characteristics of an investigational medicine change, so too does the marketing assessment of where the medicine may be successfully positioned in the market and how well it is expected to do financially. If the therapeutic value of a medicine is diminishing, at a certain point it will become unreasonable to pursue the medicine's development because of the minimal commercial potential in comparison with actual and projected costs to develop and market the medicine. An important technique to facilitate the termination of a project is to involve the people in the decision-making process who will be affected by the project's demise. By discussing the rationale and benefits of termination, the group is more likely to agree with and support the decision.

Improving the Status of a Medicine with a Marginal Efficacy or Safety Profile

There are many cases when it is not obvious if a project should be terminated or continued. It is important to guard against too rapid a termination of a project when the consensus of opinion is starting to turn against a medicine's potential for success, when some important questions have not been answered. It is possible to reduce the resources and efforts expended while the last remaining questions are addressed.

A medicine with a marginal efficacy or safety profile may or may not be able to be converted into a worthwhile medicine from medical and commercial points of view. A number of considerations that potentially may increase the therapeutic ratio of a medicine are given in Table 131.1. Some of these are intended to improve either efficacy of safety.

ALTERNATIVES TO TERMINATING A PROJECT THAT HAS PROBLEMS

Sometimes it is not clear that a project should be terminated but the original expectations are not being met. There is usually a desire to do "something." That "something" may be:

1. Convene a panel of internal and/or external consultants to review the data and perhaps suggest

TABLE 131.1 *Selected considerations that could increase the therapeutic ratio of a medicine*

1. Decrease the dosage to find the minimal effective dose
2. Modify the schedule of dose administration (e.g., use b.i.d. instead of q.d. dosing to reduce peak concentrations of the medicine in blood)
3. Change the route of administration (e.g., use a slow-release depot)
4. Have patients use another medicine concomitantly (e.g., to potentiate effects, reduce adverse reactions)
5. Use a more relevant patient population to evaluate the medicine (e.g., medicine naive, mildly ill rather than severely ill patients, severely ill rather than mildly ill patients)
6. Pursue a different indication where efficacy may be demonstrated at a lower dose
7. Determine whether an adverse reaction that is commonly observed may be used as a therapeutic goal for a new indication (e.g., sedation that is undesirable for one medicine may be used as a goal to develop the medicine as a sleep-inducing agent, emesis could be used as a goal to develop a new emetic agent)
8. Have patients take the medicine with or after meals to decrease the rate of medicine absorption

alternative development paths, clinical trial designs, formulations, indications, and so on.
2. Deemphasize the project in terms of priority and resources, while allowing it to proceed at a slower pace.
3. Redefine the objectives and redirect the project in a new direction. At some point, however, it is not fruitful to continue developing a medicine that is "looking for a disease."
4. Put a new leader on the project and possibly several new members on the team as well.
5. Reassess the feasibility of the project and the indication(s) being pursued.
6. Have an independent audit performed of specific questions relating to the project.
7. Solicit ideas for revitalizing the project.
8. Attempt to increase the therapeutic ratio (see Table 131.1) if that ratio is low.

In seeking to perform some of these steps it may become apparent that saving the project would be unwise and a more confident decision may then be reached to terminate it. It is often more palatable for a team to recommend termination than for one person to do so. Reasons for termination are usually based on failure to meet established criteria.

Extracting Lessons From a Terminated Project

When a project is terminated for negative reasons it is usually valuable to extract the lessons learned and to make them part of the institutional memory by writing them in a formal report. Collections of such lessons may provide valuable education for relevant new individuals who join the institution, and also for project leaders.

CHAPTER 132

Dissemination of Clinical Trial Results to Medical Practice

Most investigators who have completed a major clinical trial and have found a positive effect believe that the results should affect medical practice. These individual(s) usually publish their work and wait for changes in medical practice to occur. However, changes in medical practice rarely occur after a single publication, and if they do, a period of time is often required. This chapter describes a number of methods used by investigators and sponsors of clinical trials to increase the likelihood that their trial will significantly affect medical practice.

WHY IS DISSEMINATION OF CLINICAL TRIAL RESULTS SO CRITICAL?

Lack of Agreement Between Results and Medical Practice

During the early and mid-1980s, numerous well-designed and well-controlled randomized clinical trials were conducted to explore the treatment of patients who had had a myocardial infarction. The data clearly demonstrated that aspirin or beta-receptor antagonists saved patient lives when given after hospital discharge, whereas antiarrhythmic medicines and calcium channel blockers did not. Nonetheless, in most European countries, the former two treatments were little used, and the latter two treatments were much more widely used. This example in one therapeutic area (out of several that could be used) shows that the importance and relevance of clinical trial results are often not reflected in medical practice.

Why Clinical Trial Results and Medical Practice Often Do Not Agree

Clinical trial results and medical practice often do not correspond because of inadequate dissemination of the trial's results: individuals or groups with vested interests may block or challenge the newer results for personal or political reasons. Professional reputations based on the original treatment, on commercial gain, or on other motives can also interfere. More commonly, inadequate dissemination probably results from too little effort (with too few methods) to disseminate the results of a trial.

Incorporation of Clinical Trial Results Into Medical Practice

The present system of disseminating clinical trial results is largely uncontrolled and haphazard. Few studies have evaluated how well or how poorly clinical trial results are disseminated and affect medical practice. A brief review is presented by Furberg (1989). Most clinical trial results have little impact on medical practice, but of those that do, an S-shaped curve is a likely model (Fig. 132.1) to describe how incorporation occurs over time. At a certain time point (see arrow) there is a rapid increase in acceptance of a new technology or medicine. The period prior to that point may be relatively short or long, depending on many factors.

Over the last few decades, the results of some clinical trials have clearly had a rapid impact on medical practice that is not characterized by the S-shaped curve. These trials appeared to have had almost instant acceptance, but they probably represent rare exceptions to the rule.

Abandonment of Specific Medical Practices

Finkelstein and Gilbert (1985) evaluated the decline in use of eight medicines between 1964 and 1982. The pattern of abandonment did not fit an S-shaped curve, but demonstrated precipitous declines in use. This suggests that the patterns of abandonment and uptake of new technologies differ, though these eight medicines could also be exceptions to a general principle. It is possible that the precipitous declines in their use occurred because the new data from clinical trials were unequivocal and showed that severe problems were present. If the problems associated with a medicine were minor, an S-shaped decline curve would probably apply.

METHODS TO DISSEMINATE CLINICAL TRIAL RESULTS

An overall plan or strategy is essential to the goal of effectively disseminating a clinical trial's results. (Table 132.1 lists some specific methods.) The basic elements of this plan are to (1) identify the major group(s) that should be targeted, (2) discuss the possibility of editorials in major journals with the editors, (3) decide which other mechanisms in Table 132.1 are to be followed, and (4) obtain the funds and resources to accomplish these tasks.

Physician Characteristics That Affect Use of New Ideas

Some kinds of physicians are more receptive to new results or new medicines than are others. Physicians in medical specialties are reported to be more willing on average to modify their practice than are general

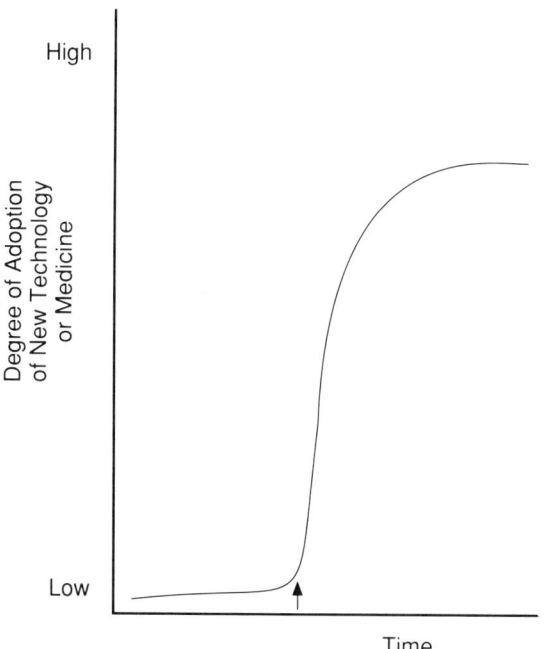

FIG. 132.1 S-shaped model of dissemination of a new technology or medicine into medical practice. The arrow indicates the point of rapid acceptance. The slope of this curve as well as its plateau height will vary greatly for different technologies or medicines that are accepted. Unaccepted technologies or medicines have a flat line near the abscissa, and resemble a terminal electroencephalogram.

TABLE 132.1 *Selected methods for disseminating clinical trial results*

1. Publication in specialized and/or general medical journals
2. Press releases to numerous types of media
3. Interviews of the principal investigators
4. Presentations at society and other professional meetings by thought leaders and other respected speakers
5. Special conferences and workshops
6. Publication of workshops
7. Consensus meetings
8. Publication of consensus meetings
9. Lecture tours by opinion leaders
10. Editorials in medical journals
11. Advertisements in major journals
12. Articles about results of a clinical trial in throwaway journals
13. Letters sent to all practicing physicians

practitioners. The age of physicians targeted is another factor: younger physicians are usually more willing to try new medicines and approaches. Physicians who have more ingrained views usually require more time and more convincing data before they are willing to modify their behavior.

The milieu of the medical practice environment (e.g., solo practice, small group practice, large group practice) often influences the speed of data dissemination. Physicians who practice with more colleagues generally learn about new results more rapidly and engage in more discussions on the pros and cons of such results.

Formats Used in Presentation of Data

The formats used to present clinical data in publications and reports often play a major role in how these data are viewed and whether they are accepted. The reader's interpretation of results is greatly influenced by the parameters or tests used (as well as the magnitude of change or difference between groups) to illustrate results. The type of table, graph, or figure used may also greatly impact the reader's interpretation. A recent book, *Presentation of Clinical Data* (Spilker and Schoenfelder, 1990), illustrates a large number of formats of differing qualities and uses.

Obtaining an Official Imprimatur

Important information about a clinical trial may reach more practitioners if it has the stamp of approval of a major society or organization. Well-respected experts may be brought together to discuss a topic for the purpose of creating a consensus statement. This consensus would then be widely distributed to major journals for publication and copies could be sent to those on various membership lists of professional societies.

Press Conferences

Investigators may call a press conference to announce the results of their latest clinical trial. This approach is usually highly frowned on by most professionals, unless the press conference is called under the aegis of a government agency or professional society. Depending on the newsworthiness of the story, a public announcement may lead to headlines in the news and medical media (plus television coverage), which in turn may lead to major changes in medical practice. Alternatively, the press conference may only cause reporters to complain about their wasted trip.

Additional Methods

For individuals or organizations with a significant amount of resources, or power to influence resources, numerous processes will increase the dissemination of clinical results. These methods include encouraging (1) an international symposium or conference on the topic(s) of interest, (2) plenary or other sessions mounted by professional societies at their annual meetings, (3) an international or national panel that will review the data or topic of the trial and arrive at a consensus, (4) supplements to major medical journals that publish meeting results, (5) satellite transmission of major meetings to hospitals and academic centers worldwide, and (6) editorials and news articles in medical journals, magazines, and newspapers.

HOW TO ASSESS THE IMPACT OF CLINICAL TRIALS ON MEDICAL PRACTICE

Factors Affecting Sales of a Medicine

Pharmaceutical companies hope that positive clinical trials conducted with their medicines (both investigational and marketed) will eventually have a positive impact on medical practice and will then result in increased sales. If a medicine's sales were at a plateau when important results of a clinical trial were promulgated, then it would be reasonable to ascribe additional sales over a defined period to the publication of results and dissemination by sales representatives, advertisements, and other means, if all other factors did not change. Of course, advertisements and increased efforts by sales representatives would probably have an effect on sales independently of the new publication.

The above situation is too simplistic to be a common occurrence. Many additional factors affect a medicine's sales, such as seasonality of the disease, intensity of the competition, new competitive products, new formulary practices to include or remove the medicine, regulatory actions, media reports, professional image of the medicine, other publications, and so on. Are there accepted methods to deal with these complexities of influencing a medicine's sales?

Methods to Evaluate the Effects of Enhanced Promotion

The first method is to evaluate the promotion of clinical trial results in a hospital. A number of hospitals that have similar patient populations may be identified and randomly divided into two groups, and a prospective study conducted. One group would continue to receive the same attention from the sales representatives, while in the other group, an intense promotion of the clinical trials' results would be conducted. The impact of a 2- to 6-month promotional effort may be followed by monitoring patient discharge medications and pharmacy sales within hospitals.

A retrospective study may be conducted within a number of hospitals; the same general assessment methods are used to evaluate the impact of the clinical data. Because of the large number of confounding factors inherent in this type of study, it would be impossible to reach as strong an interpretation as when using the prospective design. Nonetheless, changes in prescribing habits may be assessed using a retrospective analysis.

GROUPS THAT HELP TO CHANGE MEDICAL PRACTICE

Pharmaceutical manufacturers and other commercially oriented groups attempt to influence medical practice in favor of their new products. Marketed products are sometimes found to have clinical benefits that were originally unknown or were not accepted as valid. A commercially oriented group is often unavailable to pay for widespread dissemination of medical information about these benefits. Once important benefits of a new (or old) commercially valuable (or not) treatment is established, a variety of groups should play a role in changing medical practice.

Scientific Journal Editors. Scientific and clinical articles about newly discovered benefits or underutilized treatments are important sources of state-of-the-art information. Editorials, especially in prestigious journals, can be extremely important in influencing medical practice.

Professional Societies. Medical societies of all types are in a good position to evaluate the weight of evidence regarding new treatments. When they are convinced that modifying medical practice is correct, they should state this conclusion along with their reasons and the evidence to their members and to others via appropriate channels (e.g., journals, letters, press releases).

Media. Many types of media outlets may be used and many types of stories disseminated. Reaching patients with both objective and subjective stories will often lead to requests for important new treatments or information about these treatments from physicians. Reaching physicians either will encourage them to seek additional information on potentially relevant changes for their practice or will make them more receptive the next time information on the topic in question crosses their desk or is presented at a meeting.

Government Agencies. Branches of the National Institutes of Health, Centers for Disease Control, and other agencies in the United States, plus similar agencies in other countries are generally impartial and use the highest standards in judging new treatments. They usually provide well-respected opinions in cases of new treatments that influence medical practice.

Medical Societies with a Large Number of Lay Members. Medical societies with lay members create public awareness of their beliefs and sometimes agitate to bring about change in medical practice. They also are able to reach a large proportion of the relevant patient population who are to be treated.

Consumer Groups. Consumer groups include a variety of organizations of vastly different qualities and agendas. Some have the reputation of being loose cannons, but even they occasionally provide valid data.

Trade Associations. Pharmaceutical trade associations do not promote specific treatments, but do promote the atmosphere in which the seeds of information will fall on fertile soil and germinate.

Peer Pressure and Discussions at Local Medical Societies. Peer pressure is often the major influence on a physician's prescribing habits. Peers include friends, business partners, colleagues, and speakers at meetings.

Sales Representatives of Pharmaceutical Companies. Pharmaceutical sales representatives are often extremely important in influencing the prescribing habits of physicians. Their training has greatly improved over the last decade and they are treated as more credible information purveyors than in the past.

DEVELOPING A COORDINATED PLAN

Any of the groups described above that are truly committed to bringing about change in medical practice will attempt to influence the other groups. A well-orchestrated activity can have a large multiplier effect and create a bandwagon type of reaction. If the changes sought are not based on solid state-of-the-art clinical trial methods and data, then challenges will invariably be raised to question the validity of the claims. A poorly developed plan for attempting to influence medical practice or a plan based on insufficiently strong data will generally backfire, as some pharmaceutical companies found in the 1980s. The medicines were either inadequately evaluated or selected information on adverse reactions was suppressed.

EXAMPLES OF WORTHLESS TREATMENTS THAT WERE WIDELY DISSEMINATED AND TOUTED

Inadequately tested treatments and results of clinical trials that are not sound must not be allowed to be disseminated widely with fanfare and hoopla. Otherwise, the practice of medicine will be inundated with worthless treatment and fads.

Medical Treatments That Were Adopted Too Rapidly

Just as there are horror stories reported in the press of many needless deaths because of delayed acceptance of new medical treatments by physicians, regulatory authorities, or others, there are also similar horror stories of medical treatments that were adopted too readily. Medical treatments that were accepted without adequate testing include (1) the use of diethylstilbestrol (DES) to prevent premature abortion, (2) irradiation of the tonsils, (3) use of hyperbaric oxygen in children with respiratory distress, (4) freezing of gastric ulcers, and (5) a large number of surgeries that are now rejected (e.g., ligation of the internal mammary artery to treat angina).

Severe diseases for which adequate treatment does not exist have always attracted extravagant claims for cures or improved treatments that have been proved false [e.g., laetrile for cancer, krebiazin (vitamin B_{13}) for cancer]. These treatments have rarely survived the rigors of appropriate clinical tests. It is interesting that society recently entered an era in which scientifically and medically questionable treatments for acquired immunodeficiency syndrome (AIDS) were promulgated. Many treatments for AIDS were being evaluated with poor clinical trial designs and controls. Data obtained in some of these trials was not of the same high standard as those obtained in well-designed and controlled studies, and the "effectiveness" of some of those early treatments was shown to be a false-positive result. Unless high methodological standards are used to evaluate medical treatments, society will be placed in a position of having patients use ineffective medicines for serious diseases.

FACTORS THAT STIMULATE OR INHIBIT THE USE OF MEDICAL INNOVATIONS

Factors that would increase the use of medical innovations (A. Tarlov, personal communication) are listed:

1. *Admission criteria for medical school.* Individuals who should be favored for admission are those who are experimental, innovative, and willing to take risks during their careers.
2. *The learning environment.* In medical schools, teaching hospitals, and community hospitals, the learning environment should encourage the application of new techniques and procedures in medical practice.
3. *Uncertain efficacy.* The level of uncertainty or untested hypotheses that operates in ordinary medical practice encourages the use of medical innovation.
4. *Hopeless disease.* Nontraditional innovations are often acceptable and are frequently encouraged for conditions that are regarded as untreatable, terminal, or hopeless.
5. *The objectives of the medical profession.* The ultimate enemy in medical practice still is death. In the latter part of the twentieth century, the primary objectives of the medical profession in America remain to prevent disability and death. As a result, these objectives encourage the relaxation of conservative standards of practice and encourage the application of experimental innovations.
6. *Physicians' status.* Physicians with the highest status within the profession tend to be those who use high technology.
7. *Specialization.* Specialization and subspecialization in medicine and surgery also favor the application of new innovations.
8. *Medical journalism.* In December, 1983, a 5-minute film was shown on a San Francisco television station on the subject of mitral valve prolapse in women. Middle-aged women with certain symptoms were urged to see their physicians and have an echocardiogram done. The Kaiser Family Foundation monitored the subsequent rate of use of echocardiography in middle-aged women in the six counties around San Francisco. It determined that the rate of echocardiography increased threefold and was sustained at that high level for about 3 months before gradually returning to the baseline rate over the course of the next 5 months.
9. *Supplier influences.* Pharmaceutical companies and manufacturers of medical technology encourage physicians to adopt the latest innovations.
10. *Other factors.* The availability of high technology and the subsidization that hospitals provide doctors and their practices (for example, by amortizing expensive equipment) favors the application of medical innovations. Hospital administrators sometimes pressure physicians to use available and expensive equipment. The fee-for-service system favors the application of new medical technologies. Physician density results in increased competition for patients and encourages the use of sophisticated and innovative technologies.

These factors do not affect use of new technologies equally in all countries.

PROBLEMS ENCOUNTERED IN THE DISSEMINATION OF CLINICAL TRIAL RESULTS

The Game of "Telephone"

Some clinical trials are unduly praised or criticized as their results become more widely known in the medical community. The spread of information about a clinical trial is sometimes similar to the game of telephone, in which someone whispers a word, phrase, or sentence to someone, and that person in turn whispers the same statement to another person. This process continues through a number of individuals and the last person states aloud what he or she was told. It is invariably quite different from the original statement. This phenomenon occurs even when each person in the chain is doing his or her best to prevent distortion. The longer the message, the greater is the distortion in most cases.

Openness and Honesty

Physicians in general practice and elsewhere are becoming more skilled in their critical review and analysis of new information. Any group that wishes to change medical practice must convince physicians that the information being disseminated is (1) true, (2) convincing in regard to the point(s) made, and (3) relevant for the medical practice of the audience. If the value of the material being disseminated is insubstantial and incomplete (i.e., facts of importance withheld), then a backlash can be expected. Physicians who are promised more than is delivered are not easily taken a second time and become skeptical, if not cynical. This point is particularly relevant for pharmaceutical company sales representatives who attempt to influence medical practice by accentuating positive and eliminating the negative information about a new medicine. Both openness and honesty are in everyone's interest when attempting to influence the dissemination of clinical data to affect medical practice. Boissel (1989) also discusses numerous problems and issues of disseminating data from clinical trials to medical practice.

CHAPTER 133

Future Directions and Goals for Clinical Trials

INTRODUCTION

Some of the goals discussed in this chapter are realistic and readily attainable, but others are more theoretical and represent an ideal goal. Ideal goals are important to discuss because they may be used as beacons to guide and illuminate the correct path to follow in clinical trials. Goals may also be discussed in terms of short-term or long-term objectives. Most of the goals described are widely accepted by individuals involved with clinical trials and should be used as guides to affect medical practice when future clinical trials are designed, conducted, processed, analyzed, interpreted, published, and disseminated. This chapter discusses a few points of each of these seven aspects of clinical trials.

Standards for Conducting Clinical Trials

Standards of clinical trials today, compared with trials of the 1950s and 1960s, have been increased primarily by government regulations, which in turn were enacted because of public pressure. Future increases in clinical standards will hopefully come from those individuals involved in their planning and conduct rather than as a result of new regulations. Other sources of pressure that can force standards higher are journal editors and institutional ethics committees. Roles and importance of the major groups that influence standards are discussed.

DESIGN ISSUES WITHIN SINGLE CLINICAL TRIALS

The major problem in the clinical trial design arena is that suitable designs are not always utilized by investigators. Poorly designed or conducted trials virtually never yield convincing data, and patients who have participated in those trials, as well as the society that condoned those trials, have not received the full benefit for efforts and money expended. The net result of most such trials is negative (i.e., problems outweigh benefits), and the trial should be viewed as unethical. Many such unethical clinical trials may be identified prior to their initiation. It is the responsibility of ethical committees that review clinical trials to prevent the initiation of those trials that do not meet appropriate standards. A number of these weak or flawed aspects of clinical trial design are mentioned here. The particular items chosen include some that are rarely evaluated today (e.g., degree of compliance, validity of the trial blind), but will hopefully be more widely measured in the future.

Use of Open-Label (Uncontrolled) Clinical Trial Designs

There are extremely few instances in which an open-label clinical trial design is appropriate. In most instances, an open-label trial has a high likelihood of yielding false-positive results, which often creates the need for further expenditures of time, effort, and money before the true clinical situation is demonstrated and understood. Appropriate uses of open-label designs include long-term continuation studies, especially when initiated after a double-blind controlled trial of shorter duration, Phase I dose-ranging or other safety trials conducted in patients rather than volunteers, and certain pharmacokinetic trials. Open-label trial designs should not be used in Phase I trials conducted in volunteers, Phase II pilot trials, Phase II pivotal trials, or any other type of trial in which it is ethically, medically, and practically possible to use a double-blind design to achieve more reliable data.

Planned Use of an Inadequate Number of Patients

The planned use of an inadequate number of patients and the statistical concept of power are closely connected. This problem differs from the situation in which an adequate number of patients is planned, but an inadequate number is actually enrolled. Use of an inadequate number of patients often leads to an erroneous result, either false positive or false negative. Even if these results are eventually confirmed, the original data are usually unable to convince other clinicians.

Failure to Evaluate Patient Compliance

The concept of evaluating patient compliance in all appropriate studies is not yet widely accepted as important or essential. Understanding compliance, however, is essential to interpret data fully from most trials. Failure to evaluate patient compliance during a clinical trial may lead to a myriad of problems in interpreting data. For example, it is often critical to know

whether patients who did poorly in a clinical trial had problems with compliance and whether improving compliance would have improved their results. Another reason to measure compliance is to learn how it may be improved through various means (e.g., divided doses, skip doses, initiate medicine holidays, use film-coated tablets, make smaller capsules). Measuring compliance in most clinical trials will undoubtedly become an accepted standard in future years.

Failure to Validate a Clinical Trial's Blind

The degree that a trial's blind is maintained throughout a clinical trial is even less often evaluated than is patient compliance. Evaluating the integrity of a trial's blind, however, is slowly becoming more widely practiced. Clinical trials are not simply double blind, single blind, or open label. Rather, there is an entire gradient within the category of double-blind (or single-blind) trials, from those in which the blind was broken in all cases (i.e., no blind existed in practice) to those in which the integrity of the blind was completely maintained in all patients. The degree to which a blind is maintained often has a profound effect on data obtained and the interpretation of those data. It is currently both possible and important to validate the quality of a clinical trial's blind and to publish this result along with those of the study itself.

Inadequate Number or Type of Control Groups

When case-control or historical control designs are used, a single control group is often identified. One control is frequently insufficient to obtain the strongest possible results. In most situations, it would be preferable to obtain data from multiple control groups. Although more effort, time, and money are required to evaluate multiple control groups, the benefit in terms of obtaining more convincing data usually justifies the additional resources. If large automated data bases are used to obtain data (e.g., in Phase IV studies), identification of additional control groups is often a relatively easy exercise. Nonetheless, the advisability of strengthening this clinical trial design by additional resources must be carefully considered. In many cases the data obtained with case-control or historical control designs will be unconvincing, no matter how well the study is conducted and no matter how many control groups are included.

Failure to Use Validated Instruments in a Clinical Trial

As with many other aspects of clinical trials, the degree to which the instruments are validated varies along a continuum from 0 to 100%. A problem arises when investigators fail to use the most validated test instruments available. When this occurs, the data obtained are not totally convincing to readers, regardless of the time, effort, and money spent on the clinical trial. In certain trials, however, clinicians must knowingly utilize unvalidated instruments, because better validated measures do not exist or are unavailable.

A related problem arises when several validated test instruments are used in a trial but the relative importance of each is not specified in the protocol prior to initiating the trial. This gap allows any positive outcome to be interpreted as providing evidence of efficacy. The problem may be readily solved by a statement in the protocol on which is the primary efficacy variable. In addition, defining specific criteria in advance by which a patient is defined as a responder provides a precise means of differentiating statistical significance from clinical significance of the results. The magnitude of response deemed necessary to identify a patient as a responder is an indication of what change constitutes a clinically significant response.

Community-Based Clinical Trials as an Alternative to Classical Clinical Trials

At the present time there is substantial debate about the rights of patients with serious diseases to receive promising new treatments if they cannot be enrolled in clinical trials. More and more health professionals, as well as members of the public and press, are saying that these patients should not have to wait the several (or many) years it often takes before a new medicine is marketed. The solution usually proposed by proponents of expanded use of investigational medicines is to provide the new investigational medicine to virtually any patient who needs it.

Numerous mechanisms exist for widely providing investigational medicines. A medicine can be made available at points during its development (e.g., either prior to or subsequent to the establishment of efficacy). Chapter 41 on compassionate plea protocols discusses some of these issues. This section describes one of the mechanisms to provide medicines to this population of patients, i.e., via community-based clinical trials in which physicians in private practice request an investigational medicine for their patients, who are then treated on an unnamed basis (i.e., the investigator does not request medicine for each patient by name).

Sponsors who supply medicine to these physicians may or may not provide a formal protocol and data collection forms, and may or may not insist on receiving data obtained from these patients. On the other hand, sponsors have a regulatory obligation to receive data on investigational medicines, at least for safety

evaluations. Although these and numerous other issues are controversial, it seems likely that a larger number of clinical trials will be based on community practice in the future.

Greater Standardization of Informed Consents

Different countries have widely differing cultural, philosophical, and ethical views toward informed consent. Within many countries, there have been trends toward increasing standards of informed consent over the last decade. While it is unlikely (and probably undesirable) that a single worldwide standard will ever be achieved, it is desirable that efforts be made to establish standards within all countries that are consistent with their cultures and customs. Many people state that written consents are unnecessary and the physician involved in each clinical trial should be the arbiter on what information each patient needs to receive prior to obtaining their consent to enter a trial. No matter what procedures and standards are accepted within a country, the author believes it is unethical to allow individuals with vested interests in, whether or not a patient enters a clinical trial to determine (by themselves alone) what information to provide patients, without any checks or balances.

MONITORING THE CONDUCT OF CLINICAL TRIALS

An appropriate degree of monitoring should be achieved for all clinical trials. The definition of appropriate depends on the particular country, type of trial, degree of risk for patients, type of sponsor (if any), Ethics Committee requirements and roles, plus regulatory authority. Such monitoring methods must be determined and then initiated. No one involved in a clinical trial likes to have a person or group closely watch his or her every move to ensure that appropriate standards are maintained. The opposite situation (absolutely no oversight function for clinical trials) is unacceptable to society and most knowledgeable professionals in this era of heightened ethical and social awareness. If standards of unsponsored clinical trials are appropriate, as most clinical investigators believe, then investigators should have little complaint over review of their trials' conduct.

Sponsored clinical trials tend to be monitored more assiduously than unsponsored ones. Clinical investigators of unsponsored trials may lack an adequate staff who are able to monitor trials. Although this issue does not always lead to problems or difficulties, the quality of a trial's conduct is more difficult to confirm if the trial is audited at a later date. More importantly, problems that could be corrected during a trial may not be discovered until after it is complete. At that time remedial action is generally impossible. Failure to monitor a trial adequately during its conduct may also allow innumerable biases and problems to enter, through which data become irreparably flawed.

Many ethics committees outside the United States and all Ethics Committees (i.e., Institutional Review Boards) within the United States require periodic updates of a clinical trial's progress once it has been initiated. This is one means, albeit a weak one, of monitoring the trial's conduct. Reports to the Food and Drug Administration (FDA) as well as lists the FDA maintains of unacceptable investigators, are another means of monitoring trial conduct. A new and more effective method would be for trained monitors accountable to Ethics Committees to audit, at appropriate intervals, the clinical protocols approved by that committee.

Clinical trials sponsored by pharmaceutical companies in academic settings are currently monitored to high standards. Appropriate clinical standards that should be followed in designing and conducting clinical trials are described in Chapter 110.

DATA COLLECTION

Data collection in the future will probably involve more video assessments of baseline and posttreatment states. Direct visualization of clinical benefits plus interviews of patients could readily be made available on videocassettes to regulatory authorities. Audio tapes may also be more widely used. All of these methods will force professionals to think of clinical trial data in new ways. Data also may be published in new ways. One way that is already possible is to deposit tapes in registries (Chapter 107). Narratives may be linked to visual displays.

In a more speculative vein, creative methods may be developed using computers to create a document of text photos and drawings, which could be integrated through linked electronic elements in a computer without "cutting and pasting." To control our path into the future we need to focus on what to do *with* the emerging technologies rather than on the technologies themselves. The challenges of dealing with information over the next decade are (1) how to organize information better, (2) how to manage large amounts of information better, (3) how to communicate information more effectively, and (4) how to use information proactively rather than reactively.

DATA PROCESSING

The data-processing field is currently undergoing the most rapid transition of any category described in this chapter. The specific changes are primarily technical and involve new equipment and methods (i.e., hardware and software) designed to improve both the speed and accuracy of data processing. Transmission of data via telephone lines (i.e., remote data entry) may give way in the future to satellite transmission. FAX machines are being used more often to transmit data from clinical trial sites to a sponsor's home office. Processing and tracking of data are often assisted with bar coding of (1) biological samples, (2) data collection forms, or (3) clinical supplies. Communications are being enhanced with electronic and voice mail, and computer-to-computer links with laboratories. The efficiency and capacity of data storage are also rapidly improving. Despite the fact that the methods are changing, the overall goals of more simply, rapidly, and accurately assessing the data have been constant. Achievable standards of both speed and accuracy are gradually increasing.

DATA ANALYSIS

Although closely associated with data processing, the development of new or improved statistical methods of data analysis in the medical area has not been progressing at a rapid pace. More research should be undertaken to establish which existing statistical methods are suitable for currently obtained data, and in which areas new or improved methods should be developed. Statisticians at most pharmaceutical companies often have insufficient time to conduct research on new statistical methods to analyze data. The critical evaluation and assessment of basic statistical concepts is also infrequently done. Results of statistical research need to be "translated" into language that makes sense to nonstatistically trained clinicians. Contracting this research to academic statisticians is one alternative.

DATA INTERPRETATION AND EXTRAPOLATION

There is currently no means of knowing if clinicians have assessed potential biases or confounding factors that may have influenced their clinical trials' results. Even the most sophisticated clinical methodologists probably vary in the degree to which they assess these factors, but this information would be extremely valuable to have when reading a trial report or publication.

A number of currently available options could readily improve the situation. For example, a standard list of biases and confounding factors could be prepared by appropriate professional societies. One such list is in Chapter 5. Authors could then state in a published report that they have considered and evaluated all or certain relevant factors in a specific list. Another possibility is for certain journals to ask authors to consider and evaluate those factors on a standard list printed in their journal. A third possibility is for authors to enumerate or describe in a publication the factors that might have confounded or biased the clinical trial.

META-ANALYSIS

Meta-analyses provide important data and conclusions to clinical scientists and practicing physicians. The methods that have evolved over the last decade are a tribute to the thoughtfulness of those involved in developing this approach. Nonetheless, there is a great need for further refinements in both methodology and application of meta-analyses. One such refinement relates to inclusion of a greater percent of relevant trials that have been conducted. This will be achieved when prospective and (or) historical registries of clinical studies become a reality.

A second refinement required to improve meta-analysis is to combine (or evaluate individually) those clinical trials that meet a minimum or defined standard in terms of quality. Research is needed to determine which scales are best to measure to evaluate a trial's quality, what quality level is required before a trial may be included in a meta-analysis, and how this value differs for different types of trial designs, therapeutic areas, or other categories. A more accurate conclusion is not achieved by including or combining data from both poor and excellent trials. The practice of mixing data of vastly different reliability distorts the combined data and often yields misleading results.

PUBLICATIONS OF CLINICAL TRIALS

Two major problems exist with the documentation of clinical trials in most of the published literature. First, the methods section has too few details for anyone to repeat the trial. Preclinical literature, in comparison, generally provides more complete methods; most studies in biochemistry or pharmacology, for example, may be repeated based on information published in reports.

Second, the relatively few results and methods presented in most publications do not permit an adequate interpretation of the data reported. Better documentation, particularly in the results section, would enable the quality and value of each trial to be assessed better. Moreover, investigators who wish to confirm or extend results of published trials would be better able to design a comparable trial. Comparisons between published trials and existing meta-analyses would be facilitated.

Higher standards for publications, with enforcement by journal editors, would readily achieve these goals.

This process requires a decision by editors about which goals are strongly desired. Authors should be pressured to elevate standards in all aspects of the clinical trial process (i.e., trial design, conduct, analysis, and interpretation).

Information Usually Missing From a Methods Section

Numerous items should be (but often are not) included in publications of clinical trials. Most of these involve information missing from the methods section, and include the following:

1. Financial interests of the authors (if any) in the clinical trial's outcome. For example, if the trial is from academicians with a strong financial affiliation with a small biotechnology company that will benefit from results of a trial, this should be indicated in the paper. Some journals already require this information.
2. Any changes to the protocol made during the clinical trial.
3. Definition of what constitutes a positive clinical response, and/or a patient who is a responder. This information enables the reader to assess what constitutes a clinically significant response and what responses may be only statistically significant.
4. Methods of randomization used (e.g., stratification variables, blocking design) plus safeguards used to ensure the integrity of the blind.
5. Method(s) of recruiting patients, and whether it changed during the clinical trial. If so, then were results from each group of patients compared to assure homogeneity. Number of patients who were contacted or screened, who signed informed consents, and who completed each phase of the trial should be given.
6. Year(s) and months during which the clinical trial was conducted, which may indicate whether certain studies were retrospective, but presented as if they were prospective.
7. Relatively complete description of adverse reactions noted. See Tables A21 to A31 in Spilker (1984) for specific factors that should be mentioned.
8. Degree of patient compliance achieved, plus method(s) used to measure compliance.
9. Degree of blindedness achieved and method(s) used to assess and validate the clinical trial's blind.
10. Methods used in multicenter trials to ensure similar conduct of the clinical trial at different sites (e.g., roundtable meetings, exchange of investigators, rigorous monitoring, investigator's manual, training of trial coordinators).
11. Method(s) of data processing and quality control procedures used (e.g., double-entry plus computer

evaluation of differences, comparison of 10% of total raw data on data collection forms with computer printouts, site visits for auditing).

12. Other relevant details of the protocol (e.g., data monitoring committee, procedures of packaging and dispensing medicines, inclusion criteria, severity of disease).

13. When multiple endpoints are measured in a clinical trial, assurance should be given that the protocol indicated the major one(s) used to decide if the outcome was positive.

14. Many details relating to the statistical analyses (4) that should be presented in a publication are described elsewhere, but are not listed here.

ARCHIVES OF DATA

Published data usually consist of summaries of results from groups of patients. Specific data from individual patients are frequently not published. Raw, processed, or transformed data from individual patients are sometimes of great interest and importance to clinical scientists who wish to examine a clinical trial's results in detail or who desire to conduct additional analyses. For example, when new clinical or scientific questions are asked, a new clinical trial may be avoided if existing data address the question. Without the availability of raw data, most additional analyses are impossible to conduct. The present system of publishing selected summaries of medical data does not allow medical professionals (or society) to extract the full value from each clinical trial conducted. While this is not the "fault" of publishers who have limited space, it is a problem that may be addressed in several ways.

One approach for unsponsored clinical trials or for selected sponsored clinical trials is for authors to deposit their raw plus processed data in an archive. These data would preferably be deposited in the form of tapes or other electronic means, in addition to, or instead of a hard copy. These data would be made available to qualified professionals. A nominal fee could be charged to cover costs, if the government controls the archive, or allow for a reasonable profit, if a private corporation controls it. Data from well-controlled, double-blind randomized trials should primarily be stored, but data from other trials may also be similarly preserved. A time limit of 10, 15, 20, or another number of years could be used to limit the quantity of data retained.

Another approach is to require authors to agree to furnish raw data on request, as part of the acceptance for publication. If this approach were adopted, several safeguards and limitations would have to be imposed to protect the authors. For example, a simple rule would be to limit requests to the raw numbers used to create tables or figures shown in the publication.

DISSEMINATION OF CLINICAL TRIAL RESULTS

Each pharmaceutical company strives to disseminate results of their major Phase II and III clinical trials on new medicines to as wide an audience as appropriate and as rapidly as possible, through publications, symposia, scientific exhibits, advertising, and other vehicles. The increasingly competitive world that all research and development companies will face in the future means that companies must be even more effective in quickly identifying and effectively targeting their audiences. The ability of data to modify medical practice relates in part to the quality of the trial design and the protocol. New medicines are only sold and used in patients when a company is able to influence medical practice.

HOW MAY PROGRESS TOWARD THE HIGHER STANDARDS MENTIONED ABOVE BE ACHIEVED?

The major forces that will impel clinical trials toward higher standards are peer review and pressure, journal editors, Ethics Review Committees, and regulatory agencies. Pressures exerted by these groups on clinical investigators involve consideration of professional reputation, tenure, and career enhancement.

Peer Review

Peer pressure often exerts the strongest pressure on investigators to raise their standards. Many clinical trials are not planned and conducted by single investigators but by groups of professionals who collaborate as a team. These professionals usually have a variety of backgrounds and specialties. Colleagues review ideas proposed by each other at every stage of a clinical trial. This collaboration usually enhances the quality of a trial and should foster higher standards.

Journal Editors

Journal editors play a critical role in implementing higher clinical standards. The power of their influence can best be exerted when many editors adopt common standards. Only the most prestigious journals are powerful enough to have a significant independent effect on influencing clinical standards. Explicitly stating their standards in editorials and in instructions to authors is preferable to exerting their influence through comments in letters of rejection. In the latter situation, most authors merely submit their manuscript to another journal and ignore comments about increasing standards.

Peer review of relevant papers by a biostatistician should be done in addition to a clinical review. This practice would exert pressure on authors to have their data analyzed by trained statisticians. The ideal time to influence investigators is prior to initiation of a clinical trial, when their protocol is not yet 100% final.

Ethics Committees

Ethics Committees may either adopt a primarily passive role in reviewing protocols or they may be more proactive, providing input into the improvement of weak or flawed protocols and thus pressuring investigators to adopt and adhere to high standards in clinical trial design and conduct. Ethics Committees may also pressure investigators through appropriate ongoing review procedures. Thus, these committees may exert a major impact on clinical trial standards. Their roles often differ widely from institution to institution, depending largely on the views of the leaders and their members.

Regulatory Agencies

Regulatory agencies are the single most important factor in controlling and influencing standards used in clinical trials sponsored by pharmaceutical companies; it is uncertain whether they will continue to be the most important group in the future. For unsponsored academic studies, regulatory agencies have generally played a much smaller role.

The pharmaceutical industry's primary objective is to have its products reach the market as soon as possible after all necessary clinical trials are completed. Thus, it attempts to process data as rapidly and accurately as possible, and to prepare submissions expeditiously. At present, a single medicine requires a separate regulatory application for most countries in which marketing approval is sought. Each application has different requirements in terms of format, contents, and quantity of data. An important goal from the industry's perspective is that fewer applications be required worldwide. The goal of faster application review by regulatory authorities is even more important. This topic is discussed by Spilker (1989a).

Other Groups

Other groups that influence clinical standards include trade associations, professional societies, consumer groups, and the media.

CONCLUSION

In the interests of expeditiously developing new medicines for patients it is hoped that future clinical standards will achieve many of the goals described in this chapter. More accurate and precise data obtained in well-designed trials would be more credible and influential than the data from many clinical trials conducted today.

References

Abram, M.B., Chairman, Presidents Commission for the Study of Ethical Problems in Medicine and Biomedical and Behavioral Research (1981): Protecting human subjects (first biennial report on the adequacy and uniformity of Federal rules and policies, and their implementation, for the protection of human subjects in biomedical and behavioral research). No. 040-000-00452-1. U.S. Government Printing Office, Washington.

Abrams, J. (1983): Nitroglycerin and long-acting nitrates in clinical practice. *Am. J. Med.*, 74:85–94.

Abrams, W.B. (1976): The development of clinical protocols. In: *Factors Influencing Clinical Research Success.* Finkel, M.J. (Ed.), pp. 7–23. Futura, Mt. Kisco, NY.

Abramson, N.S., Meisel, A., and Safar, P. (1986): Deferred consent: A new approach for resuscitation research on comatose patients. *JAMA,* 255:2466–2471.

Abt, K., and Krupp, P. (1986): Pooling of laboratory safety data in multicenter studies. *Drug Info. J.,* 20:311–313.

Ad Hoc Committee on the Effect of Trace Anesthetics on the Health of Operating Room Personnel, American Society of Anesthesiologists. (1974): Occupational disease among operating room personnel: A national study. *Anesthesiology,* 41:321–340.

Adair, J.G., Dushenko, T.W., and Lindsay, R.C.L. (1985): Ethical regulations and their impact on research practice. *Am. Psychol.,* 40:59–72.

Adlassnig, K.-P., Kolarz, G., Scheithauer, W., and Grabner, H. (1986): Approach to a hospital-based application of a medical expert system. *Med. Inform.,* 11:205–223.

Ager, B.P., and Tickner, J.A. (1983): The control of microbiological hazards associated with air-conditioning and ventilation systems. *Ann. Occup. Hyg.,* 27:341–358.

Agras, W.S., and Bradford, R.H. (1982): Recruitment for clinical trials: The lipid research clinic's coronary primary prevention trial experience. *Circulation,* 66(Suppl. IV):1–78.

Agras, W.S., and Marshall, G. (1979): Recruitment for the coronary primary prevention trial. *Clin. Pharmacol. Ther.,* 25:688–690.

Agrimonti, F., Frairia, R., Fornaro, D., Torta, M., Borretta, G., et al. (1982): Circadian and circaseptan rhythmicities in corticosteroid-binding globulin (CBG) binding activity of human milk. *Chronobiologia,* 9:281–290.

Akers, M.J. (1984): Considerations in selecting antimicrobial preservative agents for parenteral product development. *Pharm. Tech.,* 8(May):36–46.

Alderson, M.R. (1974): Are clinical trials required. *Gerontol. Clin.,* 16:76–87.

Allehoff, W.H., Esser, G., and Schmidt, M.H. (1988): Noncompliance and dropouts as a problem of longitudinal studies in child psychology. *Soc. Psychiatr. Epidemiol.,* 23:114–120.

Allen, J.C. (1985): The design and conduct of clinical trials in childhood brain tumors. *Cancer,* 56:1827–1831.

Allen, L.V. Jr., Levinson, R.S., and Phisutsinthop, D. (1977): Compatibility of various admixtures with secondary additives at Y-injection sites of intravenous administration sets. *Am. J. Hosp. Pharm.,* 34:939–943.

Allen, P.A., and Waters, W.E. (1982): Development of an ethical committee and its effect on research design. *Lancet,* I:1233–1236.

Alperovitch, A. (1989): Clinical trials in memory disorders: Objectives and methodology. *Arch. Gerontol. Geriatr.,* Suppl. 1:207–214.

Altman, D.G. (1980): Statistics and ethics in medical research: VI. Presentation of results. *Br. Med. J.,* 281:1542–1544.

Altman, D.G. (1981): Statistics and ethics in medical research: VIII. Improving the quality of statistics in medical journals. *Br. Med. J.,* 282:44–47.

Altman, D.G., and Dore, C.J. (1990): Randomisation and baseline comparisons in clinical trials. *Lancet* 335:149–153.

Alvares, A.P., Kapelner, S., Sassa, S., and Kappas, A. (1975): Drug metabolism in normal children, lead-poisoned children, and normal adults. *Clin. Pharmacol. Ther.,* 17:179–183.

Alvares, A.P., Kappas, A., Eiseman, J.L., Anderson, K.E., Pantuck, C.B., et al. (1979): Intraindividual variation in drug disposition. *Clin. Pharmacol. Ther.,* 26:407–419.

AMA Panel on Therapeutic Plasmapheresis. (1985): Current status of therapeutic plasmapheresis and related techniques. *JAMA,* 253:819–825.

Amene, P.C. (1983): Activation of pulmonary tuberculosis following intralesional corticosteroids. *Arch. Dermatol.,* 119:361–362.

American Academy of Pediatrics Committee on Drugs. (1977): Guidelines for the ethical conduct of studies to evaluate drugs in pediatric populations. *Pediatrics,* 60:91–101.

American Medical Association. (1983): From the NIH. 1. Sensitivity to pain greater in a clinical than in a laboratory setting. *JAMA,* 250:718.

American Psychiatric Association. (1980): *Diagnostic and Statistical Manual of Mental Disorders.* 3rd edition. American Psychiatric Association, Washington.

American Psychological Association. (1982): *Ethical Principles in the Conduct of Research with Human Participants.* American Psychological Association, Washington.

Amery, W, and Dony, J. (1975): A clinical trial design avoiding undue placebo treatment. *J. Clin. Pharmacol.,* 15:674–679.

Anderson, O.W. and Andersen, R.M. (1972): Patterns of use of health services. In: *Handbook of Medical Sociology,* 2nd ed. Freeman, H.E., Levine, S. and Reeder, L.G., (Eds.). Prentice-Hall, Englewood Cliffs, NJ, pp 386–406.

Anderson, J.A., Basker, M.A., and Dalton, R. (1975): Migraine and hypnotherapy *Int. J. Clin. Exp. Hypn.,* 23:48–58.

Anderson, J.A.D., Dalton, E.R., and Basker, M.A. (1979): Insomnia and hypnotherapy. *J. R. Soc. Med.,* 72:734–739.

Andrew, E. (1984): Method for assessment of the reporting standard of clinical trials with roentgen contrast media. *Acta Radiol.* [Diagn.], 25:55–58.

Andrews, E.J., Ward, B.C., and Altman, N.H. (Eds.) (1979): *Spontaneous Animal Models of Human Disease.* Volume 1. Academic Press, New York.

Andreychuk, T., and Skriver, C. (1975): Hypnosis and biofeedback in the treatment of migraine headache. *Int. J. Clin. Exp. Hypn.,* 23:172–183.

Angell, M. (1984a): Patients' preferences in randomized clinical trials. *N. Engl. J. Med.,* 310:1385–1387.

Angell, M. (1984b): Respecting the autonomy of competent patients. *N. Engl. J. Med.*, 310:1115–1116.

Angst, J., Bech, P., Boyer, P., Bruinvels, J., Engel, R., et al. (1989): Consensus conference on the methodology of clinical trials of antidepressants, Zurich, March 1988: Report of the consensus committee. *Pharmacopsychiatry*, 22:3–7.

Anonymous. (1898): The effects of nitroglycerin upon those whose manufacture it. *JAMA*, 31:793–794.

Anonymous. (1985a): Asthma and the weather. *Lancet*, I:1079–1080.

Anonymous. (1985b): Emotion and immunity. *Lancet*, II:133–134.

Anonymous. (1987): Administration of drugs by the buccal route. *Lancet*, I:666–667.

Anonymous. (1988a): Incidence of cancer and social class. *Lancet*, I:602.

Anonymous. (1988b): Pharmacological adaptive responses to drugs. *Lancet*, I:25–26.

Anonymous. (1989a): Databases for health care outcomes. *Lancet*, II:195–196.

Anonymous. (1989b): Informing patients about clinical disagreement. *Lancet*, II:367–368.

Antrobus, J.H.L. (1988): Anxiety and informed consent. *Anaesthesia*, 43:267–269.

Anturane Reinfarction Trial Research Group (1980): Sulfinpyrazone in the prevention of sudden death after myocardial infarction. *N. Engl. J. Med.*, 302:250–256.

Appelbaum, P.S., and Grisso, T. (1988): Assessing patients' capacities to consent to treatment. *N. Engl. J. Med.*, 319:1635–1638.

Ariëns, E.J., and Wuis, E.W. (1987): Bias in pharmacokinetics and clinical pharmacology. *Clin. Pharmacol. Ther.*, 42:361–363.

Arkes, H.R. (1981): Impediments to accurate clinical judgment and possible ways to minimize their impact. *J. Consult. Clin. Psychol.*, 49:323–330.

Armitage, P. (1983): Exclusions, losses to follow-up, and withdrawals in clinical trials. In: *Clinical Trials: Issues and Approaches.* Shapiro, S.A., and Louis, T.A. (Eds.), pp. 99–113. Marcel Dekker, New York.

Armitage, P. (1989): Inference and decision in clinical trials. *J. Clin. Epidemiol.*, 42:293–299.

Aronow, W.S. (1978): Effect of passive smoking on angina pectoris. *N. Engl. J. Med.*, 299:21–24.

Asbury, C.H. (1985): *Orphan Drugs—Medical Versus Market Value.* Lexington Books, Lexington, MA.

Association of the British Pharmaceutical Industry. (1983): Compensation and drug trials. Guidelines: Clinical trials—compensation for medicine induced injury. *Br. Med. J.*, 287:675.

Atkins, F.M. (1986): A critical evaluation of clinical trials in adverse reactions to foods in adults. *J. Allergy Clin. Immunol.*, 78:174–182.

Baar, J., and Tannock, I. (1989): Analyzing the same data in two ways: A demonstration model to illustrate the reporting and misreporting of clinical trials. *J. Clin. Oncol.*, 7:969–978.

Baber, N.S., and Lewis, J.A. (1982): Confidence in results of betablocker postinfarction trials. *Br. Med. J.*, 284:1749–1750.

Bailar, J.C. III, Louis, T.A., Lavori, P.W., and Polansky, M. (1984a): Studies without internal controls *N. Engl. J. Med.*, 311:156–162.

Bailar, J.C. III, Louis, T.A., Lavori, P.W., and Polansky, M. (1984b): A classification for biomedical research reports. *N. Engl. J. Med.*, 311:1482–1487.

Bailar, J.C. III, and Mosteller, F. (Eds.) (1986): *Medical Uses of Statistics.* Massachusetts Medical Society, Waltham, MA.

Banker, G.S., and Rhodes, C.T. (1989): *Modern Pharmaceutics.* Second Edition. Marcel Dekker, New York.

Barber, B. (1980): *Informed Consent in Medical Therapy and Research.* Rutgers University Press, New Brunswick, NJ.

Barlow, D.H., and Hersen, M. (1973): Single-case experimental designs: Uses in applied clinical research. *Arch. Gen. Psychiatry*, 29:319–325.

Barlow, D.H., and Hersen, M. (1984): *Single Case Experimental Designs: Strategies for Studying Behavior Change.* Second Edition. Pergamon, New York.

Barnes, M.P., Bates, D., Cartlidge, N.E.F., French, J.M., and Shaw, D.A. (1985): Hyperbaric oxygen and multiple sclerosis: Short-term results of a placebo-controlled, double-blind trial. *Lancet*, I:297–300.

Barnett, G.O., Cimino, J.J., Hupp, J.A., and Hoffer, E.P. (1987): DXplain: An evolving diagnostic decision-support system. *JAMA*, 258:67–74.

Barofsky, I., and Sugarbaker, P.H. (1979): Health status indexes: Disease specific and general population measures. *Proceedings of the Public Health Conference on Records and Statistics*, June 1978, Washington. DHEW (PHS) 79:263–269.

Barry, D.W. (1990): A perspective on compassionate parallel category C treatment track IND procedures. *Food Drug Cosm. L. J.*, 45:347–355.

Batchelor, J.R., Welsh, K.I., Tinoco, R.M., Dollery, C.T., Hughes, G.R.V. (1980): Hydralazine-induced systemic lupus erythematosus: Influence of HLA-DR and sex on susceptibility. *Lancet*, I:1107–1109.

Bates, D. (1987): Practical problems in the organisation of clinical trials in multiple sclerosis. *Neuroepidemiology*, 6:6–16.

Bates, T.R., and Gibaldi, M. (1970): Gastrointestinal absorption of drugs. In: *Current Concepts in the Pharmaceutical Sciences: Biopharmaceutics.* Swarbrick, J. (Ed.), pp. 58–99. Lea & Febiger, Philadelphia.

Baum, M. (1983): The practical and ethical defects of surgical randomised prospective trials. Commentary. *J. Med. Ethics*, 9:92–93.

Baum, M., Kay, R., and Scheurlen, H. (Eds.). (1982): *Clinical Trials in Early Breast Cancer.* Birkhauser Verlag, Basel.

Baum, M.L., Anish, D.S., Chalmers, T.C., Sacks, H.S., Smith, H. Jr. (1981): A survey of clinical trials of antibiotic prophylaxis in colon surgery: Evidence against further use of no-treatment controls. *N. Engl. J. Med.*, 305:795–799.

Beck, J.R. (1990): How to evaluate drugs: Cost-effectiveness analysis. *JAMA*, 264:83–84.

Beecher, H.K. (1961): Surgery as placebo *JAMA*, 176:1102–1107.

Beecher, H.K. (1962): Pain, placebos and physicians. *Practitioner*, 189:141–155.

Begg, C.B., and Berlin, J.A. (1989): Publication bias and dissemination of clinical research. *JNCI*, 81:107–115.

Begg, C.B., Carbone, P.P., Elson, P.J., and Zelen, M. (1982): Participation of community hospitals in clinical trials: Analysis of five years of experience in the eastern cooperative oncology group. *N. Engl. J. Med.*, 306:1076–1080.

Bell, G.D. (1973): *The Achievers: Six Styles of Personality and Leadership.* Preston-Hill, Chapel Hill, NC.

Bellamy, N. (1984): Clinical trials: Proposal for an international coding system (ICS). *Br. J. Clin. Pharmacol.*, 17:117–123.

Belloni, G., Cerutti, R., Fiori, M.G., Moschini, L., and Porta, M. (1986): Clinical trials of contrast media in radiology (neuroradiology). *Radiol. Med.*, 72(Suppl. N2):72–76.

Belsey, R., Greene, M., and Baer, D. (1986): Managing liability risk in the office laboratory. *JAMA* 256:1338–1341.

Benedict, G.W. (1979): LRC coronary prevention trial: Baltimore. *Clin. Pharmacol. Ther.*, 25:685–687.

Benson, P.R., Roth, L.H., and Winslade, W.J. (1985): Informed consent in psychiatric research: Preliminary findings from an ongoing investigation. *Soc. Sci. Med.* 20:1331–1341.

Berkson, J. (1946): Limitations of the application of fourfold table analysis to hospital data. *Biometrics Bull.*, 2:47–53.

Berry, H., Bloom, B., Mace, B.E.W., Hamilton, E.B.D., Fernandes, L., et al. (1980): Expectation and patient preference—does it matter? *J. R. Soc. Med.*, 73:34–38.

Bertilsson, L., Alm, C., de las Carreras, C., Widen, J., Edman, G., et al. (1989): Debrisoquine hydroxylation polymorphism and personality. *Lancet*, I:555.

Besarab, A., Wesson, L., Jarrell, B., and Burke, J.F. (1983): Effect of delayed graft function and ALG on the circaseptan (about 7-day) rhythm of human renal allograft rejection. *Transplantation,* 35:562–566.

β-Blocker Heart Attack Study Group. (1981): The β-blocker heart attack trial. *JAMA,* 246:2073–2074.

β-Blocker Heart Attack Trial Research Group. (1981): Beta blocker heart attack trial: Design features. *Control. Clin. Trials,* 2:275–285.

β-Blocker Heart Attack Trial Research Group. (1982): A randomized trial of propranolol in patients with acute myocardial infarction. I. Mortality results. *JAMA,* 247:1707–1714.

Bettis, J.W. (1985): Manufacture of clinical supplies. *Drug Dev. Ind. Pharm.,* 11:1685–1702.

Bickel, P.J., Hammel, E.A., and O'Connell, J.W. (1975): Sex bias in graduate admissions: Data from Berkeley. *Science,* 187:398–404.

Bicknell, J. (1989): Consent and people with mental handicap. *Br. Med. J.,* 299:1176–1177.

Bigby, M., Stern, R.S., and Bigby, J.A. (1985): An evaluation of method reporting and use in clinical trials in dermatology. *Arch. Dermatol.,* 121:1394–1399.

Bigger, J.T. Jr. (1987): Methodology for clinical trials with antiarrhythmic drugs to prevent cardiac death: US experience. *Cardiology,* 74(Suppl. 2):40–56.

Bingham, E. (1985): Hazards to health workers from antineoplastic drugs. *N. Engl. J. Med.,* 313:1220–1221.

Birgens, H.S., Hansen, O.P., and Clausen, N.T. (1985): A methodological evaluation of 14 controlled clinical trials in myelomatosis. *Scand. J. Haematol.,* 35:26–34.

Biswas, C.K., Ramos, J.M., Agroyannis, B., and Kerr, D.N.S. (1982): Blood gas analysis: Effect of air bubbles in syringe and delay in estimation. *Br. Med. J.,* 284:923–927.

Blackburn, I.M. (1984): Setting relevant patient differences—a problem in phase-IV research. *Pharmacopsychiatry,* 17:143–147.

Blackwell, B. (1972a): For the first time in man. *Clin. Pharmacol. Ther.,* 13:812–823.

Blackwell, B. (1972b): The drug defaulter. *Clin. Pharmacol. Ther.,* 13:841–848.

Blanc, S., Leuenberger, P., Berger, J.-P., Brooke, E.M., and Schelling, J.-L. (1979): Judgments of trained observers on adverse drug reactions. *Clin. Pharmacol. Ther.,* 25:493–498.

Blanchard, E.B., and Miller, S.T. (1977): Psychological treatment of cardiovascular disease. *Arch. Gen. Psychiatry,* 34:1402–1413.

Bland, J.M., Jones, D.R., Bennett, S., Cook, D.G., Haines, A.P., et al. (1985): Is the clinical trial evidence about new drugs statistically adequate? *Br. J. Clin. Pharmacol.,* 19:155–160.

Bleich, H.L., Beckley, R.F., Horowitz, G.L., Jackson, J.D., Moody, E.S. (1985): Clinical computing in a teaching hospital. *N. Engl. J. Med.,* 312:756–764.

Bloch, R. (1987): Methodology in clinical back pain trials. *Spine,* 12:430–432.

Blois, M.S. (1988): Medicine and the nature of vertical reasoning. *N. Engl. J. Med.,* 318:847–851.

Bloom, B.S. (Ed.). (1982): *Cost-Benefit and Cost-Effectiveness Analysis in Policymaking: Cimetidine as a Model.* Biomedical Information Corporation, New York.

Blumenthal, S.J. (1989): Discovery of new drug therapies based on the study of adverse reactions. *Drug Info. J.,* 23:267–271.

Boel, J., Andersen, L.B., Rasmussen, B., Hansen, S.H., and Dossing, M. (1984): Hepatic drug metabolism and physical fitness. *Clin. Pharmacol. Ther.,* 36:121–126.

Boissel, J.-P. (1989): Impact of randomized clinical trials on medical practices. *Controlled Clin. Trials,* 10(Suppl.):120S–134S.

Boissel, J.P., and Klimt, C.R. (Eds.) (1979): *Multicenter Controlled Trials—Principles and Problems.* INSERM, Paris.

Boissel, J.-P., Blanchard, J., Panak, E., Peyrieux, J.-C., and Sacks, H. (1989): Considerations for the meta-analysis of randomized

clinical trials: Summary of a panel discussion. *Controlled Clin. Trials,* 10:254–281.

Bombardier, C., and Tugwell, P. (1982): A methodological framework to develop and select indices for clinical trials: Statistical and judgmental approaches. *J. Rheumatol.,* 9:753–757.

Bonchek, L.I. (1979): Are randomized trials appropriate for evaluating new operations? *N. Engl. J. Med.,* 301:44–45.

Bonchek, L.I. (1982): The role of the randomized clinical trial in the evaluation of new operations. *Surg. Clin. North Am.,* 62:761–769.

Bond, N.W. (Ed.) (1984): *Animal Models in Pyschopathology.* Academic Press, Sydney, Australia.

Bondi, J.V., and Pope, D.G. (1987): Drug delivery systems. In: *Drug Discovery and Development.* Williams, M., and Malick, J.B. (Eds.), pp. 291–325. Humana Press, Clifton, NJ.

Bootman, J.L., Larson, L.N., McGhan, W.F., and Townsend, R.J. (1989): Pharmacoeconomic research and clinical trials: Concepts and issues. *DICP, Ann. Pharmacother.,* 23:693–697.

Boston Interhospital Virus Study Group. NIAID-sponsored cooperative antiviral clinical study. (1975): Failure of high dose 5-iodo-2'-deoxyuridine (IDU) in the therapy of herpes simplex virus encephalitis. Evidence of unacceptable toxicity. *N. Engl. J. Med.,* 292:599–603.

Botero, D. (1976): Clinical trial methodology in intestinal parasitic diseases. *Clin. Pharmacol. Ther.,* 19:630–643.

Bounameaux, H., Holditch, T., Hellemans, H., Berent, A., and Verhaeghe, R. (1985): Placebo-controlled, double-blind, two centre trial of ketanserin in intermittent claudication. *Lancet,* II:1268–1271.

Bourne, J.G. (1971): Deaths from dental anesthesia. *Br. Med. J.,* 2:466.

Boyle, M.H., Torrance, G.W., Sinclair, J.C., and Horwood, S.P. (1983): Economic evaluation of neonatal intensive care of very-low-birth-weight infants. *N. Engl. J. Med.,* 308:1330–1337.

Braitman, L.E. (1988): Confidence intervals extract clinically useful information from data. *Ann. Intern. Med.,* 108:296–298.

Breuning, S.E., Ferguson, D.G., and Cullari, S. (1980): Analysis of single-double blind procedures, maintenance of placebo effects, and drug-induced dyskinesia with mentally retarded persons. *Appl. Res. Ment. Retard.,* 1:175–192.

Brewer, E.J. Jr., and Giannini, E.H. (1982): Standard methodology for segment I, II, and III pediatric rheumatology collaborative study group studies. I: Design. *J. Rheumatol.,* 9:109–113.

British Tuberculous Association. (1968): Hypnosis for asthma, a controlled trial. *Br. Med. J.,* 4:71–76.

Britton, J.R. (1989): Effects of social class, sex, and region of residence on age at death from cystic fibrosis. *Br. Med. J.,* 298:483–487.

Broder, S. (1989): Controlled trial methodology and progress in treatment of the acquired immunodeficiency syndrome (AIDS). *Ann. Intern. Med.,* 110:417–418.

Brodie, B.B., and Heller, W.M. (Eds.) (1972): *Bioavailability of Drugs.* S. Karger, Basel, Switzerland.

Brodie, M.J., and Feely, J. (1988): Adverse drug interactions. *Br. Med. J.,* 296:845–849.

Brosious, E.M., Schmidt, R.M., and Koepke, J.A. (1978): Hemoglobinopathy testing. A report of the 1976 and 1977 college of American pathologists surveys. *Am. J. Clin. Pathol.,* 70:563–566.

Brown, J.H.U. (1979): Functions of an institutional review board and the protection of human subjects. *Fed. Proc.,* 38:2049–2050.

Brownell, K.D., and Stunkard, A.J. (1982): The double-blind in danger: Untoward consequences of informed consent. *Am. J. Psychiatry,* 139:1487–1489.

Bruguerolle, B. (1986): Modifications de la pharmacocinétique des médicaments au cours du cycle menstruel. *Therapie,* 41:11–17.

Brundage, J.F., Scott, R.M., Lednar, W.M., Smith D.W., and Miller, R.N. (1988): Building-associated risk of febrile acute respiratory diseases in army trainees. *JAMA,* 259:2108–2112.

Bryant, G.D., and Norman, G.R. (1980): Expressions of probability: Words and numbers. *N. Engl. J. Med.,* 302:411.

Buchwald, H., Matts, J.P., Hansen, B.J., Long, J.M., Fitch, L.L., et al. (1987): Program on surgical control of the hyperlipidemias (POSCH): Recruitment experience. *Controlled Clin. Trials*, 8(Suppl.):94S-104S.

Buckalew, L.W., and Coffield, K.E. (1982a): An investigation of drug expectancy as a function of capsule color and size and preparation form. *J. Clin. Psychopharmacol.*, 2:245-248.

Buckalew, L. W., and Coffield, K.E. (1982b): Drug expectations associated with perceptual characteristics: Ethnic factors *Percept. Mot. Skills*, 55:915-918.

Bujorian, G.A. (1988): Clinical trials: Patient issues in the decision-making process. *Oncol. Nurs. Forum*, 15:779-783.

Bull, B.S., Levy, W.C., Westengard, J.C., Farr, M., Smith, P.F., et al. (1986): Ranking of laboratory tests by consensus analysis. *Lancet*, II:377-380.

Bunker, J.P. (1970): Surgical manpower: A comparison of operations and surgeons in the United States and in England and Wales. *N. Engl. J. Med.*, 282:135-144.

Burgess, E.D., and Gill, M.J. (1990): Intraperitoneal administration of acyclovir in patients receiving continuous ambulatory peritoneal dialysis. *J. Clin. Pharmacol.*, 30:997-1000.

Buros, O.K. (Ed.) (1972): *The Seventh Mental Measurements Yearbook*. Gryphon Press, Highland Park, NJ.

Bursztajn, H., and Hamm, R.M. (1982): The clinical utility of utility assessment. *Med. Decis. Making*, 2:161-165.

Busch, H., Cranach, M. V., Gulbinat, W., Renfordt, E., and Tegeler, J. (1981): Methodological and practical aspects of a multicentre study of reliability of psychopathological assessment. *Mod. Probl. Pharmacopsychiatry*, 16:37-49.

Buyse, M.E., Staquet, M.J., and Sylvester, R.J., (Eds.) (1984): *Cancer Clinical Trials. Methods and Practice*. Oxford University Press, Oxford.

Byar, D.P., and Piantadosi, S. (1985): Factorial designs for randomized clinical trials. *Cancer Treat. Rep.*, 69:1055-1063.

Byar, D.P., Simon, R.M., Friedewald, W.T., Schlesselman, J.J., DeMets, D.L., et al. (1976): Randomized clinical trials: Perspectives on some recent ideas. *N. Engl. J. Med.*, 295:74-80.

Byer, A. (1983): The practical and ethical defects of surgical randomised prospective trials. *J. Med. Ethics*, 9:90-93.

Byington, R.P., Curb, J.D., and Mattson, M.E. (1985): Assessment of double-blindness at the conclusion of the β-Blocker heart attack trial. *JAMA*, 253:1733-1736.

Byrne, D.J., Napier, A., and Cuschieri, A. (1988): How informed is signed consent? *Br. Med. J.*, 296:839-840.

Cahill, G.F., Jr., Etzwiler, D.D., and Freinkel, N. (1976): "Control" and diabetes. *New Eng. J. Med.*, 294:1004-1005.

Calabrese, E.J. (1983): *Principles of Animal Extrapolation*. John Wiley & Sons, New York.

Calabrese, E.J. (1988): Comparative biology of test species. *Environ. Health Perspect.*, 77:55-62.

Calimlim, J.F., and Weintraub, M. (1981): Selection of patients participating in a clinical trial. In: *Statistics in the Pharmaceutical Industry*. Buncher, C.R., and Tsay, J.Y. (Eds.), pp. 107-138. Marcel Dekker, New York.

Calman, K.C. (1984): Quality of life in cancer patients—an hypothesis. *J. Med. Ethics*, 10:124-127.

Campbell, S.K. (1974): *Flaws and Fallacies in Statistical Thinking*. Prentice-Hall, Englewood Cliffs, NJ.

Cancer Research Campaign Working Party. (1980): Trials and tribulations: Thoughts of the organization of multicentre clinical trials. *Br. Med. J.*, 281:918-920.

Cann, P.A. (1987): An approach to the design of therapeutic trials in IBS. *Scand. J. Gastroenterol.*, 130(Suppl.):67-76.

Canner, P.L. (1983): Brief description of the Coronary Drug Project and other studies. *Controlled Clin. Trials*, 4:273-280.

Cardon, P.V., Dommel, F.W., and Trumble, R.R.(1976): Injuries to research subjects—a survey of investigators. *N. Engl. J. Med.*, 295:650-654.

Carey, M.J., and Cordon, I. (1986): Asthma and climatic conditions: Experience from Bermuda, an isolated island community. *Br. Med. J.*, 293:843-844.

Cargill, V., Cohen, D., Kroenke, K., and Neuhauser, D. (1986): Ongoing patient randomization: An innovation in medical care research. *Health Serv. Res.*, 21:663-678.

Carpenter, W.T. Jr., Sadler, J.H., Light, P.D., Hanlon, T.E., and Kurland, A.A. (1983): The therapeutic efficacy of hemodialysis in schizophrenia. *N. Engl. J. Med.*, 308:669-675.

Carruthers, S.G., and Bailey, D.G. (1987): Tolerance and cardiovascular effects of a single dose felodipine/β-blocker combinations in healthy subjects. *J. Cardiovasc. Pharmacol.*, 10:S169-S177.

Carter, S.K. (1973): Introduction to methodology of clinical trials in the varieties of acute leukemia: Defining the numerator and denominator in leukemic trials. *Recent Results Cancer Res.*, 43:107-109.

Carter, S.K. (1979): Methodology of data reporting in advanced breast cancer trials. *Cancer Chemother. Pharmacol.*, 3:1-5.

Carter, S.K. (1980): Clinical considerations in the design of clinical trials. *Cancer Treat. Rep.*, 64:367-371.

Casale, G., and de Nicola, P. (1984): Circadian rhythms in the aged: A review. *Arch. Gerontol. Geriatr.*, 3:267-284.

Casscells, W., Schoenberger, A., and Graboys, T.B. (1978): Interpretation by physicians of clinical laboratory results. *N. Engl. J. Med.*, 299:999-1001.

Cassileth, B.R., Lusk, E.J., Miller, D.S., and Hurwitz, S. (1982): Attitudes toward clinical trials among patients and the public. *JAMA*, 248:968-970.

Cassileth, B.R., Lusk, E.J., Strouse, T.B., Miller, D.S., Brown, L.L. (1984): Psychosocial status in chronic illness. *N. Engl. J. Med.*, 311:506-511.

Cato, A. (1982): Design of clinical trials. *Drug Info. J.*, 16:44-50.

Cattaneo, A.D, Lucchelli, P.E., and Filippucci, G. (1970): Sedative effects of placebo treatment. *Eur. J. Clin. Pharmacol.*, 3:43-45.

CBE Style Manual Committee. (1983): *Council of Biology Editors Style Manual: A Guide for Authors, Editors, and Publishers in the Biological Sciences*. Fifth Edition. Council of Biology Editors, Bethesda, MD.

Challah, S., and Mays, N.B. (1986): The randomised controlled trial in the evaluation of new technology: A case study. *Br. Med. J.*, 292:877-879.

Chalmers, I., Hetherington, J., Newdick, M., Mutch, L, Grant, A., et al. (1986): The Oxford database of perinatal trials: Developing a register of published reports of controlled trials. *Controlled Clin. Trials*, 7:306-324.

Chalmers, T.C. (1974): The impact of controlled trials on the practice of medicine *Mt. Sinai J. Med.*, 41:753-759.

Chalmers, T.C. (1982): Randomized clinical trials and the consumers. In: *The Randomized Clinical Trial and Therapuetic Decisions*. Tygstrup, N., Lachin, J.M., and Juhl, E. (Eds.), pp. 257-264. Marcel Dekker, New York.

Chalmers, T.C., Levin, H., Sacks, H.S., Reitman, D., Berrier, J., et al. (1987): Meta-analysis of clinical trials as a scientific discipline. I: Control of bias and comparison with large co-operative trials. *Stat. Med.*, 6:315-328.

Chalmers, T.C., Matta, R.J., Smith, H. Jr., and Kunzler, A-M. (1977): Evidence favoring the use of anticoagulants in the hospital phase of acute myocardial infarction *N. Engl. J. Med.*, 297:1091-1096.

Chalmers, T. C., and Sacks, H. (1979): Letter to the editor. *N. Engl. J. Med.*, 301:1182.

Chalmers, T.C., Smith, H. Jr., Blackburn, B., Silverman, B., and Schroeder, B. (1981): A method for assessing the quality of a randomized control trial. *Controlled Clin. Trials*, 2:31-49.

Chan, S.S., Sacks, H.S., and Chalmers, T.C. (1982): The epidemiology of unpublished randomized control trials. *Clin. Res.*, 30:234A.

Chan, Y.K., Archibald, D.D., and Peduzzi, P.N. (1983): Management of a multicenter clinical trial. *Trends Pharmacol. Sci.*, 4:21-24.

Chaput de Saintonge, D.M. (1977): Aide-mémoire for preparing clinical trial protocols. *Br. Med. J.*, 1:1323–1324.

Chaput de Saintonge, D.M., Kirwan, J.R., Evans, S.J.W., and Crane, G.J. (1988): How can we design trials to detect clinically important changes in disease severity? *Br. J. Clin. Pharmacol.*, 26:355–362.

Charlson, M.E., and Horwitz, R.I. (1984): Applying results of randomised trials to clinical practice: Impact of losses before randomisation. *Br. Med. J.*, 289:1281–1284.

Chase, W.G., and Simon, H.A. (1973a): The mind's eye in chess. In: *Visual Information Processing*. Chase, W.G. (Ed.), pp. 215–281. Academic Press, New York.

Chase, W.G., and Simon, H.A. (1973b): Perception in chess. *Cognitive Psychol.*, 4:55–81.

Chassan, J.B. (1979): *Research Design in Clinical Psychology and Psychiatry*. John Wiley & Sons, New York.

Cheung, R., Dickins, J., Nicholson, P.W., Thomas, A.S.C., Smith, H.H., et al. (1988a): Compliance with anti-tuberculous therapy: A field trial of a pill-box with a concealed electronic recording device. *Eur. J. Clin. Pharmacol.*, 35:401–407.

Cheung, R., Sullens, C.M., Seal, D., Dickins, J., Nicholson, P.W., et al. (1988b): The paradox of using a 7 day antibacterial course to treat urinary tract infections in the community. *Br. J. Clin. Pharmacol.*, 26:391–398.

Chi, M.T.H., Feltovich, P.J., and Glaser, R. (1981): Categorization and representation of physics problems by experts and novices. *Cogn. Sci.*, 5:121–152.

Chien, Y.W. (1983): Potential developments and new approaches in oral controlled-release drug delivery systems. *Drug. Dev. Ind. Pharm.*, 9:1291–1330.

Chisholm, E.M., de Dombal, F.T., and Giles, G.R. (1985): Validation of a self administered questionnaire to elicit gastrointestinal symptoms. *Br. Med. J.*, 290:1795–1796.

Choi, S.C., Smith, P.J., and Becker, D.P. (1985): Early decision in clinical trials when the treatment differences are small. *Controlled Clin. Trials*, 6:280–288.

Churchill, L.R., and Churchill, S.W. (1989): Storytelling in medical arenas: The art of self-determination. *JAMA*, 262:1235.

CIOMS Working Group. (1990): *International Reporting of Adverse Drug Reactions: Final Report of CIOMS Working Group*. CIOMS, Geneva.

Ciuffreda, K.J., and Goldrich, S.G. (1983): Oculomotor biofeedback therapy. *Int. Rehabil. Med.*, 5:111–117.

Clark, S.J., Welling, E.C., and McCloskey D.W. (1979): The help system in the clinical laboratory: Laboratory data in drug monitoring and interpretation of drug effects on laboratory tests. In: *Proc. Third Ann. Symp. on Comput. Appl. in Med. Care.* pp. 580–582 (Cat. no. 79CH1480-3C, IEEE Service Center, Piscataway, NJ).

Clarke, A.J., Clark, B., Eason, C.T., and Parke, D.V. (1985): An assessment of a toxicological incident in a drug development program and its implications. *Regul. Toxicol. Pharmacol.*, 5:109–119.

Clarke, M., and Mason, E.S. (1985): Leatherwork: A possible hazard to reproduction. *Br. Med. J.*, 290:1235–1237.

Cleland, D.I., and King, W.R. (Eds.) (1983): *Project Management Handbook*. Van Nostrand Reinhold Co., New York.

Cleveland, W.S., and McGill, R. (1985): Graphical perception and graphical methods for analyzing scientific data. *Science*, 229:828–833.

Cobb, L.A., Thomas, G.I., Dillard, D.H., Merendino, K.A., and Bruce, R.A. (1959): An evaluation of internal-mammary-artery ligation by a double-blind technic. *N. Engl. J. Med.*, 260:1115–1118.

Cocchetto, D.M. (1986): An orientation program for new clinical trial monitors. *Clin. Res. Practices Drug Reg. Affairs*, 4:235–250.

Cohn, J.N. (1985): Clinical evaluation of cardiovascular drugs. In: *Principles and Techniques of Human Research and Therapeutics: Selected Topics*. McMahon, G. (Ed.), pp. 7–15. Futura, Mount Kisco, NY.

Colditz, G.A., Martin, P., Stampfer, M.J., Willett, W.C., Sampson, L., et al. (1986): Validation of questionnaire information on risk factors and disease outcomes in a prospective cohort study of women. *Am. J. Epidemiol.*, 123:894–900.

Coles, L.S., Fries, J.F., Kraines, R.G., and Roth, S.H. (1983): From experiment to experience: Side effects of nonsteriodal anti-inflammatory drugs. *Am. J. Med.*, 74:820–828.

Collins, J.M., Zaharko, D.S., Dedrick, R.L., and Chabner, B.A. (1986) Potential roles for preclinical pharmacology in phase I clinical trials. *Cancer Treat. Rep.*, 70:73–80.

Commission on Antiepileptic Drugs of the International League Against Epilepsy. (1989): Guidelines for clinical evaluation of antiepileptic drugs. *Epilepsia*, 30:400–408.

Committee for the Protection of Human Participants in Research. (1982): *Ethical Principles in the Conduct of Research with Human Participants*. American Psychological Association, Washington, DC.

Compston, A. (1987): Selection of patients for clinical trials. *Neuroepidemiology*, 6:34–39.

Connell, P.J., and Thompson, C.K. (1986): Flexibility of single-subject experimental designs. Part III: Using flexibility to design or modify experiments. *J. Speech Hear. Disord.*, 51:214–225.

Conners, C.K. (1976): Rating scales for use in drug studies with children. In: *ECDEU Assessment Manual for Psychopharmacology*. DHEW Pub. No. 76–338. Guy, W. (Ed.), pp. 303–312. U.S. Government Printing Office, Washington, DC.

Conney, A.H. (1967): Pharmacological implications of microsomal enzyme induction. *Pharmacol. Rev.*, 19:317–366.

Conney, A.H., Pantuck, E.J., Hsiao, K.-C., Kuntzman, R., Alvares, A.P., et al. (1977): Regulation of drug metabolism in man by environmental chemicals and diet. *Fed. Proc.*, 36:1647–1652.

Conolly, M.E., Davies, D.S., Dollery, C.T., and George, C.F. (1971): Resistance to β-adrenoceptor stimulants (a possible explanation for the rise in asthma deaths). *Br. J. Pharmacol.*, 43:389–402.

Consensus Development Panel. (1985): Drug concentrations and driving impairment. *JAMA*, 254:2618–2621.

CONSENSUS Trial Study Group. (1987): Effects of enalapril on mortality in severe congestive heart failure: Results of the cooperative north Scandinavian enalapril survival study. *N. Engl. J. Med.*, 316:1429–1435.

Cook, D.A.G., and Morgan, H.G. (1982): Families in high-rise flats. *Br. Med. J.*, 284:846.

Cooksley, W.G.E., Farrell, G.C., Cash, G.A., and Powell, L.W. (1979): The interaction of cigarette smoking and chronic drug ingestion on human drug metabolism. *Clin. Exp. Pharmacol. Physiol.*, 6:527–533.

Coppleson, L.W., Factor, R.M., Strum, S.B., Graff, P.W., and Rappaport, H. (1970): Observer disagreement in the classification and histology of Hodgkin's disease. *JNCI*, 45:731–740.

Cori, K.A. (1985): Fundamentals of master scheduling for the project manager. *Project Management J.*, 16:78–89.

Cormia, F.E., and Dougherty, J.W. (1959): Clinical evaluation of antipruritic drugs; consideration of orally or parenterally administered administered agents. *Arch. Dermatol.*, 79:172–178.

Coronary Drug Project Research Group. (1980): Influence of adherence to treatment and response of cholesterol on mortality in the coronary drug project. *N. Engl. J. Med.*, 303:1038–1041.

Costain, D. (1979): Simpson's paradox. *Br. J. Psychiatry*, 135:485.

Côté, R.A., and Robboy, S. (1980): Progress in medical information management: Systematized nomenclature of medicine (SNOMED). *JAMA*, 243:756–762.

Couch, J.R., Jr. (1987): Placebo effect and clinical trials in migraine therapy. *Neuroepidemiology*, 6:178–185.

Coulter, D.M. (1988): Eye pain with nifedipine and disturbance of taste with captopril: A mutually controlled study showing a method of postmarketing surveillance. *Br. Med. J.*, 296:1086–1088.

Council on Scientific Affairs. (1986): Lasers in medicine and surgery. *JAMA*, 256:900–907.

Cowan, C., Bourke, J., Reid, D.S., and Julian, D.G. (1987): Tolerance to glyceryl trinitrate patches: Prevention by intermittent dosing. *Br. Med. J.*, 294:544–545.

Cramer, J. and Spilker, B. (Eds.) (1991): *Patient Compliance in Medical Practice and Clinical Trials*. Raven Press, New York.

Cramer, J.A., Mattson, R.H., Prevey, M.L., Scheyer, R.D., and Ouellette, V.L. (1989): How often is medicine taken as prescribed? A novel assessment technique. *JAMA*, 261:3273–3277.

Cramer, J.A., Smith, D.B., Mattson, R.H., Delgado Escueta, A.V., Collins, J.F., et al. (1983): A method of quantification for the evaluation of antiepileptic drug therapy. *Neurology*, 33(Suppl. 1):26–37.

Crawley, R., Belsey, R., Brock, D., and Baer, D.M. (1986): Regulation of physicians' office laboratories: The Idaho experience. *JAMA*, 255:374–382.

Croke, G. (1979): Recruitment for the national cooperative gallstone study. *Clin. Pharmacol. Ther.*, 25:691–694.

Cromer, B.A., Steinberg, K., Gardner, L., Thornton, D., and Shannon, B. (1989): Psychosocial determinants of compliance in adolescents with iron deficiency. *Am. J. Dis. Child.*, 143:55–58.

Croog, S.H., Levine, S., Testa, M.A., Brown, B., Bulpitt, C.J., et al. (1986): The effects of antihypertensive therapy on the quality of life. *N. Engl. J. Med.*, 314:1657–1664.

Crooks, J., O'Malley K., and Stevenson, I.H. (1976): Pharmacokinetics in the elderly. *Clin. Pharmacokinet.*, 1:280–296.

Crouthamel, W., and Sarapu, A.C. (Eds.) (1983): *Animal Models for Oral Drug Delivery in Man: In Situ and In Vivo Approaches*. American Pharmaceutical Association, Washington, DC.

Crowe, R.R. (1984): Electroconvulsive therapy—a current perspective. *N. Engl. J. Med.*, 311:163–167.

Cullen, M.R., Cherniack, M.G., and Rosenstock, L. (1990): Occupational medicine. *N. Engl. J. Med.*, 322:594–601, 675–683.

Cummings, J.H., Sladen, G.E., James, O.F.W., Sarner, M., and Misiewicz, J.J. (1974): Laxative-induced diarrhoea: A continuing clinical problem. *Br. Med. J.*, 1:537–541.

Cunningham, A.S. (1988): Meta-analysis and methodology review: What's in a name? *J. Pediatr.*, 113:328–329.

Curson, D.A., Hirsch, S.R., Platt, S.D., Bamber, R.W., and Barnes, T.R.E. (1986): Does short term placebo treatment of chronic schizophrenia produce long term harm? *Br. Med. J.*, 293:726–728.

Cutler, P. (1985): *Problem Solving in Clinical Medicine: From Data to Diagnosis*. Second Edition. Williams & Wilkins, Baltimore.

Dahan, R., Caulin, C., Figea, L., Kanis, J.A., Caulin, F., et al. (1986): Does informed consent influence therapeutic outcome? A clinical trial of the hypnotic activity of placebo in patients admitted to hospital. *Br. Med. J.*, 293:363–364.

Dahlström, B., and Eckernas, S. (1991): Patient computers to enhance compliance with questionnaires: A challenge for the 1990's. p. 233–240. In: *Patient Compliance in Medical Practice and Clinical Trials*. Cramer, J., and Spilker, B. (Eds.). Raven Press, New York.

Dammacco, F., Campobasso, N., Altomare, E., and Iodice, G. (1984): Analogues in immunology. *Ric. Clin. Lab.*, 14:137–147.

Damrosch, S.P. (1986): Ensuring anonymity by use of subject-generated identification codes. *Res. Nurs. Health*, 9:61–63.

Dao, T.D. (1985): Cost-benefit and cost-effectiveness analysis of drug therapy. *Am. J. Hosp. Pharm.*, 42:791–802.

D'Arcy, P.F. (1984): Tobacco smoking and drugs: A clinically important interaction? *Drug Intell. Clin. Pharm.*, 18:302–307.

Darragh, A., Kenny, M., Lambe, R., and Brick, I. (1985): Sudden death of a volunteer. *Lancet*, I:93–94.

Dattilo, J., and Nelson, G.D. (1986): Single-subject evaluation in health education. *Health Educ. Q.*, 13:249–259.

Davenport, H.W. (1961): *Physiology of the Digestive Tract*. pp. 50, 149. Year Book Publishers, Chicago.

Davis, D.L., Bridbord, K., and Schneiderman, M. (1983): Cancer prevention: Assessing causes, exposures, and recent trends in mortality for U.S. males, 1968–1978. *Int. J. Health Serv.*, 13:337–372.

Davis, K.H., Hawks, R.L., and Blanke, R.V. (1988): Assessment of laboratory quality in urine drug testing: A proficiency testing pilot study. *JAMA*, 260:1749–1754.

Davis, K.V., Sprague, R., and Werry, J. (1969): Stereotyped behavior and activity level in severe retardates: The effects of drugs. *Am. J. Ment. Defic.*, 73:721–727.

Davis, M.S. (1968): Variations in patients' compliance with doctors' advice: An empirical analysis of patterns of communication. *Am. J. Public Health*, 58:274–288.

Dawes, R.M., Faust, D., and Meehl, P.E. (1989): Clinical versus actuarial judgment. *Science*, 243:1668–1674.

Dawson, G.W., and Vestal, R.E. (1982): Smoking and drug metabolism. *Pharmacol. Ther.*, 15:207–221.

Day, R.A. (1983): *How to Write and Publish a Scientific Paper*. Second Edition. ISI Press, Philadelphia.

Day, S.J., and Graham, D.F. (1989): Sample size and power for comparing two or more treatment groups in clinical trials. *Br. Med. J.*, 299:663–665.

Day, E., Maddern, L., and Wood, E. (1968): Auscultation of foetal heart rate: An assessment of its error and significance. *Brit. Med. J.*, 4:422–424.

Dayan, A.D., Clark, B., Jackson, M., Morgan, H., and Charlesworth, F.A. (1984): Role of the LD50 test in the pharmaceutical industry. *Lancet*, I:555–556.

Deabler, H.L., Fidel, E., Dillenkoffer, R.L. and Eider, S.T. (1973): The use of relaxation and hypnosis in lowering high blood pressure. *Am. J. Clin. Hypn.*, 16:75–83.

De Bono, E. (1967a): *The Five-Day Course in Thinking*. Pelican Books, Harmondsworth, Middlesex, England.

De Bono, E. (1967b): The Use of Lateral Thinking. Pelican Books, Harmondsworth, Middlesex, England.

De Bono, E. (1969): The Mechanism of Mind. Pelican Books, Harmondsworth, Middlesex, England.

DeCosse, J.J., Donegan, W.L., Sedransk, N., Jones, N.F., and Claudon, D.B. (1980): Operative procedures: Is standardization feasible or necessary? *Cancer Treat. Rep.*, 64:419–423.

de Groot, A. (1965): *Thought and Perception in Chess*. Mouton, The Hague, The Netherlands.

De Jonge, H. (1983): Deficiencies in clinical reports for registration of drugs. *Stat. Med.*, 2:155–166.

de Marr, E.W.J. (1986): The global core clinical protocol and its rational adaptations. *Drug Inf. J.*, 20:257–261.

de Marr, E.W.J., Chaudhury, R.R., Kofi Ekue, J.M., Granata, F., and Walker, A.N. (1983): Management of clinical trials in developing countries. *J. Int. Med. Res.*, 11:1–5.

DeMets, D.L., Hardy, R., Friedman, L.M., and Gordon Lan, K.K. (1984): Statistical aspects of early termination in the beta-blocker heart attack trial. *Controlled Clin. Trials*, 5:362–372.

DeMets, D.L., Williams, G.W., Brown, B.W., Jr., and the NOTT Research Group (1982): A case report of data monitoring experience: The nocturnal oxygen therapy trial. *Controlled Clin. Trials*, 3:113–124.

Department of Clinical Epidemiology and Biostatistics, McMaster University, Hamilton, Ont. (1980a): Clinical disagreement: I. How often it occurs and why. *Can. Med. Assoc. J.*, 123:499–504.

Department of Clinical Epidemiology and Biostatistics, McMaster University Health Sciences Centre, Hamilton, Ont. (1980b): Clinical disagreeement: II. How to avoid it and how to learn from one's mistakes. *Can. Med. Assoc. J.*, 123:613–617.

Department of Clinical Epidemiology and Biostatistics, McMaster University, Hamilton, Ont. (1981): How to read clinical journals: V. To distinguish useful from useless or even harmful therapy. *Can. Med. Assoc. J.*, 124:1156–1162.

Department of Clinical Epidemiology and Biostatistics, McMaster University Health Sciences Centre, Hamilton, Ont. (1984a): How to read clinical journals: VII. To understand an economic evaluation (part A). *Can. Med. Assoc. J.*, 130:1428–1433.

Department of Clinical Epidemiology and Biostatistics, McMaster University Health Sciences Centre, Hamilton, Ont. (1984b): How to read clinical journals: VII. To understand an economic evaluation (part B). *Can. Med. Assoc. J.*, 130:1542–1549.

DerSimonian, R., Charette, L.J., McPeek, B., and Mosteller, F. (1982): Reporting on methods in clinical trials. *N. Engl. J. Med.*, 306:1332–1337.

De Vecchi, A., Carandente, F., Fryd, D.S., Halberg, F., and Sutherland, E.D. (1979): Circaseptan (about 7-day) rhythm in human kidney allograft rejection in different geographic locations. In: *Proc. 7th Congress Pharmacol. Satellite Symposium on Chronopharmacology. Paris, July 21–24, 1978.* Reinberg, A., and Halberg, F. (Eds.), pp. 193–201. Pergamon Press, Oxford.

Deyo, R.A. (1984): Measuring functional outcomes in therapeutic trials for chronic disease. *Controlled Clin. Trials,* 5:223–240.

Deyo, R.A., Walsh, N.E., Schoenfeld, L.S., and Ramamurthy, S. (1990). Can trials of physical treatments be blinded? The example of transcutaneous electrical nerve stimulation for chronic pain. *Am. J. Phys. Med. Rehabil.*, 69:6–10.

Di Carlo, F.J. (1984): Carcinogenesis bioassay data: Correlation by species and sex. *Drug Metab. Rev.*, 15:409–413.

Diamond, A.L., and Laurence, D.R. (1983): Commentary. *Br. Med. J.,* 287:676–677.

Diamond, S., Solomon, G.D., Freitag, F.G., and Mehta, N. (1987): Selection of patients—critical aspects. *Neuroepidemiology,* 6: 172–177.

Diaz, F.G. (1981): Short- and long-term effects of trithiozine and cimetidine in duodenal ulcer. *Curr. Ther. Res.*, 29:853–865.

Dickersin, K., Chan, S., Chalmers, T.C., Sacks, H.S., and Smith, H. Jr. (1987): Publication bias and clinical trials. *Controlled Clin. Trials,* 8:343–353.

Dickersin, K., and Hewitt, P. (1986): Look before you quote. *Br. Med. J.,* 293:1000–1002.

Diehl, L.F., and Perry, D.J. (1986): A comparison of randomized concurrent control groups with matched historical control groups: Are historical controls valid? *J. Clin. Oncol.*, 4:1114–1120.

Dimond, E.G., Kittle, C.F., and Crockett, J.E. (1960): Comparison of internal mammary artery ligation and sham operation for angina pectoris. *Am. J. Cardiol.*, 5:483–486.

Dinman, B.D. (1980): The reality and acceptance of risk. *JAMA,* 244:1226–1228.

Dinnerstein, A.J., and Halm, J. (1970): Modification of placebo effects by means of drugs: Effects of aspirin and placebos on self-rated moods. *J. Abnorm. Psychol.*, 75:308–314.

DiPiro, J.T., Bowden, T.A., and Hooks, V.H. III. (1984): Prophylactic parenteral cephalosporins in surgery: Are the newer agents better? *JAMA,* 252:3277–3279.

Dittert, L.W., and DiSanto, A.R. (1973): The bioavailability of drug products. *J. Am. Pharm. Assoc.*, NS13:421–432.

Dixon, J.S., Smith, A., and Evans, S.J.W. (1983): Reporting clinical trials. *Br. J. Rheum.*, 22(Suppl.):74–78.

Domer, F.R. (1971): *Animal Experiments in Pharmacological Analysis.* Charles C. Thomas, Springfield, IL.

Drane, J.F. (1984): Competency to give an informed consent: A model for making clinical assessments. *JAMA,* 252:925–927.

Drayer, D.E. (1987): On the use of drugs administered as racemates. *Clin. Pharmacol. Ther.*, 42:364.

Drews, J. (1985): Judging pharmaceutical research and development from a financial point of view. *Swiss Pharm.*, 7:21–23.

Drummond, M.F., Stoddart, G.L., and Torrance, G.W. (1987): *Methods for the Economic Evaluation of Health Care Programmes.* Oxford University Press, Oxford.

Drury, M., and Hull, F.M. (1981): Prospective monitoring for adverse reactions to drugs in general practice. *Br. Med. J.,* 283:1305–1307.

Dubey, S.D. (1986): Current thoughts on crossover designs. *Clin. Res. Practices Drug Reg. Affairs,* 4:127–142.

DuChene, A.G., Hultgren, D.H., Neaton, J.D., Grambsch, P.V., Broste, S.K., et al. (1986): Forms control and error detection procedures used at the coordinating center of the multiple risk factor intervention trial (MRFIT). *Controlled Clin. Trials,* 7:34S–45S.

Duffield, C. (1988): The Delphi technique. *Aust. J. Adv. Nurs.*, 6:41–45.

Dworkin, S.F., and Chen, A.C.N. (1982): Pain in clinical and laboratory contexts. *J. Dent. Res.*, 61:772–774.

Dzierzanowski, J., Bourne, J., and Shiavi, R. (1984): Gaitspert: A knowledge-based expert system for evaluation of human gait abnormalities. In: *Sixth IEEE/Engineering in Medicine and Biology Annual Conference,* pp. 62–65. (Cat. no. 84CH2058–6, IEEE Service Center, Piscataway, NJ).

EC/IC Bypass Study Group. (1985): Failure of extracranial-intracranial arterial bypass to reduce the risk of ischematic stroke: Results of an international randomized trial. *N. Engl. J. Med.*, 313:1191–1200.

Edelson, J.T., Tosteson, A.N.A., and Sax, P. (1990): Cost-effectiveness of misoprostol for prophylaxis against nonsteroidal anti-inflammatory drug-induced gastrointestinal tract bleeding. *JAMA,* 264:41–47.

Edelstyn, G.A., MacRae, K.D., and MacDonald, F.M. (1979): Improvement of life quality in cancer patients undergoing chemotherapy. *Clin. Oncol.*, 5:43–49.

Ederer, F. (1975): Patient bias, investigator bias and the double-masked procedure in clinical trials. *Am. J. Med.*, 58:295–299.

Edlund, M.J., Craig, T.J., and Richardson, M.A. (1985): Informed consent as a form of volunteer bias. *Am. J. Psychiatry,* 142:624–627.

Ehrenkranz, N.J., and Kicklighter, J.L. (1972): Tuberculosis outbreak in a general hospital: Evidence for airborne spread of infection. *Ann. Intern. Med.*, 77:377–382.

Eisenberg, J.M. (1989): Clinical economics: A guide to the economic analysis of clinical practices. *JAMA,* 262:2879–2886.

Eisenberg, J.M., Glick, H., and Koffer, H. (1989): Pharmacoeconomics: Economic evaluation of pharmaceuticals. In: *Pharmacoepidemology.* Strom, B.L. (Ed.), pp. 325–350. Churchill Livingstone, New York.

Elin, R.J., Vesell, E.S., and Wolff, S.M. (1975): Effects of etiocholanolone-induced fever on plasma antipyrine half-lives and metabolic clearance. *Clin. Pharmacol. Ther.*, 17:447–457.

Ellenberg, J.H., and Nelson, K.B. (1980): Sample selection and the natural history of disease: Studies of febrile seizures. *JAMA,* 243:1337–1340.

Ellenberg, S.S. (1984): Randomization designs in comparative clinical trials. *N. Engl. J. Med.*, 310:1404–1408.

Ellenberg, S.S., and Eisenberger, M.A. (1985): An efficient design for phase III studies of combination chemotherapies. *Cancer Treat. Rep.*, 69:1147–1154.

Elveback, L.R., Guillier, C.L., and Keating, F.R. Jr. (1970): Health, normality, and the ghost of Gauss. *JAMA,* 211:69–75.

Emerson, J.D., McPeek, B., and Mosteller, F. (1984): Reporting clinical trials in general surgical journals. *Surgery,* 95:572–579.

EORTC Pharmacokinetics and Metabolism Group. (1987): Pharmacokinetically guided dose escalation in phase I clinical trials. Commentary and proposed guidelines. *Eur. J. Cancer. Clin. Oncol.*, 23:1083–1087.

Epidemiology Work Group of the Interagency Regulatory Liaison Group. (1981): Reviews and commentary: Guidelines for documentation of epidemiologic studies. *Am. J. Epidemiol.*, 114:609–613.

Epstein, A.M., Stern, R.S., Tognetti, J., Begg, C.B., Hartley, R.M., et al. (1988): The association of patients' socioeconomic characteristics with the length of hospital stay and hospital charges within diagnosis-related groups. *N. Engl. J. Med.*, 318:1579–1585.

Epstein, L.C., and Lasagna, L. (1969): Obtaining informed consent: Form or substance. *Arch. Intern. Med.*, 123:682–688.

Esdaile, J.M., Feinstein, A.R., and Horwitz, R.I. (1987): A reappraisal of the United Kingdom epidemic of fatal asthma: Can general mortality data implicate a therapeutic agent? *Arch. Intern. Med.*, 147:543–549.

Esdaile, J.M., and Horwitz, R.I. (1986): Observational studies of cause-effect relationships: An analysis of methodologic problems as illustrated by the conflicting data for the role of oral contraceptives in the etiology of rheumatoid arthritis. *J. Chronic Dis.*, 39:841–852.

Evans, E.F., Proctor, J.D., Fratkin, M.J., Velandia, J., and Wasserman, A.J. (1975): Blood flow in muscle groups and drug absorption. *Clin. Pharmacol. Ther.*, 17:44–47.

Evans, J.T. (1979): Internal monitoring: Patient and study management at the clinic. *Clin. Pharmacol. Ther.*, 25:712–716.

Evans, M., and Pollock, A.V. (1985): A score system for evaluating random control clinical trials of prophylaxis of abdominal surgical wound infection. *Br. J. Surg.*, 72:256–260.

Evans, R.W., Manninen, D.L., Garrison, L.P., Hart, L.G., and Blagg, C.R. (1985): The quality of life of patients with end-stage renal disease. *N. Engl. J. Med.*, 312:553–559.

Evans, S.J.W. (1982): What can we do with the data we throw away? *Br. J. Clin. Pharmacol.*, 14:653–659.

Ezdinli, E., Pocock, S., Berard, C.W., Aungst, C.W., and Silverstein, M. (1976): Comparison of intensive versus moderate chemotherapy of lymphocytic lymphomas. *Cancer*, 38:1060–1068.

Faccini, J.M., Bennett, P.N., and Reid, J.L. (1984): European ethical review committee: The experience of an international ethics committee reviewing protocols for drug trials. *Br. Med. J.*, 289:1052–1054.

Faich, G.A., and Stadel, B.V. (1989): The future of automated record linkage for postmarketing surveillance: A response to Shapiro. *Clin. Pharmacol. Ther.*, 46:387–389.

Falchuk, K.H., Peterson, L., and McNeil, B.J. (1985): Microparticulate-induced phlebitis: Its prevention by in-line filtration. *N. Engl. J. Med.*, 312:78–82.

Fanning, D.M. (1967): Families in flats. *Br. Med. J.*, 4:382–386.

Faust, R.E. (1982): Project selection factors in pharmaceutical R & D. In: *Drug Development*. Hamner, C.E. (Ed.). CRC Press, Inc., Boca Raton, FL.

Feeny, D.H., and Torrance, G.W. (1989): Incorporating utility-based quality-of-life assessment measures in clinical trials: Two examples. *Med. Care*, 3(Suppl.):S190–S204.

Feinstein, A.R. (1967): *Clinical Judgement*. Williams & Wilkins, Baltimore.

Feinstein, A.R. (1977): *Clinical Biostatistics*. The C.V. Mosby Co., St. Louis.

Feinstein, A.R. (1985a): *Clinical Epidemiology: The Architecture of Clinical Research*. W.B.Saunders, Philadelphia.

Feinstein, A. (1985b): A bibliography of publications on observer variability. *J. Chron. Dis.*, 38:619–632.

Feldman, M., Richardson, C. T., and Fordtran, J. S. (1980a): Experience with sham feeding as a test for vagotomy. *Gastroenterology*, 79:792–795.

Feldman, M., Richardson, C.T., and Fordtran, J.S. (1980b): Effect of sham feeding on gastric acid secretion in healthy subjects and duodenal ulcer patients: Evidence for increased basal vagal tone in some ulcer patients. *Gastroenterology*, 79:796–800.

Festing, M.F.W. (1990): Use of genetically heterogeneous rats and mice in toxicological research: A personal perspective. *Toxicol. Appl. Pharmacol.*, 102:197–204.

Fineberg, H.V., and Pearlman, L.A. (1981): Background paper #2: Case studies of medical technologies. Case study #11: Benefit-and-cost analysis of medical interventions: The case of cimetidine and peptic ulcer disease. The Implications of Cost-Effectiveness Analysis of Medical Technology. Congress of the U.S., Office of Technology Assessment, Washington, DC.

Finnegan, M.J., Pickering, C.A.C., and Burge, P.S. (1984): The sick building syndrome: Prevalence studies. *Br. Med. J.*, 289:1573–1575.

Finkelstein, S.N., and Gilbert, D.L. (1985): Scientific evidence and the abandonment of medical technology: A study of eight drugs. *Res. Policy*, 14:225–233.

Fisch, H-U., Hammond, K.R., Joyce, C.R.B., and O'Reilly, M. (1981): An experimental study of the clinical judgment of general physicians in evaluating and prescribing for depression. *Br. J. Psychiatry*, 138:100–109.

Fischl, M.A., Richman, D., Grieco, M.H., Gottlieb, M.S., Volberding, P.A., et al. (1987): The efficacy of azidothymidine (AZT) in the treatment of patients with AIDS and AIDS-related complex. *N. Engl. J. Med.*, 317:185–191.

Fischer, B.H., Marks, M., and Reich, T. (1983): Hyperbaric-oxygen treatment of multiple sclerosis: A randomized, placebo-controlled, double-blind study. *N. Engl. J. Med.*, 308:181–186.

Flaherty, J.A., Gaviria, F.M., Pathak, D., Mitchell, T., Wintrob, R., et al. (1988): Developing instruments for cross-cultural psychiatric research. *J. Nerv. Ment. Dis.*, 176:257–263.

Fleming, T.R., and Watelet, L.F. (1989): Approaches to monitoring clinical trials. *JNCI*, 81:188–193.

Fletcher, A.P. (1978): Drug safety tests and subsequent clinical experience. *J. R. Soc. Med.*, 71:693–696.

Fletcher, C.M., Jones, N.L., and Burrows, B., and Niden, A.H. (1964): American emphysema and British bronchitis: A standardized comparative study. *Am. Rev. Resp. Dis.*, 90:1–13.

Fletcher, R.H., and Fletcher, S.W. (1979): Clinical research in general medical journals: A 30-year perspective. *N. Engl. J. Med.*, 301:180–183.

Fletcher, R.H., Fletcher, S.W., and Wagner, E.H. (1988): *Clinical Epidemiology—The Essentials*, 2nd ed. Williams & Wilkins, Baltimore.

Fletcher, S.W., O'Malley, M.S., and Bunce, L.A. (1985): Physicians' abilities to detect lumps in silicone breast models. *JAMA*, 253:2224–2228.

Focan, C. (1979): Sequential chemotherapy and circadian rhythm in human solid tumours. A randomised trial. *Cancer Chemother. Pharmacol.*, 3:197.

Folb, P.I. (1980): *The Safety of Medicines—Evaluation and Prediction*. Springer-Verlag, New York.

Folland, E., Hammermeister, K.E., Khuri, S., Rahimtoola, S.H., and Sethi, G. (1979): Letter to the editor. *N. Engl. J. Med.*, 301:1182–1183.

Food and Drug Administration. (1974): *General guidelines for the evaluation of drugs to be approved for use during pregnancy and for treatment of infants and children: A report of the Committee on Drugs, American Academy of Pediatrics to the Food and Drug Administration*, U.S. DHEW. American Academy of Pediatrics, Evanston, IL.

Food and Drug Administration. (1977a): *FDA Bureau of Drugs Clinical Guidelines. General considerations for the clinical evaluation of drugs in infants and children*, FDA 77–3041. Superintendent of Documents, U.S. Government Printing Office, Washington, DC. (Over 24 separate guidelines are available for evaluation of different types of drugs in adults and children.).

Food and Drug Administration. (1977b): Clinical investigations: Proposed establishment of regulations on obligations of sponsors and monitors. *Fed. Reg.*, 42(187, Tuesday, September 27, 1977, Part IV):49612–49630.

Food and Drug Administration. (1978): Obligations of clinical investigators of regulated articles: Proposed establishment of regulations. *Fed. Reg.*, 43(153, Tuesday, August 8, 1878, Part V):35210–35236.

Food and Drug Administration. (1981a): Protection of human subjects; Informed consent. *Fed Reg.*, 46(17, Tuesday, January 27, 1981):8942–8958.

Food and Drug Administration. (1981b): Protection of human subjects; Standards for institutional review boards for clinical investigations. *Fed. Reg.*, 46(17, Tuesday, January 27, 1981):8958–8979.

Forbes, M.B., Perez, A.E., and Gelberg, A. (1986): FDA's adverse drug reaction drug dictionary and its role in post-marketing surveillance. *Drug Info. J.*, 20:135–145.

Ford, M.R. (1982): Biofeedback treatment for headaches, Raynaud's disease, essential hypertension, and irritable bowel syndrome: A review of the long-term follow-up literature. *Biofeedback Self Regul.*, 7:521–536.

Forrest, M., and Andersen, B. (1986): Ordinal scale and statistics in medical research. *Br. Med. J.*, 292:537–538.

Foulds, G.A. (1958): Clinical research in psychiatry. *J. Ment. Sci.,* 104:259–265.

Fourestié, V., de Lignières, B., Roudot-Thoraval, F., Fulli-Lemaire, I., Cremniter, D., et al. (1986): Suicide attempts in hypo-oestrogenic phases of the menstrual cycle. *Lancet,* II:1357–1359.

Fowler, N.O. (1979): Randomized clinical trials in surgery. *N. Engl. J. Med.,* 301:1181.

Fox, A.J., and White, G.C. (1976): Bladder cancer in rubber workers: Do screening and doctors' awareness distort the statistics? *Lancet,* 1:1009–1011.

Fraumeni, J.F. Jr., and Miller, R.W. (1972): Drug-induced cancer. *JNCI,* 48:1267–1270.

Freiman, J.A., Chalmers, T.C., Smith, H. Jr., and Kuebler, R.R. (1978): The importance of beta, the type II error and sample size in the design and interpretation of the randomized control trial. *N. Engl. J. Med.,* 299:690–694.

Freireich, E.J., Gehan, E.A., Rall, D.P., Schmidt, L.H., and Skipper, H.E. (1966): Quantitative comparison of toxicity of anticancer agents in mouse, rat, hamster, dog, monkey, and man. *Cancer Chemother. Rep.,* 50:219–244.

Frelick, R.W., and Kyle, A. (1984): Cancer clinical trial records: Physician responsibility. *Prog. Clin. Biol. Res.,* 156:369–378.

Friedewald, W.T., and Schoenberger, J.A. (1982): Overview of recent clinical and methodological advances from clinical trials of cardiovascular disease. *Controlled Clin. Trials,* 3:259–270.

Friedman, H., and Greenblatt, D.J. (1986): Rational therapeutic drug monitoring. *JAMA,* 256:2227–2233.

Friedman, L.M., Furbury, C.D., and De Mets, D.L. (1981): *Fundamentals of Clinical Trials.* J. Wright, PSG, Boston.

Friedman, R.B., Anderson, R.E., Entine, S.M., and Hirshberg, S.B. (1980): Effects of diseases on clinical laboratory tests. *Clin. Chem.,* 26:1D–476D.

Furberg, C.D. (1989): The impact of clinical trials on clinical practice. *Arzneimittelforschung/Drug Res.,* 39:986–988.

Furberg, C.D., and Black, D.M. (1988): The systolic hypertension in the elderly pilot program: Methodological issues. *Eur. Heart J.,* 9:223–227.

Furberg, C.D., and Morgan, T.M. (1987): Lessons from overviews of cardiovascular trials. *Stat. Med.,* 6:295–306.

Garattini, S. (1985): Toxic effects of chemicals: Difficulties in extrapolating data from animals to man. *CRC Crit. Rev. Toxicol.,* 16:1–29.

Gardner, M. (1982): aha! Gotcha: *Paradoxes to Puzzle and Delight.* W.H. Freeman and Company, New York.

Gardner, M.J., and Altman, D.G. (1988): Estimating with confidence. *Br. Med. J.,* 296:1210–1211.

Gardner, M.J., Altman, D.G., Jones, D.R., and Machin, D. (1983): Is the statistical assessment of papers submitted to the "British Medical Journal" effective? *Br. Med. J.,* 286:1485–1488.

Gay, W.I. (Ed.) (1965–1973): *Methods of Animal Experimentation.* Volumes I–IV. Academic Press, New York.

Gehan, E.A. (1988): Methodological issues in cancer clinical trials: The comparison of therapies. *Biomed. Pharmacother.,* 42:161–165.

Gelber, R.D. (1985): Methodological and statistical aspects in perioperative chemotherapy trials. *Recent Results Cancer Res.,* 98:53–63.

Gennaro, A.R. (1990): *Remington's Pharmaceutical Sciences.* 18th Edition. Mack, Easton, PA.

Gerbarg, Z.B., and Horwitz, R.I. (1988): Resolving conflicting clinical trials: Guidelines for meta-analysis. *J. Clin. Epidemiol.,* 41:503–509.

Gerin, M., Siemiatycki, J., Kemper, H., and Begin, D. (1985): Obtaining occupational exposure histories in epidemiologic case-control studies. *J. Occup. Med.,* 27:420–426.

Gibaldi, M., and Prescott, L. (Eds.) (1983): *Handbook of Clinical Pharmacokinetics.* ADIS Health Sciences Press, Sydney, Australia.

Gifford, R.H., and Feinstein, A.R. (1969): A critique of methodology in studies of anticoagulant therapy for acute myocardial infarction. *N. Engl. J. Med.,* 280:351–357.

Gifford, R.W., Jr. (1969): Evaluation of the hypertensive patient with emphasis on detecting curable causes. *Millbank Mem. Fund Q.,* 47:170–186.

Gilbert, J.P., McPeek, B., and Mosteller, F. (1977a): Statistics and ethics in surgery and anesthesia. *Science,* 198:684–689.

Gilbert, J.P., McPeek, B., and Mosteller, F. (1977b): Progress in surgery and anesthesia: Benefits and risks of innovative therapy. In: *Costs, Risks and Benefits of Surgery.* Bunker, J., Barnes, B., and Mosteller, F., (Eds.), pp. 124–169. Oxford University Press, New York.

Gill, P.W., Leaper, D.J., Guillou, P.J., Staniland, J.R., and Horrocks, J.C. (1973): Observer variation in clinical diagnosis—A computer-aided assessment of its magnitude and importance in 552 patients with abdominal pain. *Methods Inf. Med.,* 12:108–113.

Gillon, R. (1985): Medical oaths, declarations and codes. *Br. Med. J.,* 290:1194–1195.

Gillum, T.L. (1989): The Merck regulatory dictionary: A pragmatically developed drug effects vocabulary. *Drug Info. J.,* 23:217–220.

Girard, M. (1984): Testing the methods of assessment for adverse drug reactions. *Adv. Drug React. Acute Pois. Rev.,* 4:237–244.

Glantz, S.A. (1980): Biostatistics: How to detect, correct and prevent errors in the medical literature. *Circulation,* 61:1–7.

Glass, P., Avery, G.B., Subramanian, K.N.S., Keys, M.P., and Sostek, A.M. (1985): Effect of bright light in the hospital nursery on the incidence of retinopathy of prematurity. *N. Engl. J. Med.,* 313:401–404.

Glick, B.S., and Margolis, R. (1962): A study of the influence of experimental design on clinical outcome in drug research. *Am. J. Psychiatry,* 118:1087–1096.

Glicksman, A.S., Reinstein, L.E., Brotman, R., and McShan, D. (1980): Quality assurance programs in clinical trials. *Cancer Treat. Rep.,* 64:425–433.

Golbert, T.M., and Patterson, R. (1968): Recurrent anaphylaxis caused by a misidentified drug. *Ann. Intern. Med.,* 68:621–623.

Goldman, J., and Katz, M.D. (1982): Inconsistency and institutional review boards. *JAMA,* 248:197–202.

Goldman, L., Sia, S.T.B., Cook, E.F., Rutherford, J.D., and Weinstein, M.C. (1988): Costs and effectiveness of routine therapy with long-term beta-adrenergic antagonists after acute myocardial infarction. *N. Engl. J. Med.,* 319:152–157.

Goldsmith, M.A., Slavik, M., and Carter, S.K. (1975): Quantitative prediction of drug toxicity in humans from toxicology in small and large animals. *Cancer Res.,* 35:1354–1364.

Goldsmith, M.F. (1985): Computerized biofeedback training aids in spinal injury rehabilitation. *JAMA,* 253:1097–1099.

Goldzieher, J.W., Moses, L.E., Averkin, E., Scheel, C., and Taber, B.Z. (1971): A placebo-controlled double-blind crossover investigation of the side effects attributed to oral contraceptives. *Fertil. Steril.,* 22:609–623.

Good, I.J. (1962): A classification of fallacious arguments and interpretations. *Technometrics,* 4:125–132.

Goodman, D.G., Ward, J.M., Squire, R.A., Chu, K.C., and Linhart, M.S. (1979): Neoplastic and nonneoplastic lesions in aging F344 rats. *Toxicol. Appl. Pharmacol.,* 48:237–248.

Goodwin, J.S., Goodwin, J.M., and Vogel, A.V. (1979): Knowledge and use of placebos by house officers and nurses. *Ann. Intern. Med.,* 91:106–110.

Goodwin, J.S., Hunt, W.C., Key, C.R., and Samet, J.M. (1987): The effect of marital status on stage, treatment, and survival of cancer patients. *JAMA,* 258:3125–3130.

Gordon Lan, K.K., and Friedman, L. (1986): Monitoring boundaries for adverse effects in long-term clinical trials. *Controlled Clin. Trials,* 7:1–7.

Gore, S.M., and Altman, D.G. (1982): *Statistics in Practice*. British Medical Association, London.

Gorringe, J.A.L. (1970): Initial preparation for clinical trials. In: *The Principles and Practice of Clinical Trials*. Harris, E.L., and Fitzgerald, J.D. (Eds.), pp. 41–46. E. & S. Livingstone, Edinburgh.

Gotzsche, P.C. (1989): Methodology and overt and hidden bias in reports of 196 double-blind trials of nonsteroidal antiinflammatory drugs in rheumatoid arthritis. *Controlled Clin. Trials*, 10:31–56.

Gould, B.A., Mann, S., Davies, A.B., Altman, D.G., and Raftery, E.B. (1981): Does placebo lower blood-pressure? *Lancet*, II:1377–1381.

Gould, J.B., Davey, B., and Stafford, R.S. (1989): Socioeconomic differences in rates of cesarean sections. *N. Engl. J. Med.*, 321:233–239.

Gouvier, W.D., Richards, S., Blanton, P.D., and Fine, P.R. (1985): Dependent variables in rehabilitation research. *Arch. Phys. Med. Rehabil.*, 66:803–805.

Grabowski, H., and Vernon, J. (1982): A sensitivity analysis of expected profitability of pharmaceutical research and development. *Managerial Decision Economics*, 3:36–40.

Grabowski, H.G., and Hansen, R.W. (1990): Economic scales and tests. In: *Quality of Life Assessments in Clinical Trials*. Spilker, B. (Ed.), pp. 61–69. Raven Press, New York.

Grace, N.D., Muench, H., and Chalmers, T.C. (1966): The present status of shunts for portal hypertension in cirrhosis. *Gastroenterology*, 50:684–691.

Grage, T.B., and Zelen, M. (1982): The controlled randomized clinical trial in the evaluation of cancer treatment: The dilemma and alternative trial designs. In: *UICC Technical Report Series*. Volume 70. Flamant, R. and Fohanno, C. (Eds.), pp.23–48. International Union against Cancer, Geneva.

Graham, R.J. (1985): Project Management: *Combined Technical and Behavioral Approaches for Effective Implementation*. Van Nostrand Reinhold Co., New York.

Grahame-Smith, D.G., and Aronson, J.K. (Eds.) (1984): *Oxford Textbook of Clinical Pharmacology*. Oxford University Press, New York.

Granger, C.H. (1964): The hierarchy of objectives. *Harvard Bus. Rev.*, 42:63–74.

Gray, B.H., Cooke, R.A., and Tannenbaum, A.S. (1978): Research involving human subjects. *Science*, 201:1094–1101.

Green, S.B., Ellenberg, S.S., Finkelstein, D, Forsythe, A.B., Freedman, L.S., et al. (1990): Issues in the design of drug trials for AIDS. *Controlled Clin. Trials*, 11:80–87.

Greenberg, R.N. (1984): Overview of patient compliance with medication dosing: A literature review. *Clin. Ther.*, 6:592–599.

Greenblatt, D.J., Sellers, E.M., and Shader, R.I. (1982): Drug disposition in old age. *N. Engl. J. Med.*, 306:1081–1088.

Greenland, S., and Morgenstern, H. (1988): Classification schemes for epidemiologic research designs. *J. Clin. Epidemiol.*, 41:715–716.

Griffin, J.P. (1985): Predictive value of animal toxicity studies. *ATLA*, 12:163–170.

Griffin, J.P. (1986): Predictive value of animal toxicity studies. In: *Long-Term Animal Studies. Their Predictive Value for Man*. Walker, S.R., and Dayan, A.D. (Eds.), pp. 107–116. MTP Press, Lancaster, England.

Griffin, J.P., and Weber, J.C.P. (1985): Voluntary systems of adverse reaction reporting—Part I. *Adv. Drug React. Acute Pois. Rev.*, 4:213–230.

Griffin, J.P., and Weber, J.C.P. (1986): Voluntary systems of adverse reaction reporting—Part II. *Adv. Drug React. Acute Pois. Rev.*, 1:23–55.

Griffin, J.P., and Weber, J.C.P. (1989): Voluntary systems of adverse reaction reporting—Part III. *Adverse Drug React. Acute Pois. Rev.* (UK), 8:203–215.

Grim, P.S., Gottlieb, L.J., Boddie, A., and Batson, E. (1990): Hyperbaric oxygen therapy. *JAMA*, 263:2216–2220.

Grim, P.S., Singer, P.A., Gramelspacher, G.P., Feldman, T., Childers, R.W., et al. (1989): Informed consent in emergency research: Prehospital thrombolytic therapy for acute myocardial infarction. *JAMA*, 262:252–255.

Grimby, G., and Saltin, B. (1983): The ageing muscle. *Clin. Physiol.*, 3:209–218.

Griner, P.F., Mayewski, R.J., Mushlin, A.I., and Greenland, P. (1981): Selection and interpretation of diagnostic tests and procedures: Principles and applications. *Ann. Intern. Med.*, 94:553–600.

Grodin, M.A., Zaharoff, B.E., and Kaminow, P.V. (1986): A 12-year audit of IRB decisions. *QRB*, 12:82–86.

Gross, M. (1988): A critique of the methodologies used in clinical studies of hip-joint arthroplasty published in the English-language orthopaedic literature. *J. Bone Joint Surg.*, 70-A:1364–1371.

Gross, P.A. (1984): Collection of data documenting risk factors: Safeguards in conducting case-control studies. *Am. J. Med.*, 76(5A):28–33.

Gross, P.A., Neu, H.C., Aswapokee, P., Van Antwerpen, C., and Aswapokee, N. (1980): Deaths from nosocomial infections: Experience in a university hospital and a community hospital *Am. J. Med.*, 68:219–223.

Gundermann, K.O. (1980): Spread of microorganisms by air-conditioning systems—especially in hospitals. *Ann. N.Y. Acad. Sci.*, 353:209–217.

Gupta, M., and Chowdhuri, A.N.R. (1980): Relationship between ABO blood groups and malaria. *Bull. WHO*, 58:913–915.

Guth, W.D. (1985): *Handbook of Business Strategy*. Warren, Gorham and Lamont, Boston.

Guy, W. (1976): *ECDEU Assessment Manual for Psychopharmacology (revised)*. U.S. DHEW Pub. No. (ADM) 76–338. U.S. Government Printing Office, Washington, DC.

Guy, W. (1979): Documentation of early phase II trials. In: *Coordinating Clinical Trials in Psychopharmacology: Planning, Documentation, and Analysis*. Levine, J. (Ed.). DHEW Publication No. (ADM) 79–803, U.S. Government Printing Office, Washington, DC.

Guyatt, G.H. (1985): Methodologic problems in clinical trials in heart failure. *J. Chronic Dis.*, 38:353–363.

Guyatt, G.H., and Jaeschke, R. (1990): Measurements in clinical trials: Choosing the right approach. In: *Quality of Life Assessments in Clinical Trials*. Spilker, B. (Ed.), pp.37–47. Raven Press, New York.

Guyatt, G.H., and Newhouse, M.T. (1987): Rigorous evaluation: Greater need than ever. *Chest*, 92:580–581.

Guyatt, G., Sackett, D., Taylor, D.W., Chong, J, Roberts, R. (1986): Determining optimal therapy: Randomized trials in individual patients. *N. Engl. J. Med.*, 314:889–892.

Guyatt, G.H., Townsend, M., Berman, L.B., and Keller, J.L. (1987): A comparison of Likert and visual analogue scales for measuring change in function. *J. Chronic Dis.*, 40:1129–1133.

Guyatt, G.H., Veldhuyzen Van Zanten, S.J.O., Feeny, D.H., and Patrick, D.L. (1989): Measuring quality of life in clinical trials: A taxonomy and review. *Can. Med. Assoc. J.*, 140:1441–1448.

Haakenson, C., Fye, C.L., Sather, M.R., and Toussaint, D.J. (1987): The investigator-sponsored IND in clinical trials. *Controlled Clin. Trials*, 8:101–109.

Hagler, L., Luscombe, F., and Siegfried, J. (1987): A primer on postmarketing surveillance. *Drug Info. J.*, 21:71–107.

Hailstone, M. (1973): A case for standardization in the preparation of graphs and diagrams. *Med. Biol. Illus.*, 23:8–12.

Haines, S.J. (1983): Randomized clinical trials in neurosurgery. *Neurosurgery*, 12:259–264.

Halbreich, U., Bakhai, Y., Bacon, K.B., Goldstein, S., Asnis, G.M., et al. (1989): The normalcy of self-proclaimed "normal volunteers." *Am. J. Psychiatry*, 146:1052–1055.

Haley, R.W., Schaberg, D.R., McClish, D.K., Quade, D., Crossley, K.B., Culver, D.H., et al. (1980). The accuracy of retrospective chart review in measuring nosocomical infection rates. *Am. J. Epidemiol.* 111:516–533.

Hall, G.C., Luscombe, D.K., and Walker, S.R. (1988): Postmarketing surveillance using a computerised general practice data base. *Pharm. Med.,* 2:345–351.

Hamblin, T. (1984): Where now for therapeutic apheresis? *Br. Med. J.,* 289:779–780.

Hamilton, M., Pickering, G.W., Roberts, J.A., and Sowry, G.S. (1963): Arterial pressures of relatives of patients with secondary and malignant hypertension. *Clin. Sci.,* 24:91–108.

Hammes, C.E., and Ciccone, P.E. (Eds.) (1985): The impact of the Rx-to-OTC switch process: Present and future. *Drug. Inf. J.,* 19(2), Special Issue:85–203.

Hand, D.J. (1979): Psychiatric examples of Simpson's paradox. *Br. J. Psychiatry,* 135:90–91.

Hansen, H.J., Caudill, S.P., and Boone, J. (1985): Crisis in drug testing: Results of CDC blind study. *JAMA,* 253:2382–2387.

Hansen, R.W. (1983): International Issues of Drug Regulation. *Z. Gesamte Staatswissenchaft (J. Inst. Theor. Economics),* 139:568–577.

Harris, E.L., and Fitzgerald, J.D. (Eds.) (1970): *The Principles and Practice of Clinical Trials.* E. & S. Livingstone, Edinburgh.

Harrison, W.M., Endicott, J., Rabkin, J.G., and Nee, J. (1984): Treatment of premenstrual dysphoric changes: Clinical outcome and methodological implications. *Psychopharmacol. Bull.,* 20:118–122.

Hart, P., Farrell, G.C., Cooksley, W.G.E., and Powell, L.W. (1976): Enhanced drug metabolism in cigarette smokers. *Br. Med. J.,* 2:147–149.

Harth, S.C., and Thong, Y.H. (1990): Sociodemographic and motivational characteristics of parents who volunteer their children for clinical research: A controlled study. *Br. Med. J.,* 300:1372–1375.

Haseman, J.K., Huff, J.E., and Moore, J.A. (1983): Letter to editor (untitled). *Fundam. Appl. Toxicol.,* 3:3–5.

Haslam, K.R. (1974): Laminar air-flow air conditioning in the operating room: A review. *Anesth. Analg.,* 53:194–199.

Hassar, M., and Weintraub, M. (1976): ''Uninformed'' consent and the wealthy volunteer: An analysis of patient volunteers in a clinical trial of a new anti-inflammatory drug. *Clin. Pharmacol. Ther.,* 20:379–386.

Hatch, J.P. (1982): Controlled group designs in biofeedback research: Ask, ''what does the control group control for?'' *Biofeedback Self Regul.,* 7:377–401.

Havard, C.W.H., and Pearson, R.M. (1977): Use and effect of placebos. *Prescribers J.,* 17:94–100.

Hawkins, B.S. (1984): Evaluating the benefit of clinical trials to future patients. *Controlled Clin. Trials,* 5:13–32.

Hawkins, B.S. (1987): Perusing the literature: Generalizability of clinical trials. *Controlled Clin. Trials,* 8:255–265.

Hawkins, B.S. (1988): Selection of controls for clinical research studies in ophthalmology. *Arch. Ophthalmol.,* 106:835–840.

Hayes, R.H. (1985): Strategic planning—forward in reverse? *Harvard Bus. Rev.,* 63:111–119.

Hayes, T.M., and Harries, J. (1984): Randomised controlled trial of routine hospital clinic care versus routine general practice care for type II diabetics. *Br. Med. J.,* 289:728–730.

Haynes, R.B. (1988): Selected principles of the measurement and setting of priorities of death, disability, and suffering in clinical trials. *Am. J. Med. Sci.,* 296:364–369.

Haynes, R.B., Sackett, D.L, Gibson, E.S., Taylor, D.W., Hackett, B.C., et al. (1976): Improvement of medication compliance in uncontrolled hypertension. *Lancet,* I:1265–1268.

Haynes, R.B., Sackett, D.L., and Tugwell, P. (1983): Problems in the handling of clinical and research evidence by medical practitioners. *Arch. Intern. Med.,* 143:1971–1975.

Healy, B., Campeau, L., Gray, R., Herd, J.A., Hoogwerf, B., et al. (1989): Conflict-of-interest guidelines for a multicenter clinical trial of treatment after coronary-artery bypass-graft surgery. *N. Engl. J. Med.,* 320:949–951.

Hedman, C., Andersen, A.R., and Olesen, J. (1987): Multi-centre versus single-centre trials in migraine. *Neuroepidemiology,* 6:190–197.

Hemminki, E. (1981): Quality of reports of clinical trials submitted by the drug industry to the Finnish and Swedish control authorities. *Eur. J. Clin. Pharmacol.,* 19:157–165.

Hemminki, E. (1982): Quality of clinical trials—a concern of three decades. *Methods Inf. Med.,* 21:81–85.

Henderson-James, D., and Spilker, B. (1990): An industry perspective. In: *Quality of Life Assessments in Clinical Trials.* Spilker, B. (Ed.), pp. 183–193. Raven Press, New York.

Henkin, R.I., Schechter, P.J., Friedewald, W.T., Demets, D.L., and Raff, M. (1976): A double blind study of the effects of zinc sulfate on taste and smell dysfunction. *Am. J. Med. Sci.,* 272:285–299.

Herberman, R.B. (1985): Design of clinical trials with biological response modifiers. *Cancer Treat. Rep.,* 69:1161–1164.

Herman, P.G., and Hessel, S.J. (1975): Accuracy and its relationship to experience in the interpretation of chest radiographs. *Invest. Radiol.,* 10:62–67.

Herxheimer, H. (1972): Asthma deaths. *Lancet,* I:98.

Hetherington, J., Dickersin, K., Chalmers, I., and Meinert, C.L. (1989): Retrospective and prospective identification of unpublished controlled trials: Lessons from a survey of obstetricians and pediatricians. *Pediatrics,* 84:374–380.

Heywood, R. (1984): Prediction of adverse drug reactions from animal safety studies. In: *Detection and Prevention of Adverse Drug Reactions.* (Skandia International Symposia). Bostrom, H., and Ljungstedt, N. (Eds.), pp. 173–189. Almqvist and Wiksell International, Stockholm.

Hickam, D.H., Shortliffe, E.H., Bischoff, M.B., Scott, A.C., and Jacobs, C.D. (1985): The treatment advice of a computer-based cancer chemotherapy protocol advisor. *Ann. Intern. Med.,* 103:928–936.

Higgins, P. (1983): Can 98.6 be a fever in disguise? *Geriatr. Nurs.,* 4:101–102.

Higginson, J. (1987): Publication of ''negative'' epidemiologic studies. *J. Chronic Dis.,* 40:371–372.

Hill, A.B. (1971): Statistical evidence and inference. In: *Principles of Medical Statistics.* Ninth Edition. Oxford University Press, New York, pp. 309–323.

Hill, J.D., Hampton, J.R., and Mitchell, J.R.A. (1978): A randomised trial of home-versus-hospital management for patients with suspected myocardial infarction. *Lancet,* I:837–841.

Hines, D.C., and Goldzieher, J.W. (1969): Clinical investigation: A guide to its evaluation. *Am. J. Obstet. Gynecol.,* 105:450–487.

Hoar, S.K., Blair, A., Holmes, F.F., Boysen, C.D., Robel, R.J., et al. (1986): Agricultural herbicide use and risk of lymphoma and soft-tissue sarcoma. *JAMA,* 256:1141–1147.

Holdsworth, P.J., Thorogood, J., Benson, E.A., and Clayden, A.D. (1985): Blood group as a prognostic indicator in breast cancer. *Br. Med. J.,* 290:671–673.

Holmes, D.S., and Burish, T.G. (1983): Effectiveness of biofeedback for treating migraine and tension headaches: A review of the evidence. *J. Psychosom. Res.,* 27:515–532.

Honig, S. (1988): Clinical trials in acute musculoskeletal injury states. *Am. J. Med.,* 84(Suppl. 5A):42–44.

Hopkins, J.A., Shoemaker, W.C., Greenfield, S., Chang, P.C., and McAuliffe, T. (1980): Treatment of surgical emergencies with and without an algorithm. *Arch. Surg.,* 115:745–750.

Horwitz, R.I. (1987): Complexity and contradiction in clinical trial research. *Am. J. Med.,* 82:498–510.

Horwitz, R.I., and Feinstein, A.R. (1979): Methodologic standards and contradictory results in case-control research. *Am. J. Med.,* 66:556–564.

Hoult, J., and Reynolds, I. (1984): Schizophrenia: A comparative trial of community orientated and hospital orientated psychiatric care. *Acta Psychiatr. Scand.,* 69:359–372.

Howard, J., Whittemore, A.S., Hoover, J.J., Panos, M., and the Aspirin Myocardial Infarction Study Research Group (1982): How blind was the patient blind in AMIS? *Clin. Pharmacol. Ther.*, 32:543–553.

Howard, J.M., DeMets, D., and BHAT Research Group. (1981): How informed is informed consent? The BHAT experience. *Controlled Clin. Trials*, 2:287–303.

Howorth, F.H. (1985): Prevention of airborne infection during surgery. *Lancet*, I:386–388.

Huff, D. (1954): *How to Lie with Statistics*. First Edition. W.W. Norton & Company, New York.

Hughes, R.G. (1990): The management of third-party trials in Europe. *Drug Info. J.*, 24:169–175.

Hulley, S.B., and Cummings, S.R. (1988): *Designing Clinical Research: An Epidemiologic Approach*. Williams & Wilkins, Baltimore.

Hunninghake, D.B., Darby, C.A., and Probstfield, J.L. (1987): Recruitment experience in clinical trials: Literature summary and annotated bibliography. *Controlled Clin. Trials*, 8(Suppl.):6S–30S.

Hunt, S.M. (1986): Cross-cultural issues in the use of socio-medical indicators. *Health Policy*, 6:149–158.

Hunter, W.J., Lingk, W., and Recht, P. (1979): Intercomparison study on the determination of single administration toxicity in rats. *J. Assoc. Off. Anal Chem.*, 62:864–873.

Huskisson, E.C. (1974): Simple analgesics for arthritis. *Br. Med. J.*, 4:196–200.

Hussar, D.A. (1980): Patient compliance. In: *Remington's Pharmaceutical Sciences*. 16th Edition. Osol, A. (Ed.), pp. 1703–1713. Mack, Easton, PA.

Hutchinson, T.A., Leventhal, J.M., Kramer, M.S., Karch, F.E., Lipman, A.G., et al. (1979): An algorithm for the operational assessment of adverse drug reactions. II. Demonstration of reproducibility and validity. *JAMA*, 242:633–638.

Huth, E.J. (1982): *How to Write and Publish Papers in the Medical Sciences*. ISI Press, Philadelphia, PA.

Hypertension Prevention Trial Research Group. (1989): [Five separate articles] in *Controlled Clin. Trials*, 10(Suppl.3):1–94.

Iber, F.L. (1977): Drug metabolism in heavy consumers of ethyl alcohol. *Clin. Pharmacol. Ther.*, 22:735–742.

Ikwueke, K. (1984): The changing pattern of infectious disease. *Br. Med. J.*, 289:1355–1358.

Imperato, P.J. (1981): Legionellosis and the indoor environment. *Bull. N.Y. Acad. Med.*, 57:922–935.

Imperiale, T.F., and Horwitz, R.I. (1989): Scientific standards and the design of case-control research. *Biomed. Pharmacother.*, 43:187–196.

Ingelfinger, F.J. (1977): Debates on diabetes. *New Eng. J. Med.*, 296:1228–1230.

Ingelfinger, J.A., Mosteller, F., Thibodeau, L.A., and Ware, J.H. (1987): *Biostatistics in Clinical Medicine*. Macmillan, New York.

Inman, W.H.W. (Ed.) (1986): *Monitoring for Drug Safety*. MTP Press, Lancaster, UK.

Institute of Laboratory Animal Resources—National Research Council, and American College of Laboratory Animal Medicine—Sponsors. (1971): *Animal Models for Biomedical Research IV; Proceedings of a Symposium*. National Academy of Sciences, Washington, DC.

International Committee of Medical Journal Editors. (1982): Uniform requirements for manuscripts submitted to biomedical journals. *Ann. Intern. Med.*, 96:766–771.

Irwin, M., Lovitz, A., Marder, S.R., Mintz, J., Winslade, W.J., et al. (1985): Psychotic patients' understanding of informed consent. *Am. J. Psychiatry*, 142:1351–1354.

Jachuck, S.J., Brierley, H., Jachuck, S., and Willcox, P.M. (1982): The effect of hypotensive drugs on the quality of life. *J. R. Coll. Gen. Pract.*, 32:103–105.

Jacobs, K.W., and Nordan, F.M. (1979): Classification of placebo drugs: Effect of color. *Percept. Mot. Skills*, 49:367–372.

Jaeschke, R., and Guyatt, G.H. (1990): How to develop and validate a new quality of life instrument. In: *Quality of Life Assessments in Clinical Trials*. Spilker, B. (Ed.), pp. 47–57. Raven Press, New York.

Jaeschke, R., Singer, J., and Guyatt, G.H. (1990): A comparison of seven-point and visual analogue scales: Data from a randomized trial. *Controlled Clin. Trials*, 11:43–51.

Jamali, F. (1988): Pharmacokinetics of enantiomers of chiral non-steroidal anti-inflammatory drugs. *Eur. J. Drug Metab. Pharmacokinet.*, 13:1–9.

Jamali, F., Mehvar, R., and Pasutto, F.M. (1989): Enantioselective aspects of drug action and disposition: Therapeutic pitfalls. *J. Pharm. Sci.*, 78:695–715.

Janas, L.M., and Picciano, M.F. (1984): Human milk: A portal of drugs from mother to infant. In: *Drugs and Nutrients: The Interactive Effects*. Roe, D.A., and Campbell, T.C. (Eds.), Ch. 9, pp. 331–373. Marcel Dekker, New York.

Janicak, P.G., Davis, J.M., Gibbons, R.D., Ericksen, S., Chang, S., et al. (1985): Efficacy of ECT: A meta-analysis. *Am. J. Psychiatry*, 142:297–302.

Jarvis, M.J., Russell, M.A.H., Feyerabend, C., Eiser, J.R., Morgan, M., et al. (1985): Passive exposure to tobacco smoke: Saliva cotinine concentrations in a representative population sample of non-smoking schoolchildren. *Br. Med. J.*, 291:927–929.

Jay, A. (1976): How to run a meeting. *Harvard Bus. Rev.*, 54:43–57.

Jick, H., and Walker, A.M. (1989): Uninformed criticism of automated record linkage. *Clin. Pharmacol. Ther.*, 46:478–479.

Joffe, M. (1988): Advantages of a standard method for research on reproductive effects of occupation. *J. Epidemiol. Community Health*, 42:209–212.

Joglekar, P., and Paterson, M.L. (1986): A closer look at the returns and risks of pharmaceutical R&D. *J. Health Econ.*, 5:153–177.

Johansson, J., and Ost, L-G. (1982): Self-control procedures in biofeedback: A review of temperature biofeedback in the treatment of migraine. *Biofeedback Self Regul.*, 7:435–442.

Johnsson, G., Åblad, B., and Hansson, E. (1984): Prediction of adverse drug reactions in clinical practice from animal experiments and phase I–III studies. In: *Detection and Prevention of Adverse Drug Reactions*. (Skandia International Symposia). Boström, H., and Ljungstedt, N. (Eds.), pp. 190–199. Almqvist and Wiskell International, Stockholm.

Johnston, M. (1980): Anxiety in surgical patients. *Psychol. Med.*, 10:145–152.

Johnston, M., and Carpenter, L. (1980): Relationship between pre-operative anxiety and post-operative state. *Psychol. Med.*, 10:361–367.

Johnston-Early, A., McKenzie, M.A., Krasnow, S.H., Hood, M.A., and Cohen, M.H. (1984): Drug trapping in intravenous infusion side arms. *JAMA*, 252:2392.

Joint Committee of ABPI, BMA, CSM, and RCGP. (1988): Guidelines on post-marketing surveillance. *Br. Med. J.*, 296:399–400.

Jones, J.K. (Ed.) (1985): International adverse reaction surveillance. *Drug Info. J.*, 19:205–393.

Jordan, R.A., Seth, L., Casebolt, P., Hayes, M.J., Wilen, M.M., and Franciosa, J. (1986): Rapidly developing tolerance to trans-dermal nitroglycerin in congestive heart failure. *Ann. Intern. Med.*, 104:295–298.

Joubert, P., Rivera-Calimlim, L., and Lasagna, L. (1975): The normal volunteer in clinical investigation: How rigid should selection criteria be? *Clin. Pharmacol. Ther.*, 17:253–257.

Jusko, W.J. (1978): Role of tobacco smoking in pharmacokinetics. *J. Pharmacokinet. Biopharm.*, 6:7–39.

Kahneman, D., Slovic, P., and Tversky, A. (Eds.). (1982): *Judgement Under Uncertainty: Heuristics and Biases*. Cambridge University Press, Cambridge.

Kalow, W. (1982): Ethnic differences in drug metabolism. *Clin. Pharmacokinet.*, 7:373–400.

Karch, F.E., and Lasagna, L. (1975): Adverse drug reactions. A critical review. *JAMA*, 234:1236–1241.

Karch, F.E., Smith, C.L., Kerzner, B., Mazzullo, J.M., and Weintraub, M. (1976): Adverse drug reactions—a matter of opinion. *Clin. Pharmacol. Ther.*, 19:489–492.

Karlowski, T.R., Chalmers, T.C., Frenkel, L.D., Kapikian, A.Z., Lewis, T.L., et al. (1975): Ascorbic acid for the common cold. A prophylactic and therapeutic trial. *JAMA*, 231:1038–1042.

Kass, M.A., Meltzer, D.W., and Gordon, M. (1984): A miniature compliance monitor for eyedrop medication. *Arch. Opthalmol.*, 102:1550–1554.

Kass, M.A., Meltzer, D.W., Gordon, M., Cooper, D., and Goldberg, J. (1986): Compliance with topical pilocarpine treatment. *Am. J. Opthalmol.*, 101:515–523.

Kawamata, J., and Melby, E.C. Jr. (Eds.) (1987): *Animal Models: Assessing the Scope of Their Use in Biomedical Research.* Alan R. Liss, New York.

Kazdin, A.E. (1982): *Single-Case Research Designs. Methods for Clinical and Applied Settings.* Oxford University Press, New York.

Kearns, K.P. (1986): Flexibility of single-subject experimental designs. Part II: Design selection and arrangement of experimental phases. *J. Speech Hear. Disord.*, 51:204–214.

Keefe, D.L., Ehrreich, S.J., and Levitt, B. (1986): Problems in new-drug development: Therapeutic agents for ventricular arrhythmias. *J. Clin. Pharmacol.*, 26:562–566.

Keirse, M.J.N.C. (1984): Perinatal mortality rates do not contain what they purport to contain. *Lancet*, I:1166–1169.

Kellner, R., Rifkin, A., and Rada, R.T. (1979): The use of the intensive design in psychopharmacology. *Psychopharmacol. Bull.*, 15:35–37.

Kemp, N., Skinner, E., and Toms, J. (1984): Randomized clinical trials of cancer treatment—a public opinion survey. *Clin. Oncol.*, 10:155–161.

Kempster, P.A., Iansek, R., Balla, J.I., Dennis, P.M., and Beigler, B. (1987): Value of visual evoked response and oligoclonal bands in cerebrospinal fluid in diagnosis of spinal multiple sclerosis. *Lancet*, I:769–771.

Kenney, R.M. (1981): Between never and always. *N. Engl. J. Med.*, 305:1097–1098.

Kent, D.L., Shortliffe, E.H., Carlson, R.W., Bischoff, M.B., and Jacobs, C.D. (1985): Improvements in data collection through physician use of a computer-based chemotherapy treatment consultant. *J. Clin. Oncol.*, 3:1409–1417.

Kessler, D.A. (1989): The regulation of investigational drugs. *N. Engl. J. Med.*, 320:281–288.

Khot, A., and Burn, R. (1984): Seasonal variation and time trends of deaths from asthma in England and Wales 1960–82 *Br. Med. J.*, 289:233–234.

Khot, A., Burn, R., Evans, N., Lenney, C., and Lenney, W. (1984): Seasonal variation and time trends in childhood asthma in England and Wales 1975–81. *Br. Med. J.*, 289:235–237.

Kilo, C., Miller, J.P., and Williamson, J.R. (1980): The Achilles heel of the University Group Diabetes Program. *JAMA*, 243:450–457.

Kinane, D.F., Blackwell, C.C., Brettle, R.P., Weir, D.M., and Winstanley, F.P. (1982): ABO blood group, secretor state, and susceptibility to recurrent urinary tract infection in women. *Br. Med. J.*, 285:7–9.

King, D.W., and Fenoglio, C.M. (1983): *General Pathology: Principles and Dynamics.* Lea & Febiger, Philadelphia.

Kinosian, B.P., and Eisenberg, J.M. (1988): Cutting into cholesterol: Cost-effective alternatives for treating hypercholesterolemia. *JAMA*, 259:2249–2254.

Kirwan, J.R., and Currey, H.L.F. (1984): Clinical judgment in rheumatoid arthritis. IV. Rheumatologists' assessments of disease remain stable over long periods. *Ann. Rheum. Dis.*, 43:695–697.

Kitchen, I. (1984): *Textbook of In Vitro Practical Pharmacology.* C.V. Mosby Company, St. Louis, MO.

Kleinbloesem, C.H., van Brummelen, P., Danhof, M., Faber, H., Urquhart, J., and Breimer, D.D. (1987): Rate of increase in the plasma concentration of nifedipine as a major determinant of its

hemodynamic effects in humans. *Clin. Pharmacol. Ther.*, 41:26–30.

Klimt, C.R., and Canner, P.L. (1979): Terminating a long-term clinical trial. *Clin. Pharmacol. Ther.*, 25:641–646.

Knapp, T.R. (1983): A methodological critique of the 'ideal weight' concept. *JAMA*, 250:506–510.

Koch-Weser, J. (1974): Bioavailability of drugs. *N. Engl. J. Med.*, 291:503–506.

Koch-Weser, J., Sellers, E.M., and Zacest, R. (1977): The ambiguity of adverse drug reactions. *Eur. J. Clin. Pharmacol.*, 11:75–78.

Kolmodin, B., Azarnoff, D.L., and Sjoqvist, F. (1969): Effect of environmental factors on drug metabolism: Decreased plasma half-life of antipyrine in workers exposed to chlorinated hydrocarbon insecticides. *Clin. Pharmacol. Ther.*, 10:638–642.

Komaroff, A.L. (1982): Algorithms and the 'art' of medicine. *Am. J. Public Health*, 72:10–12.

Komaroff, A.L., Pass, T.M., McCue, J.D., Cohen, A.B., Hendricks, T.M., and Friedland, G. (1978): Management strategies for urinary and vaginal infections. *Arch. Intern. Med.*, 138:1069–1073.

Kono, K., Yoshida, Y., Watanabe, M., Watanabe, H., Inoue, S., et al. (1990): Elemental analysis of hair among hydrofluoric acid exposed workers. *Int. Arch. Occup. Environ. Health*, 62:85–88.

Koppanyi, T., and Avery, M.A. (1966): Species differences and the clinical trial of new drugs: A review. *Clin. Pharmacol. Ther.*, 7:250–270.

Koran, L.M. (1975): The reliability of clinical methods, data and judgments. *N. Engl. J. Med.*, 293:642–646, 695–701.

Kost, G.J. (1990): Critical limits for urgent clinician notification at US medical centers. *JAMA*, 263:704–707.

Kotses, H., and Glaus, K.D. (1981): Applications of biofeedback to the treatment of asthma: A critical review. *Biofeedback Self Regul.*, 6:573–593.

Koup, J.R. (1989): Disease states and drug pharmacokinetics. *J. Clin. Pharmacol.*, 29:674–679.

Kraemer, H.C. (1986): Sample size: When is enough enough? *Am. J. Med. Sci.*, 296:361.

Kramer, M.S. (1986): Assessing causality of adverse drug reactions: Global introspection and its limitations. *Drug Info. J.*, 20:433–437.

Kramer, M.S., and Boivin, J-F. (1987): Toward an "unconfounded" classification of epidemiologic research design. *J. Chronic Dis.*, 40:683–688.

Kramer, M.S., Leventhal, J.M., Hutchinson, T.A., and Feinstein, A.R. (1979): An algorithm for the operational assessment of adverse drug reactions. I. Background, description, and instructions for use. *JAMA*, 242:623–632.

Krasnow, S.H. (1989): Problems in antiemetic trial design and interpretation. *Oncology (Williston Park)*, 3 (No. 8):5–10.

Kratochwill, T.R. (Ed.) (1978): *Single Subject Research: Strategies for Evaluating Change.* Academic Press, Orlando, FL.

Krishnaswamy, K. (1983): Drug metabolism and pharmacokinetics in malnutrition. In: *Handbook of Clinical Pharmacokinetics.* Gibaldi, M., and Prescott, L. (Eds.), pp. 216–242. ADIS Health Sciences Press, New York.

Krol, W.F. (1983): Closing down the study. *Controlled Clin. Trials*, 4:505–512.

Krowczynski, L. (1987): *Extended-Release Dosage Forms.* pp. 3–5. CRC Press, Boca Raton, FL.

Krueger, D.E., and Moriyama, I.M. (1967): Mortality of the foreign born. *Am. J. Public Health*, 57:496–503.

Krupnick, J., Shea, T., and Elkin, I. (1986): Generalizability of treatment studies utilizing solicited patients. *J. Consult. Clin. Psychol.*, 54:68–78.

Kunkel, R.S. (1987): Clinical trials in migraine: Parallel versus crossover studies. *Neuroepidemiology*, 6:209–213.

Kurata, J.H., Honda, G.D., and Frankl, H. (1982): Hospitalization and mortality rates for peptic ulcers: A comparison of a large health maintenance organization and United States data. *Gastroenterology*, 83:1008–1016.

Lach, J.L. (1972): Influence of excipients and formulation factors on drug availability and toxicity. In: *Toxicological Problems of Drug Combinations. Proceedings of the European Society for the Study of Drug Toxicity,* Vol. XIII. Baker, S.B. de C., and Neuhaus, G.A., (Eds.), pp. 199–202. Excerpta Medica, Amsterdam.

Lachin, J.M., Marks, J.W., Schoenfield, L.J., NCGS Protocol Committee, and the National Cooperative Gallstone Study Group. (1981): Design and methodological considerations in the National Cooperative Gallstone Study: A multicenter trial. *Controlled Clin. Trials,* 2:177–229.

Lachman, L., Lieberman, H.A., and Kanig, J.L. (1986): *The Theory and Practice of Industrial Pharmacy.* Third Edition. Lea & Febiger, Philadelphia.

Laird, D. (1985): *Approaches to Training and Development.* Second Edition. Addison-Wesley, Reading, MA.

Lamy, P.P. (1982): Comparative pharmacokinetic changes and drug therapy in an older population. *J. Am. Geriatr. Soc.,* 30:S11–S19.

Lancaster, H.O. (1974): *An Introduction to Medical Statistics.* John Wiley & Sons, New York.

Landauer, A.A., and Pocock, D.A. (1984): Stress reduction by oxprenolol and placebo: Controlled investigation of the pharmacological and non-specific effects. *Br. Med. J.,* 289:592.

Lanes, S.F., and Walker, A.M. (1987): Do pressurized bronchodilator aerosols cause death among asthmatics? *Am. J. Epidemiol,* 125:755–760.

Lange, P.H., Limas, C., and Fraley, E.E. (1978): Tissue blood-group antigens and prognosis in low stage transitional cell carcinoma of the bladder. *J. Urol.,* 119:52–55.

La Puma, J., and Lawlor, E.F. (1990): Quality-adjusted life-years: Ethical implications for physicians and policymakers. *JAMA,* 263:2917–2921.

Larson, A.G., and Marcer, D. (1984): The who and why of pain: Analysis by social class. *Br. Med. J.,* 288:883–886.

Lasagna, L. (Ed.) (1975): *Combination Drugs: Their Use and Regulation.* Stratton Intercontinential Medical Book Corp., New York.

Lasagna, L. (1977): Prisoner subjects and drug testing. *Fed. Proc.,* 36:2349–2351.

Lasagna, L. (1979): Problems in publication of clinical trial methodology *Clin. Pharmacol. Ther.,* 25:751–753.

Lasagna, L. (1982): Historical controls. The practitioner's clinical trials. *N. Engl. J. Med.,* 307:1339–1340.

Lasagna, L. (1983): Discovering adverse drug reactions. *JAMA,* 249:2224–2225.

Lasagna, L. (1986a): Clinical testing of products prepared by biotechnology. *Regul. Toxicol. Pharmacol.,* 6:385–390.

Lasagna, L. (1986b): On reducing waste in foreign clinical trials and postregulation experience. *Clin. Pharmacol. Ther.,* 40:369–372.

Lasagna, L., Erill, S., and Naranjo, C.A. (Eds.) (1989): *Dose-Response Relationships in Clinical Pharmacology.* Excerpta Medica, Amsterdam.

Latcham, R.W., Kreitman, N., Plant, M.A., and Crawford, A. (1984): Regional variations in British alcohol morbidity rates: A myth uncovered? I: Clinical surveys. *Br. Med. J.,* 289:1341–1343.

Laupacis, A., Rorabeck, C.H., Bourne, R.B., Feeny, D., Tugwell, P., et al. (1989): Randomized trials in orthopaedics: Why, how, and when? *J. Bone Joint Surg.,* 71-A:535–543.

Laupacis, A., Sackett, D.L., and Roberts, R.S. (1988): An assessment of clinically useful measures of the consequences of treatment. *N. Engl. J. Med.,* 318:1728–1733.

Laurence, D.R. (1973): *Clinical Pharmacology.* Fourth Edition. Churchill Livingstone, Edinburgh, UK.

Laurence, D.R., and Bacharach, A.L., eds. (1964): *Evaluation of Drug Activities: Pharmacometrics.* Volumes 1 and 2. Academic Press, New York.

Laurence, D.R., McLean, A.E.M., and Weatherall, M. (Eds.) (1984): *Safety Testing of New Drugs: Laboratory Predictions and Clinical Performance.* Academic Press, London.

Lave, L.B., and Omenn, G.S. (1986): Cost-effectiveness of short-term tests for carcinogenicity. *Nature,* 324:29–34.

Lavori, P., Louis, T.A., Bailar, J.C. III, and Polansky, M. (1983): Designs for experiments—parallel comparisons of treatment. *N. Engl. J. Med.,* 309:1291–1299.

Leape, L.L., Park, R.E., Solomon, D.H., Chassin, M.R., Kosecoff, J., et al. (1989): Relation between surgeons' practice volumes and geographic variation in the rate of carotid endarterectomy. *N. Engl. J. Med.,* 321:653–657.

Lee, C., and Owen, N. (1986): Community exercise programs: Follow-up difficulty and outcome. *J. Behav. Med.,* 9:111–117.

Leikin, S.L. (1985): Beyond pro forma consent for childhood cancer research. *J. Clin. Oncol.* 3:420–428.

Leppik, I.E., Brundage, R.C., Krall, R., Cloyd, J.C., Bowman-Cloyd, T., et al. (1986): Double-blind withdrawal of phenytion and carbamazepine in patients treated with progabide for partial seizures. *Epilepsia,* 27:563–568.

Leppik, I.E., Cloyd, J.C., Sawchuk, R.J., and Pepin, S.M. (1979): Compliance and variability of plasma phenytoin levels in epileptic patients. *Ther. Drug Monitor.,* 1:475–483.

Leventhal, J.M., Hutchinson, T.A., Kramer, M.S., and Feinstein, A.R. (1979): An algorithm for the operational assessment of adverse drug reactions. III. Results of tests among clinicians. *JAMA,* 242:1991–1994.

Levine, J. (1980): Trial Assessment Procedure Scale (TAPS). Printed by Department of Health and Human Services, Public Health Service, Alcohol, Drug Abuse and Mental Health Administration, National Institute of Mental Health, Bethesda, Maryland. Available from Dr. Levine, University of Maryland, Maryland Psychiatric Research Center, P.O.Box 3235, Catonsville, MD 21228.

Levine, R.J. (1986): *Ethics and Regulation of Clinical Research.* Second Edition. Urban and Schwarzenberg, Baltimore.

Levine, R.J. (1987): The apparent incompatibility between informed consent and placebo-controlled clinical trials. *Clin. Pharmacol. Ther.,* 42:247–249.

Levine, R.J., and Lebacqz, K. (1979): Some ethical considerations in clinical trials. *Clin. Pharmacol. Ther.,* 25:728–741.

Levy, G., and Jusko, W.J. (1965): Effect of viscosity on drug absorption. *J. Pharm. Sci.,* 54:219–225.

Lewis, G.P., Jusko, W.J., and Coughlin, L.L. (1972): Cadmium accumulation in man: Influence of smoking, occupation, alcoholic habit and disease. *J. Chronic Dis.,* 25:717–726.

Lewis, J.A. (1987): Migraine trials: Crossover or parallel group? *Neuroepidemiology,* 6:198–208.

Lewis, T.L., Karlowski, T.R., Kapikian, A.Z., Lynch, J.M., Shaffer, G.W., and George, D.A. (1975): A controlled clinical trial of ascorbic acid for the common cold. *Ann. NY Acad. Sci.,* 258:505–512.

Le Witt, P.A., Miller, L.P., Levine, R.A., Lovenberg, W., Newman, R.P., et al. (1986): Tetrahydrobiopterin in dystonia: Identification of abnormal metabolism and therapeutic trials. *Neurology,* 36:760–764.

Li, V.H., Robinson, J.R., and Lee, V.H. (1987): Influence of drug properties and routes of administration on the design of restrained and controlled release system. In: *Controlled Drug Delivery: Fundamentals and Applications.* Robinson, J.R., and Lee, V.H. (Eds.), 2nd Edition. pp. 5–7. Marcel Dekker, New York.

Light, R.W., O'Hara, V.S., Moritz, T.E., McElhinney A.J., Butz, R., et al. (1990): Intrapleural tetracycline for the prevention of recurrent spontaneous pneumothorax: Results of a Department of Veterans Affairs cooperative study. *JAMA,* 264:2224–2230.

Lindahl, O., and Lindwall, L. (1982): Is all therapy just a placebo effect? *Metamedicine,* 3:255–259.

Lindeman, R.D., Tobin, J., and Shock, N.W. (1985): Longitudinal studies on the rate of decline in renal function with age. *J. Amr. Geriatr. Soc.,* 33:278–285.

Lionel, N.D.W., and Herxheimer, A. (1970): Assessing reports of therapeutic trials. *Br. Med. J.,* 3:637–640.

Lisook, A.B. (1990): FDA audits of clinical studies: Policy and procedure. *J. Clin. Pharmacol.*, 30:296–302.

Litchfield, J.T. Jr. (1961): Forecasting drug effects in man from studies in laboratory animals *JAMA*, 177:34–38.

Litchfield, J.T. Jr. (1962): Evaluation of the safety of new drugs by means of tests in animals. *Clin. Pharmacol. Ther.*, 3:665–672.

Little, J.C., McClelland, H.A., and Kerr, T.A. (1977): Videotape technique in assessing antidepressants. *Br. J. Clin. Pharmacol.*, 4(Suppl. 2):227S–232S.

Lock, S. (1984): Repetitive publication: A waste that must stop. *Br. Med. J.*, 288:661–662.

Loft, A., Andersen, T.F., and Madsen, M. (1989): A quasi-experimental design based on regional variations: Discussion of a method for evaluating outcomes of medical practice. *Soc. Sci. Med.*, 28:147–154.

Loh, I.K. (1979): Letter to the editor. *N. Engl. J. Med.*, 301:1182.

Lomas, J., Anderson, G., Enkin, M., Vayda, E., Roberts, R., et al. (1988): The role of evidence in the consensus process: Results from a Canadian consensus exercise. *JAMA*, 259:3001–3005.

London, W.P. (1987): Full-spectrum classroom light and sickness in pupils. *Lancet*, II:1205–1206.

Long, J.M., Slagle, J.R., Leon, A.S., Wick. M.W., Matts, J.P., et al. (1987): An example of expert systems applied to clinical trials: Analysis of serial graded exercise ECG test data. *Controlled Clin. Trials*, 8:136–145.

Longer, M.A., and Robinson, J.R. (1985): Sustained-release drug delivery systems. In: *Remington's Pharmaceutical Sciences.* Gennaro, A.R. (Ed.), 17th Edition, Chapter 92, pp. 1644–1661. Mack Publishing, Easton, PA.

Louik, C., Lacouture, P.G., Mitchell, A.A., Kauffman, R., and Lovejoy, F.H. Jr. (1985): A study of adverse reaction algorithms in a drug surveillance program. *Clin. Pharmacol. Ther.*, 38:183–187.

Louis, T.A., Lavori, P.W., Bailar, J.C. III, and Polansky, M. (1984): Crossover and self-controlled designs in clinical research. *N. Engl. J. Med.*, 310:24–31.

Lowrance, W.W. (1989): A broad framework for confronting health risks. In: *The Perception and Management of Drug Safety Risks.* Horisberger, B., and Dinkel, R. (Eds.), pp. 9–18. Springer-Verlag, New York.

Lucchelli, P.E., Cattaneo, A.D., and Zattoni, J. (1978): Effect of capsule colour and order of administration of hypnotic treatments. *Eur. J. Clin. Pharmacol.*, 13:153–155.

Luepker, R. V., Grimm, R. H., and Taylor, H.L. (1984): The effect of "usual care" on cardiovascular risk factors in a clinical trial. *Controlled Clin. Trials*, 5:47–53.

Lum, G., and Beeler, M.F. (1983): Reference groups: Comparing oranges with oranges and apples with apples. *JAMA*, 249:1890.

Lundberg, G.D. (1988): SI unit implementation: The next step. *JAMA*, 260:73–76.

Macera, C.A., Jackson, K.L., Farach, C., and Pate, R.R. (1988): The use of proportional hazards regression in investigating dropout rates in a longitudinal study. *J. Clin. Epidemiol.*, 41:1175–1180.

MacKenzie, C.R., and Charlson, M.E. (1986): Standards for the use of ordinal scales in clinical trials. *Br. Med. J.*, 292:40–43.

MacLeod, C., Rabin, H., Ruedy, J., Caron, M., and Zarowny, D. (1972): Comparative bioavailability of three brands of ampicillin. *Can. Med. Assoc. J.*, 107:203–209.

MacMillan, R.L., and Brown, K.W.G. (1971): Comparison of the effects of treatment of acute myocardial infarction in a coronary unit and on a general medical ward. *Can. Med. Assoc. J.*, 105:1037–1040.

Macular Photocoagulation Study Group. (1984): Changing the protocol: A case report from the macular photocoagulation study. *Controlled Clin. Trials*, 5:203–216.

Madan, P.L. (1985): Sustained-release drug delivery systems. Part. 1. Overview. *Pharm. Manuf.*, 2:22–27.

Maddox, J. (1984): Perils of too much disclosure. *Nature*, 309:665.

Maher-Loughnan, G.P. (1970): Hypnosis and autohypnosis for the treatment of asthma. *Int. J. Clin. Exp. Hypn.*, 12:1–14.

Mahon, W.A., and Daniel, E.E. (1964): A method for the assessment of reports of drug trials. *Can. Med. Assoc. J.*, 90:565–569.

Makuch, R.W., and Johnson, M.F. (1986): Some issues in the design and interpretation of "negative" clincal studies. *Arch. Intern. Med.*, 146:986–989.

Makuch, R., and Johnson, M. (1989): Issues in planning and interpreting active control equivalence studies. *J. Clin. Epidemiol.*, 42:503–511.

Malogolowkin, M.H., Horowitz, R.S., Ortega, J.A., Siegel, S.E., Hammond, G.D., et al. (1989): Tracing expert thinking in clinical trial design. *Comput. Biomed. Res.*, 22:190–208.

Margolis, C.Z. (1983): Uses of clinical algorithms. *JAMA*, 249:627–632.

Marini, J.L., Sheard, M.H., Bridges, C.I., and Wagner, E. (1976): An evaluation of the double-blind design in a study comparing lithium carbonate with placebo. *Acta. Psychiatr. Scand.*, 53:343–354.

Marks, I.M., Gelder, M.G., and Edwards, G. (1968): Hypnosis and desensitization for phobias: A controlled prospective trial. *Br. J. Psychiatry*, 114:1263–1274.

Marks, J.W., Croke, G., Gochman, N., Hofmann, A.F., Lachin, J.M., et al. (1984): Major issues in the organization and implementation of the National Cooperative Gallstone Study (NCGS). *Controlled Clin. Trials*, 5:1–12.

Martin, C.J., Platt, S.D., and Hunt, S.M. (1987): Housing conditions and ill health. *Br. Med. J.*, 294:1125–1127.

Martin, D.F., Hollanders, D., May, S.J., Ravenscroft, M.M., and Tweedle, D.E.F. (1981): Difference in relapse rates of duodenal ulcer after healing with cimetidine or tripotassium dicitrato bismuthate. *Lancet*, I:7–10.

Martin, J.E., and Epstein, L.H. (1976): Evaluating treatment effectiveness in cerebral palsy. Single subject designs. *Phys. Ther.*, 56:285–294.

Masek, B.J., Russo, D.C., and Varni, J.W. (1984): Behavioral approaches to the management of chronic pain in children. *Pediatr. Clin. North Am.*, 31:1113–1131.

Matas, A.J., Arras, J., Muyskens, J., Tellis, V., and Veith, F.J. (1985): A proposal for cadaver organ procurement: Routine removal with right of informed refusal. *J. Health Polit. Policy Law*, 10:231–244.

Mather, H.G., Morgan, D.C., Pearson, N.G., Read, K.L.Q., and Shaw, D.B. (1976): Myocardial infarction: A comparison between home and hospital care for patients. *Br. Med. J.*, 1:925–929.

Matsunga, S.K., Plezia, P.M., Karol, M.D., Katz, M.D., Camilli, A.E., et al. (1989): Effects of passive smoking on theophylline clearance. *Clin. Pharmacol. Ther.*, 46:399–407.

Mattison, N. (1988): The FDA's treatment IND: Current controversies. *Pharmaceut. Med.*, 3:159–171.

Mattson, M.E., Curb, J.D., McArdle, R., and the AMIS and BHAT Research Groups. (1985): Participation in a clinical trial: The patients' point of view. *Controlled Clin. Trials*, 6:156–167.

Mattson, R.H., Cramer, J.A., Delgado Escueta, A.V., Smith, D.B., Collins, J.F., et al. (1983): A design for the prospective evaluation of the efficacy and toxicity of antiepileptic drugs in adults. *Neurology*, 33(Suppl. 1):14–25.

Mayersohn, M. (1979): Physiological factors that modify systemic drug availability and pharmacologic response in clinical practice. In: *Principles and Perspectives in Drug Bioavailability*. Blanchard, J., Sawchuk, R.J., and Brodie, B.B. (Eds.), pp. 211–273. S. Karger, New York.

Mayes, L.C., Horwitz, R.I., and Feinstein, A.R. (1988): A collection of 56 topics with contradictory results in case-control research. *Int. J. Epidemiol.*, 17:680–685.

Mazzoni, D.J. (1972): Rx for the pharmaceutical marketer: Preventive marketing. *Med. Mark. Media*, 7:16–28.

McConnachie, R.W. (1978): The clinical assessment of brain failure in the elderly. *Pharmacology*, 16(Suppl. 1):27–35.

McGhan, W.F., Rowland, C.R., and Bootman, J.L. (1978): Cost-benefit and cost effectiveness: Methodologies for evaluating innovative pharmaceutical services. *Am. J. Hosp. Pharm.*, 35:133–140.

McGlashan, T.H., Evans, F.J., and Orne, M.T. (1969): The nature of hypnotic analgesia and placebo response to experimental pain. *Psychosom. Med.*, 31:227–246.

McKegney, F.P., and Williams, R.B. Jr. (1967): Psychological aspects of hypertension. II. The differential influence of interview variables on blood pressure. *Am. J. Psychiatry*, 123:1539–1545.

McKinney, W.P., Young, M.J., Hartz, A., and Lee, M.B.-F. (1989): The inexact use of Fisher's exact test in six major medical journals. *JAMA*, 261:3430–3433.

McLean, A.J., Harrison, P.M., Ioannides-Demos, L.L., Byrne, A.J., and McCarthy, P. (1984): Microbes, peptic ulcer, and relapse rates with different drugs. *Lancet*, II:525–526.

McLeod, R.S., Taylor, D.W., Cohen, Z., and Cullen, J.B. (1986): Single-patient randomised clinical trial: Use in determining optimum treatment for patient with inflammation of Kock continent ileostomy reservoir. *Lancet*, I:726–728.

McNamara, B.P. (1976): Concepts in health evaluation of commercial and industrial chemicals. In: *Advances In Modern Toxicology*. Mehlman, M.A., Shapiro, R., and Blumenthal, H. (Eds.). Volume 1, Part 1: pp. 61–140. New Concepts in Safety Evaluation. John Wiley & Sons, New York.

McNeil, B.J., Pauker, S.G., Sox, H.E., and Tversky, A. (1982): On the elicitation of preferences for alternative therapies. *N. Engl. J. Med.*, 306:1259–1262.

McNutt, R.A., Evans, A.T., Fletcher, R.H., and Fletcher, S.W. (1990): The effects of blinding on the quality of peer review: A randomized trial. *JAMA*, 263:1371–1376.

McPherson, F.M., and Le Gassicke, J. (1965): A single-patient, self-controlled and self-recorded trial of WY 3498. *Br. J. Psychiatry*, 111:149–154.

McPherson, F.M., and Smythies, J.R., (1969): A new antidepressent dibenzepin hydrochloride (Noveril). *Clin. Trials J.*, 1:39–43.

McPherson, K., Strong, P.M., Epstein, A., and Jones, L. (1981): Regional variations in the use of common surgical procedures: Within and between England and Wales, Canada and the United States of America. *Soc. Sci. Med.*, 15A:273–288.

McSweeny, A.J., Grant, I., Heaton, R.K., Adams, K.M., and Timms, R.M. (1982): Life quality of patients with chronic obstructive pulmonary disease. *Arch. Intern. Med.*, 142:473–478.

Meade, T.W., Gardner, M.J., Cannon, P., and Richardson, P.C. (1968): Observer variability in recording the peripheral pulses. *Br. Heart J.*, 30:661–665.

Meier, P. (1979): Terminating a trial—the ethical problem. *Clin. Pharmacol. Ther.*, 25:633–640.

Meier, P. (1980): Current research in statistical methodology for clinical trials. *Biometrics*, 38(Suppl.):141–153.

Meinert, C.L. (1986): *Clinical Trials: Design, Conduct, and Analysis*. Oxford University Press, New York.

Meinert, C.L. (1988): Toward prospective registration of clinical trials. *Controlled Clin. Trials*, 9:1–5.

Meinert, C.L., Tonascia, S., and Higgins, K. (1984): Content of reports on clinical trials: A critical review. *Controlled Clin. Trials*, 5:328–347.

Meinert, C.L., Tonascia, J., and Tonascia, S. (Eds.) (1989): The hypertension prevention trial: Design, methods, and baseline results. *Controlled Clin. Trials*, 10(Suppl.):1S–117S.

Melmon, K., Chairman, Joint Commission on Prescription Drug Use, U.S. Senate Committee on Labor and Human Resources. Subcommittee on Health and Scientific Research. (1980): Final Report. U.S. Government Printing Office, Washington.

Melzack, R. (1975): The McGill pain questionnaire: Major properties and scoring methods. *Pain*, 1:277–299.

Merz, B., Hager, T., and Macek, C. (1983): New methods of drug delivery. *JAMA*, 250:145–147, 151–153.

Metcalfe, D.D. (1989): Diseases of food hypersensitivity. *N. Engl. J. Med.*, 321:255–257.

Metz, C.A., Gutknecht, G.D., Schneider, J.C., Sheridan, A., Cross, C.J., et al. (1987): Development of a training program for new clinical research personnel. *Drug Info. J.*, 21:289–293.

Mezey, K.C. (Ed.) (1980): *Fixed Drug Combinations — Rationale and Limitations*. International Congress and Symposium Series, No. 22. Royal Society of Medicine, London; Academic Press, London; Grune & Stratton, New York.

Miller, A.B. (1980): Methodologic considerations for trials of lung cancer prophylaxis. *Can. Med. Assoc. J.*, 122:776–779.

Miller, R. L., and Melmon, K.L. (1972): Inflammatory disorders In: *Clinical Pharmacology: Basic Principles in Therapeutics*. Melmon, K.L., and Morrelli, H.F. (Eds.), p. 409. Macmillan Publishing Co., New York.

Miller, R.P. (1979): Cooling towers and evaporative condensers. *Ann. Intern. Med.*, 90:667–670.

Minatoya, H., and Spilker, B. (1975): Lack of cardiac or bronchodilator tachyphlaxis to isoprenaline in the dog. *Br. J. Pharmacol.*, 53:333–340.

Mitchell, A.S., Henry, D.A., Sanson-Fisher, R., and O'Connell, D.L. (1988): Patients as a direct source of information on adverse drug reactions. *Br. Med. J.*, 297:891–893.

Mitruka, B.M., Rawnsley, H.M., and Vadehra, D.V. (1976): *Animals for Medical Research: Models for the Study of Human Disease*. John Wiley & Sons, New York.

Moertel, C.G., and Hanley, J.A. (1976): The effect of measuring error on the results of therapeutic trials in advanced cancer. *Cancer*, 38:388–394.

Monson, R.A., and Bond, C.A. (1978): The accuracy of the medical record as an index of outpatient drug therapy. *JAMA*, 240:2182–2184.

Moore, N., Paux, G., Noblet, C., and Andrejak, M. (1988): Spouse-related drug side-effects. *Lancet*, I:468.

Moore, N.C. (1976): The personality and mental health of flat dwellers. *Br. J. Psychiatry*, 128:259–261.

Moore-Ede, M.C., Czeisler, C.A., and Richardson, G.S. (1983): Circadian timekeeping in health and disease. Part 2. Clinical implications of circadian rhythmicity. *N. Engl. J. Med.*, 309:530–536.

Morgenstern, H., and Bursic, E.S., (1982): A method for using epidemiologic data to estimate the potential impact of an intervention on the health status of a target population. *J. Community Health*, 7:292–309.

Morris, J.A., and Shapiro, D.Z. (1986): Social class and age distribution in Reye's syndrome. *Br. Med. J.*, 292:379.

Morris, R.W. (1987): Circadian and circannual rhythms of emergency room drug-overdose admissions. *Prog. Clin. Biol. Res.*, 227B:451–457.

Morrison, A.S., Jick, H., and Ory, H.W. (1977): Oral contraceptives and hepatitis. *Lancet*, 1:1142–1143.

Morrow, G.R. (1980): Clinical trials in psychosocial medicine: Methodologic and statistical considerations. Part III. Assessing measurement techniques in psychosocial oncology. *Cancer Treat. Rep.*, 64:451–456.

Morselli, P.L. (1986): Methodology of clinical trials on new drugs in epilepsy. *Funct. Neurol.*, 1:503–511.

Morton, D.J. (1984): Pharmacokinetics of twelve anticonvulsant drugs in the rat. *Neuropharmacology*, 23:1125–1127.

Moscucci, M., Byrne, L., Weintraub, M., and Cox, C. (1987): Blinding, unblinding, and the placebo effect: An analysis of patients' guesses of treatment assignment in a double-blind clinical trial. *Clin. Pharmacol. Ther.*, 41:259–265.

Moses, L.E. (1984): The series of consecutive cases as a device for assessing outcomes of intervention. *N. Engl. J. Med.*, 311:705–710.

Mosteller, F. (1979): Problems of ommission in communications. *Clin. Pharmacol. Ther.*, 25:761–764.

Mosteller, F., Gilbert, J.P., and McPeek, B. (1980): Reporting standards and research strategies for controlled trials: Agenda for the editor. *Controlled Clin. Trials*, 1:37–58.

Muggia, F.M. (1978): Clinical trials in cancer: General concepts and methodologies. *Cancer Clin. Trials*. Summer:139–144.

Muggia, F.M., Rozencweig, M., Staquet, M.J., and McGuire, W.P. Jr. (1980): Methodology of phase II clinical trial in cancer. *Recent Results Cancer Res.*, 70:53–60.

Mullen, P.D., Green, L.W., and Persinger, G.S. (1985): Clinical trials of patient education for chronic conditions: A comparative meta-analysis of intervention types. *Prev. Med.*, 14:753–781.

Munetz, M.R., Lidz, C.W., and Meisel, A. (1985): Informed consent and incompetent medical patients. *J. Fam. Pract.*, 20:273–279.

Munro, I., Fox, R., and Sharp D. (1983): Reporting on methods in clinical trials. *N. Engl. J. Med.*, 308:596–597.

Murphy, E.A. (1976): The Logic of Medicine, Johns Hopkins Univ. Press, Baltimore, pp. 249–250.

Murphy, E.A. (1982): The analysis and interpretation of experiments: Some philosophical issues. *J. Med. Philos.*, 7:307–325.

Murray, G.D., (1986): Use of an international data bank to compare outcome following severe head injury in different centres. *Stat. Med.*, 5:103–112.

Murray, G.D., Lesaffre, E., and Robertson, J.I.S. (1988): Interpreting age-related aspects of antihypertensive treatment: Statistical defects and their remedy. *J. Hypertens.*, 6(Suppl. 1):S121–S126.

Musen, M.A., Combs, D.M, Walton, J.D., Shortliffe, E.H., and Fagan, L.M. (1986): OPAL: Toward the computer-aided design of oncology advice systems. In: *Tenth Ann. Symp. on Computer Applications in Medical Care.* pp. 43–52 (Cat. no. 86CH2341-6, IEEE Service Center, Piscataway, NJ).

Myers, M.G., Cairns, J.A., and Singer, J. (1987): The consent form as a possible cause of side effects. *Clin. Pharmacol. Ther.*, 42:250–253.

Nace, E.P. (1989): The natural history of alcoholism versus treatment effectiveness: Methodological problems. *Am. J. Drug Alcohol Abuse*, 15:55–60.

Nagayama, H., Takagi, A., and Takahashi, R. (1981): Chronopharmacological studies of neuroleptics. In: *Current Developments in Psychopharmacology*. Volume VI, pp. 191–214. Spectrum Publications, Jamaica, NY.

Nakao, M.A., and Axelrod, S. (1983): Numbers are better than words: Verbal specifications of frequency have no place in medicine. *Am. J. Med.*, 74:1061–1065.

Naranjo, C.A., Busto, U., Sellers, E.M., Sandor, P., Ruiz, I., et al. (1981): A method for estimating the probability of adverse drug reactions. *Clin. Pharmacol. Ther.*, 30:239–245.

Naranjo, C.A., Lanctôt, K.L., and Lane, D.A. (1990): The Bayesian differential diagnosis of neutropenia associated with antiarrhythmic agents. *J. Clin. Pharmacol.*, 30:1120–1127.

Naranjo, C.A., Lane, D., Ho-Asjoe, M., and Lancôt, K.L. (1990): A Bayesian assessment of idiosyncratic adverse reactions to new drugs: Guillain-Barré syndrome and zimeldine. *J. Clin. Pharmacol.*, 30:174–180.

National Commission for the Protection of Human Subjects of Biomedical and Behavioral Research. (1976): *Research on the fetus (Appendix)*. DHEW Pub. No. (OS)76–128. U.S. Government Printing Office, Washington, DC.

Naylor, C.D. (1988): Two cheers for meta-analysis: Problems and opportunities in aggregating results of clinical trials. *Can. Med. Assoc. J.*, 138:891–895.

Nealon, E., Blumberg, B.D., and Brown, B. (1985): What do patients know about clinical trials? *Am. J. Nurs.*, 85:807–810.

Nelson, M.A., Allen, P., Clamp, S.E., and de Dombal, F.T. (1979): Reliability and reproducibility of clinical findings in low-back pain. *Spine*, 4:97–101.

Nestor, J.O. (1975): Results of the failure to perform adequate preclinical studies before administering new drugs to humans. *S. Afr. Med. J.*, 49:287–290.

Newcombe, R.G. (1987): Towards a reduction in publication bias. *Br. Med. J.*, 295:656–659.

Newmark, M.E., and Penry, J.K. (1980): Catamenial epilepsy: A review. *Epilepsia*, 21:281–300.

Neyman, J. (1955): Statistics-servant of all sciences. *Science*, 122:401–406.

Nicolucci, A., Grilli, R., Alexanian, A.A., Apolone, G., Torri, V., et al. (1989): Quality, evolution, and clinical implications of randomized, controlled trials on the treatment of lung cancer: A lost opportunity for meta-analysis. *JAMA*, 262:2101–2107.

Niederhuber, J.E., Ensminger, W., Gyves, J., Thrall, J., Walker, S., et al. (1984): Regional chemotherapy of colorectal cancer metastatic to the liver. *Cancer*, 53:1336–1343.

Nierenberg, A.A., and Feinstein, A.R. (1988): How to evaluate a diagnostic marker test: Lessons from the rise and fall of dexamethasone suppression test. *JAMA*, 259:1699–1702.

Nissenson, A.R., Rapaport, M., Gordon, A., and Narins, R.G. (1979): Hemodialysis in the treatment of psoriasis: A controlled trial. *Ann. Intern. Med.*, 91:218–220.

Nissman, E.F. (1987): The use of COSTART at Burroughs Wellcome Company. *Drug Info. J.*, 21:295–298.

Nobrega, F.T., Sedlack, J.D., Sedlack, R.E., Dockerty, M.B., and Ilstrup, D.M. (1983): A decline in carcinoma of the stomach: A diagnostic artifact? *Mayo Clin. Proc.*, 58:255–260.

Nodine, J., and Siegler, P. (Eds.) (1964): *Animal and Clinical Pharmacologic Techniques in Drug Evaluation*. Year Book Medical Publishers, Chicago.

Nordic Council on Medicines. (1983): *Clinical Trials of Drugs: Nordic Guidelines*. NLN publication no. 11, Nordiska Lakemedelsnamnden, Uppsala, Sweden.

Norell, S.E. (1979): Improving medication compliance: A randomised clinical trial. *Br. Med. J.*, 2:1031–1033.

Norman, C. (1984): Reduce fraud in seven easy steps. *Science*, 224:581.

Northup, S.J. (1989): Current problems associated with toxicity evaluation of medical device materials and future research needs. *Fundam. Appl. Toxicol.*, 13:196–204.

Noseworthy, J.H. (1988): There are no alternatives to double-blind, controlled trials. *Neurology*, 38(Suppl. 2):76–79.

Nussbaum, G.H. (1984): Quality assessment and assurance in clinical hyperthermia: Requirements and procedures. *Cancer Res.*, 44 (Suppl.):4811s–4817s.

Nyberg, G. (1974): Assessment of papers of clinical trials. *Med. J. Aust.*, 2:381.

Nyren, O., Gustavsson, S., Adami, H.-O., and Loof, L. (1985): Methodological aspects of clinical trials in non-ulcer dyspepsia with special reference to selectional factors. *Scand. J. Gastroenterol.*, 20(Suppl. 109):159–162.

O'Brien, W.M. (1968): Indomethacin: A survey of clinical trials. *Clin. Pharmacol. Ther.*, 9:94–107.

Obrusnik, I. (1986): Activation analysis of human hair as a tool for environmental pollution monitoring. *J. Hyg. Epidemiol. Microbiol. Immunol.*, 30:11–25.

O'Fallon, J.R., Dubey, S.D., Salsburg, D.S., Edmonson, J.H., and Soffer, A. (1978): Should there be statistical guidelines for medical research papers? *Biometrics*, 34:687–695.

Oldridge, N.B., Wicks, J.R., Hanley, C., Sutton, J.R., and Jones, N.L. (1978): Noncompliance in an exercise rehabilitation program for men who have suffered a myocardial infarction. *Can. Med. Assoc. J.*, 118:361–364.

Olive, D.L. (1986): Analysis of clinical fertility trials: A methodologic review. *Fertil. Steril.*, 45:157–171.

Olver, I.N., Simon, R.M., and Aisner, J. (1986): Antiemetic studies: A methodological discussion. *Cancer Treat. Rep.*, 70:555–563.

Ott, J.N. (1976): *Health and Light*. Pocket Books, New York.

Ottenbacher, K.J. (1986): Reliability and accuracy of visually analyzing graphed data from single-subject designs. *Am. J. Occup. Ther.*, 40:464–469.

Ouslander, J.G. (1981): Drug therapy in the elderly. *Ann. Intern. Med.*, 95:711–722.

Overall, J.E., and Rhoades, H.M. (1984): Are there two studies that clearly reveal superiority of drug over placebo? *Psychopharmacol. Bull.*, 20:64–67.

Owen, R. (1982): Reader bias. *JAMA*, 247:2533–2534.

Oye, R.K., and Shapiro, M.F. (1984): Reporting results from chemotherapy trials: Does response make a difference in patient survival? *JAMA*, 252:2722–2725.

Paccaud, F., Martin-Beran, B., and Gutzwiller, F. (1988): Hour of birth as a prognostic factor for perinatal death. *Lancet*, I:340–342.

Packe, G.E., and Ayres, J.G. (1985): Asthma outbreak during a thunderstorm. *Lancet*, II:199–204.

Packer, M. (1988): Clinical trials in congestive heart failure: Why do studies report conflicting results? *Ann. Intern. Med.*, 109:3–5.

Pantuck, E.J., Pantuck, C.B., Garland, W.A., Min, B.H., and Wattenberg, L.W. (1979): Stimulatory effect of brussels sprouts and cabbage on human drug metabolism. *Clin. Pharmacol. Ther.*, 25:88–95.

Parkinson Study Group. (1989): Effect of deprenyl on the progression of disability in early Parkinson's disease. *N. Engl. J. Med.*, 321:1364–1371.

Pater, J.L., and Willan, A.R. (1984): Methodologic issues in trials of antiemetics. *J. Clin. Oncol.*, 2:484–487.

Payer, L. (1988): *Medicine and Culture*. H. Holt, New York.

Payne, J.E., Pheils, M.T., Chapuis, P.H., and Macpherson, J.G. (1981): The effect of fluorouracil on survival in metastatic colorectal cancer: Fluorouracil response improves survival. *Aust. N.Z. J. Surg.*, 51:12–15.

Pearl, J., Spilker, B.A., Woodward, W.A., and Bentley, R.G. (1976): Anticholinergic activity of antipsychotic drugs in relation to their extrapyramidal effects. *J. Pharm. Pharmacol.*, 28:302–304.

Pearn, J.H. (1984): The child and clinical research. *Lancet*, II:510–512.

Pearson, R.M. (1982): Who is taking their tablets? *Br. Med. J.*, 285:757–758.

Peck, C.L., and King, N.J. (1982): Increasing patient compliance with prescriptions. *JAMA*, 248:2874–2877.

Pediatric Rheumatology Collaborative Study Group. (1982): Methodology and studies of children with juvenile rheumatoid arthritis. *J. Rheumatol.*, 9:107–155.

Pelikan, E.W. (1989): Racial differences in drug response. *N. Engl. J. Med.*, 321:257–158.

Penn, R.G., and Griffin, J.P. (1982): Adverse reactions to nitrofurantoin in the United Kingdom, Sweden, and Holland. *Br. Med. J.*, 284:1440–1445.

Penta, J.S., Rozencweig, M., Guarino, A.M., and Muggia, F.M. (1979): Mouse and large-animal toxicology studies of twelve antitumor agents: Relevance to starting dose for phase I clinical tirals. *Cancer Chemother. Pharmacol.*, 3:97–101.

Perez, C.A., Gardner, P., and Glasgow, G.P. (1984): Radiotherapy quality assurance in clinical trials. *Int. J. Radiat. Oncol. Biol. Phys.*, 10:119–125.

Peto, R., Gray, R., Collins, R., Wheatley, K., Hennekens, C., et al. (1988): Randomised trial of prophylactic daily aspirin in British male doctors. *Br. Med. J.*, 296:313–316.

Petri, H., De Vet, H.C.W., Naus, J., and Urquhart, J. (1988): Prescription sequence analysis: A new and fast method for assessing certain adverse reactions of prescription drugs in large populations. *Stat. Med.*, 7:1171–1175.

Pharma Corporation and the Degge Group Ltd. (1988) *International Drug Benefit/Risk Assessment Data Resource Handbook*. Ciba-Geigy, Ltd., Basel, Switzerland.

Pietzcker, A., and Muller-Oerlinghausen, B. (1984): The outpatient clinic for patients under chronic lithium or neuroleptic treatment as a phase-IV research tool. *Pharmacopsychiatry*, 17:162–167.

Pinkel, D. (1958): The use of body surface area as a criterion of drug dosage in cancer chemotherapy. *Cancer Res.*, 18:853–856.

Pinsky, C.M. (1985): Applicability of phase I trial results in the design of phase II and III biological response modifier trials. *Cancer Treat. Rep.*, 69:1171–1173.

Pitt, H.A., and Costrini, A.M. (1979): Vitamin C prophylaxis in marine recruits. *JAMA*, 241:908–911.

Platt, R. (1963): Heredity in hypertension. *Lancet*, 1:899–904.

Pochin, E.E. (1975): The acceptance of risk. *Br. Med. Bull.*, 31:184–190.

Pochin, E.E. (1981): Risk-benefit in medicine. In: *Risk-Benefit Analysis in Drug Research*. Cavalla, J.F. (Ed.), pp. 1–16. MTP Press, Lancaster, UK.

Pocock, S.J. (1985): Current issues in the design and interpretation of clinical trials. *Br. Med. J.*, 290:39–42.

Pocock, S.J., Hughes, M.D., and Lee, R.J. (1987): Statistical problems in the reporting of clinical trials: A survey of three medical journals. *N. Engl. J. Med.*, 317:426–432.

Poland, A., Smith, D., Kuntzman, R., Jacobson, M., and Conney, A.H. (1970): Effect of intensive occupational exposure to DDT on phenylbutazone and cortisol metabolism in human subjects. *Clin. Pharmacol. Ther.*, 11:724–732.

Pöllmann, L. (1983): Long-term follow-up of postoperative swelling. *Int. J. Oral Surg.*, 12:90–94.

Pollock, I., Young, E., Stoneham, M., Slater, N., Wilkinson, J.D., et al. (1989): Survey of colourings and preservatives in drugs. *Br. Med. J.*, 299:649–651.

Potter, L.S. (1991): Oral contraceptive compliance and its role in the effectiveness of the method. In: Cramer, J., and Spilker, B. (Eds.), *Patient Compliance in Medical Practice and Clinical Trials*, pp. 195–207. Raven Press, New York.

Poynard, T., Pignon, J.P., Mory, B., Naveau, S., and Chaput, J.C. (1989): Methodological problems of randomized clinical trials in the treatment of duodenal ulcer, "gastritis" and *Campylobacter pylori* infection. *Gastroenterol. Clin. Biol.*, 13:112B–115B.

Prentice, R.A., and Walker, S.R. (1986): Trends in the development of new medicines by UK-owned pharmaceutical companies (1964–1980). *Br. J. Clin. Pharmacol.*, 21:437–443.

Probstfield, J.L., Russell, M.L., Henske, J.C., Reardon, R.J., and Insull, W., Jr. (1986): Successful program for recovery of dropouts to a clinical trial. *Am. J. Med.*, 80:777–784.

Prout, T.E. (1979): Other examples of recruitment problems and solutions. *Clin. Pharmacol. Ther.*, 25:695–698.

Pullar, T., Birtwell, A.J., Wiles, P.G., Hay, A., and Feely, M.P. (1988): Use of a pharmacologic indicator to compare compliance with tablets prescribed to be taken once, twice, or three times daily. *Clin. Pharmacol. Ther.*, 44:540–545.

Pullar, T., Kumar, S., Tindall, H., and Feely, M. (1989): Time to stop counting tablets? *Clin. Pharmacol. Ther.*, 46:163–168.

Purchase, I.F.H. (1980): Inter-species comparisons of carcinogenicity. *Br. J. Cancer*, 41:454–468.

Pye, G., Christie, M., Chamberlain, J.O., Moss, S.M., and Hardcastle, J.D. (1988): A comparison of methods for increasing compliance within a general practitioner based screening project for colorectal cancer and the effect on practitioner workload. *J. Epidemiol Community Health*. 42:66–71.

Qureshi, B. (1989): Eye, eye. *Br. Med. J.*, 298:1230.

Rabkin, J.G., Markowitz, J.S., Stewart, J., McGrath, P., Harrison, W., et al. (1986): How blind is blind? Assessment of patient and doctor medication guesses in a placebo-controlled trial of imipramine and phenelzine. *Psychiatry Res.*, 19:75–86.

Rabkin, S.W., Boyko, E., Shane, F., and Kaufert, J. (1984): A randomized trial comparing smoking cessation programs utilizing behaviour modification, health education or hypnosis. *Addict. Behav.*, 9:157–173.

Rahman, M., Rahaman, M.M., Wojtyniak, B., and Aziz, K.M.S. (1985): Impact of environmental sanitation and crowding on infant mortality in rural Bangladesh. *Lancet*, II:28–30.

Ransil, B.J., Greenblatt, D.J., and Koch-Weser, J. (1977): Evidence for systematic temporal variation in 24-hour urinary creatinine excretion. *J. Clin. Pharmacol.*, 17:108–119.

Ravikiran, T.N., Datta, H., and Chaudhury, R.R. (1980): Critical analysis of clinical trials. *Indian J. Med. Res.*, 71:460–464.

Raymond, C. (1989): Nagging doubt, public opinion offer obstacles to ending 'cluster' studies. *JAMA*, 261:2297–2298.

Rechnitzer, P.A., Pickard, H.A., Paivio, A.U., Yuhasz, M.S., and Cunningham, D. (1972): Long-term follow-up study of survival and recurrence rates following myocardial infarction in exercising and control subjects. *Circulation*, 45:853–857.

Redwood, D.R., Rosing, D.R., Goldstein, R.E., Beiser, G.D., and Epstein, S.E. (1971): Importance of the design of an exercise protocol in the evaluation of patients with angina pectoris. *Circulation*, 43:618–628.

Registry of Comparative Pathology. (1973): *Animal Models of Human Disease*. Second Fascicle. T.C. Jones, D.B. Hackel, and G. Migaki (Eds.). Information Services, Bethesda, MD.

Reich, J.W., and Hilleman, D.E. (1985): A geocentric approach to pharmaceutical research and development and drug regulatory affairs. *Clin. Res. Pract. Drug Reg. Affairs*, 3:1–22.

Reid, W.H., Ahmed, I., and Levie, C.A. (1981): Treatment of sleepwalking: A controlled study. *Am. J. Psychother.*, 35:27–37.

Reidenberg, M. M. (1977): Obesity and fasting—effects on drug metabolism and drug action in man *Clin. Pharmacol. Ther.*, 22:729–734.

Reidenberg, M.M., and Lowenthal, D.T. (1968): Adverse nondrug reactions. *N. Engl. J. Med.*, 279:678–679.

Reiffenstein, R.J., Schiltroth, A.J., and Todd, D.M. (1968): Current standards in reported drug trials. *Can. Med. Assoc. J.*, 99:1134–1135.

Reinberg, A., and Halberg, F. (1971): Circadian Chronopharmacology. *Annu. Rev. Pharmacol.*, 11:455–492.

Reinberg, A. and Smolensky, M.H. (1982): Circadian changes of drug disposition in man *Clin. Pharmacokinet.*, 7:401–420.

Reines, S.A., and Fong, D. (1987): Clinical evaluation of drug candidates. In: *Drug Discovery and Development*. Williams, M., and Malick, J.B. (Eds.), pp. 327–352, Humana Press, Clifton, NJ.

Reiser, J., and Warner, J.O. (1985): The value of participating in an asthma trial. *Lancet*, I:206–207.

Relman, A.S. (1989): Economic incentives in clinical investigation. *N. Engl. J. Med.*, 320:933–934.

Remington, P.L., Hall, W.N., Davis, I.H., Herald, A., and Gunn, R.A. (1985): Airborne transmission of measles in a physician's office. *JAMA*, 253:1574–1577.

Remington, R.D. (1979): Research related to validation of treatment modalities by large-scale clinical trials. *Circulation*, 60:1605–1608.

Rennels, G.D., and Miller, P.L. (1988): Artificial intelligence research in anesthesia and intensive care. *J. Clin. Monit.*, 4:274–289.

Rennels, G.D., Shortliffe, E.H., Stockdale, F.E., and Miller, P.L. (1987): A computational model of reasoning from the clinical literature. *Comput. Methods Programs*, 24:139–149.

Rennie, D. (1989): Editors and auditors. *JAMA*, 261:2543–2545.

Revill, J.P. (Ed.) (1978): *Drug Information Sources: A Worldwide Annotated Survey*. Gothard House Publications, Oxon, UK.

Reynolds, I., and Hoult, J.E. (1984): The relatives of the mentally ill: A comparative trial of community-oriented and hospital-oriented psychiatric care. *J. Nerv. Ment. Dis.*, 172:480–489.

Riecken, H.W., and Ravich, R. (1982): Informed consent to biomedical research in Veterans Administration hospitals. *JAMA*, 248:344–348.

Riegelman, R.K. (1981): *Studying a Study and Testing a Test: How to Read the Medical Literature*. Little, Brown and Company, Boston.

Riesenberg, D.E., and Arehart-Treichel, J. (1986): "Sick building" syndrome plagues workers, dwellers. *JAMA*, 255:3063.

Riley, T.L., Porter, R.J., White, B.G., and Penry, J.K. (1981): The hospital experience and seizure control. *Neurology*, 31:912–915.

Ring-Larsen, H., Henriksen, J.H., Wilken, C., Clausen, J., Pals, H., et al. (1986): Diuretic treatment in decompensated cirrhosis and congestive heart failure: Effect of posture. *Br. Med. J.*, 292:1351–1353.

Roberts, R.S., Spitzer, W.O., Delmore, T., and Sackett, D.L. (1978): An empirical demonstration of Berkson's bias. *J. Chronic Dis.*, 31:119–128.

Roberts, R.J. (1984): *Drug Therapy in Infants: Pharmacologic Principles and Clinical Experience*. W.B. Saunders Company, Philadelphia.

Robertson, D.M., and Ilstrup, D. (1983): Direct, indirect, and sham laser photocoagulation in the management of central serous chorioretinopathy. *Am. J. Ophthalmol.*, 95:457–466.

Robertson, E.A., Zweig, M.H., and Van Steirteghem, A.C. (1983): Evaluating the clinical efficacy of laboratory tests. *Am. J. Clin. Pathol.*, 79:78–86.

Robertson, W.O. (1983): Quantifying the meanings of words. *JAMA*, 249:2631–2632.

Robinson, I. (1987): Analysing the structure of 23 clinical trials in multiple sclerosis. *Neuroepidemiology*, 6:46–76.

Rodda, B.E. (1974): Sequential analysis in phase I and phase II clinical trials. In: *Importance of Experimental Design and Biostatistics*. McMahon, F.G. (Ed.), pp. 19–27. Futura, Mt. Kisco, NY.

Roe, D.A. (1984): Risk factors in drug-induced nutritional deficiencies. In: *Drugs And Nutrients: The Interactive Effects*. Roe, D.A, and Campbell, T.C. (Eds.), pp. 505–523. Marcel Dekker, New York.

Rooney, S.M., Jain, S., and Goldiner, P.L. (1983): Effect of transcutaneous nerve stimulation on postoperative pain after thoracotomy. *Anesth. Analg.*, 62:1010–1012.

Roscoe, R.J., Steenland, K., Halperin, W.E., Beaumont, J.J., and Waxweiler, R.J. (1989): Lung cancer mortality among nonsmoking uranium miners exposed to radon daughters. *JAMA*, 262:629–633.

Rose, G.A. (1965): Ischemic heart disease: Chest pain questionnaire. *Milbank Mem. Fund Q.*, 43:32–39.

Rose, G.A., Holland, W.W., and Crowley, E.A. (1964): A sphygmomanometer for epidemiologists. *Lancet*, 1:296–300.

Rosengren, A., Wedel, H., and Wilhelmsen, L. (1988): Coronary heart disease and mortality in middle aged men from different occupational classes in Sweden. *Br. Med. J.*, 297:1497–1500.

Rosengren, A., Wilhelmsen, L., Berglund, G., and Elmfeldt, D. (1987): Non-participants in a general population study of men, with special reference to social and alcoholic problems. *Acta Med. Scand.*, 221:243–251.

Ross, D.F., and Pihl, R.O. (1989): Modification of the balanced-placebo design for use at high blood alcohol levels. *Addict. Behav.*, 14:91–97.

Rossi, A.C., Knapp, D.E., Anello, C., O'Neill, R.T., Graham, C.F., et al. (1983): Discovery of adverse drug reactions—a comparison of selected phase IV studies with spontaneous reporting methods. *JAMA*, 249:2226–2228.

Rossi, A.C., Knapp, D.E., Anello, C., O'Neill, R.T., and Graham, C.F. (1984): Postmarketing drug surveillance. *JAMA*, 251:729–730.

Rotberg, M.H., and Surwit, R.S. (1981): Biofeedback techniques in the treatment of visual and ophthalmologic disorders: A review of the literature. *Biofeedback Self Regul.*, 6:375–388.

Rotmensz, N. (Ed.) (1989): *Data Management and Clinical Trials*. EORTC Study Group on Data Management. Elsevier, Amsterdam.

Rouzioux, J.M. (1979): The ethical problems of human therapeutic trials. In: *Multicenter Controlled Trials—Principles and Problems*. pp. 253–264. INSERM, Paris.

Rowe, J.W. (1977): Clinical research on aging: Strategies and directions. *N. Engl. J. Med.*, 297:1332–1336.

Rowe, J.W. (1985): Health care of the elderly *N. Engl. J. Med.*, 312:827–835.

Rozencweig, M., Von Hoff, D.D., Staquet, M.J., Schein, P.S., Penta, J.S., et al. (1981): Animal toxicology for early clinical trials with anticancer agents. *Cancer Clin. Trials*, 4:21–28.

Rubin, E., and Lieber, C.S. (1968): Hepatic microsomal enzymes in man and rat: Induction and inhibition by ethanol. *Science*, 162:690–691.

Rudd, P., Byyny, R.L., Zachary, V., LoVerde, M.E., Titus, C., et al. (1989): The natural history of medication compliance in a drug trial: Limitations of pill counts. *Clin. Pharmacol. Ther.*, 46:169–176.

Ruelius, H.W. (1987): Extrapolation from animals to man: Predictions, pitfalls and perspectives. *Xenobiotica*, 17:255–265.

Ruffin, J.M., Grizzle, J.E., Hightower, N.C., McHardy, G., Shull,

H., et al. (1969): A co-operative double-blind evaluation of gastric "freezing" in the treatment of duodenal ulcer. *N. Engl. J. Med.,* 281:16–19.

Russell, L.B. (1985): Issues in the design of future preventive medicine studies. *Ciba Found. Symp.,* 110:203–217.

Ryan, K.J., Chairman, National Commission for the Protection of Human Subjects of Biomedical and Behavioral Research. (1977): Research involving children. DHEW Pub. No. (OS)77–0004. U.S. Government Printing Office, Washington, DC.

Sackett, D.L. (1976): Priorities and methods for future research. In: *Compliance with Therapeutic Regimens.* Sackett, D.L. and Haynes, R.B. (Eds.). Johns Hopkins Univ. Press, Baltimore, pp. 169–189.

Sackett, D.L. (1978): Clinical diagnosis and the clinical laboratory. Clin. Invest. Med., 1:37–43.

Sackett, D.L. (1979): Bias in analytic research. *J. Chronic Dis.,* 32:51–63.

Sackett, D.L. (1980): How can we improve patient compliance? In: *Controversies in Therapeutics,* Lasagna, L. (Ed.). W.B. Saunders, Philadelphia, pp. 552–558.

Sackett, D.L., Haynes, R.B., Gent, M., and Taylor, D.W. (1980): Compliance. In: *Monitoring for Drug Safety.* Inman, W.H.W. (Ed.), pp. 427–438. MTP Press, Lancaster, UK.

Sackett, D.L., Haynes, R.B., and Tugwell, P. (1985): *Clinical Epidemiology: A Basic Science for Clinical Medicine.* Little, Brown and Company, Boston.

Sackett, D.L., and Snow, J.C. (1979): The magnitude of compliance and noncompliance. In: *Compliance in Health Care.* Haynes, R.B., Taylor, D.W., and Sackett, D.L. (Eds.). Johns Hopkins University Press, Baltimore.

Sacks, H., Chalmers, T.C., and Smith, H. Jr. (1982): Randomized versus historical controls for clinical trials. *Am. J. Med.,* 72:233–240.

Sacks, H.S., Berrier, J., Reitman, D., Ancona-Berk, V.A., and Chalmers, T.C. (1987): Meta-analyses of randomized controlled trials. *N. Engl. J. Med.,* 316:450–455.

Sacks, H.S., Chalmers, T.C., and Smith, H. Jr. (1983): Sensitivity and specificity of clinical trials: Randomized v historical controls. *Arch. Intern. Med.,* 143:753–755.

Salsburg, D. (1983): The lifetime feeding study in mice and rats—an examination of its validity as a bioassay for human carcinogens. *Fundam. Appl. Toxicol.,* 3:63–67.

Saltzman, A. (1985): Adverse reaction terminology standardization: A report on Schering-Plough's use of the WHO dictionary and the formation of the WHO adverse reaction terminology users group (WUG) consortium. *Drug Info. J.,* 19:35–41.

Samra, J.S., Iqbal, P.K., Tang, L.C.H., Shafi, M., Obhrai, M.S., et al. (1988): Bilingual consultation. *Lancet,* I:648.

Sanderson, I.M., Kennerley, J.W., and Parr, G.D. (1984): An evaluation of the relative importance of formulation and process variables using factorial design. *J. Pharm. Pharmacol.,* 36:789–795.

Sartwell, P.E. (1974): Retrospective studies: A review for the clinician. *Ann. Intern. Med.,* 81:381–386.

Saudek, C.D., Selam, J-L., Pitt, H.A., Waxman, K., Rubio, M., et al. (1989): A preliminary trial of the programmable implantable medication system for insulin delivery. *N. Engl. J. Med.,* 321:574–579.

Saurbrey, N., Jensen, J., Rasmussen, P.E., Gjorup, T., Guldager, H., et al. (1984): Danish patients' attitudes toward scientific-ethical questions: An interview study focusing therapeutic trials. *Acta Med. Scand.,* 215:99–104.

Sayers, J.A., and Blake, P. (1989): An alternative approach to clinical research associate training. *Drug Info. J.,* 23:321–326.

Schafer, A. (1982): The ethics of the randomized clinical trial. *N. Engl. J. Med.,* 307:719–724.

Schalling, D., Asberg, M., Edman, G, and Oreland, L. (1987): Markers for vulnerability to psychopathology: Temperament traits associated with platelet MAO activity. *Acta Psychiatr. Scand.,* 76:172–182.

Schapira, K., McClelland, H.A., Griffiths, N.R., and Newell, D.J. (1970): Study on the effects of tablet colour in the treatment of anxiety states. *Br. Med. J.,* 2:446–449.

Schechter, P.J., Friedewald, W.T., Bronzert, D.A., Raff, M.S., and Henkin, R.I. (1972): Idiopathic hypogeusia: A description of the syndrome and a single blind study with zinc sulfate. *Int. Rev. Neurobiol.(Suppl.),* 1:125–140.

Schein, P.S., Davis, R.D., Carter, S., Newman, J., and Schein, D.R. (1970): The evaluation of anticancer drugs in dogs and monkeys for the prediction of qualitative toxicities in man. *Clin. Pharmacol. Ther.,* 11:3–40.

Scheline, R.R. (1972): Toxicological implications of drug metabolism by intestinal bacteria. In: *Toxicological Problems of Drug Combinations.* Proceedings of the European Society for the Study of Drug Toxicity, Vol. XIII. Baker, S.B. de C., and Neuhaus, G.A., (Eds.), pp. 35–43. Excerpta Medica, Amsterdam.

Scheurlen, H., Kay, R., and Baum, M. (Eds.) (1988): *Cancer Clinical Trials: A Critical Appraisal.* Springer-Verlag, Berlin.

Schiavo, D.M., Sinha, D.P., Black, H.E., Arthaud, L., Massa, T., et al. (1984): Tapetal changes in beagle dogs. *Toxicol. Appl. Pharmacol.,* 72:187–194.

Schindel, L. (1968): Placebo-induced side-effects. In: *Drug Induced Diseases.* Meyler, L., and Peck, H.M. (Eds.), Volume 3, pp. 323–330. Excerpta Medica, Amsterdam.

Schipper, H., Clinch, J., and Powell, V. (1990): Definitions and conceptual issues. In: *Quality of Life Assessments in Clinical Trials.* Spilker, B. (Ed.), pp. 11–25. Raven Press, New York.

Schneider, M. (1974): An environmental study of mercury contamination in dental offices. *J. Am. Dent. Assoc.,* 89:1092–1098.

Schoenberger, J.A. (1979): Recruitment in the coronary drug project and the aspirin myocardial infarction study. *Clin. Pharmacol. Ther.,* 25:681–684.

Schor, S., and Karten, I. (1966): Statistical evaluation of medical journal manuscripts. *JAMA,* 195:1123–1128.

Schull, W.J., and Cobb, S. (1969): The intrafamilial transmission of rheumatoid arthritis. 3. The lack of support for a genetic hypothesis. *J. Chronic Dis.,* 22:217–222.

Schulz, S.C., van Kammen, D.P., Balow, J.E., Flye, M.W., and Bunney, W.E. Jr. (1981): Dialysis in schizophrenia: A double-blind evaluation. *Science,* 211:1066–1068.

Schumacher, H.R., Klippel, J.H., and Robinson, D.R. (Eds.) (1988): *Primer on the Rheumatic Diseases.* Ninth Edition. Arthritis Foundation. Atlanta.

Schwartz, A. (Ed.) (1971): *Methods in Pharmacology.* Volume I. Plenum Press, New York.

Schwartz, M.L., Meyer, M.B., Covino, B.G., Narang, R.M., Sethi, V., et al. (1974): Antiarrhythmic effectiveness of intramuscular lidocaine: Influence of different injection sites. *J. Clin. Pharmacol.,* 14:77–83.

Schwartz, S., and Griffin, T. (1986): *Medical Thinking: The Psychology of Medical Judgment and Decision Making.* Springer-Verlag, New York.

Scott, H.D., Thacher-Renshaw, A., Rosenbaum, S.E., Waters, W.J. Jr., Green, M., et al. (1990): Physician reporting of adverse drug reactions: Results of the Rhode Island adverse drug reaction reporting project. *JAMA,* 263:1785–1788.

Sedransk, N. and Carter, S. (Eds.) (1980): Proceedings of the symposium on designs for clinical cancer research. *Cancer Treat. Rep.,* 64:363–538.

Segal, D.L., Lisook, A.B., and Currier, C. (1985): FDA audits of clinical investigators. *Clin. Res. Pract. Drug Reg. Affairs,* 3:265–293.

Segall, H.N. (1960): The electrocardiogram and its interpretation: A study of reports by 20 physicians on a set of 100 electrocardiograms. *Can. Med. Assoc. J.,* 82:2–6.

Seigel, D. (1984): Clinical trials. In: *Handbook of Experimental Pharmacology.* Volume 69, Sears, M.L. (Ed.), pp. 687–697. Springer-Verlag, Berlin.

Selevan, S.G., Lindbohm, M.-L., Hornung, R.W., and Hemminki,

K. (1985): A study of occupational exposure to antineoplastic drugs and fetal loss in nurses. *N. Engl. J. Med.*, 313:1173–1178.

Seltzer, H.S. (1972): A summary of criticisms of the findings and conclusions of the University Group Diabetes Program (UGDP). *Diabetes*, 21:976–979.

Seltzer, C.C., Bosse, R., and Garvey A.J. (1974): Mail survey response by smoking status. *Am. J. Epidemiol.*, 100:453–457.

Sexton, D.L. (1983): Some methodological issues in chronic illness research. *Nurs. Res.*, 32:378–380.

Shand, D.G. (1982): Biological determinants of altered pharmacokinetics in the elderly. *Gerontology*, 28(Suppl. 1):8–17.

Shapiro, A.K. (1969): Iatroplacebogenics. *Int. Pharmacopsychiatry*, 2:215–248.

Shapiro, M.F., and Charrow, R.P. (1985): Scientific misconduct in investigational drug trials. *N. Engl. J. Med.*, 312:731–736.

Shapiro, M.F., and Charrow, R.P. (1989): The role of data audits in detecting scientific misconduct: Results of the FDA program. *JAMA*, 261:2505–2511.

Shapiro, S., Strax, P. and Venet, L. (1971): Periodic breast cancer screening in reducing mortality from breast cancer. *JAMA*, 215:1777–1785.

Shaw, C.D., and Costain, D.W. (1989): Guidelines for medical audit: Seven principles. *Br. Med. J.*, 299:498–499.

Sheiner, L.B., and Benet, L.Z. (1985): Premarketing observational studies of population pharmacokinetics of new drugs. *Clin. Pharmacol. Ther.*, 38:481–487.

Shepard, T.H. (1986): Teratogenesis: General principles. In: *Drug and Chemical Action in Pregnancy*. Fabro, S., and Scialli, A.R. (Eds.), pp. 237–250. Marcel Dekker, New York.

Sheps, S.B., and Schechter, M.T. (1984): The assessment of diagnostic tests: A survey of current medical research. *JAMA*, 252:2418–2422.

Shortliffe, E.H. (1987): Computer programs to support clinical decision making. *JAMA*, 258:61–66.

Shubin, S. (1981): Research behind bars. Prisoners as experimental subjects. *The Sciences*, 21:10–13, 29.

Shulman, S.R., and Raiford, D.S. (1990): FDA regulations provide broader access to unapproved drugs. *J. Clin. Pharmacol.*, 30:585–587.

Sills, J.M., Faich, G.A., Milstien, J.B., and Turner, W.M. (1986): Postmarketing reporting of adverse drug reactions to the FDA: An overview of the 1985 FDA guideline. *Drug Info. J.*, 20:151–156.

Silverstein, M.D., Mulley, A.G., and Dienstag, J.L. (1984): Should donor blood be screened for elevated alanine aminotransferase levels? *JAMA*, 252:2839–2845.

Simes, R.J. (1986): Publication bias: The case for an international registry of clinical trials. *J. Clin. Oncol.*, 4:1529–1541.

Simes, R.J. (1987): Confronting publication bias: A cohort design for meta-analysis. *Stat. Med.*, 6:11–29.

Simon, R. (1987a): How large should a phase II trial of a new drug be? *Cancer Treat. Rep.*, 71:1079–1085.

Simon, R. (1987b): Overviews of randomized clinical trials. *Cancer Treat. Rep.*, 71:3–5.

Simon, R., and Wittes, R.E. (1985): Methodologic guidelines for reports of clinical trials. *Cancer Treat. Rep.*, 69:1–3.

Sinclair, J.C. (1966): Prevention and treatment of the respiratory distress syndrome. *Pediatr. Clin. North Am.*, 13:711–730.

Singh, B.M., Holland, M.R., and Thorn, P.A. (1984): Metabolic control of diabetes in general practice clinics: Comparison with a hospital clinic. *Br. Med. J.*, 289:726–728.

Slatter, S. St. P. (1977): *Competition and Marketing Strategies in the Pharmaceutical Industry*. Holmes and Meier Publishers, New York.

Sloboda, W., and Currier, C. (1985): FDA's monitoring of clinical trials. *Psychopharmacol. Bull.*, 21:105–106.

Sloboda, W., and Lisook, A.B. (1987): Food and drug administration audit of foreign clinical trials. *Psychopharmacol. Bull.*, 23:193–195.

Slovic, P., Fischhoff, B., and Lichtenstein, S. (1982): Facts versus fears: Understanding perceived risk. In: *Judgment Under Uncertainty: Heuristics and Biases*. Kahneman, D., Slovic, P., and Tversky, A. (Eds.). Cambridge University Press, Cambridge, England.

Slovic, P., Kraus, N.N., Lappe, H., Letzel, H., and Malmfors, T. (1989): Risk perception of prescription drugs: Report on a survey in Sweden. *Pharmaceut. Med.*, 4:43–65.

Smith, A., Traganza, E., and Harrison, G. (1969): Studies on the effectiveness of antidepressant drugs. *Psychopharmacol. Bull.*, 5(Suppl. 1):1–53.

Smith, D.G., Clemens, J., Crede, W., Harvey, M., and Gracely, E.J. (1987): Impact of multiple comparisons in randomized clinical trials. *Am. J. Med.*, 83:545–550.

Smith, E.B. (1989): Effect of investigator bias on clinical trials. *Arch. Dermatol.*, 125:216–218.

Smith, K., and O'Day, J. (1982): Simpson's paradox: An example using accident data from the state of Texas. *Accid. Anal. Prev.*, 14:131–133.

Smith, R. (1984): Medical journals in the third world: Problems and possibilities. *Br. Med. J.*, 289:1684–1685.

Smith, T.W., Haber, E., Yeatman, L., and Butler, V.P. Jr. (1976): Reversal of advanced digoxin intoxication with Fab fragments of digoxin-specific antibodies. *N. Engl. J. Med.*, 294:797–800.

Snoddy, C.S., Jr. Michalak, R.A., and Kaufman, L.S. (1985): The pyramid concept. *Drug Info. J.*, 19:27–33.

Snowden, R., and Pearson, B. (1984): Pelvic infection: A comparison of the Dalkon shield and three other intrauterine devices. *Br. Med. J.*, 288:1570–1573.

Society of Toxicological Pathologists. (1986): Society of Toxicological Pathologists' position paper on blinded slide reading. *Toxicol. Pathol.*, 14:493–494.

Sogliero-Gilbert, G., Mosher, K., and Zubkoff, L. (1986): A procedure for the simplification and assessment of lab parameters in clinical trials. *Drug Info. J.*, 20:279–296.

Solomon, S. (1987): Selection of patients for clinical drug trials in migraine. *Neuroepidemiology*, 6:164–171.

Sotto, A., Cabrera, S., Castro, J., Borbolla, E., and Gonzalez, N. (1983): Blood groups in recurrent giardiasis. *Lancet*, II:1312–1313.

Southam, C.M. (1973): Varieties of significance. *N. Engl. J. Med.*, 289:924.

Spector, S.L., Kinsman, R., Mawhinney, H., Siegel, S.C., Rachelefsky, G.S., et al. (1986): Compliance of patients with asthma with an experimental aerosolized medication: Implications for controlled clinical trials. *J. Allergy Clin. Immunol.*, 77:65–70.

Speer, F. (1968): Tobacco and the nonsmoker: A study of subjective symptoms. *Arch. Environ. Health*, 16:443–446.

Spielberg, S.P. (1984): In vitro assessment of pharmacogenetic susceptibility to toxic drug metabolites in humans. *Fed. Proc.*, 43:2308–2313.

Spilker, A.V., and Kessler, J.M. (1987): Comparison of symptoms elicited by checklist and fill-in-the blank questionnaires. *Pharmacoepidemiol. Newslett.*, 3:8–13.

Spilker, B. (1970): Comparison of the inotropic response to glucagon, ouabain and noradrenaline. *Br. J. Pharmacol.*, 40:382–395.

Spilker, B. (1973a): A comparative description of inotropic agents in vitro. *Arch. Int. Pharmacodyn. Ther.*, 202:325–341.

Spilker, B. (1973b): Increase in asthma mortality. *Br. Med. J.*, 4:171–172.

Spilker, B. (1978): Medication records. *JAMA*, 239:929.

Spilker, B. (1983): Practical considerations in planning and conducting clinical trials with investigational or marketed drugs. *Clin. Neuropharmacol.*, 6:325–347.

Spilker, B. (1984): *Guide to Clinical Studies and Developing Protocols*. Raven Press, New York.

Spilker, B. (1985): Development of orphan drugs. *Trends Pharmacol. Sci.*, 6:185–188.

Spilker, B. (1986): *Guide to Clinical Interpretation of Data*. Raven Press, New York.

Spilker, B. (1987a): *Guide to Planning and Managing Multiple Clinical Studies*. Raven Press, New York.

Spilker, B. (1987b): Practical considerations in the clinical development of CNS drugs. In: *Psychopharmacology: The Third Generation of Progress*. Meltzer, H.Y. (Ed.), pp. 1659–1666. Raven Press, New York.

Spilker, B. (1987c): Clinical evaluation of topical antipruritics and antihistimines. In: *Models in Dermatology*. Volume 3. Lowe, N.J. and Maibach, H.I. (Ed.), pp. 55–61. S. Karger, Basel.

Spilker, B. (1989a): *Multinational Drug Companies: Issues in Drug Development and Discovery*. Raven Press, New York.

Spilker, B. (1989b): Golden rules of drug discovery. *Drug News Perspect.*, 2:26–30.

Spilker, B. (1989c): Career opportunities for physicians in the pharmaceutical industry. *J. Clin. Pharmacol.*, 29:1069–1076.

Spilker, B. (1989d): Career opportunities in fields related to drugs. *Drug News Perspect.*, 2:389–396.

Spilker, B. (Ed.). (1990a): *Quality of Life Assessments in Clinical Trials*. Raven Press, New York.

Spilker, B. (1990b): Orphan drugs. In Volume 1 (*General Introduction*) of the six volume series: *Comprehensive Medicinal Chemistry*. Kennewell, P.D. (Ed.) and Hansch, C. (Series Ed.), pp. 667–674. Pergamon Press, Oxford.

Spilker, B. (1991): Teaching courses in clinical trial research methods. *J. Clin. Pharmacol.*, 31:(In press).

Spilker, B., Bruni, J., Jones, M., Upton, A., Cato, A., et al. (1983): A double-blind crossover study of cinromide versus placebo in epileptic outpatients with partial seizures. *Epilepsia*, 24:410–421.

Spilker, B., and Cuatrecasas, P. (1988): Changing images of the American drug industry. *Drug News Perspect.*, 1:325–328.

Spilker, B., and Cuatrecasas, P. (1989): Assessing risks. *Drug News Perspect.*, 2:69–73.

Spilker, B., and Cuatrecasas, P. (1990): *Inside the Drug Industry*. R.J. Prous, Barcelona, Spain.

Spilker, B. Kamiya, J., Callaway, E., and Yeager, C. (1969): Visual evoked responses in subjects trained to control alpha rhythms. *Psychophysiology*, 5:683–695.

Spilker, B., and Maugh, T.H. (1980): How useful is hair analysis? *Energy Med.*, 1:5–9.

Spilker, B., Minatoya, H., and McKeon, W.B. Jr. (1975a): Comparison of animal models for predicting bronchodilator efficacy in man. *Arch. Int. Pharmacodyn. Ther.*, 217:218–235.

Spilker, B., Schargel, L., Koss, R.F., and Minatoya, H. (1975b): Cardiovascular effects and blood concentrations of ajmaline and its 17-monochloroacetate ester in cats. *Arch. Int. Pharmacodyn.*, 216:63–78.

Spilker, B., Molinek, F.R. Jr., Johnston, K.A., Simpson, R.L. Jr., and Tilson, H.H. (1990): Quality of life bibliography and indexes. *Med. Care*, 28(Suppl.):DS1–DS77.

Spilker, B., and Schoenfelder, J. (1990): *Presentation of Clinical Data*. Raven Press, New York.

Spilker, B., and Schoenfelder, J. (1991): *Data Collection Forms in Clinical Trials*. Raven Press, New York.

Spilker, B., and Segreti, A. (1984): Validation of the phenomenon of regression of seizure frequency in epilepsy *Epilepsia*, 25:443–449.

Spilker, B., and Tyll, J. (1976): On the question of tachyphylaxis to isoproterenol in guinea pigs. *Eur. J. Pharmacol.* 36:283–288.

Spodick, D.H. (1973): The surgical mystique and the double standard. Controlled trials of medical and surgical therapy for cardiac diseases: Analysis, hypothesis, proposal. *Am. Heart J.*, 85:579–583.

Spodick, D.H., Aronow, W., Lown, B., Barber, B., and Mathur, V.S. (1978): Equal standards for medical and surgical treatments: Responsibility for reviewers and editors. *Br. Heart J.*, 40:1429.

Sriwatanakul, K., Kelvie, W., Lasagna, L., Calimlin, J.F., Weis, O.F., et al. (1983a): Studies with different types of visual analog scales for measurement of pain. *Clin. Pharmacol. Ther.*, 34:234–239.

Sriwatanakul, K., Lasagna, L., and Cox, C. (1983b): Evaluation of current clinical trial methodology in analgesimetry based on experts' opinions and analysis of several analgesic studies. *Clin. Pharmacol. Ther.*, 34:277–283.

Stanley, B., Stanley, M., Stein, J., Guido, L., and Transit, R.-P. (1985): Psychopharmacologic treatment and informed consent: Empirical research. *Psychopharmacol. Bull.*, 21:110–113.

Stanley, K., Stjernsward, J., and Isley, M. (1981): *Recent Results in Cancer Research, Volume 77: The Conduct of a Cooperative Clinical Trial*. Springer-Verlag, New York.

Statland, B.E. (1983): *Clinical Decision Levels for Lab Tests*. Medical Economics Books, Oradell, NJ.

Steering Committee of the Physicians' Health Study Research Group. (1988): Preliminary report: Findings from the aspirin component of the ongoing physicians' health study. *N. Engl. J. Med.*, 318:262–264.

Steinberg, W.M., Goldstein, S.S., Davis, N.D., Shamma'a, J., and Anderson, K. (1985): Diagnostic assays in acute pancreatitis: A study of sensitivity and specificity. *Ann. Intern. Med.*, 102:576–580.

Steiner, S.S., and Dince, W.M. (1981): Biofeedback efficacy studies. *Biofeedback Self Regul.*, 6:275–288.

Stellar, S., Ahrens, S.P., Meibohm, A.R., and Reines, S.A. (1984): Migraine prevention with timolol: A double-blind crossover study. *JAMA*, 252:2576–2580.

Stephens, M.D.B. (1985a): Postmarketing surveillance (PMS). In: *The Detection of New Adverse Drug Reactions*. pp. 81–124. Stockton Press, New York.

Stephens, M.D.B. (1985b): *The Detection of New Adverse Drug Reactions*. Stockton Press, New York.

Stephenson, J.B.P. (1978): Reversal of hypnosis-induced analgesia by naloxone. *Lancet*, II:991–992.

Stolley, P.D. (1990): How to interpret studies of adverse drug reactions. *Clin. Pharmacol. Ther.*, 48:337–339.

Sterling, E., and Sterling, T. (1983): The impact of different ventilation levels and fluorescent lighting types on building illness: An experimental study. *Can. J. Public Health*, 74:385–392.

Sterling, T.D., and Kobayashi, D.M. (1977): Exposure to pollutants in enclosed "living spaces." *Environ. Res.*, 13:1–35.

Strachan, C.J.L., and Oates, G.D. (1977): Surgical trials. In: *Clinical Trials*. Johnson, F.N., and Johnson, S. (Eds.), pp. 188–198. Blackwell Scientific Publications, Oxford, England.

Strom, B.L. (Ed.) (1989): *Pharmacoepidemiology*. Churchill Livingstone, New York.

Strom, B.L., and Carson, J.L. (1989): Automated data bases used for pharmacoepidemiology research. *Clin. Pharmacol. Ther.*, 46:390–394.

Strom, B.L., Miettinen, O.S., and Melmon, K.L. (1983): Postmarketing studies of drug efficacy: When must they be randomized? *Clin. Pharmacol. Ther.*, 34:1–7.

Stuart, I. (1985): Do patients cash prescriptions? *Br. Med. J.* 291:1246.

Stupfel, M. (1975): Biorhythms in toxicology and pharmacology: I. Generalities, ultradian and circadian biorhythms. *Biomedicine*, 22:18–24.

Sturdevant, R.A.L., Isenberg, J.I., Secrist, D., and Ansfield, J. (1977): Antacid and placebo produced similar pain relief in duodenal ulcer patients. *Gastroenterology*, 72:1–5.

Sugarbaker, P.H., Barofsky, I., Rosenberg, S.A., and Gianola, F.J. (1982): Quality of life assessment of patients in extremity sarcoma clinical trials. *Surgery*, 91:17–23.

Sundaresan, N., Voorhies, R., Kwok, K-L, and Thaler, H.T. (1981): Hypothesis testing in neurosurgical trials. *J. Neurosurg.*, 54:468–472.

Sunderman, F.W. Jr. (1975): Current concepts of "normal values," "reference values," and "discrimination values" in clinical chemistry. *Clin. Chem.*, 21:1873–1877.

Sundram, C.J. (1988): Informed consent for major medical treatment of mentally disabled people. *N. Engl. J. Med.*, 318:1368–1373.

Susser, M.W. (1973): *Causal Thinking in the Health Sciences.* Oxford University Press, New York.

Sutton, G.C. (1989): How accurate is computer-aided diagnosis? *Lancet,* II:905–908.

Svensson, C.K. (1989): Representation of American blacks in clinical trials of new drugs. *JAMA,* 261:263–265.

Swain, J.F., Rouse, I.L., Curley, C.B., and Sacks, F.M. (1990) Comparison of the effects of oat bran and low-fiber wheat on serum lipoprotein levels and blood pressure. *N. Engl. J. Med.*, 322:147–152.

Swinbanks, D. (1989): Japanese doctors keep quiet. *Nature,* 339:409.

Tallarida, R.J., Murray, R.B., and Eiben, C. (1979): A scale for assessing the severity of diseases and adverse drug reactions: Application to drug benefit and risk. *Clin. Pharmacol. Ther.,* 25:381–390.

Tannock, I., and Murphy, K. (1983): Reflections on medical oncology: An appeal for better clinical trials and improved reporting of their results. *J. Clin. Oncol.,* 1:66–70.

Taub, E., and School, P.J. (1978): Some methodological considerations in thermal biofeedback training. *Behav. Res. Meth. Instru.,* 10:617–622.

Taves, D.R. (1974): Minimization: A new method of assigning patients to treatment and control groups. *Clin. Pharmacol. Ther.,* 15:443–453.

Taylor, B., Wadsworth, J., Wadsworth, M., and Peckham, C. (1984): Changes in the reported prevalence of childhood eczema since the 1939–45 war. *Lancet,* II:1255–1257.

Taylor, K.M., Margolese, R.G., and Soskolne, C.L. (1984): Physicians' reasons for not entering eligible patients in a randomized clinical trial of surgery for breast cancer. *N. Engl. J. Med.,* 310:1363–1367.

Teal, T.W., and Dimmig, A.L. (1985): Adverse drug experience management: A brief review of the McNeil pharmaceutical system. *Drug Info. J.,* 19:17–25.

Temple, R. (1982): Government viewpoint of clinical trials. *Drug Info. J.,* 16:10–17.

Temple, R. (1987): The clinical investigation of drugs for use by the elderly: Food and Drug guidelines. *Clin. Pharmacol. Ther.,* 42:681–685.

Temple, R., and Pledger, G.W. (1980): The FDA's critique of the Anturane reinfarction trial. *N. Engl. J. Med.,* 303:1488–1492.

Tfelt-Hansen, P., and Nielsen, S.L. (1986): Methodology of drug trials in migraine. *Funct. Neurol.,* 1:499–502.

Thacker, S.B. (1988): Meta-analysis: A quantative approach to research integration. *JAMA,* 259:1685–1689.

Thatcher, R.M. (1983): 98.6 F: What is normal? *J. Gerontol. Nurs.,* 9:23–27.

Thiede, T., Chievitz, E., and Christensen, B.C. (1964): Chlornaphazine as a bladder carcinogen. *Acta Med. Scand.,* 175:721–725.

Thompson, E.I. (1980): Application of restricted sequential design in a clinical protocol. *Cancer Treat. Rep.,* 64:399–403.

Thompson, J.K., Raczynski, J.M., Haber, J.D., and Sturgis, E.T. (1983): The control issue in biofeedback training. *Biofeedback Self Regul.,* 8:153–164.

Thomson, M.E., and Kramer, M.S. (1984): Methodologic standards for controlled clinical trials of early contact and maternal-infant behavior. *Pediatrics,* 73:294–300.

Todd, B.S. (1987): A model-based diagnostic program. *Software Eng. J.,* May:54–63.

Tomlin, P.J. (1979): Health problems of anaesthetists and their families in the West Midlands. *Br. Med. J.,* 1:779–784.

Toogood, J.H. (1980): What do we mean by ''usually''? *Lancet,* I:1094.

Trombitas, I.D., and Simpson, R.L. Jr. (1986): Monitoring the world's published literature for adverse drug experiences. *Drug Info. J.,* 20:57–62.

Tufte, E.R. (1983): *The Visual Display of Quantitative Information.* Graphics Press, Cheshire, CT.

Tugwell, P., and Bombardier, C. (1982): A methodologic framework for developing and selecting endpoints in clinical trials. *J. Rheumatol.,* 9:758–762.

Tunnessen, W.W. Jr., and Feinstein, A.R. (1980): The steroid-croup controversy: An analytic review of methodologic problems. *J. Pediatr.,* 96:751–756.

Turner, G., Lisook, A.B., and Delman, D.P. (1987): FDA's conduct, review, and evaluation of inspections of clinical investigators. *Drug Info. J.,* 21:117–125.

Turner, R.A. (1965): *Screening Methods in Pharmacology.* Academic Press, New York.

Turner, R.A., and Hebborn, P. (Eds.) (1971): *Screening Methods in Pharmacology.* Volume II. Academic Press, New York.

Turner, W.M., Milstien, J.B., Faich, G.A., and Armstrong, G.D. (1986): The processing of adverse reaction reports at FDA. *Drug Info. J.,* 20:147–150.

Tversky, A., and Kahneman, D. (1981): The framing of decisions and the psychology of choice. *Science,* 211:453–458.

Tyrer, P.J., and Remington, M. (1979): Controlled comparison of day-hospital and outpatient treatment for neurotic disorders. *Lancet,* I:1014–1016.

Tyson, J.E., Furzan, J.A., Reisch., J.S., and Mize, S.G. (1983): An evaluation of the quality of therapeutic studies in perinatal medicine. *Obstet. Gynecol.,* 62:99–102.

U.S. Department of Health and Human Services, Public Health Service (1980): A Compilation of Journal Instructions to Authors. NIH Publication No. 80–1991, Bethesda, MD.

U.S. Department of Health and Human Services, Public Health Service (1983): Bibliography on Health Indexes. Clearinghouse on Health Indexes. 1:DHHS Pub. No. (PHS) 83–1250.

University of Edinburgh, Department of Pharmacology staff, and McLeod, L.J. (1970): *Pharmacological Experiments on Intact Preparations.* E & S Livingstone, Edinburgh, UK.

University of Edinburgh, Department of Pharmacology staff. (1968): *Pharmacological Experiments on Isolated Preparations.* E & S Livingstone, Edinburgh, UK.

Urquhart, J. (1989): Noncompliance: The ultimate absorption barrier. In: *Novel Drug Delivery and Its Therapeutic Application.* Prescott, L.F., and Nimmo, W.S. (Eds.), pp. 127–137. John Wiley & Sons, Chichester.

Vaisrub, N. (1985): Manuscript review from a statistician's perspective. *JAMA,* 253:3145–3147.

van der Linden, W. (1980a): Pitfalls in randomized surgical trials. *Surgery,* 87:258–262.

van der Linden, W. (1980b): On the generalization of surgical trial results. *Acta Chir. Scand.,* 146:229–234.

Vayda, E. (1973): A comparison of surgical rates in Canada and in England and Wales. *N. Engl. J. Med.,* 289:1224–1229.

Veatch, R.M. (1977): *Case Studies in Medical Ethics.* Harvard University Press, Cambridge, MA.

Venning, G.R. (1982): Validity of anecdotal reports of suspected adverse drug reactions: The problem of false alarms *Br. Med. J.,* 284:249–252.

Venning, G.R. (1983a): Identification of adverse reactions to new drugs. III: Alerting processes and early warning systems. *Br. Med. J.,* 286:458–460.

Venning, G.R. (1983b): Identification of adverse reactions to new drugs. IV: Verification of suspected adverse reactions. *Br. Med. J.,* 286:544–547.

Venulet, J. (1985): Informativity of adverse drug reactions data in medical publications. *Drug Info. J.,* 19:357–365.

Venulet, J., Blattner, R., von Bulow, J., and Berneker, G.C. (1982): How good are articles on adverse drug reactions? *Br. Med. J.,* 284:252–254.

Venulet, J., Ciucci, A., and Berneker, G.C. (1980): Standardized assessment of drug-adverse reaction associations—rationale and experience. *Int. J. Clin. Pharmacol. Ther. Toxicol.,* 18:381–388.

Vere, D.W. (1976): Risks of everyday life. *Proc. R. Soc. Med.*, 69:105–107.

Vesell, E.S. (1978): Disease as one of many variables affecting drug disposition and response: Alterations of drug disposition in liver disease *Drug Metab. Rev.*, 8:265–291.

Vesell, E.S. (1984a): New directions in pharmacogenetics *Fed. Proc.*, 43:2319–2325.

Vesell, E.S. (1984b): Complex effects of diet on drug disposition. *Clin. Pharmacol. Ther.*, 36:285–296.

Vesell, E.S., and Penno, M.B. (1984): A new polymorphism of hepatic drug oxidation in humans: Family studies of antipyrine metabolites. *Fed. Proc.*, 43:2342–2347.

Vesell, E.S., Shively, C.A., and Passananti, G.T. (1977): Temporal variations of antipyrine half-life in man. *Clin. Pharmacol. Ther.*, 22:843–852.

Vestal, R.E. (1978): Drug use in the elderly: A review of problems and special considerations *Drugs*, 16:358–382.

Vestal, R.E., Norris, A.H., Tobin, J.D., Cohen, B.H., and Shock, N.W. (1975): Antipyrine metabolism in man: Influence of age, alcohol, caffeine, and smoking. *Clin. Pharmacol. Ther.*, 18:425–432.

Vestal, R.E., Wood, A.J.J., Branch, R.A., Shand, D.G., and Wilkinson, G.R. (1979): Effects of age and cigarette smoking on propranolol disposition *Clin. Pharmacol. Ther.*, 26:8–15.

Viamontes, J.A. (1972): Review of drug effectiveness in the treatment of alcoholism. *Am. J. Psychiatry*, 128:1570–1571.

Vogel, A.V., Goodwin, J.S., and Goodwin, J.M. (1980): The therapeutics of placebo. *Am. Fam. Physician*, 22:105–109.

von Kerekjarto, M. (1982): Considerations for the impact of medical therapy on quality of life. In: *Clinical Trials in Early Breast Cancer.* Baum, M., Kay, R., and Scheurlen, H. (Eds.), pp. 388–396. Birkhauser Verlag, Boston.

von Wartburg, W.P. (1989): Overview of the drug safety issue and Ciba Geigy's response: RAD-AR. In: *The Perception and Management of Drug Safety Risks.* Horisberger, B., and Dinkel, R. (Eds.), pp.37–45. Springer-Verlag, Berlin.

von Wittenau, M.S., and LeBeau, J.E. (1982): The role of genetic toxicology in drug safety evaluation. *Regul. Toxicol. Pharmacol.*, 2:177–183.

Vul, F.R. (1976): "Lunar rhythms" in the course of the epileptic process. *Zh. Nevropatol. Psikhiatr.*, 76:1875–1879.

Wachter, K.W. (1988): Disturbed by meta-analysis? *Science*, 241:1407–1408.

Waddell, G., Main, C.J., Morris, E.W., Venner, R.M., Rae, P.S., et al. (1982): Normality and reliability in the clinical assessment of backache. *Br. Med. J.*, 284:1519–1523.

Waitzkin, H. (1984): Doctor-patient communication: Clinical implications of social scientific research. *JAMA*, 252:2441–2446.

Walker, S.R., and Griffin, J.P., (Eds.) (1989): *International Medicines Regulations: A Forward Look to 1992.* Kluwer Academic Publishers, Dordrecht, The Netherlands.

Walker, S.R., and Lumley, C.E. (1986): Regulatory requirements for the preclinical safety testing of pharmaceuticals. In: *Development of Drugs & Modern Medicines.* Gorrod, J.W., Gibson, G.G., and Mitchard, M. (Eds.), pp. 615–626. Ellis Horwood Limited, Chichester, England.

Wallach, J.B. (1978): *Interpretation of Diagnostic Tests: A Handbook Synopsis of Laboratory Medicine.* Third Edition. Little, Brown and Co., Boston.

Wang, R.I.H., Wiesen, R.L., Stockdale, S., and Hieb, E. (1977): A method for evaluating anxiolytic sedatives. *J. Clin. Pharmacol.*, 17:269–275.

Ware, J.H., Muller, J.E., and Braunwald, E. (1985): The futility index: An approach to the cost-effective termination of randomized clinical trials. *Am. J. Med.*, 78:635–643.

Warr, D., McKinney, S., and Tannock, I. (1984): Influence of measurement error on assessment of response to anticancer chemotherapy: Proposal for new criteria of tumor response. *J. Clin. Oncol.*, 2:1040–1046.

Warrell, D.A., Looareesuwan, S., Warrell, M.J., Kasemsarn, P., and Intaraprasert, R. (1982): Dexamethasone proves deleterious in cerebral malaria: A double-blind trial in 100 comatose patients. *N. Engl. J. Med.*, 306:313–319.

Wasson, J.H., Sauvigne, A.E., Mogielnicki, R.P., Frey, W.G., and Sox, C.H. (1984): Continuity of outpatient medical care in elderly men: A randomized trial. *JAMA*, 252:2413–2417.

Weber, A., and Fischer, T. (1980): Passive smoking at work. *Int. Arch. Occup. Environ. Health*, 47:209–221.

Webster, J., Newnham, D., Petrie, J.C., and Lovell, H.G. (1984): Influence of arm position on measurement of blood pressure. *Br. Med. J.*, 288:1574–1575.

Wechsler, H., Grosser, G.H., and Greenblatt, M. (1965): Research evaluating antidepressant medications on hospitalized mental patients: A survey of published reports during a five-year period. *J. Nerv. Ment. Dis.*, 141:231–239.

Wehr, T.A., and Wirz-Justice, A. (1982): Circadian rhythm mechanisms in affective illness and in antidepressant drug action. *Pharmacopsychiatria*, 15:31–39.

Weinshilboum, R.M. (1984): Human pharmacogenetics. *Fed. Proc.*, 43:2295–2297.

Weinstein, M.C. (1974): Allocation of subjects in medical experiments. *N. Engl. J. Med.*, 291:1278–1285.

Weintraub, M. (1982): How to critically assess clinical drug trials. *Drug Ther.*, 12:131–148.

Weintraub, M., Francetic, I., Hasday, J.D., Jacox, R.F., and Atwater, E.C. (1980): Tiopinac in rheumatoid arthritis: A three-phase dose-ranging, efficacy, and aspirin-withdrawal protocol. *Clin. Pharmacol. Ther.*, 27:579–585.

Weintraub, M., and Northington, F.K. (1986): Drugs that wouldn't die. *JAMA*, 255:2327–2328.

Weintraub, M., Sriwatanakul, K., Sundaresan, P.R., Weis, O.F., and Dorn, M. (1983): Extended-release fenfluramine: Patient acceptance and efficacy of evening dosing. *Clin. Pharmacol. Ther.*, 33:621–627.

Weiss, G.B., Bunce, H. III, and Hokanson, J.A. (1983): Comparing survival of responders and nonresponders after treatment: A potential source of confusion in interpreting cancer clinical trials. *Controlled Clin. Trials*, 4:43–52.

Weiss, K.B. (1990): Seasonal trends in US asthma hospitalizations and mortality. *JAMA*, 263:2323–2328.

Weiss, W., Bornstein, M.B., Miller, A., and Slagle, S. (1988): Clinical trial design in multiple sclerosis therapy. *Neurology*, 38(Suppl. 2):80–81.

Weissman, L. (1981): Multiple dose phase I trials—normal volunteers or patients? One viewpoint. *J. Clin. Pharmacol.*, 21:385–387.

Welch, R.M., and Findlay, J.W.A. (1981): Excretion of drugs in human breast milk. *Drug Metab. Rev.*, 12:261–277.

Welling, P.G. (1977): Influence of food and diet on gastrointestinal drug absorption: A review. *J. Pharmacokinet. Biopharm.*, 5:291–334.

Wells, F.O., and Griffin, J.P. (1989): Ethics committees for clinical research experience in the United Kingdom. *Drugs*, 37:229–232.

Wenger, N.K., Mattson, M.E., Furberg, C.D., and Elinson, J. (1984): Assessment of quality of life in clinical trials of cardiovascular therapies. *Am. J. Cardiol.*, 54:908–913.

West, S., Brandon, B., Stolley, P., and Rumrill, R. (1975): A review of antihistamines and the common cold. *Pediatrics*, 56:100–107.

White, C. (1953): Sampling in medical research. *Brit. Med. J.*, 2:1284–1288.

White, D.R., Jackson, D.V., Muss, H.B., Richards, F. II, Michielutte, R., et al. (1984): Informed consent: Patient information forms in chemotherapy trials. *Am. J. Clin. Oncol.*, 7:183–190.

White, W.B. (1989): Methods of blood pressure determination to assess antihypertensive agents: Are casual measurements enough? *Clin. Pharmacol. Ther.*, 45:581–586.

Whitehead, C.C., Polsky, R.H., Crookshank, C., and Fik, E. (1984):

Objective and subjective evaluation of psychiatric ward redesign. *Am. J. Psychiatry*, 141:639–644.

Whittier, F.C., Evans, D.H., Anderson, P.C., and Nolph, K.D. (1983): Peritoneal dialysis for psoriasis: A controlled study. *Ann. Intern. Med.*, 99:165–168.

Whorwell, P.J., Prior, A., and Faragher, E.B. (1984): Controlled trial of hypnotherapy in the treatment of severe refractory irritable-bowel syndrome. *Lancet*, II:1232–1234.

Widmann, F.K. (1983): *Clinical Interpretation of Laboratory Tests*. Ninth Edition. F.A. Davis Co., Philadelphia.

Wilbourn, J., Haroun, L., Heseltine, E., Kaldor, J., Partensky, C., and Vainio, H. (1986): Response of experimental animals to human carcinogens: An analysis based upon the IARC monographs programme. *Carcinogenesis*, 7:1853–1863.

Wiles, C.M., Clarke, C.R.A., Irwin, H.P., Edgar, E.F., and Swan, A.V. (1986): Hyperbaric oxygen in multiple sclerosis: A double blind trial. *Br. Med. J.*, 292:367–371.

Wilhelmsen, L. (1979): Ethics of clinical trials—the use of placebo. *Eur. J. Clin. Pharmacol.*, 16:295–297.

Williams, M.E. (1985): Electronic databases. *Science*, 228:445–456.

Williams, T.F. (1987): Aging or disease? *Clin. Pharmacol. Ther.*, 42:663–665.

Williford, W.O., Bingham, S.F., Weiss, D.G., Collins, J.F., Rains, K.T., et al. (1987): The "constant intake rate" assumption in interim recruitment goal methodology for multicenter clinical trials. *J. Chron. Dis.*, 40:297–307.

Wilson, K., Oram, M., Horth, C.E., and Burnett, D. (1982): The influence of the menstrual cycle on the metabolism and clearance of methaqualone. *Br. J. Clin. Pharmacol.*, 14:333–339.

Winship, D.H., Summers, R.W., Singleton, J.W., Best, W.R., Becktel, J.M., et al. (1979): National cooperative Crohn's disease study: Study design and conduct of the study. *Gastroenterology*, 77:829–842.

Wisser, H., and Breuer, H. (1981): Circadian changes of clinical chemical and endocrinological parameters. *J. Clin. Chem. Clin. Biochem.*, 19:323–337.

Wittes, R.E. (1987): Antineoplastic agents and FDA regulations: Square pegs for round holes? *Cancer Treat. Rep.*, 71:795–806.

Wolery, M., and Harris, S.R. (1982): Interpreting results of single-subject research designs. *Phys. Ther.*, 62:445–452.

Wolfrum, C., Klieser, E., and Lehmann, E. (1984): Single case experiments in psychopharmacological trials. *Neuropsychobiology*, 12:152–157.

Wong, E.T., and Lincoln, T.L. (1983): Ready! fire!...aim!: An inquiry into laboratory test ordering. *JAMA*, 250:2510–2513.

Wood, T.A. (1989): The cost to patients of participating in clinical trials. *JAMA*, 261:1150–1151.

Woody, R.H. (1968): Inter-judge reliability in clinical electroencephalography. *J. Clin. Psychol.*, 24:251–256.

Working Party on Ethics of Research in Children—British Paediatric Association. (1980): Guidelines to aid ethical committees considering research involving children. *Arch. Dis. Child.*, 55:75–77.

Worthen, D.B. (1988): Drug is a four letter word. *Int. Pharm. J.*, 2:136–137.

Worthington, H. (1984): Statistical methodology for clinical trials of caries prophylactic agents—current knowledge. *Int. Dent. J.*, 34:278–284.

Wright, I.S. (1987): Drug or medication. *Clin. Pharmacol. Ther.*, 42:245.

Wrong, O., Metcalfe-Gibson, A., Morrison, R.B.I., Ng, S.T., and Howard, A.V. (1965): In vivo dialysis of faeces as a method of stool analysis. *Clin. Sci.*, 28:357–375.

Wyld, R., and Nimmo, W.S. (1988): Do patients fasting before and after operation receive their prescribed drug treatment? *Br. Med. J.*, 296:744.

Yankelowitz, B.Y. (1980): Making visual aids work for you. *Br. Med. J.*, 281:1718.

Yerushalmy, J. (1966): On inferring causality from observed associations. In: *Controversy in Internal Medicine*. Ingelfinger, F.J., Relman, A.S. and Finland, M. (Eds.). W.B. Saunders, Philadelphia, pp. 659–668.

Yorkshire Breast Cancer Group. (1977): Observer variation in recording clinical data from women presenting with breast lesions. *Br. Med. J.*, 2:1196–1199.

Young, D.S., Pestaner, L.C., and Gibberman, V. (1975): Effects of drugs on clinical laboratory tests. *Clin. Chem.*, 21:1D–432D.

Young, M.J., Bresnitz, E.A., and Strom, B.L. (1983): Sample size nomograms for interpreting negative clinical studies. *Ann. Intern. Med.*, 99:248–251.

Yu, G.C.S. (1986): Remote data entry and retrieval: The human and administrative aspects. *Drug Inf. J.*, 20:103–107.

Yusuf, S., Simon, R., and Ellenberg, S. (1987): Workshop on methodologic issues in overviews of randomized clinical trials, May 1986. *Stat. Med.*, 6:221–409.

Zaharko, D.S., Dedrick, R.L., Bischoff, K.B., Longstreth, J.A., and Oliverio, V.T. (1971): Methotrexate tissue distribution: Prediction by a mathematical model. *JNCI*, 46:775–784.

Zarafonetes, C.J.D., Riley, P.A. Jr., Willis, P.W. III., Power, L.H., et al. (1978): Clinically significant adverse events in a Phase 1 testing program. *Clin. Pharmacol. Ther.*, 24:127–132.

Zbinden, G., and Flury-Roversi, M. (1981): Significance of the LD50-test for toxicological evaluation of chemical substances. *Arch. Toxicol.*, 47:77–99.

Zelen, M. (1979): A new design for randomized clinical trials. *N. Engl. J. Med.*, 300:1242–1245.

Zelen, M. (1983): Guidelines for publishing papers on cancer clinical trials: Responsibilities of editors and authors. *J. Clin. Oncol.*, 1:164–169.

Zelen, M. (1982): Strategy and alternate randomized designs in cancer clinical trials. *Cancer Treat. Rep.*, 66:1095–1100.

Zhou, H.H., Koshakji, R.P., Silberstein, D.J., Wilkinson, G.R., and Wood, A.J. (1989): Altered sensitivity to and clearance of propranolol in men of Chinese descent as compared with American whites. *N. Engl. J. Med.*, 320:565–570.

Ziessman, H.A., Thrall, J.H., Yang, P.J., Walker, S.C., Cozzi, E.A., et al. (1984): Hepatic arterial perfusion scintigraphy with Tc-99m-MAA: Use of a totally implanted drug delivery system. *Radiology*, 152:167–172.

Zimmerman, M. (1983): Weighted versus unweighted life event scores: Is there a difference? *J. Hum. Stress*, 9:30–35.

Zussman, B.M. (1974): Tobacco sensitivity in the allergic population. *J. Asthma Res.*, 11:159–167.

Subject Index

1116 / SUBJECT INDEX

Crossover design (*contd.*)
period effect, 32
requirements, 29–30
saving flawed, 32
schemata, 33
suitable diseases, 32
timing crossover, 32
types of data obtained, 34
washout period, 32

D

Data
amount, data collection form, 265
archive. *See* Archive
baseline period, 76
elimination, 475–476
examination in monitoring, 437–438
types, 161–162
Data access, archive, 821
Data analysis, 476
abnormal
categorizing, 897
clinical significance, 897
auditing, 455
bias, 25
blind, 476
compliance, 113
data extrapolation, differentiating between, 507
data interpretation, differentiating between, 507
eliminating patients, 476–477
future, 1075
last observation carried forward, 478
model report, 476
multiple, 478
statistical test, 476
statistician, 476
Data base. *See also* Automated multipurpose data base
electronic computer search, 1005
ideal, 54
Data base release, data processing 488
Data clumping, 541
Data coding system, 267–270
postcoding data, 267–270,271
precoding data, 267,268
Data collection
abnormal data, 539
adverse reaction, 569

source, 586,587
future, 1075
patient group, 241
protocol, 233
Data collection form, 262–271
adverse reaction
Food and Drug
Administration 1639 form, 1018
United Kingdom, 1019
approaches, 262
binders, 265–266
checklist, 1002
closed system, 264–265
combining similar, 262–263
completing, 270–271
data amount, 265
data flow, 485
designing, 263–266
flow chart, 271
generic, 264
information, standardized, 263
monitor's review, 1002
one set/patient, 271
open system, 264–265
options, 268,269
organization, 262–263
paper, 265–266
partial sets, 271
pitfalls, 264
posttreatment data, 266
pretrial roundtable meeting, 421
review by investigator, 997
signature, 271
specialized, 266
table of contents, 1002
time of day recording, 266
two sets/patient, 271
visit-by-visit format, 262
Data dredging bias, 25
Data editing, 473,489
computer entry, 487
Data entry
computer entry
corrections, 488
programming, 487
models, 486
remote. *See* Remote data entry
Data extrapolation
bias, 22
data analysis differentiating between, 507
data interpretation, differentiating between, 507

dimensions, 508
discontinued patient, 700
disease model, 697–698
extrapolation direction, 702
future, 1075–1076
generalizability, 702
Hawthorne effect, 699–700
medical practice effect, 555
normal volunteers, 702
real world difference, 695–697
representativeness, 700–702
assessment methods, 701–702
trial artificiality, 698–699
types, 695
Data flow, 482,483,484
data collection form, 485
Data handling, 412–413
computer, 1005
Data imputation, 500–501
definition, 500
guidelines, 501
method, 500
Data interpretation, 635–636. *See also* Clinical significance
active medicine control group, 720–722
administration route, 628
age, 620
alternative, 704–705
analogy, 522
anecdotal observation, 708
axiom, 506
baseline, 618
bias, 21,25,629
blind, 616
blood group, 623
blood level, 646–647
diminished, 646
high, 646
orally administered medicine, 646
parenterally administered medicine, 646
body surface, 620
caffeine, 672
circadian rhythm, 622
circaseptan rhythm, 622
clinical significance, 507
clinical trial conduct, 632
clinical trial design, 614
clinical trial duration, 617
clinical trial staff, 630
combination medicine, 721
concomitant medicine, 672
conservative, 517
control group, 720–722

Author Index